To my son David

TABLE OF CONTENTS

CONTRIBUTORS

Joann Albright, PhD
Chief Clinician
SVP Quality Management
Magellan Health Services
Avon, CT

Kelli D. Back
Law Offices of Mark S. Joffe
Washington, DC

Elizabeth Bierbower
Vice President
Product Innovation
Humana Inc.
Louisville, KY

Richard F. Birhanzel, MBA
Senior Executive
Accenture
Minneapolis, MN

Kelly Hanratty Butler
Senior Manager
Health Care Service Corp.
Chicago, IL

Dale F. Cook
Northeast Region Small Group Business
Division CFO
Aetna, Inc.

M. Nicholas Coppola, PhD, MHA, MSA, FACHE
Lieutenant Colonel, U.S. Army, Medical Service
Associate Professor, & Director, Army-Baylor University Graduate Program in Health & Business Administration, Dept of Health Administration (MCCS-HFB)
Army Medical Department Center & School
Ft. Sam Houston, TX

Gregg H. Dooge, Esq.
Foley & Lardner LLP
Milwaukee, WI

Dawn Erckenbrack, EdD, MHA, FACHE
Lieutenant Colonel, U.S. Army, Medical Service
Health Program Analysis & Evaluation
Office of the Assistant Secretary of Defense (Health Affairs)/TMA
Falls Church, VA

Joanna Case Famadas
Baltimore, MD

Troy M. Filipek, FSA, FCA, MAAA
Actuary
Milliman, Inc.
Brookfield, WI

Peter D. Fox
Independent Managed Care Consultant
Denver and Breckenridge, CO

Donald L. Fowler, Jr.
Senior Executive
Accenture
Raleigh, NC

Djordje Gikic, MD, MPH
Johns Hopkins Bloomberg School of Public
    Health,Preventive Medicine Program
Baltimore, MD

Nancy Garrett, PhD
Director
Healthcare Informatics
BlueCross BlueShield of Minnesota
Eagan, MN

Rusty Hailey, PharmD, DPh, MBA, FAMCP
Chief Pharmacy Officer and Senior Vice
    President, Pharmacy Services
Coventry Health Care, Inc.
Franklin, TN

Jeffrey P. Harrison, PhD, MBA, MHA, FACHE
Assistant Professor
Health Administration
University of North Florida
Jacksonville, FL

Deborah Heggie, PhD
Chief Clinician
SVP Clinical Operations
Magellan Health Services
Avon, CT

Donna Horoschak, JD
Vice President
State Policy
America's Health Insurance Plans
Washington, DC

Robert E. Hurley, PhD
Associate Professor
Department of Health Administration
Virginia Commonwealth University
Richmond, VA

Mark S. Joffe
Law Offices of Mark S. Joffe
Washington, DC

Bernie Kerr, EdD, MPH, MHA, MIM, FACHE
Associate Professor
Central Michigan University
Doctor of Health Administration Program
Mount Pleasant, MI

Kevin Knarr
Senior Executive
Accenture
Reston, VA

Anthony M. Kotin, MD
Chief Clinical Officer
Magellan Health Services
Avon, CT

Sidney J. Lindenberg
Technical Advisor
CMS, Center for Beneficiary Choice
Medicare Advantage Group, Division of
    Qualification and Plan Management
Baltimore, MD

Marc Manley, MD, MPH,
Vice President and Medical Director
Population Health
BlueCross BlueShield of Minnesota
Eagan, MN

Brian J. McKenna
Strategic Communications
America's Health Insurance Plans
Washington, DC

Kimberley A. Mentzer
Senior Executive
Accenture
Reston, VA

Patricia Metzger
Memorial Herman Healthcare System
Houston, TX

Lawrence Nardozzi, MD
National Psychiatric Officer
Magellan Health Services
Avon, CT

Robert P. Navarro, PharmD
President, NavarroPharma, LLC
Raleigh, NC

Margaret E. O'Kane
President
National Committee for Quality Assurance
    (NCQA)
Washington, DC

Elizabeth Pascuzzi, EdD
President and Principal Consultant
Managed Care Learning
Bradfordwoods, PA

David W. Plocher, MD
Chief Medical Officer and Sr. Vice President
    of Health Management and Informatics
BlueCross BlueShield of Minnesota
Eagan, MN

Leigh C. Riley, Esq.
Foley and Lardner LLP
Milwaukee, WI

Thomas Riley
Vice President of e-Solutions and Strategic
    Relationships
Health Care Service Corp.
Chicago, IL

Jacqueline M. Saue, Esq.
Foley and Lardner LLP
Washington, DC

Samantha Silva, MHA
Director, State Policy
America's Health Insurance Plans
Washington, DC

Pamela B. Siren
Neighborhood Health Plan
Vice President, Quality and Compliance
Boston, MA

Stephen A. Somers, PhD
President
Center for Health Care Strategies, Inc.
Hamilton, NJ

Michael G. Sturm, FSA, MAAA
Principal and Consulting Actuary
Milliman, Inc.
Brookfield, WI

Michael J. Taylor
Principal
Towers Perrin
Boston, MA

Eric R. Wagner
Senior Vice President
MedStar Health, Inc.
Columbia, MD

Fred Waxenberg, PhD
VP Clinical Operations
Magellan Health Services
Avon, CT

Hugh Waters
Johns Hopkins Bloomberg School of Public
    Health, Preventive Medicine Program
Baltimore, MD

Jonathan P. Weiner
Johns Hopkins Bloomberg School of Public
    Health, Preventive Medicine Program
Baltimore, MD

Carlos J. Zarabozo
formerly with the Office of Policy of the
    Centers for Medicare and Medicaid
    Services
Washington, DC

ABOUT THE AUTHOR

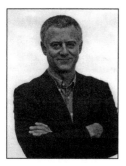 Dr. Peter R. Kongstvedt is a senior executive at the global consulting firm Accenture, based in their Reston, VA office. He has over 12 years consulting experience and almost 20 years of experience at the senior-most levels of health plans, including managed care, health insurance, and BlueCross BlueShield plans. Dr. Kongstvedt's primary focus is in strategic planning and in performance metrics and measurement, and he serves as Accenture's primary thought leader in this industry sector. In addition to being an author and editor of this book, Dr. Kongstvedt is the primary author of *Managed Care: What It Is and How It Works,* also published by Jones and Bartlett.

ACKNOWLEDGMENTS

I wish to acknowledge and thank Russ Nash, and other senior leaders and colleagues at the consulting firm Accenture, for their support during the creation of this book. Balancing the day-to-day needs of the firm with the extra-curricular writing and editing of a book is not for the faint of heart, and their support was crucial to my being able to undertake it at all. Individuals at the Sanofi-Aventis Managed Care Digest Series as well as at Health Leaders/Interstudy kindly allowed me access to their data, including pre-publication data, while the Johns Hopkins Welch Medical Library kindly provided me with a temporary account, allowing me the use of their resources.

Although I cannot name them all, since to do so would double the size of this book, I thank my many colleagues and friends in the managed care and consulting industries beside whom I have had the pleasure to work with over the years. Lastly, I want to give sincere thanks to the many readers of previous editions of this book for their support, kind words, observations, and suggestions that have helped to keep me current.

PREFACE

Up until now, there have always been two related books, both of which were released as fourth editions in 2000 and 2001, respectively: *The Managed Health Care Handbook* and *The Essentials of Managed Health Care,* derived from the *Handbook*. This *Fifth Edition* serves to replace both of those prior books. Where once the *Handbook* strove to provide substantial detail on a comprehensive array of subjects, the need for that level of detail has paradoxically dropped as consolidation in the industry, as well as maturation of management, has decreased the number of individuals desiring such additional information. Conversely, the value of a comprehensive and robustly detailed overview of the basic aspects of managed health care remains high, both for individuals new to the industry as well as for academic departments and courses. The result is this *Fifth Edition* of the *Essentials,* modestly expanded in scope from prior editions, but still focused primarily on the fundamentals of the industry.

Turbulence remains a prominent dynamic of managed health care. Physicians do not exhibit the same types of practice behaviors prevalent one and two decades ago, though there remain high levels of variability in practice overall. New diagnostic and therapeutic interventions continually appear, providing ever-expanding opportunities for medical interventions. The response of the marketplace to what is now considered traditional managed health care (and it was only 15 years ago that the words "traditional" and "managed health care" would never have been linked) has led to new innovations that were not part of the healthcare environment when the last edition was published.

This edition contains very substantial revisions as well as new material. The introduction of new types of consumer-based health plans and services has practical implications throughout the book. Approaches to provider networks have been revised to take into account not only new types of products but new approaches to reimbursement and incentive systems. Care management continues to evolve, leading to a heavily revised chapter on basic utilization management and entirely new chapters on disease management, case management, pharmacy benefits management, behavioral health management, prevention, and the use of data and analysis in care management. Operations in managed care have likewise evolved, leading to a substantial revision of the chapter on member services and entirely new chapters on claims administration, sales and marketing, healthcare consumerism, and the employer's view of managed health care. External accreditation has become more sophisticated, requiring considerable revisions in that chapter as well. New laws and programs in Medicare required a complete rewriting of that chapter, and new approaches to Medicaid likewise led to important revisions. Entirely new chapters on the military health system and managed care in a global context have been added. Changes in federal laws and regulations meant considerable updates and revisions were required of applicable chapters; while in the case of the Health Insurance Portability and Accountability Act (HIPAA), an entirely new chapter was created. Lastly, even the glossary was revised, dropping some obsolete terms, but also increasing the number of terms by over 25 percent.

The path chosen by the United States, combining single payer systems (i.e., Medicare, Medicaid, and other federal health programs) with a heavy reliance on private health insurance is unique in the industrialized world. The result includes high healthcare costs as a percentage of the gross domestic product, seen by most as a severe failing; but the result also includes advanced medical interventions and high access to care (i.e., little queuing and early treatment) that leads much of the rest of the world. The current system has also resulted in the greatest percentage of uninsured or underinsured citizens of any industrialized nation, and access to health care by the poor remains a problem. No simple solution exists to maintain the good while eliminating the bad.

The reality is that the healthcare delivery and financing system existing in the United States is incredibly complex, and that complexity is always accelerating, never slowing, or even increasing at a steady pace. As a result, it is neither possible to describe a steady state nor even a reliably predictable state. In a word, the health care system is chaotic—not using a dictionary definition of chaos as meaning total disorder, but using the word chaos in terms of the science of chaos theory. More accurately stated, the delivery, organization, and financing of health care is a complexly adapting system. The concept of complexity is useful to bear in mind throughout the book. By doing so, the reader will maintain a sense of the true vibrancy of managed health care and will not fall into the trap of thinking that managed health care is monolithic, simplistic, or that there is only one way to do something.

Everything you read here is a reflection of managed health care in 2006. An immediate and practical effect of the complex health care environment is that changes will continue to occur in this industry, and some of those changes will not have been anticipated in this book. Therefore, it is incumbent on the reader to ascertain for herself or himself the applicability and accuracy of the information presented in the *Essentials,* particularly in regard to federal and state laws. The fundamental concepts and attributes of managed health care nonetheless remain, regardless of such changes. The environmental forces that led to the creation and continued evolution of managed health care still exist and are in many ways even greater than in the past.

The two primary missions of the predecessor books remain unchanged: To provide a strategic and operational resource for managers in the field and to provide a comprehensive resource for advanced academic programs. It is also intended to be of value to a wider audience, such as regulators, law professionals, policy makers, practicing physicians, and managers of most types of healthcare organizations. It is based as much as possible on actual operations of managed care plans, rather than on purely theoretical models. Finally, material is presented in as accessible a style as possible for each subject area, so as to facilitate its use by any reader.

While the best approach for understanding the information contained in the *Essentials* is to proceed in the order in which it is presented, this is not a requirement. In addition to its primary roles as a resource to managers and academic programs, it is also a reference text. That means that material is included which will likely be of lesser importance to some readers. As such, it is clearly not necessary that all chapters be read by all readers in order to gain a practical level of understanding, and to aid the reader, chapters cross-reference each other when necessary. There is also a glossary in the back of the book for those times when the acronyms run heavy, the terms are obtuse, or fresh neologisms are blithely used.

The intent to provide practical knowledge necessitates that some of what is presented is also biased: my biases as well as those of contributing authors. There is no shortage of impassioned opinions in this industry, and many of those opinions are held with near-religious zeal. That means that there will be some who have differing opinions or experiences than what is found here. Specific efforts, therefore, have been made to present varying opinions when appropriate, along with the occasional editorial comment when such is warranted. Still, the information in this book has been created with an overriding single and consistent focus: to enable the reader, regardless of their place in the healthcare system, to better understand and to succeed in the world of managed health care.

Peter Reid Kongstvedt
Mclean, VA

KEEPING CURRENT

Keeping current on trends and data presents significant challenges, particularly in regard to trends and data presented in a book. However, there are several useful resources accessible via the Internet that periodically provide updated data and trend information, as well as discussion on important health policy issues relevant to managed health care. The most useful of these are as follows.

(Note that all Web addresses and associated costs are current at the time of publication but are always subject to change)

The Center for Medicare and Medicaid Services (CMS): http://www.cms.org. (Free)

The Office of the Actuary at CMS: http://www.cms.hhs.gov/NationalHealthExpendData/. (Free)

The Centers for Disease Control and Prevention, National Center for Health Statistics: http:// www.cdc.gov/nchs/. (Free)

The Center for Studying Health System Change: http://www.hschange.com/. (Free)

The Henry J. Kaiser Family Foundation (particularly their annual series on health insurance and healthcare marketplace trends): http://www.kff.org. (Free)

The annually updated Sanofi-Aventis Managed Care Digest Series: http://www.managedcaredigest. com. (Free with registration)

HealthLeaders–InterStudy: http://home.healthleaders-interstudy.com. (Requires purchase)

Health Affairs: http://www.healthaffairs.org/. (Requires subscription)

Part 1

INTRODUCTION TO MANAGED HEALTH CARE

"You know more than you think you do."

—Benjamin Spock, MD
(1903–1998)
Baby and Child Care [1945]

THE ORIGINS OF MANAGED HEALTH CARE

Peter D. Fox and Peter R. Kongstvedt

Study Objectives

- Understand the evolution of managed care, including the forces that have driven this evolution.
- Understand current trends in managed care, including how market dynamics continue to change over time.
- Understand the public policy and market performance issues facing managed care.

Discussion Topics

1. Discuss why HMOs were formed in the first place.
2. Discuss what some of the managed care steps are that employers can take to constrain health care costs and promote wellness besides contracting with HMOs.
3. Discuss how important to employers it generally is that managed care plans demonstrate that they offer quality care.
4. Discuss the salient forces leading to the rise and fall of various types of managed care plans. Speculate on how current and future forces might lead to further changes.
5. Discuss how the relationship between the government and the managed care industry has changed over the years.

MANAGED CARE:
THE EARLY YEARS (PRE-1970)

This chapter addresses the development of health maintenance organizations (HMOs) and other managed care organizations (MCOs) rather than focusing on the operational issues found in the other chapters of this book. The historical roots are presented, and some of the major dynamics involved in the evolution of the managed health care industry are discussed.

The Western Clinic in Tacoma, Washington is sometimes cited as the first example of an HMO, or prepaid group practice, as it was known until the early 1970s. Starting in 1910, the Western Clinic offered, exclusively through its own providers, a broad range of medical services in return for a premium payment of $0.50 per member per month.[1] The program was available to lumber mill owners and their employees and served to assure the clinic a flow of patients and revenues. A similar program was developed by a Dr. Bridge, who started a clinic in Tacoma that later expanded to 20 sites in Oregon and Washington.

In 1929, Michael Shadid, MD, established a rural farmers' cooperative health plan in Elk City, Oklahoma, by forming a lay organization of leading farmers in the community. Participating farmers purchased shares for $50 each to raise capital for a new hospital in return for receiving medical care at a discount.[2] For his trouble, Dr. Shadid lost his membership in the county medical society and was threatened with having his license to practice suspended. Some 20 years later, however, he was vindicated through the out-of-court settlement in his favor of an antitrust suit against the county and state medical societies. In 1934, the Farmers Union assumed control of both the hospital and the health plan.

Health insurance itself is of relatively recent origin.[3] In 1929, Baylor Hospital in Texas agreed to provide some 1,500 teachers prepaid care at its hospital, an arrangement that represented the origins of Blue Cross. The program was subsequently expanded to include the participation of other employers and hospitals, initially as single hospital plans. Starting in 1939, state medical societies in California and elsewhere created, generally statewide, Blue Shield plans, which reimbursed for physician services. At the time, commercial health insurance was not a factor.

The formation of the various Blue Cross and Blue Shield plans in the midst of the Great Depression, as well as that of many HMOs, reflected not consumers' demanding coverage or nonphysician entrepreneurs seeking to establish a business but rather providers' wanting to protect and enhance patient revenues. Many of these developments were threatening to organized medicine. In 1932, the American Medical Association (AMA) adopted a strong stance against prepaid group practices, favoring, instead, indemnity type insurance. The AMA's position was in response to both the small number of prepaid group practices in existence at the time and the findings in 1932 of the Committee on the Cost of Medical Care—a highly visible private group of leaders from medicine, dentistry, public health, consumers, and so forth—that recommended the expansion of group practice as an efficient delivery system. The AMA's stance at the national level set the tone for continued state and local medical society opposition to prepaid group practice.

The period immediately around World War II saw the formation of several HMOs, some of which remain prominent today. These HMOs represent a diversity of origins with the initial impetus coming, variously, from employers, providers seeking patient revenues, consumers seeking access to improved and affordable health care, and even a housing lending agency seeking to reduce the number of foreclosures. They encountered varying degrees of opposition from local medical societies. The following are examples of early HMOs:

- The Kaiser Foundation Health Plan was started in 1937 by Dr. Sidney Garfield at the behest of the Kaiser construction company, which sought to finance medical care, initially for workers and families who were building an aqueduct in the southern California desert to transport water from the Colorado River to Los Angeles and, subsequently, for workers who were constructing the Grand Coulee Dam in Washington State. A similar program was established in 1942 at Kaiser ship-building plants in the San Francisco Bay area.

- In 1937, the Group Health Association (GHA) was started in Washington, DC at the behest of the Home Owner's Loan Corporation to reduce the number of mortgage defaults that resulted from large medical expenses. It was created as a nonprofit consumer cooperative, with the board elected periodically by the enrollees. The District of Columbia Medical Society opposed the formation of GHA. It sought to restrict hospital admitting privileges for GHA physicians and threatened expulsion from the medical society. A bitter antitrust battle ensued that culminated in the U.S. Supreme Court's ruling in favor of GHA. In 1994, faced with insolvency despite an enrollment of some 128,000, GHA was acquired by Humana Health Plans, a for-profit, publicly traded corporation. Since that time, it has been divested by Humana and the membership incorporated into Kaiser Foundation Health Plan of the Mid-Atlantic.
- In 1944, at the behest of New York City, which was seeking coverage for its employees, the Health Insurance Plan (HIP) of Greater New York was formed.
- In 1947, consumers in Seattle organized 400 families who contributed $100 each to form the Group Health Cooperative of Puget Sound. Predictably, opposition was encountered from the Kings County Medical Society.

Only in later years did nonprovider entrepreneurs form for-profit HMOs in significant numbers.

The early independent practice association (IPA) type of HMO, which contract with physi-

cians in independent fee-for-service practice, was a competitive reaction to group practice–based HMOs. The basic structure was created in 1954 when the San Joaquin County Medical Society in California formed the San Joaquin Medical Foundation in response to competition from Kaiser. The foundation established a relative value fee schedule for paying physicians, heard grievances against physicians, and monitored quality of care. It became licensed by the state to accept capitation payment, making it the first IPA model HMO.

The Adolescent Years: 1970–1985

Through the 1960s and into the early 1970s, HMOs played only a modest role in the financing and delivery of health care, although they were a significant presence in a few communities such as the Seattle area and parts of California. In 1970, the total number of HMOs was in the 30s, the exact number depending on the definition used. From then until the early to mid-1990s, HMOs expanded at an ever-increasing rate. However, beginning in the early to mid-1990s, HMOs consolidated through mergers and acquisitions, resulting in a decline in the number of such plans beginning in the late 1990s, as discussed later in this chapter.

The major boost to the HMO movement during the early period of growth was the enactment in 1973 of the federal HMO Act. That act, as described later, both authorized start-up funding and, more important, ensured access to the employer-based insurance market. It evolved from discussions that Paul Ellwood, MD had in 1970 with the political leadership of the U.S. Department of Health, Education, and Welfare (which later became the Department of Health and Human Services).[4] Ellwood had been personally close to Philip Lee, MD, Assistant Secretary for Health during the presidency of Lyndon Johnson, and participated in designing the Health Planning Act of 1966.

Ellwood, sometimes referred to as the father of the modern HMO movement, was asked in the early Nixon years to devise ways of constraining the rise in the Medicare budget. Out of those discussions evolved both a proposal to capitate HMOs for Medicare beneficiaries (which was not enacted until 1982) and the laying of the groundwork for what became the HMO Act of 1973. The desire to foster HMOs reflected the perspective that the fee-for-service system, by paying physicians based on their volume of services, incorporated the wrong incentives. Also, the term *health maintenance organization* was coined as a substitute for *prepaid group practice,* principally because it had greater public appeal.

The main features of the HMO Act were the following:

- Grants and loans were available for the planning and start-up phases of new HMOs as well as for service area expansions for existing HMOs.
- State laws that restricted the development of HMOs were overridden for HMOs that were federally qualified, as described later.
- Most important of all were the "dual choice" provisions, which required employers with 25 or more employees that offered indemnity coverage also to offer two federally qualified HMOs, one of each type: (1) the closed panel or group or staff model and (2) the open panel or IPA/network model, if the plans made a formal request* (the different model types are discussed in Chapter 2). Some HMOs were reluctant to exercise the mandate, fearing that doing so would antagonize employers, who would in turn discourage employees from enrolling. However, the dual choice mandates were used by other HMOs to get in the door of employer groups to at least become established.

---

*For workers under collective bargaining agreements, the union had to agree to the offering.

The statute established a process under which HMOs could elect to be federally qualified. Plans had to satisfy a series of requirements, such as meeting minimum benefit package standards set forth in the act, demonstrating that their provider networks were adequate, having a quality assurance system, meeting standards of financial stability, and having an enrollee grievance process. Some states emulated these requirements and adopted them for all HMOs that were licensed in the state regardless of federal qualification status.

Obtaining federal qualification had always been at the discretion of the individual HMO, unlike state licensure, which is mandatory. Plans that requested federal qualification did so for four principal reasons. First, it represented a "Good Housekeeping Seal of Approval" that was helpful in marketing. Second, the dual choice requirements ensured access to the employer market. Third, the override of state laws—important in some states but not others—applied only to federally qualified HMOs. Fourth, federal qualification was required for the receipt of federal grants and loans that were available during the early years of the act. Federal qualification is no longer in existence, but it was important when managed care was in its infancy and HMOs were struggling for inclusion in employment-based health benefit programs, which account for most private insurance in the United States.

The HMO Act also contained provisions that were seen by some as retarding the growth of HMOs. This stemmed from a compromise in Congress between members having differing objectives. One camp was principally interested in fostering competition in the health care marketplace by promoting plans that incorporated incentives for providers to constrain costs. The second camp, although perhaps sharing the first objective, principally saw the HMO Act as a precursor to health reform and sought a vehicle to expand access to coverage for individuals who were without insurance or who had limited benefits. Imposing requirements on HMOs but not on indemnity carriers, however, reduced the ability of HMOs to compete.

Of particular note were requirements with regard to the comprehensiveness of the benefit package* as well as open enrollment and community rating. The open enrollment provision required that plans accept individuals and groups without regard to their health status. The requirement for community rating of premiums (see Chapter 25 for a discussion of community rating) limited the ability of plans to relate premium levels to the health status of the individual enrollee or employer group. Both provisions represented laudable public policy goals; the problem was that they had the potential for making federally qualified HMOs noncompetitive because the same requirements did not apply to the traditional insurance plans against which they competed. This situation was largely corrected in the late 1970s with the enactment of amendments to the HMO Act that reduced some of the more onerous requirements. The federal dual choice provisions were "sunsetted," that is, expired, in 1995 and are no longer in effect. Further, many states require forms of community rating for the small group market from all carriers now, not just HMOs; a few states, however, continue to have differing rating requirements for HMOs than they do for indemnity plans.

Another reason that HMO development was retarded was the slowness of the federal government in issuing regulations implementing the act. Employers knew that they would have to contract with federally qualified plans. Even those who were supportive of the mandate, however, delayed until the government both determined which plans would be qualified and established the processes for the implementation of the dual choice provisions. The Carter administration, which assumed office in 1977, was supportive of HMOs. In particular, Hale Champion as undersecretary of the U.S. Department of Health and Human Services, made issuance of the regulations a priority, and rapid growth ensued.

Politically, several aspects of this history are interesting. First, although differences arose on specifics, the congressional support for legislation promoting HMO development came from both political parties. Also, there was not widespread state opposition to the override of restrictive state laws. In addition, most employers did not actively oppose the dual choice requirements, although many disliked the federal government in effect telling them to contract with HMOs. Perhaps most interesting of all was the generally positive interaction between the public sector and the private sector, with government fostering HMO development both through its regulatory processes and also as a purchaser under its employee benefits programs.

Other managed care developments also occurred during the 1970s and early 1980s. Of note was the evolution of preferred provider organizations (PPOs). PPOs are generally regarded as originating in Denver, where in the early 1970s Samuel Jenkins, a vice president of the benefits consulting firm of the Martin E. Segal Company, negotiated discounts with hospitals on behalf of the company's Taft–Hartley trust fund clients.[5] Hospitals did so in return for the health plans having lower cost sharing for its users, thereby generating patient volume at the expense of its competitors.

Service plans (defined in Chapter 2), of which the Blue Cross and Blue Shield plans predominate, placed limits on maximum

---

*The ripple effects of the early HMO benefits requirements affect the health insurance and managed health care market even today. Prior to the comprehensive benefits that HMOs provided, indemnity health insurance and service plans (such as Blue Cross and Blue Shield plans) typically did not cover preventive care such as well child visits, routine health exams, or immunizations, and rarely provided coverage for outpatient drugs. HMOs were not required to offer drugs either but commonly did so to entice individuals to join. Soon the drug benefit became commonplace in all types of health plans.

charges of physicians; those limits reflected a composite of actual charges using a methodology known as "usual and customary" fee calculation, that is, based on statistical profiles of what physicians actually charged for individual services. They also had limits on payments to hospitals, in some cases paying them based on their actual costs. As PPOs grew in the market, the service plans began to adopt new methods of calculating payment maximums. By the late 1980s, however, even the service plans had created PPOs in response to market pressures, with the primary difference being a greater level of discount paid to providers. (Reimbursement is discussed in detail in Chapters 6 and 7.) Finally, as noted in Chapter 2 and elsewhere in this book, there are no clear distinctions between managed health care plan types anymore, though various attributes are discussed further throughout this text.

Utilization review expanded outside the HMO setting between 1970 and 1985, although it has earlier origins:

- In 1959, Blue Cross of Western Pennsylvania, the Allegheny County Medical Society Foundation, and the Hospital Council of Western Pennsylvania performed retrospective analyses of hospital claims to identify utilization that was significantly above the average.[6]
- Around 1970, California's Medicaid program initiated hospital precertification and concurrent review in conjunction with medical care foundations in that state, typically county-based associations of physicians who elected to participate, starting with the Sacramento Foundation for Medical Care.
- The 1972 Social Security Amendments authorized the federal Professional Standards Review Organization (PSRO) to review the appropriateness of care provided to Medicare and Medicaid beneficiaries. Although the effectiveness of the PSRO program has been debated, the PSRO program established an orga-

nizational infrastructure and data capacity upon which both the public and private sectors could rely. In time the PSRO was replaced by the Peer Review Organization (PRO), itself in turn replaced by the Quality Improvement Organization (QIO), which continues to provide oversight of clinical services on behalf of the federal and many state governments. Although the methods used by these organizations evolved along with their acronyms, their focus remained essentially the same.
- In the 1970s, a handful of large corporations initiated precertification and concurrent review for inpatient care, much to the dismay of the provider community.

Developments in indemnity insurance, mostly during the 1980s, included encouraging persons with conventional insurance to obtain second opinions before undergoing elective surgery and the widespread adoption of large case management—that is, the coordination of services for persons with expensive conditions, such as selected accident patients, cancer cases, and very low birthweight infants. Utilization review, the encouragement of second opinions, and instituting large case management all entailed at times questioning physicians' medical judgments, something that had been rare outside of the HMO setting. These activities, further discussed in Part III of this book, were crude by today's standards of medical management but represented a radically new role of insurance companies in managing the cost of health care at the time.

Also during the 1980s, worksite wellness programs became more prevalent as employers, in varying degrees and varying ways, instituted such programs as the following:

- Screening (for hypertension and diabetes)
- Health risk appraisal
- Promotion of exercise (whether through having gyms, conveniently located showers, or running paths; providing subsi-

dies for health club memberships; or simply by providing information)

- Stress reduction
- Classes (smoking cessation, lifting of heavy weights, and the benefits of - exercise)
- Nutritional efforts, including serving healthy food in the cafeteria
- Weight loss programs
- Mental health counseling

MANAGED CARE GROWS UP: 1985 TO 1995

The period between 1985 and 1995 saw a combination of innovation, maturation, and restructuring, each of which is discussed in the following sections.

Innovation

In many communities, hospitals and physicians collaborated to form integrated delivery systems (IDSs). These had two principal forms. The first entailed mergers or acquisitions that resulted in the creation of single legal entities, for example, of hospitals and group practices. The second was the formation of physician–hospital organizations (PHOs), principally as vehicles for contracting with MCOs. Typically, PHOs are separately incorporated, with the hospital and the physicians each having the right to designate half the members of the board. Most PHOs sought to enter into fee-for-service arrangements with HMOs and PPOs, although some accepted shared or full capitation risk. IDSs are discussed further in Chapter 2.

IDSs did not become important elements of the managed health care environment for a number of reasons, including provider participation requirements and reimbursement systems that did not support managed care goals. For example, most IDSs allowed all physicians with admitting privileges at the hospital in question to participate rather than selecting the more efficient ones. Also, the physicians were commonly required to use

the hospital for outpatient services (for laboratory tests) that might be obtained at lower cost elsewhere, hence hurting the ability of the PHO to be price competitive. Finally, some IDSs suffered from organizational fragmentation, reimbursement systems to individual doctors who were misaligned with the goals of the PHO, inadequate information systems, management that was inexperienced, and a lack of capital. In the end, most PHOs in particular were unable to sustain the financial risk for medical expenses.

A second innovation was the growth of carve-outs, which are organizations that have specialized provider networks and are paid on a capitation or other basis for a specific service, such as mental health (see Chapter 13), specialty disease management (see Chapter 10), chiropractic, and dental. The carve-out companies market their services principally to HMOs and large self-insured employers. In recent years, some of the large health plans that contracted for such specialty services have reintegrated them into the main company (so-called carve-in or insourcing arrangements). One reason for the reintegration was the view that carved-out services made it difficult to coordinate services, for example, between physical and mental health. Similar in concept are groups of specialists, such as ophthalmologists or radiologists, who accept capitation risk for their services (sometimes referred to as sub-capitation) through contracts with health plans and employer groups. Capitation is not the only method of reimbursement to carve-outs or specialty groups; discounted fee-for-service payments may also be used (see Chapter 6).

A third set of innovations are those made possible by advances in computer technology. Vastly improved computer programs, marketed by private firms or developed by managed care plans for internal use, that generate statistical profiles of the use of services rendered by physicians have become available. These profiles serve to assess efficiency and quality and may also serve to adjust payment levels to providers who are paid under capitation or risk-sharing arrangements to reflect patient severity. Chapters 16 and 17 discuss further the uses of medical infomatics.

Another example of the impact of computer technology is a virtual revolution in the processing of medical and drug claims, which is now much more commonly performed electronically rather than by paper submission and manual entry.* The result has been lower administrative costs and superior information, with the most prevalent and technologically advanced systems being the processing of prescription drug claims, enabling the pharmacist at the time a prescription is dispensed to receive information about eligibility of the member for coverage, amount of copay or co-insurance required on a drug-by-drug basis (real-time access to a health plan's formulary; see Chapter 12), and potential adverse effects. Management information systems can be expected to improve dramatically over the next few years as providers, almost universally, submit claims electronically. This impact from information technology is now being furthered by the requirements and mandated standards under the Health Insurance Portability and Accountability Act of 1996 (HIPAA) for administrative simplification, accelerating the movement toward inexpensive electronic interchange for the basic health insurance transactions, including the following:

- Claims
- Claims status
- Authorizations
- Eligibility checking
- Payment

---

*GF Anderson *et al* argue that "the United States lags as much as a dozen years beyond other industrialized countries" in the implementation of computer-based health information systems. See Anderson GF *et al*. Health care spending and use of information technology in OECD countries. *Health Affairs.* May/June 2006;XXV(3):819–829.

Maturation

Maturation can be seen from several vantage points. The first is the extent of HMO and PPO growth, with HMO enrollment increasing from 15.1 million in 1984 to 63 million in 1996; HMO enrollment reached 78.9 million in 2000, and then declined to 66.1 million in 2004.[7] This market dynamic is discussed further in following sections. However, insurance carriers are selling hybrid products that combine elements of HMOs and PPOs, making statistical compilations difficult. For example, there are health plans that have two networks, a narrow network and a broader one, with high cost sharing when the broader one is used, and yet even higher when a non-network provider is used. Such a plan functions virtually like an HMO with a POS plan and may be licensed as such, but could also be classified and/or licensed as a PPO.

Medicare and Medicaid (see Chapters 26 and 27) have also increasingly relied on managed care. Whereas Medicaid managed care has enjoyed relatively steady growth, Medicare managed care is another story. After rising from 1.3 to 6.3 million between 1990 and 1999, Medicare managed care enrollment reversed itself and declined to 4.6 million in 2003.[8] This decline has widely been attributed to changes in federal law enacted in 1997 governing reimbursement to Medicare managed care plans, resulting in financial losses and withdrawal of such care plans from many markets. However, analysis by Robert Berenson concludes that the law's provision that guaranteed annual increases, at a minimum of 2%, resulted in plans getting paid more than they would have received under the previous reimbursement formula.[9] Other contributing factors besides reimbursement changes may have been health plans' lacking the care management systems necessary to care for a senior and disabled population and in some cases the plans having reduced premiums below, or increased benefits above, levels that were sustainable in the long term to acquire market share early.

The Medicare Modernization Act, discussed in Chapter 26, contains many provisions that are likely to lead to a return of growth for Medicare managed care in both HMOs and PPOs. Most notable are the provisions that result in plans' being paid at rates that are, on average, above Medicare fee-for-service costs.[10] How Medicare managed health care evolves is not easily predicted, however, in light of the history over the past 20 years, particularly given the propensity of the federal government to alter reimbursement periodically.

Another phenomenon is the maturation of external quality oversight activities. Starting in 1991, the National Committee for Quality Assurance (NCQA; see Chapter 23) began to accredit HMOs. The NCQA was launched by the HMOs' trade association in 1979 but became independent in 1991, with the majority of board seats being held by employer, union, and consumer representatives. Many employers are requiring or strongly encouraging NCQA accreditation of the HMOs with which they contract, and accreditation came to replace federal qualification as the seal of approval. NCQA, which initially focused only on HMOs, has evolved with the market, for example, to encompass mental health carveouts, PPOs, physician credentialing verification organizations, and others. In addition to NCQA, other bodies that accredit managed care plans have also developed, as described in Chapter 23.

Performance measurement systems (report cards) continue to evolve, the most prominent being the Health Plan Employer Data and Information Set (HEDIS), which was developed by the NCQA at the behest of several large employers and health plans. The HEDIS data set has evolved and grown on a regular basis; the HEDIS data set that is current at the time of publication may be found in Chapter 23. Other forms of report cards have appeared since then and continue to develop as the market demands increasing levels of sophistication.

Another form of maturation is the focus of cost management efforts, which used to be almost exclusively inpatient hospital utilization. Practice patterns have changed dramatically in the last 25 years, however, and inpatient utilization has declined significantly. As illustration, hospital care as a percentage of national personal health care expenditures declined from 46.9% to 36.6%, whereas physician and other clinical services increased from 21.8% to 25.6%, and prescription drugs rose from 5.6% to 12.1%.[11] Although hospital utilization still receives considerable scrutiny, greater attention is being paid to ambulatory services such as prescription drugs, diagnostics, and care by specialists. Perhaps even more important is that the high concentration of costs in a small number of patients with chronic conditions has resulted in significantly more attention being paid to disease management, as discussed in Chapter 10.

Restructuring

Perhaps the most dramatic development is the restructuring that began in the late 1980s, reflecting the interplay between managed care, the health care delivery system, and the overall health care marketplace. The definitional distinctions have blurred as MCOs underwent a process of hybridization, making meaningful statistics difficult to collect. Staff and group model HMOs, declining in number and faced with limited capital and a need to expand geographically, formed IPA components, and in some cases (*eg,* Health-America of Pennsylvania's Pittsburgh plan, Harvard Pilgrim [née Harvard Community] Health Plan) even divested the medical group or staff model component. HMOs expanded their offerings to include PPO and point-of-service (POS) products, and some PPOs obtained HMO licenses. HMOs also found themselves contracting with employers on a self-funded rather than a capitated basis whereby the risk for medical costs remains with the employer, and a variety of hybrid arrangements has also emerged. The major commercial health insurance companies also dramatically increased their involvement in managed care by both acquiring local health plans and starting up HMOs and PPOs. In short, the managed care environment became even more complicated.

Another change is role of the primary care physician (PCP), who assumed responsibility for overseeing the allocation of resources. Most MCOs regard gaining the loyalty of PCPs as critical to their success. In a traditional HMO, the role of the PCP has been to manage a patient's medical care, including access to specialty care. This proved to be a mixed blessing for PCPs, who sometimes felt caught between pressures to reduce costs on the one hand and, on the other hand, the need to satisfy the desires of consumers who may question whether the physician has their best interests at heart in light of the financial incentives to limit resource consumption. The growing popularity of PPOs as compared to HMOs appears to have led to a shift away from PCP-based plans in recent years, for example, the requirement for authorization to access specialty services, known as the "gatekeeper" requirement. That being said, many plans (including PPOs) require lower copays if a member receives care from a PCP than if the member receives care from a specialist, thus retaining a primary care focus.

Finally, consolidation is notable among both health care plans and providers. Among physicians there continues a slow but discernable movement away from solo practice and toward group practice. As for hospitals, a substantial amount of consolidation on a regional or local level occurred, creating large local and regional systems. This consolidation occurred largely in the mid- to late-1990s and continues today, although at a much slower rate. National consolidation of hospitals has not been a significant factor in recent years, however. Hospital consolidation was commonly justified in terms of its potential for rationalizing clinical and support systems. A clearer impact, however, has been the enhanced ability to negotiate favorable payment terms, often to the chagrin of the health plans with which they contract[12] (see Chapter 7).

Health plan consolidation has also been robust and continues today. Smaller local health plans have been acquired or in some cases ceased operations because of a number of forces. Large employers with employees who are spread geographically have generally been moving toward national companies at the expense of local health plans. For smaller plans, the financial strain of having to continually upgrade computer systems and other technology can become excessive. Smaller plans may also find themselves unable to negotiate the same discounts as larger competitors, exacerbating the financial strain. Smaller plans in unique markets such as in rural areas or where physician loyalty is high (as may be found in one of the few successful provider-sponsored health plans; see Chapter 2) may continue to thrive, but that is the exception.

Even larger health plans have been targets for acquisition, primarily in the for-profit sector. Indeed, as of 2006 all of the Blue Cross Blue Shield plans that had converted to for-profit status have been amalgamated into a single company: Anthem (sometimes referred to as Anthem/WellPoint, reflecting the names of the two large predecessors). At the time of publication, four commercial for-profit companies accounted for the majority of covered lives: CIGNA, Aetna, United Health Care, and Anthem/WellPoint. Consolidation has not only occurred in the for-profit sector but also in the non-investor-owned (NIO)* sector, primarily in Blue Cross and Blue Shield plans. Market growth in the Blue Cross Blue Shield system has been considerable as a result of many factors, including its generally broad provider networks, the managed care backlash, and the Blue's improved ability to offer national accounts when compared to the

---

*NIO is a term preferred by a number of not-for-profit health plans because Blue Cross and Blue Shield plans in particular are taxed as though they are for-profit health insurance companies, not as though they are charitable organizations.

prior decade. In any given state, the Blue plan often has the highest market penetration of any health plan.

MANAGED CARE IN RECENT TIMES: 1995–2005

The economic boom of the mid- to late-1990s changed the dynamics in the managed health care industry. As a result of unemployment dropping below 4%, corporate profits becoming robust, and the economy growing, employers found it increasingly necessary to compete for employees. The anti-managed care rhetoric of political campaigns, combined with media "horror stories," helped fuel negative public sentiment about managed care. Despite generally positive perceptions of their own health plans, most consumers have negative perceptions about managed care in general.

The Managed Care Backlash

Anti-managed care sentiment, commonly referred to as the "managed care backlash," became a defining force in the industry. Political speeches, movies and television shows, news articles, and even cartoons increasingly began to portray managed care in an unflattering light.

In some respects, this is not surprising. Because managed care had significantly lower costs than traditional health plans did, it became a dominant form of health care coverage when many employers put their employees (and dependents) into managed care as their only type of coverage. When the number of individuals in managed care became substantial, the number of problems rose as well, including individuals who did not want to be in a managed care plan. Some of the problems were mostly irritants, such as mistakes in paperwork or claims processing in health plans with information technology (IT) systems that were unable to handle the load. Commonly, the consumer associated such problems with managed care even

though they were really part of health insurance in general. Other problems were highly emotional though not actually a threat to health, such as denial of coverage for care that was genuinely not medically necessary; for example, an unnecessary diagnostic test. Finally, a major source of contention with many consumers was the requirement that they obtain prior authorization from their primary care physician to access specialty care, although arguably this provision both reduces costs and increases quality by ensuring primary care physicians are fully apprised of the care that their patients receive.

A few problems, however, were real or—at least potential—threats to health, such as denial of coverage for truly necessary medical care or difficulties in accessing care resulting in subsequent ill effects on health. Although quite uncommon in practice (although not statistically studied), isolated problems of this nature could generate adverse publicity. The emotional overlay accompanying health care outstrips almost any other aspect of life. The loss of life or limb in a spouse or child causes grief in ways that a house fire or losing one's employment does not.

The managed care industry was not simply an innocent victim of bad publicity. As health plans and managed care companies grew, their ability to actually manage the delivery system was severely tested and frequently found wanting. Where clinically oriented decisions on coverage were once done with active involvement of medical managers, the rapidly growing health plans became increasingly bureaucratic and distant from their members and providers. Rapid growth also led to greater inconsistencies in decision making regarding coverage for clinical services. The public's perception that decisions regarding coverage of clinical care being made by "bean counters" or other faceless clerks may not have been fair or accurate in the opinion of managed care executives, but neither was it without merit. Decision-making authority was often delegated and applied using general policies and not necessarily with a sense of compassion or flexibility.

When enough instances of serious problems occur, they make good fodder for news that uses the well-proven reporting technique of "identifiable victim" stories in which actual names and faces are associated with anecdotes of poor care or other very real problems. Whether problems portrayed in the news may or may not have been represented fairly from the viewpoint of the health plan was irrelevant. When added on top of disgruntlement caused by minor or upsetting (though not dangerous) irritants caused by health plan operations, the public is not liable to be sympathetic to managed care, particularly with the backdrop of few insurance companies being loved.

Perhaps the most serious charge leveled against the managed care industry was the accusation that health plans *deliberately* refused to pay for necessary care to generate profits and enrich executives and shareholders. The negative reaction was enhanced by media stories of multi million dollar compensation packages of senior executives. Putting aside the fact that financial incentives drive almost all aspects of health care to varying degrees, this was a particularly pernicious charge that health plans faced, specifically the increasing number of for-profit plans.

One result of the backlash was new consumer protections at the state and/or federal level, or at least the threat of such legislation. For example, many states have passed legislation—the so-called prudent lay person rule—guaranteeing payment for emergency services if the precipitating symptoms could reasonably have been interpreted as an emergency, for example, chest pain that subsequently turned out to be indigestion. States have also passed bills instituting state-supervised independent appeals processes in the event of a medical denial. Finally, several unsuccessful attempts were made at the federal level to pass a so-called Patient Bill of Rights, which would have mirrored at a na-

tional level provisions that many states had adopted.

Last, a frequently cited reason for the managed care backlash is American's desire for choice. People simply did not want to be told that they could not go to any provider and still receive full coverage for their care. This attitude caused many HMOs to expand their networks aggressively and fueled the shift from traditional HMOs to less restrictive forms of coverage. For example, whereas enrollment in HMOs decreased from 24% in 1998 to 15% in 2005, PPO enrollment increased from 35% to 61%. Also noteworthy is that traditional insurance has become of only minor importance, with the percentage of enrollment in traditional plans. That is, those without contracted networks or other forms of managed care, which stood at 73% of employer-sponsored plans in 1988, declining to only 3% in 2005.[13]

Another example of the movement toward less restrictive forms of coverage is that a number of HMOs abandoned the primary care physician model (the so-called gatekeeper model discussed in Chapter 2) to one of "open access," allowing members to access any provider in the network (though usually with lower copays for primary care than for specialty care).[14] During this time, the managed care industry kept pointing out the good things it was doing for members such as coverage for preventive services and drugs, the absence of lifetime coverage limits, coverage of highly expensive care, and so forth, but to no avail.

The managed care backlash has become mostly an echo. The volume of HMO jokes has declined, news stories about coverage restrictions or withheld care are now uncommon, and there is little or no state or federal attention paid to placing restrictions on managed care plans. The HMO's legacy of richer benefits, combined with the general loosening of medical management and broad access to providers, collided with other forces by the end of the millennium, and health care costs once again shot up.

The Return of Health Cost Inflation

The rapid increases in health care costs experienced in the late 1980s and early 1990s had slowed considerably by the mid-1990s, but health cost inflation returned by the turn of the century. Managed care had been a significant contributor to holding down the rate of rise, but many of the fundamental reasons for increased health care costs remain today. It is worth noting that although the percentage of the gross domestic product (GDP) consumed by health costs throughout much of the 1990s remained steady at around 13.2%, this was only partially because of lower health cost inflation. The other reason was the robust growth of the GDP itself; in other words, health cost inflation slowed while the overall GDP grew at a higher rate than it had for many years.

The health economy is too complex to ascribe inflationary pressures to any single attribute, or even a small constellation of attributes. Where health cost inflation was once caused as much by unnecessary utilization as by anything else, other forces have always been present. The lessening of some of the controls traditionally associated with managed health care combined with a richer benefit package has certainly contributed to rising health costs, but numerous other factors have also been in play. Examples of other such factors are the following:

- Drug therapy advances and prescription drug prices
- Shifting demographics, including the aging of the population
- Expectations for a long and healthy life, regardless of costs
- Greater consumer demands upon the health care system
- The litigiousness of our society, leading physicians to practice defensive medicine
- High administrative costs related to the care that is delivered
- Inefficient or poor quality care rendered by some providers (professional and institutional) as evidenced by continuing large variations in practice behavior and insufficient adherence to evidence-based medical practice
- High incomes for some types of providers (regardless of efficiency or quality)
- The cost of complying with government mandates

These usual suspects are not the only ones pushing health cost inflation, however. Two relatively new categories are establishing themselves as major drivers of cost inflation: (1) rapidly developing (and usually expensive) medical technology, in some cases diffused widely with minimal evidence of effectiveness, and (2) genomics. Examples of new medical technology are the implantable cardiac defibrillator, drug-eluting vascular stents, new orthopedic implants, and miniaturization of devices, to name a few. In the arena of genomics, the appearance of so-called specialty pharmacy, injectable drugs that are proteins manufactured through DNA replication, has led to treatments that may not be used frequently but that are hugely expensive when they are used, commonly costing in excess of $10,000 per patient per year or more. The discovery of various alleles (*ie,* genes) for cancer that help guide physicians as to the best therapy depending on the genetic profile (*eg,* for breast cancer) are all adding to cost inflation. On a more positive note, although stem cell research has yet to result in concrete therapies, such new approaches to treating disease could be discovered and result in both improved treatment and lower cost.

Managed Health Care in Mid-Decade

At the same time health benefits costs began rising, the economy began to soften, and increasingly U.S. companies have become confronted with competition from abroad from companies that do not face the insurance costs of their American counterparts. These two forces led not to a return to traditional managed care but rather to an increase in cost sharing with consumers through higher payroll deductions for health benefits coverage and, more important, in the form of changes in the benefits. Levels of copayments and co-insurance have been rising and in many cases have become more complex. For example, physician office visit copays that were once most commonly $5.00 are now $20.00 or higher, and pharmacy benefits that were once simple copays now have widely differing levels of copayment tiering as well as significant deductibles. Ironically, cost sharing was the primary method of cost control available to indemnity insurance prior to the advent of managed health care.

The most recent significant development is the rise of the consumer-directed health plan (CDHP), including such variants as health savings accounts (HSAs) and other types of high-deductible health plans. CDHPs are described in Chapter 2, and issues associated with consumerism are more fully discussed in Chapter 20. A hallmark of a CDHP, though, is the notion that consumer choice and consumer accountability have substantially increased in importance. Health plans are improving the ability of members to choose physicians, hospitals, benefits plans, and so forth easily, using technology such as the Internet. They are also providing members with better information regarding the quality and cost of the care they are seeking along with information to help them understand their health care options. Aspects of informing consumers through data or information transparency, decision support tools, financial budgeting tools, and the like are currently the focus of much effort in all health plans, not just CDHPs.

The other aspect of CDHPs in their various forms is a benefits design that depends on greater cost sharing with consumers, a dynamic also observed with almost all benefits designs whether considered CDHPs or "traditional" managed care products. Through the existence of a gap in coverage between the pre-tax savings and when the high-deductible health plan coverage comes into play, the consumer is responsible for expenses. It is not yet clear whether CDHPs as they exist at the time of publication actually require more cost sharing by consumers than do other plan designs because of the rapid increases in cost sharing in all benefits designs. In fact, one study reports that CDHPs actually reduce cost sharing for many groups, in particular the small group of members responsible for half of all medical spending.[15]

Managed care has not ceded the field to the imposition of higher cost sharing combined with improved information to assist in decision making. For example, new pay-for-performance programs are being tested and implemented to align financial incentives for roviders with quality goals, as discussed fully in Chapter 8. Practice behavior by physicians has evolved, and as care management becomes more sophisticated, managed care companies have placed more emphasis on chronic and/or highly expensive medical conditions, with less focus on routine care, as discussed in detail in Part III of this book.

CONCLUSION

The health care sector in the United States is highly dynamic. The roots of managed health care, and health insurance in general, are many. The continued growth and evolution of managed health care is affected by the health sector economy, marketplace needs, legal and regulatory requirements, changes in health care delivery, consumer demands, politics, and a myriad of other forces, many of which interact with each other. What started out with simple roots has become complex and robust and will only become more so.

ADDITIONAL RESOURCES

Following is a list of several good sources on managed care trends. (Note: All Web addresses are current as of August 2006, but are subject to change.)

1. The Center for Medicare and Medicaid Services (CMS), especially the Office of the Actuary; navigate to http://www.cms

.org, or more specifically to http://www.cms.hhs.gov/NationalHealthExpendData/(free).

2. The Henry J. Kaiser Family Foundation (http://www.kff.org), particularly the series on the health care marketplace trends (free).

3. The Sanofi-Aventis Managed Care Digest Series, updated annually and accessible at http://www.managedcaredigest.com (free with registration).

4. HealthLeaders–InterStudy, accessible at http://home.healthleaders-interstudy.com (requires purchase).

References and Notes

1. Mayer TR, Mayer GG. HMOs: Origins and development. *N Engl J Med.* 1985:312,590–594.

2. MacLeod GK. An overview of managed care. In: Kongstvedt PR, ed. *The Managed Care Handbook,* 2nd ed. Gaithersburg, Md: Aspen, 1993:3–11.

3. Starr P. *The Social Transformation of American Medicine.* New York, NY: Basic Books, 1982: 295–310.

4. Strumpf GB. Historical evolution and political process. In: Mackie DL, Decker DK, eds. *Group and IPA HMOs.* Gaithersburg, Md: Aspen, 1981:17–36.

5. Spies JJ, Friedland J, and Fox PD. Alternative health care delivery systems: HMOs and PPOs. In: Fox PD, Goldbeck W, and Spies, JJ, eds. *Health Care Cost Management: Private Sector Initiatives.* Ann Arbor, Mich: Health Administration Press, 1984:43–68.

6. Fielding JE. *Corporate Cost Management.* Reading, Mass: Addison-Wesley, 1984.

7. Kaiser Family Foundation. *Trends and Indicators in the Changing Health Care Marketplace.* Place TK: Kaiser Family Foundation, 2005, Menlo Park, CA:Exhibit 2.13.

8. Data available from the Office of the Actuary, Centers for Medicare and Medicaid Services, and Kaiser Family Foundation, *op cit*, Exhibit 2.17.

9. Berenson RA. Medicare disadvantages and the search for the elusive "level playing field." *Health Affairs Web Exclusive.* December 15, 2004:W4.

10. Biles B, Nicholas LH, and Cooper BS. The cost of privatization: Extra payments to Medicare advantage plans—2005 update. *Common Wealth Fund Issue Brief.* December 2004.

11. Smith C, Cowan C, Heffler S, *et al.* National health spending in 2004: Recent slowdown led by prescription drug spending. *Health Affairs.* January/February 2006;XXV(1):186–196.

12. Devers KJ, Casalino LP, Rudell L, *et al.* Hospitals' negotiating leverage with health plans: How and why has it changed. Part II. *Health Services Res.* February 2003;XXXVIII (1):419–446.

13. Kaiser Family Fund. *Op cit*, Exhibit 2.3.

14. For additional discussion of some of the changes that HMOs and other managed care plans have made, see Draper DA, *et al.* The changing face of managed care. *Health Affairs.* January/February 2002;XXI(1):11–23.

15. Remler DK, Glied SA. How much more cost sharing will health savings accounts bring? *Health Affairs.* 2006;25(4):1070–1078.

2

Types of Managed Care Organizations and Integrated Health Care Delivery Systems

Eric R. Wagner and Peter R. Kongstvedt

Study Objectives

- Understand the different types of managed care organizations.
- Understand key differences between managed care organizations.
- Understand the inherent strengths and weaknesses of each model type.
- Understand the basic forms of Integrated Delivery Systems (IDSs) and how they are evolving.
- Understand the major strengths and weakness of each type of IDS, initially, and how they have played out as the markets developed.
- Understand the roles of physicians and hospitals in each type of IDS.

Discussion Topics

1. Describe the continuum of managed health care plans and key differences for each, using examples of each.
2. Discuss the principle elements of control found in each type of managed care plan. In which plans do those elements appear?
3. Discuss the primary strengths and advantages, and weaknesses and disadvantages, of each type of managed care plan.
4. Discuss in what type of market situations each type of managed care plan might be the preferred model.
5. Describe how a managed care plan of one type might evolve into another type of plan over time.
6. Discuss the key elements of the different types of integrated delivery systems.

7. Describe the conditions under which a managed care plan would desire to contract with an integrated delivery system; describe these conditions for each model type.
8. Describe the conditions under which a managed care plan would actively avoid contracting with an integrated delivery system; describe these conditions for each model type.

INTRODUCTION

Serious challenges are associated with attempting to describe the types of organizations in a field as dynamic as managed care. The health care system in the United States has been continually evolving and change is the only constant. Nevertheless, distinctions remain between different managed care organizations (MCOs), though many of those distinctions are rooted in the historic classifications that separated different forms of managed care, particularly during its time of rapid growth (see also Chapter 1). Despite the continual blurring of types of health care plans, it is useful to understand the different types of organization even though the pure form may only rarely be observed. It also is worth noting that research done in 1999 suggested that most of the U.S. public, the majority of whom were enrolled in a managed care organization, did not believe that they received their health care coverage through managed care.*

A decade ago or longer, the various types of MCOs were reasonably distinct. Since then the differences between traditional forms of health insurance and managed care organizations have narrowed to the point where it is very difficult to tell whether an entity is an insurance company or an MCO. In contrast to the situation 20 years ago, when managed care organizations were often referred to as

"alternative delivery systems," managed care in various forms is now the dominant form of health insurance coverage in the United States, and relatively few people receive their health insurance through the once traditional form of indemnity health insurance coverage. In other words, regardless of organizational type, many of the aspects of managed health care migrated into other forms of coverage and continue to evolve and migrate all the time.

Originally, health maintenance organizations (HMOs), preferred provider organizations (PPOs), and traditional forms of indemnity health insurance were distinct, mutually exclusive products and mechanisms for providing health care coverage. Today, an observer may be hard-pressed to uncover the differences between products that bill themselves as HMOs, PPOs, or managed care overlays to health insurance. The advent of consumer-directed health plans (CDHPs) beginning in the early part of 2000 does provide a greater difference when compared to other types of health plans, however, and these will be discussed later in this chapter as well as in Chapter 20, though even then, many aspects of managed health care are found in such plans.

For other types of health plans (ie, non-CDHPs), differences in plan type may be hard to distinguish. For example, many HMOs, which traditionally limit their members to a designated set of participating providers, now allow their members to use nonparticipating providers at a reduced coverage level. Such point-of-service (POS) plans combine HMO-like systems with indemnity systems, allowing individual members to choose which systems they wish to access at

---

*According to the 1999 Health Confidence Survey conducted by the Employee Benefit Research Institute, almost two-thirds of the 87% of workers who are covered by managed care think they have never been in a managed care plan. See September 21, 1999, EBRI News Release.

the time they need the medical service. POS rose and fell in popularity as a plan design, however, and is no longer as prevalent as it once was. Similarly, a few PPOs, which historically provided unrestricted access to physicians and other health care providers (albeit at different coverage levels), implemented primary care physician (PCP) case management or gatekeeper systems and even added elements of financial risk to their reimbursement systems. The majority of PPOs did not implement a PCP case management system, but even then often do provide for lower required copayments by members to see a PCP and higher copayments to see a specialty physician, thus encouraging a de facto form of PCP care management. Finally, almost all indemnity insurance (or self-insurance) plans now include utilization management (UM) features and provider networks in their plans that were once found only in HMOs or PPOs, though indemnity insurance is now a quite rare form of coverage.

As a result of these changes, the descriptions of the different types of managed care systems that follow provide only a guideline for determining the form of MCO that is observed. In many cases (or in most cases in some markets), the MCO will be a hybrid of several specific types.

Further confusing this is the existence of integrated health care delivery systems (IDSs)* that were created by providers in response to managed care. In the never-ending movement to render a taxonomy of MCOs, some of these types of IDSs even require licensure from the state if they accept risk for medical costs (*eg*, a "limited Knox-Keene" license in California) or from the federal government (*eg*, a provider-sponsored organization [PSO] contracting with Medicare on a financial risk basis and that does not already have state licensure). IDSs are briefly discussed later in this chapter.

Some disagreement exists about whether the term *managed care* accurately describes the new generation of health care delivery and financing mechanisms. Those commentators who object to the term raise questions about what exactly it is that MCOs are managing. These commentators ask: Is the individual patient's medical care being managed or is the organization simply managing the composition and reimbursement of the provider delivery system?

Observers who favor the term *managed care* believe that managing the provider delivery system can be equivalent in its outcomes to managing the medical care delivered to the patient. In contrast to historical methods of financing health care delivery in the United States, the current generation of financing mechanisms includes far more active management of both the delivery system through which care is provided and the medical care that is actually delivered to individual patients.

Perhaps the strongest reason that many in the industry have for not using the term *managed care* is the negative perceptions now associated with it. As managed care became the dominant model for health coverage in the United States during the 1990s, there was a strong public backlash against the restrictive features that were part of many managed care plans. The backlash, discussed in Chapter 1, may also have been driven to a certain extent by the change in focus as the large, old-line insurance companies entered the managed care market. Their focus shifted more heavily toward cost control and away from the old concepts of health maintenance, preventive care, and managing care by providing it in the most appropriate settings. In addition, many consumers were "forced" into managed care as the new managed care plans became the sole health benefit offering for many employers. American consumers value choice in most of their economic transactions, and health care is no exception.

Many health plans now simply call themselves that: health plans, or in the case of

---

*No reason that the *H* doesn't get use in this acronym other than "IDS" rolls off the tongue better, but IDS is the term commonly used.

the larger commercial companies, health insurance plans. Although the term *managed care* may not perfectly describe the current generation of financing and health care management vehicles, it continues to provide a convenient shorthand description for the range of alternatives to be discussed in this book and will therefore continue to be used.

A simplistic but useful concept regarding managed care is the continuum illustrated in Figure 2–1. On one end of the continuum is managed indemnity with simple precertification of elective admissions and large case management of catastrophic cases, superimposed on a traditional indemnity insurance plan. Similar to indemnity is the service plan, which has contractual relationships with providers addressing maximum fee allowances, prohibiting balance billing, and using the same utilization management techniques as managed indemnity (the nearly universal examples of service plans are traditional Blue Cross and Blue Shield plans). Further along the continuum are PPOs, POS, open panel (both direct contract and individual practice association [IPA] type) HMOs, and finally closed panel (group and staff model) HMOs. As you progress from one end of the continuum to the other, you add new and greater elements of control and accountability, you tend to increase both the complexity and the overhead required to operate the plan, and you achieve greater potential control of cost and quality.

CDHPs, which combine a high-deductible insurance policy with a PPO network and a unique pre-tax "up-front" financing mechanism, do not fit neatly on this continuum, however. Because of that, as well as their continued highly rapid evolution, they are described later in the chapter, separate from the more traditional types of managed care plans.

This chapter provides a description of the different types of managed health care organizations and the common acronyms used to represent them. A brief explanation is provided for each type of organization. In addition, this chapter includes descriptions of the basic forms of HMOs—the original types of managed care organizations—and their relationships with physicians.

TYPES OF MANAGED CARE ORGANIZATIONS

With the clear understanding that there are really no firm distinctions or boundaries between them, what follows is a discussion of the broad types of MCOs. Throughout this book, these types of MCOs may be referred to in such a way as to conform to what follows in this chapter; in other cases, a chapter author might simply throw in the towel and use the term *MCO* or *health plan* to cover the whole array of plan types. But distinctions between types of MCOs are not mere historic relics; there are differences that matter, and the terms themselves still enjoy wide usage (or misusage in some cases).

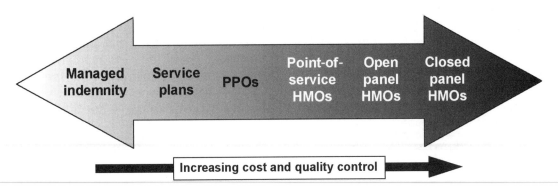

Figure 2–1 Continuum of Managed Care

Indemnity Insurance

Indemnity type of health insurance is simply that: It indemnifies the beneficiary from financial costs associated with health care. Indemnity insurance and service plans were the main type of health plan prior to the advent of managed health care, with notable exceptions as discussed in Chapter 1. Originally, few controls were in place to manage cost, and coverage was only for illness, not for wellness, preventive services (immunizations), or prescription drugs. The insurance company would also determine what the maximum appropriate charge should be for a procedure or professional visit, and that was all that was paid. A provider was then free to bill the beneficiary for anything not paid by the insurance company. In some cases, the insurance company paid the money directly to the beneficiary and the provider needed to then get paid by the beneficiary if it had not already collected its charges.

Rising health care costs hit indemnity insurance hard during the 1980s and early 1990s, and as managed care grew, indemnity insurance shrank. Indemnity insurance is now relatively rare, though not extinct. Where it does exist, it frequently has managed care approaches applied.

Service Plans

Service plans, the majority of which (though not exclusively so) are Blue Cross and Blue Shield (BCBS) plans, are similar in their basics to indemnity insurance with a very important difference: the existence of a contracted provider network. This contracted network provides for several highly important elements that carry throughout managed care in general:

- The plan contracts directly with providers (physicians, hospitals, and so forth).
- Provider contracts specify that the plan will pay them directly, and they may only bill the patient (member) for coinsurance, copays, or deductibles.

- As long as a member (beneficiary) receives services from a contracted provider, the member is protected from balance billing; that is, a provider cannot bill the patient for charges denied by the plan (see chapter 30).
- The plan has a method of calculating what maximum fee will be paid for all procedures or provider visits as regards professional services.
- The plan has a method for determining appropriate payments to hospitals.

Unmanaged service plans were subject to the same pressures as indemnity insurance in regards to medical costs with the same result. The difference is that the service plan has not disappeared from the landscape to the same degree as indemnity insurance and is often a part of another type of offering. For example, a PPO offered by a Blue Cross Blue Shield plan provides a degree of network coverage even if the member does not go to a PPO-contracted provider.

Managed Care Applied to Indemnity Insurance and Service Plans

The perceived success of HMOs and other types of managed care organizations in controlling the utilization and cost of health services prompted the development of managed care overlays that could be combined with traditional indemnity insurance, service plan insurance, or indemnity-like self-insurance (the term *indemnity insurance* is used to refer to all three forms of coverage in this context). These managed care overlays are intended to provide cost control for insured plans while retaining the individual's freedom of choice of provider and coverage for out-of-plan services. Though traditional indemnity insurance is now uncommon because of the high cost, it is still worthwhile understanding how these overlays are applied.

The following types of managed care overlays came into existence:

- *General utilization management.* These companies offer a complete menu of utilization management activities that can be selected by individual employers or insurers. Some offer or can develop panels of participating providers within individual markets and bear strong resemblances to PPOs.

- *Specialty utilization management.* Firms that focus on utilization review for specialty services have become common. Behavioral health (see chapter 13) and dental care are two common types of specialty utilization management overlays.
- *Disease management.* Free-standing disease management companies or an insurer's internal program may focus on specific common and costly diseases (*eg,* diabetes) rather than on utilization more broadly. See Chapter 10 for a detailed discussion on disease management.
- *Catastrophic or large case management.* Some firms have developed to assist employers and insurers with managing catastrophic cases regardless of the specialty involved. This service includes screening to identify cases that will become catastrophic, negotiation of services and reimbursement with providers who can treat the patient's condition, development of a treatment protocol for the patient, and ongoing monitoring of the treatment. See chapter 11 for a detailed discussion of case management.
- *Workers' compensation utilization management.* In response to the rapid increases in the cost of workers' compensation insurance, firms have developed managed care overlays to address what they claim are the unique needs of patients covered under workers' compensation benefits. Workers' compensation insurance is actually property-casualty insurance, not health insurance. Nevertheless, managed care methods may be applied in some cases.

Many indemnity insurance companies have carried these concepts several steps farther along the continuum by transforming themselves into MCOs through acquisitions of HMOs and other managed care companies. In fact, all of the major indemnity insurance companies that existed at the beginning of the 1990s have either sold their health insurance business lines to other companies or acquired major managed care companies. As noted in Chapter 1, as of 2006 four companies have become the largest MCOs in the country, surpassing the original managed care companies or free-standing HMOs in size and geographic coverage. One of those companies began its life in managed care, one company had its origins in the Blue Cross Blue Shield system of service plans, and two began as indemnity insurers. All four now operate in the same markets and offer similar types of services. At least in the case of these four large commercial companies, it is less an issue of blurring and more an issue of being able to offer almost all types of health plans, with plenty of hybridization.

Preferred Provider Organizations

PPOs are entities through which employer health benefit plans and health insurance carriers contract to purchase health care services for covered beneficiaries from a selected network of participating providers. Typically, participating providers in PPOs agree to abide by utilization management and other procedures implemented by the PPO and agree to accept the PPO's reimbursement structure and payment levels. In return, PPOs may limit the size of their participating provider panels and provide incentives for their covered individuals to use participating providers instead of other providers. In contrast to traditional HMO coverage, individuals with PPO coverage are permitted to use non-PPO providers, although higher levels of coinsurance or deductibles routinely apply to services provided by these nonparticipating providers. PPOs can be broad or they can be specialty-only (*eg,* behavioral health, chiropractic, dental).

The key common characteristics of PPOs include the following:

- *Provider network.* PPOs typically establish a network by contracting with selected providers in a community to provide health services for covered individuals. Most PPOs contract directly with hospitals, physicians, and other diagnostic facilities. Providers can be selected to participate on the basis of their cost efficiency, community reputation, and scope of services. Some PPOs assemble massive databases of information about potential providers, including costs by diagnostic category, before they make their contracting decisions. As a practical matter, however, PPOs now rarely deliberately limit the size of their network but rather contract with any provider willing to accept the terms and conditions of the PPO contract (and who meet screening criteria as discussed in Chapter 5).
- *Negotiated payment rates.* Most PPO participation agreements require participating providers to accept the PPO's payments as payment in full for covered services (except for applicable copays, coinsurance, or deductibles). Although negotiating payment rates with physicians and other professional providers may take place, it is more common for the PPO simply to inform the physician of what payment rates will be, which the physician can either agree to and contract with the PPO, or not agree to in which case they do not become a PPO provider. PPOs attempt to negotiate payment rates with hospitals that provide them with a competitive cost advantage relative to charge-based payment systems. These payment rates usually take the form of discounts from charges, fixed fee schedules, all-inclusive per diem rates, or payments based on diagnosis-related groups. Some PPOs have established bundled pricing arrangements for certain services, including normal delivery, open-heart surgery, and some types of oncology.
- *Utilization management.* Many PPOs implement utilization management programs to control the utilization and cost of health services provided to their covered beneficiaries. In the more sophisticated PPOs, these utilization management programs resemble the programs operated by HMOs.
- *Consumer choice.* Unlike traditional HMOs, PPOs generally allow covered beneficiaries to use non-PPO providers instead of PPO providers when they need health services. Higher levels of beneficiary cost sharing, often in the form of higher copayments, typically are imposed when PPO beneficiaries use non-PPO providers.

PPOs may be owned by many different types of organizations, as illustrated in Table 2–1. Furthermore, a PPO may be operated solely for the benefit of its owner (*eg*, a PPO created by a Blue Cross Blue Shield plan that provides services only to BCBS members), or it may be so-called rental PPO that was formed to offer services to any health plan under an administrative fee agreement (which may be limited to an access fee alone, or may include fees for other activities such as UM, claims repricing, and so forth).

Exclusive Provider Organizations

Exclusive provider organizations (EPOs) are similar to PPOs in their organization and purpose. Unlike PPOs, however, EPOs limit their beneficiaries to participating providers for any health care services. In other words, beneficiaries covered by an EPO are required to receive all their covered health care services from providers that participate with the EPO. The EPO generally does not cover services received from other providers, although there may be exceptions.

Some EPOs parallel HMOs in that they not only require exclusive use of the EPO provider

Table 2–1 PPO Ownership Models—2004

Type of Owner	Number of Eligible Employees (millions)	Percentage of Eligible Employees	Number of PPOs
Employer/employer coalition	0.3	0.3	4
HMO	2.4	2.2	60
Hospital	0.3	0.3	6
Hospital alliance	5.0	4.7	55
Independent investor	43.6	40.4	59
Insurance company	51.7	47.9	415
Multiownership	2.0	1.9	34
Physician/hospital joint venture	1.4	1.3	15
Physician/medical group	0.5	0.5	7
Third-party administrator	0.6	0.6	6
Other	0.08	0.1	5
Total	**107.9**	**100%**	**666**

Source: Sanofi-Aventis Managed Care Digest Series. *HMO-PPO/Medicare-Medicaid Digest 2005.* Available at: http://www.managedcaredigest.com.

network but also use a gatekeeper approach to authorizing non–primary care services. In these cases, the primary difference between an HMO and an EPO is that the former is regulated under HMO laws and regulations, whereas the latter is regulated under insurance laws and regulations or the Employee Retirement Income Security Act (ERISA; see Chapter 31) in the case of self-funded plans. Most EPOs are actually offered by PPOs, not HMOs.

EPOs usually are implemented by employers whose primary motivation is cost saving. These employers are less concerned about the reaction of their employees to severe restrictions on the choice of health care provider and offer the EPO as a replacement for traditional indemnity health insurance coverage. Because of the severe restrictions on provider choice, only a few large employers have been willing to convert their entire health benefits programs to an EPO format. When EPOs originally surfaced as a form of health coverage, some

observers predicted that they were the wave of the future and would be adopted by many large employers. In reality, some of those who established EPOs have abandoned them in favor of insurance vehicles that offer more choice to beneficiaries. In any case, although the number of PPOs that offer an EPO option to employers has grown, the actual number of individuals enrolled in EPOs has been declining.

Point-of-Service Plans

POS plans essentially combine an HMO or HMO-like health plan with indemnity (or service plan) coverage for care received outside of the HMO. Once touted as yet another wave of the future, they grew in the mid-1990s only to decline in popularity as their hoped-for cost savings failed to materialize. There are two ways in which POS plans were organized, depending on the vehicle to provide the HMO or HMO-like services.

Primary Care Preferred Provider Organizations

These types of POS plans are hybrids of more traditional HMO and PPO models, though they are licensed as PPOs.

The following are characteristics of these types of plans:

- Primary care physicians may be reimbursed through capitation payments (*ie*, a fixed payment per member per month) or other performance-based reimbursement methods (see Chapters 6 and 8).
- There may be an amount withheld from physician compensation that is paid contingent upon achievement of utilization or cost targets. Some states restrict the ability of managed care organizations to establish withholds, and they have become less common over time.
- The primary care physician acts as a gatekeeper for referral and institutional medical services.
- The member retains some coverage for services rendered that either are not authorized by the primary care physician or are delivered by nonparticipating providers. Such coverage is typically significantly lower than coverage for authorized services delivered by participating providers is (*eg*, 100% compared to 60%).

Point-of-Service Health Maintenance Organizations

As POS plans grew, some HMOs recognized that the major impediment to enrolling additional members and expanding market share was the reluctance of individuals to forfeit completely their ability to receive reimbursement for using nonparticipating providers. These individuals consider the possibility that they would need the services of a renowned specialist for a rare (and expensive to treat) disorder and believe that the HMO would not refer them for care or reimburse their expenses. This possibility, no matter how unlikely, overshadows all the other benefits of HMO coverage in the minds of many individuals. It also precluded most employers from limiting health benefit choice to a single HMO.

A number of HMOs (and insurance carriers with both HMOs and indemnity operations) adopted a solution to this problem: They provide some level of indemnity-type coverage for their members. HMO members covered under these types of benefit plans may decide whether to use HMO benefits or indemnity-style benefits for each instance of care. In other words, the member is allowed to make a coverage choice at the *point of service* when medical care is needed.

The indemnity coverage available under point-of-service options from HMOs typically incorporates high deductibles and coinsurance to encourage members to use HMO services within network instead of out-of-plan services. Members who use the non-HMO benefit portion of the benefit plan may also be subject to utilization review (*eg*, preadmission certification and continued stay review).

Health Maintenance Organizations

HMOs are organized health care systems that are responsible for both the financing and the delivery of a broad range of comprehensive health services to an enrolled population. The original definition of an HMO also included the aspect of financing health care for a prepaid fixed fee (hence the term *prepaid health plan*), but that portion of the definition is no longer absolute, although it is still common.

In many ways, an HMO can be viewed as a combination of a health insurer and a health care delivery management system. Whereas traditional health care insurance companies are responsible for reimbursing covered individuals for the cost of their health care, HMOs are responsible for providing or coordinating health care services to their covered members through affiliated providers who are reimbursed under various methods (see Chapters 6 and 7).

As a result of their responsibility for providing covered health services to their members, HMOs must ensure that their members have access to covered health care services. In addition, HMOs generally are responsible for ensuring the quality and appropriateness of the health services they provide to their members.

Health Maintenance Organization Models

The commonly recognized models of HMOs are staff, group, network, independent (or individual) practice association (IPA), and direct contract. An additional model is the open access plan, which has characteristics of an HMO and a PPO. The major differences among these models pertain to the relationship between the HMO and its participating physicians. At one time, individual HMOs could be neatly categorized into a single model type for descriptive purposes. Currently, many (if not most) HMOs have different relationships with different groups of physicians. As a result, many HMOs cannot easily be classified as a single model type, although such plans are occasionally referred to as mixed models. The HMO model type descriptions now may be more appropriately used to describe an HMO's relationship with certain segments of its physicians.

The following paragraphs provide brief descriptions of the five traditional HMO model types, followed by a brief description of the open access model.

Staff Model

In a staff model HMO, the physicians who serve the HMO's covered beneficiaries are employed by the HMO. These physicians typically are paid on a salary basis and may also receive bonus or incentive payments that are based on their performance and productivity. Staff model HMOs must employ physicians in all the most common specialties to provide for the health care needs of their members. These HMOs often contract with selected subspecialists in the community for infrequently needed health services.

Staff model HMOs may also be known as closed panel HMOs because most participating physicians are employees of the HMO, and community physicians are unable to participate. There have been many well-known examples of staff model HMOs in the past, but most of them have since shed the physician components. Examples included Harvard-Pilgrim Health Plan (the physicians became an independent medical group that is no longer exclusive to Harvard-Pilgrim), Group Health Association of Washington, DC (no longer in existence), FHP (no longer in existence), and others. In most cases, these plans "spun off" the physician component as a private medical group, though initially subsidized by the HMO parent. The track records of these suddenly free-standing groups were not always good, and some of them are now gone. Those staff model HMOs that still exist are incorporating other types of physician relationships into their delivery system. And although insurance companies that dabbled in the creation of staff model systems (*eg,* Aetna's Healthways) have abandoned them, some integrated delivery systems still use a staff model approach (for example, in the Twin Cities).

Physicians in staff model HMOs usually practice in one or more centralized ambulatory care facilities. These facilities, which often resemble outpatient clinics, contain physician offices and ancillary support facilities (*eg,* laboratory and radiology) to support the health care needs of the HMO's beneficiaries. Staff model HMOs usually contract with hospitals and other inpatient facilities in the community to provide nonphysician services for their members.

Staff model HMOs have a theoretical advantage relative to other HMO models in managing health care delivery because they have a greater degree of control over the practice patterns of their physicians. As a result, it can be easier for staff model HMOs to manage and control the utilization of health services. They also offer the convenience of one-stop shopping for their members because the HMO's facilities tend to be full service (*ie*, they have laboratory, radiology, and other departments).

Offsetting this advantage are several disadvantages for staff model HMOs. First, staff model HMOs are usually more costly to develop and implement because of the small membership and the large fixed salary expenses the HMO must incur for staff physicians and support staff. Second, staff model HMOs provide a limited choice of participating physicians from which potential HMO members may select. Many potential members are reluctant to change from their current physician and find the idea of a clinic setting uncomfortable. Third, many staff model HMOs experienced productivity problems with their staff physicians, which raised their costs for providing care. For example, the former Group Health Association in Washington, DC was forced to sell itself to Humana and convert to a group model plan partially because of physician productivity concerns; eventually, Humana in turn sold its entire DC plan to Kaiser (a group model plan, not a staff model). Finally, it is expensive for staff model HMOs to expand their services into new areas because of the need to construct new ambulatory care facilities. These disadvantages have led to steadily eroding presence in the market to the point where they are only present in a few locations in the country.

Group Model

In pure group model HMOs, the HMO contracts with a multispecialty physician group practice to provide all physician services to the HMO's members. The physicians in the group practice are employed by the group practice and not by the HMO. In some cases, these physicians may be allowed to see both HMO patients and other patients, although their primary function may be to treat HMO members.

Physicians in a group practice share facilities, equipment, medical records, and support staff. The group may contract with the HMO on an all-inclusive capitation basis to provide physician services to HMO members. Alternatively, the group may contract on a cost basis to provide its services, in which case it shares attributes of a staff model described earlier.

There are two broad categories of group model HMOs as described in the following subsections.

Captive Group. In the captive group model, the physician group practice exists solely to provide services to the HMO's beneficiaries. In most cases, the HMO formed the group practice to serve its members and recruited physicians and now provides administrative services to the group. The most prominent example of this type of HMO is the Kaiser Foundation Health Plan, where the Permanente Medical Groups provide all physician services for Kaiser's members. The Kaiser Foundation Health Plan, as the licensed HMO, is responsible for marketing the benefit plans, enrolling members, collecting premium payments, and performing other HMO functions. The Permanente Medical Groups are responsible for rendering physician services to Kaiser's members under an exclusive contractual relationship with Kaiser. Kaiser is sometimes mistakenly thought to be a staff model HMO because of the close relationship between it and the Permanente Medical Groups. Although not the only example, Kaiser is clearly the most robust, particularly in California.

Independent Group. In the independent group model HMO, the HMO contracts with an existing, independent, multispecialty physician group to provide physician services to its members. In some cases, the independent physician group is the sponsor or owner of the HMO. An example of the independent group model HMO is Geisinger Health Plan of Danville, Pennsylvania. The Geisinger Clinic, which is a large, multispecialty physician group practice, is the independent group associated with the Geisinger Health Plan (though the health plan also contracts with independent physicians to ensure adequate coverage of its entire service area).

Typically, the physician group in an independent group model HMO continues to provide services to non-HMO patients while it participates in the HMO. Although the group may have an exclusive relationship with the HMO, this relationship usually does not prevent the group from engaging in non-HMO business. These types of group models may or may not also contract with other, independent physicians in the community to broaden the network for marketing reasons.

Common Features of Group Models. Both types of group model HMOs may also be referred to as closed panel HMOs because physicians must be members of the group practice to participate in the HMO; as a result, the HMO is considered closed to physicians who are not part of the group. This may not necessarily be the case if the HMO also contracts with community physicians, though that is most likely to occur when the medical group does not cover all parts of the service area.

Both types of group model HMOs share the advantages of staff model HMOs of making it somewhat easier to conduct utilization management because of the integration of physician practices and of providing broad services at its facilities. In addition, group practice HMOs may have lower capital needs than staff model HMOs do because the HMO itself does not have to support the large fixed salary costs associated with staff physicians. Related to that, group model HMOs often report very low administrative costs because some of the activities of the HMO (*eg*, care management) are done by the medical group and not the HMO and are therefore considered part of the medical expense, not an administrative expense.

Group model HMOs have several disadvantages in common with staff model HMOs. Like staff model HMOs, group model HMOs provide a limited choice of participating physicians from which potential HMO members can select. The limited physician panel can be a disadvantage in marketing the

HMO. The limited number of office locations for the participating medical groups may also restrict the geographic accessibility of physicians for the HMO's members. The lack of accessibility can make it difficult for the HMO to market its coverage to a wide geographic area. Finally, certain group practices may be perceived by some potential HMO members as offering an undesirable clinic setting. Offsetting this disadvantage may be the perception of high quality associated with many of the physician group practices that are affiliated with HMOs. These disadvantages become less of a problem if the medical group(s) are quite large as is the case with Kaiser Permanente in California.

Network Model

In network model HMOs, the HMO contracts with more than one group practice to provide physician services to the HMO's members. These group practices may be broad-based, multispecialty groups, in which case the HMO resembles the group practice model described earlier. An example of this type of HMO is Health Insurance Plan (HIP) of Greater New York,* which contracts with many multispecialty physician group practices in the New York area. Network models also predominate in California where there are a number of existing large medical groups, unlike most other parts of the country where groups tend to be smaller.

Alternatively, the HMO may contract with several small groups of primary care physicians (*ie*, family practice, internal medicine, pediatrics, and obstetrics/gynecology), in which case the HMO can be classified as a primary care network model. In the primary care network model, the HMO contracts with several groups consisting of 7 to 15 primary care physicians representing the specialties of family practice and/or internal medicine, pediatrics, and obstetrics/gynecology to provide

---

*In 2006, HIP merged with Group Health Inc., a non-Blue Cross Blue Shield service plan, thus hybridizing the model to a significant degree.

physician services to its members. The HMO may compensate these groups on an all-inclusive physician capitation basis or on a partial capitation basis, but rarely on a fee-for-service basis (see Chapter 6). The group is responsible for providing all physician services to the HMO's members assigned to the group and may refer to other physicians as necessary. In the case of all-inclusive physician capitation, the group is financially responsible for reimbursing other physicians for any referrals it makes. In some cases, the HMO may negotiate participation arrangements with specialist physicians to make it easier for its primary care groups to manage their referrals.

In contrast to the staff and group model HMOs described previously, network models may be either closed or open panel plans. If the network model HMO is a closed panel plan, it will only contract with a limited number of existing group practices. If it is an open panel plan, participation in the group practices will be open to any physician who meets the HMO's and group's credentials criteria. In some cases, network model HMOs will assist independent primary care physicians with the formation of primary care groups for the sole purpose of participating in the HMO's network.

Network model HMOs address many of the disadvantages associated with staff and group model HMOs. In particular, the broader physician participation that is usually identified with network model HMOs helps overcome the marketing disadvantage associated with the closed panel staff and group model plans. Nevertheless, network model HMOs usually have more limited physician participation than either Independent Practice Association (IPA) model or direct contract model plans do if for no other reason than the fact that there are simply not that many large medical groups.

Independent (or Individual) Practice Association Model

Independent (or individual) practice association (IPA) model HMOs contract with an association of physicians—the IPA—to provide physician services to their members. The physicians are members of the IPA, which is a separate legal entity, but they remain independent practitioners and retain their separate offices and identities. IPA physicians continue to see their non-HMO patients and maintain their own offices, medical records, and support staff. IPA model HMOs are open panel plans because participation is open to all community physicians who meet the HMO's and IPA's selection criteria.

Generally, IPAs attempt to recruit physicians from all specialties to participate in their plans. Broad participation of physicians allows the IPA to provide all necessary physician services through participating physicians and minimizes the need for IPA physicians to refer HMO members to nonparticipating physicians to obtain services. In addition, broad physician participation can help make the IPA model HMO more attractive to potential HMO members.

IPA model HMOs usually follow one of two different methods of establishing relationships with their IPAs. In the first method, the HMO contracts with an IPA that has been independently established by community physicians. These types of IPAs often have contracts with more than one HMO on a nonexclusive basis. In the second method, the HMO works with community physicians to create an IPA and to recruit physicians to participate in it. The HMO's contract with these types of IPAs is usually on an exclusive basis because of the HMO's leading role in forming the IPA.

IPAs may be formed as large community-wide entities where physicians can participate without regard to the hospital with which they are affiliated. Alternatively, IPAs may be hospital-based and formed so that only physicians from one or two hospitals are eligible to participate in the IPA.

Most, though not all HMOs, compensate their IPAs on an all-inclusive physician capitation basis to provide services to the HMO's members. The IPA then compensates its participating physicians on either a fee-for-service basis or a combination of fee-for-service and capitation. In the fee-for-service variation,

IPAs pay all their participating physicians on the basis of a fee schedule, and the IPA withholds a portion of each payment for incentive and risk-sharing purposes.

Under the primary care capitation approach, IPAs pay their participating primary care physicians on a capitation basis and pay their specialist physicians on the basis of a fee schedule. The IPA may withhold a portion of both the capitation and fee-for-service payments for risk-sharing and incentive purposes.

IPA model HMOs overcome the disadvantages associated with staff, group, and network model HMOs. They require less capital to establish and operate. In addition, they can provide a broad choice of participating physicians who practice in their private offices. As a result, IPA model HMOs offer marketing advantages in comparison to the staff and group model plans.

There are two major disadvantages of IPA model HMOs from the HMO's perspective. First, the development of an IPA creates an organized forum for physicians to negotiate as a group with the HMO. The organized forum of an IPA can help its physician members achieve some of the negotiating benefits of belonging to a group practice. Unlike the situation with a group practice, however, individual members of an IPA retain their ability to negotiate and contract directly with managed care plans. Because of their acceptance of combined risk through capitation payments, IPAs are generally immune from antitrust restrictions on group activities by physicians as long as they do not prevent or prohibit their member physicians from participating directly with an HMO.

Second, the process of utilization management can be more difficult in an IPA model HMO than it is in staff and group model plans because physicians remain individual practitioners with little sense of being a part of the HMO. As a result, IPA model HMOs may devote more administrative resources to managing inpatient and outpatient utilization than their staff and group model counterparts do. Notwithstanding this historical disadvantage, many IPA model HMOs have overcome the challenge and succeeded in managing utilization at least as well as their closed panel counterparts.

Direct Contract Model

As the name implies, direct contract model HMOs contract directly with individual physicians to provide physician services to their members. With the exception of their direct contractual relationship with participating physicians, direct contract model HMOs are similar to IPA model plans. Direct contracting is the most common type of HMO model.

It is also common for this type of model also to be referred to as an IPA, despite the lack of the legal entity of an IPA. It is not the intent of this chapter, or this book, to proselytize purity of terminology. If individuals wish to refer to this as an IPA, that's their business. But the reader should be aware of the differences because the presence or absence of an actual IPA has an effect on the HMO and its management needs.

Direct contract model HMOs attempt to recruit broad panels of community physicians to provide physician services as participating providers. These HMOs usually recruit both primary care and specialist physicians and typically use a primary care case management approach (also known as a gatekeeper system).

Like IPA model plans, direct contract model HMOs compensate their physicians on either a fee-for-service basis or a primary care capitation basis. Primary care capitation historically was more commonly used by direct contract model HMOs because it helps limit the financial risk assumed by the HMO.* Unlike IPA model HMOs, direct con-

---

*As is noted in Chapter 6, many health plans have moved away from primary care capitation in recent years. Although there are several reasons for this change, one of the most compelling reasons has been the need to get accurate encounter reporting from physicians for quality measurement purposes; fee-for-service reimbursement facilitates such reporting.

tract model HMOs retain most of the financial risk for providing physician services; IPA model plans transfer this risk to their IPAs.

Direct contract model HMOs have most of the same advantages as IPA model HMOs. In addition, direct model HMOs eliminate the potential of a physician bargaining unit by contracting directly with individual physicians. This contracting model reduces the possibility of mass termination of physician participation agreements.

Direct contract model HMOs have several disadvantages. First, the HMO may assume additional financial risk for physician services relative to an IPA model HMO, as noted earlier. This additional risk exposure can be expensive if primary care physicians generate excessive referrals to specialist physicians.

Second, it can be more difficult and time-consuming for a direct contract model HMO to recruit physicians and manage the network because it lacks the physician leadership inherent in an IPA model plan. It is more difficult for nonphysicians to recruit physicians, as several direct contract model HMOs discovered in their attempts to expand into new markets. This disadvantage is now primarily of historical interest only because there is little or no new HMO market expansion anymore.

Finally, utilization management may be more difficult in direct contract model HMOs because all contact with physicians is on an individual basis and there may be little incentive for physicians to participate in the utilization management programs.

Mixed Model
As the term describes, many HMOs or MCOs are actually mixes of different model types. It is far more common for closed panel types of MCOs to add open panel components to their health plan than the reverse, but there are examples of large open panel HMOs adding a staff model component through a contract with an IDS, for example.

Open Access HMO
The oxymoronic term *open access HMO* is an HMO that does not use a PCP or "gatekeeper"

approach to managing access and utilization. In other words, though licensed as an HMO, there is no requirement at all to go through a PCP to access a specialist. It is common for the copayment to be different (*ie*, lower to see a PCP, higher to see a specialist), and there may be other mild economic incentives to use PCPs preferentially, but it is not required.

In this regard, they bear some resemblance to PPOs, except that a PPO may not differentiate copayment or co-insurance based on specialty type, though many certainly do. Open access plans may also put the physicians at some level of financial risk for medical costs, as discussed in Chapter 6. Last, these types of plans reportedly depend heavily on their ability to create meaningful physician practice profiles to allow medical managers to focus on problem areas (see Chapter 16).

Open access HMOs are not as common as PCP-based HMOs. Many were created and then failed in the 1970s and 1980s. However, new ones appeared in the late 1990s and appear to be reasonably successful. It is fair to say that the environment that physicians practice in at the present is substantially different from that of 1980, but it is not clear if that is the reason these new open access plans appear to be succeeding. Nevertheless, by the early-2000s, most HMOs that were going to become open access had done so.

Self-Insured and Experience-Rated Health Maintenance Organizations

Historically, HMOs offered community-rated premiums to all employers and individuals who enrolled for HMO coverage. The federal HMO Act (no longer in force) originally mandated community rating for all HMOs that decided to pursue federal qualification. Many states had similar requirements.

Community rating was eventually expanded to include rating by class, where premium rates for an individual employer group could be adjusted prospectively on the basis of demographic characteristics that were associated with utilization differences. Such characteristics often included the age and sex distributions of the employer's workforce and the standard industrial classification of the employer.

Although community rating by class provided HMOs with some flexibility to offer more attractive rates to selected employer groups, many employers continued to believe that their group-specific experience would be better than the rates offered by HMOs. Some HMOs developed self-insured or experience-rated options in response to the needs expressed by these employers.

Under a typical self-insured benefit option, an HMO receives a fixed monthly payment to cover administrative services (and profit) and variable payments that are based on the actual or incurred expenses made by the HMO for health services. There is usually a settlement process at the end of a specified period, during which a final payment is calculated (either to the HMO by the employer or to the employer by the HMO). Variations in the payment arrangement exist and are similar in structure to the different forms of self-funded insurance programs.

Under experience-rated benefit options, an HMO receives monthly premium payments much as it would under traditional premium-based plans. There typically is a settlement process where the employer is credited with some portion (or all) of the actual utilization and cost of its group to arrive at a final premium rate. Refunds or additional payments are then calculated and made to the appropriate party.

The HMO regulations of some states preclude HMOs from offering self-insured or experience-rated benefit plans. HMOs avoid these prohibitions by incorporating related corporate entities that use the HMO's negotiated provider agreements, management systems, utilization protocols, and personnel to service the self-insured line of business.

Rating methodologies are discussed in Chapter 25.

CONSUMER-DIRECTED HEALTH PLANS

CDHPs combine a high-deductible insurance plan with some form of pre-tax savings account. They are often associated with a PPO network as well. At its most basic, health care costs are paid first from the pre-tax account and when that is exhausted, any additional costs up to the deductible are paid out-of-pocket by the member (this gap is sometimes referred to as a bridge or, less charitably, as a doughnut hole). Preventive services are usually covered outside of this system, however. The definition of preventive services is not uniform among plan sponsors. Any funds left over in the savings account may roll over to be used in following years as needed.

There are two basic forms of CDHPs: commercial CDHPs that use Health Reimbursement Accounts (HRAs) and plans associated with Health Savings Accounts (HSAs). HSAs were created as part of the Medicare Modernization Act and are a more rigid form of CDHP in how they are constructed, with guidance provided by the Treasury Department (because the HSA is funded with pretax dollars), including such definitions as what constitutes preventive care. Commercial CDHPs and their associated HRAs are also subject to Treasury Department regulation, but that applies only to the HRA itself, while the plan design is otherwise more flexible, subject to state insurance regulations or, in the case of self-funded business under ERISA (see Chapter 31), the Labor Department. As a practical matter, the differences are not especially important to understanding the basics of CDHPs for purposes of this overview.

An example of a simplistic schematic of a CDHP is illustrated in Figure 2–2.

CDHPs are not considered managed health care plans by some who consider them as more akin to simpler indemnity-type insurance plans from the past. This is because of the presence of a high-deductible health insurance policy as the primary product, with

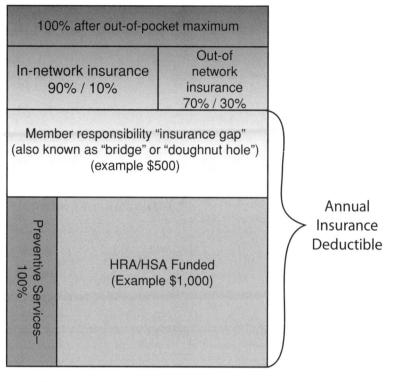

Figure 2–2 Example of Basic Construct of a CDHP

new benefits in the form of preventive services combined with new pre-tax funding mechanisms for at least a portion of the costs. Furthermore, one of the primary tenets behind CDHPs is that the consumer has become shielded by traditional managed care plans as to how much health really costs; in other words, consumers have come to believe that an office visit really only costs $10 or that a sophisticated diagnostic test only costs $20. The CDHP is therefore constructed to make cost a factor in consumer decision making through the use of both the pre-tax fund and the bridge, with the CDHP providing information to consumers to help them make decisions based on cost and quality of services. Because consumerism and aspects of CDHPs are discussed in greater detail in Chapter 20, the method of providing that information will not be discussed here.

CDHPs have not entirely shed all aspects of managed health care, however. Most are associated with a PPO to provide the value of the negotiated discount to the consumer. From the provider viewpoint, this is a mixed blessing at best because providers may find that it is difficult to collect all of the money owed to them when they must bill the member directly. Integrating the functions of the HRAs or HSAs through debit cards, and even finding ways of providing a credit facility so as to improve the provider's ability to collect what it is due, is a major focus of effort at the time of publication and is discussed further in Chapter 20.

Simply integrating with an existing PPO is the most common but not the only aspect of managed care that CDHPs retain. Integration of medical management into the new plan designs remains an evolving aspect as well, particularly with CDHPs offered by the larger and more established companies. Disease management (DM; see Chapter 10) and case management (CM; see Chapter 11) are most frequently applied because a small proportion of the population accounts for a disproportionately high percentage of medical costs. In those cases, medical costs can quickly move past the pre-tax fund and the bridge and trigger the high-deductible insurance, where focus on managing chronic disease is exactly the same as it is for any other type of managed health care plan. Having said that, how a CDHP applies DM in the early stages of a chronic disease, when costs are still applicable to the pre-tax fund and the bridge, is still evolving.

INTEGRATED HEALTH CARE DELIVERY SYSTEMS*

There are myriad types of IDSs, and some of the more common forms are discussed briefly in this chapter. At the very least, an IDS represents providers coming together in some type of legal structure for purposes of managing health care and contracting with health plans such as HMOs, PPOs, or health insurance companies. The IPA as discussed earlier is an IDS, and some IDSs combine different types of providers as well. The common denominator, however, is the physician; many types of organizations can exist in health care for purposes of managing health care and contracting with health plans that do not involve physicians (*eg*, a multifacility hospital system with affiliated ancillary services), but unless there is a significant physician component (specifically, physicians other than the paid hospital staff), it would not be considered an IDS.

---

*Portions of this section were adapted from Chapter 4: "Integrated Health Care Delivery Systems," by Peter R. Kongstvedt, David W. Plocher, and Jean Stanford. *The Managed Health Care Handbook*, 4th ed. New York, NY: Aspen Publishers, 2000.

Although neither this chapter nor this book focus on creating and operating an IDS, it is worthwhile to have at least a passing acquaintance with them. The most common IDSs are briefly described as follows.

Independent Practice Association

IPAs have been discussed earlier and that discussion will not be repeated here.

Physician Practice Management Companies

Physician practice management companies (PPMCs) arrived on the integration scene in the mid-1990s. PPMCs may in some ways be viewed as variants in management services organizations, but unlike the MSO, PPMCs are physician only. In other words, there is no involvement by the hospital. PPMCs were usually publicly traded companies as well, placing great pressure on the need to report positive earnings.

Most major PPMCs have failed—either going through bankruptcy or exiting the business altogether, though a few do remain in existence. Several reasons contributed to their failure. One common problem was decreased productivity because the PPMCs purchased physician practices only to find that once the physician had "cashed out" his or her practice, there was no longer sufficient incentive for the physician to be highly productive. PPMCs also found that there was in fact little profit margin to be had in practices in which the primary cost was for compensation, despite small improvements in practice overhead costs as a result of economies of scale. Last, many PPMCs entered into full-risk capitation arrangements with HMOs and found themselves unable to manage them profitably. Since the failures of the late 1990s, there has been little PPMC activity other than some specialty PPMCs that are part of an approach to highly specialized care management (*eg*, pediatric intensive care.

Group Practice Without Walls

The group practice without walls (GPWW), also known as the clinic without walls, is a step toward greater integration of physician services. The GPWW does not require the participation of a hospital and, indeed, is often formed as a vehicle for physicians to organize without being dependent on a hospital for services or support. In some cases, GPWW formation has occurred to leverage negotiating strength not only with MCOs but with hospitals as well.

The GPWW is composed of private practice physicians who agree to aggregate their practices into a single legal entity, but the physicians continue to practice medicine in their independent locations. In other words, the physicians appear to be independent from the view of their patients, but from the view of a contracting entity (usually an MCO) they are a single group. This is differentiated from the for-profit, physician-only MSOs described later by two salient features: first, the GPWW is owned solely by the member physicians and not by any outside investors, and second, the GPWW is a legal merging of all assets of the physicians' practices rather than the acquisition of only the tangible assets (as is often the case in an MSO).

To be considered a medical group, the physicians must have their personal income affected by the performance of the group as a whole. Although an IPA will place a defined portion of a physician's income at risk (that portion related to the managed care contract held by the IPA), the group's income from any source has an effect on the physician's income and on profit sharing in the group; that being said, it is common in this model for an individual physician's income to be affected most by individual productivity.

The GPWW is owned by the member physicians, and governance is by the physicians. The GPWW may contract with an outside organization to provide business support services. Office support services are generally provided through the group, although as a practical matter the practicing physicians may notice little difference in what they are used to receiving.

The GPWW model continues to exist in markets with a sufficient amount of full-risk capitation or other strongly managed health care. Full-risk capitation may still represent a significant amount of revenue in such markets, but even when capitation is for the direct services only, the GPWW can potentially achieve enhanced revenues through pay-for-performance programs which will be discussed further in Chapter 8. Outside of such markets, however, the GPWW model is much less common.

Physician-Hospital Organizations

The physician-hospital organization (PHO) is an entity that, at a minimum, allows a hospital and its physicians to negotiate with third-party payers. PHOs may do little more than provide for such a negotiating vehicle, although this could raise the risk of antitrust. PHOs may actively manage the relationship between the providers and MCOs, or they may provide more services, to the point where they may more aptly be considered MSOs (see discussion later).

PHOs often formed as a reaction to market forces from managed care. PHOs are considered the easiest type of vertically integrated system to develop (although they are not actually that easy, at least if done well). They also are a vehicle to provide some integration while preserving the independence and autonomy of the physicians.

By definition, a PHO requires the participation of a hospital and at least some portion of the admitting physicians. In the mid-1990s, PHOs were formed primarily as a defense mechanism to deal with an increase in managed care contracting activity. Even then, it was not uncommon for the same physicians who join the PHO already to be under contract with one or more managed care plans. Since then, fewer PHOs were created, though existing ones continue to operate.

In its weakest form, the PHO is considered a messenger model. This means that the PHO analyzes the terms and conditions offered by an MCO and transmits its analysis and the contract to each physician, who then decides on an individual basis whether to participate.

In its simplest and more common version, the participating physicians and the hospital develop model contract terms and reimbursement levels and use those terms to negotiate with MCOs. The PHO usually has a limited amount of time to negotiate the contract successfully (eg, 90 days). If that time limit passes, then the participating physicians are free to contract directly with the MCO; if the PHO successfully reaches an agreement with the MCO, then the physicians agree to be bound by those terms. The contract is still between the physician and the MCO and between the hospital and the MCO. In some cases, the contract between the physicians and the MCO is relatively brief and may reference a contract between the PHO and the MCO.

The reader should note that the "PO" portion of a PHO may be a different model entirely. As an example, a GPWW or an IPA could represent the physician portion of the PHO, although most commonly the physicians remain independent and contract individually with the PHO.

One final note concerning PHOs and other types of physician organizations: the Federal Trade Commission (FTC) has toughened its scrutiny of such organizations during the last few years. Physician organizations that are not paid on a capitation basis, and that do not accept substantial financial risk through some other mechanism, now find it much more difficult to operate within the FTC's antitrust safety zone. Although it is beyond the scope of this introductory chapter, those interested in physician organizations are urged to consult with competent antitrust counsel during the formation and operational stages.*

---

*Interested readers may also want to review the full FTC's opinion in the *Matter of North Texas Specialty Physicians* and other resources on this recent case.

Management Services Organizations

An MSO represents the evolution of the PHO into an entity that provides more services to the physicians. Not only does the MSO provide a vehicle for negotiating with MCOs, but it also provides additional services to support the physicians' practices. The physician, however, usually remains an independent private practitioner. The MSO is based around one or more hospitals.

In its simplest form, the MSO operates as a service bureau, providing basic practice support services to member physicians. These services include such activities as billing and collection, administrative support in certain areas, electronic data interchange (such as electronic billing), and other services. Recently, existing MSOs are being considered as excellent vehicles to provide the electronic backbone for the electronic medical record and other forms of electronic connectivity (see Chapter 17).

The physician can remain an independent practitioner, under no legal obligation to use the services of the hospital on an exclusive basis. The MSO must receive compensation from the physician at fair market value, or the hospital and physician could incur legal problems. The MSO should, through economies of scale as well as good management, be able to provide those services at a reasonable rate.

An MSO may also be considerably broader in scope. In addition to providing all the services described earlier, the MSO may actually purchase many of the assets of the physician's practice; for example, the MSO may purchase the physician's office space or office equipment (at fair market value). The MSO can employ the office support staff of the physician as well. MSOs can further incorporate functions such as quality management, utilization management (UM), provider relations, member services, and even claims processing in those markets where there is significant full-risk capitation. This form of MSO is usually constructed as a unique business entity, separate from a PHO.

The MSO does not always have direct contracts with health plans for two reasons: many plans insist on having the provider be the contracting agent, and many states will not allow health plans (especially HMOs) to have contracts with any entity that does not have the power to bind the provider. The physician may remain an independent private practitioner under no contractual obligation to use the hospital on an exclusive basis.

Foundation Model

A foundation model IDS is one in which a hospital creates a not-for-profit foundation and actually purchases physicians' practices (both tangible and intangible assets) and puts those practices into the foundation. This model usually occurs when, for some legal reason (*eg*, the hospital is a not-for-profit entity that cannot own a for-profit subsidiary, or there is a state law against the corporate practice of medicine), the hospital cannot employ the physicians directly or use hospital funds to purchase the practices directly. It must be noted that to qualify for and maintain its not-for-profit status, the foundation must prove that it provides substantial community benefit.

A second form of foundation model does not involve a hospital. In that model, the foundation is an entity that exists on its own and contracts for services with a medical group and a hospital. On a historical note, in the early days of HMOs many open panel types of plans that were not formed as IPAs were formed as foundations; the foundation held the HMO license and contracted with one or more IPAs and hospitals for services.

The foundation itself is governed by a board that is not dominated by either the hospital or the physicians (in fact, physicians may represent no more than 20% of the board) and includes lay members. The foundation owns and manages the practices, but the physicians become members of a medical group that, in turn, has an exclusive contract for services with the foundation; in other words, the foundation is the only source of revenue to the medical group. The physicians have contracts with the medical group that are long term and contain non-compete clauses.

Although the physicians are in an independent group, and the foundation is also independent from the hospital, the relationship in fact is close among all members of the triad. The medical group, however, retains a significant measure of autonomy regarding its own business affairs, and the foundation has no control over certain aspects, such as individual physician compensation.

Provider-Sponsored Organization

Provider-sponsored organization (PSO) is a term used to describe a cooperative venture of a group of providers who control an integrated provider system engaged in *both* delivery and financing of health care services. PSOs were part of the federal Balanced Budget Act of 1997 and were created so as to allow provider organizations to contract directly with Medicare on an at-risk basis for all medical services, bypassing existing Medicare HMOs (called Medicare+Choice at that time, and Medicare Advantage now) entirely. Though PSO activity was focused on the Medicare population, it could theoretically have expanded to include commercial and Medicaid initiatives as well. As a grand experiment, however, it failed miserably.

Providers found to their detriment that taking on full risk for the health care costs of the elderly involved more than taking the money and providing the services. In other words, "cutting out the middleman" in the form of bypassing experienced Medicare HMOs was a fast route to deep financial losses. Medical costs were made up of more than the services delivered by members of the PSO; considerable expense was also associated with care delivered by non-PSO providers, medical technology costs, and so forth. Furthermore, many PSOs tried to maintain existing fee-for-service reimbursement or otherwise failed to spread the financial risk sufficiently.

Last, PSOs found it difficult in many cases to practice the type of care management that was required to keep costs under control because the providers themselves rebelled at such constraints.

The failure of so many PSOs when they were first introduced meant that they essentially disappeared from the managed care landscape. Medicare still has provisions for how PSOs may accept risk for Medicare members, and it is possible that there may be a cautious reappearance of them, particularly in light of the new acuity-based premium payment being implemented (see Chapter 26).

CONCLUSION

Managed care is on a continuum, with a number of plan types offering an array of features that vary in their abilities to balance access to care, cost, quality control, benefit design, and flexibility, and the rise and, evolution of integrated health care delivery systems has paralleled the industry. During the last two decades, managed care has gone from being a relatively small part of the health care system synonymous with "alternative delivery system" to being a mainstream manner in which employer-insured individuals obtain their care. Managed care organizations will continue to evolve, with features from one type of plan appearing in others and new features continually being developed. As consolidation in the marketplace continues, it will blur the lines further. The recent appearance of new designs such as consumer-directed health plans makes taxonomy an even greater challenge than it was before. And although there is no one single definition of the term *managed care* that has endured in the past or will survive into the future, the basic tenets of managed health care will continue to evolve in pace with market demands and requirements.

3

ELEMENTS OF THE MANAGEMENT CONTROL AND GOVERNANCE STRUCTURE

Peter R. Kongstvedt

Study Objectives

- Understand the basic elements of governance and control of a managed care organization.
- Understand the typical key executive roles in an MCO.
- Understand risk management at the board level.

Discussion Topics

1. Describe and discuss the most important functions of a board of directors.
2. Describe and discuss how a typical board can lower their risk profile.
3. Describe and discuss the key executive positions and their functions.
4. Describe and discuss typical operating committees of the board and their functions.

It is not really possible to deal comprehensively with the topic of the elements of governance and management control structure in one chapter of a book. Myriad courses, texts, and other learning resources are available to the reader that deal with the basic elements of management. For the purposes of this chapter, it is assumed that the reader has a working knowledge of business and management, so certain fundamental aspects of management will not be discussed here (*eg*, how to read a balance sheet, write a job description, or construct an organizational chart).

There is no standardization of management governance or control structure in managed care; for example, the function, or even the very presence, of a board of directors varies from plan to plan. The function of key officers or managers, as well as of committees, likewise varies depending on the type of organization, the ownership, and the motivations and skills of the individuals involved. Because each plan constructs its own management control structure to suit its needs, only a few of the most common elements are described in this chapter. Further, many legal and regulatory requirements (state and federal) vary depending on many other aspects of a health plan (*eg*, for-profit; not-for-profit; state of domicile; provider-owned; product types such as commercially insured, self-funded, Medicare, Medicaid; and so forth).

The legal and regulatory aspects are discussed in the appropriate chapters elsewhere in this book and are not broken out here. Detailed discussions of operational activities are likewise the topics of most chapters in this book. What follows in this chapter is a brief overview of certain management control elements as they pertain specifically to managed health care.

In the existing market in which consolidation has been a major factor (see Chapter 1), governance and management control do not exist for most health plans on a free-standing basis. State laws and regulations may require certain governance structures, but that does not translate into a free-standing board, for example. Likewise, management control in national companies is far more likely to be exerted at the national or regional level than at a local level. Nevertheless, it is important to understand this aspect of how a health plan works. Therefore, the following discussion occurs in the context of an independent, free-standing managed health care plan for purposes of descriptions.

BOARD OF DIRECTORS

Many, although not all, types of managed care plans have a board of directors. The makeup and function of the board are influenced by many factors, but the board has the final responsibility for governance of the operation.

Examples of plans or managed care operations that would not necessarily have their own boards include the following:

- Preadmission certification and medical case management operations of insurance companies
- Preferred provider organizations (PPOs) developed by large insurance companies
- PPOs developed for single employers by an insurance company
- A health maintenance organization (HMO) set up by a single company for purposes of serving only the employees of that company
- Employer-sponsored/developed plans (PPOs, precertification operations)
- HMOs or exclusive provider organizations (EPOs) set up as a line of business of an insurance company

With one exception, these operations or plans are subsidiaries of larger companies; those companies do have boards of directors, but their boards are involved with oversight of the entire company and not the subsidiary operation. PPOs or HMOs that are divisions of insurance companies may be required to list a board on their licensure forms, but that board may have little real operational role. The one exception noted earlier is an HMO set up by a single company for purposes of serving only the employees of that company; that is considered a form of self-funding and is regulated by labor laws, not insurance laws.

Board Makeup

All HMOs have boards (except the one type noted earlier, and that type will not be discussed further), although not all those boards are particularly functional. This is especially true for HMOs that are part of large national companies or even subsidiaries of large regional plans (*eg*, the HMO subsidiary of a large Blue Cross and Blue Shield plan). Each local HMO is incorporated and required to have a board, but it is not uncommon for the chains to use the same two corporate officers (perhaps with one local representative) as the board for every HMO. Again, the board fulfills its legal function and obligation, but the actual operation of the HMO is controlled through the management structure of the company rather than through a direct relationship between the plan director and the board.

The legal requirements for boards, particularly for HMOs, are spelled out in each state's laws and regulations. In the past, it was common for states to require an HMO to have at least one-third of the board be consumer representatives, but this is no longer necessarily the case. The same requirement used to exist for federal qualification, but that no longer exists either.

Board makeup also varies depending on whether the plan is for-profit, in which case the owners' or shareholders' representatives may hold the majority of seats, or not-for-profit, in which case there will be broader community representation. A very few not-for-profit health plans are organized as cooperatives, in which case the board members are all members of the plan. Not-for-profit plans that are not cooperatives are generally best served by board members who are truly independent and who have no potential conflicts of interest; provider-sponsored not-for-profit plans may be restricted to no more than 20% of board seats being held by providers. The use of outside directors rather than plan officers as directors in any case is dictated by local events, company bylaws, and laws and regulations (including the tax code for not-for-profit health plans). Provider-sponsored for-profit plans may have majority representation by providers and so must take special precautions to avoid antitrust problems.

Function of the Board

As stated earlier, the function of the board is governance: overseeing and maintaining final responsibility for the plan. In a real sense, the buck stops with the board. Final approval authority of corporate bylaws rests with the board. It is the bylaws that govern the basic structure of power and control not only of the plan officers but of the board itself.

The fiduciary responsibility of the board in an operating plan is clear. General oversight of the profitability or reserve status rests with the board, as does oversight and approval of significant fiscal events such as a major acquisition or a significant expenditure. In a for-profit plan, the board has fiduciary responsibility to protect the interests of the stockholders. In the wake of recent accounting scandals such as the Enron debacle, the congress enacted the Sarbanes–Oxley Act of 2002* to significantly tighten accounting standards as well as provide for far greater accountability on the part of both boards of directors (the audit committee in particular) and senior management for financial reporting. The Sarbanes–Oakley Act is discussed further in Chapter 24.

---

*Pub. L. No. 107-204, 116 Stat. 745, also known as the Public Company Accounting Reform and Investor Protection Act of 2002 and commonly called SOX or SarbOx.

Legal responsibilities of the board also may include review of reports and document signing. For example, a board officer may be required to sign the quarterly financial report to the state regulatory agency, the board chairperson may be required to sign any acquisition documents, and the board is responsible for the veracity of financial statements to stockholders.

Setting and approving policy is another common function of an active board. This may be as broad as determining the overall policy of using a gatekeeper system, or it may be as detailed as approving organizational charts and reporting structures. Although most policies and procedures are the responsibility of the plan officers, an active board may set a policy regarding what operational policies must be brought to the board for approval or change.

In HMOs and many other types of managed care plans, the board has a special responsibility for oversight of the quality management (QM) program and for the quality of care delivered to members. Usually this responsibility is discharged through board (or board subcommittee) review of the QM documentation (including the overall QM plan and regular reports on findings and activities) and through feedback to the medical director and plan QM committee.

In free-standing plans, the board also has responsibility for hiring the chief executive officer (CEO) of the plan and for reviewing that officer's performance. The board in such plans often sets the CEO's compensation package, and the CEO reports to the board.

Active boards generally have committees to take up certain functions. Common board committees may include an executive committee (for rapid access to decision making and confidential discussions), a compensation committee (to set general compensation guidelines for the plan, set the CEO's compensation, and approve and issue stock options), a finance committee or audit committee (to review financial results, approve budgets, set and approve spending authorities, review the

annual audit, review and approve outside funding sources, and so forth), and a QM committee (as noted earlier).

Board Liability Issues

Any board faces the problem of liability for its actions. This is especially so in a board made up of outside directors and in a board of a not-for-profit organization. This is not to say that a board must always make correct decisions (it may make an incorrect decision, but do so in good faith), although being right is often considered better than being wrong. Rather, it is to say that a board should act in ways to reduce its own liability, and such actions will also be consistent with good governance. It is beyond the scope of this chapter to fully discuss board liability and prevention, but a few general comments may be made. Examples given in this section do not constitute legal opinions but are simply provided to help illustrate possible issues. The reader is urged to consult competent legal counsel as needed to understand board liability fully.

It is of paramount importance that board members exercise their duties to the benefit of the plan and not in their own self-interest. Conflict of interest is a very difficult problem and can surface more readily than one might suppose. Examples of such conflicts would include actions that preferentially profit the board member, actions that are more in the interest of the board member than the plan (*eg*, influencing how services are purchased by the plan), taking advantage of proprietary information to profit, and so forth. It is certainly possible for an action to benefit both the plan and the board member, but extra care must be taken to ensure that the action is first in the interest of the plan. In many cases, a board member with an obvious conflict of interest will abstain from voting on an issue or may even absent herself from discussing the issue at all.

The board must also take care that it operates within the confines of the plan bylaws. In other words, the board cannot take any action that is not allowed in the bylaws of the organization. Examples of such actions might include payment to an individual beyond the normal reimbursement policies, entering into an unrelated line of business, and so forth.

Board members must also perform their duties with some measure of diligence. For example, if plan management provides board members with information needed to properly decide on a course of action or a policy, it is incumbent on the board members to understand what is being provided and to ask the necessary questions to gain an adequate understanding to make an informed decision. Related to this is a duty to actually attend board meetings; although this might seem obvious, some board members may be so lax in their attendance as to provide virtually no governance or oversight. In all events, thorough documentation of the decision-making process is valuable, and those records should be maintained for an appropriate length of time. And as noted earlier, the audit committee in particular has added responsibility as a result of the Sarbanes–Oxley Act of 2002.

The board's primary responsibility is to the plan or organization and to the shareholders in the event that the plan is for-profit. The board may also have some measure of responsibility to other individuals or organizations if the plan acts in such a way as to harm the other party illegally. For example, if a health plan knowingly sets a policy not to credential physicians, and a panel physician commits malpractice, it is possible that the board (which either agreed to the policy or failed to change it) may have some liability.

Regardless of how the board is made up, it is important for there to be adequate director and officer liability insurance as well as insurance for errors and omissions. The need for such insurance may be attenuated by certain provisions in the company's or plan's bylaws holding the board members and officers harmless from liability. This issue requires review by legal counsel.

KEY MANAGEMENT POSITIONS

The roles and titles of the key managers in any plan vary depending on the type of plan, its legal organization, its line of business, its complexity, whether it is free-standing or a satellite of another operation, and the local needs and talent. There is little consistency in this area from plan to plan. How each key role is defined (or even whether it will be present at all) is strictly up to the management of each plan. What follows, then, is a general overview of certain key roles.

Executive Director/ Chief Executive Officer

Most plans have at least one key manager. Whether that individual is called a CEO, an executive director, a general manager, or a plan manager is a function of the items mentioned earlier in this chapter (*eg*, scope of authority, reporting structure of the company, and the like). In a free-standing health plan, that individual is truly the chief executive officer with significant authority and responsibility. In most cases, that of a health plan being the subsidiary of a larger company, this key manager will often be referred to as an executive director.

The executive director is usually responsible for all the operational aspects of the plan, although that is not always the case. For example, some large companies (*eg*, insurance companies or national HMO chains) have marketing reporting vertically to a regional marketing director rather than through the plan manager. A few companies take that to the extreme of having each functional area reporting vertically to regional managers rather than having all operations coordinated at the local level by a single manager; thus, reporting is a function of the overall environment, and there is little standardization in the industry. The executive director also has responsibility for general administrative operations and public affairs.

In free-standing plans such as a traditional HMO, the CEO is responsible for all areas.

The other officers and key managers report to the CEO, who in turn reports to the board (or to a regional manager in the case of national companies that have relatively autonomous HMO subsidiaries). In a freestanding plan, the CEO also has heightened responsibilities for financial reporting under the Sarbanes–Oxley Act of 2002, including personally attesting to the accuracy of the financial statements (along with the chief financial officer).

Medical Director/ Chief Medical Officer

Almost by definition, managed care plans will have a medical director or chief medical officer. Whether that position is a full-time manager or a community physician who comes in a few hours per week is determined by the needs of the plan. Although part-time medical directors were once common in the early period of managed care, that is now relatively uncommon. Medical or care management may also be performed for a health plan through a more centralized or regionalized approach for plans that are subsidiaries of national or regional companies. In that case, care management functions, including that of the medical director, are provided through a centralized organization; even then, there is a medical director, and in the case of large health plans, multiple medical directors who in turn report to a chief medical officer.

The medical director usually has responsibility for provider relations, provider recruiting, QM, utilization management, and medical policy. Some health plans have chosen to place network management activities under an officer who is not the medical director, however, under the belief that network contracting and management is less a clinical function than it is a business function. Some plans (eg, simple PPOs) may use the medical director, or a medical consultant, only to review claims or perhaps to approve physician applications and to review patterns of utilization. The spectrum of medical director involvement parallels the intensity of medical management activities. Usually the medical director reports to the executive director but may report through another senior officer in the case of some of the national or large regional companies.

As a plan grows in size, particularly if it is a complex plan, the need for the medical director to leverage time becomes crucial. If the medical director gets bogged down in day-to-day minutiae, the ability to provide leadership in the critical areas of utilization, quality, network management, and medical policy becomes dramatically reduced. Two approaches are commonly employed to deal with this problem. The most common is bringing in an associate medical director, and in fact there may be many associate medical directors in large plans. The role of the associate medical director is then defined as a subset of the overall duties of the medical director; for example, this person may focus primarily on utilization management or QM. In the larger companies, what is referred to here as an associate medical director is actually called a medical director, but for one of those specific functions. This concept of adding qualified staff is not different from basic management practices for any specialized activity, but health plan managers are occasionally slow to realize the value of adding physician managers when they may be quick to realize the value of adding multiple layers of management in other operational areas.

The second approach to the issue of dealing with medical management in a large plan is to decentralize certain functions. For example, in a closed panel plan (eg, a staff model HMO or a multisite group practice) it is common practice to assign management responsibilities to a physician at each geographic site. This on-site physician manager may have responsibility for utilization and staffing at the site or other duties as necessary. In an open panel setting (eg, an open panel HMO), the network may be divided up into regions, and associate medical directors may be assigned responsibilities for designated regions. In either case, management must be realistic about the time and resources required for these associate medical directors to do their jobs. The skills, motivations, and compensation for decentralized or delegated medical management must be carefully thought through, and of course the medical director retains ultimate accountability.

Finance Director/ Chief Financial Officer

In freestanding plans or large operations, it is common to have a finance director or chief financial officer. That individual is generally responsible for oversight of all financial and accounting operations, fiscal reporting, and budget preparation. In some plans, rating and underwriting also report to this function. This position usually reports to the executive director, although once again some national companies use vertical reporting.

Marketing Director

This person is responsible for marketing the plan. Responsibility generally includes oversight of marketing representatives, advertising, client relations, and enrollment forecasting. A few plans have marketing generating initial premium rates, which are then sent to finance or underwriting for review, but that is uncommon. This position reports to the executive director or vertically, depending on the company.

Operations Director

In larger plans, it is not uncommon to have an operations director. This position usually oversees claims, enrollment, underwriting (unless finance is doing so), member services, office management, and any other traditional back room functions. In small plans, the management information systems (MIS) or information technology (IT) may also be overseen by the operations director. This position usually reports to the executive director.

Chief Information Officer

Most plans separate out this function from operations, since IT supports virtually all other functions. This officer is responsible for all of the computer hardware and software and often other technology support systems as well such as telecommunications. This position may also be called a Chief Technology Officer.

Corporate Compliance Officer

Because of the requirements under Medicare and the Health Insurance Portability and Accountability Act (HIPAA; see Chapter 32), health plans must have a corporate compliance officer. This officer's responsibility is to ensure that the plan operates in compliance with applicable regulatory requirements for Medicare (in the case of the plan having a Medicare contract) and for compliance with privacy requirements under HIPAA for all health plans. In the case of HIPAA, the corporate compliance responsibilities for the privacy policies and procedures include the following:

- Designation of a privacy official who is responsible for the development and implementation of the privacy policies and procedures
- Training for all members of the workforce who obtain protected health information (PHI), including an attestation every 3 years that the employee will honor the covered entity's privacy policies
- Administrative, technical, and physical safeguards to protect the privacy of PHI, including procedures for verifying the identity and authority of requestors of information
- Detailed specifications of what must be documented to ensure compliance with the regulation

COMMITTEES

Again, there is little consistency from plan to plan regarding committees, especially in the case of managed care subsidiaries of national or large regional companies. Nonmedical committees are often ad hoc, convened to meet a specific need and then dissolved. Most plans tend to have standing committees to address management issues in defined areas, but that is idiosyncratic from plan to plan. An example of a common type of nonmedical committee in a not-for-profit HMO might be a consumer or member advisory committee; though having no voting rights or governance powers, this committee provides consumer or member input to plan managers.

In the medical management area, committees serve to diffuse some elements of responsibility (which can be beneficial for medical-legal reasons) and allow important input from the field into procedure and policy or even into case-specific interpretation of existing policy. Some examples of common medical management committees are given here. The actual formation, role, responsibility, and activity of any committee vary from plan to plan. These examples of committees are from the viewpoint of an HMO and are less likely to apply to another form of managed health care plan, though they certainly do exist. More information about each of these areas may be found in the pertinent chapters of this book.

Quality Management Committee

This is one area where a committee is essential for oversight of the QM activity, setting of standards, review of data, feedback to providers, follow-up, and approval of sanctions. A peer review committee may be a subset of the QM committee or it may be separate.

Credentialing Committee

This committee may also be a subset of the QM committee or it may be separate. In new plans with heavy credentialing needs, it is probably best for the committee to be separate. In states that require "due process" for provider termination, this is the committee most likely to take on that responsibility.

Medical Advisory Committee

Many plans have a medical advisory committee whose purpose is to review general medical management issues brought to it by the medical director. Such issues may include changes in the contract with providers, compensation, changes in authorization procedures, and so on. This committee serves as a sounding board for the medical director. Occasionally it has voting authority, but that is rare because such authority is really vested with the board. In national companies, this committee may have input to local medical management issues, but medical issues that cross all plans (*eg*, medical policy for new technology) are generally provided from a corporate-level medical policy committee.

Utilization Review Committee

This committee reviews utilization issues brought to it by the medical director. Often this committee approves or reviews policy regarding coverage. This committee is also the one that reviews utilization patterns of providers and approves or reviews the sanctioning process (for utilization reasons) against providers.

Sometimes this committee gets involved in resolving disputes between the plan and a provider regarding utilization approval and may be involved in reviewing cases for medical necessity. In large plans, this function may be further subdivided into various specialty panels for review of consultant utilization. This committee may be a subset of the medical advisory committee or it may be free-standing. It is an example of a committee that is far more likely to exist in a free-standing health plan than in a national company in which other approaches are taken to address utilization issues.

Pharmacy and Therapeutics Committee

Plans with significant pharmacy benefits often have a pharmacy and therapeutics (P&T) committee. This committee is usually charged with developing a formulary, reviewing changes to that formulary, and reviewing abnormal prescription utilization patterns by providers. This committee is usually freestanding. In national plans, the formulary may or may not be subject to local input, depending on the type of plan benefit (*eg*, tiered copayments).

Medical Grievance Review Committee

In most states, a separate committee must be established to review member grievances regarding medical management or coverage determinations. This committee must be made up mostly of health professionals of a specialty appropriate to the medical condition under review. This means that most health professional members of this committee will attend meetings only if their specialty is related to the type of grievance being reviewed. The medical professionals should not have been involved in the member's medical care, and if the grievance is significant, they may also be required to not be participating physicians in the plan.

Related to this is the process for external review of appeals. In those states that do not require it, this may be a contracted group of independent physicians. In those states that require such an appeal process, an independent review organization is usually defined by the state and is not part of the plan's committee structure.

Corporate Compliance Committee

This committee is a function of the plan's corporate compliance program as noted earlier in the description of the corporate compliance officer.

MANAGEMENT CONTROL STRUCTURE

Control structure refers to issues such as reporting responsibility, spending (and other commitment) authority, hiring and firing, the conduct of performance evaluations of employees, and so forth. Each plan will set these up to fit its situation and needs. Although these issues are too diverse to be addressed in this chapter, a wealth of material on all of these functions can be found in the general management literature.

One item that is of special significance is the monthly operating report (MOR), though it may be called by a variety of terms (*eg*, an executive dashboard). Most tightly run managed care plans develop an MOR to use as the basic management tool. The typical MOR reports the month- and year-to-date financial status of the plan. Those data are backed up with details regarding membership, premium revenue, other revenue, medical costs (usually total and broken out into categories, such as hospital, primary care, referral care, ancillary services, and so forth), marketing costs, administrative costs (including key operating metrics), other expenses, taxes (if appropriate), and the bottom line. Results are generally reported in terms of whole dollars and per member per month. If the plan is not producing an MOR, it is probably not managing optimally.

How much detail is reported routinely or on an ad hoc basis is a local call. The point here is that managed care, especially in tightly run plans, is so dynamic that managers cannot wait for quarterly results. Managers must have current and reliable data from which to manage. Sutton's Law dictates that you must "go where the money is," and that can only be done if the MOR tells you where to look.

As discussed in Chapter 16, many plans are now using a data warehouse or other forms of collecting data and converting it into information. The data warehouse provides an accessible repository of data (both raw data and information that has been created from that data) to managers so as to allow them to understand the metrics of the plan without continually having to order special reports to be run at the expense of other necessary systems activities. To paraphrase J. Edwards Deming, you can't manage what you can't measure.

Related to this is a type of reporting system often referred to as an executive information system, or EIS. The EIS allows executives to obtain reports from a large selection of available information. Again, this does not require special reports to be run on the main system, nor does it require the executive to design a report or choose the data to populate the report. Various other types of reports are described throughout this book. Which reports and routine reviews a manager needs to run the business is a decision each plan must make.

CONCLUSION

The basic functions of governance and control in HMOs and other managed care plans are similar to those in any business, although the specifics regarding the board of directors, plan officers, and responsibilities of key managers vary tremendously from plan to plan. With the market consolidation of the managed health care industry, governance and management control functions that were routine in free-standing health plans have now become more vertical, coming together not at the local level but rather at the level of regional or corporate officers. Nevertheless, the management and governance needs remain, even if the form and structure continues to evolve under legal, regulatory, and market pressures.

4

Common Myths and Assertions about Health Insurance Plans

Brian McKenna

Study Objectives

- Understand how anecdotal evidence has affected the public and political debate surrounding managed care.
- Understand common misconceptions about managed care and provide evidence to clarify and correct these misconceptions.
- Understand managed care's impact on the affordability and quality of health care.
- Understand how managed care has affected access to health care services.
- Understand the relationship between managed care and physicians and the impact managed care has had on physician/patient interaction.

Discussion Topics

1. Discuss why it is important to examine scientific evidence rather than anecdotal evidence when making assertions about managed care, and why the use of such evidence may or may not occur.
2. Discuss the role of anecdotal evidence in forming public opinion and policy.
3. Describe at least four managed care myths. Discuss if these myths are true or false and why.
4. Discuss managed care's impact on the cost/affordability of health coverage and the quality of health care delivered. How does this compare to quality and cost under the fee-for-service system?

5. Identify at least three areas in which managed care has improved access to different types of health care services. Do the same exercise applied to areas where access to different types of health care services may have been hindered.
6. Give three examples of common assertions about managed care's impact on physicians and physician/patient interaction. Explain how these assertions are proven true or false by evidence.

INTRODUCTION

U.S. health care has experienced dramatic changes in the past two decades, with managed health care principles and organizations leading the way toward a system based on new concepts in care management and service delivery. Some view managed health care as the response to the health care cost crisis that would not go away and whose persistence threatened the viability of the U.S. economy. Others view managed care as the response to serious, well-documented quality problems—specifically, prevalent patterns of underuse, overuse, misuse, and geographic variation in medical services—that characterized much of U.S. health care.

Although both statements accurately portray the factors that brought about the widespread adoption of managed health care in the United States, they don't capture the countless institutional and personal adjustments that have been required to accommodate such change. Although change is a necessary response to a faltering system, it rarely is easy. As the leading agent of change in the U.S. health care system, managed care has made health coverage more affordable and created a new emphasis on quality but not without attendant controversy.

Changing the health care system by questioning longstanding practices, asking physicians to become more accountable, and asking patients to become active participants in their care led to what some term the "managed care backlash," also discussed in Chapter 1. This phenomenon became evi-

dent in the old political debates, though not in the numerous studies of consumer satisfaction with health plans or in patterns of consumer choice among health plans.

Interestingly, when consumers are asked directly about the quality of their personal health care, they express positive attitudes. National surveys have reported high levels of consumer satisfaction with managed care health plans. In a 1998 analysis of public attitudes, the president of the Roper Center for Public Opinion Research at the University of Connecticut stated that "huge majorities say they are satisfied with their health care, including their ability to get a doctor's appointment and the most sophisticated medical treatment."[1] A 1998 comprehensive review of surveys on public attitudes toward managed care concluded that "there is little evidence of widespread or serious dissatisfaction with health care arrangements among those who have coverage."[2] The same review also found that the vast majority of people enrolled in managed care would recommend their plan to others. Since that time, most Americans continue to be satisfied with their health plan. A 2002 Harris Interactive Survey found that 67% of adults with employer-sponsored health plans give their plan a grade of A or B, and only 8% rate their plans as a D or an F. Most people would recommend their own health plan to family members or friends.[3] Most recently, data from 2005 show that more than half of Americans are extremely satisfied (17%) or are very satisfied (37%) with their current health plan, and more than one-third are somewhat satisfied

(35%). Moreover, the percentage of Americans who are extremely satisfied has grown for 4 straight years.[4]

Much of the debate about managed care has been conducted around claims about how particular individuals' cases were handled. In the late 1990s, some media organizations started to more closely examine these claims. For instance, in August 1998, the *Washington Post* ran a front-page article by Howard Kurtz, the *Post's* media critic, that recounts several of the stories that were being covered by multiple national news organizations, including the *Washington Post,* and reported that upon further examination "such stories are often more complicated than they seem at first."[5]

In a similar vein, the author of the Harris Interactive survey noted earlier discussed the impact of the media on Harris's survey results as follows:

> The contrast between these numbers—with well over 60% of the public giving their own plans generally positive ratings—and the negative image of health insurance and managed care, as shown by other Harris Interactive surveys, is very striking. . . . These differences obviously reflect in part the difference between personal experiences and the impact of negative media reporting. The personal experiences of the public with their own health plans are not nearly as bad as their beliefs about health insurance and managed care, which in many cases come from what they see on TV, in movies, or in magazines and newspapers.[3]

As the debate over the direction of our nation's health care system continues, it is essential that claims about how the system is working be subjected to critical analysis. If our understanding of health care in the United States is allowed to be based on unsubstantiated assertions and incomplete information, both the problems we define and the solutions we devise will be wrong. In this chapter, we seek to advance the discussion about managed care by examining just a few of the claims commonly heard in debates.

HEALTH INSURANCE CHOICES

Critics of managed care claim that the growth of managed care health systems in the United States has restricted choice. In fact, managed care has expanded health insurance coverage options available to consumers. Prior to the advent of health maintenance organizations (HMOs), preferred provider organizations (PPOs), and other managed care plans, as described in Chapters 1 and 2, individuals were limited to traditional indemnity coverage. Health plans developed as a new choice for consumers, providing them access to coverage with features such as preventive care, low cost sharing (deductibles and copayments), credentialed practitioners, and quality assurance programs.

In a report commissioned by the American Association of Health Plans (AAHP), data gathered by the Barents Group in 1996 show that almost two-thirds of employees offered health coverage had a choice of more than one health plan.[6] This number continues to remain stable today.[7] Furthermore, 82% of U.S. workers were offered a PPO plan that covered care provided by out-of-network physicians and hospitals.[7]

HEALTH CARE QUALITY

In the public debate, managed care plan members often are portrayed as receiving lower quality care than is available through traditional indemnity coverage. Notwithstanding this portrayal, a pattern of generally positive findings about quality of care in HMOs has been documented in comprehensive literature reviews published in 1994, 1997, and 2002.[8,9]

These research findings generally show that HMO members receive care that is comparable to, or better than, care provided in indemnity plans. Furthermore, the success of health plans in providing quality care has not compromised their ability to provide more affordable care through efficient and appropriate use of resources. Among the numerous studies (in addition to the literature reviews mentioned earlier) documenting that consumers with health plan coverage receive better or comparable quality care than those with fee-for-service coverage are the following:

- A large-scale study comparing the quality of care for elderly heart attack patients found that HMO patients were significantly more likely than fee-for-service (FFS) patients to receive aspirin therapy (88% vs. 83%) and beta-blocker therapy (73% vs. 62%), and the use of anti-clotting drugs was almost identical among HMO and FFS patients (64% vs. 66%). Aspirin, beta-blockers, and anti-clotting drugs are effective and clinically proven therapies for the treatment of patients experiencing acute myocardial infarction.[7]
- A study examining diagnosis and treatment of breast cancer found that Medicare HMO enrollees were more likely than Medicare FFS patients to have their breast cancer diagnosed at an earlier stage. HMO enrollees diagnosed at early stages were more likely to receive breast-conserving surgery as opposed to mastectomy (38.4% vs. 36.8%). HMO enrollees receiving breast-conserving surgery were significantly more likely than FFS patients to obtain the radiation therapy recommended by their oncologists (69% vs. 63.7%).[8]
- Seniors enrolled in Medicare HMOs were more likely than those with FFS insurance to receive influenza vaccinations (71.2% vs. 65.5%). The study further found that of all seniors, HMO enrollees were more likely than those with FFS insurance to have had a physician office visit (87.3% vs. 84.9%).[9]

UTILIZATION REVIEW AND MEDICAL NECESSITY

Critics of managed care claim that utilization review personnel routinely overrule doctors' decisions on necessary treatment. In fact, coverage denial rates for physician recommendations are very low. Refuting these oft-repeated claims is a national survey of over 2,000 physicians caring for patients in plans that utilize managed care techniques that revealed the *final* coverage denial rate for physician recommendations within eight categories of care was at most 3%, and much less for most categories of care.[10] *Initial* denial rates were somewhat higher, but between one-half and two-thirds of initial denials were reversed by the health plan, resulting in the lower rates. Coverage for hospitalization was denied only 1% of the time; surgical procedures, 1.2%; and specialist referrals, 2.6%.[14]

In recent years, many states have implemented "external review" programs to resolve coverage disputes between health plans and consumers. External review, also known as independent medical review, is a process that enables consumers to appeal coverage decisions to a third party, typically once the internal appeals process has been completed. By the end of 2005, 44 states and the District of Columbia had implemented external review programs. These programs typically involve review by one or more independent physicians of specific coverage disputes. The reviewer or panel of reviewers then makes a decision as to whether the service in question should be covered by the health plan. Consistent with the low coverage denial rates cited previously, the number of coverage disputes brought before external review panels is relatively small. The aggregate rate of appeal across all external review programs in 2003 and 2004 was approximately one appeal per 12,000 eligible individuals. Although the results of these external reviews vary from state to state, a study examining 2003 and 2004 data found that external reviewers agreed with health plan coverage decisions 60% of the time and reversed health plan decisions in favor of the consumer 40% of the time.[15]

HEALTH STATUS OF MANAGED CARE ENROLLEES

Critics of managed care contended that health plans achieved the quality and positive outcomes they did because they enrolled a healthier population; in other words, managed care plans avoided enrolling sick patients. Research, however, shows that HMOs and indemnity plans enrolled similar proportions of members who were in poor health. For example, a survey of 59,000 households in 1998 and 1999 found that, among the privately insured, HMOs did not enroll a healthier population. In fact, the survey found that HMOs actually tended to have more enrollees in poor health. In particular, the survey found that HMOs enrolled a higher percentage of individuals in poor physical health than non-HMOs (14.3% vs. 13.6%). Additionally, HMOs enrolled a higher percentage of individuals with an expensive chronic condition than non-HMOs (14.4% vs. 13.0%).[16]

ACCESS TO CLINICAL TRIALS

A prominent report released by the U.S. Government Accounting Office (GAO) in September 1999 highlighted the current state of affairs affecting patient participation in National Institutes of Health–sponsored clinical trials.[17] Findings in this report are contrary to prevalent assertions that health plans are the cause of poor enrollment in clinical trials. In general, research shows that health plans often cover the routine patient care costs of clinical trials and enrollment in these trials typically meets or exceeds expectations.

The GAO report found that almost all of the insurers surveyed examine the appropriateness of coverage for such trials on a case-by-case basis. When insurers determine that coverage is in a patient's best interest, they typically cover the cost of the routine care as-

sociated with the trial and care that would have been otherwise provided. In fact, the Congressional Budget Office estimates that health plans currently pay at least 90% of clinical trial–related patient care costs.[18] In concluding that it found no evidence to support claims that managed care has impeded participation in clinical trials, the GAO noted that a number of impediments to the enrollment process are independent of how care is financed.

Despite the increase in the number of trials, the GAO noted in its report that enrollment in these trials often meets or exceeds expectations. Given that managed care enrollment has grown over time, current clinical trial enrollment trends demonstrate that patient access to such trials has not been reduced by the growth in managed care

INDUSTRY PROFITS AND ADMINISTRATIVE COSTS

The public debate often includes claims that managed care plans' profits are largely responsible for the rising cost of health insurance. But a close examination of how the health care premium dollar is spent shows that health plan profits are a very small component of the total premium dollar. An analysis by PricewaterhouseCoopers (PwC), conducted for America's Health Insurance Plans, found that health plan profits accounted for only 3 cents of every premium dollar paid in 2005.[19] This analysis is consistent with data from other sources showing an average profit margin during the first quarter of each of the last 5 years of 3.2%.*

---

*Based on an America's Health Insurance Plans (AHIP) calculation of data included in a news release dated October 24, 2005, by Weiss Ratings that noted that the industry profit margin was 4.6% in the first quarter of 2005, compared with 4.2% in the first quarter of 2004; 3.5% in the first quarter of 2003; 2.4% in the first quarter of 2002; and 1.1% in the first quarter of 2001. An average profit margin for these 5 years is 3.2%.

A related popular misconception is that managed care plan administrative costs make up a large component of the premium dollar while adding little value to consumers. First, it is important to note that a portion of health plan administrative costs are nondiscretionary. For example, the cost of complying with government laws and regulations are considered administrative costs and, in fact, account for a significant portion of overall administrative costs. In addition, health plan administrative costs typically include the cost of programs that clearly benefit consumers, such as disease management, health promotion, and disease prevention programs. Investments in health information technologies, such as those that allow consumers to access information about specific medical conditions and communicate with providers via computer are also considered administrative costs. Other administrative activities integral to health plan operations include processing claims, guarding against fraudulent billing practices, and communicating with consumers regarding their existing and new benefits. The PwC analysis found that the administrative costs associated with complying with government laws and regulations, processing claims, and fraud detection accounted for 6% of health care costs. Disease management, health promotion, disease prevention, and investment in information technology accounted for another 5% of health care costs. It is important to point out that, by far the largest portion of the health care dollar goes toward paying for medical services such as physician services, outpatient costs, inpatient costs, and prescription drugs.[19]

A statistic that often gets lost in the managed care debate, and one that is perhaps a far more deserving culprit in the rise of health care costs, concerns the underlying and pervasive costs associated with our medical liability system. The medical services mentioned earlier, for which the bulk of the premium dollar is being paid, unfortunately include the cost of medical liability and defensive medicine. Defensive medicine refers to the behavior where providers, in an effort to protect themselves from litigation, order tests and procedures they believe are not medically necessary. A recent survey of Pennsylvania providers across six medical specialties found that 93% reported practicing defensive medicine.[20] PwC estimates that "approximately 10% of the costs of medical services are attributed to the cost of litigation and defensive medicine."*[19,21,22] A Tillinghast-Towers Perrin study estimated that the direct costs of medical liability in 2004 alone were $28.7 billion.[23]

A second contributor to health care costs that is often overlooked is the aggregate impact of government coverage mandates. A recent study determined that there are more than 1,800 mandated health benefits in effect across the states. The study concluded that these mandates increase the cost of health coverage anywhere from just under 20% to more than 50%, depending on the state.[24]

DISEASE MANAGEMENT

Some critics of managed care contend that health plans fail to add any value to the health care system and play a small role in improving the health of Americans. Yet there is widespread evidence that one of the hallmarks of managed care—disease management—significantly benefits consumers with chronic illnesses by improving health out-

---

*As cited in PricewaterhouseCoopers, January 2006. The 10% was adapted from Kessler and McClellan and CMS's Medical Economic Indices. Kessler and McClellan estimate that the cost of defensive medicine was in the range of 5% to 9% of medical costs. The direct cost of medical liability insurance is roughly 2%. This suggests that total medical liability costs are in the 7% to 11% range.

comes, avoiding unnecessary hospitalizations, and saving money. For example:

- One study evaluating the effectiveness of disease management for patients with end-stage renal disease (ESRD) found that Medicare HMO enrollees had better outcomes than Medicare FFS ESRD patients did. Researches found a 45% to 54% lower hospitalization rate and a 19% to 35% better overall survival rate for the Medicare HMO ESRD patients enrolled in disease management program.[25]
- A study of diabetes disease management programs found that participants experienced improvements associated with significantly fewer long-term complications for the eyes, kidneys, cardiovascular system, and the nervous system (*ie*, patients' average hemoglobin level—a measure of diabetic control—decreased, moving it closer to the nondiabetic level). Additionally, the study found that the longer the involvement in the program, the better the health outcome for the participants.[26]
- A study of individuals having, or being at a high risk for, one or more of 17 chronic conditions or diseases found increased savings, fewer hospital admissions, fewer emergency room visits, reduced absenteeism from school or work, and a significant improvement in diabetics' hemoglobin A1c levels.[27]

HEALTH CARE COSTS

As health care costs continue to rise, some have placed the blame on managed care, claiming that managed care hasn't lived up to its promise to control skyrocketing health care costs. In fact, managed care has contributed to slowing down the growth in health premiums on more than one occasion over the past two decades. During the late 1980s, growth in health spending rose to unprecedented levels, peaking in 1989 at 16.5%.[19] For much of the

1990s, health care costs rose at a much slower rate, and many experts agreed that the declining growth in health spending could be attributed to managed care plans. In the late 1990s, health spending began to increase by again, peaking around 2002, when it was estimated that premiums increased 13.7%.[28] Health care costs have slowed once again, rising by about 8.8% from 2004 to 2005,[19] though in truth it is difficult to predict the rate of growth in the future.

Although the initial success of managed care plans in slowing the growth of health spending was largely attributed to plans' use of provider networks and other managed care techniques, consumer and purchaser preferences and government regulation have resulted in health plans becoming more innovative in designing strategies to control rising health care costs. For example, health plans' use of drug formularies, tiered formularies in particular, have played a significant role in slowing the growth of prescription drug spending, which represents one of the fastest growing areas of health care spending.

From 1995 to 2002, prescription drug spending increased by more than 10% each year.[29] However, in recent years, prescription drug spending increases have slowed significantly from their recent peak increase of 18.1% in 1999. Prescription drug spending increased by 7.2% in 2004—less than half the increase of 1999.[28] In its report, PwC addresses the various reasons for the recent deceleration of prescription drug spending increases, noting:

> [O]ne of the most striking reasons is that many health plans are shifting to two-, three-, and most recently four-tiered formularies that make beneficiaries more cost conscious when they choose preferred prescription drugs. The number of employers with at least three tiers of copayments has increased from 27% in 2000 to 68% in 2004.[29]

This view tracks other findings as well. An article examining health care cost trends noted that slower growth in drug spending "likely reflects, in part, the movement toward three-tier copayments, which have now become common in health benefit offerings, as well as the continuing growth in those copayments across all of the three tiers."[30]

Health plans' use of tiered formularies to help control prescription drug costs is just one recent example of how managed care has contributed to stemming the tide of rising costs. As the health care marketplace continues to evolve and mature, plans will continue to explore new, innovative strategies to make health coverage more affordable for consumers.

CONCLUSION

Critics of managed care still make antiquated arguments from the perceived managed care backlash of years ago. Many of the claims made by opponents of managed care are simply wrong or even outdated; whereas others are provided without any of the context needed to evaluate them properly. By examining some of the more common assertions about managed care, it becomes clear that an informed debate cannot take place without a fair discussion of all of the facts and a thorough evaluation of not only managed care but of the other components of the U.S. health care system.

References

1. Ladd E. Health care hysteria, part II. Op ed. *New York Times.* July 23, 1998.
2. Bowman K. *Health Care Attitudes Today.* American Enterprise Institute, 1998, http://aei.org/publications/pubID.9180,filter.social/pub_detail.asp. Accessed April 15, 2006.
3. Harris Interactive. *The Harris Poll #3.* January 16, 2002.
4. Employee Benefit Research Institute. *2005 Health Confidence Survey Notes.* November 2005;26(11), http://www.ebri.org/publications/notes/index.cfm?fa = notesDisp&content_id = 3596. Accessed March 31, 2006.
5. H. Kurtz. Some managed-care sagas need second exam. *Washington Post.* August 10, 1998, Page A01.
6. Barents Group. *Characteristics of Health Plan Choices Available to Employees Through Employer-Based Health Benefits 1996.* June 1997.
7. Kaiser Family Foundation. *Employer Health Benefits 2005 Annual Survey.* September 14, 2005, http://www.kff.org/insurance/7315.cfm. Accessed April 1, 2006.
8. RH Miller and HS Luft. Managed care plan performance since 1980: A literature analysis. *Journal of the American Medical Association* 271, no. 19 (1994): 1512–1519.
9. RH Miller and HS Luft. Does managed care lead to better or worse quality of care? *Health Affairs* (Sep/Oct 1997): 7–25.
10. RH Miller and HS Luft. HMO plan performance update: An analysis of the literature, 1997–2001. *Health Affairs* (July/Aug 2002) 63–86.
11. Soumerai SB, McLaughlin TJ, Gurwitz JH, et al. Timeliness and quality of care for elderly patients with acute myocardial infarction under health maintenance organization vs. fee-for-service insurance. Archives *Internal Med* 1999,159(17):2013–2020.
12. Riley, Gerald F, Potosky, Arnold L, Klabunde, Carrie N. *et al.* Stage at diagnosis and treatment patterns among older women with breast cancer: An HMO and FFS comparison. 1999, 281:720–726.
13. Schneider EC, Cleary, PD, Zaslavsky, AM, and Epstein, AM. Racial disparity in influenza vaccination: Does managed care narrow the gap between African Americans and whites? *Journal of the American Medical Association* 286(12), 2001, 1455–1460.
14. Remler DK, Donelan K, Blendon RJ, Lundberg GD, Leape LL, Calkins DR, Binns K, Newhouse JP. What do managed care plans do to affect care? Results from a survey of physicians. *Inquiry.* 1997, 34(3):196–204.
15. America's Health Insurance Plans (AHIP). *Update on State External Review Programs.* January 2006, www.ahipresearch.org/pdfs/External_ReviewJan06.pdf. Accessed May 1, 2006.

16. Schaefer E, Reschovsky JD. Are HMO en-rollees healthier than others? Results from the *Community Tracking Study. Health Affairs.* May/June 2002, 21(3): 249–258.

17. US General Accounting Office (GAO). *NIH Clinical Trials: Various Factors Affect Patient Participation.* September 1999. www.gao.gov/cgi-bin/getrpt?GAO/HEHS-99-182, Accessed 5/1/2006.

18. Congressional Budget Office. *Cost Estimate for H.R.3605/S.1890, the Patients' Bill of Rights Act of 1998.* July 16, 1998, http://www.cbo.gov/showdoc.cfm?index = 667&sequence = 0; Accessed May 1, 2006.

19. PricewaterhouseCoopers. *The Factors Fueling Rising Healthcare Costs 2006.* Report prepared for America's Health Insurance Plans. January 2006.

20. Studdert, David M. Defensive medicine among high-risk specialist physicians in a volatile malpractice environment, *JAMA* 293 (1 June 2005): 2609–2617.

21. Kessler, McClellan. Addressing the new health care crisis: Reforming the medical litigation system to improve the quality of health care. Washington, DC: Department of Health and Human Services, Office of the Assistant Secretary for Planning and Evaluation. March 2003.

22. CMS. *Medical Economic Indices.*

23. Tillinghast-Towers Perrin. *US Tort Costs and Cross-Border Perspectives: 2005 Update.* March 13, 2006, www.towersperrin.com/tp/getweb cachedoc?webc = TILL/USA/2006/200603/2005_Tort.pdf. Accessed May 1, 2006.

24. Council for Affordable Health Insurance. *Health Insurance Mandates in the States 2006.* March 7, 2006, www.cahi.org. Accessed May 1, 2006.

25. Nissenson AR, Collins AJ, Dickmeyer J, et al: Evaluation of disease-state management of dialysis patients. *Am J Kidney Dis* 2001, 37: 938–944.

26. Sidorov J, Gabbay R, Harris R, et al. Disease management for diabetes mellitus: Impact on hemoglobin A1c. *Am J Managed Care.* 2000, 6: 1217–1226.

27. Gold WR and Kongstvedt, P. How broadening DM's focus helped shrink one plan's costs. *Managed Care 12*(11):33–39, November 2003.

28. PricewaterhouseCoopers. *The Factors Fueling Rising Healthcare Costs.* Report prepared for the American Association of Health Plans. April 2002, January 2006, http://www.pwcglobal.com/extweb/pwcpublications.nsf/docid/E4C0FC004429297A852571090065A70B. Accessed April 14, 2006.

29. Center for Studying Health Systems Change. *Tracking Health Care Costs: Spending Growth Stabilizes at High Rate in 2004.* June 2005, Data Bulletin No. 29.

30. Strunk, Bradley C, Ginsburg, Paul B and John P Cookson. Tracking health care costs: Declining growth trend pauses in 2004 (June 21, 2005). Health Affairs Web Exclusive. (www.healthaffairs.org).

Part 2

THE HEALTH CARE DELIVERY SYSTEM

*When one's all right, he's prone to spite
The doctor's peaceful mission.
But when he's sick, it's loud and quick
He bawls for a physician.*

—Eugene Field
(1850–1895)
Doctors, st. 2 [1890]

5

PHYSICIAN NETWORKS IN MANAGED HEALTH CARE

Peter R. Kongstvedt

Study Objectives

- Understand the role of the primary care physician (PCP) in different types of managed care plans.
- Understand the role of different types of specialty care physician in different types of managed care plans.
- Understand the unique attributes of hospital-based physicians.
- Understand the role of nonphysician providers of medical care.
- Understand network development methodologies.
- Understand different types of physician contracting approaches or methods.
- Understand basic credentialing.
- Understand how physicians may view the health plan.
- Understand issues of network maintenance.
- Understand issues of sanctioning and removal of physicians from the network.

Discussion Topics

1. Describe a typical credentialing process, indicating which steps are required and for which reasons. Discuss possible problems that may arise for any steps that are not completed.
2. Discuss the pros and cons of contracting with faculty practice plans, and how a managed care plan addresses those issues. Discuss the same issues as regards other types of physician organizations.
3. What are the most important issues to focus on in network maintenance?

4. What proactive steps can a managed care plan take to improve provider relations? How might these steps differ between different types of health plans?
5. Discuss different approaches a health plan might take to developing and maintaining a network under differing conditions such as a rural area, a medically underserved area, or a community in which there is little competition between certain types of specialists.

INTRODUCTION

The backbone of any managed health care plan is the physician network. Hospitals, ancillary services, and nonphysician professional health care providers are also critical to a health plan, but nothing is as important as the physician network. Overall, the majority of practicing physicians in the United States does contract with managed care plans to varying degrees. Tracking Report 14[1] issued in May 2006 by the Center for Studying Health System Change* provides the following data illustrated in Tables 5-1 and 5-2.

*Center for Studying Health System Change, 600 Maryland Avenue, SW, Suite 550, Washington, DC 20024-2512.

What is not apparent from this report, however, are the percentages of physicians who do not contract with managed care plans by choice versus the percentage of physicians with whom the plan chooses not to contract with. One can conjecture that the high proportion of both senior physicians and solo or small group practice physicians who do not contract represent the physician's decisions regarding contracting, whereas the high proportion of non-board-certified physicians who do not contract may represent the plan's criteria not to contract with physicians who do not meet credentialing standards. Voluntary and involuntary physician turnover is generally low, however. In 2002, for example, the trade association for the industry, America's Health Insurance Plans (AHIP) reported a 3%

Table 5–1 Trends in Physician Contracting and Managed Care Revenue, 1996 through 2005

	1996–1997	1998–1999	2000–2001	2004–2005
Physicians with No Managed Care Contracts	9.4%	8.6%	9.2%	11.5%*
Average number of managed care contracts among physicians with > 1 managed care contract	12	13	13	13
Physicians with No Managed Care Revenue	5.7%	5.2%	5.8%	8.6%*
Revenue from managed care among physicians with > 1% managed care revenue (mean)	42%	45%	45%	44%

*Change from 2000–2001 is statistically significant at $p < .001$.
Source: Center for Studying Health System Change. Community Tracking Study Physician Survey. Reprinted with permission of the Center for Studying Health System Change, Washington, DC, http://www.hschange.org.

Table 5–2 Physicians with No Managed Care Contracts, 2004–2005

PHYSICIAN CHARACTERISTICS

Gender

Female (R)	11.4%
Male	11.5

Race

White (R)	11.1
Black	11.6
Other	9.0

Hours Worked in Previous Week

Part Time (1–39 hours) (R)	15.3
Full Time (40 hours)	9.8**

Years in Practice

0–10 Years (R)	10.6
11–20 Years	9.6
21+ Years	14.3**

Specialty

Primary Care Physicians (R)	9.4
Medical Specialists	10.5
Surgical Specialists	8.8
OB-GYN	11.8
Psychiatrists	34.6**

Board Certification

Board Certified (R)	10.7
Not Board Certified	19.6**

PRACTICE CHARACTERISTICS

Practice Size

Solo/2 Physicians (R)	15.2
3 or More Physicians	7.4**
Institutional Practice	11.7**

Census Region

West (R)	14.8
Northeast	10.5*
South	11.5*
Midwest	8.6**

continues

Table 5–2 Physicians with No Managed Care Contracts, 2004–2005—continued

MARKET CHARACTERISTICS	
Competitive Situation Practice Faces[†]	
Not at All Competitive (R)	15.6
Somewhat Competitive	8.6**
Very Competitive	10.1**

Difference from reference group, as indicated by (R), is statistically significant at *$p < .05$ and **$p < .01$.
[†]Physician respondents were asked to describe the competitive situation that their practice faced from other physicians.
Source: Center for Studying Health System Change. *Community Tracking Study Physician Survey*. Reprinted with permission of the Center for Studying Health System Change, Washington, DC, http://www.hschange.org.

involuntary and a 6% voluntary turnover rate in its member plans.[2]

PRIMARY CARE AND SPECIALTY CARE

Most managed care organizations (MCOs) divide the physician network into primary care physicians (PCPs) and specialty care physicians (SCPs), though in reality such distinctions are not always clear. This is because in all types of health care delivery and health plans, the role of the PCP is important. Even in the absence of a health plan design that requires enrollees to access their PCP to obtain either direct care or referral authorization for specialty care (so-called gatekeeper types of health plans), a great deal of the regular health care of Americans is via PCPs.

The first place to begin is with what specialties are generally considered primary care. In virtually all systems, care rendered by physicians in the specialties of family practice, internal medicine, and pediatrics are considered primary care. It is worth noting that the supply of new PCPs appears to be declining, with the number of graduating medical students matching to primary care residencies declining every year since 1998, which could portend greater difficulties in having primary care access in the future.[3] General practitioners (*ie*, physicians who have not obtained full residency training beyond their internships) may also be considered PCPs, but their use by

MCOs is quite low except in rural or underserved areas where there may not be sufficient residency-trained PCPs.

Many obstetrics/gynecology (OB/Gyn) specialists feel that they too deliver primary care to their patients. They argue that they are often the only physician a young woman sees for many years. This is certainly true in the case of generally healthy young women, but it is not always so when medical problems not involving the female reproductive tract occur. In the early 1990s, there was at least one program designed to retrain OB/Gyn physicians to provide a broader range of primary care, but the results were quite disappointing, with a very high dropout rate and a high level of dissatisfaction with broad primary care expressed by the OB/Gyns.[4] Notwithstanding that failed experiment, as of 2002 59% of reporting health maintenance organizations (HMO) and point-of-service (POS) plans allowed members to use OB/Gyns as their primary care coordinator, though it is not clear if those same numbers would apply to HMO-only health plans.[2]

Regardless, most all plans, including HMOs, allow direct access to OB/Gyn for female members,* even HMOs that capitate primary

---

*It should be noted that in addition to simple marketplace demands, many states have passed laws requiring health plans to allow direct access to OB/Gyns.

care (discussed in Chapter 6) or otherwise use PCPs as case managers (*ie*, use a gatekeeper system). In that case, the PCP and the OB/Gyn share the clinical care (and perhaps the capitation, if that is the reimbursement system in use) between the OB/Gyn and the internist or family practitioner. HMOs that do capitate must define which services are to be delivered by each. For example, the OB/Gyn may be seen without referral for Pap smears and pelvic examinations, for pregnancy, for sterilization procedures, and so forth. For clinical care that is out of the scope of normal OB/Gyn practice, the member must see the PCP for either treatment by or referral to any other specialist.

Although it is most common for PCPs to be trained in primary care, many internists are also trained in an additional specialty, for example, pulmonary medicine or gastroenterology. Unless such a specialist restricts his or her practice only to specialized conditions or procedures (*eg*, a gastroenterologist who focuses primarily on invasive procedures), it is common to have a practice mix of both specialty patients and primary care. In the early days of managed care, it was more common for MCOs to adhere more strictly to a definition of primary care than it is now when most health plans consider most internists with specialties to also act as PCPs. This theoretically could lead to adverse selection in which the sicker patients of that specialist actively seek to join an MCO that allows them to access the specialist as a PCP, but as a practical matter that is no longer an issue given the broad nature of most networks and the fact that physicians generally participate with multiple plans if they participate at all.

Specialty physicians may be thought of as those physicians who are not PCPs, except in the case of internal medicine specialists who may be considered both. Certainly all surgical specialties are SCPs, as are the hospital-based specialties such as pathology, radiology, and anesthesia. Internal medicine subspecialists, as noted earlier, may be considered both SCPs and PCPs when providing both specialized and primary clinical care, or may have practices that are in fact restricted to specialized care. In some cases, the distinction is easy (*eg*, neurology or invasive cardiology), while in other cases the MCO must make the distinction on a physician-by-physician basis.

For traditional HMOs, the distinction between PCP designation and SCP designation is very important as regards how specialty services are authorized and paid for. In a traditional HMO in which the PCP acts as the care coordinator and must authorize any visits to a specialist (a gatekeeper type of HMO), the HMO cannot allow a specialist to be able to see a member for primary care, then refer that member back to himself or herself at a later time for specialty services (*ie*, get paid first to see the member as a PCP, and then get paid a second time to see the same member as an SCP). It is uncommon and foolhardy to allow a physician to be able to authorize referrals back to themselves and get paid twice to provide care for the same member. It is possible, though, for a physician to be a PCP for his or her own panel of members, but take referrals as a SCP from other PCPs who are not associated with that physician in some way, such as in the same multispecialty group.

In those MCOs that provide for open access (*ie*, do not require a member to receive authorization from his or her PCP to see a specialist), it is enough to determine whether or not the SCP meets the credentialing criteria (discussed later) and to simply ask the physician if he or she would like to be included in the directory as both general internal medicine and as the specialty or as the specialty alone.

HOSPITAL-BASED PHYSICIANS

A very unique type of specialist is the hospital-based physician (HBP). Broadly speaking, HBPs fall into one of four specialties:

- Radiology
- Anesthesiology
- Pathology
- Hospitalist

All acute-care medical/surgical hospitals have the first three, and many teaching hospitals have the fourth as well. There are two defining features of an HBP. The first is that there is usually no competition within a hospital for their particular specialty. For example, one single radiology group may provide all professional services for inpatient and outpatient radiology provided at the hospital. Even in the rare instances when there is more than one group, or different private practitioners, providing services (more common for anesthesia than for the other three specialties), some system is in place to determine how services will be divided up, and in no case does the patient (*ie*, member) have any choice. The second defining feature is that it is essentially not possible to receive inpatient care without incurring charges from one or more of the first three types of HBP.

Outpatient radiology, as well as elective ambulatory procedures that require anesthesia, may be done on a more selective basis, however. Pathology fees associated with elective outpatient laboratory and pathology may likewise be more selective by requiring only the use of contracted providers. In these cases, the approach to contracting is basically the same as that used for ancillary services as discussed in Chapter 7.

Hospitalists are different from the other three types of HBPs. Hospitalists are physicians who concentrate solely on the day-to-day management of inpatient care. In some cases, the hospitalist may concentrate solely on critical care and is also then referred to as an intensivist. In other cases, the hospitalist manages most types of inpatient cases, excluding certain focused types of cases such as childbirth or transplantation. The use of hospitalists is associated with both decreased costs and improved outcomes, and contracting between MCOs and hospitalists is not only readily done, but many MCOs seek ways of providing extra financial support for their use. Further discussion of hospitalists may be found in Chapter 9 as part of the broader issue of utilization management.

Contracting with the other types of HBPs as regards hospital-associated care can present challenges to an MCO because they hold what amounts to a monopoly for their particular types of inpatient services. Lack of a contract may even create a barrier to contracting with a hospital that is otherwise willing to agree to terms (hospital contracting is discussed in Chapter 7). This, of course, represents a serious problem for both the hospital and the other physicians that use the hospital. It is therefore important to work with the leadership of a hospital, both clinical and administrative leadership, as part of the process of recruiting and contracting with HBPs.

RECRUITING

Young or newly forming plans will concentrate primarily on initial network development. Mature plans will concentrate more on network maintenance (discussed later in this chapter), although recruiting to fill in areas with suboptimal access will always be an ongoing process, particularly during periods of high growth or expansion into a new service area. As the market has matured and consolidated (see Chapter 1), there are now few if any new start-ups, at least for commercial products. However, a health plan newly entering into the Medicare market through Medicare Advantage (see Chapter 26) or a start-up of a Medicare or Medicaid (see Chapter 27) plan may find that it needs to create a new network to cover parts of the service area in which it currently is not present. In any case, it is worthwhile to understand the processes and dynamics of building a network.

Access Needs

Consider geographic needs first. This generally breaks down into three main considerations: the need to target potential new members, the need to provide good access to areas with high concentrations of members, and the need to use contracted hospitals.

Primary target markets should be identified (*eg*, a large and growing suburban-industrial community or in the case of Medicare, a large concentration of seniors). Even when the plan is not looking to expand, it should be analyzing access needs on a regular basis as noted later. Physicians should be recruited from that medical staff of a contracting hospital, rather than physicians who practice only at a noncontracting hospital, even if it is in the targeted area. Priorities will also be affected by the availability, acceptability (to plan managers, to potential members, and to the rest of the medical panel), scope of practice, and practice capacities of physicians in target areas.

In addition to the broad geographic needs and hospital-related needs, it is important to assess accessibility in general. There are a number of ways to do this. One method is to look at the number of physicians per 1,000 members. The composition of a health plan's provider network is determined by marketing considerations and by need for coverage. In the past, very tight staffing ratios were considered optimal for management and control, but marketplace demands for broad networks have essentially dictated that except for group and staff model plans, broad networks are far more desirable than narrow networks are.

Provider networks' need may also be calculated using specialty-specific ratios of physicians per 1,000 enrollees. Such ratios have changed over time. A 1991 source suggested that plan networks typically had a physician-to-enrollee ratio of 0.8 primary care physicians per 1,000 enrollees and 1.3 total physicians per 1,000 enrollees.[5] Another source a few years later cited two mature staff model HMOs with 1.8 total physicians per 1,000 enrollees, which was a significantly more generous level of staffing than earlier "lean" staffing of HMOs and was close to the national average physician-to-population ratios.[6]

More recently, in one large report using 2004 data,[7] HMOs nationally reported 179 members per PCP on average, with a range of 125 members per PCP in open panel or independent (or individual) practice association (IPA) HMOs, 426 members per PCP for group model plans, and up to 722 members per PCP in staff model plans. By way of comparison, the ratio of specialty physicians was approximately double that of PCPs for all HMOs except staff model in which the ratio was almost tripled (likely as a reflection of the higher concentration of members per PCP in staff models). The average HMO had 6,263 physicians in total; however, ratios vary widely by plan model type, scope of physician practice, and plan size.

Staffing ratios for preferred provider organizations (PPOs) are much harder to determine for several reasons. First, PPOs that are owned for exclusive use by an insurer will be somewhat different than so-called rental PPOs (see Chapter 2). Second, many or even most PPOs serve customers that, through the nature of the managed care product itself, often do not know how many actual members are eligible for coverage. These companies know how many employees are covered, but although dependents with coverage are known to the health plan, no actual data is created until that dependent actually incurs a service. In other words, an HMO always knows how many members (both employee and dependents) are covered, whereas many or most PPOs only know for certain how many employees are covered, making comparisons between HMOs and PPOs difficult. Having said that, national staffing trends indicate an average of 101.6 PCPs and 188.1 specialty physicians per 1,000 employees, and an average of 3,041 PCPs and 5,921 specialists per PPO.[8] However, there is extremely high variation across all PPOs as regards these numbers.

For HMOs at least, it is more useful to look at the number of members whom each physician must accept (on the basis of contractual terms, see Chapter 30), such as 200 members per PCP. The ratios of physicians to members in open panels can vary tremendously depending on age of the plan, geographic access needs, the product lines being sold (eg, a Medicare risk product may require a higher number of physicians per 1,000 Medicare members than will a commercial), maturity of the marketplace in general, number of open practices, and marketing needs. One can also look at staffing needs by comparing average encounter data for Medicare and non-Medicare enrollees, as illustrated in Table 5-3, and extrapolating need from that.

For PCPs, another useful measure is geographic accessibility. This is generally calculated through one of two methods: drive time and number of PCPs by geographic availability. Drive time refers to how long members in the plan's service area have to drive to reach a PCP (or a PCP with an open practice, that is, one still accepting new patients). In general, drive time should be no more than 15 minutes, although 30 minutes may be appropriate for certain rural areas. Although a drive time of 20 minutes may be acceptable for access from a purely medical viewpoint, it will not be so acceptable in a heavily urbanized market.

The Centers for Medicare and Medicaid Services (CMS) also provides examples of minimum access standards for Medicare Advantage "at-risk," or coordinated care plans (Chapter 26).[9] For example, CMS states that for commonly used services, a 30-minute drive time (may be longer in rural areas) is required. CMS further states that a plan:

> must also ensure that, when medically necessary, services are available 24 hours a day, 7 days a week. This includes requiring primary care physicians to have appropriate backup for absences. The standards should consider the member's need and common waiting times for comparable services in the community. (Examples of reasonable standards for primary care services are: (1) Urgent but non-emergent—within 24 hours; (2) Non-urgent, but in need of attention—within 1 week; and (3) Routine and preventive care—within 30 days.).

Analyzing the number of PCPs by geographic availability is also useful. Generally, the plan will want to be able to provide at least two PCPs within 2 or 3 miles of each ZIP code from which the plan will be drawing members (the density is usually greater in urban areas and less in rural areas). Another measure of geographic availability is the radius from where the members live (eg, two PCPs within an 8-mile radius for urban areas and two PCPs within a 20-mile ra-

Table 5–3 HMO Utilization

	Hospital Days per 1,000 Members		Physician Encounters per Member		Ambulatory Visits per Member	
	2003	2004	2003	2004	2003	2004
PAYER TYPE						
Non-Medicare	220.1	224.0	3.2	3.4	1.8	1.7
Medicare	1,456.7	1,485.3	7.1	8.4	2.8	3.4
Medicaid	348.3	329.0	3.7	3.7	2.0	1.7

Source: Sanofi-Aventis. HMO-PPO/Medicare-Medicaid Managed Care Digest Series. Digest 2005. Available at: http://www.managedcaredigest.com.

dius for rural areas). Again, these ratios may represent a minimum configuration and will not necessarily be acceptable in any given marketplace.

Closed Panel Access Needs

Although the focus of this chapter is on open panel MCOs, it is still worthwhile noting some data from closed panel plans, even if these data are now over a decade old. These data help illustrate the types of access needs found in the most saturated type of managed care setting (*ie*, the physicians only see members of the HMO, and do not see other patients as well).

Based on research published in 1995, there appears to be some differences in staffing ratios between "large" and "small" closed panel HMOs, with the difference occurring at approximately 80,000 members. In plans with less than 80,000 members, the weighted mean PCP staffing ratio (rounded) was 0.89:1,000, with a standard deviation of 0.68; for plans with more than 80,000 members, the weighted mean PCP staffing ratio (rounded) was 0.66:1,000, with a standard deviation of 0.51. The weighted mean staffing ratio for all physicians (not just PCPs) was 2.8:1,000 for small plans, and 1.2:1,000 for large plans. The majority of closed panel HMOs increased their staffing ratios for Medicare members to a mean of 1.6:1,000 Medicare enrollees.[10]

These data compare with data published in 1992 obtained at an earlier point in time from essentially the same sources, in which large, closed panel plans that served a primarily commercial population had an average PCP staffing ratio of 0.8:1,000 and an average physician staffing ratio of 1.3:1,000. Plans that were smaller had more than twice those ratios. In the 1992 data, the ratios per 1,000 members, by specialty type, were 0.3 for full-time general/family practice, 0.3 for internal medicine, 0.2 for pediatrics, and 0.1 for OB/Gyn.[5] When looking solely at general

pediatricians for *pediatric* enrollees (as opposed to all enrollees, which is what the other ratios look at), recent data reports 0.54:1,000 for large plans, and 0.79:1,000 for small plans.[10] These 1992 and 1995 numbers generally represent how the HMO industry looked in its heyday (at least for closed panel plans), and as illustrated earlier regarding the average number of members for PCPs in group and staff model plans, staffing ratios have become more relaxed in recent years even for closed panel plans.

Closed panel plans such as staff or group model HMOs (or large group practices with a significant at-risk managed care practice) must carefully weigh the advantages and disadvantages of bringing an SCP in-house to join the medical staff rather than contracting out for services. The need to bring an SCP in-house may arise if the volume of referrals is high, if the plan is unable to obtain satisfactory contracts outside, if there are questions about the quality of care being delivered by outside SCPs and there are no good alternatives, if there is patient dissatisfaction, or if there are problems with proper utilization management.

Balanced against this are issues that may militate against the decision to bring an SCP in-house. Providing adequate on-call coverage could be a problem. If there is only one of that type of SCP and cross-coverage with another in-house SCP is not possible, the SCP could burn out; if coverage previously had been provided by outside SCPs who now no longer receive referrals, they may be less than cooperative about sharing calls. Related to that is the issue of needing to cover a large geographic area. If the plan uses multiple hospitals covering a wide territory, or if there are multiple medical centers, the SCP may not be able to provide sufficient coverage and the volume of referrals coming back inside may decrease. Even if referrals can be tightened up on an outpatient basis, attention must be paid to emergency care, especially for surgery, obstetrics, orthopedics, and cardiology.

NONPHYSICIAN OR MIDLEVEL PRACTITIONERS

Nonphysician clinicians (NPCs) or midlevel practitioners (MLPs) in primary care include physician assistants (PAs) and nurse practitioners (NPs). There are several different types of NP designations, each having a different focus and training; those include advanced practice nurses (APNs), nurse-midwives (NMs), nurse anesthetists (NAs), and clinical nurse specialists (CNSs). The use of NPCs in health care is quite widespread, with one study reporting an increase in the proportion of patients who saw NCPs from 30.6% to 36.1%; this includes a mix of patients who saw both an NCP and a physician along with patients who saw only an NCP for care, and includes types of NCPs such as psychologists, optometrists, and chiropractors who are not generally considered MLPs.[11]

Staffing rations vary in managed care plans as regards the use of such NCPs. For example, in 1995 Dial *et al* reported:

> The median enrollment-weighted ratio of FTE APNs per 100,000 members in those plans was 19.7, with an interquartile range of 15.9 to 21.5. Almost two-thirds (63.4%) of responding HMOs employed PAs. With two exceptions, these were the same HMOs that reported having APNs on staff. The median weighted ratio of FTE PAs per 100,000 members was 8.1, with an interquartile range of 8.1 to 14.8.[10]

Specifically regarding NPs, more than 106,000 practice in 48 states and the District of Columbia, 39% hold hospital privileges, 13% have long-term care privileges, more than 96% prescribe medications, and 20% practice in rural or frontier areas.[12] Specifically regarding PAs, there are approximately 66,500 PAs of whom approximately 89% are in active practice, with 43% employed by a single or multispecialty physician group prac-

tice while 22% are employed by hospitals and 14% are employed by solo physician offices, and work settings included hospital inpatient units, physician offices, emergency departments, and operating rooms.[13]

Although the data are old, closed panel (group and staff model) health plans are more likely to use nonphysician providers to deliver some medical care to their members. In a previously cited study, 65% of closed panel plans reported the use of nonphysician providers, with a mean ratio of 0.08:1,000.10 In a 1992 report, 86% of closed panel plans reported using nonphysician providers (compared with 48% of open panel plans), 52% of plans used PAs, 52% of plans used NPs, and 28% of plans used certified nurse-midwives.[14]

Well-qualified NCPs are generally found to be a great asset in managed care in that they are able to deliver excellent primary care, provide more health maintenance and health promotion services, tend to spend more time with patients, and receive generally good acceptance from most members. NCPs may also play an important role in the management of chronically ill patients. They may provide the primary locus of coordination of care or case management for patients with diseases such as chronic asthma, diabetes, and the like. In a similar vein, NCPs may take a key role in managing high-risk patients, using practice protocols for prevention and health maintenance in this population. Certified nurse-midwives may not only provide services for routine deliveries, but may in fact provide primary gynecological care using practice guidelines and protocols.

The availability of NCPs varies widely from state to state and is strongly correlated with a "favorable state practice environment."[15] The practice environment includes such variables as the ability to write prescriptions, the ability to practice in a (relatively) autonomous manner for certain situations, and the ability to receive direct reimbursement. In some locations, MCOs are contracting directly with NPs for primary care services, although that remains relatively infrequent.

Tiered Specialty Physician Networks

Although relatively uncommon, some large national health insurance companies are using data from their disease management activities, claims data, and quality management data to develop tiered networks of specialists. In other words, the health plan identifies specialists who appear to provide high-quality care, good outcomes, and efficiency as regards the total cost of care (not just the SCP's own charges). That list of specialists is made available to members and to other providers. Similar to tiering programs for hospitals as discussed in Chapter 7, these programs provide better benefits coverage to those members who choose to receive selected types of specialty care from those SCPs considered to be in the highest tier.

TYPES OF CONTRACTING SITUATIONS

In developing a network, an open panel may have to deal with a number of possible types of contracting situations. The subject of the contract itself is addressed in Chapter 30, and reimbursement is discussed in Chapters 6 and 8. This discussion focuses on the types of situations that may present themselves, regardless of specific contracting and reimbursement issues.

Individual Physicians

This is the most common category of contracting in open panels, which is not surprising given the large number of solo practitioners in many parts of the country. In this model, the physician contracts directly with the health plan and not through any third party or intermediary. The advantage to the plan is that there is a direct relationship with the physician, which makes it cleaner and simpler to interact. The disadvantage is that it is only one physician, and therefore the effort to obtain and maintain that relationship is disproportionately great.

Medical Groups

Not substantially different from individual physicians, small groups (ie, 2–10 physicians) usually operate relatively cohesively. The advantage to the plan is that the same amount of effort to obtain and maintain a small group yields a higher number of physicians. Plans generally prefer to contract with small groups for that reason. The disadvantage is that, if the relationship with the group needs to be terminated (for whatever reason, theirs or the health plan's), there is greater disruption in patient care.

Medical groups can be single specialty (eg, all primary care internists or all orthopedic surgeons), or multispecialty. Relatively uncommon in certain parts of the country, medical groups in general and multispecialty groups in particular are occasionally the dominant practices in certain areas. The advantage of contracting with multispecialty groups is that the plan obtains not only PCPs but SCPs as well. This provides for broader access (including specialists to whom other PCPs may refer) and allows for existing referral patterns to continue.

One potential disadvantage of multispecialty groups is that sometimes they are dominated by the SCPs in the group, which may lead to inappropriate overutilization of referral services. Another potential disadvantage is the case where, by accepting the group, the plan is forced to accept a specialist whose cost or quality is not what is desired (although not so bad as to prevent contracting with the group).

Independent Practice Associations

The independent practice association (IPA) is the original form of open panel plan. In the early 1970s, it was envisioned that open panel plans would all be IPA model plans. In this situation, there is actually a legal entity of an IPA, which contracts with physicians, and the IPA in turn contracts with the health plan. The advantage to the plan is that a large number of providers come along with the contract. Furthermore, if relations between the IPA and the health plan are close, there may be a confluence of goals, which benefits all parties. An integrated delivery system (IDS; see Chapter 2) may also use an IPA for the physician portion of the integrated delivery system. Most IPAs encompass all or most specialties, including primary care, but some single specialty IPAs do exist. An MCO may need to contract with more than one IPA to provide adequate coverage for the entire service area. Last, some relationships between MCOs and IPAs are exclusive, whereas others are not.

The primary value to contract with an IPA is that it brings a large number of physicians into the health plan at one time. Only one negotiating focus is required because the IPA physicians all agree to abide by terms agreed to between the IPA and the MCO. The IPA may also be willing and able to accept more financial risk than could a solo physician or small group (compensation is discussed in Chapters 6 and 8). In addition, some IPAs also carry out functions such as network management, credentialing, and even medical management (both utilization and quality management) on behalf of the MCO, thereby allowing for lower administrative costs at the MCO.

There are two primary disadvantages to contracting with IPAs. The first is that an IPA can function somewhat as a union. If relations between the IPA and the health plan are arm's length or problematic, the IPA can hold a considerable portion (or perhaps all) of the delivery system hostage to negotiations. This fact has not been lost on the Justice Department of the federal government. IPAs that function as anticompetitive forces may encounter difficulties with the law.

The second disadvantage is that the plan's ability to select and deselect individual physicians is much more limited when contracting through an IPA than when contracting directly with the providers. If the IPA is at risk for medical expenses, there may be a confluence of objectives between the plan and the IPA to bring in cost-effective and high-quality providers and to remove those providers whose cost or quality is not acceptable. Unfortunately, the IPA has its own internal political structure, so that defining who is cost effective or high quality, as well as dealing with outliers, may not match exactly between the plan and the IPA. If the plan has the contractual right to refuse to accept or to departicipate (ie, remove) individual providers in the IPA, that obstacle may be avoided, although the purely political obstacles remain.

Specialty Management Companies

Though not common, there exist companies that focus on managing very specialized services using physicians. In some cases, these companies are physician practice management companies (PPMCs; see Chapter 2) that manage the specialty medical group, and technically it is the medical group that contracts with the MCO even though it is managed by the PPMC. In other cases, the physicians work for the specialty management company, and it is the company that contracts with the MCO.

Two examples out of many are single specialty case management such as neonatal care, and emergency and critical care using non-hospital-based physicians. The physicians working for these companies obtain privileges at all hospitals in a defined service area and are then responsible for providing care for all of the MCO's cases that fall within certain criteria; for example, in the neonatal intensive care unit, or patients seen in the emergency department who must be evaluated for possible hospital admission.

Integrated Delivery Systems

Many hospitals have been exploring methods of developing organizations that will legally and structurally bond the physicians to the hospital. Sometimes these are referred to as physician-hospital organizations (PHOs) or management service organizations (MSOs). In addition to hospital-based IDSs, there are physician-only MSOs. These and other forms of integrated delivery systems are discussed in Chapter 2. The positive and negative ramifications that apply to IPAs are similar to those for IDSs (including their antitrust risk) and have been discussed previously. In addition to those issues, there are two other broad issues that relate specifically to hospital-based organizations.

First is the link between a hospital's own willingness to do business with a plan and the plan's willingness to do business with the PHO or MSO. In other words, the hospital may refuse to contract with the plan or may not provide favorable terms unless the plan brings in the PHO, perhaps even on an exclusive basis. That obviously removes control of that entire portion of the delivery system (physicians and hospital), leaving the plan at the mercy (or abilities) of the PHO or MSO to achieve the goals of the plan. If the PHO or MSO is at significant risk for medical expenses, there may be a confluence of goals.

The second issue relates to the reasons that the PHO formed in the first place. If the hospital has the goals of keeping beds filled and keeping the medical staff happy (and busy), the selection process for choosing which providers are in the PHO may be weighted toward those physicians who admit a lot of patients to the hospital, a criterion that may not be ideal from the plan's perspective. Another reason that the PHO may have formed was to circle the wagons, that is, to resist aggressive managed care. In that event, there may be a real mismatch between how the plan wants to perform medical management and how the PHO will allow it to occur. Issues of control of utilization management, quality management, and provider selection become difficult to resolve.

Nonetheless, hospital-centered organizations can function effectively. If the organization is formed with a genuine understanding of the goals of managed care, a genuine willingness to deal with difficult issues of utilization, quality, and provider selection, and a willingness to share control with the health plan, it is possible to work together.

As discussed more fully in Chapter 2, large PPMCs were for a brief period a viable contracting entity. PPMCs accepted global risk from the MCO, with the intent of managing utilization and keeping the savings rather than sharing with a hospital system. Most general PPMCs have since failed, many in a spectacular display of self-immolation by entering bankruptcy, not paying physicians, and simply ceasing to exist. PPMCs have become largely irrelevant for contracting except for some specialty services as noted earlier.

The primary advantage to a health plan in contracting with an IDS is the ability to have a network in rapid order. This is similar to the advantage in contracting with an IPA, but also includes (at least) hospital services. This may be a primary driver in the case of a plan entering into a new market, or one which is already competitive, and may in fact be the only way an MCO can get a network. A plan that needs to expand its medical service area quickly, that is offering an entirely new managed care product such as Medicare Advantage (Chapter 26) or Medicaid Managed Care (Chapter 27), or that is expanding into entirely new geographic areas may find that contracting through IDSs enables it to achieve its expansion goals and be first to market. An additional advantage may occur if the IDS is willing to provide a substantial savings to the plan, better than that which would be available on a direct contract basis.

It should be noted that in certain states, HMOs are not allowed to contract solely with the IDS, but must have contracts directly with the physicians. The individual physician contract may be brief and encompass no more than standard "hold harmless" language (see Chapter 30) and then reference the contract between the IDS and the physician and, in turn, the contract between the IDS and the plan. This requirement is meant to ensure that each and every individual physician understands and agrees to certain provisions required under state law, such as the prohibition on balance billing (discussed in Chapters 1 and 30).

Faculty Practice Plans

Faculty practice plans (FPPs) are medical groups that are organized around teaching programs, primarily at university hospitals. An FPP may be a single entity or may encompass multiple entities defined along specialty lines (*eg*, cardiology or anesthesiology). Plans generally contract with the legal group representing the FPP rather than with individual physicians within the FPP, although that varies from plan to plan.

FPPs represent special challenges for various reasons. First, many teaching institutions and FPPs tend to be less cost-effective in their practice styles than private physicians. This probably relates to the primary missions of the teaching program: to teach and to perform research. Cost-effectiveness is a secondary goal only (if a goal at all).

A second challenge is that an FPP, like a medical group, comes all together or not at all. This again means that the plan has little ability to select or deselect the individual physicians within the FPP. Related to that is the lack of detail regarding claims and encounter data. Many FPPs simply bill the plan, accept capitation, or collect encounter data in the name of the FPP rather than in the name of the individual provider who performed the service. This means that the plan has little ability to analyze data to the same level of detail that is afforded in the rest of the network. At least theoretically this issue could be addressed through the use of the new National Provider Identifier (NPI), which was required by the Health Insurance Portability and Accountability Act of 1996 (HIPAA) in which each provider is issued a single identifier; however, because HIPAA allows a medical group to use a single NPI for all services, there will likely be little change to this issue.

A third major challenge is the use of house officers (interns and residents in training) and medical students to deliver care. In teaching hospitals, the day-to-day care is actually delivered by house officers, rather than by the attending faculty physician, who functions as teachers and supervisors. House officers and medical students, because they are learning how to practice medicine, tend to be profligate in their use of medical resources; they are there to learn medicine, not simply to perform direct service to patients. Furthermore, experience does allow physicians to learn what is cost-effective, and house officers and medical students have yet to gain such experience. Nevertheless, there is some evidence that intensive attention to utilization management by faculty can have a highly beneficial effect on house staff.[16] That type of focus remains the exception and not the rule, but there has been a slow acceptance of the need to manage utilization even within teaching programs.

The last major issue with teaching programs and FPPs is the nature of how they deliver services. Most teaching programs are not really set up for case management. It is far more common to have multiple specialty clinics (*eg*, pulmonary, cardiology, or vascular surgery) to which patients are referred for each specific problem. Such a system takes on characteristics of a medical pinball machine, where the members ricochet from clinic to clinic, having each organ system attended to with little regard for the totality of care. This can lead to run-ups in cost as well as continuity problems and a clear lack of control or accountability, though proponents of the electronic medical record hope that this will diminish as real-time access to all clinical information becomes available.

Despite these difficulties, there are good reasons for health plans to contract with teaching programs and FPPs other than the societal good derived from the training of medical practitioners. Teaching programs and FPPs provide not only routine care but tertiary and highly specialized care as well, care that the plan will have to find means to provide in any event. Teaching programs also add prestige to the plan by virtue of their reputation for providing high-quality care, although that can be a two-edged sword in that the participation of a teaching program may draw adverse selection in membership.* Most teaching programs and FPPs recognize the problems cited previously and are willing to work with plans to ameliorate them.

Retail Health Clinics

Retail health clinics are essentially small clinics, usually associated with a retail store such as a grocery store or pharmacy. Unlike traditional urgent care centers, retail clinics are staffed by PAs or NPs, not physicians, and they exist solely to provide services for relatively minor medical conditions such as minor infections. They provide convenience to consumers because they are readily accessible, and the consumer can shop at the retail store while waiting for test results or for a prescription to be filled. They are also less expensive than a visit to a physician is. Many MCOs are contracting with retail health clinics so as to provide access to members on a more convenient and less expensive basis for minor illnesses.

Because it costs the MCO or employer less for a retail health clinic visit than a physician visit for a minor condition, MCOs are taking two approaches to steering members in that direction. The first is to have less cost sharing when the member uses the clinic; for example, a $5 or $10 copay to access the clinic vs. a $20 copay to see a physician and a $100 co-

pay to use the emergency department. With the advent of consumer-directed health plans (CDHPs; see Chapters 2 and 20) and the need to provide information to consumers so as to allow them to make informed choices about obtaining the most cost-effective health care, pricing and cost information is being made available via the Web, thus allowing consumers in CDHPs to spend less money to receive care for minor illnesses.

Physicians, particularly PCPs, have mixed attitudes regarding retail health clinics. On the one hand, it may ease some capacity pressures on a very busy practice. On the other hand, it is lost revenue to the PCP (or the emergency department, but that is not really of concern to either the MCO or to PCPs). Additionally, physicians raise the concern that use of retail health clinics does not provide for continuity of care and contain the possibility of missing a serious condition. However, there is no research to indicate the overall impact on health by the use of retail health clinics.

CREDENTIALING

It is not enough to get physicians to sign contracts. Without performing proper credentialing, the plan has no knowledge of the quality or acceptability of physicians. Furthermore, in the event of a legal action against a physician, the plan may expose itself to some liability by having failed to carry out proper credentialing. In the past, for example, one well-known study reported that up to 5% of physicians applying for positions in ambulatory care clinics had misrepresented their credentials in their applications.[17] Because of changes in reporting boards (discussed later) and in how sophisticated credentialing verification organizations (CVOs) operate as discussed later, the problem of fraudulent credentials has been diminished, though not eliminated.

Regulatory requirements for credentialing are highly variable. At the state level, some states prescribe the minimum requirements to credential physicians, while other states simply require MCOs to conduct credentialing

---

*In other words, if there is more than one health plan competing in a single group account (ie an employer group) for membership, members with serious illnesses may choose the health plan affiliated with a teaching program to ensure access to high-quality tertiary care. That means that sicker members join that health plan and less-sick members join the health plan that does not have such an affiliation. This issue does not come up if the plan is the sole carrier in an account or if all the competing plans use the teaching program, but it is a clear problem if there are multiple plans competing freely for members in a single account.

and recredentialing without specifying what data are to be collected and/or verified. Accreditation bodies in managed health care (see Chapter 23) have listed the minimum required credentialing data and processes for the health plan to be accredited. Credentialing requirements may also vary depending on the type of MCO, with HMO credentialing requirements usually being more stringent than other types of health plans. Some have even argued that with markets shifting to a greater focus on the consumer (see Chapter 20), existing credentialing programs should be abandoned for all but the most basic data required to conduct business and should be replaced with consumer-centric data such as cost, outcomes, and consumer-oriented services.[18] That approach cannot be endorsed because regardless of the type of health plan, there is implied a certain responsibility that if the MCO offers a network to its members, that network meets at least minimum standards. This chapter discusses credentialing primarily as it currently applies to most managed care plans.

In most HMOs, the medical director bears ultimate responsibility for credentialing along with a credentialing committee, although the activities of credentialing are usually carried out by the provider relations department. In a few HMOs and in most other types of MCOs, responsibility for credentialing may be the responsibility of either the medical director or else another officer who does not report to the medical director. The latter situation reflects how many large health plans, particularly national companies, have divided up responsibilities and functions, with network management being an activity independent of medical management. Regardless of where the responsibility lies, the requirements are the same.

Three broad activities are involved in credentialing: data collection, verification, and finally review and decision. Data collection may come from a variety of sources and is much more extensive during the initial credentialing than it is for recredentialing. Verification of education and training is re-

quired only for initial credentialing, whereas verification of other data may be required during recredentialing as well. Final review and decision refers to the health plan's ultimate decision, based on the data, as to whether to contract with the physician (or other type of provider).

The credentialing process should be carried out during the recruiting process, or rarely, after a contract or letter of intent is signed. MCOs with Medicare Advantage plans must also determine whether a physician has been sanctioned by Medicare. Periodic recredentialing (usually every 24 to 36 months) should also take place. Recredentialing may be less extensive than primary credentialing, but more sophisticated plans are adding new elements to the recredentialing process, including looking at measures of quality of care, member satisfaction, compliance with plan policies and procedures, and utilization management.

In the past, some regulators and outside accreditation agencies required that the health plan (in particular HMOs) conduct primary source verification, that is, obtain the information directly rather than relying on another party to obtain it. Fortunately, the industry has evolved, and accredited CVOs (ie, CVOs accredited by an accreditation organization; see Chapter 23) may be relied upon to conduct much of the data collection and verification on behalf of a health plan.

In 2002, in response to the ever-growing burden on both health plans and (especially) providers created by the credentialing process, as well as increasing and increasingly complex new sources of data, a coalition representing the health plans, the providers, and others created the Council for Affordable Quality Health Care (CAQH).* While also undertaking some

---

*In fact, at the time of publication, CAQH is housed in the same offices as the industry's trade association, America's Health Insurance Plans (AHIP) at 601 Pennsylvania Ave. NW, South Building Suite 500, Washington, DC 20004.

other initiatives, CAQH created the Universal Credentialing DataSource (UCD) to provide significant improvements in efficiency and efficacy of the credentialing process. Although the UCD is not used by every MCO in the United States, it is used by a substantial number of them, including most of the major commercial companies and a number of Blue Cross Blue Shield plans. Not all MCOs use a CVO and there are other CVOs in operation (and CAQH does more than function as a CVO), but given the scope and size of the UCD it is worth making note of it and briefly describing what it does in regards to credentialing.

Like most CVOs, the UCD enables a provider to provide the required credentialing data to one source, either online or via fax or mail, at no cost; the cost to access the UCD is borne by the health plans. Similar to other CVOs, the CAQH then performs primary source verification of that data. The CAQH also obtains data from other sources such as the two federal databases: the National Practitioner Data Bank (NPDB) and the Healthcare Integrity and Protection Data Bank (HIPDB). These two databanks are discussed later.

In addition to these data, the CAQH also monitors data from other important sources that are not usually routinely sampled by most MCOs or even CVOs: data regarding sanctions and discipline actions. Not all sanctions and disciplinary actions merit action on the part of the plan, but either a pattern of sanctions or disciplinary actions or an egregious problem, including deceiving the plan regarding such actions, would result in the plan terminating that physician's contract. Ongoing monitoring of this type of information is important for maintaining the quality and integrity of the network.

Table 5-4 lists the elements of a typical credentialing application. Table 5-5 lists credentialing verification sources (to be used by the MCO or by the CVO). Table 5-6 lists elements for ongoing monitoring as conducted by the CAQH.

Table 5–4 Elements of a Typical Credentialing Application

- Demographics, Licenses, and Other Identifiers
  - Full name
  - Date of birth, place of birth, gender
  - Social security number
  - Home address
  - Medical license
  - Drug Enforcement Agency (DEA) registration
  - State controlled substance registration
  - National Provider Identifier (NPI)—to be phased in 2007–2008
  - Universal Provider Identification Number (UPIN) for Medicare
  - Medicaid number
- Education, Training, and Specialties
  - Professional education
  - Undergraduate education
  - Internship, residency, fellowship
  - Primary specialty, secondary specialty
  - Certifications
  - Other Interests
- Practice Details
  - Credentialing, business, billing office contact information
  - Practice general information
  - Office hours
  - Covering colleagues
  - Phone coverage
  - Practice limitations, age limitations, handicap accessibility
  - Practice services
- Billing and Remittance Information
- Hospital Privileges
  - Hospital contact information
  - Admitting privilege

continues

Table 5–4 Elements of a Typical Credentialing Application—continued

- Professional Liability Insurance
  - Carrier contact information
  - Coverage
- Work History and References
  - Current and previous work history (past 10 years or since graduation)
  - Gaps in work history (3 months or more)
  - Military service
  - Professional references
- Disclosure Questions
  - Limitations of suspension of privileges
  - Suspension from government programs
  - Malpractice cancellation
  - Felony conviction
  - Drug and alcohol abuse
  - Chronic or debilitating illness
- Images of Supporting Documents
  - Current professional liability insurance policy fact sheet
  - DEA registration
  - Educational Commission for Foreign Medical Graduates (ECFMG) certificate
  - State controlled dangerous substance certificate
  - State license certificate
  - Internal Revenue Service form W-9: request of taxpayer identification
  - Number and certification

*Medicare and Medicaid identifiers, despite being replaced by the NPI in 2007–2008, may still need to be obtained for any providers being newly credentialed to determine sanctions by those government payers. This would not apply, however, to a provider newly in practice once the NPI has been fully implemented.
Source: CAQH, used with permission.

Federal Databases

Special types of credentialing checks have been created by the federal government. The NPDB has been in existence since 1989, whereas the HIPDB was created in 1999. Both data banks have an impact on how health plans credential providers.

The National Practitioner Data Bank

The NPDB was created by the Health Care Quality Improvement Act of 1986 (HCQIA),[19] with final regulations published in 1989.[20] In March 2006, further revisions to the regulation of the NPDB were proposed under section 1921 of the Social Security Act,[21] which, if adopted, would add adverse action reports beyond issues related to professional competence and conduct on all licensed practitioners. Also it would add adverse action reports relative to certain negative actions or findings, mainly those taken by private accrediting organizations (*eg*, the Joint Commission on Accreditation of Healthcare Organizations, The National Committee for Quality Assurance (NCQA), URAC, and others). It would also allow access to the NPDB by a substantial number of non-health-plan organizations. At the time of publication, it is not known what final revisions were adopted, so the interested reader is referred to the official Web site for the HCQIA as listed later.

The HCQIA provides for qualified immunity from antitrust lawsuits for credentialing activities as well as professional medical staff sanctions when the terms of the act are followed. Information reported to the NPDB is considered confidential and may not be disclosed except as specified in the regulations. The NPDB itself requires reporting of and serves as a central repository of information for:

1. Malpractice payments made for the benefit of physicians, dentists, and other health care practitioners
2. Licensure actions taken by state medical boards and state boards of dentistry against physicians and dentists and

Table 5–5 Credentialing Data Verification Sources

Graduation from medical school (any one of the following):

- Confirmation from the medical school
- American Medical Association Master File of Physicians in the United States
- Confirmation from the Association of American Medical Colleges
- Confirmation from the Educational Commission for Foreign Medical Graduates for international medical graduates licensed after 1986
- Confirmation from state licensure agency if the agency performs primary verification of medical school graduation

Valid license to practice medicine (any one of the following):

- State licensure agency
- Federation of State Medical Boards
- Primary admitting facility if the facility performs primary verification of licensure

Completion of residency training (any one of the following):

- Confirmation from the residency training program
- American Medical Association Master File of Physicians in the United States
- Confirmation from the Association of American Medical Colleges
- Confirmation from state licensure agency if the agency performs primary verification of residency training

Board certification (any one of the following):

- American Board of Medical Specialties Compendium of Certified Medical Specialists
- American Osteopathic Association Directory of Osteopathic Physicians
- Confirmation from the appropriate specialty board
- American Medical Association Master File of Physicians in the United States
- Confirmation from state licensure agency if the agency performs primary verification of board status

other health care practitioners who are licensed or otherwise authorized by a state to provide health care services

3. Professional review actions primarily taken against physicians and dentists by hospitals and other health care entities, including health maintenance organizations, group practices, and professional societies
4. Actions taken by the Drug Enforcement Agency (DEA)
5. Medicare/Medicaid exclusions

Hospitals are required to query the NPDB every 2 years. Health care entities such as HMOs, preferred provider organizations, and group practices may query under the following circumstances:

1. When entering an employment or affiliation arrangement with a physician, dentist, or other health care practitioner
2. When considering an applicant for medical staff appointment or clinical privileges
3. When conducting peer review activity

Table 5–6 Elements for Ongoing Network Monitoring

Elements	Examples of External Sources
• Disciplinary actions from licensing boards	• State licensing boards
• Expiration of specialty certification	• HHS Office of Inspector General Exclusions Database
• Malpractice events	• Office of Personnel Management Debarment List
• Medicare debarment	• NPDB/HIPBD
• Member complaints and grievances	• Universal Credentialing DataSource
• Utilization review	• American Board of Medical Specialties
	• Federation of State Medical Boards
	• Office of Foreign Assets Control

Source: CAQH, used with permission

To be eligible, such entities must both provide health care services and have a formal peer review process for the purpose of furthering the quality of health care. The act also states that any hospital, HMO, preferred provider organization, or group practice may contact the NPDB to obtain information about a physician and that, if the hospital or health plan fails to do so, it will be assumed that it did so anyway. In other words, there is a potential for liability on the part of the plan if it fails to check with the NPDB and contracts with a physician who has a poor record as reported in the NPDB and there is a malpractice problem later on.

Healthcare Integrity and Protection Data Bank

The Secretary of the U.S. Department of Health and Human Services (DHHS), acting through the Office of Inspector General (OIG), was directed by HIPAA (see also Chapter 32) to create the HIPDB to combat fraud and abuse in health insurance and health care delivery. The HIPDB is a national health care fraud and abuse data collection program for the reporting and disclosure of certain final adverse actions (excluding settlements in which no findings of liability have been made) taken against health care providers, suppliers, or practitioners. It is to contain the following types of information:

- Civil judgments against health care providers, suppliers, or practitioners in federal or state courts related to the delivery of health care items or services
- Federal or state criminal convictions against health care providers, suppliers, or practitioners related to the delivery of health care items or services
- Injunctions
- Actions by federal or state agencies responsible for the licensing and certification of health care providers, suppliers, or practitioners
- Exclusion of health care providers, suppliers, or practitioners from participation in federal or state health care programs
- Any other adjudicated actions or decisions that the secretary establishes by regulations[22]

The HIPDB is a tracking system that serves as an alert function to users, indicating that a comprehensive review of the practitioner's, provider's, or supplier's past actions may be prudent. HIPDB information should be used in combination with information from other sources to make determinations on acceptance or rejection of a provider into the network. In addition to federal and state agencies that purchase health care services (*eg*, Medicare, Medicaid, the Department of Defense), health plans are also eligible to query the HIPDB. For purposes of this database, a health plan is defined as follows:

- A policy of health insurance
- A contract of a service benefit organization
- A membership agreement with a health maintenance organization or other prepaid health plan
- A plan, program, agreement, or other mechanism established, maintained, or made available by a self-insured employer or group of self-insured employers, a practitioner, provider or supplier group, third-party administrator, integrated health care delivery system, employee welfare association, public service group or organization, or professional association
- An insurance company, insurance service, or insurance organization licensed to engage in the business of selling health care insurance in a state and that is subject to state law that regulates health insurance[23]

The U.S. Department of Health and Human Services (HHS), Health Resources and Services Administration (HRSA), Bureau of Health Professions (BHP), Office of Workforce Evaluation and Quality Assurance (OWEQA), Practitioner Data Banks Branch (PDBB) is responsible for the management of the National Practitioner Data Bank and the Healthcare Integrity and Protection Data Bank. At the time of publication, general information about both data banks may be found at http://www.npdb-hipdb.com. The data banks themselves are located at http://www.npdb-hipdb.hrsa.gov, though neither data bank is accessible to the general public, and only qualified organizations may query them. Information may be obtained via the Internet site noted earlier or by writing to the following address:

National Practitioner Data Bank
Healthcare Integrity and Protection Data Bank
P.O. Box 10832
Chantilly, VA 20153-0832
Phone: 1-800-767-6732 (outside the United States: 703-802-9395)
Web site: http://www.npdb-hipdb.com/custsrv.html

Office Evaluation

If a tightly managed plan such as an HMO is contracting directly with physicians, it will likely desire to perform a direct evaluation of the physician's office; in fact, as noted in Chapter 23, on-site office evaluation is required for accreditation of HMOs. If the plan has contracted through an IDS, it may forgo such a review if the IDS has already performed the review to the satisfaction of the plan; in other words, delegated that activity to the IDS, though still requiring that accreditation standards be met. Plans that are less closely managed (*eg*, a loosely managed PPO) may not perform an office evaluation simply because it is interested only in contractual terms and having a physician meet minimum credentialing requirements (see earlier discussion), not because it truly intends to manage health care. Even then, conducting an office evaluation is worthwhile if for no other reason than to determine the overall acceptability of the practice environment to members.

There are two main items to evaluate in a physician's office: capacity to accept new members and office ambiance. In addition, the plan or IDS may review the office from the standpoint of a quality management process, compliance with Occupational Safety and Health Administration (OSHA) guidelines, presence of certain types of equipment (*eg*, a defibrillator), and so forth. If capacity and ambiance are the only review areas, the evaluation is best accomplished by having the recruiter visit the office and may be performed in one fairly short visit. A more detailed review requires a trained health professional, usually a nurse, and may take an hour or two.

In addition to asking physicians directly how many new members they will accept (and usually including that in the contract; see Chapter 30), the recruiter should ask to examine the appointment system (or appointment book in some small offices). In this way, the recruiter can get a reasonably good idea of how much appointment availability the physician has. For example, if there are no available appointment slots for a physical examination for 6 weeks or more, the physician may be overestimating his or her ability to accept more work.

The recruiter can also get an idea of how easy it is for a patient with an acute problem to be put on the schedule. This may be examined by looking at the number of acute slots left open each day and by looking at the number of double-booked appointments that were put in at the end of each day. In addition, the recruiter can assess less tangible items such as cleanliness of the office, friendliness of the staff toward patients, and general atmosphere. Hours of operation can be verified, as can provisions for emergency care and in-office equipment capabilities.

Medical Record Review

It was common in the past for the medical director of an HMO to review a sample of the physician's medical records. The purpose of this was to assure the medical director that physicians did indeed practice high-quality medicine and that their practice was already cost-effective. This practice is now rarely done for a variety or reasons. The most important reason is the privacy requirements under HIPAA (Chapter 32) have made such reviews more difficult, though not impossible. Prior to HIPAA it was still the standard for medical record review of cases that were not about HMO members to be masked as to personal identity; under HIPAA, however, what constitutes protected health informa-

tion is extensive, the requirements are stricter, and the penalties are certainly substantial. Furthermore, health plans are now so large that it is simply impractical to conduct wide-scale record reviews in the absence of an indication of a problem.

Electronic Connectivity

Many MCOs are beginning to consider electronic connectivity as a crucial aspect of recredentialing and renewal of provider contracts. Although still not common, as pressures to lower administrative costs continue and as the need for more accurate and efficient business transactions becomes acute, some MCOs are considering requiring electronic communication of basic transactions (*eg*, claims billing and authorizations) as a condition of contract renewal. This is not dissimilar to the requirements that CMS currently has for participating providers to submit claims electronically for Medicare (requirements that are largely met via the use of third-party billing services). Because of HIPAA, there are now electronic standards in existence for these types of electronic transactions.

THE NATIONAL PROVIDER IDENTIFIER

Among the requirements of HIPAA is the phase-in and use of the National Provider Identifier (NPI). On June 23, 2004, the Department of Health and Human Services published its final rule, and the NPI is scheduled to be phased in by the end by May 23, 2007 (May 23, 2008 for small health plans). The NPI will replace all other forms of provider identifiers such as the Medicare universal provider identification numbers (UPIN), Blue Cross and Blue Shield numbers, health plan provider numbers, TRICARE (see Chapter 28) numbers, Medicaid numbers, and so forth. The only provider numbers that are not affected are the taxpayer identifying number and the Drug Enforcement Administration number for providers who prescribe or administer prescription drugs. The employer identification number is not affected either, to the extent that a provider is also an employer. The NPI is unique and never-ending in that once assigned an NPI, the provider will use that identifier for all transactions regardless of location, plan type, or anything else.

Eventually the NPI will vastly simplify the ability of an MCO or CVO to keep track of information related to an individual physician or other provider, but it will take many years for that to occur. Because of that, MCOs will still need to know the Medicare UPIN and any Medicaid identifiers for credentialing purposes, at least for physicians new to the network. The reason is that there remains a need to determine whether a physician has been sanctioned by Medicare or Medicaid.* This will not apply to any physicians new to practice after the NPI has been fully phased in.

The NPI is a 10-digit number, with the tenth digit being a checksum. There is no embedded intelligence in the NPI. Nothing in the 10 digits will provide any additional information about the provider other than identifying who or what the provider is. As discussed in Chapter 18, for organizations that depend on embedded intelligence, this could pose a major problem. For example, if the plan has been using special characters or digits in the physician identifier to determine which payment schedule to use, which products the physician participates in, and so forth, the plan will need to find another way to do that; this particular issue is highly technical, idiosyncratic to any particular MCO, and beyond the scope of this discussion.

What the NPI will do is create a need to update the provider database. The MCO will need to obtain the NPI for all participating providers and map that to the existing database. In many if not most MCOs and health insurance companies, the provider database contains numerous duplications, and multiple entries for individual providers are not uncommon and may actually have been done deliberately for some reason (to allow them to bill differently for certain services in different situations).

COMPENSATION

Compensation of physicians is discussed in Chapters 6 and 8.

ORIENTATION

In all enterprises, time invested in the beginning to ensure real understanding is time well spent. In a strongly managed health plan such as an HMO, a planned approach to orientation of a newly added physician will pay off in improved compliance with the plan's procedures and policies, in increased professional satisfaction on the part of the physician and in increased member satisfaction. Orientation is aimed at two audiences: the physician and the physician's office staff. Table 5-7 lists some topics to consider in orienting physicians, and Table 5-8 lists some topics for orienting their office staff.

NETWORK MAINTENANCE

Maintenance of the professional relationship with physicians in the network recently has assumed a far greater role in managed care than at any previous time in the industry's history. The saturation of managed care plans in some communities, coupled with increasing interventions by third-party payers (commercial, Medicare, and Medicaid) limiting providers' ability to cost shift to other fee-for-service payers, has placed increasing strain on physicians and has clearly colored how they view participation with managed care plans. Failure to service the network properly can lead to defections or closure of practices to the plan, difficulty with new

---

*It is not known at the time of publication whether any cross-walks between the UPIN and the NPI will be available for use in credentialing. If such a cross-walk were available, it would obviate the need to obtain the UPIN during credentialing.

Table 5–7 Suggested Topics for Physician Orientation

- Plan subscription agreement and schedule of benefits
- Authorization policies and procedures
- Forms and paperwork
- Utilization and financial data supplied by plan
- Committees and meetings
- Quality management program and peer review
- Recredentialing requirements
- Member transfer in or out of practice
  - Member initiated
  - Physician initiated
- Plan member grievance procedure
- Schedule of compensation from plan
- Contact persons in plan
- Affiliated providers
  - Primary care
  - Consultants
  - Institutions
  - Ancillary services

Table 5–8 Suggested Topics for Orientation of Office Staff

- Plan subscription agreement and schedule of benefits
- Authorization policies and procedures
- Forms and paperwork
- Member transfer in or out of practice
  - Member initiated
  - Physician initiated
- Plan member grievance procedure
- Member eligibility verification
- Member identification card
- Current member list and eligibility verification
- Affiliated providers
  - Primary care
  - Consultants
  - Institutions
  - Ancillary services
- Contact persons in plan
  - Names
  - Telephone numbers
  - Hours of operation

recruiting, and a slow downward spiral. Even for those plans that have not properly maintained their networks, however, it is never too late to put in the effort because it is certainly possible to recover from a poor history.

Network maintenance as addressed in this section refers to managing the network from a business point of view, not from a clinical one, though there are obvious overlaps. If medical management is broadly considered to be onerous by the physicians, for example, no amount of efficient business transactions will completely make up for generated ill will. Management issues that are unique to a particular physician and do not represent larger management issues—inappropriate behavior, for example—would not create broad management intervention across the network.

In most plans, there are individuals who are solely responsible for maintaining communications with the physician panel, both PCPs and consultants, and both the physicians and their office staff. The roles of these provider relations representatives are to elicit feedback from the physicians and office staff, to update them on changes, to troubleshoot, maintain, and manage the contracts and other required documents, and generally to keep things running smoothly.

The importance of this function cannot be overstated. Some care must be taken in selecting the individuals who will fill this role. Unless provider relations staff are mature and experienced, they may be prone to forgetting for whom they are actually working. It is appropriate and necessary for them to represent the PCPs' point of view to plan management, but it is inappropriate if they find themselves siding against the health plan in the event of a dispute unless the plan is truly at fault. The provider relations staff must seek to prevent rifts, not to foster them.

Managing provider relations has also been aided through the use of information technology (IT) by the appearance of contract management systems and customer relationship management (CRM) systems. These systems are related to the IT support systems in use for managing customer relations in general for the MCO, allowing for tracking of issues, maintenance of contact information, recording all contacts, storing images of paper documents (*eg*, contracts and correspondence), and the like.

The provider relations function is similar to customer relations (see Chapter 19); but an even better metaphor is that of business partner. In a customer relation, the customer is always right; in a health plan, neither the plan nor the physician is always right. It is perhaps more useful to strive to be seen as a reliable and desirable business partner to the providers with whom the plan does business under contracts and agreements. Provider relations must therefore be proactive rather than simply reactive.

The plan should have a well-developed early warning system for troubleshooting. Such a system could include regular on-site visits by provider relations staff (and occasionally by the medical director, at least in the case of larger medical groups) and regular two-way communications vehicles. Regular meetings with groups of participating physicians, attended by senior-level representatives (possibly including physicians representing the health plan), are also good vehicles for keeping current with network attitudes and issues.

At the level of individual physicians, changes in patterns, particularly patterns in utilization and compliance with plan policy and procedure, will often be a sign that the relationship is going awry. Last, close monitoring of the member services complaints report can yield crucial information; physicians will often tell their patients what they think and what they intend to do long before they tell the plan.

If the plan contracts with an IDS for its network, that does not mean that obligations to maintain the network cease. Many of the issues discussed here remain under the control of the plan and will continue to exert a strong influence over the physicians in the contracted network. The IDS will have the burden of responsibility for network maintenance and must therefore also pay attention to these issues. It is imperative that both the plan and the IDS pay close attention to network maintenance and not rely solely on one party for this vital function. If both parties are not actively involved, there is the strong possibility of network problems degenerating into finger-pointing, in which case both parties lose.

Electronic Connectivity

Electronic commerce (e-commerce) and electronic connectivity, discussed in greater depth in Chapter 17, can also be considered an important part of maintaining and managing the network. The more that the Internet can be used for activities that currently either require a lot of time-consuming effort or that don't exist at all, the more the MCO has to offer to the physicians. Two of the most common categories of MCO–physician e-commerce are discussed in the following subsections.

Physician Directories

It has become common for MCOs to provide access to provider directories to members via the Internet, using the World Wide Web (the Web). In the simplest case, this means a static lookup function whereby a member can search the directory to find a physician who meets specialty and geographic needs. In more advanced settings, this may include more detailed information such as a photo, a brief curriculum vitae, cultural information (*eg*, languages spoken or a special focus on certain cultural needs), the ability to create and print out a map to the office, and other useful information. Such advanced systems also allow members to choose or change their PCP. All of these functions, although member oriented, also provide greater opportunities for the physicians to gain membership from the health plan.

Although still uncommon, some MCOs are also providing consumers with a rating of a medical group via the Web based on several criteria. These may be criteria created by the MCO itself, such as reported member satisfaction rates, compliance with certain clinical protocols for common conditions, and other measures. In other cases, MCOs are contracting with third parties to provide such information as can be compiled from public sources and are providing members access to that information via the Web. In either case, the general term data transparency is being used to denote the ability of a member to access more than just basic information about a provider; this is also discussed in Chapter 20 as part of the overall issue of consumerism. And it is not only MCOs that have such Web sites. Any number of private sites provide directories of physicians to consumers. Many of these sites include information similar to that noted previously, as well as a listing of the health plans in which the physician participates.

Physician Interaction with the Plan

The Internet is also being used in network maintenance and management by allowing physicians and the health plan to communicate electronically. This does not refer to simple e-mail, but to greater interactions. The most common types of interactions include claims submissions, referral authorization submissions, electronic payments, and so forth. But more advanced capabilities also exist, such as the ability to look up the status of individual claims, to check member/patient eligibility, and access drug formularies.

Regardless of whether electronic connectivity is done via the Web or through other means (*eg*, dedicated data lines for high-volume providers, clearinghouses, or service bureaus), certain business-related electronic transactions have been standardized as part of the Administrative Simplification section of HIPAA and have been in place since 2002. HIPAA does not mandate that physicians or other providers use electronic connectivity, but it does mandate that if they do use electronic connectivity for these transactions, they must conform to the standards.

The electronic standards were set by the American National Standards Institute (ANSI) with considerable input from other standard-making organizations (most importantly Health Level 7, or HL7) and are collectively referred to as ANSI X12 (or sometimes X12N) standards, referring to an ANSI-accredited group that defines electronic data interchange (EDI) standards for many U.S. industries, including health care insurance. When the mandated standards went into effect in 2002, version 4010 of these X12 standards was the one chosen. Newer versions now exist, but because of the need to maintain stability in standards so as to encourage adoption, the 4010 versions remain the standard at the time of publication; migration to the 5010 version is expected to occur at some point in the future, but exactly when is unknown. The exception is for required standards that have not yet been finalized; for example, at the time of publication, the standard for the claims attachment was proposed to be the 4050 version, whereas the standards for First Report of Injury were not yet proposed at all.

Table 5-9 lists the ANSI X12 standard electronic transactions under HIPAA.

The existence of these standards has gone a long way toward increasing adoption of electronic transactions. Regrettably, full use of these transactions is not made by most physicians. Electronic claims submission is the most common transaction, but use of the other transactions remains relatively low at the time of publication. As practice management software evolves and physicians continue to put newer practice management systems in place, greater use of all the transactions will take place, with attendant im-

Table 5–9 HIPAA Standardized Electronic Transactions

Transaction	ANSI X12 Standard
Claims submission	837
Eligibility	270 (inquiry) 271 (response)
Claim status	276 (inquiry) 277 (response)
Referral certification and authorization	278
Health care payment to provider, with remittance advice	835
Claims attachment (additional clinical information from provider to health plan, used for claims adjudication)	275 (not finalized at the time of publication), and HL7 Clinical Architecture Document (CDA)
Enrollment and disenrollment in health plan*	834
Premium payment to health plan*	820
First report of injury	148 (not yet issued)

*These are for voluntarily but not mandatory use by employers, unions, or associations that pay premiums to the health plan on behalf of members.
Source: Compiled by author based on 45 CFR §160.920 and other sources at CMS. Available at: http://www.cms.gov.

provements in administrative efficiencies by both physicians and MCOs.

Removing Physicians from the Network

Beyond the elements referred to earlier, another function of network maintenance is the determination of who not to keep in the plan. In any managed care plan, there will be physicians who simply cannot or will not work within the system and whose practice style is clearly cost-ineffective or of poor quality. As noted in the introduction to this chapter, voluntary and involuntary physician turnover is generally low, with the most recent data from 2002 reporting a 3% involuntary and 6% voluntary turnover rate in reporting health plans.[2]

Sanctions for reasons of poor quality are the most serious, and MCOs must work closely with legal counsel to establish proper processes for sanctioning. Removal of a physician from the network for quality reasons must also follow the process described in the HCQIA, including reporting such removal to the NPDB as well as the medical licensure boards in many states.

A plan may also choose to terminate physicians because the physician panel is too large, but this is rarely an issue for PCPs because most plans can always use wider access to primary care for both medical delivery and marketing reasons. The exception in primary care is likely to occur when a plan makes a wholesale commitment to an IDS and, as part of that commitment, agrees to terminate any PCPs that are not part of the IDS. In this situation, plans will usually resist terminating existing PCP relationships but may agree to no longer recruit new PCPs that are not part of the IDS (unless the IDS cannot provide sufficient PCPs in a geographic region).

Regarding the issue of unacceptably costly practice style, the plan must develop a mechanism for identification of such practitioners that uses a combination of claims and utilization data (see Chapter 16) and some type of formal performance evaluation system. If identified providers are reluctant to change, even after the medical director has worked closely with them, then serious consideration should be given to terminating them from the network.

There are several common objections to removing a physician from the network. Asking the members to change physicians is not easy or pleasant, benefits managers get upset, and invariably it seems the physician in question is in a strategic location. The decision often comes down to whether the plan wants to continue to subsidize that physician's poor practice behavior from the earnings of the other physicians (in capitated or risk/bonus types of reimbursement systems) and from the plan's earnings, or drive the rates up to uncompetitive levels. If those are unacceptable alternatives, then the separation must occur.

Various states, though not all, have enacted legislation that requires "due process" or "fair procedure" protection for instances when a provider is terminated from participating in a health plan. This type of legislation also requires health plans to show cause, provide reasons in writing, and/or allow for appeal or review of criteria for practice profiling or utilization/cost performance when providers are terminated from participation in a health plan's network. There is little uniformity, however, from state to state as regards such laws.

Some HMOs contractually require a physician to participate until the entire membership has had a chance to change plans (which may take a year unless the physician's member panel is small), but that option can be quite costly because the physician will have no incentive to control cost once he or she has been notified of termination. In those cases, the contract usually also allows the plan to increase the amount of withhold (*eg*, from 20% up to 50%) to cover excess costs. In preferred provider organizations, there is usually no need for such arrangements because the member may still see that physician, albeit at a higher level of co-insurance.

CONCLUSION

Network development requires an orderly project management approach, whether such development is undertaken by a health plan or by an integrated delivery system. It is equally important to invest in proper orientation of new physicians and their office staff. Maintenance of the relationship between the physicians and the plan is a key element of success that is gaining increasing importance as plans become ever more competitive in the marketplace. The plan or IDS must be willing to terminate a provider's contract in certain circumstances to deliver the proper combination of quality and cost-effectiveness that is a requirement of managed care.

References

1. O'Malley AS, Reschovsky JD. No exodus: Physicians and managed care networks. *Tracking Report 14*. Available at: http://www.hschange.com/CONTENT/838/. Accessed September 7, 2006.

2. America's Health Insurance Plans. *2002 AHIP Survey of Health Insurance Plans: Chartbook of Findings*. Washington, DC: America's Health Insurance Plans; 2004. Available at: http://www.ahipresearch.org/pdfs/2_2002SurvChartBook.pdf. Accessed September 7, 2006.

3. Whitcomb ME, Cohen JJ. The future of primary care medicine. *N Engl J Med*. 2004, 351 (7):710–712.

4. Defina T. Educating physicians in managed care. *Health System Leader*. May 1995, 2(4):4–11.

5. Group Health Association of America (GHAA). *HMO Industry Profile. Vol. 2, Physician Staffing*

and Utilization Patterns. Washington, DC: Group Health Association of America, 1991.

6. Hart LG, Wagner E. Physician staffing ratios in staff-model HMOs: A cautionary tale. *Health Affairs.* January–February 1997:55–70.

7. Sanofi-Aventis. HMO-PPO/Medicare-Medicaid Digest 2005. Managed Care Digest Series. Available at: http://www.managedcaredigest. com. Accessed September 7, 2006.

8. Sanofi-Aventis. HMO-PPO/Medicare/Medicaid Digest 2005. Managed Care Digest Series. Available at: http://www.managedcaredigest. com. Accessed September 7, 2006.

9. Centers for Medicare and Medicaid Services. Benefits and beneficiary protections. In: *Medicare Managed Care Manual.* 2005. Available at: http://www.cms.hhs.gov/manuals/ downloads/mc86c04.pdf. Accessed July 14, 2006.

10. Dial TH, Palsbo SE, Bergsten C, Gabel JR, Weiner J. Clinical staffing in staff- and group-model HMOs. *Health Affairs.* Summer 1995 14(2):168–80.

11. Druss BG, Marcus SC, Olfson M, TanielianT, Pincus HA. Trends in care by nonphysician clinicians in the United States. *Engl J Med.* 2003, 348:130–137.

12. American Academy of Nurse Practitioners. *US Nurse Practitioner Work Force, 2004.* Available at: http://www.aanp.org. Accessed September 7, 2006.

13. American Academy of Physician Assistants. *2005 AAPA Physician Assistant Census Report.* Available at: http://www.aapa.org. Accessed September 7, 2006.

14. Packer-Thursman J. The role of midlevel practitioners. *HMO Magazine.* March/April 1992: 28–34.

15. Sekscenski ES, Sansom S, Bazell C, *et al.* State practice environments and the supply of physician assistants, nurse practitioners, and certified nurse-midwives. *N Engl J Med.* 1994, 331(19): 1266–1271.

16. Woodside JR, Bodne R, Tonnesen AS, Frazier J. Intensive, focused utilization management in a teaching hospital: An exploratory study. *Qual Assur Util Rev.* 1991, 6:47–50.

17. Schaffer, Rollo FD, Holt CA. Falsification of clinical credentials by physicians applying for ambulatory staff privileges. *N Engl J Med.* 1988, 318:356–357.

18. Amerongen D. Physician credentialing in a consumer centric world. *Health Affairs.* September–October 2002, 21(5):152-6.

19. Health Care Quality Improvement Act of 1986, Public Law 99-660, November 14, 1986.

20. Code of Federal Regulations, Title 45, Part 60, Revised as of October 1, 2005.

21. Proposed rules. *Federal Register.* March 21, 2006, 71(54).

22. Code of Federal Regulations, Title 45, Part 61, Revised as of October 26, 1999.

23. Health Insurance Portability and Accountability Act of 1996 (P.L. 104-191). § 1128E of Social Security Act, 1996.

6

BASIC COMPENSATION OF PHYSICIANS IN MANAGED HEALTH CARE

Peter R. Kongstvedt

Study Objectives

- Understand the different methods of compensating primary care physicians (PCPs) and specialty care physicians (SCPs) in health plans.
- Understand the variations of the most common forms of each method.
- Understand the strengths and weaknesses of each method and each variation.
- Understand under what circumstances a health plan would desire to use each method over the others.
- Understand under what circumstances a PCP would prefer each method over the others.
- Understand regulatory constraints on reimbursement methodologies and the circumstances that bring those constraints into affect.

Discussion Topics

1. Discuss the key differences between different types of reimbursement models, and when each type of model would be the preferred approach.
2. Discuss what conditions would make a particular type of reimbursement model either undesirable or prohibited.
3. Describe the key elements in most capitation programs in open panel HMOs.
4. Describe the difference between service risk and financial risk in capitation.
5. Describe how an IPA might accept capitation, reimburse its member physicians on a fee-for-service basis, and still be considered as a risk-bearing entity. How might the IPA operate to lower its risk profile?

6. Describe the market and/or network environment that would favor using capitation vs. FFS, and vice versa.

INTRODUCTION

This chapter provides an overview of the most common methods managed care organizations (MCOs) use to reimburse physicians. Some methods are common to both primary care physicians* (PCPs) and to specialty care physicians (SCPs). Other methods are specific to each category or even specialty. Categorization of PCPs and SCPs is discussed in Chapter 5.

MCOs, primarily health maintenance organizations (HMOs), frequently use some form of risk-based reimbursement to pay physicians, especially PCPs. SCPs may also be paid under some form of risk-based reimbursement, although with less frequency than occurs with PCPs. Risk-based reimbursement, both financial risk and service risk as described later, are discussed in this chapter.

Broader types of MCOs, including HMOs and preferred provider organizations (PPOs), are also now beginning to incorporate some form of performance-based incentive compensation as well, and that topic is discussed separately in Chapter 8. It can be confusing to separate these two forms of financial incentives, especially because performance-based incentive programs frequently contain measures similar to those found in risk-based reimbursement (*eg*, utilization measures). For purposes of this discussion, risk-based reimbursement focuses primarily on medical costs and utilization and is an integral part of the reimbursement system, whereas performance-based incentives encompass (or even focus solely on) other performance measures and are not necessarily a basic aspect of physician reimbursement.

The primary focus here is on how the MCO pays the contracted entity (see Chapter 2). Although this means the direct payment to a physician is by the MCO in most cases, in some cases it is between the MCO and an intermediate organization such as an independent practice association (IPA) or integrated delivery system (IDS). It is possible and even common to use these methods of reimbursement on an individual physician basis in such groups, but not necessarily so. Since the creation of managed care, many medical groups and independent practice associations (IPAs) have blended forms of capitation, fee-for-service (FFS), and salary for the compensation of individual physicians even though the IPA accepts capitation. In the case of such organized groups, this chapter discusses only the reimbursement of the group by the MCO, rather than reimbursement of any one physician in that group. Having said that, it remains important to consider compensation to individual physicians rather than a medical group as a whole when looking at the effect of financial incentives on behavior.

A reimbursement system is simply one of the many tools available in managed care and has limited ability to achieve desired goals in the absence of other tools such as competent management of utilization and quality. In decades past, commentators whose knowledge about managed health care was superficial often made the erroneous assumption that managed care equaled capitation. This was never the case, and reimbursement of physicians and hospitals in managed health care was and is anything but homogeneous. The objective of any of these reimbursement

---

*Physician extenders such as physicians assistants and clinical nurse practitioners are generally treated as being associated with primary care physicians and bill as such so are not discussed separately.

systems is to better align the compensation of physicians with the overall goals of managed health care. By itself, however, it is unlikely that any compensation system will have much of an impact.[3]

Managed care is marked by a high degree of continual change and variation, and that has always been the case, including at the time of publication. Change occurs through market forces, changes in managed health care practices, new laws or regulations (especially in Medicare and Medicaid), and uncountable other forces. As a result, the divisions by provider type and the reimbursement mechanisms described here are rarely found in a pure state.

BASIC MODELS OF REIMBURSEMENT

At a simplistic level, there are two basic ways to compensate open panel physicians for services: capitation and FFS. There are many varieties of these two ways, as is discussed. Physicians are also paid on salary, but that is generally administered within a medical group and not by an MCO; therefore, salary is not discussed in this chapter. There are also other methods of reimbursement that are discussed just as there are surely ways of

paying doctors that defy any easy explanation. This chapter focuses on the types of reimbursement methods used by the majority of MCOs.* Where appropriate, distinctions between reimbursement systems for PCPs and for SCPs are made.

All types of MCOs other than HMOs use FFS or one of its variations as is discussed later in this chapter, though there are some exceptions as are noted in turn. HMOs use a far greater variety of reimbursement methodologies. Figure 6-1 illustrates the prevalence of the most common types of physician reimbursement by HMOs in the aggregate, reflecting the fact that HMOs may use overlapping types of reimbursement. Tables 6-1 and 6-2 (using data from a different source and time period) illustrate the most common methods of reimbursing primary care versus specialty care physicians.

In past years, HMOs tended to use one form of reimbursement or the other. Now,

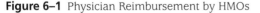

*A recent addition to managed care reimbursement of all types has been pay-for-performance (P4P), which is considered distinct from risk/bonus arrangements and is discussed in Chapter 8.

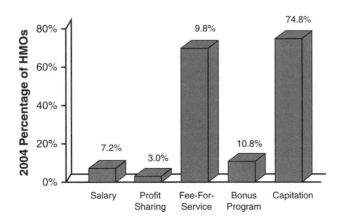

Figure 6–1 Physician Reimbursement by HMOs

Source: Sanofi-Aventis. *HMO-PPO/Medicare-Medicaid Digest 2005.* Managed Care Digest Series. Available at: http://www.managedcaredigest.com.

Table 6–1 Primary Care Physician Reimbursement Methodologies by HMOs—July 1, 2003

Reimbursement Type	National Average (%)
Capitation	29.8
Fee-for-service	46.2
Relative value scale	30.8
Salary	2.1

Source: HealthLeaders-InterStudy, used with Permission. http://www.healthleaders-interstudy.com/.

the opposite is more frequently the case. There are many reasons for this, including the following:

- Consolidation of health plans has led to broader geographic coverage, requiring different reimbursement methods in differing locales based on local norms.
- Consolidation has also led to the combination of different reimbursement methods used by formerly separate but now merged HMOs.
- Different products offered by the same MCO might use the same physicians but require different reimbursement methods (*eg*, capitation for an HMO or Medicare risk product, FFS for a PPO product, and performance-based FFS for a point-of-service product).

Table 6–2 Specialty Care Physician Reimbursement Methodologies by HMOs—July 1, 2003

Reimbursement Type	National Average
Capitation	18.7
Fee-for-service	56.2
Relative value scale	33.7
Salary	1.3

Source: HealthLeaders-InterStudy, used with Permission. http://www.healthleaders-interstudy.com/.

- Self-funded employer health plans (see Chapter 31) might prefer FFS so as to better capture utilization data and only pay for what they need.
- A mixture of capitation for some services and FFS for other services might be used.
- Physicians might desire one form of reimbursement over another, such as a large medical group desiring capitation, while independent physicians in a particular location prefer FFS.
- As a result of the so-called managed care backlash (see Chapter 1) some years ago, changes in the regulatory and legal climate occurred that had and are having an impact, as is discussed briefly later in this chapter.

RISK

Risk means that a physician's income from an MCO can vary based on utilization and/or medical care cost. Capitation is considered risk-based compensation, but there are risk-based FFS reimbursement systems as well, all of which are discussed in this chapter. There are two broad categories of risk for capitated physicians: financial risk and service risk.

Financial risk refers to actual income placed at risk, regardless of whether the physician has a service risk as well. Financial risk is usually confined to capitated PCPs, though it can easily be applied to performance-based FFS as well. Furthermore, an identical system may be put in place for a capitated contract with an IPA in which all participating physicians, PCPs, and SCPs bear an equal amount of financial risk. There are two common forms of financial risk: withholds and capitated pools for nonprimary care services.

Service risk refers to the physician receiving a fixed payment for his or her own professional services, but not being at risk in the sense of having to potentially pay money out (or conversely, not receive money owed to them). In other words, service risk is essentially the fact that if service volume is high, then the physician receives relatively lower income per encounter, and vice versa. Although the physician may not be at obvious financial risk, the physician does lose the ability to sell services to someone else for additional income in the event that the physician's schedule fills up with capitated patients at a rate higher than that used to calculate the capitation. This issue is irrelevant if the physician has slack time in the schedule, but can be an issue if the physician is extremely busy. It is common for physicians, primarily PCPs with large panels of capitated members, to feel that their capitation patients are "abusing" the service by coming in too frequently, but the perception is always more grievous than the reality.

CAPITATION

Capitation is prepayment for services on a per-member per-month (PMPM) basis. In other words, a physician is paid the same amount of money every month for a member regardless of whether that member receives services or not and regardless of how expensive those services are. There are many different forms and variants of capitation, the most common of which are discussed in the sections that follow. Capitation may be used to reimburse either PCPs or SCPs but is far more commonly used for PCPs. There are also differences in capitation methodologies between PCP and SCP capitation. Therefore, PCP capitation is discussed in some detail, and SCP capitation is discussed following that. Figure 6-2 illustrates the average percentage of capitated contracts by HMO size.

Primary Care Capitation

Used almost exclusively by HMOs (or the now uncommon type of plan known as a capitated PPO; see Chapter 2), PCP capitation is used only when a so-called gatekeeper structure is in place. In other words, the member may access the PCP whenever he or she needs to do so but is only covered for services

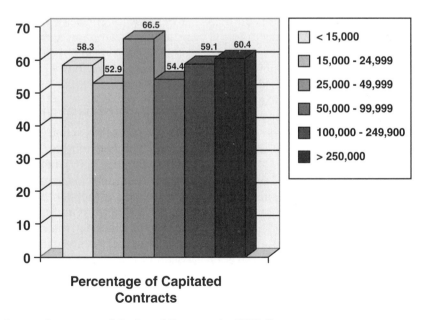

Figure 6–2 Average Percentage of Capitated Contracts by HMO Size

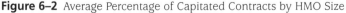

Source: Sanofi-Aventis. *HMO-PPO/Medicare-Medicaid Digest 2005.* Managed Care Digest Series. Available at: http://www.managedcaredigest.com.

by SCPs upon referral by the PCP, with notable exceptions such as direct access to OB/Gyn as discussed in Chapter 5. As noted earlier, capitation is used for primary care by HMOs to a significant degree. Although there are broad similarities with capitation as applied to SCPs and other types of providers, including hospitals, there are many commonly present features unique to PCPs. These features are discussed as follows.

Scope of Covered Services

To determine an appropriate capitation, it must first be defined what will be covered in the scope of primary care services and what will not. Defining the scope of covered services forms the basis for estimating the total costs of primary care. If a plan is unable to define primary care services easily, a national actuarial firm* can provide the necessary detail as well as help calculate capitation rates.

All services that the PCP is expected to deliver, including preventive services, outpatient care, and hospital visits (as appropriate), must be defined, as illustrated in Chapter 30 regarding contracting. Certain areas require special attention in defining, such as diagnostic testing, prescriptions, and surgical procedures. For example, selected diagnostic testing (eg, office urinalysis or electrocardiograms) may be included in the capitation, but other lab testing must be sent out to an outside reference lab (see Chapter 7) and the capitation covers only the blood drawing (unless, as is common, the patient is sent to a freestanding outside reference lab for all routine services, including blood drawing).

The cost of prescription drugs is an area that experienced great pressure in recent years, with differing opinions about whether to include that cost in the capitation amount. Because prescription drugs are not a service delivered directly by the PCP, those costs are considered financial risk and are discussed

separately from service risk later in this section.

Surgical and scoping (eg, flexible sigmoidoscopy) procedures are a particularly difficult area to define, especially if the same procedure is performed by the PCP and by an SCP. Under capitation, the PCP may be encouraged to refer the patient out rather than incur the expense, however, paying the PCP FFS for that procedure (referred to as a carve-out, and discussed later) also carries the risk of overutilization.

Other services such as immunizations are easy to define but still may or may not be covered by the capitation payment if the cost of the service is volatile. In the case of immunizations, the schedule of immunizations is frequently changed because new vaccines are released, and the cost of the vaccine may fluctuate as well.

Many capitation systems also hold the PCP accountable for nonprimary care services, either through risk programs or through positive incentive programs, both of which are discussed later in this chapter. For such programs, the same exercise of categorizing what and how services are defined should be carried out for specialty or referral services, institutional care, and ancillary services. Essentially, costs need to be estimated for each of the categories that will be capitated or tracked for at-risk PCPs.

Calculation of Capitation Payments

Most plans use an actuary to set these cost categories initially on the basis of the plan's geographic area, the benefits plans in place, and the medical management and cost controls in place. If the plan has been in operation for some time and has a data system capable of tracking the detail, estimating costs in categories is a matter of collating the existing data, though even then most MCOs use an actuary to calculate the amounts.

As a rough example, if a physician receives approximately $50 per visit (collected, not just billed) and a reasonable estimated visitation rate is 3.6 primary care visits per member per year (PMPY), then multiplying 3.6 by

---

*For example, Milliman at http://www.milliman. com, or Reden & Anders at http://www.reden-anders.com, and others.

$50 and dividing the result by 12 (to get the revenue per month) yields $15 PMPM. That could approximate the capitation rate. This example is crude and does not take into account any particular definition of scope of covered services, actual visitation rates for an area, visit rate differences by age and sex, average collections by a physician, effect of co-pays (discussed later), or differences in mean fees among different specialties, so this figure should not be used in capitating primary care services.

If the plan uses a risk/bonus arrangement, it is useful to be able to demonstrate to physicians that if utilization is managed, they will receive more than they would have under FFS. For example, if the plan uses a blended capitation rate of $15 PMPM and there are in fact 3.6 visits PMPY, and if good utilization management yields a bonus of $3 PMPM from the risk pools (discussed later), then the physician receives a year-end reconciliation that blends out to $18 PMPM, or $60 per visit. Also, pure luck (good or bad) will have an effect on the ultimate per-visit payment, as discussed later.

Variations by Age and Gender

Capitation systems routinely vary payments by the age and gender of the enrolled member to take into account the differences in average utilization of medical services in those categories. For example,* the capitation rate for a member younger than 18 months of age might be $50 PMPM to reflect the high utilization of services by newborns. The capitation rate may then fall to $10 PMPM for members 1 to 2 years of age, $8 PMPM for members 2 to 18 years of age, $7 PMPM for male members 18 to 45 years of age, and $20 PMPM for female members 18 to 45 years of age (reflecting the higher costs for women in their childbearing years), and so forth. As an end result of this, the actual PMPM payment

to a physician may fluctuate each month depending on the demographics of their enrolled panel of members. As with most factors that are used to vary capitation amounts, the larger the enrolled panel of capitated members a physician has, the more likely that adjustments will accurately reflect expected utilization.

Variation by Case-Mix Adjustment

It is possible, although still not yet common, to vary capitation by factors other than age and sex. The most important is an adjustment based on health status or clinical acuity. As discussed in Chapter 16, it is possible to profile patient panels in such a way as to adjust for health status or clinical acuity, generally referred to as a case-mix adjustment. As Medicare has moved to a risk/case-mix-adjusted methodology of paying risk-bearing MCOs (see Chapter 26), this becomes at least theoretically more important to deal with when capitating PCPs.

Even within a commercial enrolled membership, variations in health status and clinical acuity will exist. In the commercial population, it is a relatively small subset of the enrolled membership that would be categorized as very high risk and high cost. Many MCOs identify those patients and either make special provisions for payment of the PCP, or do not even include those patients in the PCP's panel because the care of such complex patients is usually best done by a specialist and/or a disease management or case management function (this issue is further discussed in Chapters 10 and 11). However, in that case, no actual adjustment to the capitation is made, but rather the highly complex patient is removed from the panel of patients covered by capitation.

As MCOs are better able to use technology to stratify members by clinical acuity, case-mix adjustments to capitation payments may be made. It must be noted, however, that in a recent study small sample sizes for individual physicians compounded generic problems in performance measurement related to case-mix adjustment, size of treatment effects,

---

*All capitation examples are presented for illustrative purposes and do *not* represent accurate capitation rates.

availability of adequate standards and metrics, and more.[4]

Variations by Other Factors

Another relatively easily analyzed factor is geography. Even in the same statistical metropolitan area, there may be considerable differences in utilization. For example, in the Baltimore–Washington, DC, MSA, significant differences in utilization exist among some counties in Maryland, northern Virginia, and the District of Columbia.* In such situations, it may be appropriate to factor in geographic location when capitation payments are calculated.

Practice type may occasionally be a legitimate capitation factor. As an example, internists argue that the case mix they get is different from the case mix family practitioners get. This has not generally been borne out in any studies, but there is some evidence that even in the same stratum of age and sex, specialty internists (*eg*, cardiologists) have sicker patients than general internists do.[5]

Straightforward business adjustments to capitation may be made as well. One example that occurs in certain plans is an adjustment for exclusivity. In this case, the plan pays a higher capitation rate to those providers who do not sign up with any other managed care plans (there are usually no restrictions against participating with government programs or indemnity carriers). Such arrangements may raise the potential for antitrust actions, but that is dependent on the particular situation.

In any event, if factors other than age and sex are to be used to adjust capitation, the calculations become more complex, and communicating these factors to the participating providers becomes far more difficult. The plan must also guard against an imbalance in factors that leads to a higher than expected (or rated for) capitation payout over the entire network. In other words, adjustments should lead not only to increases in capitation but to decreases as well; that is, it must be a zero-sum situation because the amount of premium being collected is fixed for the duration of the benefits contract.

Carve-Outs

Capitation systems usually allow for certain services delivered by the PCP to be carved out of the capitation payment. The most common example as noted earlier are immunizations, which are not paid under capitation but instead are reimbursed on a fee schedule. As a general rule, carve-outs should only be used for those services that are not subject to discretionary utilization. In the case of immunizations, the medical guidelines for administering them are clear-cut but subject to change (*eg*, there may be an increase in the number of immunizations that are to be given in the first years of life or new vaccines are approved for use), and there is little question about their use. That would not be the case, for example, for office-based laboratory testing in which there is a high degree of discretion about how much testing is necessary, and which may be considered a profit center by the practice.

Withholds and Physician Risk Pools

In health plans that capitate PCPs, additional forms of financial risk and reward to the PCP may also exist. The two common forms are withholds and capitation pools for nonprimary care, and both are discussed here. Precise data on the combination or lack thereof of these two additional forms of PCP risk are lacking, but from a practical standpoint it is far easier to combine the two or to have only physician risk pools than it is to have a withhold without the existence of risk pools. In any event, the prevalence of both withholds and physician risk pools has declined in recent years and now represents approximately one-third of all HMOs, or roughly half as prevalent as capitation of PCPs for direct services. Table 6-3 illustrates

---

*Author's experience at Blue Cross Blue Shield of the National Capital Area, unpublished data, 1989–1992.

Table 6–3 HMO Use of Physician Withholds and Risk Pools—2004

Model Type	Percentage of HMOs	HMO Enrollment
IPA	31.4	13,626,286
Network	32.2	8,835,060
Group	35.0	7,159,058
Staff	26.7	818,475
Ownership		
Corporate owned	29.0	23,055,690
Corporate managed	66.7	76,991
Corporate affiliated	42.9	3,340,411
Hospital owned	55.6	346,363
Independent	38.8	3,619,424
Tax Status		
Not-for-profit	36.4	14,833,495
For-profit	29.6	15,605,384
Average/Total	**31.8%**	**30,438,879**

Source: Sanofi-Aventis. *HMO-PPO/Medicare-Medicaid Digest 2005.* Managed Care Digest Series. Available at: http://www.managedcaredigest.com.

the prevalence of the use of withholds and physician risk pools in HMOs.

Withholds

A *withhold* is simply a percentage, for example, 20%, of the primary care capitation that is withheld every month and used to pay for cost overruns in referral or institutional services. In the earlier example of $15 PMPM, a 20% withhold would be $3. The PCP would actually receive a check each month for the difference between the capitation rate and the withhold, in this case $12; the withhold is held by the plan and used at year-end (or whenever) for reconciliation of cost overruns, with the remainder returned to the PCP as discussed later. The amount of payment withheld generally varies from 5% to 20%, rarely more.

Although rare (and even more rarely used), some plans also have a clause in their physician's contract that states that the plan may increase the amount of withhold beyond what is already being withheld in the event of cost excesses. For example, the withhold can be increased from 20% to 30% if referral costs are out of control. This method is ill-advised because it has little positive effect on utilization and only serves to reallocate a small amount of money from payment of a PCP to payment of specialists. Although generating a great deal of ill will, the total dollars saved by the plan in such cases are best described as "decimal dust." Because MCOs have become more sophisticated in medical management, there is far less reliance on financial incentives to control or influence utilization.

Physician Risk Pools

When capitation exists for primary care services and the PCP is also on a bonus/risk program for other medical costs, payment for referral services and institutional services is often made from capitation funds or pools as well. The services themselves may be paid for under a number of mechanisms (FFS, per diem, capitation, and the like), but the expense is drawn against a capitated fund or pool. HMOs handle these types of risk pools in a variety of ways, and some common methods are described.

It must be stressed that the illustration that follows generally no longer exists in the real world exactly as it appears here. In HMOs that use this approach, there is considerable variation, and there is no uniformity as to whether an HMO will put the PCP at some level of risk for either or both of these types of service. The illustration also reflects models that were more prevalent roughly a decade ago, while mature HMOs have undergone considerable changes since then. Nevertheless, the illustration provides a common basis for understanding this type of model. Figure 6-3 illustrates schematically how some of these risk pools operate.

There are three broad classes of nonprimary care risk pools: referral (or specialty care), hospital (or institutional care, regardless of whether it is inpatient, outpatient, or emergency department), and ancillary services (*eg*, laboratory, radiology, pharmacy, and so forth, though pharmacy may also be

considered a separate risk pool). Many HMOs also have a fourth pool, usually called "other," in which they accrue liabilities for such things as stop loss or malpractice, and in which the physicians have no stake (see discussion later). Some HMOs combine the ancillary services into the "other" pool, which is the model illustrated in Figure 6-3. It is not uncommon for these risk pools to be handled in different ways regarding the flow of funds and levels of risk and reward for the physicians and the plan.

As an example, the PCP receives a $15 PMPM blended capitation rate for primary care services (in other words, the blend of all the age and sex capitation rates for that physician's membership base comes out to $15 PMPM). For each member, $40 PMPM is added to a capitated pool for all specialty referral services, and $100 PMPM is added to a capitated pool for hospital or institutional inpatient and outpatient services.* The PCP

---

*Once again the reader is reminded that these numbers are presented for illustrative purposes and do *not* represent accurate capitation rates.

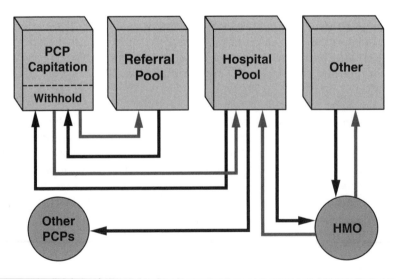

Figure 6–3 Capitation Risk Pools

does not actually receive the money in those pools; the plan holds on to it. Any medical expenses incurred by members in that PCP's panel are counted against the appropriate pool of funds. At the end of the year, a reconciliation of the various pools is made (see discussion later).

As with primary care, the scope of covered services must first be defined. For example, will home health be covered under institutional or referral (probably institutional because it reduces institutional costs), and will hospital-based professionals (radiology, pathology, and anesthesia) be covered under institutional or referral? The same exercise is carried out with any category for which capitated funds will be accrued. Specific carve-out services such as behavioral health (Chapter 13) must also be accounted for because the PCP should not stand any financial risk for such services because the health plan has either taken responsibility itself or else put another entity at financial risk for those services.

If all of the withhold is not used or there is a surplus in either the referral pool or the institutional services pool, often any surplus in a pool is first used to pay for any excess expenses in the other pool. For example, if there is money left in the referral pool but the institutional pool has cost overruns, the extra funds in the referral pool are first applied against the excessive expenses in the hospital pool, and vice versa.

After both funds are covered, any excess money is shared with or paid to the physicians. In some cases, only those physicians with positive balances in their own risk pools receive any money. For example, a PCP has referral services funds tracked for his or her own patients. If the cost of services for those members leaves a positive balance in the referral pool, and if there is money left in the institutional services pool on a plan-wide basis, the PCP receives a pro rata share of the money. In other words, risk is shared with all physicians in the plan, but reward may be tracked individually. In another example, some plans disburse positive balances in re-

ferral and institutional funds on the basis of both utilization and measures of quality and member satisfaction.

The degree to which an individual PCP's pools will have an impact on year-end bonus disbursements may vary. If the decision is to minimize risk to individual PCPs but not eliminate the risk pools entirely, then a low stop-loss protection level must be set (see discussion later) to minimize or even stop tracking expenses against an individual PCP's pools while those expenses are still low.

For example, if a PCP has a member with an expensive chronic disease, the referral expenses will be paid either out of the plan-wide referral capitation pool, out of a separate fund for disease management costs, or out of a separate stop-loss fund and will not count against the individual PCP's referral risk fund after referral expenses have reached, for example, $5,000. In this way, high-cost cases, which could wipe out an individual PCP's risk pool, will have less effect than that PCP's ability to manage overall referral expenses in the rest of the member panel.

In plans in which both referral and hospital risk pools are used, some plans pay out all extra funds in the referral pool but only half of the funds in the hospital pool. In other cases, there may be an upper limit on the amount of bonus a PCP can receive from the hospital pool. The justification for this is that the plan stands a considerably greater degree of risk for hospital services and therefore deserves a greater degree of reward. Furthermore, it is often a combination of utilization management (UM) and effective negotiating that yields a positive result, and the plan does most or all of the negotiating and usually manages utilization as well.

Pharmacy Costs

A specific category of expense is an area of both focus and disagreement: the risk for the cost of pharmaceuticals. MCOs have employed a variety of means to manage drug costs. Examples include changing the benefit to a three-tier or four-tier copay, replacing copays with deductibles and/or co-insurance, increasing use of drug utilization review, precertifying selected drugs, using formularies, contracting for favorable terms, and other techniques as discussed in detail in Chapter 12. Pertinent to this chapter, though, is a brief discussion about the use of financial risk/incentives based on drug costs. As noted earlier, some MCOs do not include drug costs in any financial risk/incentive programs, though most do at least provide data and feedback to network physicians on drug utilization and cost.

There is no evidence that the presence or absence of financial incentives has a negative effect on quality or has led to inappropriate prescribing. One can debate whether the use of financial risk/incentives has any real effect on drug costs, but two older studies failed to show such an association.[6,7] With the high levels of variation in prescribing patterns and habits, it is theoretically sound to place drug costs into a risk/incentive program along with the other aspects of managing this benefit cost because it is the physician who prescribes the drug. Unfortunately, it may not be the PCP but rather the SCP who writes the prescription, though that issue is not markedly different from any diagnostic or other therapeutic interventions by an SCP.

However, as new and superior pharmaceuticals are released into the market, the number of medications taken by Americans increases, the cost of those new drugs increases (though countered by movement of drugs off-patent and to generic status), the risk of litigation increases (see the example cited in the section titled "Civil Liability for Physician Compensation Programs" later in this chapter), and pressure from patients increases, physicians argue that the level of cost volatility is simply too high. If the health plan is including the cost of specialty pharmaceuticals that are extremely expensive if rarely used types of injectibles (see Chapter 12 for a discussion of this specific issue),

then the volatility can be even higher. For all of these reasons, many health plans have chosen not to include pharmacy costs under any of the physician risk pools.

Medical Expenses for which the Primary Care Physician is Not at Risk

As noted earlier, even in plans that use withholds and physician risk pools, PCPs will not be at-risk for certain medical expenses. For example, a plan may negotiate a capitated laboratory contract; laboratory capitation is then backed out of the referral and primary care capitation amounts and accounted for separately. If the PCP orders laboratory services from another vendor, that cost is deducted from his or her referral pool; otherwise, lab cost and use has no effect on the PCP's compensation.

Other examples of such nonrisk services might include any type of rider benefit (eg, vision or dental) or services over which PCPs have no control, such as obstetrics. Another example would be defined as catastrophic conditions (eg, persistent vegetative state or certain chronic diseases as discussed in Chapter 11) if the PCP is taken out of the case management function by the plan and the plan's case management system takes over the coordination of care. It is important to use clear and consistent definitions of what types of cases will be treated this way. Otherwise, there will be pressure from PCPs to include too much in this category, thereby eroding the entire concept of capitation. Once a service has been taken out of the at-risk category, it is exceedingly difficult to put it back in.

Reinsurance and Stop-Loss Protection

The degree of risk to which any physician is exposed needs to be defined. As mentioned earlier, it is common for a plan to stop deducting expenses against an individual PCP's pool after a certain threshold is reached for purposes of the year-end reconciliation. There are two forms of stop-loss protection: costs for individual members and aggregate cost protection.

As an example of individual case cost protection, if a PCP has a member with leukemia, after the referral expenses reach $3,000, it will no longer be counted against the PCP's referral pool, or perhaps only 20% of expenses in excess of $2,500 will be counted against the referral pool; the uncounted expenses will be paid either from an aggregate pool or from a specially allocated stop-loss fund.

It is possible to vary the amount of stop-loss protection by the size of a PCP's member base to reduce the element of chance. For example, if a PCP has fewer than 300 members, the stop loss is $2,000; if the PCP has more than 800 members, the stop loss is $4,000. It is equally common for a stop loss to exist for hospital services, although the level is much higher, for example, $40,000. As alluded to earlier, the lower the stop loss, the less the effect of high-cost cases on individual capitation funds and the greater the effect of overall medical management by the PCP. On the other hand, if it is too low, there may be a perverse incentive to run up expenses to get them past the stop loss. Multitiered stop loss also creates an artificial barrier to the PCPs' acceptance of new members. For example, if the stop loss for 300 members or fewer is less than that for 301 members or more, PCPs may resist adding members above the 300 limit so as to protect the lower stop-loss level. Tiered stop loss can be time-limited to prevent this problem.

As an example of aggregate protection, the plan may reduce deductions to 20% or even stop deducting referral expenses after total expenses for an individual PCP reach 150% of the capitation risk pool amount. Providing aggregate stop-loss protection on the basis of a percentage of total capitation enables such protection to be tied to the membership base of the PCP. Because most MCOs limit the total risk at which a PCP is placed (*eg*, 20% of the PCP's capitation amount as noted previously), as well as regulatory limits in Medicare and Medicaid MCOs as noted later, aggregate stop loss is useful primarily in large groups or IDSs.

The combination of stop-loss protection and risk sharing across the physician panel (discussed later) serves to reduce any individual PCP's exposure to events outside his or her control. It is frustrating for a PCP to manage all his or her cases properly but receive no incentive because one seriously ill patient had high expenses.

In any case, providing stop-loss protection to an individual physician is important, and the plan must budget for its cost. Although such stop-loss protection can be paid from the aggregate of all the physician's referral funds, that ensures that there will be a draw on the withhold (if there is one). Because positive referral balances are paid back to PCPs, negative balances need to be funded through the withhold, so there can never be a full return of the withhold. Therefore, it is preferable to budget a line item for stop-loss expense and to reduce the referral allocations by that amount.

It is likewise important for there to exist a mechanism for peer review of excess expenses to determine whether they were caused by bad luck or poor case management. In the latter situation, the plan should have recourse to recovering all or part (up to the contractually agreed upon maximum individual physician risk) of the excess costs from a physician who failed to provide proper case management.

Last, only the largest MCOs can afford to carry the total cost of stop-loss protection, and provider groups that accept full or global risk (discussed later) are rarely able to do so. Provider groups at full risk (or IDSs at global risk) as well as small to midsized MCOs therefore purchase commercially available stop-loss insurance, also known as reinsurance. *Reinsurance* is actually an insurance policy that protects the health plan or provider organization from catastrophic claims, also referred to as shock claims. Reinsurance is usually for both individual highly expensive claims and for excessively high aggregate costs. Accounting for both the cost and for recoveries under reinsurance is noted in Chapter 24.

Individual versus Pooled Risk

All forms of financial risk are affected by how the HMO handles the issue of individual risk versus pooled risk. In other words, to what degree is an individual physician at risk for his or her own performance versus the degree that that risk is shared with some or all other PCPs? It is human nature to wish to share the downside risk (and pain) with others, but keep the upside (profit) for oneself. In those plans that do track risk pools individually, it is more common for only one pool (usually referral), if any, to be tracked on an individual basis while the withhold, if any, and hospital pool are aggregate. It is very rare for the hospital risk pool, when it exists, to be at the individual physician level.

Although many HMOs contract directly with PCPs, many contract through the vehicle of the IPA,* physician hospital organization (PHO) or management services organization (MSO), or other form of IDS (see Chapter 2 for discussions of these organizations). The HMO capitates the IPA, or IDS, but that organization may or may not capitate the PCPs. In fact, some of these organizations pay the PCPs on an FFS basis, using one or more of the FFS reimbursement methods (performance-based or not) described later.

Even when there is no intervening organization, the issue of who is actually being capitated, and for what, still remains. Is it the individual PCP? A subset of the total network of PCPs (ie, pools of doctors [PODs])? Is it the entire network of PCPs? The answers may not be the same for each category or risk. For example, a plan may wish to capitate PCPs individually for their own services, combine them into PODs for purposes of referral services, and use the performance of the entire network for purposes of hospital services.

A plan can also choose to use different categories for risk and for reward. For example, a plan may spread risk across the entire network, but only reward a subset of PCPs. An example was given earlier in which positive balances in withholds or referral pools were used to offset deficits in the hospital pool; any remaining surplus balance would be paid only to those PCPs with a positive balance.

There are common and predictable problems with individual risk. The majority of those problems relate to the issue of small numbers. As noted earlier, luck can have as much or more of an impact on utilization as does good management, at least in small member panels. As a PCP's panel grows to more than 500 members, this problem starts to lessen, but still persists. This is one of the most important reasons that an HMO would contractually require PCPs not to close their practice to the HMO until a PCP has at least 250 or more members (see Chapter 30); it is also the identical reason that a PCP should desire to have a large panel enrolled. When a PCP has good utilization results, that PCP generally desires to keep the reward for those hard labors; when results are poor, PCPs frequently feel that they have been dealt an abnormally sick population of members and should not be held accountable for the high medical costs. This is a common and usually unfounded complaint, but a sophisticated practice profiling system (see Chapter 16) is able to quantify this.

The larger the dollars at stake, the more danger the problem of small numbers becomes to an individual PCP. Although stop loss and reinsurance somewhat ameliorate the problem, the problem remains. This is the very reason that plans may be willing to use individual pools for referral services, but will not do so for hospital services, where the dollars are substantially higher.

The other major problem with individual risk is the ability of some PCPs to game the system. In other words, to enhance income, the PCP manages to get the sickest patients to transfer out of the practice, with a result-

---

*The term *IPA* is often used to describe any HMO that uses private physicians practicing in their own offices (as opposed to a group or staff model HMO), but in fact, the term *IPA* technically refers to an actual legal entity. See Chapter 2.

ing improvement in that individual PCP's medical costs. Although all plans prohibit a PCP from kicking a member out of his or her practice because of medical condition, the rare unethical PCP can find a way to do so and remain undetected.

Related to that last issue is the concern that individual risk incites a PCP to withhold necessary medical care. Although this charge has been leveled at the HMO industry for many years, it has never been demonstrated and is discussed later.

Last, in the past in several cases, HMOs have required an individual PCP (or small group) actually to write a check to the plan to cover cost overruns in medical expenses (as opposed to simple reconciliation of accidental overpayments). This usually occurred when the plan had agreed to not actually keep the withhold (in response to the PCP's plea to improve cash flow), but to track it nonetheless. Whenever a PCP is required to pay money back to the plan because of medical costs, a severe problem in provider relations is likely to occur, and it is a poor idea that is bound to lead to trouble.

If the plan chooses to pool risk across the entire network, then the flip side of individual risk occurs: the impact of any individual PCP's actions are diluted so much as to be undetectable. If a PCP is having good results, then that PCP may resent having to cover for the problems of colleagues with poor results (of course, no one objects to being helped out when one's own results are poor). If the plan does not track individual results, it will have little capability of providing meaningful data to individual physicians to help them better manage medical resources.

Because of these two extremes, many plans have chosen to use PODs for at least some financial risk management. PODs are a subset of the entire network, although there is no standard size. PODs may be a large medical group, an aggregation of 10 to 15 physicians, or may be made up of all participating PCPs in an entire geographic area. A POD could also be made up of the physicians in a PHO

or MSO that accepts risk. The common denominator is that sufficient members are enrolled in practices in the POD to allow for statistical integrity, but membership is still small enough to allow the POD to make changes that can affect utilization results. The chief risk is that PODs require support from the plan in the form of data and utilization management.

It should not be assumed that PODs are a panacea; they are not. If a POD fails, the repercussions are greater than if an individual physician fails because far more members are affected and the dollars are higher. There are times when individual risk and reward are best, times when the entire network should be treated as a single entity, and times when PODs make sense. Medical managers should be aware that there is some evidence from older studies that individual risk/bonus arrangements elicit behavior changes, whereas aggregated risk/bonus arrangements do not.[8]

Point-of-Service Plans

For the purposes of this discussion, POS plans are those that allow members to obtain a high level of benefits by using the HMO or gatekeeper system while still having insurance-type benefits available if they choose to use providers without going through the managed care system. POS plans were very popular when they were first introduced and grew rapidly. Because they essentially failed to prove superior to other designs, they have been in decline, as discussed in Chapter 2 (along with a more detailed discussion of how a POS plan is designed). Nevertheless, POS plans became a reality for most HMOs and still exist in more than two-thirds of them even if actual enrollment of members in the POS option has shrunk to approximately 16% of total HMO enrollment.[9]

Because members with POS benefits are not totally locked into the managed care plan, medical services can be received both in-network and out-of-network. Although the plan can actuarially determine the level of in-network and out-of-network use for the entire enrolled group, that cannot be said for an individual physician's member panel. This has an obvious impact on capitation rates.

When POS plans were first introduced in the 1980s, some plans attempted to adjust capitation rates on the basis of prospective in-network utilization. The capitation rate was thus reduced, further exacerbating the problem of luck (good or bad). Because of the problem of small numbers noted earlier, when the probability of out-of-network usage is added, chance becomes an even greater force. One PCP might find that all of her or his members access services exclusively through the PCP (resulting in severe underpayment because of the reduced capitation amount), while another PCP may find that the majority of his or her members go out-of-network (resulting in overpayment because of the low visit rate). In those MCOs that place the PCP at some level of financial risk for specialty services, the same problem existed, though in reverse (members staying in-network resulted in better financial results in the risk pool than occurred when members went out-of-network).

Other plans attempted to make adjustments on a retrospective basis, actually asking a PCP to refund a percentage of the capitation payment they had received all year (corresponding to the percentage of out-of-network costs that predicted actuarially) or increasing the withhold to high levels to recover the money. The ability of the PCP to write that check was usually poor because of the chronic cash flow problems that most physicians face (they need to pay their staff, the rent, supplies costs, insurance, and so forth); even if they did pay back the MCO, it meant financial hardship. These two approaches created terribly difficult exercises in provider relations, were generally perceived as unfair (a perception shared by this author), and are now uncommon or perhaps nonexistent (data are not available to verify that claim, however).

An alternative approach was not to reduce the capitation rate. That meant that the MCO paid twice for some out-of-network costs (specifically those services for which the PCP was capitated but which were delivered by out-of-network physicians). It also created windfall profits for the PCP whose POS members never came in for services (or, on a more pernicious note, for the PCP who did not provide adequate access for POS members, thereby driving them out-of-network for services). As noted earlier, if the PCP also was at some level of risk/incentive for nonprimary services, the reverse dynamic occurred.

The problem of using capitation with POS has become so difficult that many plans choose to capitate PCPs for pure HMO (ie, not POS) members and pay FFS (without using any risk pool) for POS members. This creates new problems as a result of the schizophrenic reimbursement systems and results in what psychologists refer to as cognitive dissonance. But it is viable and is used. Many MCOs with high levels of POS membership preferred simply not to capitate all, and they use FFS exclusively.

As stated earlier, POS makes it difficult to measure utilization performance of PCPs. For example, if performance is based only on in-network utilization, one good way to look like a stellar performer is subtly to encourage POS members to seek services out-of-network. If PCPs are held accountable for all services, both in-network and out-of-network, they may argue that it is not fair that they are held accountable for cost and utilization that are completely out of their control.

Although this issue is not easily resolved, some plans have chosen simply not to include POS in any utilization-based performance measures, while others fold out-of-network utilization into the utilization performance-based reimbursement system, whether capitation or FFS. To attenuate the problem of lack of control by an individual PCP, the risk or reward system is spread out among groups of

PCPs or the entire network, thereby maintaining actuarial integrity. In other MCOs that choose to maintain a performance-based reimbursement system that includes POS, the incentive may be based primarily on nonutilization factors (*eg*, quality measures, member satisfaction, efficient use of electronic commerce, and other measures) and only secondarily on cost or utilization measures. In these programs, though, the funding for nonutilization incentives may be derived from medical cost savings, in which case incentives are paid only if surpluses are generated. Performance-based (*ie*, non-utilization-based) incentive programs are the focus of Chapter 8.

Specialty Physician Capitation

Basic Specialty Physician Capitation

SCP capitation is, in general, simpler than PCP capitation. As with PCP capitation, it is a fixed payment PMPM for services. The capitation payment may be adjusted for age, sex, and product type, but this is not done as universally as is found in PCP capitation. Severity adjustment as discussed earlier is also possible and may become more prevalent in Medicare Advantage plans (see Chapter 26) that have changed over to acuity-based prospective premium payments. In all events, the capitation amount is calculated based on the expected volume of referrals, the average cost, the ability to manage utilization, and the relative negotiating strengths of each party. A large plan may have past data to guide it, but even then it is common to use an outside actuary to derive the correct capitation amount.

As with PCP capitation, the services covered by the capitation payment must be clearly defined. It is not uncommon for certain procedures to be carved out of the capitation consideration. The reason for this is that those SCPs who perform high-cost procedures will be relatively disadvantaged compared to SCPs who perform only less expensive office-based care, even if both SCPs

are in the same specialty. The risk of such carve-outs is obvious: there is no incentive not to perform the procedure and every financial incentive to do it. Alternatively, the capitation of an SCP who performs such procedures may be adjusted upward to reflect the additional capability, while also allowing that SCP to bill the plan FFS when performing the procedure upon referral from another physician.

Though no longer as common as it was in past years, the capitation amount may be based on a percentage of premium revenue, rather than a hard PMPM dollar amount. In Medicare and Medicaid plans, this is not unreasonable because the premium revenue is set by the government and presumably has the appropriate mix of specialty services already in the total. For commercial plans, however, this is not as clear. Premiums are set as much by marketplace pressures as they are by actuarial buildup, and a plan forced to market low premiums ends up passing along that reduced income in exact proportion to the percentage of premium payment the SCP group has negotiated. In addition, if the MCO has poor underwriting procedures (see Chapter 25), a PMPM premium shortfall may occur, which is also passed on to SCPs under a percentage of premium arrangement. In other words, true capitation is a fixed amount, whereas percentage of premium varies based on the amount of premium the MCO actually collects.

Although theoretically the same utilization issues apply to specialty care as well as primary care, the numbers involved in SCP capitation are often significantly smaller for any given specialty (even though specialty PMPM costs as a whole are usually one and a half to two times higher than primary care). For example, PCP capitation may average $15 PMPM, whereas the capitation for neurology may be $0.55. Thus, adjustments based on demographic variables become very small indeed and may not be worth the effort. Because the numbers can be smaller, an SCP requires a much higher number of members for capitation to have meaning. Where a PCP may achieve relative stability in capitation at a membership level of 400 to 600, an SCP may require triple that number or more to avoid the problem of random chance having more effect than medical management has on utilization.

Directly capitating SCPs as individuals or as specialty groups (or multispecialty groups) is the easiest approach, though a specialty IPA or a single-specialty management company may also be the vehicle for contracting and capitating, as noted in Chapter 5. Unless the SCP group, IPA, or other contracting vehicle is able to cover the entire service area, however, the plan must create procedures for the PCPs to know to which SCP they should refer those patients who are actually covered under the capitation.

Contact Capitation

Contact capitation is an odd and uncommonly used form of SCP capitation, but it warrants brief discussion because it has been used in the past and retains a small degree of allure to some managers. Like any other form of reimbursement, contact capitation does not have a single definition of how it works and is subject to a variety of local variations. Further, although it once elicited interest (at least on the West Coast) as a sophisticated way of capitating, it turned out to be too complex to be widely adopted.

Contact capitation begins with a capitated (ie, budgeted based on PMPM calculations) pool of money for each major specialty. Like other forms of capitation, provisions in the calculations are made for product design, the effect of copays and co-insurance, the effect of stop-loss insurance for catastrophic cases, and the effect of other-party liability offsets, as discussed earlier as well as later.

The plan then tracks each unique member contact with each specialist; that is, regardless of whether that member/patient sees the SCP once or 100 times, it is counted as a single contact. This is tracked over a set period

of time, such as a year, a quarter, or semi-annually. Once the period is over, the counters are reset to zero and the count begins again. The plan pays out the total capitated pool of money to the SCPs based on the distribution of the contacts. For example, if one cardiologist has 8% of the total number of cardiology contacts (ie, unique, nonduplicated patients), that cardiologist receives 8% of the total capitation pool. It is usually assumed that once a patient makes contact with that SCP, the patient will remain with that SCP. Of course, this is not something that can be guaranteed, and so provision must be made for patients who change SCPs during the course of the tracking period.

The timing of payouts under contact capitation is highly variable, unlike more common forms of capitation. Because the payout is a factor of the total percentage of contacts in a period of time, it cannot occur until adequate encounters have occurred to allow for a calculation. The few systems that still use contact capitation usually use an entire 12-month period to make the adjustments, though some may do so on a quarterly or semiannual basis. In any case, some form of interim payment mechanism must therefore be in place because even an IPA run by Darth Vader would not expect physicians to receive no reimbursement for a year. This interim payment may be a form of discounted FFS, it may be a monthly "capitation" payment based on the distribution of contacts each month or to-date, or some other means. In all cases, this adds a layer of complexity to the ultimate calculation; and in the dread event it requires an actual refund of money from an SCP, very hard feelings will follow.

Single-Specialty Management or Specialty Network Manager Capitation

This method is uncommon, but still exists for a few focused types of services. In this case, the HMO contracts with one single entity to provide all services within a single specialty, but that entity does not actually provide all of the services. There are two basic approaches.

In one approach, an HMO capitates a single specialist (*ie*, an individual physician) to manage all services in that specialty for all HMO members, even though the SCP cannot personally provide the services. This contracted SCP, the specialty network manager, must then subcontract with other specialists to provide services throughout the medical service area. The specialty network manager either makes or loses money depending on how efficiently specialty services are managed. The specialty network manager may subcapitate with other SCPs as discussed later or may pay FFS. In all events, the primary SCP acts like a second gatekeeper in that PCPs need to work through the primary SCP to access specialty care for members. Sometimes the primary SCP receives the full capitation payment and must pay the other SCPs directly, or the HMO may administer the claims payments and provide the accounting and reporting for the primary contract holder. In fact, the HMO may wish to do so to track performance on a real-time basis, as well as protect members from possible nonpayment of claims by the primary contract holder.

In the other approach, an HMO contracts with a single institution for single-specialty services (*eg*, the HMO contracts with a local university faculty practice plan for all cardiology services). The contracted institution is then responsible for arranging for specialty services that it cannot provide itself. The primary specialty contract holder receives the capitation payment and must then administer payment to subcontractors. In some cases, the administrative cost to the primary contractor may be greater than the total capitation payment because it is often a manual process.

Disease Management Organizations

Another variation on single group capitation is capitation for single-specialty services to a specialty organization (*eg*, a vendor that spe-

cializes in cancer services or cardiac care). As discussed in Chapter 5, this is most commonly a company or corporation that employs physicians and support staff and provides facilities and ancillary services, or it may be a professional group in those states that have corporate practice of medicine acts prohibiting physicians from being employees of corporations for purposes of practicing medicine. It can also be an organization created by a large, comprehensive provider system as an internal unit.

In this variation on capitation, the organization is then responsible for providing all specialty services within the MCO's medical service area. This approach may also be applied to emergency department care if the vendor's physicians are on staff at all of the HMO's participating hospitals.

In this situation, the disease management organization focuses on those chronic conditions in which a broad, integrated approach can make a difference in outcomes and/or cost of care. Because they are more comprehensive, the capitation calculation must take into account a somewhat larger set of factors, such as the following:

- Inpatient cost and utilization
- Outpatient costs and utilization
  - By service type
  - By location
- Physician costs and utilization
- Nonacute care costs
  - Inpatient facilities such as skilled nursing facilities
  - Outpatient or alternative settings such as hospice
- Pharmaceutical costs and utilization
  - Those agents included as a routine part of medical surgical benefits such as injectibles
  - The cost of outpatient or chronic drugs if the disease management organization is to be at risk for their use
- Frequency of the disease state
  - New occurrences expected by age and sex categories
  - Existing cases[10]

Full Professional Risk Capitation

Full professional risk capitation* as applied to PCPs refers to the PCP receiving money for all professional services: primary and specialty but not hospital services although the group may still be on an incentive program regarding hospital utilization management. This should be distinguished from global capitation, which is discussed briefly later and in Chapter 2 regarding IDSs, and which refers to capitation for all medical costs, not just professional. In either case, the amount of full professional risk capitation and global capitation has always been concentrated in the western United States, particularly in California, though even that region of the country has experienced a decline in such capitation arrangements.[11]

It is also worth noting that in California, where there is the greatest concentration of such arrangements, when such large intermediary physician organizations accepted full professional capitation, most of the risk was retained at the group or organization level. In such organizations, it was common to capitate PCPs for primary care services but pay FFS for specialty services. In addition, only 13% of medical groups and 19% of IPAs provided bonuses or withholds based on utilization or cost performance, which averaged 10% of base compensation.[12]

In a few situations in decades past, the PCP not only authorized the referral, but also had to write checks to SCPs for specialty services. Although once marginally popular, it is currently rare if it even exists at all anymore because there were problems when the PCPs were unable to pay for specialty costs and members were exposed to balance billing. This was because the capitation funds arrived on a prepaid basis, but costs were not incurred until sometime later (*ie*, the cash arrives on day 1, but the expenses do not occur

until sometime well after day 1). As cash built up, PCPs sometimes failed to understand that the bulk of that cash was actually a liability (for specialty services to be incurred sometime in the future) and needed to be treated as such. So, they used the cash and had insufficient funds when they needed to write the checks to the SCPs. Also, if they had not purchased adequate stop-loss insurance (see earlier discussion), they were exposed to the cost of catastrophic cases.

There was a resurgence of interest in this form of capitation as PCPs banded together into large groups or other forms of collective activity such as IPAs, PHOs, and MSOs. In some cases, the medical organizations in turn negotiated capitation agreements with specialists or other provider organizations; in other words, the organization accepting full professional risk capitation "down-streamed" some of that risk through subcapitation agreements with SCPs or other providers. It should be noted that many state insurance departments do not allow a provider to subcapitate without a special license; that is, the insurance department believes that only a licensed HMO or specialty HMO and not another provider may capitate a provider; for example, in California this would take the form of a "Limited Knox-Keene License."

Multispecialty medical groups, if they are large enough and are made up of a sufficient number of PCPs and SCPs to provide most of the service, can also accept full professional risk capitation. In other words, full professional risk capitation is generally not supportable by other than a large group (either PCPs or a multispecialty group) or a large organized system of PCPs, but even then only if the organized group is large, well capitalized, has good information systems, and is able to manage the funds and risk-based accounting (see Chapter 24) through their business office.

It should be noted that many HMOs are reluctant to enter into such arrangements unless they are convinced that the physicians will be able to manage utilization because they do not wish to be exposed to the risk of failure such as occurred with the physician

---

*The term *full professional risk* capitation is one of convenience in this chapter. There is no consistent term for this in the real world.

practice management companies (PPMCs). At an individual or small group level, full professional risk capitation is unacceptable, though to the degree that the primary care group can capitate SCPs for services, the less the danger of having insufficient funds.

Any group accepting full professional risk capitation needs strong financial management skills and good computer systems support. Of considerable interest, one substantial study looked at how physicians at such a form of financial risk managed their own utilization: the physicians employed techniques identical to traditional HMO UM, including the use of a PCP gatekeeper, an authorization system, practice profiling, clinical guidelines, and managed care education.[13] In another study focusing on two very large medical groups in California (where full risk and global risk contracts are concentrated), the groups were quite consistent in their approach to managing utilization and were fairly rigorous in their denials of coverage (though most consistently because of requests for clinical services that were outside of the scope of benefits covered by the member's policy).[14]

Although capitation is a challenge with POS plans as noted earlier, it is possible to capitate a large group or an IDS even for POS. In most cases, a prospective adjustment is made to the capitation rate based on the actuary's best estimate of in-network versus out-of-network utilization. Out-of-network claims are paid by the plan from the funds that had been backed out of the capitation rate. Surpluses (or a percentage of surpluses) in that pool of funds may be returned to the group or IDS to encourage it to find ways of getting the enrolled members to seek care in-network, thus reducing out-of-network utilization.

Global Capitation

One of the most significant changes occurred in the late 1990s, when many physician practice management companies (PPMCs) and IDSs sought out global risk capitation (*ie*, capitation for *all* medical costs) with the belief

that substantial profits were to be had by "cutting out the middleman." But they found that it is not called "risk" for nothing, and most of these PPMCs failed (as discussed in Chapter 2). A few IDSs failed as well, but more often they suffered substantial losses and now no longer accept global risk. There remain exceptions, mostly in California, but it is no longer as prevalent as it once was, though it was never a dominant form of reimbursement.

The difficulties associated with global capitation in the past affected managed care reimbursement in several ways. First and most obvious, fewer provider organizations seek or accept global risk. Second, when those PPMCs failed, the MCOs had to pay the physicians and cover the loss to keep the network intact, and that resulted in a higher degree of hesitation by HMOs in even considering delegation of global risk. Third, individual physicians had to recontract with the MCOs once the PPMC went out of business or the IDS stopped accepting capitation, and this new and direct contract may have been through capitation or FFS (and may account for some of the variation in levels of capitation reported in past years by physicians who were formerly paid FFS or salary by the PPMC or IDS).

Effect of Benefits Design on Capitation

Benefits design may have a great effect on reimbursement to physicians in capitated programs, although the effect is felt in any reimbursement system that relies on performance. The two major categories of benefits design that have such an impact are reductions in benefits and changes in copayment levels. The presence of the POS plan benefit design has already been discussed.

Benefits Reductions

Because many managed care plans have adopted greater flexibility in benefits design in response to marketplace demands, the underpinnings of actuarial assumptions that are used to build capitation rates have become more variable and complex. The impact of a reduction of types of services covered for nonroutine care (*eg*, limitations on infertility treatments or on durable medical equipment) is usually not so great as to warrant changing previously acceptable capitation rates, but that is not an absolute.

Benefits changes can have a greater impact on risk pools. For example, if mental health and chemical dependency coverage are carved out of the PCP managing system and turned over to a dedicated management function (a common occurrence in managed care; see Chapter 13), then concomitant reductions in the referral and hospital risk pools are warranted. The same is true if an account wanted to carve out pharmacy services to another vendor (*eg*, a national company that administers a card and mail-order program; see Chapter 12).

Copayment Levels

Copayment levels can have an immediate impact on capitation rates, both for direct physician capitation and for risk pool allocations. The amount of capitation due a physician could be different with a $10 copay compared to a $20 copay. For example, if a PCP capitation rate were calculated to be $15 on the basis of 3.6 visits PMPY at $50 per visit plus a $10 copay, then application of a $20 copay could reduce the capitation amount to $12 [$50 − ($20 − $10) = $40; 3.6 visits × $40 = $144; $144 ÷ 12 months = $12 PMPM].

Although copayment amounts are routinely used to calculate initial capitation amounts, as a practical matter, some health plans do not actually reduce the capitation amount when they increase required copays, preferring instead to inform the physicians that instead of an adjustment to their capitation, they are getting a fee increase through the ability to double the amount of copayment collected at the time of service. This, ironically, reintroduces an element of FFS into a capitated system, though not so much as to necessarily have any effect as such.

The same issue applies for calculating contributions to referral risk pools and hospital risk pools. For example, if consultant care has a $30 copay, then estimated consultant visit costs would have to take the copay into account. The same is true for hospital care if copays of $100 or $200 are applied. For that matter, deductibles (*ie*, a flat amount of money that the member must pay the provider for services before any coverage is provided; a $500 deductible for a hospital admission, for example) can have the same effect on calculating the amount to fund a physician risk pool.*

The effect of copays and cost sharing on utilization is real, though most of the data on the effect of cost sharing on utilization is relatively old now. Based on that older data, it appears that cost sharing does not necessarily selectively reduce inappropriate hospitalization (in other words, although total utilization may be reduced with cost sharing, the change in utilization may not reflect a change in whether the utilization was appropriate in the first place).[15] The impact of increased cost sharing also appears to differ with respect to the health status of an individual as well as the amount of out-of-pocket expense to which the member is exposed.[16-18] It does appear to have a disproportionately negative effect on low-income individuals who may not always seek out necessary care[19] and on access to at least some, but not all preventive screening services such as colorectal screening[20] and prostate antigen screening though not mammography.[21]

Commercial actuaries have proprietary models for what they term "behavioral shift," which refers to members altering their use of medical (or any other) services in response to economic stimuli or barriers. Those models are not generally available in the public literature, however. Unless a health plan uses

---

*It is difficult at best to apply a deductible for capitated services, so it is rarely if ever seen.

an actuary for this purpose, deciding whether to adjust capitation rates on the basis of expected utilization differences from copays is difficult. Explaining such adjustments to physicians is no easy task either because changes in utilization are population based, and any individual member may or may not change his or her behavior.

Last, adjusting capitation rates for copays is not easily done if there are widespread differences in copay amounts among different accounts. For example, if 50% of the members have a $10 copay, 35% have a $20 copay, and 15% have a $40 copay for primary care services (not to mention differential copays for referral services), calculating the appropriate capitation will be a challenge both to carry out and to explain to the physicians. Even so, it is worth doing unless the variations are minor or infrequent, and automated tools can make the calculations painless.

Reasons to Capitate

The first and most powerful reason for an HMO to capitate providers is that capitation puts the provider at some level of risk or incentive for medical expenses and utilization. Capitation eliminates the FFS incentive to overutilize and brings the financial incentives of the capitated provider in line with the financial incentives of the HMO. Under capitation, costs are more easily predicted by the health plan (though not absolutely predictable because of problems of out-of-network care). Capitation is also easier and less costly to administer than FFS is (*eg*, fewer claims to adjudicate), thus resulting in lower administrative costs in the HMO and potentially lower premium rates to the member.

The most powerful reasons for a provider to accept capitation from an HMO are financial. Capitation ensures good cash flow: the capitation money comes in at a predictable rate, regardless of services rendered, and comes in as prepayment, thus providing positive cash flow. Also, for physicians who are effective medical case managers as well as cost-effective providers of direct patient care, the profit margins under capitation can exceed those found in FFS, especially as FFS fees come under continued pressure.

Problems with Capitation Systems

The most common problem with capitation involves chance. As mentioned earlier, a significant element of chance is involved when too few members are in an enrolled base to make up for bad luck (or good luck, but nobody ever complains about that). Physicians with fewer than 100 members may find that the dice simply roll against them, and they will have members who need bypass surgery or have cancer, AIDS, or a host of other expensive medical problems. The only way to assuage that is to spread the risk for expensive cases through common risk-sharing pools for referral and institutional expenses and to provide stop-loss protection for expensive cases.

The problem of small numbers is especially acute in the early period of a PCP's participation with the MCO, unless the MCO is failing to grow. To deal with this, as well as a way to entice PCPs to participate, some HMOs have offered to pay the PCP on an FFS basis for the first 6 months, or until the PCP has more than 50 enrollees, whichever comes first. A few HMOs have offered to pay capitation, but have guaranteed that the PCP would receive the higher of capitation or FFS in that first 6 months. A few HMOs have even agreed to pay FFS until the PCP has more than 50 members without any time limit, but that is unwise because it may act as a disincentive to the PCP to enroll an adequate number of members.

Another problem that can occur is in the perception of the physicians and their office staff. Although many practices have now acclimated to capitation, there is a feeling that capitation is really funny money. When PCPs are receiving a capitation payment of $15, this is sometimes unconsciously (or consciously) confused with the office charge. In their minds, it appears as though everyone is coming in for service and demanding the most expensive care possible, all for an office charge of $15 It is easy to forget that many of the members who have signed up with that physician are not even coming in at all. It only takes 10% of the members to come in once per month to make it seem as if there is a never-ending stream of entitled demanders in the waiting room. The best approach to this is to make sure that the plan collects data on encounters so that the actual reimbursement per visit can be calculated.

The last major perceived problem is inappropriate underutilization. Once a very hot topic, the argument was made against capitation in general and risk/bonus arrangements in particular because it seemed the HMO was paying physicians to not do something, and that was dangerous.[22-32] Despite these concerns, the preponderance of the literature demonstrated that managed care systems provided equal or better care to members than uncontrolled FFS systems did, even while lowering costs.[33-55] As experience with capitation grew while at the same time the market penetration of HMOs declined, this argument against capitation lost any real sense of urgency. Even so, research published in 2001 shows that when consumers were asked if a 10% cost control/quality physician incentive program was a good or bad idea, 73% said that a cost control incentive was a bad idea and only half responded that a quality incentive program was a good idea,[56] demonstrating that the public remains relatively negative about capitation and/or incentive programs.

In an unmanaged FFS system, there is a direct and immediate relationship between doing something and getting paid for it; under capitation, the reward is temporally remote from the action. In other words, the capitation check does not change each month depending on services. Furthermore, by carefully constructing a stop-loss protection program, the effect of high-cost cases on capitation funds is attenuated. Spreading the risk over more than

one physician can lower the effect of single cases on a physician's reimbursement, but at the cost of not recognizing individual performance. In addition, it must be kept in mind that HMOs, with their lack of deductibles and high levels of co-insurance, lower economic barriers to care, thus improving access to care.

One last issue should be raised, although it is not a problem per se but something to be aware of. In a capitated system, savings from decreased utilization may not always result in direct savings to the plan. In other words, if primary care services undergo a reduction in utilization, the capitation payments will not go down, just as they will not go up when there is increased utilization.

FEE-FOR-SERVICE

Some veterans of managed health care hold that the FFS system of U.S. medicine is the root of all the problems we have historically faced with high costs. Although that is simplistic, there is some truth to it, particularly when there were no controls in place. In a system where economic reward is predicated on how much one does, particularly if procedural services pay more than cognitive ones (eg, reimbursement for a 15 minute procedure may be three to five times higher than reimbursement for a 15 minute office visit), it is only human nature to do more because it pays more. The reward is immediate and tangible: a bill is made out, and it usually gets paid (though often at a discount if paid by a health plan). Doing less results in getting paid less.

On the other side of the argument, FFS results in distribution of payment on the basis of expenditure of resources. In other words, a physician who is caring for sicker patients is paid more, reflecting that physician's greater investment of time, energy, and skills.

In a managed health care plan, FFS may be used to compensate physicians and may be the method of choice in many situations. For example, in a consumer-directed health plan (CDHP) or a preferred provider organization (PPO; see Chapter 2 for definitions of both), FFS is virtually the only option available (except in the unusual and oxymoronic "capitated PPO"). An HMO might also use FFS reimbursement for many professional services that are not capitated and may use FFS instead of capitation even for PCPs. As noted earlier, HMOs may capitate IPAs, medical groups, or PHOs, but those organizations actually pay FFS to the physicians. Also as noted earlier, certain products such as POSs are difficult to capitate and lead many MCOs with a large POS enrollment to use FFS. Last, some HMOs simply believe that FFS is the best way to reimburse PCPs, and they have operated that way for decades.

Categories of Fee-for-Service

There are two broad categories of FFS: straight FFS and performance-based FFS. Performance-based incentive programs unrelated to cost or utilization are discussed separately in Chapter 8.

The first category, straight FFS, is less common in HMOs, although nearly universal in PPOs, CDHPs, and Blue Cross Blue Shield (BCBS) service plans. In some cases, an HMO may not even be allowed to use straight FFS because the PCPs are required to be at some level of financial risk for the HMO to qualify for licensure.

Performance-based FFS simply refers to the fact that the fees the physicians ultimately receive are influenced to some degree by performance and may be applied to all physicians in the network, or only to PCPs. Whether *performance* refers to overall plan performance, performance of only one segment of medical costs (professional costs, for example), or performance of the individual physician is quite variable. How performance affects the fees is likewise variable. The no-balance-billing clause (see Chapter 30) is critically important to the use of performance-based FFS. This clause states that the physician will only look to the plan for payment of services and will accept pay-

ment by the plan as payment in full. In other words, if the plan has to reduce or otherwise alter the amount of payment, the physician will not look to the member for any additional fees.

Determination of Fees

There are several approaches a health plan may use to determine what is an appropriate fee for any specific type of procedure, rather than simply paying a charge as billed. These approaches are described as follows. Whether or not the plan pays the provider directly, whether or not the provider can demand payment from the member for any differences between what the plan pays and what the charges were, or whether or not the plan reimburses the member who is in turn responsible for paying the provider are all aspects of how the network and benefits designs are created and managed, as discussed in Chapters 2 and 5.

▪ Prevailing Fees

Prevailing fees refers to the fact that the fees billed for professional services are not uniform across geographic areas or physician specialty type. Health plans that cover a wide geographic area often choose to alter their fee schedules (discussed later) based on such discrepancies if there is a logical reason; for example, it is costlier to practice in an urban area than to practice in a rural one. It is necessary for a health plan to know what the prevailing fees are to determine its own fee schedule, as well as when paying for care delivered by out-of-network physicians, as discussed later.

Usual, Customary, or Reasonable
The historical method of determining prevailing fees was known as the usual, customary, or reasonable (UCR) fee. To the extent that *UCR* is referred to at all anymore, the exact definition of the term *UCR* underwent a significant change approximately 20 years ago. Where once it was defined as "usual, cus-

tomary, *and* reasonable," it is now defined as "usual, customary, *or* reasonable." The definition of reasonable is one made by the payor, not the provider, and is usually quite a bit lower than any of the prevailing charges for certain procedures that the payors determine to be grossly overpriced. For example, when the charges for a procedure such as cataract removal and lens implantation were first set, it was a new and complex procedure, took a long time to do, and required skills in rare supply. Now it is a highly routine and high-volume procedure, takes little time, and is performed by a great number of ophthalmologists; the historical basis for the charge is therefore no longer valid. In consequence, payors (MCOs, health insurance companies, and governmental agencies) pay less than the billed charges.

Determination of Prevailing Fees in the Commercial Sector

As noted, there is little uniformity in prevailing fees across the country and there can be tremendous discrepancies among physicians' fees for the same service. One common methodology for determining prevailing fees is to collect data for charges by current procedural terminology (CPT) code, calculate the charges that represent the 25th, 50th, 90th, and 95th percentiles, and then choose which percentile represents a reasonable prevailing fee. Other common types of codes that are used are the HCFA* Common Procedural Coding System (HCPCS) and anesthesia billing units.

It is uncommon for plans to generate all of the prevailing fee data themselves unless they are very large in a geographic area, such as a BCBS plan with a high market penetra-

tion in a single state, in which case they can achieve statistically meaningful numbers. Many plans do not have that amount of concentrated data, however. Even large national health insurance companies may have a large amount of data, but it is spread across wide geographic areas and there may be sufficient data to set the maximum for certain CPT codes, but not others.

For this reason, many health plans purchase a commercially available database. Two commonly used commercial databases are owned by Ingenix*: the MDR database and the Prevailing Healthcare Charges System. Both databases provide information based on actual charge data in various geographic regions as well as additional information, including conversion factors based on a relative value scale (discussed later). Actuarial firms also commonly use proprietary prevailing fee databases.

As with UCR, the simple existence of a wide spread of prevailing fees, including high fees, does not necessarily lead to ever-increasing fee payments, even to noncontracted providers as discussed later. The issue of reasonableness is still present and may offset the existence of high fees charged for particular types of services as illustrated with the example of cataract surgery provided earlier. This is the very reason prevailing fee databases are now no longer simple surveys of charges submitted to payors, but are also combined with other approaches to determine reasonableness, such as a relative value scale. In all events, there must be a mechanism to determine what a reasonable fee is and not subject the health plan and its customers to unwarranted fee inflation.

Rarely, the health plan's customer, that is, an employer contracting with the health plan, determines the percentile used, and the customer may even choose different percentiles for different types of services (*eg*, basic medical/surgical, behavioral health, preventive care, and so forth). It is by far most

---

*HCFA stands for Health Care Financing Administration—the old name of the Centers for Medicare and Medicaid Services. HCPCS include some CPT codes, but also include codes for billing for other types of services such as ambulance and durable medical equipment.

*See http://www.ingenix.com.

common, however, for the MCO to make the determination.

The Centers for Medicare and Medicaid Services (CMS) created the resource-based relative value scale (RBRVS) that is discussed later in this section. Based on CMS's use of that scale to pay physicians for services to Medicare beneficiaries, a de facto set of prevailing fees is created and many commercial companies use that information to help providers to ensure that they are charging the most they are entitled to charge under Medicare. Some health plans also look at these prevailing CMS fees when the goal is to pay no more or no less than does Medicare, though that may not be acceptable in many markets.

In the simplest form of indemnity insurance, when a claim is submitted, it is paid in full (subject to co-insurance, deductibles, and overall benefits determination) if it is lower than the UCR or maximum reasonable prevailing fee. If the claim is higher, it is paid at the UCR or maximum reasonable prevailing fee. Of course, this simplest form of indemnity insurance is now exceedingly rare, and the determination of prevailing fees is used in conjunction with other reimbursement methodologies as discussed in this section.

A Special Requirement for Reimbursement When Co-insurance is in Place

For any benefits plan in which the member must pay co-insurance (a percentage of the total) to a contracted FFS provider, an important policy must be put in place. This policy is the result of numerous lawsuits by state's attorneys general and concerns the base on which the co-insurance is calculated. It applies to any charges from any types of providers but not to capitation systems, nor to benefits plans that use copays rather than co-insurance.

In the prior decade, some insurance companies (*eg*, some BCBS plans or other predominantly non-HMO plans) that contracted with providers for reduced fees or charges calculated the member's co-insurance requirement on the charged amount, not on the negotiated amount. For example, if a member was subject to a 20% co-insurance requirement and a physician charged $100 but the plan's negotiated fee was $75, the member had to pay 20% of $100 (or $20), not 20% of $75 (or $15).

This was determined to be fraudulent by the courts because the member was required to pay a percentage of the total cost, not of charges that exceeded the total. As illustrated, the member was in fact paying more than the designated percentage of the total payment to the contracted provider. Since then, any plan using FFS or charge-based reimbursement (including many of the forms of reimbursement of hospitals and institutions discussed in Chapter 7) must apply the co-insurance percentage to the actual total reimbursement amount to contracted providers, not the charge. The net effect of this was to reduce the total amount of money received by the providers, but it provided better protection for the members.

This issue applies only to payments to contracted providers whose charges are higher than the total payment they agree to accept as payment in full. It does not apply to any charges by noncontracted providers, even when the plan's payment is less than the charges, as discussed next.

Out-of-Network Fees

The way a health plan determines fees to be paid to noncontracting physicians, although not the direct focus of this chapter, is a topic that deserves brief mention. In any service plan, PPO, POS, CDHP, or even HMO, members will incur charges out-of-network (*ie*, from providers that do not contract with the health plan). In the case of HMOs, that will generally occur only in emergencies or when the member is traveling far from the service area and needs care. For other types of plans, out-of-network care is expected and is part of the benefits package. In the case of HMOs that do not have out-of-network benefits, costs for true emergencies or out-of-network care authorized by the HMO are usually paid in full.

Other than for pure HMO products, what an MCO actually pays for out-of-network charges is not as simple as it appears on its face. For example, a POS plan may provide for a 30% co-insurance for out-of-network care, but that does not mean that the plan will actually pay 70% of the charge. Unless the benefits state specifically that the plan will pay at those levels, the most common approach is to pay at 70% of what the POS plan considers reasonable using the prevailing fee or UCR schedule as described earlier. In other cases, *reasonable* is defined using the fee schedule that the plan uses to reimburse in-network providers. In the latter case, depending on the level of discount the plan has with contracting providers, the difference between the "allowed" charge and what the patient was charged can be considerably less than 70%. Because the out-of-network provider is not subject to no-balance billing, the patient is liable for the difference between what the plan pays and what the provider charged.

Almost all large health plans have a unit that is responsible for negotiating with non-contracted providers for individual, highly expensive cases. Usually the focus of that negotiation is with a hospital because that is where the largest charges are incurred, but in some cases it involves negotiating with a physician or physicians as well. For example, while away from home a member may incur serious trauma, or a woman may give premature birth to a gravely ill infant. The health plan clearly has an obligation to provide coverage, but it is in the financial interest of both the health plan and the member for the plan and the provider to agree to what will be charged and what will be paid. This lowers the financial exposure of the health plan for obvious reasons, but it also lowers the member's financial exposure to balance billing for any charges not covered by the plan, either as a result of having to pay a percentage co-insurance or to the plan capping payments based on the reasonableness of the charges.

The provider in turn is paid quickly and directly, which is of great benefit; however, the topic of revenue cycle for providers is beyond this book.

Because the focus of this chapter is not on benefits design, further discussion of coverage issues is not warranted.

Electronic Visits

Electronic visits, or e-visits, are also known as online visits. This refers to a clinical interaction between a physician and a patient that takes place over the Internet, not on a face-to-face basis. This is usually done through a specialized form of secure e-mail or through the use of a more structured application that automatically filters requests for e-visits through branched chain algorithms and access to medical self-help. Some MCOs are now reimbursing physicians for providing care by e-visits, though at a rate usually lower than that of a standard office visit. The member is usually also required to pay the copayment based on plan design and is so informed prior to using the service.

Because e-visits are still relatively new at the time of publication, they are singled out for mention here. There is no uniformity of either fees or coding for such visits, but if the practice of reimbursing for e-visits grows, that will change.

Fee Schedules

A fee schedule is simply a list of the maximum amount that a health plan will pay for each and every type of encounter or procedure based on the coding methodologies noted earlier. If the plan is using its own historical payment schedules, or is relying on a prevailing fee database and simply selecting a percentile to use, then each encounter or procedure will be associated with a maximum payment amount.

In some plans, the negotiated payment rate to contracted providers is simply a percentage discount off of the reasonable prevailing fee or the submitted claim, whichever is lower. The advantage to using this approach is that it is extremely easy to obtain. Most physicians will gladly accept a discount on fees if it ensures rapid and guaranteed payment. The problem is that there is nothing to prevent a physician whose fees are below the maximum from increasing their fees up to the maximum, which they will promptly do unless they are totally asleep at the wheel. Having said that, it is now rare for any physician to charge less than the maximum allowed as a result of the pressure they face on income, leading them to raise their fees to a level that ensures they will always receive the maximum payment.

In other cases, a plan may negotiate with a physician organization (*eg*, an IPA) around specific types of codes, such as the evaluation and management codes associated with office visits. It is rare to negotiate with individual physicians unless the physician is a subspecialist that the plan specifically needs in its service area (*eg*, a neurosurgeon in a mid-sized town). In provider-sponsored MCOs or IDSs, it is important that the physicians who participate in the plan not be the ones to set the fee schedules or relative value scales (RVS). To do so courts an antitrust violation. In such organizations, it is necessary to employ an outside firm to create the fee schedules and/or RVS scales.

Relative Value Scales

The use of an RVS has gained widespread popularity in FFS plans. In this system, each procedure, as defined in CPT, has a relative value associated with it. The plan pays the physician on the basis of a monetary multiplier for the RVS value. For example, if a procedure has a value of 4 and the multiplier is $12, the payment is $48. In the past, RVSs merely reflected prevailing fees or UCRs, but had the advantage of allowing for easy modifications to the fees overall by simply changing the multiplier. This could be done uniformly for all types of procedures or differently for classes of procedures (*eg*, the multiplier for office visits could be raised more than the multiplier for cataract removal and lens implantation).

A classic problem in using a simple RVS and negotiating the value of the multiplier has been the imbalance between procedural and cognitive services. As in FFS in general, procedures have higher charges than cognitive services. In other words, there is less payment to a physician for performing a careful history and physical examination and thinking about the patient's problem than for doing a procedure involving needles, scalpels, or machines.

This is why the use of a simple RVS based solely on historical prevailing fees has given way to the resource-based relative value scale (RBRVS).

Resource-Based Relative Value Scale

The most well known RBRVS was developed for Medicare on behalf of the Health Care Financing Administration (HCFA, now CMS). By looking at the amount of resources actually required to provide each service (including not only tangible resources such as materials, clinical settings, and time, but also the resources invested by the physician in training), a relative value was assigned to each CPT code in use by Medicare. That meant that many CPT codes not commonly used by Medicare (*eg*, for pediatric procedures) were not originally affected by RBRVS, but it has since broadened to cover more codes.

RBRVS has addressed to some extent the imbalance between cognitive and procedural services noted earlier, lowering the value of invasive procedures (*eg*, cardiac surgery) and raising the value of cognitive ones (*eg*, office visits). CMS has imposed this on all physicians for Medicare recipients and uses it to limit the amount that nonparticipating physicians may charge Medicare beneficiaries, using a complicated formula not germane to this discussion.

The Medicare RBRVS is not the only one in use. Some other RBRVS systems (*eg*, the one used for determining fees in workers' compensation programs in California) modified their approach to leaven the effect of historical charges with other factors such as the amount of time, effort, and technical skill required to provide a service, the cost of malpractice insurance for each specialty, and even the physician psychological stress when a bad outcome has serious consequences. Commercial RBRVS systems are also available.

Most large insurers and MCOs have followed suit in setting their determination of reasonable fees. They usually do not pay the same amount as Medicare, but frequently use the same RBRVS schedules. The percentage above or below a Medicare payment is partly determined by geography and partly by competition.

Global Fees

A variation on FFS is the global fee. A global fee is a single fee that encompasses all services delivered in an episode. Common examples of global fees include obstetrics, in which a single fee is supposed to cover all prenatal visits, the delivery itself, and at least one postnatal visit and certain surgical procedures, in which a single surgical fee pays for preoperative care, the surgery itself, and postoperative care.

Global fees may encompass more than one provider if the providers themselves are organized to manage it. The most common example of this is the management of a patient with coronary artery disease. The MCO and providers negotiate a global fee that covers multiple services for this disease. For example, cardiac testing, coronary angiography, and the coronary surgical procedure are all part of the single global fee. In some cases, the diagnostic workup is uncomplicated and the patient will have a stent placed or perhaps transluminal coronary angioplasty; in other cases, the patient has complex disease and requires multivessel coronary artery bypass surgery. Unless the volume of such cases referred to the contracted providers is high and therefore evens out (actuarially speaking), it is common to also negotiate an outlier "trim point" where the costs so exceed the global fee that the MCO pays an additional amount, usually a fixed amount per day or some form of fee schedule.

The concept is applicable to chronic, nonsurgical care as well, though not as often as for surgical care. The most common examples are in diseases such as insulin-dependent diabetes, acquired immunodeficiency syndrome (AIDS), end stage renal disease, and others that are similar in their chronicity. In these types of situations, the SCP or the organized provider system (*eg*, a nephrologist, a dialysis center, and other physicians such as ophthalmologists and podiatrists) are paid a fixed fee on a regular basis. This can be monthly or quarterly, but it is not advisable to lengthen the time period beyond that because these patients are not necessarily stable. For this type of global fee to work, the services must be well-defined, similar to what is done under capitation. Services beyond what are included in the global fee (*eg*, acute hospitalizations) are paid separately by the MCO. This approach is very well-suited to disease management programs (see Chapter 10), especially in HMOs that remove such chronically ill patients from a PCP's member panel so that care is managed by an SCP of the appropriate specialty.

It is possible, though not common, to use a form of global fees to cover primary care as well. To do so, the plan must statistically analyze what goes into the average primary care visit to calculate the global fee. That analysis must include the range of visit codes as well as all covered services that occur during primary care visits (*eg*, electrocardiography, simple laboratory tests, spirometry, and so forth). The analysis will vary by specialty type (*ie*, internal medicine, family practice, and pediatrics). The analysis then builds (by specialty) a composite type of visit. The average type of visit for internal medicine, for example, may be an intermediate visit, and 10% of the time an electrocardiogram is performed, 20% of the time a urinalysis is performed, and so forth (these figures are fictitious and should not be used for actual fee calculations). The plan then builds up the global fee by putting together the pieces, for example, $50 for the office visit, $5 for the electrocardiogram ($50 × 0.1), and so forth.

Regardless of specialty type, the chief value of a global fee is that it protects against problems of unbundling and upcoding. With *unbundling,* the physician bills separate charges for services once included in a single fee; for example, the office visit is $45, the bandage is $10, starch in the nurse's uniform is $3, and so forth. *Upcoding* refers to billing for a procedure that yields greater revenue than that actually performed; an example is coding for an office visit that was longer than the time actually spent with the patient. In the primary care setting, however, global fees offer no protection against *churning,* which is the practice of seeing patients more often than is medically necessary to generate more bills. In fact, global fees, if not managed correctly, may exacerbate a problem with churning, and that is a form of utilization that requires monitoring by the MCO.

A global fee system is really a hybrid of capitation and FFS. Like capitation, PMPM targets in all categories of medical expense are monitored, and there is a statistical buildup to determine the global fee. Also like capitation, it transfers some level of risk to the provider and provides for some stability in costs to the MCO. Unlike capitation, there are generally no payouts from capitated risk pools (*eg,* referral pools), so there is no dollar-for-dollar relationship between utilization and reimbursement. Like FFS, payment is only made if services are rendered, and no payments are made if there are no services. Thus, even though some level of risk has been transferred to the provider, it is based on known medical conditions that are more clearly within the purview of the contracted provider(s).

Bundled Case Rates or Package Pricing

Bundled case rates refer to a reimbursement that combines both the institutional and the professional charges into a single payment. For example, a plan may negotiate a bundled case rate of $30,000 for cardiac bypass surgery. That fee covers the charges from the hospital, the surgeon, the pump technician, and the anesthesiologist as well as all preoperative and postoperative care. Bundled case rates sometimes have outlier provisions for cases that become catastrophic and grossly exceed expected utilization.

Variation Based on Location of Service

Because the facility costs make up part of the total cost of a procedure, many health plans pay attention to where a procedure is performed. Commonly, the same procedure performed in a hospital facility is far more expensive than when performed in a free-standing ambulatory surgical center, solely because of the differences in what each type of facility charges (unless the plan has negotiated equivalent charges for each type of location). To lower the aggregate cost of the procedure, therefore, the plan may reduce the fees paid to the physician if the procedure is performed in a hospital or other high-cost location but increase the fees paid if the physician uses a low-cost facility.

Withholds

As with capitation, some plans that use FFS to reimburse PCPs withhold a certain percentage of the fee to cover medical cost overruns. For example, the plan may be using a negotiated fee schedule that amounts to a 20% discount for most physician fees. The plan then withholds an additional 20% in a risk pool until the end of the year. In effect, physicians receive what amounts to 60% of their usual fee but may receive an additional 20% at the end of the year if there were no excess medical costs.

It is possible to create profiles of physicians' utilization patterns to distribute more equitably the withhold funds in the event that some, but not all, of the withhold is used to cover extra medical costs. This is difficult in an FFS system using a withhold if there is no gatekeeper model in place. In that case, most plans simply return remaining withhold funds on a straight pro rata basis, although some plans return withhold on a preferential basis to PCPs as opposed to SCPs.

Mandatory Reductions in All Fees

In an HMO where risk for medical cost is shared with all the physicians and reimbursement is on an FFS basis, there must be a mechanism whereby fees may be reduced unilaterally by the HMO in the event of serious cost overruns. This Draconian measure is no longer found in HMOs that are not provider-sponsored because such plans long ago failed and either disappeared or were acquired by healthier plans. A provider-sponsored plan usually does not have access to deep financial resources, however, so cannot allow itself to drop into a serious financial deficit.

For example, the plan may be using a fee schedule that is equivalent to a 20% discount on the most common fees in the area. In the event that medical expenses are over budget and there is not enough money in the risk withhold fund to cover them, all physician fees are reduced by a further percentage, say an additional 10%, to cover the expenses. At this point, the effective discount is 30%, although this would really be 50% in the event that a withhold system was in place, all of the withhold funds had been used, and there were still excess medical liabilities. The major policy decision to be made when things go south is setting how low fee reductions will go before they will not be further reduced. For example, the plan may set the lowest possible fees at 60% of Medicare, though if the plan reaches that point, there may not be many physicians left in the network to pay.

Budgeted FFS

Related to mandatory fee reductions, budgeted FFS is used in a few plans. In this variation, which is much like contact capitation briefly discussed earlier, the plan budgets a maximum amount of money that may be spent in each specialty category. This maximum may be expressed either as a PMPM amount (eg, $7.50 PMPM) or as a percentage of revenue (eg, 5.6% of premium revenue). As costs in that specialty category approach or exceed the budgeted amount, the withhold in that specialty, but not across all specialties, is increased. In addition, the fees for that specialty, but not all specialties, may be reduced.

This approach has the advantage of focusing the reimbursement changes on those specialties in which excess costs occur rather than on all specialties in the network. The disadvantage is that this is not individual provider specific; in other words, all specialists are treated the same, and there is no specific focus on individual outliers. This approach was once somewhat popular in HMOs that did not use PCPs to manage care but is now uncommon.

Point-of-Service and Performance-Based FFS

As discussed earlier, a central issue facing plan management in applying performance-based reimbursement under POS is determining whether to include out-of-network costs in the performance evaluation of PCPs. The issues are identical no matter if capitation is being used or performance-based FFS is used.

Price Transparency

The term *price transparency* or *pricing transparency,* sometimes also referred to as cost transparency, simply refers to making information about the cost or price of health care services available to consumers. This is a central tenet of CDHPs: inform consumers about the cost and quality of services and empower them to make their own decisions. As a practical matter there are some difficulties with doing this, such as needing services on an urgent or acute basis, whether a consumer is capable of distinguishing between differing services, and so forth. But the concept has taken root, and at the time of publication, it is beginning to be implemented, both by health plans and by some providers as well.

Pricing transparency is usually done by posting pricing information on the Internet, usually by the health plan. In some cases, this might be available only to registered members of the plan; in other cases, it is simply being put out there. What information is actually being posted is not necessarily straightforward, however.

As regards physician pricing, what is usually posted is information about how much the plan pays contracted physicians for certain things (*eg*, office visits, delivering a baby) and what the local prevailing charges are. This enables consumers to understand how much more they will have to pay if they see a noncontracting physician. At the time of publication, most health plans that post information at all are not posting pricing information specific to individual physicians, but rather using aggregate type data; however, at the time of publication, one major national company has announced that it plans to make available information about cost, quality, and service at the level of individual physicians.[57]

Many CDHPs and health plans also provide assistance with a type of calculator that enables consumers to figure out what their out-of-pocket responsibility will be and the effect on their Health Reimbursement Account Health Savings Accounts (discussed in Chapters 2 and 20). What the ultimate impact of this approach will be is not known.

Problems with FFS in Managed Health Care Plans

There are two significant problems with using FFS in managed health care plans. These problems can become markedly exacerbated if the plan starts to get into financial trouble. The best approach to both of these problems requires the MCO to have excellent data management and profiling capabilities (see Chapter 16). Without good profiling and data management capabilities to identify and manage issues early, as well as provide feedback to the PCPs, managers are more likely than not to experience these problems.

The first problem is churning. This simply means that physicians perform more procedures than are really necessary and schedule patient revisits at frequent intervals. Because most patients depend on the physician to recommend when they should come back and what tests should be done, it is easy to have a patient come back for a blood pressure check in 2 weeks instead of a month and to have serum electrolytes measured (unless laboratory services are capitated) in the physician's office at the same time. Few patients will argue, and the physician collects for the work.

Few physicians consciously churn, but it does happen, even if unconsciously. The serious problem comes when the plan reduces the fees because of medical expense overruns. When this happens, a feeding frenzy can occur. In effect, physicians start to feel that they have to get theirs first. If the fees are lowered 10% this month, what might happen next month? Better to get in as many visits as possible this month because next month may bring a 20% fee reduction. This creates a self-fulfilling prophecy, and the inevitable downward spiral begins.

For an HMO, the only effective approach to churning is tight management (or switching to capitation). Some HMOs develop physician peer review committees to review utilization. These committees have the authority to sanction physicians who abuse the system. This has some slowing effect if there are enough reviewers and not too many physicians to review. The actions of such committees should follow a process that includes warnings and a probationary period in which expectations for improvement are clearly outlined. Other plans apply differential withholds selectively on those providers whose utilization is clearly out of line, although defining that takes some care.

The second major problem is upcoding (sometimes referred to as CPT creep) and unbundling. As mentioned earlier, upcoding refers to a slow creeping upward of CPT codes that pay more; for example, a routine office visit becomes an extended one, a Pap smear and pelvic examination become a full physical examination, or a cholecystectomy becomes a laparotomy. Unbundling refers to charging for services that were previously included in a single fee without lowering (or lowering sufficiently) the original fee.

These problems are best monitored by the claims department in coordination with whichever department is responsible for data analysis. There are two useful approaches. The first is to look for trends by providers. Individuals who are trying to game the system will usually stand out. If there is one physician who has 40% extended visits compared to 20% for all the other physicians in the panel, it may be worth further review. The second approach is to automate the claims system to rebundle unbundled claims and to separate for review any claims that appear to have a gross mismatch between services rendered and the clinical reason for the visit.

There are also software programs in existence that automatically recode claims based on statistical norms. Using the preceding example, a PCP with 40% extended visits may have 20% of them lowered to routine visits by the system, using some type of criteria to choose which visits get lowered. The use of these programs has been tempered by lawsuits filed against the MCOs that used them, charging that the MCOs were arbitrarily refusing to pay for the care that was actually rendered. In the end, the large MCOs settled and compensated the physicians using a settlement fund. The software programs are still used, but automatically recoding claims has given way to using the results to determine who to audit.

The net result of these pressures has resulted in the primary approach to escalating costs caused by FFS being one of simply paying low fees. The advent of CDHPs, with their higher levels of consumer cost sharing and responsibility, combined with increasing price

transparency, is also beginning to build, with the intent of having consumers become informed purchasers of health care with price being one of the things they are informed about. Whether this will actually have an impact is unknown at this time.

LEGISLATION AND REGULATION APPLICABLE TO PHYSICIAN INCENTIVE PROGRAMS

Beginning in the 1990s, many states and the federal government passed laws and created regulations that affect physician incentive programs. These apply primarily to capitation programs and to incentive programs under which a physician's income may be affected by performance, particularly utilization and medical cost performance. Although capitation and/or incentive programs have not been found to have a negative effect on quality as addressed earlier, the intent was to protect beneficiaries from the potential harm that the politicians and regulators perceived existed. In general, while adding an extra layer of bureaucracy (and therefore a bit of extra cost), health plans have had little or no problem complying.

It is very difficult to discuss state laws and regulations that apply to physician compensation and incentives under managed health care. Not all states have passed such laws or promulgated such regulations, and those that have show little consistency from one state to another. In general, when states do have such laws, they focus on disclosure of financial incentives. For a discussion of state regulation in general, the reader is referred to Chapter 33; though that chapter does not specifically address physician incentives, it does help illustrate the inconsistent environment at the state level. Because of this lack of consistency and stability at the state level, little discussion of state issues is included in this section and the reader will be required to research each state individually as needed.

The remainder of this section focuses on the federal regulations because those are consistent and also serve to illustrate the approaches taken by some states. Beginning in 1987, CMS (then called HCFA) implemented regulations that placed limits on physician incentive programs in Medicare and Medicaid MCOs. These regulations have been modified several times, and as of the time of publication, the most recent revision was 67, issued August 12, 2005.

The reader is also referred to Chapter 26 for further discussion of Medicare and managed health care, and to Chapter 27 for a discussion of Medicaid and managed health care.

Significant Financial Risk

CMS first determines whether a physician or medical group is at "significant financial risk"* (SFR) for medical costs. For purposes of this regulation, medical costs are only those costs applicable to Medicare or Medicaid beneficiaries. The determination of SFR is as follows:

> The amount at risk for referral services is the difference between the maximum potential referral payments and the minimum potential referral payments. Bonuses unrelated to utilization (*eg*, quality bonuses such as those related to member satisfaction or open physician panels) should not be counted toward referral payments. Maximum potential payments is defined as the maximum *anticipated* total payments that the physician/group could receive. If there is no specific dollar or percentage amount noted in the incentive arrangement, then the PIP should be considered as potentially putting 100% of the potential payments at risk for referral services. The SFR threshold is set at 25% of

"potential payments" for covered services, regardless of the frequency of assessment (*ie*, collection) or distribution of payments. SFR is present when the 25% threshold is exceeded.

The following incentive arrangements should be considered as SFR:

- Withholds greater than 25% of potential payments.
- Withholds less than 25% of potential payments if the physician or physician group is potentially liable for amounts exceeding 25% of potential payments.
- Bonuses that are greater than 33% of potential payments minus the bonus.
- Withholds plus bonuses if the withholds plus bonuses equal more than 25% of potential payments. The threshold bonus percentage for a particular withhold percentage may be calculated using the formula: Withhold % = -0.75 (Bonus %) + 25%.
- Capitation arrangements, if the difference between the maximum potential payments and the minimum potential payments is more than 25% of the maximum potential payments; or the maximum and minimum potential payments are not clearly explained in the physician's or physician group's contract.
- Any other incentive arrangements that have the potential to hold a physician or physician group liable for more than 25% of potential payments.[58]

Any service that a physician does not provide herself or that is not provided by another member of the physician's group, should be considered a referral service. If the physician group refers patients to other providers (including independent contractors to the group) to perform the ancillary services, then those services are considered referral services. If the physician group performs ancillary services, then those services are not considered referral services. Whether such referrals contribute to the financial risk borne by the physician depend on whether his or her compensation arrangements are such that referrals for those services or supplies could affect the physician's income.

Stop-Loss Protection

Stop-loss protection must be in place to protect physicians and/or physician groups to whom SFR has been transferred by an MCO. Either aggregate or per-patient stop loss may be acquired. The rule specifies that if aggregate stop loss is provided, it must cover 90% of the cost of referral services that exceed 25% of potential payments; physicians and groups can be held liable for only 10%. If per-patient stop loss is acquired, it must be determined based on the physician or physician group's patient panel size and cover 90% of the referral costs that exceed the per-patient limits noted in Table 6-4.

CMS has also set criteria for when an MCO, physician, or physician group may pool their patients for purposes of determining stop-loss levels. To determine the patient panel size in Table 6-4, specific criteria are stated in the regulations. Any entity that meets all five criteria required for the pooling of risk is allowed to pool that risk to determine the amount of stop loss required by the regulation. Those five criteria are as follows:

- Pooling of patients is otherwise consistent with the relevant contracts governing the compensation arrangements for the physician or group (ie, no contracts can require that risk be segmented by MCO or patient category).
- The physician or group is at risk for referral services with respect to each of the categories of patients being pooled.
- The terms of the compensation arrangements permit the physician or group to spread the risk across the categories of patients being pooled (ie, payments must be held in a common risk pool).
- The distribution of payments to physicians from the risk pool is not calculated separately by patient category (either by MCO or by Medicaid, Medicare, or commercial).

Table 6–4 Limits on Referral Costs Based on Patient Panel Size in Medicare or Medicaid MCOs

Patient Panel Size	Single Combined Limit	Separate Institutional Limit	Separate Professional Limit
1–1,000	$6,000	$10,000	$3,000
1,001–5,000	$30,000	$40,000	$10,000
5,001–8.000	$40,000	$60,000	$15,000
8,001–10,000	$75,000	$100,000	$20,000
10,001–25,000	$150,000	$200,000	$25,000
> 25,000	None	None	None

Source: Centers for Medicare and Medicaid Services. *CMS Medicare Managed Care Manual.* 2006. Publication 100-16. Available at: http://www.cms.hhs.gov/manuals/.

- The terms of the risk borne by the physician or group are comparable for all categories of patients being pooled.[58]

Pooling and stop-loss requirements applicable to a group cannot be extended to a subcontracting level. In other words, if a group meets pooling requirements for a high stop loss, but subcontracts with physicians who are at SFR with smaller patient panels, then the stop-loss requirements for the smaller panels apply to those subcontracted physicians. If an MCO uses PODs as described earlier in this chapter, then the pooling criteria may still be met by the POD if the incentive program for the POD physicians meets the criteria noted earlier, even though the POD is not an actual legal entity. In other words, the concept of sharing risk and reward through a POD system may be considered pooling for this purpose.

An MCO, medical group, or physician may combine commercial membership with Medicare and Medicaid membership for purposes of pooling if the financial risk is applicable to all members, but may not do so if the risk arrangements are different between those types of patients. If such pooling is appropriate but stop loss is still required, then the stop-loss arrangement need only cover Medicare and Medicaid members, not commercial members.

Although Table 6-4 does indicate what constitutes SFR for small panel sizes (*ie*, 500 to 1,000 members), a health plan should really avoid putting a physician at that level of risk. As discussed earlier in this chapter, the degree of financial risk for medical costs that a physician with a small panel would face is usually limited by the MCO in any event. In cases where a physician with a small panel might be placed at SFR, the MCO can provide stop-loss protection by adjusting the capitation payment or fee schedule so as to budget for the cost of the stop loss (in other words, treat it as an insurance premium).

Finally, for those medical groups with large panels of enrollees, or for IDSs that pool risk,

either the MCO may provide stop-loss coverage at a competitive premium rate, or commercial stop-loss insurance is available from third parties.

Disclosure Requirements

CMS requires disclosure to both CMS itself and to members or beneficiaries of the Medicare or Medicaid MCO. This disclosure applies to all providers in the network if they are at any financial risk. For example, if an MCO capitates an IPA, and the IPA in turn capitates a medical group, then both financial arrangements are subject to disclosure. If that medical group in turn subcapitates other medical groups, that too is subject to disclosure. IPAs that contract only with individual physicians and not with physician groups are considered physician groups under this rule.

The following pieces of information are required by the regulation to be provided to CMS:

- Whether referral services are covered by the physician incentive program (PIP). If only services furnished directly by the physician or group are addressed by the PIP, then there's no need for disclosure of other aspects of the PIP.
- Type of incentive arrangement (*eg*, withhold, bonus, capitation).
- Percentage of total income at risk for referrals.
- Amount and type of stop-loss protection.
- Panel size and whether enrollees were pooled to achieve the panel size.
- If the MCO is required by this regulation to conduct a customer satisfaction survey, a summary of the survey results.[58]

At Medicare or Medicaid beneficiaries' request, MCOs must provide information indicating whether the MCO or any of its contractors or subcontractors use a PIP that may affect the use of referral services, the type of incentive arrangement(s) used, and whether stop-loss protection is provided. If the MCO is required to conduct a survey, it must also provide beneficiary requestors with a summary of survey results.

Formerly, CMS (when it was called HCFA) required the use of the Consumer Assessment of Health Plans Study (CAHPS), which was focused solely on Medicare-managed care plans for any plan that put physicians at SFR. That has since evolved, however, and CAHPS now stands for Consumer Assessment of Healthcare Providers and Systems and is designed to look at Medicare-managed care, Medicare FFS, Medicare providers, and Medicare drug plans. It is under the purview of the Agency for Healthcare Research and Quality (AHRQ*) and is far more broadly administered. In fact, many health plans use it to meet one of the requirements for external accreditation (see Chapter 23).

The MCO is required to provide to a beneficiary only a summary statement or letter outlining all of the incentive arrangements in place throughout the MCO. A beneficiary won't necessarily be able to tell from the required MCO disclosure whether a specific physician has a PIP or the amount or type of risk that individual physician might experience. However, there is nothing in federal statute or regulation to prevent an MCO or individual physician from providing physician-specific information to a beneficiary who requests it.

CIVIL LIABILITY FOR PHYSICIAN COMPENSATION PROGRAMS

In cases where an MCO, IDS, or medical group does not have Medicare or Medicaid risk business, and there are no state laws or regulations governing physician compensation or incentives, managers should note that potential liability still remains in civil court. Physician incentives in managed health care have largely withstood legal challenges in the past, but that is no guarantee that they cannot be successfully challenged at all. Regardless of the facts or merits of

incentive systems, some judges and juries have expressed their opinion in judgment that financial incentives to management utilization or cost are injurious to patients. This is a different issue from utilization management and does not even require that a member be injured for a plaintiff's attorney to file a suit; the very existence of an incentive program is reason enough.

For example, in 1999, two states, Texas and Georgia, had passed legislation to make it easier for members to sue MCOs. In another example, in October of 1999, Harris Methodist Health Plan in Texas reached a $4.7 million settlement with plaintiff's attorneys who had filed two class-action lawsuits against the HMO because it did not disclose that capitation payments included prescription costs, thus, they argued, incenting physicians to limit prescribing. The settlement is believed to be the first in the nation in which uninjured patients recovered cash (approximately $50 per member) because the HMO failed to disclose such incentives.[59]

Exposure to lawsuits regarding financial incentives is not necessarily confined solely to individual plaintiffs. In 1998, the former attorney general of Texas, citing a 1997 state law prohibiting financial incentives "that act directly or indirectly as an inducement to limit medically necessary services," filed a suit in a state district court, asking the court to fine six HMOs and prevent them from offering financial incentives to physicians. Harris Methodist Health Plan of Texas, the same HMO cited earlier, was fined $3.5 million in that action. On the other hand, other lawsuits have rejected any linkage between physician incentives and the care provided.[60] For self-funded plans under the Employee Retirement Income Security Act (ERISA; see Chapter 31), the Supreme Court recently provided limits against lawsuits against managed care companies for incentive programs and other activities.[61]

CONCLUSION

To be effective, an MCO (HMO, IDS, or any type of risk-assuming managed care system)

_____

*See https://www.cahps.ahrq.gov.

must align the financial incentives and goals of all the parties: the health plan and the providers who deliver the care. Capitation, and to a somewhat lesser extent, performance-based fee-for-service, do that in ways that traditional fee-for-service do not.

In a closely managed plan such as an HMO, capitation is often considered to be more consistent with the overall goal of managing costs. Although capitation is initially harder to calculate, and is sometimes harder to gain acceptance from physicians, this system has less likelihood of leading to overutilization than FFS does. Problems of inappropriate underutilization must be guarded against with effective monitoring and an effective quality management system.

FFS can be used as well but requires a different set of management skills and good data and profiling systems. It is easier to install and is often more acceptable to physi-cians, but can quickly get out of control unless it is managed carefully. New products such as POS are better suited to FFS than is capitation. Global fees offer a middle ground, at least in some circumstances. New products also require new approaches to reimbursement because classic approaches are not ideally suited. As managed care evolves, reimbursement may be expected to evolve further.

The reimbursement system is a tool, and like any tool it has limitations. Just as a hammer is the correct tool for pounding and removing nails, it is poor for cutting wood and drilling holes. A reimbursement system is a powerful and effective tool but can be effective only in conjunction with other managed care functions: utilization management, quality management, network contracting, provider relations, and the many other activities of a well-run managed care organization.

References

1. Robinson JC. Blended payment methods in physician organizations under managed care. *JAMA*. 1999, 282:1258–1263.
2. Hillman AL, Welch WP, Pauly MV. Contractual arrangements between HMOs and primary care physicians: Three-tiered HMOs and risk pools. *Med Care*. 1992, 30:136–148.
3. Conrad DA, Maynard C, Cheadle A, *et al*. Primary care physician compensation method in medical groups: Does it influence the use and cost of health services for enrollees in managed care organizations? *JAMA*. 1998, 279(11):853–858.
4. Landon BE, Normand SL, Blumenthal D, Daley J. Physician clinical performance assessment: Prospects and barriers. *JAMA*. 2003, 290(9): 1183–1189.
5. Kravitz RL, Greenfield S, Rogers W, *et al*. Differences in the mix of patients among medical specialties and systems of care: Results from the medical outcomes study. *JAMA*. 1992, 267:1617–1623.
6. Popovian R, Johnson K, Nichol M, Liu G. The impact of pharmaceutical capitation to primary medical groups on the health-care expenditures of Medicare HMO enrollees. *J Managed Care Pharmacy*. September/October 1999, Vol 5, Number 5: 438-441.
7. Hillman AL, Pauly MV, Escarce JJ, Ribley K, Gaynor M, Clouse J, Ross R. Financial incentives and drug spending in managed care. *Health Affairs*. March/April 1999, 18(2):189–200.
8. Debrock L, Arnould RJ. Utilization control in HMOs. *Quarterly Review of Economics and Finance*. Autumn 1992, 32(3):31–53.
9. Sanofi-Aventis. HMO-PPO/Medicare-Medicaid Digest 2005. Managed Care Digest Series. Available at: http://www.managedcaredigest.com. Accessed June 21, 2006.
10. LaPensee KT. Pricing specialty carve-outs and disease management programs under managed care. *Managed Care Q*. 1997, 5(2): 10–19.
11. Hurly R, Grossman J, Lake T, Casaline L. A longitudinal perspective on health plan—Provider risk contracting. *Health Affairs*. July/August 2002, 21(4):144–153.
12. Rosenthal MB, Frank RG, Buchanan JL, Epstein AM. Transmission of financial incentives to physicians by intermediary organiza-

tions in California. *Health Affairs*. 2002, 21(4): 197–205.

13. Kerr EA, Mittman BS, Hays RD, *et al.* Managed care and capitation in California: How do physicians at financial risk control their own utilization? *Ann Intern Med*. 1995, 123:500–504.

14. Kapur K, Gresenz C, Studdert D. Managing care: Utilization review in action at two capitated medical groups. Web Exclusive. *Health Affairs*. June 18, 2003, W3:275–282.

15. Siu AL, Sonnenberg FA, Manning WG, Goldberg GA, Bloomfield ES, Newhouse JP, Brook RH. Inappropriate use of hospitals in a randomized trial of health insurance plans. *N Engl J Med*. 1986, 315:1259–1266.

16. Shapiro MF, Hayward RA, Freeman HE, Sudman S, Corey CR. Out-of-pocket payments and use of care for serious and minor symptoms. *Arch Intern Med*. 1989, 149:1645–1648.

17. Newhouse JP, Manning WG, Morris CN, *et al.* Some interim results from a controlled trial of cost sharing in health insurance. *N Engl J Med*. 1981, 305:1501–1507.

18. O'Grady KF, Manning WG, Newhouse JP, Brook RH. The impact of cost sharing on emergency department use. *N Engl J Med*. 1985, 313:484–490.

19. Federman A, Vladeck B, Siu A. Avoidance of health care services because of cost: Impact of the Medicare Savings Program. *Health Affairs*. January/February 2005, 24(1):263–270.

20. Varghese RK, Friedman C, Ahmed F, Franks AL, Manning M, Seeff LC. Does health insurance coverage of office visits influence colorectal cancer testing? *Cancer Epidemiol Biomarkers Prev*. March 2005, 14(3):744–747.

21. Liang SY, Phillips KA, Tye S, Haas JS, Sakowski J. Does patient cost sharing matter? Its impact on recommended versus controversial cancer screening services. *Am J Manag Care*. February 2004, 10(2 Pt 1):99–107.

22. Hillman AL. Health maintenance organizations, financial incentives, and physician's judgments. *Ann Intern Med*. 1990, 112:891–893.

23. Hillman AL. Financial incentives for physicians in HMOs—Is there a conflict of interest? *N Engl J Med*. 1987, 317:1743–1748.

24. Hillman AL, Pauly MV, Kerstein JJ. How do financial incentives affect physicians' clinical decisions and the financial performance of health maintenance organizations? *N Engl J Med*. 1989, 321:86–92.

25. Reagan MD. Toward full disclosure of referral restrictions and financial incentives by pre-paid health plans. *N Engl J Med*. 1987, 317: 1729–1734.

26. *Medicare: Physician Incentive Payments by Prepaid Health Plans Could Lower Quality of Care*. Washington, DC: General Accounting Office. 1988. General Accounting Office publication GAO/HRD-89-29.

27. Pearson SD, Sabin JE, Emanuel EJ. Ethical guidelines for physician compensation based on capitation. *N Eng J Med*. 1998, 339(10): 689–93.

28. Chauffler H, McMenamin S. Reforms are needed to increase quality of care and health plan accountability in California. University of California Berkley School of Public Health. California Managed Health Care Improvement Task Force Survey 1997. Reported on Managed Care at: http://www.mcol.com. Accessed May 15, 2000.

29. Grumbach K, Osmond D, Vranizan K, *et al.* Primary care physicians' experience of financial incentives in managed care systems. *NEJM*. 1998, 339(21):1516–1521.

30. Escarce JJ, Shea JA, Chen W. Segmentation of hospital markets: Where do HMO enrollees get care? *Health Affairs*. November–December 1997:186–187.

31. Miller TE, Sage WS. Disclosing physician financial incentives. *JAMA*. 1999, 281:1424–1430.

32. Simon CJ, Emmons DW. Physicians earnings at risk: What physicians don't know about managed care capitated contracts could place them—and their patients—at risk. *Health Affairs*. 1997, 16:120–126.

33. Ware JE, Brook RH, Rogers WH *et al.* Comparison of health outcomes at a health maintenance organization with those of FFS care. *Lancet*. May 3, 1986, 1(8488):1017–1022.

34. Udvarhelyi IS, Jennison K, Phillips RS, Epstein AM. Comparison of the quality of ambulatory care for FFS and prepaid patients. *Ann Intern Med*. 1991, 115:394–400.

35. Sloss EM, Keeler EB, *et al.* Effect of a health maintenance organization on physiologic health. *Ann Intern Med*. 1987, 106:130–138.

36. Clancy CM, Hillner BE. Physicians as gatekeepers—The impact of financial incentives. *Arch Intern Med*. 1989, 149:917–920.

37. Lurie N, Christianson J, Finch M, Moscovice I. The effects of capitation on health and functional status of the Medicaid elderly: A ran-

domized trial. *Ann Intern Med.* 1994, 120: 506–511.

38. Braveman P, Schaaf M, Egerter S, *et al.* Insurance-related differences in the risk of ruptured appendix. *N Engl J Med.* 1994, 331 (7):444–449.

39. Relman A. Medical insurance and health: What about managed care? *N Engl J Med.* 1994, 331(7):471–472.

40. Murray JP, Greenfield S, Kaplan SH, Yano EM. Ambulatory testing for capitation and FFS patients in the same practice setting: relationship to outcomes. *Med Care.* March 1992, 30 (3):252–261.

41. Dudley RA, Miller RH, Korenbrot TY, Luft HS. The impact of financial incentives on quality of health care. *Milbank Q.* 1998, 76(4):649–86.

42. Brook RH. Managed care is not the problem, quality is. *JAMA.*1997 November 19, 278:19: 1612–1614.

43. Baker LC, Cantor JC. Physician satisfaction under managed care. *Health Affairs.* 1993 (suppl):258–270.

44. Weiss MD. Capitation can be beneficial to providers and patients. *Maryland Med J.* 1997, 46:4:170–171.

45. Miller RH, Luft HS. Does managed care lead to better or worse quality of care? *Health Affairs.* September/October 1997, 16(5):7–25.

46. Seidman JJ, Bass EP, Rubin HR. Review of studies that compare the quality of cardiovascular care in HMO versus non-HMO settings. *Med Care.* 1998, 36:1607–25.

47. Bruno R, Gilbert B. In California, Medi-Cal managed care is superior to Medi-Cal fee-for-service. *Managed Care Q.* 1998, 6:4:7–14.

48. Whitmore H. Comparing outcomes in managed care. *HMO Magazine.* January–February 1996:75.

49. Hellinger FJ. The effect of managed care on quality: a review of recent evidence. *Arch Int Med.* April 27, 1998, 158(8):833–41.

50. Berwick DM. Quality of health care, V: Payment by capitation and the quality of care. *N Eng J Med.* 1996, 335:1227–1231.

51. Riely G, Potosky AL, Lubitz JD, Brown ML. Stage of cancer at diagnosis for Medicare

HMO and fee-for-service enrollees. *Am J Public Health.* October 1994, 84(10):1598–604.

52. Carlisle D, Siu AL, Keeler EB, McGlynn EA, et al. HMO vs. fee-for-service care of older persons with acute myocardial infarction. *Am J Public Health.* December 1992, 82(12):1626–30.

53. Carey TS, Garret J, Jackman A, et al. The outcomes and costs of care for acute low back pain among patients seen by primary care practitioners, chiropractors, and orthopedic surgeons. *N Eng J Med.* October 5, 1995, 333 (14):914–916.

54. Yelin EH, Criswell LA, FeigenbaumPG. Health care utilization and outcomes among persons with rheumatoid arthritis in fee-for-service and prepaid group practice settings. *JAMA.* October 2, 1996, 276(13):1048–53.

55. Collaborating with managed care organizations for mammogram screening and rescreening. Center for Disease Control. 1997. Available at: http://www.cdc.gov/cancer/ nbccedp/bccpdfs/mcobook.pdf. Accessed September 15, 2006.

56. Gallagher TH, St. Peter RF, Chesney M, Lo B. Cost control bonuses for managed care physicians. *Health Affairs.* March/April 2001, 20(2): 186–192.

57. Aetna. *Aetna Expands Efforts to Provide Consumers with a Transparent View of Health Care Costs and Quality.* June 13, 2006; Aetna press release. Available at: http://www.aetna. com/news/2006/pr_20060613.htm. Accessed July 17, 2006.

58. *Federal Register* 42 CFR 422.208/210. June 26, 1998.

59. *Ingram vs. Harris Health Plan*, No. 98-CV-179 (USDC E.D. Texas, settlement filed Oct. 12, 1999).

60. *Shea v. Esensten*, Minn. Ct. App. No. 949878. February 6, 2001.

61. Jost TS. The Supreme Court limits lawsuits against managed care organizations. *Health Affairs,* 2004. Available at: http://content. healthaffairs.org/cgi/reprint/hlthaff.w4.417v1. Accessed July 28, 2006.

7

HOSPITALS, FACILITIES, AND ANCILLARY SERVICES

Peter R. Kongstvedt

Study Objectives

- Understand the basic approaches to contracting for hospital services.
- Understand critical differences between inpatient and outpatient services and how that relates to contracting.
- Understand the basic forms of reimbursement for hospital and ambulatory facility services—inpatient and outpatient.
- Understand what circumstances make certain forms of reimbursement more favorable than other forms—inpatient and outpatient.
- Understand what is meant by ancillary services.
- Understand basic contracting approaches to different types of ancillary services and which approaches work best under what circumstances.

Discussion Topics

1. Discuss market attributes that might make contracting with a hospital more or less difficult for a health plan.
2. Discuss the key advantages and disadvantages of the various reimbursement systems for hospitals from the point of view of a managed care plan, by type of plan. Perform the same exercise, but from the point of view of the hospital.
3. Discuss under what circumstances an HMO would use the following types of hospital reimbursement: capitation, DRGs, per diem, APCs or APGs, charge-based.

4. What management tools would a hospital need in order to be able to effectively operate in a heavily capitated environment?
5. Discuss various policies and procedures for managing ancillary utilization in different types of managed care plans; be specific regarding the type of ancillary service.

INTRODUCTION

Hospital contracting is one of the most important tasks that an executive director and other appropriate health plan managers face. Hospital executives likewise need a thorough understanding of the issues involved in contracting with managed care organizations (MCOs). In the United States (other than in Maryland in which hospital payment rates are regulated and there is little or no latitude allowed in reimbursing hospitals), this represents an area of great potential for creativity, though that creativity has in the past not always been successful.

Considerable consolidation in the hospital industry occurred in the late 1990s and beyond, and this led to the creation of systems with multiple hospitals. The MCO is then in a position of negotiating a broader contract with the system for services at multiple sites. Theoretically, consolidation brought the potential of cost reduction and rationalization of clinical services that could allow the new system to provide care far more efficiently than individual hospitals could, thus allowing for a considerable price advantage. In practice, however, the opposite occurred, with hospital price increases consistently in the mid to high double digits in those markets where hospital systems exhibited market power.[1,2]

In addition to consolidation by hospitals, other factors have led to aggressive price inflation by hospitals.[1] As the number of excess beds decreased across the country, hospital capacity began to be strained as inpatient occupancy increased. Examples of average hospital occupancy rates in 2004 are illustrated in Figure 7-1. In the past, hospitals were of-ten willing to contract at aggressive reimbursement rates to cover excess overhead associated with a low inpatient census; the cost of keeping the facility open, cost of clinical personnel, cost of equipment, and so forth existed whether or not a hospital bed was occupied, so a hospital was glad to get whatever revenue it could. A hospital that runs a consistently high census does not have that excess overhead, so there is little pressure to look for low-margin, incremental revenue.

The relative decline in the number of commercial lives covered under health maintenance organizations (HMOs; see Chapter 1) also meant less potential ability for an aggressive HMO to shift from one hospital to another, though in reality market forces hinder that as well. Vertical integration by hospital-based integrated delivery systems (IDSs) also meant potentially tighter affiliations between physicians and a hospital system, making it difficult for an MCO to drop a hospital.

Hospital costs have also been subject to inflationary pressures. Staffing shortages, particularly for nurses and other skilled individuals, have led to substantial increases in payroll costs. Physical plant upgrades, new clinical equipment, high-cost medical technology (eg, drug-eluting vascular stents) that a hospital must purchase, and the like all contribute to high cost inflation. Hospitals analyze their reimbursement from all sources, and with public sector reimbursement (Medicare and Medicaid) often failing to even cover costs, cost shifting to private payers takes place. A hospital that is running a high occupancy and enjoys market power simply does not need to contract with an MCO at an unprofitable level of reimbursement, whereas

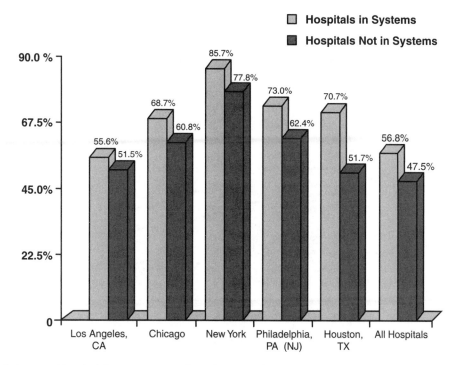

Figure 7-1 Average Hospital Occupancy in Selected Metropolitan Statistical Areas,* 2004

*Average occupancy represents only the acute-care portion of the hospitals' occupancy.

Source: Sanofi-Aventis. *Integrated Health Systems Digest.* Managed Care Digest Series. Available at: http://www. managedcaredigest.com.

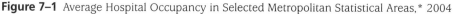

an MCO may not be viable without having an important hospital system in its network.

Hospital utilization has been decreasing for many years, though there has been a rise in the admission rate for individuals over the age of 65, as illustrated in Figure 7-2. Furthermore, the average length of stay has also been in decline, as illustrated in Figure 7-3 (which uses data from an earlier time period, however). Much of this is a result of the effect of managed care over the past few decades as well as advances in medical technology that enable care that once required an inpatient stay to be delivered in the outpatient setting. Furthermore, decreasing hospital capacity also has a strong effect because fewer beds mean tighter criteria for admission. In all events, the net result is that when patients are admitted to the hospital, they are considerably sicker than they were 20 years ago,

and they require concomitantly higher levels of clinical resources.

The net effect of all of these factors is an increase in the difficulty and complexity of negotiating and contracting between MCOs and hospitals since the beginning of the new millennium.

HOSPITAL NETWORK DEVELOPMENT AND MAINTENANCE

The development of a hospital network can be viewed from two primary perspectives: new network development and renegotiation with existing network participants. In the past, new network development was a common occurrence as new MCOs entered the marketplace. Now, however, relatively few MCOs are starting up as new organizations because of the already high number of exist-

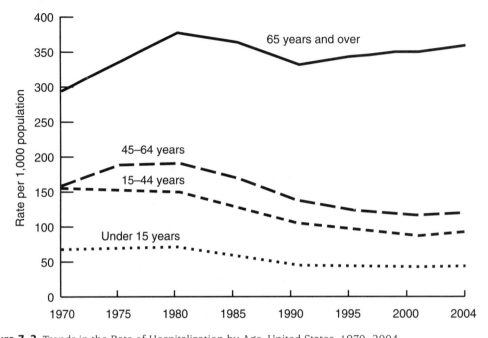

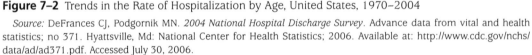

Figure 7–2 Trends in the Rate of Hospitalization by Age, United States, 1970–2004

Source: DeFrances CJ, Podgornik MN. *2004 National Hospital Discharge Survey.* Advance data from vital and health statistics; no 371. Hyattsville, Md: National Center for Health Statistics; 2006. Available at: http://www.cdc.gov/nchs/data/ad/ad371.pdf. Accessed July 30, 2006.

ing plans and the consolidation that has and is continuing to occur. New start-ups still do take place but are confined to completely new product types such as Medicare Advantage (see Chapter 26).

In all cases, whether a start-up or an existing plan, an MCO must have adequate hospital coverage in its service area, at least in the cases of HMOs, Medicare, and Medicaid managed care plans as a condition of licensure, to say nothing of marketplace acceptability. Standards for accessibility vary, but a common standard is access to a hospital with no more than a 30-minute drive time, with allowances for variables such as being in a rural area.

Maintaining the network and periodic renegotiation of existing contracts is the most common event that any MCO will face. This occurs most commonly through the regular contracting cycle, but may also be instigated by one party or the other as a result of a change in circumstances. Consolidation in the

health plan industry provides a common cause for renegotiation. If two MCOs merge, their legacy networks may not be compatible, there may be contractual clauses in existing contracts that automatically terminate the contract in the event of a change of control, or negotiating leverage may have changed. In almost all cases of consolidation, the reimbursement terms are not exact matches; that is, the terms between the premerged MCOs are not the same for the same hospital.

The same principle applies to the creation of a large hospital system through mergers or affiliations. Prior to a merger or consolidation of hospitals, the terms between the premerger hospitals and an MCO are unlikely to be the same. As noted earlier, although the new system may rationalize clinical services and provide for more inclusive contracting, it also has more negotiating leverage, which it will use.

The approach to hospital network development and maintenance will be affected to some degree by the type of MCO. A health

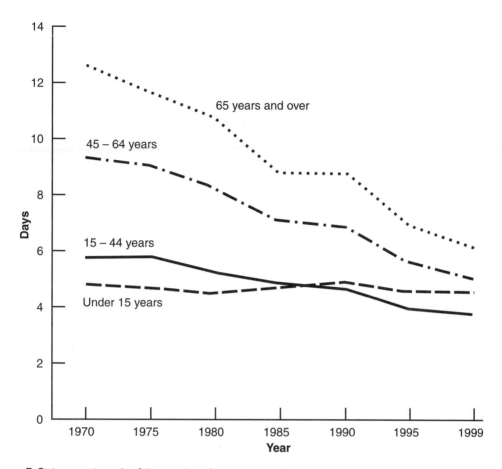

Figure 7-3 Average Length of Stay in Days by Age, United States, 1970–1999

Source: Popovic JR. *1999 National Hospital Discharge Survey: Annual Summary with Detailed Diagnosis and Procedure Data.* National Center for Health Statistics. *Vital Health Stat.* 2001;13(151). Available at: http://www.cdc.gov/nchs/data/series/sr_13/sr13_151.pdf. Accessed July 16, 2006.

maintenance organization (HMO) has potentially greater ability to have a more restricted network than would a preferred provider organization (PPO) or other non-HMO type of health plan. In past decades, HMOs did indeed seek to contract with a sharply limited number of hospitals so as to best obtain significant discounts in return for channeling patients. In the past decade, however, that dynamic has eroded as a result of market desires for broad networks. Nevertheless, HMOs still are most likely to contract with fewer hospitals than other types of health plans, if not to the same degree as in the past. PPOs generally seek to contract with as many hospitals as possible, though if reimbursement

terms are considered inadequate, a PPO could in fact have fewer hospitals in a market than might a large HMO as a result of hospitals' declining to contract.

Credentialing or Privileging

Hospital credentialing refers to the requirement that the hospital meets applicable accreditation standards. Hospital accreditation is almost always carried out by the Joint Commission on Accreditation of Health Care Organizations* (JCAHO; see also Chapter 23

———————

*See http://www.jointcommission.org.

regarding accreditation). For community hospitals, this is usually sufficient, and no further credentialing is done.

In other cases, an MCO will take further steps in this process as it applies to certain types of care; for example, cardiac surgery, bariatric surgery, and so forth. A hospital would need to meet certain criteria for the MCO to provide benefits for those specific services; for example, a hospital must do a minimum number of cardiac bypass operations each year and meet defined outcomes criteria, or it must meet certain staffing criteria for the intensive care unit, and the like. If a hospital meets the specific criteria for a defined set of procedures, it may be considered a "center of excellence" and the MCO will selectively refer those types of cases to it.

Evaluating Hospitals

Evaluating hospitals for an MCO is done by balancing a number of variables. In a small or rural market there may be limited or even no choices. In many urban and suburban locations, local and regional hospital consolidation has led to a significant rise in market power by the hospital systems, leading to fewer or no alternatives as regards what hospitals an MCO must have in its network. In some cases, there will be some level of competition between relatively equal hospital choices, providing some degree of latitude in the contracting process.

Before beginning the selection process, plan management must first decide how much they are willing to limit the choices in the plan. Generally, the more the MCO is willing to limit the number of participating hospitals, the greater the leverage in negotiating. Limiting the number has significant disadvantages as well. If the MCO strictly limits itself to just a few hospitals, it will have a competitive disadvantage in the marketplace because prospective members and accounts often use hospitals as a means of judging whether to join an MCO; therefore, if the plan fails to include a sufficient selection of hospitals, it will see disappointing marketing results.

The first step in the contracting process is the creation of information from a combination of hard data—such as occupancy and cost, as discussed later, and services offered—as well as judgment about the hospital's willingness to negotiate and the perception of the public and physician community about the hospital's quality. It does little good for an MCO to make an agreement with a hospital that is perceived as inferior. Likewise, it is less than optimal to contract with a hospital that does not do high-volume obstetrics if there is a regional competitor that does because the plan will be less attractive to young families.

In some instances, the presence of a well-run integrated delivery system (see Chapter 2) makes a particular hospital attractive. This is most likely to be the case if a plan is a new entrant to the market, is introducing a new service line, or has been unable to create an attractive network from a marketing standpoint. The IDS may be in a position to accept considerable financial risk, such as total capitation, which may be desirable to an HMO that wishes to limit financial risk; such risk arrangements have become far less common in recent years, however, as discussed in Chapter 2.

If the hospital is a sponsor or joint venture partner in an MCO, the choice factors become rather clear. If a hospital is an enthusiastic supporter of the MCO, or if there is a long history of a good working relationship, that should also be taken into consideration. Of course, the reverse is equally true: If a hospital or IDS owns a health plan that competes, an MCO may choose not to subsidize that competitor by channeling business to the parent hospital or IDS.

General Negotiating Strategy

Setting an overall strategy is important to the ultimate success of an MCO's hospital network. It is certainly possible to approach the project of hospital negotiations by using the managerial equivalent of Brownian motion, but the end results will be tepid. An MCO's ability to negotiate successfully with the hospitals in its area depends on a number of things. Chief among them are the personal abilities of the negotiator, the size of the plan, the MCO's ability to actually shift patient care, the MCO's past payment history regarding both timeliness of payment and policies regarding recoding submitted claims, and the past track record of the MCO in delivering what was promised.

The strategy should address both regional and plan-wide issues. There may be one set of criteria for primary care services in a service area and a different set for tertiary services; for example, an MCO may want to approach some hospitals for tertiary services on a much wider regional basis than it does for primary care. Hospitals and systems also need to be prioritized as to importance to the MCO. If the MCO does not intend to restrict its hospital panel significantly, then first priority would go to those hospitals with the most marketing value. An MCO that is willing to restrict its network must also develop a "best alternative to negotiated agreement," or BATNA. The BATNA will vary widely across an MCO's service area depending on the degree of competition between hospitals and the necessity of having a particular hospital or system in the network viable in the market.

Medicare Advantage

A special situation exists as regards Medicare Advantage (MA), the Medicare risk-based managed care program (see Chapter 26). All of the reimbursement options discussed later in this chapter may be used, but in the event that a hospital refuses to contract with a Medicare Advantage plan and that hospital is essential to meet access requirements, then the plan may essentially include the hospital in its network and reimburse it using Medicare's traditional reimbursement terms. Specifically:

- Additionally, an MA regional plan, upon CMS [Centers for Medicare and Medicaid Services] preapproval, can use

methods other than written agreements to establish that access requirements are met.

- An MA regional plan may seek reimbursement upon application to CMS and upon the following requirements being met and demonstrated to CMS:

1. The plan needs to contract with a general acute hospital to meet access requirements;
2. The plan has first made a good faith effort to contract with this hospital;
3. There are no competing Medicare participating hospitals in the area to which MA regional plan enrollees could reasonably be referred for inpatient hospital services;
4. The plan designates this hospital for all in-network inpatient hospital services; and
5. All requirements in 42 CFR 422.112(c)(1)-(4) are satisfied then the plan may designate this hospital as an essential hospital with normal in-network cost sharing levels applying to all plan members.[3]

Data Development

In most cases, an MCO will have considerable history regarding its own payments to the hospital, and in the case of a relatively sophisticated MCO, analysis will provide data that incorporates severity adjustments and other modifiers to enable accurate comparisons between hospitals for similar types of care. In the absence of historical data, an MCO will want to see a hospital's chargemaster (also called a charge master).

The chargemaster is simply a list of what the hospital charges for each and every thing it bills for, and it can contain between 15,000 and 25,000 items, each item represented by a type of nomenclature or code. The Health Insurance Portability and Accountability Act (HIPAA; see Chapter 32) requires that any hospital that uses electronic billing (which is all of them) must use standard code sets: the International Classification of Disease, 9th Revision, Clinical Modification (ICD-9-CM),* Healthcare (previously HCFA) Common Procedural Coding System (HCPCS), and Current Procedural Technology, 4th Revision (CPT-4), though these are generally included in the HCPCS codes when used by hospitals. There is no uniformity from hospital to hospital regarding charges for the same procedures, with even the federal government reporting pricing variances of 259% across the United States.[4]

The chargemaster does not represent what the hospital is actually paid for all of those billable procedures; it is the maximum that a hospital will charge. In the aggregate, the ratio of gross charges to payments received is 2.6; in other words, hospitals on average are paid roughly 38% of charges from private and government payers.[5] Only the uninsured routinely face having to pay the full charges reflected in the chargemaster because they do not have coverage from a health plan that has negotiated reimbursement at levels below full charges; though some hospitals are now accepting less than full charges from some uninsured patients, this is always on a case-by-case basis. Health plans, too, can face full charges when members incur emergency services outside of the service area, and that is discussed separately later.

It is important to know the hospital's occupancy rate (these data may be available from the local or state health department, the American Hospital Association,[6] or in the hospital's annual report) and operating margin (this too may be available at the health department or may be published in the hos-

pital's annual report). These have an obvious direct bearing on the willingness of a hospital to negotiate. An MCO will also need to quantify how many bed days the plan incurs at the hospital during the year and the types of services for those days, for example, medical/surgical, obstetrics, intensive care, mental health, and so forth. An often overlooked aspect of the financial analysis is the cost of outpatient procedures. As discussed more fully later in this chapter, performing a procedure on an outpatient basis is not necessarily less costly than doing it as an inpatient.

In addition to the actual reimbursement, it is important for an MCO to know how quickly it pays the hospital. Hospitals are very sensitive to cash flow, particularly because government payers are not always prompt. If an MCO does not pay promptly (eg, within 30 days), that is sure to be a contentious issue regardless of the cause of slow payments. The other important issue to document is how often the MCO makes downward adjustments to bills and why because those too are frequent issues in negotiations. Although payment timeliness and charge recoding are not the topic of this chapter, these are issues important to any hospital and will be addressed during any negotiation. Related to this, the ability of a hospital and MCO to interact administratively and the ability to resolve operating problems on an ongoing basis play heavily in the negotiating strategy.

The last thing the plan must do is to make a realistic assessment of its ability to shift patients from the hospital in the event of a highly unfavorable negotiation. This is not a BATNA that can be taken lightly, of course, because of the disruption that would occur for both members and network physicians. It also may not be an all-or-none approach but rather one of shifting a portion; for example, shifting routine cases away but still using the hospital for complex cases or shifting away all elective outpatient procedures (which tend to be highly profitable). In some cases, there is no alternative because of market consolidation, or the MCO is simply not

---

*ICD-9-CM will eventually be replaced by ICD-10, but the timing of that is not known at the time of publication.

predicated on a model that provides for shifting cases (for example, a PPO that does not employ significant medical management).

Many other variables can affect a negotiation, but the preceding should be considered the minimum that needs to be understood prior to commencing a negotiation regarding reimbursement.

TIERED NETWORKS

As discussed earlier, there is great variability in cost between hospitals. There is also variability in quality. Though that is somewhat more difficult to measure on a broad basis, it is possible to measure quality of selected processes and outcomes. The MCO can ameliorate that difference to some degree, or considerable degree, through its negotiating and contracting process as discussed later. If a substantial difference in cost between hospitals for similar services remains even after best efforts at negotiation, the MCO has a limited set of responses.

One response is to terminate or let lapse the contract, requiring members and physicians to use alternative hospitals. This is a worst-case scenario and may not be possible in many situations in which a hospital or hospital system is required to provide adequate access, and even when it is possible, it is highly disruptive. The second alternative is to endure substantial cost increases, passing those costs on to the MCO's customers when rate renewals occur, adding more fuel to the inflationary fires. The third option is to accept the high cost increases but attempt to selectively shift cases away from the high-cost hospital when possible.

The basic benefits design prevalent throughout the past two decades has been one of identical coverage to a member, regardless of in which hospital care was received. For example, a member may pay no deductible or else a modest fixed deductible such as $200 per admission, whether admitted to a high-cost or a low-cost hospital. Members whose benefits provided for co-insurance as well as a deductible, for example, 20% of allowed charges* after the deductible has been met, did share some of the added financial burden when using a high-cost hospital, though it was and is rare that the member knows ahead of time what that amount will be.

A tightly managed HMO may address the problem of high-cost hospitals primarily through medical management, aggressively shifting nonemergency admissions from a high-cost to a low-cost hospital at the time of precertification (see Chapter 9). All other types of MCOs, including many HMOs, may also consider modifying the benefits design so as to facilitate the use of lower cost hospitals by clearly differentiating an out-of-pocket financial cost to the member; that is, it will cost the member more out-of-pocket to use a high-cost hospital than it will to use a low-cost one. This is simply applying an economic barrier (or conversely, supplying an economic enabler) to influence where a member chooses to go for elective admissions; this also requires cooperation on the part of the admitting physician. Put in less harsh terms, tiered networks encourage consumers to participate actively in managing their own health care costs.

This is approach is known as tiering. Hospitals that are in the first or core tier require the member to pay the lowest deductible and/or copayment or co-insurance, if the member even needs to pay anything at all. A hospital in the second or premium tier would require the member to pay a higher deductible and/or copayment or co-insurance. It is also possible though not common to have a third tier requiring an even higher out-

---

*Allowed charges refer to what the MCO and hospital have agreed to contractually, not necessarily what the nondiscounted charges are. For example, the hospital may bill $10,000 for an inpatient stay, but the plan has negotiated a 20% discount, so the allowed charges are $8,000 and the member is responsible for 20% of the $8,000, not of the $10,000; for simplicity's sake, this example does not include the effect of a deductible.

of-pocket payment by members; a third tier may also refer to out-of-network or noncontracted hospitals. Differentials in out-of-pocket are usually not applied to emergency services because by definition such services are not elective. Tiering may also be applied only to a subset of routine services, such as routine elective surgery or obstetrics. Last, as noted in Chapter 5, tiering may also be applied to specialty physicians, though that is less common than it is for hospitals.

The presence of tiering in a marketplace is highly variable. In 2003, for example, the Center for Studying Health System Change reported that in 12 representative communities, half had at least launched a tiered network and most of the rest were considering it, though several that did launch a tiered network abandoned it.[7] The differences in out-of-pocket costs to members between tiers are also quite variable, at least in the 2002/2003 period, with additional cost per day varying between $100.00 and $750.00, or 10% to 30% co-insurance.[8,3] Last, hospital tiers need not be applied evenly across the MCO. In some cases, tiers are created at the request of specific employers rather than being applied to all products; in other cases, tiers are only applied to products that specifically incorporate hospital tiering into their benefit structure.

Cost is not necessarily the sole criteria used. Although cost considerations are usually present, quality and outcome measures are also incorporated by some health plans that have created hospital tiers. Quality measures may be part of a national initiative such as the Leapfrog Group* or CMS. Measures can also be specific to the health plan and look at measures such as compliance with treatment protocols for acute myocardial infarction, patient safety, and other measures. In many markets, such measures are being used more for performance-based incentives or so-called pay for performance, rather than tiering, as discussed fully in Chapter 8.

High-cost hospitals tend to resist tiering for the obvious reason that it steers patients

*See http://www.leapfroggroup.org.

away. In markets where high-cost hospitals are part of a larger and desirable system, it is not uncommon for the system to require the MCO to put all of the system's hospitals in the network at the lower tier or else lose the system entirely. This becomes an even greater threat if the system is an IDS and the MCO would lose not only the hospital system, but a considerable part of the physician network as well. Alternatively, an expensive tertiary hospital may make it clear that if patients are steered away, the hospital will refuse to participate at all, subjecting the plan and its members (if co-insurance is present) to a high degree of financial exposure.

SUBACUTE CARE: SKILLED OR INTERMEDIATE NURSING FACILITIES

In addition to contracting with acute care hospitals, MCOs need to contract with at least one subacute facility (ie, a skilled or intermediate nursing facility) and/or rehabilitation facility within the service area. Subacute facilities are well suited for prolonged convalescence or recovery cases (eg, a patient requiring prolonged traction, a frail patient requiring prolonged intravenous antibiotics for a deeply seated infection, or a patient requiring prolonged stroke rehabilitation), if home therapy is not appropriate for some reason, because the cost for a bed-day in a subacute facility is much less than it is in an acute care hospital. In other cases, a patient may be able to be cared for at home, but it is still more cost-effective to deliver the therapy in the subacute facility because of more favorable pricing achievable through economies of scale.

The MCO should contract only with those subacute facilities that meet the plan's (and implicitly the plan members') needs for pleasant surroundings, even if there may be a better price elsewhere. For example, the facility might ensure that the plan's members are given a private room or are placed in a room with a patient with a similar functional status, and in a section of the facility that has a clean and pleasant environment.

TYPES OF REIMBURSEMENT ARRANGEMENTS

A number of reimbursement methodologies are available in contracting with hospitals, except in those rare states where regulations diminish or prohibit creativity. Table 7-1 lists a number of methods that have been used by plans, but it is not exhaustive. Table 7-2 illus-

Table 7–1 Models for Reimbursing Hospitals

- Charges
- Discounts
- Per diems
- Sliding scales for discounts and per diems
- Differential by day in hospital
- Diagnosis-related groups (DRGs) and Medicare Severity DRGs (MS-DRGs)
- Differential by service type
- Case rates
  - Institutional only
  - Package pricing or bundled rates
- Capitation
- Percentage of premium revenue
- Contact capitation (uncommon)
- Bed leasing (very uncommon)
- Periodic interim payments or cash advances
- Performance-based incentives
  - Quality and service incentives
  - Penalties and withholds
- Ambulatory patient groups (APGs) and ambulatory payment classifications (APCs) for outpatient care

Table 7–2 Hospital Reimbursement Methodologies by HMOs, July 1, 2003

Capitation	12.0%
Per diems	44.1
DRGs	24.1
Fee schedules	24.3

Source: HealthLeaders-InterStudy, Used with Permission from http://www.healthleaders-interstudy.com/.

trates the average distribution of hospital reimbursement methodologies by HMOs as of July 1, 2003; distribution of methodologies by MCOs other than HMOs would not include capitation.

Management on either side of the equation must account for their internal ability to manage these financial terms in their information systems. The more one is dependent on manual intervention and adjustment, the higher the error rate, the higher the cost of administration of the contract, and the greater the need for reconciliations.

Under HIPAA, transactions and code sets were standardized, as discussed in Chapters 17 and 32. An unintended consequence of this was a diminution of variety in reimbursement arrangements. Creative arrangements such as certain types of package pricing (discussed later) were administered through the use of unique, nonstandard billing codes that were programmed by the MCO's claims system to pay based on the negotiated terms. With the elimination of any use of nonstandard codes, MCOs either had to find different ways to support the logic or else eliminate creative arrangements in favor of more straightforward reimbursement methods.

Ad Hoc Negotiations

Before discussing contractually agreed upon reimbursement methodologies, it is worthwhile briefly discussing the role of ad hoc negotiations. This simply refers to the fact that members sometimes receive care from a hospital that does not have a contract with the health plan. For example, a member may have a heart attack or a motor vehicle accident while outside the plan's service area. When that happens, the MCO is potentially exposed to the full brunt of the fees associated with the hospital's chargemaster.

Most MCOs these days contract with so-called rental PPOs (see Chapter 2) to provide for contractual reimbursement terms for care provided outside the MCO's own contracted network. In other words, if a member receives services from a hospital that is not in the MCO's own network but is in another PPO, and if the MCO has a contract with that other PPO, then the reimbursement terms of the rental PPO are in force. In past years, health plans did not always make it clear that they had such contracts with rental PPOs, and a hospital that contracted with the PPO but not the MCO itself would find itself receiving the PPO reimbursement and not the billed charges, requiring it to write down the difference. This situation was called a "stealth PPO" and is now uncommon, with MCOs that have such rental PPO agreements in place ensuring that someplace on the member's identification card is a logo of the rental PPO.

In the absence of a rental PPO arrangement for out-of-network services, health plans have a unit that is responsible for negotiating with noncontracted providers for individual, highly expensive cases. In the case of emergency care, the health plan clearly has an obligation to provide coverage, but it is in the financial interest of the health plan, the member, and the provider to agree to what will be charged and what will be paid. This lowers the financial exposure of the health plan for obvious reasons, but it also lowers the member's financial exposure to balance billing for any charges not covered by the plan or as a result of having to pay a percentage co-insurance. The provider in turn is paid quickly and directly, which is of great benefit as noted earlier.

Straight Charges

The simplest (albeit least desirable) payment mechanism in health care is straight charges. It is also obviously the most expensive, after the option of no contract at all. This is a fallback position to be agreed to only in the event that the MCO is unable to obtain any form of discount at all because it is still desirable to have a contract with a no balance billing clause in it (see Chapter 30) for purposes of reserve requirements and licensure. Straight charges are very uncommon in managed care.

Straight Discount on Charges

Another possible arrangement with a hospital is a straight percentage discount on charges. In this case, the hospital submits its claim in full and the plan discounts it by the agreed-to percentage and then pays it. The hospital accepts this amount as payment in full. The amount of discount that can be obtained depends on the factors discussed earlier. This type of arrangement is not infrequent in markets with low levels of managed care penetration and in rural markets, but it is very uncommon in markets with high levels of managed care. When this type of arrangement does exist, an MCO usually at the least requires that no single charge from the chargemaster can exceed a certain degree of inflation from year to year.

Sliding Scale Discount on Charges

Sliding scale discounts are an option, particularly in markets with low managed care penetration but some level of competitiveness between hospitals. With a sliding scale, the percentage discount is reflective of total volume of admissions and outpatient procedures. Whether to lump the two categories together or deal with them separately is not as important as making sure that the parties deal with them both. With the rapidly climbing cost of outpatient charges, savings from reduction of inpatient utilization could be negated by an unanticipated overrun in outpatient charges.

An example of a sliding scale is a 20% reduction in charges for 0 to 200 total bed days per year with incremental increases in the discount up to a maximum percentage. An interim percentage discount is usually negotiated, and the parties reconcile at the end of the year based on the final total volume. The time periods for measurement are also negotiable. For example, the discount could vary on a month-to-month basis rather than yearly. The sliding scale could track total bed days, number of admissions, or whole dollars spent. The most important thing is to be sure that it is a clearly defined and easily measurable objective.

As noted earlier, an important issue to look at in a sliding scale is timeliness of payment. It is likely that the hospital will demand a clause in the contract spelling out the plan's requirement to process claims in a timely manner, usually 30 days or sooner. In some cases, it may negotiate a sliding scale, or a modifier to the main sliding scale, that applies a further reduction based on the plan's ability to turn a clean claim around quickly; for example, an additional 4% discount for paying a clean claim within 7 days of receipt. Conversely, the hospital may demand a penalty for clean claims that are not processed within 30 days. Many states have laws and regulations that require timely payment before the imposition of penalties and interest payments (see Chapter 33), and so the additional discount based on rapid payment must be negotiated using that as the base level.

Straight Per Diem Charges

Unlike straight charges, a negotiated per diem is a single charge for a day in the hospital regardless of any actual charges or costs incurred. In this very common type of arrangement, the plan negotiates a per diem rate with the hospital and pays that rate without adjustments. For example, the plan will pay $1,000 for each day regardless of the actual cost of the service.

Hospital administrators are often reluctant to add days in the intensive care unit or obstetrics to the base per diem unless there is sufficient volume of regular medical-surgical cases to make the ultimate cost predictable. In a small plan, or in a midsized plan with a large number of participating hospitals, the hospital administrator is concerned that the hospital will be used for expensive cases at a low per diem while competitors will be used for less costly cases. In such cases, a good option is to negotiate multiple sets of per diem charges based on service type (*eg*, medical-surgical, obstetrics, intensive care, neonatal intensive care, rehabilitation, and so forth) or a combination of per diems and a flat case rate (see later discussion) for obstetrics.

The key to making a per diem work is predictability. If the plan and hospital can accurately predict the number and mix of cases, then they can accurately calculate a per diem. The per diem is simply an estimate of the charges or costs for an average day in that hospital minus the level of discount. The larger the volume of business between the hospital and the MCO, the more predictable the average daily cost will be.

Although very unusual in actuality, a theoretical disadvantage of the per diem approach is that the per diem must be paid even if the billed charges are less than the per diem rate. For example, if the plan has a per diem arrangement that pays $1,000 per day for medical admissions and the total allowable charges (billed charges less charges for noncovered items provided during the admission) for a 5-day admission are $6,200, the hospital is reimbursed $5,000 for the admission ($1,000 per day × 5 days). This is acceptable as long as the average per diem represents an acceptable discount, but it has been anecdotally reported that some large, self-insured accounts have demanded the lesser of the charges or the per diems for each case (*ie*, laying off the upper end of the risk but harvesting the reward). Such demands are to be avoided because they corrupt the integrity of the per diem calculation.

A plan may also negotiate to reimburse the hospital for expensive surgical implants provided at the hospital's actual cost of the implant. Such reimbursement would be limited to a defined list of implants (*eg*, cochlear implants) where the cost to the hospital for the implant is far greater than is recoverable under the per diem or outpatient arrangement.

Sliding Scale Per Diem

Like the sliding scale discount on charges discussed previously, the sliding scale per diem is also based on total volume. In this case, the plan negotiates an interim per diem that it will pay for each day in the hospital. Depending on the total number of bed days or admissions in the year, the plan will either pay a lump sum settlement at the end of the year or withhold an amount from the final payment for the year to adjust for an additional reduction in the per diem from an increase in total bed days or admissions. It may be preferable to make an arrangement whereby on a quarterly or semiannual basis the plan adjusts the interim per diem so as to reduce any disparities caused by unexpected changes in utilization patterns.

Differential by Day in Hospital

This simply refers to the fact that most hospitalizations are more expensive on the first day. For example, the first day for surgical cases includes operating suite costs, the operating surgical team costs (nurses and recovery), and so forth. This type of reimbursement method is generally combined with a per diem approach, but the first day is paid at a higher rate. For example, the first day may be $1,500 and each subsequent day is $750.

Observation Stays

As a result of commercial and government payers refusing to pay for an overnight stay for certain conditions, most hospitals have created observation stays. Such stays are usually 23 hours or less, though it is possible to twist the definition at times to cover more than that. The purpose of the observation stay is just what it implies: to keep an eye on a patient to determine if full admission is warranted. On the one hand, the resources used for an observation stay are similar to those used for a single day of an inpatient stay (usually the first day, which is front-loaded with costs as noted earlier), so the MCO and the hospital may choose to treat it as a single day under the reimbursement methodology. On

the other hand, it may be argued that the patient is not as sick as one that clearly requires admission and therefore an observation stay should be reimbursed at a lesser rate. The latter is more commonly the case when negotiating payment for observation stays.

Step-Down Units

A step-down unit is a ward or section of a ward in an acute-care hospital that is used in much the same way as a subacute nursing facility. A patient who requires less care and monitoring, such as someone recovering from a hip replacement (after all the drains have been removed), may need only bed rest, traction, and minimal nursing care. In recognition of the lesser resource needs, the charge per day should be less.

Refusal to Pay for Serious Errors or Internal Inefficiencies

In any reimbursement method that is based on charges and/or days in the hospital, many MCOs refuse to pay for services that are incurred either as a result of hospital errors or inefficiencies. For example, if a patient is admitted for a routine surgical procedure, but surgery is delayed because of scheduling problems, the MCO will not pay for the extra day. Similarly, if a patient is admitted on a weekend and the hospital is unable to perform certain necessary diagnostic tests (*eg*, radiology specialty procedures are not open on weekends), the MCO will not pay for the weekend days that the patient spends.

More serious are medical errors, sometimes referred to as "never events" because they are events that should never happen to a patient in the hospital. In 2002, the National Quality Forum* defined 27 such never events in six categories: "Surgical events (*eg*, surgery being performed on the wrong patient or wrong body part), product or device events (*eg*, using contaminated drugs), patient pro-

---

*See http://www.qualityforum.org.

tection events (*eg*, an infant discharged to the wrong person), care management events (*eg*, a medication error), environmental events (*eg*, electric shock or burn), and criminal events (*eg*, sexual assault of a patient)."[10] The MCO would not pay any costs associated with such never events,[†] and indeed the hospital should not charge for them.

Somewhat less clear as an example would be a patient that receives the wrong medication, leading to a significant complication. The MCO may refuse to pay for those added days because they were caused by errors by the hospital or its staff. Medication errors that do not lead to significant costs may be subject to performance-based incentive programs as described in Chapter 8.

Diagnosis-Related Groups

Used by Medicare, a common reimbursement methodology also used by commercial health plans is by diagnosis-related groups (DRGs). There are publications of DRG categories, criteria, outliers, and trim points (*ie*, the cost or length of stay that causes the DRG payment to be supplemented or supplanted by another payment mechanism) to enable the plan to negotiate a payment mechanism for DRGs based on Medicare rates or, in some cases, state-regulated rates. DRGs serve to share risk with the hospital, thus making the hospital an active partner in controlling utilization and making plan expenses more manageable. Beginning in 2008 and scheduled for completion in 2009, Medicare will replace standard DRGs with Medicare Severity DRGs (MS-DRGs). MS-DRGs collapse some existing DRGs into fewer categories, while adding DRG codes to account for patients with existing complications or co-morbidities (CCs), or major complications or

co-morbidities (MCCs). This will better align payment to the actual costs to care for such complicated patients.

DRGs are created by CMS or by the commercial payer based on what the hospital bills for the case using the standardized code sets described earlier as well as diagnostic codes. That information is put through a "grouper" who puts the case into the appropriate DRG based on the average use of resources for similar cases. In the case of CMS, actual payments are also adjusted for labor and nonlabor variables, including disproportionate share of low-income patients, indirect teaching costs (for teaching hospitals), cost of living for labor costs, and a few other variables.[11] Trim points are simply the point at which a very complicated and expensive case exceeds the average for the DRG by such a high degree that it is considered an outlier and additional payment is made. With the implementation of MS-DRGs, fewer cases will qualify as outliers.

Service-Related Case Rates

Similar to DRGs, service-related case rates are a cruder cut. In this reimbursement mechanism, various service types are defined (*eg*, medicine, surgery, intensive care, neonatal intensive care, psychiatry, obstetrics, and the like), and the hospital receives a flat per-admission reimbursement for whatever type of service the patient is admitted to (*eg*, all surgical admissions cost $8,100). If services are mixed, a prorated payment may be made (*eg*, 50% of surgical and 50% of intensive care). Never used widely, service-related case rates have largely been supplanted by DRGs.

Case Rates and Package Pricing

Whatever mechanism a plan uses for hospital reimbursement, it may still need to address certain categories of procedures and negotiate special rates. The most common of these is obstetrics. It is common to negotiate a flat rate or case rate for a normal

---

[†]Gail M. Amundson, MD, FACP; Medical Director, Quality, Measurement and Provider Incentives, HealthPartners, Inc. Personal communication, July 21, 2006.

vaginal delivery and a flat rate or case rate for a cesarean section or a blended rate for both. In the case of blended case rates (which are much preferred over separate rates for the two types of deliveries), the expected reimbursement for each type of delivery is multiplied by the expected (or desired) percentage of utilization. For example, a case rate for vaginal delivery is $3,500, and for cesarean section it is $5,000. Utilization is expected to be 80% vaginal and 20% cesarean section, and therefore the case rate is $3,800 ($3,500 × 0.8 = $2,800; $5,000 × 0.2 = $1,000; $2,800 + $1,000 = $3,800).

Other common areas for which case rates are used are specialty procedures at tertiary hospitals, for example, coronary artery bypass surgery, heart transplants, or certain types of cancer treatment. These procedures, although relatively infrequent, are tremendously costly.

A broader variation is package pricing or bundled case rates. As discussed in Chapter 6, the package price or bundled case rate refers to an all-inclusive rate paid for both institutional and professional services. The plan negotiates a flat rate for a procedure (eg, coronary artery bypass surgery or cataract surgery), and that rate is used to pay all parties who provide services connected with that procedure, including preadmission and postdischarge care. Bundled case rates are not uncommon in teaching facilities where there is a faculty practice plan that works closely with the hospital.

Capitation or Percentage of Revenue

Capitation refers to reimbursing the hospital on a per member per month (PMPM) basis to cover all institutional costs for a defined population of members. The use of capitation is generally restricted to HMOs, though HMOs do not use capitation exclusively. The payment may be varied by age and sex but does not fluctuate with premium revenue. Severity-adjusted capitation is still relatively uncommon, but as CMS fully converts to severity-adjusted payments for Medicare Advantage plans (see Chapter 26), those plans may also begin to adjust capitation payments to hospitals. Severity adjustments for commercial members are also feasible using existing methodologies.

Percentage of revenue refers to a fixed percentage of premium revenue (ie, a percentage of the collected premium rate) being paid to the hospital, again to cover all institutional services. The difference between percentage of revenue and capitation is that percentage of revenue may vary with the premium rate charged and the actual revenue yield. Although capitation and percentage of premium revenue are essentially the same for public sector programs (ie, risk contracts for Medicare and Medicaid), that is not the case for the commercial sector. For commercial products, percentages vary most commonly based on benefit plan design (eg, the level of copayments the member must make), but there are other reasons as well. In the event the plan fails to develop rates or perform underwriting properly (or gets caught up in a price war), a proportionate percentage of that shortfall is passed directly to the hospital.

In all cases, the hospital bears the entire risk for institutional services for the defined membership base; if the hospital cannot provide the services itself, the cost for such care is deducted from the capitation payment. For this type of arrangement to work, a hospital must know that it will serve a clearly defined segment of a plan's enrollment and that it can provide most of the necessary services to those members. In these cases, the primary care physician is clearly associated with just one hospital. Alternatively, if the plan is dealing with a multihospital system with multiple facilities in the plan's service area, it may be reasonable to expect that the hospitals in the system can care for the plan's members on an exclusive basis.

As for physician capitation (see Chapter 6), there needs to be a clear definition of what is covered under the capitation and what is not. For example, the capitation may include outpatient procedures, but the plan and hospital need to account for outpatient procedures that are being performed outside of the hospital's domain. Will home health be part of the capitation, and if so, what agency? It is preferable to not place the hospital at-risk for services it cannot control, as long as there is a clear definition of what those services are.

The hospital must also perform aggressive utilization management (UM) to see any margin from capitation; if UM is carried out so as to ruffle the least number of feathers of attending staff, the hospital will pay a stiff price since it is the hospital, not the physicians, that is at financial risk for inpatient costs. More advanced methods of managing utilization are also clearly in the hospital's financial benefit. For example, advanced disease management results in a general reduction of inpatient hospital stays. It is therefore in the interests of the hospital to ensure that such programs exist and are optimally managed. The various forms of medical management are discussed in detail in Chapters 9 through 11.

The hospital also needs to have stop-loss insurance to protect it against catastrophic cases. This stop-loss coverage may be provided by the MCO; for example, the plan may reimburse the hospital at a low per diem for all days of a case after it has been in the hospital for a number of days (*eg*, beyond 30 days in a year). Alternatively, the plan may pay a percentage of charges after a certain charge level has been reached and the plan's own reinsurance comes into play. For capitated hospitals, if the MCO does not provide the stop loss, then the hospital should purchase it from an outside company specializing in such products.

Point-of-service (POS) plans with an out-of-network benefit make capitation methods difficult to use. As discussed in Chapter 6, capitation in POS may mean having to pay twice for a service, once under capitation and again if the member seeks service outside the network. In areas where there are no real alternatives to a certain hospital (*eg*, a rural

area or an area where a hospital enjoys a monopoly), this problem may not be material, but that is the exception. Contact capitation, as noted later, may also attenuate this problem. The alternative is to deduct out-of-area costs from the capitation payment.

The advantage of capitation to an MCO is that it is not only budgetable but results in laying off all or most of the risk for institutional expenses. The hospital becomes a full partner in controlling utilization, and the plan has less need to try to control utilization. A problem is that the plan realizes none of the savings for improved utilization control. Another problem can arise if the hospital refuses to share any of the savings (calculated as though there were a per diem or discounted charges model) with the physicians who are controlling the cases.

The most important problem to note is that some hospitals are simply not able to manage the financial risk associated with capitation. The financial management tools and expertise, utilization management, and data requirements in a hospital may not be adequate to manage the risk associated with a broad population of members. In situations where there is a small base of capitated lives, chance becomes equally or even more important than clinical management. In the event that capitation results in severe financial results, nothing but harm and poor future relations will result. It should therefore be a requirement that when an MCO capitates a hospital or IDS, the MCO is able to ascertain whether the provider system has the necessary capabilities, and a mechanism for regular monitoring of results must be in place. Because of this risk of financial loss, the use of capitation has been declining in recent years.

Closely related to hospital capitation is the idea of global capitation, in which an IDS accepts capitation or percentage of premium revenue in exchange for total risk for medical services, as is discussed in Chapter 5. In the past, for-profit physician practice management companies also accepted global capitation but were unable to manage costs successfully, leading to massive failures as described in Chapter 2. Global capitation still does exist in some pockets around the country (primarily California) but is now relatively uncommon.

Contact Capitation

Contact capitation of hospitals is similar to contact capitation for specialty physicians as discussed in Chapter 6. Like contact capitation for specialty physicians, this method of reimbursement is not common. In short, the capitation is tied to the percentage of admissions to a hospital, with adjustments made for the type of service provided. As an example (not adjusting for service type), the capitation rate is $80 PMPM.* The plan has 500,000 members, and 50% of admissions go to that hospital system that month. The payment therefore is $80 × (500,000 × 0.5) = $20,000,000.

Adjusting for service type is usually required, however, unless it is clear to all parties that there is no relevant reason for such an adjustment (eg, the population covered by capitation is large, the number of hospitals participating is low, and the services offered are equal between the different hospitals). *Type-of-service adjustment* simply means more categories in which the percentages must be calculated or an adjustment takes place in the payment by some factor that accounts for the acuity. As an example, using the same base capitation and population size noted previously, if hospital A has 10% more intensive care days in its mix than does hospital B, and intensive care days are considered twice as costly as other days, then the percentage of the capitation payment is adjusted by that amount; in this case, hospital A receives $24,000,000, and hospital B receives $16,000,000. This adjusted percentage = the actual percentage plus or minus

the percentage adjustment. For hospital A, it is ($80 × 500,000) × [(0.5 + (0.5 × 0.1)] = $80 × (500,000 × 0.6) = $24,000,000. For hospital B, it is ($80 × 500,000) × [0.5 − (0.5 × 0.1)] = $80 × (500,000 × 0.4) = $16,000,000.)

Such adjustments can quickly become complicated, particularly when there are more than two types of service-type adjustments to be made. And like contact capitation for specialty physicians, this system requires sophisticated information systems and is often not an automated function, thus requiring manual administration. Unlike specialty physician contact capitation, though, the number of participants is lower and therefore at least theoretically more manageable.

As noted earlier, this form of reimbursement can also be combined with case rates or other capitation rates. Obstetrics is the most common reason for having an additional reimbursement system, with the cost of obstetrics being carved out of the basic capitation rate and payment for obstetrical services occurring either through case rates or a separate capitation.

Periodic Interim Payments and Cash Advances

Once common but now less so, periodic interim payments (PIPs) and cash advances are methods whereby the plan advances to a hospital cash to cover expected claims. This cash advance is periodically replenished if it gets below a certain amount. Claims may be applied directly against the cash advance or may be paid outside it, in which case the cash advance serves as an advance deposit. The value of this to a hospital is obvious: positive cash flow. PIPs and cash advances are quite valuable to a hospital and can generate a discount in and of themselves.

This is also a mechanism that has great application in those cases where an MCO's claims systems are overwhelmed or the MCO is otherwise unable to process payments in a timely manner. The cash advance enables

---

*As always, example capitation numbers are fictitious and used solely for illustrative purposes.

the MCO to meet timely payment provisions and keeps the hospital financially sound, while allowing additional time for the MCO to clean up its payment systems.

Performance-Based Reimbursement Service and Quality Incentives

The largest portion of reimbursement to hospitals is likely to be done under one or more of the methods described earlier. Capitation is clearly an example of performance-based reimbursement in that the hospital only profits if it can provide services at a low cost and a high level of quality but is based solely on utilization. MCOs can also apply performance-based financial incentives to hospitals, so-called pay-for-performance, regardless of whether capitation is involved. This topic is discussed in Chapter 8.

Penalties and Withholds

As with physician services (see Chapter 6), penalties or withholds occasionally are used in hospital reimbursement methods. As an example, a plan may negotiate with a hospital to allow the hospital's own utilization management department to perform all the basic utilization and case management functions (see Chapters 9 and 11). As part of that negotiation, goals are set for average length of stay and average admission rate. Part of the payment to the hospital may be withheld, or conversely the plan may set aside a bonus pool. In any event, if the goals are met or exceeded, the hospital receives its withhold or bonus, and vice versa. One complication with this is the possibility that a hospital can make its statistics look good by simply sending patients to other hospitals; this is similar to problems encountered with physician capitation. If a service area is clearly defined, or if the hospital is capitated, then it may be easier to apply a risk or reward program. The reader should be aware, however, that there is evidence from at least one older study that financial penalty models applied to hospitals have little or no effect on utilization or physician performance.[12] The use of penalties and withholds is now very uncommon.

SINGLE-SPECIALTY HOSPITALS

A single-specialty hospital is one that focuses solely on a restricted set of procedures that are performed in an inpatient setting (though the hospital also provides services for outpatient procedures as well). Examples include hospitals that do only cardiac procedures or orthopedic procedures. Because they restrict themselves to elective procedures within a single specialty, these hospitals do not have emergency departments nor are they equipped to handle patients with multiple and severe medical conditions; for example, a cardiac patient with poorly controlled diabetes that might require a fully staffed medical intensive care unit.

Almost always investor-owned, single-specialty hospitals have been subject to criticism, especially by community and tertiary hospitals who accuse them of "skimming" off the most lucrative cases (*ie*, relatively healthy patients requiring fewer resources who are also covered by either private insurance or Medicare), leaving the regular hospitals to deal with sicker patients, less remuneration, and a requirement to provide a broad array of services.[13]

Some MCOs have criticized them based on a frequent ownership model in which the physicians who admit patients to the single-specialty hospital are also investors in it. The argument is similar to that expressed later in this chapter about physician ownership of ancillary services: If the physician has a financial interest in increasing utilization, such increases will occur. According to the General Accounting Office (GAO) of the federal government, 70% of specialty hospitals (either existing or under development) that reported ownership data to the GAO had some physician ownership, and the average rate of physician ownership was just over 50%.[14]

At the time of publication, the legal and regulatory prohibitions against physician ownership that are discussed under ancillary services did not apply because there is an exemption for "whole hospitals" because they are freestanding facilities. Subsequent to the growth of single-specialty hospitals, the Medicare Modernization Act (MMA; see also Chapter 26) placed a moratorium on allowing physicians to self-refer to *new* single-specialty hospitals (existing ones were not included) in which they had an equity interest;[15] that moratorium was to expire June 2005 but was extended by a year, however on May 18, 2006, CMS lifted the moratorium. In that same press release, CMS* stated that it intends to alter its reimbursement methodologies for both inpatient care and ambulatory surgical centers to account for differences in severity of illness and other cost factors in comparison to community and tertiary hospitals[16] and that effort remains a work in progress.

MCOs differ widely in their approach to single-specialty hospitals. Some avoid them because of the physician equity issue, as noted. Others choose to contract with them because of lower costs. When an MCO does contract with a single-specialty hospital, it is common for the general and tertiary hospitals in the MCO's network to demand an increase in reimbursement because presumably those cases not serviced at the single-specialty hospital will be sicker and require more resources, or at the least a general and tertiary hospital must maintain the capability of caring for severely ill patients.

EMERGENCY DEPARTMENT

Except in some cases of capitation, how the MCO reimburses the hospital for inpatient services differs from how it reimburses for emergency department (ED) services. Methodologies for reimbursing for ED services are similar to those discussed later for outpatient procedures, though ED reimbursement and elective outpatient procedure reimbursement may be dealt with differently from each other. Utilization of the ED has been increasing even as the number of EDs decreased, as illustrated in Figure 7-4 (the data represents all payers, not just MCOs), with ED utilization increasing by 14% from 1997 to 2000, from 94.9 million to 108.0 million visits annually, while the number of hospital EDs in the United States decreased from 4,005 to 3,934.[17]

How an ED is used by patients is variable, as would be expected. For ED use overall (not specific to managed care), the reported percentage distribution of emergency department visits, by immediacy with which patient should be seen, in 2004 was as follows:

- Urgent: 37.8%
- Semiurgent: 21.8%
- No triage or unknown: 15.1%
- Emergent: 12.9%
- Nonurgent: 12.5%[18]

Unlike other services, hospitals have a legal requirement regarding emergency services. In 1986, the federal government passed the Emergency Medical Treatment and Active Labor Act (EMTALA) to prevent transfer or "dumping" of uninsured patients by private hospitals to public hospitals.[19] EMTALA requires that all patients presenting to any hospital ED must have a medical screening exam performed by qualified personnel, usually the emergency physician. The medical screening exam cannot be delayed for insurance reasons: either to obtain insurance information or to obtain preauthorization for examination. Although theoretically an MCO could deny payment even though the ED was required by law to provide services, hospitals rightly refused to agree to those terms.

To address inappropriate use of the ED by members for what should be routine care, it is

---

*CMS Press Release, May 18, 2006. http://www.cms.hhs.gov/apps/media/press/release.asp?Counter = 1860. Accessed September 15, 2006.

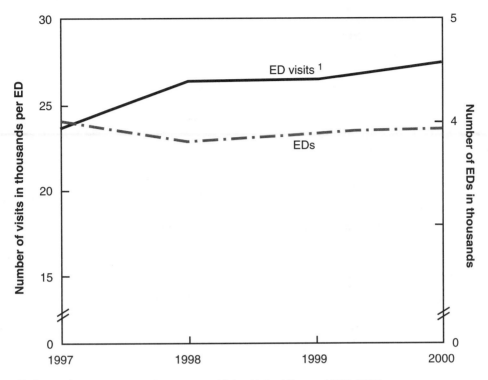

Figure 7–4 Trends in Emergency Department Visits, United States, 1997–2000

Source: McCaig LF, Ly N. *National Hospital Ambulatory Medical Care Survey: 2000 Emergency Department Summary.* Advance data from vital and health statistics; no. 326. Hyattsville, Md: National Center for Health Statistics; 2002. Available at: http://www.cdc.gov/nchs/data/ad/ad326.pdf. Accessed July 16, 2006.

not uncommon for an MCO to impose higher copayments or co-insurance on ED visits that do not lead to hospitalization. This does not in itself differentiate between appropriate and inappropriate use of the ED, but in past studies it does appear that increased cost sharing does lower the use of inappropriate use, as is discussed (and appropriately referenced) in Chapter 9 regarding utilization management.

One unique aspect of the ED is its function as a gateway to admission to the hospital. In the case of trauma or other obvious significant medical conditions, this is a proper and expected use of the ED. But because of concerns about legal liability, many EDs have established chest pain protocols that result either in an admission to the cardiac care unit, or in an observation stay, regardless of how serious the patient's condition appears

to be. This results in substantially increased costs to the plan, as well as to the member if the member has co-insurance. Some plans have addressed this problem by negotiating special rates for such admissions when there is no subsequent evidence of a heart attack. Other plans actually contract with specialty management companies to assume responsibility for the evaluation and disposition of these cases at each hospital's ED, as discussed briefly in Chapter 5.

OUTPATIENT PROCEDURES

As mentioned earlier, the shift from inpatient to outpatient care has been dramatic. As care has shifted, so have charges. It is not uncommon to see outpatient charges exceeding the cost of an inpatient day unless steps are taken to address that imbalance. Outpatient procedures may also be conducted in free-standing ambulatory surgery centers (ASCs), which are often owned in whole or in part by physicians; physicians had equity interests in 83% of ASCs, and hospitals have equity interest in 44%.[20] Arguments about ASCs in which physicians hold equity are identical to those discussed under single-specialty hospitals.

Discounts on Charges

Either straight discounts or sliding scale discounts may be applied to outpatient procedures. Some hospitals argue that the cost to deliver highly technical outpatient procedures actually is greater than an average per diem, primarily because the per diem assumes more than a single day in the hospital, thereby spreading the costs over a greater number of reimbursable days. In the past, some plans have responded by simply admitting patients for their outpatient surgery, paying the per diem, and sending the patient home, but as hospitals capacity has declined and there are fewer available beds, as well as the hospital objecting to this practice, this tactic has become uncommon.

Many plans negotiate the cost of outpatient surgery to never exceed the cost of an inpatient day, whereas other plans concede the problem of front-loading surgical services and agree to cap outpatient charges at a fixed percentage of the per diem (eg, 125% of the average per diem).

Many outpatient procedures can also be done at locations other than a hospital, and because such procedures are generally more lucrative than are inpatient stays, hospitals do not want to lose them to competing free-standing sites. This provides an incentive for the hospital to negotiate competitively, but that is not always the case. When cost disparities between hospital-based outpatient procedures and freestanding surgi-center sites are high, MCOs find ways to steer patients to the less costly location. One common approach is tiering as discussed earlier in this

chapter. Another approach is to reimburse physicians differentially based on location of service; in other words, the physician receives a higher fee if the procedure is performed in a low-cost location.

Package Pricing or Bundled Charges

Plans may negotiate package pricing or bundled charges for outpatient procedures. In this method of reimbursement, all the various charges are bundled into one single charge, thereby reducing the problem of unbundling and exploding (ie, charging for multiple codes or brand-new codes where previously only one code was used). Plans may use their own data to develop the bundled charges, or they may use outside data (one commonly used source is the Milliman Care Guidelines*). Bundled charges are generally tied to the principal procedure code used by the facility. Bundled charges may also be added together in the event that more than one procedure is performed, although the second procedure is discounted because the patient was already in the facility and using services.

Related to this approach is tiered rates (not to be confused with tiering as discussed earlier in this chapter). In this case, the outpatient department categorizes all procedures into several different categories. The plan then pays a different rate for each category, but that rate covers all services performed in the outpatient department, and only one category is used at a time (ie, the hospital cannot add several categories together for a single patient encounter).

Ambulatory Visits

Two classification systems have been developed and used in the reimbursement of ambulatory visits or encounters: ambulatory patient groups (APGs) and ambulatory pay-

---

*See http://www.milliman.com.

ment classification (APCs). APGs were developed by 3M[21] as a forerunner and are quite similar to APCs. Both are in the public domain. The APCs have been and are still being implemented by CMS for outpatient prospective payment in hospital outpatient departments and ambulatory surgery centers for Medicare patients.[22] APCs (and less commonly APGs) are also used by a variety of MCOs and Medicaid agencies.

APGs and ACGs are to outpatient services what DRGs are to inpatient ones, although APGs and APCs are based on procedures rather than simply on diagnoses, contain a greater degree of adjustment for severity, and are considerably more complex. They are superior to using charges as a basis of reimbursement for outpatient services because they are inherently less subject to price inflation. Now several commercial systems support these for both MCOs and provider systems.

PRICING TRANSPARENCY

Just as discussed in Chapter 6, the term *price transparency* or *pricing transparency*, sometimes also referred to as cost transparency, simply refers to making information about the cost or price of health care services available to consumers. This is a central tenet of consumer-directed health plans (CDHPs; see Chapters 2 and 20): inform consumers about the cost and quality of services and empower them to make their own decisions. As a practical matter there are some difficulties with doing this, such as needing services on an urgent or acute basis, whether a consumer is capable of distinguishing between differing services, and so forth. But the concept has taken root, and at the time of publication, it is beginning to be implemented, both by health plans and by some providers as well.

Pricing transparency is usually done by posting pricing information on the Internet, usually by the health plan. In some cases this might be available only to registered members of the plan, in other cases it is simply being put out there. At the time of publica-

tion, at least one major hospital chain, HCA, has committed to making its pricing transparent and available to all consumers[23] and others may follow. Whether such posted information will include selected charges from the hospital's chargemaster or will also provide specific information as it applies to various private and governmental payers is not known at the time of publication.

Health plans, too, have made commitments to making cost information available to members. Although the trend is just beginning, a number of health plans provide hospital-specific cost information to members, not only in CDHP products but in all products. This enables consumers to understand how much they will have to pay depending on which particular hospital they go to for selected services. Many CDHPs and health plans also provide assistance with a type of calculator that enables consumers to figure out what their out-of-pocket responsibility will be and the effect on their Health Reimbursement Account or Health Savings Accounts (also discussed in Chapters 2 and 20). What the ultimate impact of this approach will be is not known.

ANCILLARY SERVICES

Ancillary services are those services that are provided as an adjunct to basic primary or specialty services and include most everything other than institutional services (although institutions can provide ancillary services). Ancillary services are broadly divided into diagnostic and therapeutic services. Examples of ancillary diagnostic services include laboratory, routine radiology, nuclear testing, computed tomography (CT), magnetic resonance imaging (MRI), magnetic resonance angiography (MRA), positron emission tomography (PET) scans, electrocardiography, cardiac testing (including plain and nuclear stress testing, other cardiac nuclear imaging, other invasive imaging, echocardiography, and Holter monitoring), and so forth. Examples of ancillary therapeutic services include cardiac rehabilitation, noncardiac rehabilitation, physical therapy (PT), occupational therapy (OT), speech therapy, and so forth.

Pharmacy services are a special form of ancillary services that account for a significant measure of cost, and this topic is discussed in detail in Chapter 12. Mental health and substance abuse services may also be considered ancillary from a health plan's standpoint, but are really core services, albeit discreetly defined; those services are discussed in Chapter 13.

Ancillary services are unique in that they are rarely sought out by the patient unless ordered by a physician (with some notable exceptions such as freestanding cardiac diagnostic centers, but those may be treated like any other specialty service). Because most ancillary services generally require an order from a physician, it is logical that managing the cost of such services is dependent on either changing the utilization patterns of physicians or on directly managing utilization. The other primary method of controlling costs of ancillary services is to contract for such services in such a way as to make costs predictable. In fact, many MCOs rely far more heavily on favorable contracting terms to manage the cost of these services than they do on managing utilization. Even with favorable contracts, however, managing utilization of ancillary services remains an important ingredient to long-term cost control.

Credentialing and Privileging

Providers of ancillary services must be credentialed just as physicians and hospitals are. For some MCOs, it may be sufficient that the provider is licensed by the state, implying that all basic clinical requirements are being met. Some MCOs go a step further and evaluate the provider for aspects of service such as accessibility and availability, adequate office space, ability to produce reports on quality, and so forth; this is referred to as *privileging*. This approach may also be taken for ancillary services provided in physicians' offices, such as radiology; offices failing to meet privileging criteria do not receive reimbursement for those services.

Contracting and Reimbursement for Ancillary Services

Contracting and ancillary services network development is one of the most important approaches an MCO takes to dealing with costs in this area. Many ancillary services are among the first to be "carved out" of the main medical delivery system, sometimes with the financial risk transferred to another organization that is able to achieve economies of scale and manage the overall cost and quality. A plan usually has its choice of hospital-based (sometimes that is the only choice), freestanding or independent, or office-based service. The choice can be made on the basis of a combination of quality, cost, access, service (*eg*, turnaround time for testing), and convenience for members. Unlike physician services, ancillary services usually may be limited to a small subset of providers. This allows for greater leverage in negotiating as well as greater control of quality and service.

For routine types of ancillary services such as laboratory, the exception to being able to obtain substantial discounts and savings is when a limited number of providers offer the service, as might occur in a rural area. For certain types of specialized diagnostic services such as specialty radiology and others, contracting is useful, but equally important is the focus on utilization because the cost of each procedure is high even with a favorable rate.

Depending on the benefits design, this is an area where the MCO may be relatively strict about coverage issues. It may, for example, reimburse the member at the negotiated rate for services incurred out-of-network except for emergency care; the differences between charges and negotiated rates can be ten-fold or higher.

Discounts on Fee-for-Service

Many routine diagnostic ancillary services such as laboratory are high-volume services, so it is not difficult to obtain reasonable discounts or to have a negotiated fee schedule. As services get more complex and less frequent (relatively speaking), the ability to achieve a significant discount becomes less at least theoretically. In actuality, however, if there is any level of competition from providers of ancillary services, reasonable discounts may be obtained. The reason is that in most cases, the use of ancillary services is nonemergent; in other words, it is reasonable to expect that members may have to travel to particular locations to receive the services, or at least to receive them with a higher level of benefits. Similar to any PPO, a member who receives services from a noncontracted or nonpreferred provider of ancillary services would be expected to shoulder a higher portion, or even all, of the cost. Such economic steering provides for volume increases to the contracting provider.

Flat Rates

Similar to per diem payments to hospitals, flat rates simply mean that the ancillary provider is paid a fixed single payment rate regardless of the number of visits or resources used in providing services. For common services such as laboratory or routine radiology, this would mean a fixed fee that does not change regardless of what is ordered.

For therapeutic ancillary providers, case rates can be tiered, similar to differing per diem rates based on type of service in a hospital. For example, for home health care that is inclusive of high-intensity services such as chemotherapy or other high-technology services, the plan may pay different levels of case rates depending on which category of complexity the case falls into.

Capitation

In HMOs or plans that have absolute limitations on out-of-network benefits, ancillary services lend themselves to capitation. HMOs that provide benefits for out-of-network use (*ie*, a POS plan) may still capitate and may simply provide no coverage benefit for nonemergency services from a noncontracted provider (if it provides some level of coverage for out-of-network services, it will likely use an approach other than capitation). However, if a capitated provider strictly limits access or cannot meet demand, the plan will end up paying twice—once through capitation and a second time through fee-for-service. If the MCO has a large membership base, the ability to forecast cost and usage even under POS may be possible, but if the MCO has a small enrollment base, capitation for benefits plans other than a pure HMO plan may not be feasible.

Capitating for ancillary services clearly makes the provider of the service a partner in controlling costs and helps the MCO budget and forecast more accurately. The benefit to the provider of the service is a guaranteed source of referrals and a steady income. In diagnostic services, great economies of scale often are present (this is especially true for diagnostic laboratory services). In those services for which the provider delivering the service may be determining the need for continued services (*eg*, PT), capitation removes the fee-for-service incentives that may lead to inappropriately increased utilization. As with all capitation contracts, medical managers must be sure that they can direct all (or at least a defined portion) of the care to the capitated provider and not allow referrals to noncontracted providers.

Certain types of ancillary services require greater skill in capitating than others do. If an ancillary service is highly self-contained, then it is easier to capitate; for example, PT usually is limited to therapy given by the physical therapists and does not involve other types of ancillary providers. Home health, on the other hand, is often a combination of home health nurses and clinical aids, durable medical equipment (DME), home infusion and medication delivery (which includes the cost of the drug or intravenous substance as well as the cost to deliver it), home physical therapy, and so forth. A number of plans have successfully capitated for home health services, although those have tended to be larger plans with sufficient volume to be able to accurately predict costs in all of these different areas. Other plans have been able to capitate only parts of home health (*eg*, home respiratory therapy), but have had less success in other forms. In those cases, a combination of capitation and fixed case rates (*eg*, for a course of chemotherapy) may yield positive results.

A relatively uncommon variant on capitation is similar to the single-specialty management organization or specialty network manager, as discussed in Chapters 5 and 6. In this case, a single entity accepts capitation from the plan for all of a particular ancillary service (*eg*, PT). That organization then serves as a network manager or even an independent practice association (IPA). The participating ancillary providers may be subcontractors to the network manager and may be paid either through subcapitation or through a form of fee-for-service, but in all events, the network manager is at-risk for the total costs of the capitated service (the participating ancillary providers may be at-risk as well through capitation, fee adjustments, withholds, and so forth).

Some plans that capitate for ancillary services are employing risk and reward systems to ensure high levels of quality and satisfaction. For example, a plan may withhold 10% of the capitation or set up an incentive pool to ensure compliance with service standards such as accessibility, member satisfaction, turnaround time for results, responsiveness to referring physicians, documentation, and so forth.

Physician-Owned Ancillary Services

Compelling evidence shows that physician ownership of diagnostic or therapeutic equipment or services, whether owned individually or through joint ventures or partnerships, can lead to significant increases in utilization of those services. Several studies documented this phenomenon in diagnostic imaging,[24] laboratory,[25] and a remarkably wide range of other services.[26] Physician self-

referral has been restricted by CMS for Medicare services.[27] MCOs that enroll public sector members (*ie*, Medicare or Medicaid) must adhere to CMS requirements as well. Most MCOs have followed suit and restrict physician self-referral as a routine requirement of plan participation by physicians, clearly prohibiting physician self-referral in their provider contracts (unless expressly allowed by the plan). The MCO contract also requires the physician to disclose any fiduciary relationship with such ancillary service providers.

Actually tracing ownership or fiduciary relationships is not always easy to do, however. The ancillary services may have a completely separate provider name and tax identification number, may have a separate billing address (perhaps not even in the same geographic area), and may otherwise appear to be an independent vendor. Tracking unusually high rates of referral to a given provider of ancillary services may be the only clue to such potential utilization abuse.

Another source of information is the national Healthcare Integrity and Protection Data Bank (HIPDB). The Secretary of the U.S. Department of Health and Human Services (DHHS), acting through the Office of Inspector General (OIG), was directed by the Health Insurance Portability and Accountability Act of 1996 (HIPAA; see Chapter 32) to create the HIPDB to combat fraud and abuse in health insurance and health care delivery. The HIPDB is a national health care fraud and abuse data collection program for the reporting and disclosure of certain final adverse actions (excluding settlements in which no findings of liability have been made) taken against health care providers, suppliers, or practitioners. Although focused primarily on actions such as fraud convictions and exclusion from state or federal programs, actions taken by CMS around physician self-referral would be included. The reader is referred to Chapter 5 for additional discussion about the HIPDB.

Having said this, it is neither practical nor desirable to place too heavy a restriction on physicians' ability to use appropriate services or equipment that they own to deliver routine care within their specialty. For example, orthopedists cannot properly care for their patients if they cannot take radiographs. In some cases, a physician may be the only available provider of a given service (*eg*, in a rural area). In other cases, it may actually be more cost-effective to allow physicians to use their own facility. The point here is that physician-owned services must not be allowed to become a lucrative profit center, one that is subject to abuse.

Managed care plans deal with this issue in a number of ways. One method is to have an outright contractual ban on self-referral other than for specifically designated services. For example, a cardiologist may be reimbursed for performing in-office exercise tolerance testing but be prohibited from referring to a freestanding cardiac diagnostic center in which he or she has a fiduciary relationship. Another method is to reimburse for such physician self-referred services at a low margin (not so low as to cause the physician to lose money but low enough to prevent any profit) or to include it in the capitation payment. The last common method is to contract for all ancillary services through a very limited network of providers and to require the physicians and members to use only those contracted providers for ancillary services; this is discussed later in this chapter.

Management of Ancillary Services Utilization

Utilization management is not the topic of this chapter, but rather that of Chapter 9. However, there are several specific approaches to managing the use of ancillary services, and those are briefly discussed as follows.

Data Capture

The ability to manage utilization of ancillary services is directly related to the ability to capture accurate and timely data. If there is no way to capture data regarding ancillary services, there will be difficulty controlling utilization. Lack of data will also make contracting problematic because no vendor will be willing to contract aggressively without having some idea of projected utilization (at least not on terms that will be beneficial to the plan or medical group responsible for the cost).

Data elements that need to be captured include who ordered the service (this is sometimes different from the physician of record; for example, a member may have signed up with a primary care physician [PCP], but the referral physician ordered the tests), what was ordered, what is being paid for (in other words, is the plan paying for more than was ordered?), and how much it is costing. Data issues are discussed in Chapter 16.

Financial Incentives

Ancillary services utilization is commonly incorporated into primary care reimbursement systems that are performance based (*eg*, capitation or performance-based fee-for-service; see Chapter 6). In one older study, capitation with risk sharing, combined with education and feedback (see discussion later) led to a clear reduction in the use of ambulatory testing, while having no adverse impact on outcomes.[28] This approach applies primarily to HMOs with such risk-based reimbursement methodologies.

Use of ancillary services can also be incorporated in performance-based incentive programs (see Chapter 8) in other types of MCOs as well. For example, PPOs that use a preauthorization approach to selected imaging studies (see discussion later) may incorporate compliance with the program into a performance-based incentive system. Overall costs for ancillary services may likewise be a measure in such programs.

Feedback

The issue of monetary gain leading to excessive use of ancillary services has been discussed earlier in this chapter, but there are a number of nonmonetary causes of excessive testing; such causes include the quest for diagnostic certainty, peer pressure, convenience, patient demands, and fear of malpractice claims.[29]

There is evidence that physicians will modify their use of ancillary services when given feedback on their performance. Simple feedback regarding test-ordering behavior has led to modest reductions in use.[30] This response has been confirmed for simple feedback, and somewhat greater decreases have been seen when feedback was combined with other written guidelines or peer review.[31,32]

Feedback to physicians regarding their use of ancillary services is therefore a worthwhile endeavor. Feedback should include comparisons to their peers and should be properly adjusted for factors that affect utilization (*eg,* age and sex of patients, specialty type, adjustments for acuity or severity, and the like). Feedback should also contain adequate data to enable a physician to know where performance may be improved.

Focused Utilization Management

Certain types of highly costly ancillary services may be subject to a focused effort to manage utilization. Using techniques similar to those applied in some types of HMOs (see Chapter 9), precertification or preauthorization has made its appearance. This may be carried out by the MCO, or it may be contracted out to a specialized company in a manner similar to behavioral health (Chapter 13). In any case, the ordering physician must obtain preauthorization from the plan for selected services or else the MCO does not cover the cost.

The initial focus of this approach has been on specialized diagnostic studies, in particular, MRI, MRA, and PET scans, and nuclear stress testing, though other specialty imaging procedures may also be subject to preauthorization. Some MCOs take this approach to CT scanning as well if data analysis indicates apparent overutilization. The preauthorization process is designed to see that certain clinical criteria are met, clinically appropriate

alternatives are considered, unnecessary duplicate testing is not performed, and so forth.

Outsourcing

The advent of digitization of data has created the opportunity to outsource certain aspects of ancillary services. The most common of these is radiology; specifically interpretation, not the actual physical procedure itself. Interpretation of electrocardiograms, routine pathology readings, and some other types of services (*eg,* monitoring readings from an intensive care unit, though not the subject of this section) also lend themselves to potential outsourcing.

This is principally done by provider systems rather than health plans, though it can be applicable to MCOs either directly or indirectly through contracts with systems that use it. For example, a hospital system contracts with radiologists in another country such as India, Australia, or Israel, to read x- rays, CT scans, or other types of images (as long as the image can be digitized) when the local radiologists are asleep at night.[33] This provides for a better quality of life for the local radiologist, certainly.* But it also provides a venue for lower costs for radiology, though one that is not commonly used by MCOs.

CONCLUSION

As with all provider payment systems, reimbursement mechanisms and contracts with hospitals are tools. The importance of these tools cannot be overestimated, and managed care executives must craft these tools with all the skills they have available. It is possible and desirable to develop win-win situations with hospitals, and that can be a pivotal issue in the ultimate success of a plan.

---

*For Medicare, CMS prohibits payments for care provided outside of the United States so the hospital pays the overseas radiologist while the local radiologist "reviews" the interpretation and then charges Medicare.

References

1. Devers KJ, Casalino LP, Rudell LS, Stoddard JJ, Brewster LR, Lake TK. Hospitals' negotiation leverage with health plans: How and why has it changed. *Health Serv Res*. February 2003, 38:1(Part 2):419-46.

2. US Government Accountability Office. *Differences in Health Care Prices Across Metropolitan Areas Linked to Competition and Other Factors*. December 2005. Publication #GAO-06-281T. Available at: http://www.gao.gov/new.items/d06281t.pdf. Accessed July 14, 2006.

3. Centers for Medicare and Medicaid Services. *Medicare Managed Care Manual*. 2005. Available at: http://www.cms.hhs.gov/manuals/downloads/mc86c04.pdf. Accessed July 14, 2006.

4. U.S. Government Accountability Office. *Federal Employees Health Benefits Program: Competition and Other Factors Linked to Wide Variation in Health Care Prices*. August 2005. Publication #GAO-05-856. Available at: http://www. gao.gov/new.items/d05856.pdf. Accessed July 14, 2006.

5. Tompkins CP, Altman SH, Eilat E. The precarious pricing system of hospital services. *Health Affairs*. 2006, 25(1):45–56.

6. American Hospital Association. *American Hospital Association Guide to the Health Care Field*. American Hospital Association. Published annually and available at: http://www.aha.org/.

7. Mays G, Claxton G, Strunk B. Tiered-provider networks: Patients face cost-choice trade-offs. Center for Studying Health System Change. November 2003. Issue Brief #71.

8. Yegian JM. Tiered hospital networks. *Health Affairs*. March 19, 2003. Web Exclusive, W3-147–153.Available at: http://content.healthafairs.org/cgi/reprint/hlthaff.w3.147v1.pdf. Accessed July 27, 2006.

9. Robinson JC. Hospital tiers in health insurance: balancing consumer choice with financial incentives. *Health Affairs*. March 19, 2003. Web Exclusive, W3-135–146. Available at: http://content.healthaffairs.org/cgi/reprint/hlthaff.w3.135v1.pdf. Accessed July 29, 2006.

10. Leapfrog Group. The Leapfrog Group statement on "never events" in health care. May 18, 2006. Available at: http://www.leapfroggroup. org/news/leapfrog_news/2330901. Accessed July 22, 2006.

11. Centers for Medicare and Medicaid Services. Acute inpatient PPS. May 2006. Available at: http://www.cms.hhs.gov/AcuteInpatientPPS/01_overview.asp. Accessed July 16, 2006.

12. Debrock L, Arnould RJ. Utilization control in HMOs. *Quarterly Review of Economics and Finance*. Autumn 1992, 32(3):31–53.

13. Greenwald L, Cromwell J, Adamache W, *et al*. Specialty versus community hospitals: Referrals, quality and community benefits. *Health Affairs*. 2006, 25(1):106–118.

14. U.S. Government Accountability Office. *Specialty Hospitals: Geographic Location, Services Provided and Financial Performance*. Washington, DC: U.S. Government Accountability Office. October 2003. Publication no. GAO-04-167.

15. 42 USC, sec. 1395nn (d)(3)(B).

16. Report to the Congress: Physician-owned specialty hospitals. *MedPAC*. March 2005. Available at: http://www.medpac.gov/publications/congressional_reports/Mar05_SpecHospitals.pdf. Accessed July 28, 2006.

17. McCaig LF, Ly N. National hospital ambulatory medical care survey: 2000 emergency department summary. Advance data from vital and health statistics; no. 326. Hyattsville, Md: National Center Health Statistics. 2002. Available at: http://www.cdc.gov/nchs/data/ad/ad326.pdf. Accessed July 16, 2006.

18. McCaig LF, Nawar EN. National hospital ambulatory medical care survey: 2004 emergency department summary. Advance data from vital and health statistics; no 372. Hyattsville, Md: National Center for Health Statistics. 2006. Available at: http://www.cdc. gov/nchs/data/ad/ad372.pdf. Accessed July 16, 2006.

19. 42, USC, sec. 1395 dd (1986). Pub. L. No. 99-272.

20. American Association of Ambulatory Surgery Centers. *ASC Ownership Survey*. February 2004. Available at: http://www.aaasc.org/advocacy/documents/ASCOwnership.pdf. Accessed July 16, 2006.

21. Available via the 3M Health Information Systems site. Available at: http://www.3m.com/us/healthcare/his/products/outpatient/ambulatory.jhtml. Accessed July 16, 2006.

22. Centers for Medicare and Medicaid Services. Hospital outpatient PPS. May 2006. Available at: http://www.cms.hhs.gov/HospitalOutpatient PPS/01_overview.asp. Accessed July 16, 2006.

23. Hospital Corporation of America. *HCA CEO makes commitment to pricing transparency.* May 1, 2006. HCA press release. Available at: http://phx.corporate-ir.net/phoenix.zhtml?c = 63489&p = irol-newsArticle&ID = 849984& highlight = . Accessed July 17, 2006.

24. Hillman BJ, Joseph CA, Mabry MR, *et al.* Frequency and costs of diagnostic imaging in office practice—A comparison of self-referring and radiologist-referring physicians. *N Engl J Med.* 1990, 323:1604–1608.

25. Office of the Inspector General. *Financial Arrangements between Physicians and Health Care Businesses: Report to Congress.* Washington, DC: Department of Health and Human Services, 1989. Department of Health and Human Services Publication no. OAI-12-88-01410.

26. State of Florida Health Care Cost Containment Board. *Joint Ventures among Health Care Providers in Florida.* Tallahassee, Fla: State of Florida. 1991:2.

27. The Ethics in Patient Referrals Act—Omnibus Budget Reconciliation Act of 1989.

28. Murray JP, Greenfield S, Kaplan SH, Yano EM. Ambulatory testing for capitation and fee-for-service patients in the same practice setting: relationship to outcomes. *Medical Care.* March 1992, 30(3):252–261.

29. Kassirer JP. Our stubborn quest for diagnostic certainty: A cause of excessive testing. *N Engl J Med.* 1989, 320:1489–1491.

30. Berwick DM, Coltin KL. Feedback reduces test use in a health maintenance organization. *JAMA.* 1986, 255:1450–1454.

31. Marton KI, Tul V, Sox HC. Modifying test-ordering behavior in the outpatient medical clinic. *Arch Intern Med.* 1985, 145:816–821.

32. Martin AR, Wolf MA, Thibodeau LA, *et al.* A trial of two strategies to modify the test-ordering behavior of medical residents. *N Engl J Med.* 1980, 303:1330–1336.

33. Wachter RM. The "dis-location" of U.S. medicine—The implications of medical outsourcing. *N Engl J Med.* February 16, 2006, 354:7.

8

Performance-Based Incentives in Managed Health Care: Pay-for-Performance

Peter R. Kongstvedt

Study Objectives

- Understand the basic approaches to pay-for-performance (P4P).
- Understand critical differences between hospital- and physician-focused P4P programs.
- Understand the common performance measures used for hospitals and for physicians.
- Understand the challenges in administering such programs.
- Understand current approaches being used by employers, health plans, and Medicare in P4P.

Discussion Topics

1. Discuss market forces that are creating an increased interest in P4P programs.
2. Discuss what a health plan must do to increase the effectiveness of a P4P program.
3. Discuss how P4P programs might evolve in the future.
4. Discuss various means of realistically funding P4P and what market and regulatory forces might affect such funding.

INTRODUCTION

Performance-based incentives, now commonly referred to as pay-for-performance or P4P (or less commonly, PFP), is an encompassing term that describes methods that a managed care organization (MCO) or government payer such as Medicare (administered by the Centers for Medicare and Medicaid Services—CMS) uses to offer incentives to providers for issues other than managing utilization (though a few MCOs do combine utilization-based incentives into their P4P programs). Rewards or incentives are primarily financial, either directly or indirectly, as is described later in this chapter. The preponderance of P4P programs are in health maintenance organizations (HMOs),* but that is changing with the appearance of robust programs in preferred provider organizations (PPOs) by regional and national companies. Demonstration programs by CMS for use in fee-for-service (FFS) Medicare, as described later in this chapter, will accelerate its adoption outside of the HMO model.

One reasonable definition developed at a P4P Design Principles conference in November 2004, sponsored by American Healthways, Inc. and Johns Hopkins University, is: "The use of incentives to encourage and reinforce the delivery of evidence-based practices and health care system transformation that promote better outcomes as efficiently as possible."[1] Another useful description that was written as P4P applies to physicians but is relevant to hospitals as well is: "The goal of incorporating financial incentives for quality into physicians' payments is not simply to reward 'good' physicians or punish 'bad' ones. The goal is to change the status quo by stimulating both immediate and long term improvements in performance."[2]

Nonutilization-based performance is most often clinical, but not exclusively so. Examples of nonclinical (or more accurately, not

overtly and directly clinical) performance might include electronic connectivity, electronic decision support, and patient satisfaction. Clinical performance essentially means adherence to evidence-based clinical practice as well as performance around patient safety. Clinical performance may also be thought of within the classic approach to measure quality first described by Avedis Donabedian[3] and paraphrased here:

Structure: The physical and programatic support for care. Examples would include existence of computerized order entry systems, appointment availability, electronic medical records (EMRs) or electronic health records (EHRs), and the like. The financial incentive system itself is also an example of structure. Many performance measures that are considered nonclinical fall into this category, though some clinical ones do as well.

Process: How care is actually delivered, regardless of the outcome of that care. Examples include adherence to evidence-based clinical protocols, the processes used by hospital nursing staff to dispense medications, and so forth.

Outcome: The clinical outcome of how care is delivered. Examples include improved blood test results for diabetics, fewer safety errors in a hospital, improved quality of life for a patient with a chronic and debilitating disease, and patient satisfaction with care.

Performance-based incentives in managed health care have existed off and on for at least two decades. For example, in group and staff model HMOs where it is easier to observe behavior, formal performance evaluations of physicians were in use in the 1970s.[4] In open panel HMOs, including direct contract model and independent practice association (IPA) models, incentive programs that included quality-based goals (but also included utilization-based goals) such as compliance with clinical protocols have existed since the 1980s.[5,6] Performance-based contracting for hospitals has likewise existed

---

*See Chapter 2 for a description of the various models or types of health plans.

since the late 1980s.[7] All of these early programs were HMO-based, though a quality-based evaluation system for PPOs was described in the 1980s that had the implicit effect of rewarding performance through selective contracting.[8]

Approaches to P4P expanded in the 1990s. A large study published in 1995 reported that 36% of MCOs used member satisfaction surveys for purposes of adjusting physician payments, and 56% of MCOs used quality measures.[9] Looking at the same issue from the perspective of physicians who receive income from MCOs, another study, using 1996 and 1997 data, reported 23% of physicians (mostly primary care physicians rather than specialists) had financial incentives based on patient satisfaction, and 18% had incentives based on quality of care such as preventive care measures.[10] Tables 8-1 and 8-2 illustrate

levels of incentive-based financial impact on physician practices in HMOs in 1999.

Beginning in 2002, P4P expanded in a major way when under the auspices of the Integrated Healthcare Association (IHA; a California association with representation by health plans, physicians, hospitals, pharmaceutical companies, purchasers, and consumers), six MCOs operating in California (Aetna, Blue Cross of California, Blue Shield of California, CIGNA, Health Net, and PacifiCare) agreed to a program in which measures were collaboratively developed with IHA, and those measures were used by all six of the MCOs for their respective physician P4P programs.[11] Performance for 2003 was measured and $37.4 million in financial incentives were paid in 2004;[12] Blue Cross of California alone paid out $72 million to physicians in 2005.[13] This particular program continues to evolve

Table 8–1 Percentage of Physicians whose Compensation is Affected by Selected Financial Incentives by Practice Arrangement, 1999

Practice Arrangement	Percentage of Physicians in Practices of Two or More, by Practice Arrangement	Incentives Based on Individual Physician Performance		
		Performance-Based		Productivity
		Profiling	Patient Satisfaction and/or Quality	
Small group (2–9 physicians)	42	10%	16%	72%
Medium group (10–29 physicians)	10	10	18	70
Large group (30+ physicians)	8	14*	32**	81**
Staff/group HMO	7	33**	70**	65*
Hospital-owned, medical school, or other	33	16**	37**	72
All	100	14	29	72

* Significantly different from small groups at $P < .05$.
** Significantly different from small groups at $P < .001$.
Note: Sample excludes full owners of solo practices, physicians spending less than 60% of their time in patient care, and physicians practicing in community health centers and city-, county-, or state-owned hospitals and clinics. Physicians may be subject to more than one incentive.
Source: Center for Studying Health System Change. *Community Tracking Study Physician Survey, 1998–99.*
Source: Stoddard J, Grossman JM, Rudell L. *Physicians More Likely to Face Quality Incentives Than Incentives That May Restrain Care.* Center for Studying Health System Change; January 2002. Issue Brief #48. Reprinted with permission of the Center for Studying Health System Change, Washington, DC, http://www.hschange.org.

Table 8–2 Percentage of Physicians whose Compensation is Affected by Selected Financial Incentives, by Percentage of Practice Revenue from Capitation, 1999

Size of Practice	Percentage of Practice Revenue from Capitation	Incentives Based on Individual Physician Performance		Productivity*
		Performance-Based		
		Profiling*	Patient Satisfaction and/or Quality*	
None	39%	8%	19%	71%
1–24	30	13	27	74
25–49	14	22	34	77
50+	17	25	50	67
All	100	14	29	72

* All comparisons are significant for linear trend at $P < .001$.
Note: Sample excludes full owners of solo practices, physicians spending less than 60% of their time in patient care, and physicians practicing in community health centers and city-, county-, or state-owned hospitals and clinics. Physicians may be subject to more than one incentive.
Source: Center for Studying Health System Change. *Community Tracking Study Physician Survey, 1998–99.*
Source: Stoddard J, Grossman JM, Rudell L. *Physicians More Likely to Face Quality Incentives Than Incentives That May Restrain Care.* Center for Studying Health System Change; January 2002. Issue Brief #48. Reprinted with permission of the Center for Studying Health System Change, Washington, DC, http://www.hschange.org.

and now covers 35,000 physicians and 6.2 million members participating in HMOs in California.[14] The magnitude of this program as well as the experiences gained and reported have led to a sharp increase in interest in P4P.

It is also worthy to note that P4P is being used outside of the United States; most notably by the United Kingdom's National Health Service (NHS). An attempt by the NHS to introduce a quality-based financial incentive program for general practitioners in the mid-1980s was rejected by the physicians, and modest programs oriented toward preventive services in the 1990s were abandoned for lack of effectiveness. However, beginning in 2004 (and still expanding at the time of publication), the NHS is implementing a complex P4P program for general practitioners in which approximately one-quarter of the income of the general practitioner will be based on 146 differentially weighted quality indicators covering clinical care for 10 chronic diseases, organization of care, and patient experience, supported by a new EHR that is being nationally instituted.[15,16]

Because there is neither stability nor commonality in how these P4P programs are created and applied by health plans and governmental payers, what follows describes only those that are most commonly in use for hospitals and physicians at the time of publication.

BASIC APPROACH TO PAY-FOR-PERFORMANCE

Relationship with Providers

Participation by providers in a P4P program is almost always voluntary. Involuntary participation is possible, and the use of tiering as it applies to hospitals and described later in this chapter is one example, though tiering usually also has an element of cost associated with it as described in Chapter 7. It is also possible to apply other approaches to P4P without the agreement of the providers if the data sources are soley from the MCO and require no cooperation from the providers, or if the MCO requires cooperation with the program as part of the contractual process. Imposing a P4P program through the contractual process may force the provider to agree, though perhaps not if a hospital system has sufficient market power to force the MCO to back down. But such an imposition is clearly at odds with eliciting positive changes in behavior that will lead to improvement in outcomes and member satisfaction. Furthermore, gaining the cooperation of the providers enables the P4P program to study measures that require the provider to collect and report the data.

To gain support, the providers need to buy-in to the program. This is done through involvement of the providers through their appropriate representatives. The use of nationally recognized standards as described later in this chapter also makes it more appealing to providers, though local issues should not necessarily be neglected. Last, to the extent possible the P4P program should be perceived as a positive one, not a punitive one.

Measures

A plethora of measures are used in P4P programs across the country. No one program uses all possible measures because that would be overwhelming and would also dilute the effect of measurement on any individual type of care. Measures may be complex or they may be simple, though as a general rule simpler measures are both more understandable, more likely to be implemented, and more likely to be accepted (measures must also be seen as valid by the providers). It is possible to be too simple, however, and the program will need to contain sufficient complexity to account for variations that are outside the abilities of the providers to control.

Severity adjustments as described in Chapter 16 are sometimes applied to data when looking at outcomes measures, but except for the new MCO payment approach instituted by CMS (see Chapter 26), the severity adjusting systems themselves were never designed specifically to support financial incentive programs. Until further development of severity adjustment systems that are specifically oriented toward incentive programs, measurements that do not require severity adjustments are preferrable.

Last, parameters must be set around the population of members for which data will be collected. For example, a member may be required to be continuously enrolled with the MCO for at least 2 years for data regarding breast cancer screening to be used.* So-called anchor dates must be set so that identical time periods are used for certain measures. The program may also choose not to even collect data from a provider if the number of members subject to the measure is too small; for example, 30 or fewer members. Of course, data should only be collected for clinical services that are covered by the MCO's schedule of benefits.

Sources of Data

Data must be reliable, consistent, and valid. In other words, data collected to create measurement results need to mean what the program understands it to mean, the data need to mean the same thing when reported by different providers, and the data need to actually represent what happened. They should be as easy to collect and report as possible, though the more sophisticated the program becomes, the more complex the data-reporting aspect becomes. Hospitals that have installed highly functional clinical support systems are more able to report more complex data, and the advent of the EHR should

---

*Short gaps in enrollment may be allowed; for example, 45 days or less in a year and only one such gap.

provide markedly enhanced capabilities for data reporting for physicians.

The typical sources of data used to create performance measures are as follows:

- Medical claims
- Pharmacy claims
- Laboratory results
- Clinical chart or medical record audits
  - Inpatient episodes
  - Outpatient procedures
  - Medical office chart reviews
- Facility or medical office audits
- Patient surveys

Most MCOs use data from care delivered only to their own members, though this can create a problem of small numbers. Unless there is a significant concentration of an MCO's members with an individual provider, there may be insufficent events to allow for statistical integrity. Certainly, many health plans such as large Blue Cross and Blue Shield plans or large regional HMOs have such high concentrations, but many national plans do not as regards a single provider. When insufficient data are available, pooling data together from multiple plans provides for greater integrity of results, though how the data are then used in each MCO's P4P program would be unique to each MCO.

Ultimately, what data are collected is driven by two considerations: what data are obtainable (even if not routinely created or reported, data may still be obtainable with some effort), and what the P4P program wants to measure.

Sources of Applicable Measures

Measures used in a P4P program may be created by the MCO (preferably with the input of the providers) or may be obtained from nationally recognized programs. In reality, it is usually a mix of both because nationally recognized programs base their measures on evidence-based medicine and accepted patient safety requirements. Table 8-3 provides a partial listing of nationally recognized sources for measurements at the time of publication.

Many of the organizations listed in Table 8-3 participate cooperatively, and there is frequent overlap between them. One specific nationally recognized set of measures, the Health Plan Employer Data Information Set (HEDIS; see also Chapter 23), is worth singling out. HEDIS was created and is continually upgraded by NCQA, is a mature and widely accepted set of measures that are commonly used by MCOs, and is often incorporated, in whole or in part, in a P4P program. The entire HEDIS data set can be found in Chapter 23.

Clinical process and outcomes measures that are created by the MCO focusing on local needs must be based on evidence-based medicine and clearly supported in the medical literature. The measures must be for events that happen in sufficient volume so as to make measurement both possible and meaningful or else be so significant that occurances of any kind warrant attention (for example, medication errors in hospitals). Input and acceptance from the providers that will be affected by the program should be part of the process of creating MCO-specific measures.

Audits of facilities and medical offices may be created by the MCO or may be based on nationally recognized sources. For example, JCAHO has standards for facilities, though as a practical matter all hospitals with which the MCO will contract will already be accredited by JCAHO. Structural measures such as the use of electronic prescribing (e-prescribing) or use of the EHR may be audited or self-reported.

Incorporation of consumer perspectives on quality can be relatively complex,[17] though very simple measures such as overall satisfaction, although not as useful as more rigourously constructed survey instruments, at least have the advantage of ease of administration. One commonly used and well-constructed set of measures is the Consumer Assessment of Healthcare Providers and Systems (CAHPS), available from the AHRQ;[18] the CAHPS initial focus was (and still is) on

Table 8–3 Partial List of National Sources for Measurements

Organization	Web Address
National Committee on Quality Assurance (NCQA)	http://www.ncqa.org/
Joint Commission on Accreditation of Healthcare Organizations (JCAHO)	http://www.jointcommission.org/
Bridges to Excellence	http://www.bridgestoexcellence.org/
Leap Frog Group	http://www.leapfroggroup.org/
Integrated Healthcare Association (IHA)	http://www.iha.org/
Ambulatory Care Quality Alliance (AQA)	http://www.ambulatoryqualityalliance.org/
Hospital Quality Alliance (HQA; sponsored by the American Hospital Association)	http://www.aha.org/aha/key_issues/ qualityalliance/index.html
National Quality Forum (NQF)	http://www.qualityforum.org/
Institute for Health Care Improvement (IHI)	http://www.ihi.org/ihi
Agency for Healthcare Research and Quality	http://www.ahrq.gov/
National Guidelines Clearinghouse	http://www.guideline.gov/
CMS	http://www.cms.hhs.gov
State-based organizations; for example, the Massachusetts Health Quality Partnership	http://www.mhqp.org
Professional associations such as American College of Surgeons National Surgical Quality Improvement Program and American College of Cardiology	Various

Source: Compiled by author from various Web sites. Accessed June and July, 2006.

health plans, but versions focusing on hospitals and on ambulatory care are being tested at the time of publication.

Rewarding Provider Performance

How measurements are used to reward provider performance is highly variable from MCO to MCO. It is also different for hospitals than it is for physicians.* Therefore, the broad concepts are discussed here, whereas

---

*P4P programs for providers other than hospitals and physicians programs are certainly possible but are very uncommon at the time of publication and therefore are not discussed further in the chapter.

issues specific to hospitals and to physicians are discussed separately later in the chapter.

Tiering

Discussed more fully in Chapter 7 and briefly in Chapter 5, tiering refers to when the MCO creates different tiers of a provider network such that a member's coverage for services differs depending on which tier a provider is in. For example, benefits coverage at a Tier 1 hospital would be subject to a $100 copay, whereas coverage at a Tier 2 hospital would be subject to a $500 copay. Though less common, specialty physicians may also be the focus of a tiered network. Cost for services is most frequently the reason behind placing a provider into a tier, but quality of care may also factor into the decision. This is particularly the case when tiering the physician network.

Reimbursement Adjustments

An MCO can use a P4P program to adjust reimbursement to providers. Such adjustments would come in the form of higher payment for similar services to those providers that meet or exceed measurement goals. Reimbursement adjustments are most easily done by adjusting the multipliers for either diagnosis-related groups (DRGs) for hospitals or a relative value scale (RVS) for physicians. Adjustments to other types of reimbursement systems are certainly possible as well. If an MCO uses a withhold in its reimbursement methodology, part of the return of that withhold may be based on meeting goals based on quality, not just utilization. The timing of when to make such adjustments must also be taken into consideration; annual adjustments are the most common, but it is possible to make adjustments on a more frequent basis. Basic reimbursement methodologies are discussed more fully in Chapters 6 (physicians) and 7 (hospitals).

Bonus Payments

Bonus payments are just that: payments to providers separate from any direct reimbursement for services. Bonus payments may be paid out in full for meeting a threshold, may be graduated based on the degree to which a goal has been met, or may be a combination of the two.

Timing of bonus payments varies from program to program. Paying incentives on a frequent basis, quarterly, for example, may be problematic for several reasons. There may be insufficient data to provide meaningful results, there may be too much variation within short periods of time that tend to level out when using longer time periods, and the amount of the bonus may be perceived as too small to have a significant impact. These three issues are ameliorated when longer time periods, such as annual periods, are used. Annual bonus payments have the problems of being more remote from the events that are being measured and of not occuring frequently enough to provide the actual incentive to change. These may be overcome by providing regular performance reports (for those measures that are applicable to regular reporting, such as preventive services) on a frequent basis, even if the incentives are paid annually.

Funding Bonus Payments

There are several issues to consider when addressing the source of funding for bonus payments. The first of these concerns the differences between fully insured products and self-funded products. For fully insured products, the MCO receives a premium payment and is then responsible for medical costs; any variation in claims costs results in profits or losses to the MCO, not the employer or member paying the premium. For self-funded or administrative services only (ASO) products, the employer is responsible for the medical claims cost, even though the MCO is performing the administration, including processing the claims payment; any variations in predicted claims costs affect the employer, not the MCO. Self-funding is discussed more fully in Chapter 31 because it is the result of the Employee Retirement Income and Security Act (ERISA).

An MCO is free to do what it wants with funds derived from insured products, but because it is paid for administrative services only under an ASO agreement, it does not have that latitude. Most ASO arrangements are negotiated between the employer and the MCO (really between the employer's benefits management consultants and the MCO) on a service-specific basis; that is, each type of service is priced separately, as discussed in Chapter 22. The practical result is that in an ASO arrangement, the MCO must negotiate with the employer to fund a P4P program as a separate item. This may be done as a discrete fund, or it may be done as a function of medical costs that the employer is responsible for paying. Either way, the MCO and the employer must agree on the funding approach as part of the contract between the employer and the MCO.

The simplist approach to funding is to budget for the program and include the cost in the premiums charged to employers; such costs are legitimately considered medical benefits costs since they are paid to providers based on care delivered. This same approach may be used in ASO products, though as noted earlier may be the subject of negotiation, with some employers not wanting to pay in to the program.

Funding can also be made through holding back on the amount of fee increases that the MCO would have made in provider payments. This can be done across the board, budgeting for a 4% increase but only paying a 2% increase for actual claims and diverting the other 2% to be paid out under the P4P program. Bonus payments still represent claims costs but are paid under the P4P program rather than as FFS. As discussed earlier, differential payments of fees to higher performers rather than bonus payments may also be done using this approach.

For fully insured products at least, funding for the program can also derive either in part or in full from savings based on reduced utilization and/or medical costs when compared to budget. This has the benefit of funding the program through savings, but it also has the potential to result in low or no payments made despite achieving quality goals if medical costs are high.

DATA TRANSPARENCY TO CONSUMERS

Data transparency to consumers refers to making the results of the program public or at least available to members of the MCO, as discussed more fully in Chapter 20. Reports could represent aggregate results for the entire program, could be provider-specific, or a mix of both. Reports may also translate specific results into simple graphics (*eg,* three stars out of four). Results made available might not represent all measures. For example, some measures may be new to the program and untested; in other cases, the MCO or providers may perceive the potential for increased liability resulting from such reporting.

Providing data transparency may be done by the MCO itself or the MCO may outsource that function to a commercial company that specializes in providing such data to consumers. In the case of Medicare, CMS makes available to the public comparisons between hospitals using the quality measures described later in this chapter.[19] In at least one state, California, results are made public by a state agency—the California Office of Patient Advocate.[20]

Although it may seem that providing the public with quality information should be a laudable and unmitigated good, some thoughtful policy analysts raise the concern that such public reporting of quality information at the level of individual physcians could have unintended negative consequences, such as physicians avoiding caring for difficult patients, focusing on the performance measures to the neglect of other aspects of care, and neglecting the roles of patient preferences and clinical judgment.[21] Such concerns are certainly warranted, but it is unknown whether such negative consequences actually occur, and there is little doubt that the public desires access to information about providers' quality of care.

PAY-FOR-PERFORMANCE FOR HOSPITALS

A P4P program may be focused only on hospitals, only on physicians, or have both components. Even when a program does have both hospital and physician components, it is very uncommon for there to be much overlap. This section describes common measures and types of hospital-focused P4P programs, representing a composite of programs that are in place at the time of publication.* In addition, CMS has launched P4P for Medicare, including a demonstration project, which is briefly described.

Common Measures

Measures commonly applied to hospitals fall into four general categories: clinical measures, patient safety, the use of information technology (IT), and patient satisfaction. There is considerable overlap between these types of measures, and one can reasonably argue that this is more of a continuum than it is a set of categories.

Clinical Measures

The most commony used clinical measures are for care that is delivered in sufficient frequency so as to be measurable, and for which easily measured evidence-based clinical practices exist. The most common of these is for acute myocardial infarction (AMI) or heart attack, and the common measures are the administration of beta blockers and asprin upon admission and prescribing antiplatelet medication and beta blockers upon discharge, unless clinically contraindicated. Some programs include measures for prescription of lipid-lowering agents as well.

Other cardiac care may also be addressed, most commonly focusing on bypass surgery and percutaneous coronary interventions (PCI); for example, PCI being performed within 90 minutes of arrival. Processes for the treatment of congestive heart failure may be measured; for example, the percentage of patients with left ventricular systolic dysfunction that are given an angiotensin converting

---

*Examples in this section were compiled by the author based on review of numerous existing programs, with both overlap and variations existing in program design, source of the measures, and setting of standards.

enzyme (ACE) inhibitor or an angiotensin receptor blocker (ARB).

Noncardiac care may be measured, and one of the most common measures is the administration of appropriate antibiotics within 4 hours of arrival for a patient with a community-acquired pneumonia. Processes involved in labor and delivery may be part of the program, as could processes for any particular high-volume service.

Patient Safety

Patient safety is really a subset of clinical measures, but is frequently the focus of clearly identified sections of a P4P program. As discussed in Chapter 7, many MCOs actually refuse to reimburse hospitals for errors that are considered "never events" in that they should never occur, for example, operating on the wrong body part, and all never events may be considered patient safety issues. This section is focused less on never events than it is on more common patient safety measures, though there is some overlap in the area of medication errors.

Safety measures may also be indirect. An example of an indirect measure of safety is simply the volume of a particular procedure that a hospital does on an annual basis; for example, 400 or more cardiac bypass grafts or PCI procedures per year.

Medication errors are a common focus of patient safety measures. According to a report issued by the Institute of Medicine in 2006, between 380,000 and 450,000 preventable medication errors occur in acute care hospitals each year, and each preventable medication error adds approximately $8,750 (in 2006 adjusted dollars) to the cost of the admission.[22] Preventable medication errors for any reason should never occur, but the P4P program may need to set goals that change over time to actually help fund the changes in processes and technology required to achieve a zero percentage of preventable medication errors.

Hospital-acquired infections, another common focus of safety measures, are a serious complication because the bacteria involved are frequently resistant to most antibiotics. Therefore, it is appropriate to set performance goals to induce changes in processes to reduce the rate of hospital-acquired infections, with the ultimate goal being zero. Surgical complications are likewise subject to performance measures, though most programs focus on specific types of surgery such as cardiac surgery and selected high-volume orthopedic procedures.

Patient Satisfaction

Patient satisfaction is a combination of survey results and any complaints or grievances that a member may file with the MCO regarding a hospital. The MCO may routinely survey all members who receive care at a hospital or only a statistically significant subset. Return rates on surveys that are simply mailed to members are notoriously low, however, so the MCO may choose to perform telephone surveys to increase the number of data. A standardized survey, the Hospital Consumer Assessment of Health Providers and Systems (H-CAHPS) is being created for CMS that may also lend itself to use in P4P programs; H-CAHPS is still being field tested at the time of publication, but should be available in the near future.

The Use of Information Technology

The use of IT may be an adjunct to patient safety, but it may also be broader. It is an area of performance that is far more subject to revision over time than are the clinical measures discussed earlier. Certainly, clinical measures can and will change as medical science evolves and superior approaches to intervetions and safety emerge. But changes in IT occur as functionality is improved in systems and demonstrated to contribute to clinical processes and outcomes, and those innovations do not require painstaking clinical research.

One frequent measure in the use of IT is the existence and use of a computerized physician order entry (CPOE) system.[23,24]

CPOE improves safety by reducing medication errors caused by illegible handwriting or a misreading of written orders. A CPOE system can also be programmed to create standard orders for certain diagnoses (an AMI for example) automatically, though always subject to final review and authorization by a physician. Last, a CPOE can reduce medication errors caused by improper dosing, that is, prescribing an inappropriately high or low dose of a medication.

The existence of an EHR is another common measure for hospital P4P programs, though there are gradations as a result of the term EHR being used to describe electronic record systems of variable scope. A sophisticated P4P program defines the essential and desired (though not necessarily essential) attributes of the EHR that would result in performance incentives as well as requirements around actually using it.

In September 2005, the Department of Health and Human Services awarded a 3-year contract to the Certification Commission for Healthcare Information Technology (CCHIT) to develop and evaluate certification criteria and create an inspection process for health care information technology in three areas:

- Ambulatory EHRs for the office-based physician or provider
- Inpatient EHRs for hospitals and health systems
- The network components through which they interoperate and share information[25]

At the time of publication, CCHIT announced that certification of inpatient EHR applications will be available in 2007.[26] Use of a CCHIT-certified EHR could therefore serve as the goal.

The last common area of IT performance is the existence and use of clinical decision support systems. Such systems support not only the physicians but other professionals caring for patients. Clinical decision support systems may provide access to clinical data and support in information management, but most important they provide access to "expert systems" that support clinical care such as aiding in diagnosis or the provision of treatment protocols.

Incentives

Incentives to hospitals fall along the entire array discussed earlier: adjustments to payments made for services, bonus payments, and tiering.

Financial Incentives

Financial incentives may be either adjustments to payment rates or bonus payments. Adjustments to payment rates are most easily accomplished by adjusting the multiplier for DRGs, though adjustments to per diem rates are also feasible. Bonus payments are the other common approach to providing financial incentives to hospitals in P4P programs. In either case, the degree of incentive commonly ranges from 1% up to 5% of total payments to the hospital.*

Tiering

Tiering is briefly described earlier in the chapter, and more fully in Chapter 7. As noted, cost considerations are usually the primary drivers of tiering, but quality measures may be included or even used exclusively. Exclusive use of quality measures would most likely occur when pricing differences are relatively modest but differences in quality measures are not. Volume on selected procedures as noted earlier is another common measure used for tiering, at least as regards those specific procedures.

Medicare

CMS has begun to apply P4P to hospitals participating in Medicare (which is pretty much all hospitals in the country, though there are some rare exceptions for specialized private hospitals). Because of both the magnitude of impact that Medicare has on any hospital's revenues as well as the propensity of the commercial sector to take advantage of initiatives that CMS creates, it is briefly described as it exists at the time of publication. CMS does routinely modify and improve such types of programs, however, so any interested reader will want to stay current by reviewing the program at CMS's Web site.* Medicare-managed care is discussed in detail in Chapter 26.

Hospital Quality Initiative

The Hospital Quality Initiative program was created through the Medicare Modernization Act of 2003 (MMA), section 501(b), and applies to all hospitals that participate in Medicare. In this program, hospitals were required to report a "starter set" of 10 quality-related measures. Hospitals that did not comply with providing the measures would face a 0.4% reduction in their annual payment update. According to CMS, 98.3% of hospitals successfully reported the measures.[27] In addition to the 10 starter set measures, hospitals may report 10 more measures to CMS on a voluntary basis. The entire measure set is illustrated in Table 8-4.

Premier Hospital Quality Incentive Demonstration

In addition to the broad program for all hospitals participating in Medicare, and under MMA section 501(b), CMS launched a 3-year demonstration project: the Premier Hospital system, covering 270 participating hospitals. In this demonstration, CMS is collecting data on 34 quality measures relating to five clinical conditions. Hospitals scoring in the top 10% for a given set of quality measures will receive a 2% bonus payment on top of the standard DRG payment for the relevant dis-

---

*Source of this information is the author's review of multiple programs described in public documents.

---

*See http://www.cms.hhs.gov/. Accessed July 22, 2006.

Table 8–4 CMS Hospital Quality Measures

Measure	Condition
Aspirin at arrival	**Acute myocardial infarction (AMI)/heart attack**
Aspirin at discharge	
Beta blocker at arrival	
Beta blocker at discharge	
ACE inhibitor or angiotensin receptor blocker (ARB) for left ventricular systolic dysfunction	
Smoking cessation	
Thrombolytic agent received within 30 minutes of hospital arrival	
Percutaneous coronary intervention (PCI) received within 120 minutes of hospital arrival	
Left ventricular function assessment	**Heart failure**
ACE inhibitor or angiotensin receptor blocker (ARB) for left ventricular systolic dysfunction	
Comprehensive discharge instructions	
Smoking cessation	
Initial antibiotic received within 4 hours of hospital arrival	**Pneumonia**
Pneumococcal vaccination status	
Blood culture performed before first antibiotic received	
Smoking cessation	
Oxygenation assessment	
Appropriate initial antibiotic selection	
Prophylactic antibiotic received within 1 hour prior to surgical incision	**Surgical infection prevention**
Prophylactic antibiotics discontinued within 24 hours after surgery end time	

Source: CMS. Hospital Quality Initiative Overview, 2005. Available at: http://www.cms.hhs.gov/ HospitalQualityInits/downloads/HospitalOverview200512.pdf. Accessed July 23, 2006.

charges. Those scoring in the next highest 10% will receive a 1% bonus. In the third year of the demonstration, those hospitals that do not meet a predetermined threshold score on quality measures will be subject to reductions in payment. Hospital-specific performance will be publicly reported on CMS's Web site.[27] The project has not concluded at the time of publication, but according to the administra-tor for CMS, in 2005 there were significant improvements in all clinical categories.[28]

PAY-FOR-PERFORMANCE FOR PHYSICIANS

Physician P4P programs are generally more complex than are those for hospitals. They have historically been oriented toward primary care physicians, with measures focusing on prevention and certain common conditions. Although a few measures focused on care that may be delivered by either primary care or specialty physicians (*eg* diabetes), measures that focus explicitly on specialists have generally not been used. That will change; NCQA, working with several other organizations including CMS, is currently creating and testing specialist-specific measures.*

There is great variation in physician P4P program design, scope, source of the measures, and setting of standards; far more variation than is found in hospital-focused programs. This section discusses issues that are unique to any physician perormance measures and describes common measures and types of physician-focused P4P programs, representing a composite of programs that are in place at the time of publication.† Also, CMS has launched several physician P4P demonstation projects that are briefly described.

Measuring Individual versus Group Performance

The traditional complaint about performance measures as applied to individual physicians is that more than one physician may be involved with the care of any particular patient; for example, a cardiologist and a family practitioner may both provide care to a patient with coronary artery disease. Weaknesses in measures can also arise as a result of the small numbers of events that occur. For example, a physician may have only 120 patients with a particular health plan, many of whom do not have signficant medical problems and seek little care; those that do seek care have a variety of conditions, so only a handful of patients receive care that is the focus of the P4P program. One well-constructed study of a common chronic condition (diabetes) projected that a physician would need to have more than 100 patients with that diagnosis before the reliability of an individual physician report card would be 80%.[29] Last, is the problem one of patient compliance? A physician may practice with strict adherence to evidence-based medicine, but if he or she has patients that are asbestos-smoking, motorcycle-riding drug dealers with authority problems, compliance on the part of the patient may produce poor outcomes that are not the result of physician performance.

There are two basic approaches to addressing these inherent weaknesses in physician P4P programs. The first is to incite performance of a large group of physicians such as a large medical group, an IPA, or the entire local network, but not the individual physicians themselves (though of course individual physicians still need to submit their data as needed); in other words, collect the data from each physician, but measure performance in the aggregate. This addresses the weaknesses noted previously because the numbers are sufficiently large to be statistically significant (assuming that the type of care being provided is commonly rendered), any physicians involved in the care of the patient are likely to be in the group being measured, and patient compliance traits even out. The weakness of measuring the group is that the impact on individual performance is only indirect. How the group distributes the incentive compensation to individual physicians is likely to be unrelated to individual performance.

The second basic approach to addressing the weaknesses inherent in measuring the performance of individual physicians is to focus on process and structure but not outcomes. Examples of measurable processes might include documenting that appropriate tests, prescriptions, or preventive services

---

*John Freeman of NCQA, personal communication, July 24, 2006.

†Examples in this section were compiled by the author based on review of numerous existing programs, with both overlap and variations existing in program design, source of the measures, and setting of standards.

were ordered, even if the patient fails to follow through. Examples of measurable structure might include the use of e-prescribing or an EHR. CMS is currently experimenting with just such measures that could be applied to individual physicians caring for Medicare beneficiaries. The only type of outcome study that would at least theoretically be valid at the level of individual physicians would be measures related to patient satisfaction.

Ease of Data Collection and Reporting

Although most hospitals have some level of automation, as well as personnel to perform the work, most physician practices outside of large medical groups have neither. The more work required on the part of the physician or the office staff to collect and report the data, the more resistance the MCO will encounter. Data from sources outside of the office, such as claims data or pharmacy data, do not create any extra burden on the physician. Office-based data such as compliance with clinical protocols or reporting laboratory results (unless the MCO can obtain such data directly from reference labs, something that is possible using existing electronic standards) may be reported by the physician or may require the MCO to send in auditors. This is not to say that office-based data should not be obtained and used; rather, the MCO must take into account physician time, effort, and cost considerations when designing the program.

The Role of Feedback

For any P4P program to work, and especially so for a physician program, regular, accurate, and useful feedback must be provided. A hospital may be capable of creating internal reports that track to a P4P program (such internally generated reports may in fact be what is used for the program itself), but physicians usually have less capability to do so. Also, even when they carefully document

all aspects of care that they deliver, certain measures may simply not be available to them. When introducing new measures and goals, it is useful to collect data and generate feedback reports and comparisons against those new goals prior to actually using the measures for any financial incentives. Last, for feedback to be effective, it is also necessary that the goals that are set are actually achievable. Under those conditions, it is likely to be effective in improving performance, even in the absence of financial incentives.[30,31]

Common Measures

Measures commonly applied to physicians fall into three general categories: clinical measures, the use of IT, and patient satisfaction. And as noted earlier regarding hospitals, there is considerable overlap between these types of measures, and one can reasonably argue that this is more of a continuum than it is a set of categories. There are also some accreditation-based certifications for which some programs are providing financial incentives.

Clinical Measures

Few if any programs look at all of the clinical conditions that are commonly addressed under P4P, and the actual measures used vary considerably from program to program. Measures and goals are also periodically updated and modified. Examples of clinical conditions and measurements commonly addressed in P4P programs are as follows:

- Congestive heart failure (CHF); for example:
  - Appropriate medication use, such as an ACE inhibitor or ARB for patients with left ventricular systolic dysfunction
  - Dietary counseling
  - Smoking cessation
- Coronary artery disease (CAD); for example:
  - Management of hyperlipidemia

- ○ LDL cholesterol < 130
- ○ Use of asprin or other antithrombotic
- ○ Blood pressure control
- ○ Smoking cessation
- Diabetes; for example:
  - ○ Evidence of retinal and neuropathy exams
  - ○ Dietary counseling
  - ○ Smoking cessation
  - ○ Blood pressure control
  - ○ Hemoglobin A1c levels*
  - ○ LDL cholesterol < 130
- Asthma; for example:
  - ○ Appropriate use of medications, such as
    - – Maintenance inhaled corticosteriods
    - – Urgent-only use of bronchodilators
  - ○ Lung function testing
  - ○ Counseling to remove environmental triggers (smoke, dust mites, etc.)
  - ○ Smoking cessation
- Chronic obstructive pulmonary disease (COPD); for example:
  - ○ Smoking cessation
  - ○ Spirometry testing
  - ○ Calculation of body mass index
  - ○ Appropriate uses of medications
- Obesity
- Preventive services; for example:
  - ○ Immunizations
  - ○ Cervical cancer screening
  - ○ Breast cancer screening
  - ○ Colorectal screening
  - ○ Chlamydia screening in women
  - ○ Blood pressure control
  - ○ Detection and treatment of hyperlipidemia

Although utilization measures are not generally used in P4P programs, a large number of them do measure the use of generic prescriptions by the physicians and incorporate that measure into the incentive structure.

---

*A common blood test, correlating with the degree of control of blood sugar levels.

Patient Satisfaction

Patient satisfaction is a combination of survey results and any complaints or grievances that a member may file with the MCO regarding a physician. Financial incentives resulting from patient satisfaction may be applied at the level of the entire group of physicians or may be individually applied.

It is not practical for an MCO to survey all members who receive care from a physician. Web-based access to surveys may be offered to members, but the weakness of that approach is that it is far more likely for disgruntled or upset members to access the survey than for satisfied members who see no reason to take the time (though one can argue that there's nothing wrong with that—the MCO needs to know when members are unhappy).

More commonly, a statistically significant number of members are surveyed. As noted earlier, return rates on surveys that are simply mailed to members are notoriously low, however, so the MCO may choose to perform telephone surveys to increase the number of data or employ other methods to improve response rates. A standardized survey, the Ambulatory Consumer Assessment of Health Providers and Systems (A-CAHPS) is being created for CMS by AHRQ,[32] and that will also lend itself to use in P4P programs. A-CAHPS is still being field tested at the time of publication but should be available in the near future.

The other routine sets of measures in this category are access and waiting times. Access simply refers to appointment availability: how long does it take to get a routine appointment or an urgent appointment. Access may be measured through self-reporting or may be audited by the MCO. Waiting times are simply the average amount of time patients have to wait from when their appointment was scheduled to when the physician actually sees them. Waiting times are frequently measured through the use of simple cards that the office staff write both numbers on (or the patient may fill it out). At some point in the future, sophisticated scheduling and EHR systems may track this.

The Use of Information Technology

One frequent measure in the use of IT is for e-prescribing, not simply having access to it, but actually using it. Another measure is the existence and use of an EHR. As with hospitals, there are gradations as a result of the term *EHR* being used to describe electronic record systems of variable scope. A sophisticated P4P program defines the essential and desired (though not necessarily essential) attributes of the EHR that would result in performance incentives. An easier alternative, however, is to use external accreditation that certifies that the EHR meets appropriate standards; for example, the Physician Recognition Software Certification by NCQA.[33] In addition, certification for ambulatory EHR products by the CCHIT became available in 2006;[26] therefore, use of a CCHIT-certified application could also be an appropriate goal around the EHR.

Another common measure of IT use is a patient registry. This refers to a registry of patients arrayed by clinical condition, for example, a registry of all patients with CHF. This enables the physician to track those patients, their treatments, and their conditions in an organized fashion. It is certainly possible to do this using paper, but that is not commonly accepted as having met the goal. An EHR is not required to create a patient registry; commonly used programs for the personal computer (PC) may be adequate, if not optimal.

Some programs incorporate measures around the use of electronic connectivity between the physician and the MCO. The most common of these is electronic claims submission. Additional standards for common types of electronic data exchange as well (*eg,* authorizations, eligibilty verification, and others) are described in Chapter 17.

The last area of IT performance is less commonly measured: the existence and use of point-of-care clinical decision support systems. As used in many P4P programs, this refers primarily to computerized "expert systems" that support clinical care such as aiding in diagnosis or the provision of treatment protocols and may be either PC-based, network-based, or under certain conditions, accessed on the Internet.

NCQA Physician Recognition Program

Some P4P programs have specific financial rewards for those physicians who are successfully accredited by NCQA under the Physician Recognition Program. In addition to the Software Certification Program, at the time of publication there are three other certification programs:

- The Diabetes Physician Recognition Program[34] (DPRP), developed by NCQA and the American Diabetes Association, awards recognition to physicians who demonstrate that they provide high-quality care to patients with diabetes.
- The Heart/Stroke Physician Recognition Program[35] (HSRP), developed by NCQA and the American Heart Association/ American Stroke Association (AHA/ASA), awards recognition to physicians who demonstrate that they provide high-quality care to patients with cardiac conditions or who have had a stroke.
- The Physician Practice Connections[36] (PPC), which NCQA developed in collaboration with Bridges to Excellence, awards recognition to physician practices that use up-to-date information and systems to enhance patient care. All of the elements described in the preceding section on the use of IT are scored, and physicians may be certified at one of three possible levels; incentives are tied to the level of certification.

Incentives

Incentives to physicians fall along the entire array discussed earlier. The most common forms of incentives are adjustments to payments made for services and bonus payments, though tiering is also making an appearance.

Financial Incentives

Financial incentives may be either adjustments to payment rates or as bonus payments. There is no good data available as to the prevelance of these two types of incentives, but a review of publicly available information suggests that bonus payments are more common.* Adjustments to payment rates are most easily accomplished by adjusting the multiplier for an RVS. Bonus payments may be paid quarterly or semi-annually but are most commonly paid annually. Bonus payment may be paid based on meeting certain threshhold levels (*ie,* the bonus is paid out at 100% if a goal is met or exceeded), or it may be graduated (*ie,* the percentage paid is related to the percentage of the goal that is achieved). It is also possible to combine threshold and graduated bonus payments for different types of measures. In any case, the amount of incentive commonly ranges from 5% up to 10% of total payments, but there are a few programs that reach 20%.†

Tiering

Tiering is applied only to specialty physicians and is briefly described earlier in this chapter and in Chapter 5. Although still relatively uncommon, specialist tiering programs are based primarily on quality measures, though volume on selected procedures is another common measure incorporated into tiering decisions, at least in regards to select procedures such as transplants and certain types of cardiac procedures. Of course, a specialty physician also needs to agree to the reimbursement and other contractual terms to be selected for inclusion.

---

*Source of this information is the author's review of multiple programs described in public documents.

†Source of this information is the author's review of multiple programs described in public documents.

Medicare

Unlike the Hospital Quality Initiative that CMS is applying to all hospitals as described earlier, at the time of publication CMS is approaching P4P for physicians solely on the basis of demonstration projects, not imposing any specific program on all participating physicians. Each project is at a different stage in its life cycle and results are not known.

CMS describes these projects as follows.[27]

Physician Group Practice Demonstration

Mandated by the Benefits Improvement and Protection Act of 2000 (BIPA 2000), this demonstration is the first pay-for-performance initiative for physicians under the Medicare program. The demonstration rewards physicians for improving the quality and efficiency of health care services delivered to Medicare fee-for-service beneficiaries. The demonstration seeks to encourage coordination of Part A and Part B services, promote efficiency through investment in administrative structure and process, and reward physicians for improving health outcomes.

Ten large (200+ physicians) group practices across the country are participating in this demonstration, which began in April 2005. The physician group practices will be able to earn performance-based payments after achieving savings in comparison to a control group. The performance payment is largely based on various quality results.

Medicare Care Management Performance Demonstration

Provided for under the MMA, section 649, this program is modeled on the Bridges to Excellence program, and is a 3-year pay-for-performance demonstration with physicians to promote the adoption and use of health information technology to improve the quality of patient care for chronically ill Medicare patients. Doctors who meet or exceed performance standards established by CMS in clinical delivery systems and patient outcomes will receive bonus payments for managing the care of eligible Medicare beneficiaries.

In contrast to the Physician Group Practice Demonstration, this demonstration, which is under development at the time of publication, is focused on small and medium-sized physician practices. It will be implemented in four states, Arkansas, California, Massachusetts, and Utah, with the support of the Quality Improvement Organizations in those states.

Medicare Health Care Quality Demonstration

This demonstration, which also was mandated by section 646 of the MMA, will be a 5-year demonstration program under which projects enhance quality by improving patient safety, reducing variations in utilization by appropriate use of evidence-based care and best practice guidelines, encouraging shared decision making, and using culturally and ethnically appropriate care. Eligible entities include physician groups, integrated health systems, or regional coalitions of the same.

RESULTS OF PAY-FOR-PERFORMANCE PROGRAMS

Because P4P has actually been in existence for many years, results about the effectiveness should be clear. Unfortunately, at least for the earlier programs the results are not clear that performance incentives have a long-term effect.[37] Since that study, however, approaches to P4P have improved considerably, at least as regards the ability to capture necessary data, though scientifically rigorous studies showing positive results remain ambigous, at least on a broad basis.[38,39] More recent reports tend to be positive. The announcement by CMS of positive results in hospitals noted earlier in the chapter is one such example. Another example is a report of very positive results from the IHA for the large physician-focused program in California.[40]

Remarkably, there is one study published in 2005 that is cited by proponents of P4P as demonstrating superior metrics for providers under P4P than for a similar set of providers that were not under P4P. That same study is cited by critics of P4P as showing that most of the incentives went to providers that were already providing better quality of care, thus concluding that P4P did not actually change any behavior.[41] In any event, even when incentive programs are used, they undergo continual retooling in a quest to improve their effectiveness, however that might be measured.[42]

CONCLUSION

P4P programs are one more set of tools used in managed health care, and as such, should not be considered a panacea to managing the quality of health care. Like financial incentives based on utilization described in Chapter 6, P4P programs align financial incentives with the overall goals of the MCO and its customers; in the case of P4P, it also more easily aligns to the goals of the providers themselves who generally do appreciate being rewarded based on quality. How P4P will evolve is difficult to predict, though with the advent of the EHR such programs should gain a new ability to further improve the quality of health care.

References

1. American Healthways. *Outcomes-Based Compensation: Pay-for-Performance Design Principles.* 2005. Available at: http://www. rewarding quality.com/. Accessed July 18, 2006.
2. Epstein AM, Lee TH, Hamel MB. Paying physicians for high-quality care. *N Engl J Med.* January 22, 2004, 350;(4):406–410.
3. Donabedian A. *The Definition of Quality and Approaches to Its Assessment.* Ann Arbor, Mich: Health Administration Press, 1980.
4. Cooper RM. Formal physician performance evaluations. *J Ambulatory Care Manage.* 1980, 3:19–33.

5. Schlackman N. Integrating quality assessment and physician incentive payment. *Qual Rev Bull.* August 1989, 15(8):234–237.

6. Traska MR. HMO uses quality measures to pays its physicians. *Hospitals.* July 5, 1988, 62(13):34, 36.

7. Sennett C, Legorreta AP, Zata SL. Performance-based hospital contracting for quality improvement. *J Quality Improvement.* 1993, 19 (9):374–383.

8. McGuirk-Porell M, Goldberg GA, Goldin D, *et al.* A performance-based quality evaluation system for preferred provider organizations. *Qual Rev Bull.* November 1991:365–373.

9. Gold MR, Hurley R, Lake T, Ensor T, Berenson R. A national survey of the arrangements managed-care plans make with physicians. *N Engl J Med.* 1995, 333(25):1678–1683.

10. Lake TK, St. Peter RF. *Payment Arrangements and Financial Incentives for Physicians. Community Tracking Study.* Washington, DC: Center for Studying Health System Change. Fall 1997. Data Bulletin #8.

11. Integrated Healthcare Association. *History of IHA's Pay for Performance Initiative.* Available at: http://www.iha.org/payfprfd.htm. Accessed July 21, 2006.

12. Integrated Healthcare Association. *Advancing Quality Through Collaboration: The California Pay for Performance Program.* February 2006. Available at: http://www.iha.org/wp020606. pdf. Accessed July 21, 2006.

13. Blue Cross of California. Blue Cross of California pays out $72 million in physician bonus incentives. Press release. Available at: http://www.bluecrossca.com. Accessed July 23, 2006.

14. Integrated Healthcare Association. Integrated Healthcare Association shares five years of experience in pay for performance with healthcare leaders at national conference. February 6, 2006. Press release. Available at: http://www.iha.org/020606.htm. Accessed July 21, 2006.

15. Roland M. Linking physician's pay to the quality of care—A major experiment in the United Kingdom. *N Engl J Med.* September 30, 2004, 351(14):1448–1454.

16. Doran T, Fullwood C, Gravelle H, *et al.* Pay-for-performance in family practices in the United Kingdom. *N Engl J Med.* 2006, 355:375–384.

17. Cleary PD, Edgman-Levitan S. Health care quality: Incorporating consumer perspectives. *JAMA.* 1997, 278:1608–1612.

18. Available at: https://www.cahps.ahrq.gov/ default.asp. Accessed July 21, 2006.

19. Available at: http://www.hospitalcompare.hhs. gov/hospital/home2.asp. Accessed July 23, 2006.

20. Available at: http://www.opa.ca.gov/report_ card/med_groups/display_counties.asp? target = /report_card/med_groups/rating_ summary_report.asp. Accessed July 18, 2006.

21. Werner RM, Asch RA. The unintended consequences of publicly reported quality information. *JAMA.* 2005, 293:1239–1244.

22. Aspden P, Wolcott J, Bootman J, Cronenwett L, eds. *Preventing Medication Errors: Quality Chasm Series.* Washington, DC: National Academies Press, 2006. Available at: http://www. nap.edu/catalog/11623.html#toc. Accessed July 23, 2006.

23. Bates DW, Leape LL, Cullen DJ, *et al.* Effect of computerized physician order entry and a team intervention on prevention of serious medication errors. *JAMA.* 1998, 280: 1311–1316.

24. Bates DW, Teich JM, Merchia PR, Schmiz BS, Kuperman GJ, Spurr CD. Effects of computerized physician order entry on prescribing practices. *Arch Int Med.* 2000, 160:2741–2747.

25. Certification Commission for Healthcare Information Technology. Overview. 2006. Available at: http://www.cchit.org/about/ overview.htm. Accessed July 24, 2006.

26. Certification Commissionfor Healthcare Information Technology. Certifying your Electronic Health Record (EHR) product. 2006. Available at: http://www.cchit.org/vendors/. Accessed July 24, 2006.

27. Centers for Medicare and Medicaid Services. Medicare "Pay-for-Performance (P4P)" initiatives. January 31, 2005. Press release. Available at: http://www.cms.hhs.gov/apps/media/press/ release.asp. Accessed July 23, 2006.

28. Centers for Medicare and Medicaid Services. Medicare pay-for-performance demonstration shows significant quality of care improvement at participating hospitals. May 4, 2005. Press release. Available at: http://www.cms. hhs.gov/apps/media/press/release.asp. Accessed July 23, 2006.

29. Hofer TP, Hayward RA, Greenfield S, Wagner EH, Kaplan SH, Manning WG. The unreliability of individual physician "report cards" for assessing the costs and quality of care of a chronic disease. *JAMA*. 1999, 281:2098–2105.

30. Kiefe CI, Allison JJ, Williams OD, *et al*. Improving quality improvement using achievable benchmarks for physician feedback: a randomized controlled trial. *JAMA*. 2001, 285: 2871–2879.

31. Bordley WC, Chelminski A, Margolis PA, Kraus R, Szilagyi PG, Vann JJ. The effect of audit and feedback on immunization delivery. *Am J Prev Med*. May 2000, 18(4):343–350.

32. *Agency for Healthcare Research and Quality*. The CAHPS connection. June 2006: 2(3). AHRQ Publication No. 06-0015-3-EF. Available at: https://www.cahps.ahrq.gov/content/CAHPS Connection/files/CAHPSConnectionVolume2 Issue3.html#cgsurvey. Accessed July 22, 2006.

33. National Committee for Quality Assurance. Physician recognition software certification. Available at: http://www.ncqa.org/Programs/ PRSC/index.htm. Accessed July 23, 2006.

34. National Committee for Quality Assurance. DPRP. Available at: http://www.ncqa.org/dprp/. Accessed July 23, 2006.

35. National Committee for Quality Assurance. Heart/Stroke Recognition Program. Available at: http://www.ncqa.org/hsrp/. Accessed July 23, 2006.

36. National Committee for Quality Assurance. Physician Practice Connections. Available at: http://www.ncqa.org/ppc/. Accessed July 23, 2006.

37. Dudley RA, Miller RH, Korenbrot TY, Luft HS. The impact of financial incentives on quality of health care. *Millbank Quarterly*. 1998, 76(4): 649–685.

38. Dudley RA. Pay-for-performance research: how to learn what clinicians and policy makers need to know. *JAMA*. 2005, 294(14):1821–1823.

39. Rosenthal MB, Frank RG. What is the empirical basis for paying for quality in health care? *Med Care Res Rev*. 2006, 63(2):135–157.

40. Integrated Healthcare Association. Continued quality improvement in California health care announced by Integrated Healthcare Association. July 13, 2006. Press release. Available at: http://www.iha.org/071306.htm. Accessed July 23, 2006.

41. Rosenthal MB, Frank RG, Epstein AM. Early experience with pay-for-performance, from concept to practice. *JAMA*. 2005, 294: 1788–1793.

42. Ogrod ES. Compensation and quality: A physician's view. *Health Affairs*. 1997, 16(3):82–86.

Part 3

MEDICAL MANAGEMENT

You can't always get what you want.
But if you try sometimes
You just might find
You get what you need.

—Mick Jagger [1969]

9

MANAGING BASIC MEDICAL-SURGICAL UTILIZATION

Peter R. Kongstvedt and Kimberley A. Mentzer

Study Objectives

- Understand what managing utilization means.
- Understand the basic categories of medical-surgical utilization management.
- Understand basic differences between managing utilization in the inpatient, outpatient, and specialty services categories.
- Understand what basic utilization management techniques are most useful in different situations.
- Understand basic measurements of utilization.
- Understand basic roles for different types of professionals in managing utilization.
- Understand how approaches to managing utilization have changed over the years and why those changes have occurred.

Discussion Topics

1. Discuss the key attributes of managing basic medical-surgical utilization in different types of managed care plans.
2. Discuss how basic utilization management has changed over the years and why.
3. Discuss how utilization management might change in the future and why.
4. Briefly describe differences in managing utilization of acute care versus chronic care.

5. Discuss the unique challenges a provider or hospital-sponsored HMO has in managing utilization and how those challenges might realistically be met.
6. Discuss the hospitalist approach in inpatient care, and when such an approach is appropriate and when it is not.
7. Discuss the types of data and reports that would be useful to the medical director for managing specialist utilization; discuss how this might differ in different types of plans.

INTRODUCTION

Evidence demonstrates that a high degree of unwarranted variation exists in the practice of medicine: patients may be overtreated, undertreated, or treated with the wrong interventions. This unwarranted care can be further categorized into three situations:

- **Use or lack of use of evidence-based medicine:** In this situation, a care plan is proven to be effective, and there are no significant "trade-offs." For example, use of a beta blocker for patients post heart attack varies widely,[1] although it should be nearly 100% because clinical contraindications are rare.
- **Preference—sensitive care:** In this situation, a choice is involved (trade-offs) because at least two valid alternative treatments are available. For example, in southern California, a patient is six times more likely to have back surgery for a herniated disk than in New York.*
- **Supply—sensitive care:** In this situation, the more available a treatment is, the more often it is used. For example, per capita spending per Medicare enrollee in Florida is more than twice that seen in Minnesota.[2]

A principal objective of the management of utilization is the reduction of unwarranted practice variation by establishing parameters for cost-effective utilization of health care resources. The techniques used in utilization management (UM) programs serve to manage resource utilization within those parameters to contain cost while ensuring appropriate care is provided.[3] Where utilization guidelines, case management, condition management, and wellness/behavior modification health coaching are incorporated into health delivery, the degree of practice variation and the amount of inappropriate care are reduced. This affects even the nonmanaged-care patients of physicians who have significant managed care practices; for example, inpatient utilization in nonmanaged-care patients is observed when managed care presence is high.[4]

Utilization management has evolved along with the market. In the early managed care era when unnecessary utilization was high basic approaches to UM produced strong financial results, with a several-fold return on investment.[3,5–10] As discussed in Chapter 1, however, a combination of the so-called managed care backlash against health maintenance organizations (HMOs) and the desire of consumers to have both broad access to providers and fewer restrictions on access to care (by eliminating, for example, the primary care physician "gatekeeper" model) led many managed care organizations (MCOs) to reduce or even eliminate many UM activities. At the same time, other health plan types such as preferred provider organizations (PPOs) grew, and consumer-directed health plans (CDH or CDHPs) have recently been introduced,* both

---

*Private communication from proprietary disease management vendor and author, May 2006.

*See Chapter 2 for descriptions of these various health plan types.

of which are less likely to approach UM in as comprehensive an approach as a traditional HMO. Last, the provider environment changed as well over the years, with providers realizing that unnecessary utilization can and should be eliminated.

For the many reasons listed in Chapter 1, health care costs once again began to rise around the turn of the millennium. Attendant increases in health care costs were met with a combination of higher cost sharing by consumers, more sophisticated approaches to managing the costs of only the most expensive types of care through disease management (DM; see Chapter 10), and selective use of the traditional approaches to UM.[11] In some cases, traditional forms of UM that had been abandoned by MCOs because of market pressures are starting to reappear because of increased cost pressures.[12] In other words, managing utilization remains a highly dynamic and changing activity.

Regardless of plan type or benefit design, there are many facets to the management of utilization. Even accounting for new product and health plan designs, managed care has become prevalent, and the divisions between the management of specialty physician care, inpatient care, outpatient care, case and condition management, preventive care, and indeed all aspects of health care delivery have become progressively blurred. Furthermore, the applications and tools that health plans utilize to facilitate these functions are more integrated and are shifting to the creation of longitudinal, member-centric records.

Many aspects of utilization and care management are discussed in this book in separate chapters; however, a core set of activities may be considered fundamental to managing utilization of medical and surgical services. This chapter's purpose is to provide an overview of that core set. The topics addressed in this chapter overlap information presented in greater detail in other chapters; if anything, this attribute helps to underscore the fact that management of medical services is not made up of discrete activities unrelated to each other. Interested readers should understand that although other chapters of this book go into depth on some of the other activities of care management, many more cannot be addressed in this text because of practical limitations on space. It is also important to understand that not all MCOs use all approaches to UM as described in this chapter.

DEMAND MANAGEMENT

Demand management refers to activities of a health plan designed to direct necessary health care services to the most appropriate level of care (*eg,* direct away from expensive emergency department setting) and potentially reduce the overall requirement for health care services by members. In addition to helping to lower health care costs, these services also may provide a competitive advantage to a health plan by enhancing its reputation for service and giving members additional value for their premium dollar. Demand management services fall into five broad categories that are briefly discussed in the following subsections to place them in context with the basic medical-surgical UM functions.

Nurse Advice Lines

Nurse advice lines provide members with access to advice regarding medical conditions, the need for medical care, health promotion and preventive care, and numerous other advice-related activities. Such advice lines have been in use in closed-panel HMOs for many years, where they were once (and occasionally still are) referred to as "triage"* nurse lines but are now common in most MCOs. Plans may staff these lines with their

---

*The use of the term *triage nurse* is not recommended if for no other reason than its military history. *Triage* is a term used in battlefield medicine that refers to the separation of casualties into three categories: immediate attention required, attention can be delayed, and casualty is beyond hope and will only be given palliative care. Use of the term *advice* nurse is more appropriate.

own nurses, or they may purchase the service from any one of a number of commercial vendors. Hours of operation are commonly 24 hours per day, 7 days per week, and a toll-free line makes it easy for members to access the service.

Special market segments such as Medicare and Medicaid (see Chapters 26 and 27) benefit from dedicated programs and have become contractual requirements in certain geographies. Attention to the special problems and concerns of seniors will go a long way toward improving health status and can be a major contributor to the overall management of care in this population. Easy access to medical advice in the Medicaid population may enable these members to avoid a trip to the emergency department.

Self-Care and Medical Consumerism Programs

This activity refers to the provision of information to members to enable them to provide care for themselves, or to better evaluate when they need to seek care from a professional. With the increased focus on CDH and the objective of making the health care consumer a more informed consumer, this capability has increased in importance for health plans, and by the time of publication will be an accreditation standard by the National Committee for Quality Assurance (NCQA; see Chapter 23).[13] In the past, member newsletters with medical advice were used extensively by HMOs. Because health plans have determined that members have different preferred communication channels, the information is typically now made available through a multichannel tool set (eg, Web-based, phone, mailings).

The most common example of a proactive approach is a self-care guide provided by the plan. These guides are generally written in an easy-to-understand manner, and they provide step-by-step advice for common medical conditions and preventive care. Information about the wise use of medical services or

how to be an informed consumer would fall into this category as well. With the increasing use of the Internet and the increase in availability of new health information, the Web-based channel has become preferred by health plans. From an administrative perspective, it is a cheaper per-transaction cost, and it supports more personalization for each member.

Self-care programs have been evaluated since the early 1980s. Typical results have shown $2.50 to $3.50 saved for every $1 invested.[14] In one structured study in a staff model HMO, the targeted use of self-care manuals resulted in decreased outpatient visits and a 2:1 return on the cost of the program.[15] Another study on a fever health education program decreased pediatric clinic utilization by 35% for fever visits and 25% for all acute visits.[16]

Shared Decision-Making Programs

This activity refers to making the member an active participant in choosing a course of care. Although this general philosophy may be prevalent in the routine interactions between patients and physicians, shared decision programs are more focused. They provide patients in-depth information on specific procedures. By providing this information, patients gain a deeper understanding of not only the disease process, but also the treatment alternatives. In a few cases, MCOs employing this type of program will not finalize authorization for certain elective procedures (eg, transurethral resection of the prostate) until the member has completed the shared decision-making program. The value of shared decision-making programs is well documented.[17–20]

A number of commercial services produce these programs, some with innovative business model designs.[21] Many use interactive CD-ROMs, videotapes or DVDs, computer programs, and Internet Web sites to provide information. Supplemental access to a nurse advice line, as well as the ability to discuss the alternatives with the physician after the patient has reviewed the material, is also routine.

Medical Informatics

Medical informatics is a broad term that applies to the use of information technology in the management of health care delivery, and the use of data in medical management is discussed in greater detail in Chapter 16. For purposes of this chapter, *medical informatics* refers to the use of information technology in helping to manage demand for services. An MCO may use information systems to anticipate demand for services or to analyze how demand for services can be better managed. For example, an analysis of the use of urgent care or emergency services may be related to hours of operation, location of primary care, work patterns at a large employer, and so forth. By looking for patterns, the plan may be able to develop strategies for lowering demand for one type of service by substituting another type of service.

Most MCOs now provide services to members through their Web sites on the Internet, including health assessments (discussed later), wellness, behavior modification, and self-care information, in addition to some administrative capabilities (*eg,* obtaining a new identification card). MCOs and health care delivery systems are also using the Internet to support medical education and management of utilization and quality. Most MCOs provide members with access to health information from reputable and recognized external sources rather than attempt to create such content on their own.

The Internet also has become a source of health-related information that is totally unregulated or monitored for quality. The constitutional right to free speech is silent about the issue of publishing drivel, even potentially dangerous drivel. Therefore, medical managers will want to stay abreast of at least the most popular health information Web sites and make the locations of high-quality sites known to the plan's membership (along with a note that advice can vary from one source to another and still be of good quality).

Preventive Services and Health Risk Appraisals

Preventive services, which are a hallmark of the HMO industry but which are also gaining importance in other types of health plans, are discussed in detail in Chapter 14. Therefore, only a brief mention of some of these activities is provided here. Because of the increased capabilities in health plan informatics to identify target members and the lower cost of multiple outreach channels, preventive services are being rolled out to all product types, including HMOs, PPOs, and CDHPs.

Common preventive services include immunizations, mammograms, routine physical examinations, and counseling regarding behaviors that members can undertake to lower their risk of ill health. Counseling and education also may be directed toward specific clinical conditions. For example, several years ago one managed indemnity plan studied an employer's on-site prenatal education program. The study found that participants had an average cost per delivery that was $3,200 less than that of nonparticipants.[22]

The health risk appraisal (HRA)* is a tool designed to elicit information from a member regarding certain activities and behaviors that can influence health status. HRAs are administered in multiple formats (*eg,* paper, phone, Web) and are becoming more common for employer groups to support during the open-enrollment process. To obtain compliance by members, some employers are offering incentives for completion (*eg,* bonus dollars in flexible spending account or coupons for health services).

The objective of the HRA is to collect information and, through analysis, create a mem-

---

*An MCO may use the term *health appraisal* so as to eliminate any perceived negative connotations of the word *risk,* but this is purely cosmetic.

ber profile of an individual's health risks and needs for behavior modification that may improve a member's health outcomes. Ultimately, the health appraisal findings trigger applicable care management programs, including wellness and behavior modification programs (*eg*, smoking cessation, stress reduction, or weight management).

The use of such behavior modification programs can provide even a near-term benefit. For example, a study of modifiable health risks (*eg*, tobacco use, physical activity, and so forth) and short-term health care costs found higher health care costs over an 18-month period, ranging from $1,500 to $2,500 per patient, when comparing low-risk behavior to high-risk behavior.[23] Disease-specific HRAs also exist and may be incorporated into a disease management program. In all cases, the health appraisal findings are typically shared with the member and may be used by the MCO's care management department. Results may also be shared with the member's physician in some cases.

HRAs may be broadly classified into three categories:

1. **Risk-based HRA:** It is the earliest type of HRA. It focuses on patient behavior and its effect on health risk.
2. **Habit-based HRA:** It is similar to the risk-based HRA. It not only looks at habits that create increased health risk but also incorporates elements of health education and behavioral change.
3. **Utilization-based HRA:** A form of HRA that focuses on predictors of utilization. It has not been as predictive as expected.[24]

In plans that have a large Medicare enrollment, the plan may take extra steps in performing an initial assessment. The most common extra activity is an in-home assessment of the new Medicare member. A trained nurse or medical social worker may determine, for example, that if the plan gives the new Medicare enrollee a bath mat or shower chair, it will significantly reduce the

risk of a hip fracture as a result of the person falling in the bathtub. An inventory of the member's diet also may yield valuable information that will enable the new member's provider to improve health status by lowering sodium intake or consumption of saturated fats. This activity not only improves the quality of care for these members, but also yields considerable savings. For example, Kaiser Permanente in Denver reported a $70 per member per month (PMPM) drop in cost within 6 months of implementing a Medicare health status and risk screening program.[25] In another example, HealthPartners of Southern Arizona* reported savings of $6,500 per Medicare patient from its screening and early intervention program.[26]

Personal Health Record and Personal Health Manager Tools

As health care in the United States continues to move to a more consumer-driven model where the member is expected to be more involved in health care decisions, a trend has evolved in the creation of personal health records (PHR). Personal health management involves activities such as tracking and monitoring personal health measures (*eg*, blood pressure, cholesterol), selecting health providers, managing health dollars (*eg*, flexible spending, health spending, and health reimbursement accounts), and understanding/influencing care treatments. It is important to note that a PHR is not the same as an electronic health record (EHR). Personal health management tools enable the data to be shared in multiple directions, and business rules can drive key messages, actions, reminders, and content. The information is personalized (and may be controlled by the individual), secure, interoperable (includes multiple data sources such as claims, authorizations, and even results from an HRA), and interactive. A rules-based messaging capabil-

---

*Since acquired by UnitedHealth Group.

ity includes health reminders (*eg,* appointments, prescription refills), compliance reminders (*eg,* mammogram), and helpful suggestions (*eg,* availability of generic option). At the time of publication, the primary trade association for the health insurance industry, American's Health Insurance Plans (AHIP), was in the process of standardizing the core data elements of the PHR so as to improve interoperability between health plans, and Medicare is planning to launch a PHR pilot program.

MEASUREMENTS OF UTILIZATION

It is not possible to manage utilization well unless there is a means to measure it. Although the topic of using data and information for medical management is discussed in depth in Chapter 16, some basic measurements need to be noted here to bring per-

spective to basic medical-surgical utilization management. This brief discussion can illustrate only the broadest types of utilization measurements, but these measures are the ones commonly reported by MCOs and reviewed by both medical managers and other senior executives.

Table 9-1 illustrates some common utilization metrics for HMOs, and Table 9-2 provides comparative data on PPOs, though only for commercial utilization. The meaning of these measures is either self-evident or will be described later in the chapter. It is important to bear in mind that utilization data reported by PPOs are likely to have far less precision than those reported by HMOs primarily because of two reasons. The first is that there are occasional deficiencies in a PPO's ability to capture membership numbers accurately because of reliance on old processing systems that do not record a de-

Table 9–1 Annual Utilization Rates of HMOs, 2004

HMO Utilization Measure	Average for HMOs in Systems	Average for HMOs Not in Systems	Average for All HMOs
Number of HMO enrollees per plan	217,083	156,479	168,991
Hospital days per 1,000 non-Medicare members	218.5	225.7	224.0
Hospital days per 1,000 Medicare members	1,349.6	1,545.9	1,485.4
Hospital admissions per 1,000 non-Medicare members	59.7	60.5	60.3
Hospital admissions per 1,000 Medicare members	265.2	274.0	271.1
Physician encounters per non-Medicare member	3.2	3.5	3.4
Physician encounters per Medicare member	7.0	8.5	8.0
Ambulatory visits per non-Medicare member	1.5	1.8	1.7
Ambulatory visits per Medicare member	2.7	3.8	3.4
Average length of stay (ALOS) per non-Medicare hospital admission	3.6	3.7	3.7
ALOS per Medicare hospital admission	5.7	5.7	5.7

Source: Sanofi-Aventis. *HMO-PPO/Medicare-Medicaid Digest 2005.* Managed Care Digest Series. Available at: http://www.managedcaredigest.com.

Table 9–2 Annual Utilization Rates of PPOs, 2004,* Commercial PPO Members

PPO Size	Hospital Days per 1,000 Members	Average Length of Stay (days)	Physician Encounters per Member
Under 19,000	230.3	3.9	3.6
20,000–99,999	231.5	4.0	4.6
100,000–499,999	216.3	3.9	4.2
500,000–999,999	255.7	3.9	4.0
1,000,000+	242.7	3.5	3.2
Overall Average	229.7	3.9	4.2

*Excluding psychiatric/substance abuse.
Source: Sanofi-Aventis. *HMO-PPO/Medicare-Medicaid Digest 2005.* Managed Care Digest Series. Available at: http://www.managedcaredigest.com.

pendent* as even existing until that dependent actually incurs services. The second reason is that PPOs are not uniform in their design, with many PPOs not offering full services. Thus, the data in Table 9-2 must be viewed with a bit of caution.

Physician Utilization Data

A basic tenet of managed health care is to provide low cost and easy access to primary care, though not always to specialty care services, at least in HMOs. Legislation in several states requires open access to a variety of specialty providers even in HMOs, but there is little uniformity between states about which types of providers are given such privileges. Obstetrics/gynecology (OB/Gyn) is the only specialty that is commonly granted open access by HMOs. With the shift to PPOs and CDHPs, the premise is to allow consumer choice to specialty services while applying and increasing the financial impact of more cost sharing on specialty service choices.

Measurement of physician visits, or encounters, as illustrated in Tables 9-1 and 9-2 are not

separated by primary or specialty care. With the steady blurring of managed care models, the increase in specialty-specific open access requirements under state laws, and the fact that many physicians perform both roles, it is difficult to make these distinctions.

In those plans that use a primary care physician (PCP) referral authorization system for specialty care as discussed later in this chapter, measurement of referral rates may be useful. There is no set standard for reporting data on referral utilization as there is for hospital utilization. Nevertheless, managers use certain measures frequently and find them useful. In HMOs that do not pay benefits for services provided without an authorization from a PCP, a useful and common measure is the referral rate per 1,000 members per year (how to calculate that type of rate is described later). Like the measurement of hospitalization rate, this figure looks at an annualized referral rate for every 1,000 members. Some HMOs also track referrals per 100 encounters per PCP, that is, a referral percentage.

When calculating referral rates in an HMO, it is important to know what is being counted: initial referrals or total visits to a referral specialist. In other words, counting only the initial referral or authorization may result in missing a large portion of the actual utiliza-

*An employee is the subscriber, but a spouse or child covered under the subscriber's policy is considered a dependent; both subscriber and dependents are considered members.

tion. It is not uncommon, especially in loosely managed HMOs, for a single referral to generate multiple visits to a specialist. For example, if a PCP refers a member with the request to evaluate and treat, it is really a request for the specialist to take over the care of the patient. Succeeding visits will be to the specialist, not to the PCP. Such types of measurements do not apply to MCOs that are not HMOs, of course, because there is no specialty authorization process.

Hospital Utilization Data

One cannot manage hospital utilization using intuition and unsupported estimates. Data is required, just as it is in managing any other aspect of a health plan. The most common high level data are measurements around so-called bed days per thousand, which is defined and illustrated as follows.

Definition of the Numbers

It is important to choose what is to be measured and to define that measurement precisely. Most plans measure bed days per 1,000 plan members per year (the formula is given later). Deciding what to count as a bed day is not always straightforward, however.

Outpatient surgery should not be counted as a single day in the hospital on the assumption that an outpatient procedure will cost the plan nearly the same as or sometimes more than a single inpatient day. With the heavy shift from inpatient to outpatient for surgical procedures and because reimbursement for outpatient procedures is almost always different from that for inpatient days (see Chapter 7), it is more appropriate to count outpatient procedures separately, though using the same approach to the calculation.

A few plans count skilled nursing home days in the total, though most do not. Although plans may add commercial, Medicare, Medicaid, and fee-for-service into the total calculation, it is most common to separate those very different types of businesses and patient populations. In some plans, the day of dis-

charge is counted; in most it is not unless the hospital charges for it.

How to count nursery days is not straightforward, and a decision must be reached on whether to count nursery days in the total when the mother is still in the hospital or only if the newborn is boarding over or in intensive care. Under the assumption that skilled nursing days are not counted as hospital days because the cost is so much less, the same assumption may be made for nursery days while the mother is in the hospital. In most hospitals, the nursery charges for a normal newborn are relatively low. If the newborn requires a stay beyond the mother's discharge, the charges usually are higher. If the neonate is in the intensive care unit, charges will be quite high. If the MCO has negotiated an all-inclusive per diem rate or a case rate that takes normal nursery days into account while the mother is in the hospital, there may be no need to count them separately. If the MCO must pay a high rate for nursery, then it should count them in the total.

Formulas to Calculate Institutional Utilization

The standard formula to calculate bed days per 1,000 members per year (BD/K) is relatively straightforward. It may be used to calculate the annualized bed days per 1,000 members for any chosen time period (*eg,* for the day, the month to date, the year to date, and so forth). The exact same formula is applicable to calculating ambulatory procedures per 1,000 members per year.

The calculation of bed days per 1,000 uses the assumption of a 365-day year as opposed to a 12-month year to prevent variations that are caused solely by the length of the month. The formula is as follows:

$$[A \div (B \div 365)] \div (C \div 1,000)$$

where A is gross bed days per time unit, B is days per time unit, and C is plan membership.

This calculation may be broken into steps. Table 9-3 illustrates the calculation for bed days per 1,000 on a single day, while Table 9-4

Table 9–3 Sample Calculation of Bed Days for a Single Day

Assume: Current hospital census = 60
Plan membership = 100,000

Step 1: Gross days $= 60 \div (1 \div 365)$
                          $= 60 \div 0.00274$
                          $= 21,897.81$

Step 2: Days per 1,000 $= 21,897.81 \div (100,000 \div 1,000)$
                          $= 3,649.635 \div 100$
                          $= 219 \text{ (rounded)}$

Therefore, the days per 1,000 for that single day is 219.

illustrates the calculation for bed days per 1,000 for a month to date. Small numbers are used in these illustrations so as to provide clarity to the example.

VARIATIONS IN UTILIZATION

A substantial body of evidence points to the fact that hospital utilization and procedure rates vary significantly from one geographic area of the country to another in the absence of explanations as a result of sociodemographic or morbidity factors. As far back as 1982, Wennberg and Gittelsohn coined the term "surgical signature" to describe a regional practice pattern of surgical rates within an area that cannot be explained by differences in population morbidity or other market phenomena.[27] According to Wennberg and Caper, the rate of some treatments did not vary much from one market to the next; however, the variations in rates across markets was four- to fivefold for other treatments with no population-based explanation for the differences.[28] Variations on utilization continued to be reported throughout the 1980s and 1990s,[29-35] including research that revealed geographic variations in the type and use of different treatments by physicians across the country. The phenomenon can be explained in various ways, including the hypothesis that variations in health care and treatment are "caused by variability in prevalence of physicians who are enthusiasts about the use of the services whose use varies."[36] In addition, other evidence supports the theory that those health care markets with a higher than average number of hospital beds and physicians tend to have correspondingly higher utilization rates.[37,38] Such variations were not

Table 9–4 Sample Calculation of Bed Days for the Month to Date (MTD)

Assume: Total gross hospital bed days MTD = 1,200
Plan membership = 100,000
Days in MTD = 21

Step 1: Gross days MTD $= 1,200 \div (21 \div 365)$
                              $= 1,200 \div 0.0575$
                              $= 20,869.565$

Step 2: Days per 1,000 in MTD $= 20,869.565 \div (100,000 \div 1,000)$
                              $= 20,869.565 \div 100$
                              $= 209 \text{ (rounded)}$

Therefore, the days per 1,000 for the MTD is 209.

limited to private health care. Medicare routinely reports substantial variations in costs and utilization by geographic area,[2] and substantial geographic variations in inpatient and ambulatory utilization in the Veterans Affairs hospitals and clinics have also been reported, even though physician income was unaffected by utilization.[39]

The National Center for Health Statistics, Centers for Disease Control and Prevention, performed a study of variance in hospitalizations and reported that 12% of all hospitalizations in the United States were avoidable.[40] Unlike other studies, the hospitalizations in that study did not vary greatly by region (*ie,* range of 11% to 13%); differences were primarily tied to sociodemographic factors. Low- to middle-income and minority segments of the study population had higher hospitalization rates, and admissions of people age 65 and older accounted for almost half of the avoidable hospitalizations. The authors suggest that this variation was linked to disparities in access to primary care that might have prevented acute disease and subsequent hospitalization.

Research continues to demonstrate that significant variations exist in utilization not only by region of the country, but even on a hospital-to-hospital basis, including variations between academic facilities.[41,42] In fact, the regularly updated *Dartmouth Atlas of Health Care** continues to report high levels of variation in utilization across the country.

Practice variation also is evident in the management of various diseases. Several research findings (not focused specifically on managed care) present evidence that although medically accepted approaches for the management of particular diseases exist, the implementation of these approaches varies widely. Examples include the following:

- Treatment of pneumonia in the elderly indicates administration of antibiotics

---

*See http://www.dartmouthatlas.org/.

within 8 hours of admission and blood cultures within 24 hours of admission are related to higher patient survival rates. Actual practice differs significantly across geographic areas, with a variance of 49% to 90% for antibiotics given within the 8-hour guideline and a variance of 46% to 83% for the blood culture guideline.[43]

- Rates of prescribing beta blockers after acute myocardial infarction (AMI, also known as a heart attack) remain low despite widespread education efforts. One study comparing regional variation in the management of cardiovascular patients showed that patients receiving prescriptions for beta blockers post AMI ranged from 55% to 81%.[1]

- Variations in the use of procedures are also high, with wide differences in the application of clinical indications for various procedures as well as rates of use.[44-51]

Variations reflecting inappropriate overtreatment or undertreatment may be attributable to multiple factors, including the practice of "defensive medicine," training biases, and lack of access to the most current medical practice information. Variations also may occur because of fee-for-service incentives that reimburse providers for more care or financial incentives under capitation that reward providers for less care. In addition, variations may result when there is an oversupply of providers trying to do more for fewer patients. Sex, race, insurance status of patients, and access to technology also contribute to variation.[52,53]

THE ROLE OF ELECTRONIC CONNECTIVITY

Electronic connectivity is an area that has not been exploited to any substantial degree for purposes of utilization management. Other than basic transactions such as authorizations and claims, electronic connectivity for UM has been largely restricted to the provision of clinical protocols, directories of providers, formularies, and other such static "look-up" functions. The use of an electronic medical record (EMR) or an electronic health record (EHR), which are similar but not identical (the EMR may be thought of as an electronic version of a physician's paper record, and the EHR may be thought of as a more comprehensive record containing additional data from other sources), is still not prevalent at the time of publication, though the use of the PHR as described earlier is starting to pick up.

Those EMRs/EHRs that do exist face the challenge of standardizing nomenclature, electronic field definitions, and interoperability. Those challenges are being addressed, but the fact is that in 2006, there is still relatively little use of the EMR or EHR outside of some large, organized medical groups and health systems. This will change as standards are set and the EMR and EHR become more widely adopted. In addition, as discussed in Chapter 8, some MCOs are providing various forms of financial incentives to promote the adoption of EMRs and EHRs by physicians and hospitals.

Greater use of EMRs/EHRs will also have an impact on utilization. For example, based on a 2006 study by HealthCore (a subsidiary of the national health insurance company WellPoint), it appears that the sharing of data using the Web during the emergency department (ED) and admission process may have significant effects on overall costs, with the impact on outcomes still under study. In this study, a health plan-based record of a member (Patient Clinical Summary) similar to a PHR was accessed on the Web at the point of triage in the ED and utilized in the evaluation process. For those admitted by the ED, an overall $545 savings was observed for those patients with a Patient Clinical Summary versus the control group.[54] It is anticipated that access to the EMR or EHR by providers will provide for greater continuity, elimination of duplicate or unnecessary testing, and better decision making by providers.

LINKAGE OF EVIDENCE-BASED MEDICINE TO PAY-FOR-PERFORMANCE

Many variations in medical practice are caused by lack of adherence to evidence-based medical practice. This refers to well-understood approaches to the treatment of common diseases. The examples listed earlier regarding the hospital treatments of community-acquired pneumonia and of AMI are examples: for uncomplicated cases, the diagnostic and treatment protocols are clear, but compliance is not uniform. Similar examples of evidence-based medical protocols may be found for other common conditions such as congestive heart failure (CHF), diabetes, and chronic obstructive pulmonary disease (COPD).

To increase the use of evidence-based medical protocols as well as align financial incentives to reward improvements in clinical quality, many MCOs are instituting pay-for-performance programs in which a financial incentive is provided for increasing the use of those protocols. These programs are discussed in detail in Chapter 8 and may be thought of as an adjunct to managing both utilization and quality because improvements in quality also decrease utilization associated with suboptimal clinical outcomes.

AUTHORIZATION AND PRECERTIFICATION SYSTEMS

One of the (relatively) definitive elements in managed health care is the presence of authorization and precertification (also known as "pre-cert" and occasionally as "pre-auth") systems. This may be as simple as precertification of elective hospitalizations in an indemnity plan or PPO or as complex as mandatory authorization for all nonprimary care services in an HMO. Although there are no official definitions and the use of these two terms varies, the term *authorization* is usually applied to services provided by specialists and other health professionals, whereas precertification is usually applied to nonprofessional services such as hospitalization or drug therapy. Authorization also implies that it is the PCP that authorizes coverage (subject to the service actually being a covered benefit), whereas precertification implies that it is the health plan that authorizes coverage, though there is some overlap in how the terms are actually used. This is how the terms are used for purposes of this chapter.

There are multiple reasons for authorization and precertification systems. One is to enable the medical management functions of the plan to review a case for medical necessity. A second reason is to channel care to the most appropriate location (*eg,* the outpatient setting or to a participating specialist rather than a nonparticipating one). Third, the precertification system may be used to provide timely information to the concurrent utilization review system and to the large case management function of the health plan. Fourth, the system may help the finance department to estimate the accruals for medical expenditures each month.

There is a caveat regarding authorization and precertification systems, however: most of the time, the necessary information comes from the treating physician. On its surface, this would seem to pose no reason for caution, but a study reported in 2000 demonstrated that 39% of practicing physicians had used one tactic or another to manipulate reimbursement or coverage rules so as to obtain coverage for care that they deemed was necessary for their patients and that 54% of them reported doing this more than they did 5 years prior. The researchers also concluded that financial gain was not the primary motivator for such "gaming" of the system.[56] Therefore, the utility of authorization and precertification systems may be diminished in comparison to its use in prior years.

Definition of Services Requiring Authorization and Precertification

The first requirement in an authorization system is to define what will require authorization and what will not. This is obviously tied to the benefits design and type of health plan. No managed care systems require authorization for primary care services. Most HMOs require members to choose a single PCP* to coordinate care (except for so-called open access HMOs that operate more like PPOs), and accessing the PCP never requires any form of authorization. As discussed in Chapter 5, most HMOs also provide access to certain specialties, such as obstetrics and gynecology (OB/Gyn) or optometry, without the need for an authorization as well. Some states have also passed special laws allowing HMO members access to an even greater array of providers such as chiropractors. It is also common for all MCOs, including HMOs, to provide for direct access to behavioral health providers as discussed in Chapter 13, though such direct access may be limited to contracted behavioral health providers.

Most MCOs seek in some way to encourage or even require the use of PCPs for routine services for reasons that are discussed in a later section. In HMOs that use PCPs to coordinate and authorize services, so-called gatekeeper plans, most services not rendered by the PCP require authorization. In other words, any service from a referral specialist, any hospitalization, any procedure, and so forth requires specific authorization by the PCP. PPOs and other types of MCOs that are not HMOs do not require authorization to see a specialist but may instead use differential copay requirements so as to encourage members to access PCPs preferentially; for example, a $10 copay to see a PCP and a $25 copay to see a specialist. The exception to this is the oxymoronically labeled "gatekeeper PPO" that is licensed as a PPO but operates like an HMO; these were never common and are now quite rare if they even exist at all anymore. For purposes of this discussion, it is assumed that HMOs use PCP

---

*As discussed in Chapter 5, there are also circumstances when a medical specialist (*eg,* a cardiologist) may act as a PCP.

gatekeeper models, whereas PPOs and other types of MCOs do not.

In all MCOs, including HMOs, PPOs, CDHPs, and managed indemnity plans, it is common for precertification to be required for elective hospitalizations. Depending on the type of plan, precertification may also be required for selected or even all ambulatory procedures other than routine screening tests such as colonoscopy or mammography. Precertification is discussed in more detail in a later section of this chapter.

In any plan, there will be times when a member is unable to obtain prior authorization. This is usually because of an emergency or an urgent problem that occurs out of area. In those cases, the plan must make provision for the retrospective review of the case to determine whether authorization may be granted after the fact. Certain rules may also be defined regarding the member's obligation in those circumstances (*eg,* notification within 24 hours of the emergency). Such requirements do not allow for automatic authorization if the plan is notified within 24 hours but only for automatic review of the case to determine medical necessity, even when the plan uses a "reasonable layperson's standard" (see Chapter 33).

Definition of Who Can Authorize Services

A required policy for authorization and precertification systems is to define who has the ability to authorize services and to what extent. This varies considerably depending on the type of plan and the degree to which it is medically managed. In most PPOs, there is usually only a requirement for precertification for elective hospitalizations and procedures, but that type of authorization comes from plan personnel and not from the PCP or any other physician.

For example, if a participating surgeon in a PPO wishes to admit a patient for surgery, the surgeon (or more likely the surgeon's assistant) first calls a central telephone number and speaks with a plan representative, usually a nurse. That representative then asks a number of questions about the patient's condition, and if predetermined criteria are met, and after the member's eligibility is confirmed, an authorization is issued. In most cases, the surgery must take place on the day of admission, and certain procedures may only be done on an outpatient basis. Many MCOs are experimenting with automating this activity, at least for common and routine services such as a biopsy on a breast lump. In addition, because labor and delivery are not elective, most MCOs (including most HMOs) do not require precertification at all but do require notification at the time of admission.

As noted earlier, most HMOs use PCPs to coordinate and authorize services not rendered by the PCP; that is, any service from a referral specialist, any hospitalization, any procedure, and so forth. Even in HMOs, however, there can be some dispute. For example, if a PCP authorizes a member to see a referral specialist, does that specialist have the ability to authorize tests, surgery, or another referral to himself or herself or to another specialist? Does a PCP require authorization to hospitalize one of his or her own patients?

Another exception to the PCP-only concept occurs in HMOs that allow specialists to contact the plan directly about hospitalizations. In these cases, the referral to the specialist must have been made by the PCP in the first place, but the specialist may determine that hospitalization is required and obtain authorization directly from the plan's medical management department. Plans that operate this way generally do so because the PCPs have no real involvement in hospital cases anyway and because there is no utility in involving them in that decision.

There was once a fundamental split in HMOs that required PCP authorization for nonprimary care services: whether or not the PCP's authorization needed secondary review by a utilization management committee

(UMC). From the mid-1980s until the mid-1990s, it was common for many HMOs to require that the PCP's authorization first go to a UMC for additional review. If the UMC approved the authorization request, then it was valid and the member and the PCP were so notified (or just the PCP was notified) and the referral went forward; if the UMC decided that the referral was medically unnecessary, investigational, or not a covered benefit, then the authorization would be denied and the PCP so notified. The PCP then had the much coveted task of explaining that decision to the member. Although this type of secondary review system still exists in some HMOs and some capitated medical groups, most have abandoned it in favor of a model in which the PCP's authorization is valid immediately. This is a result of improvements in information systems and data analytics (see Chapter 16), because PCPs have become much more experienced with managed care, to improve relations between the HMO and the physician network, to improve member satisfaction, and also because of liability concerns by the members of the UMC.

In any type of managed care plan, there may be services that require specific authorization from the plan's medical director or a specialized department within medical management rather than from the PCP. This is usually the case for expensive procedures such as transplants and for controversial procedures or treatments that may be considered experimental or of limited value except in particular circumstances. This is also necessary when the plan has negotiated a special arrangement for high-cost services. The authorization system not only serves to review the medical necessity of the service but ensures that the care will be delivered at an institution that has contracted with the plan.

The last area that commonly requires authorization or precertification from the plan is the use of certain pharmaceutical agents. As discussed in Chapter 12, it is common for any type of MCO that provides drug benefits (which almost all do) to have a list of drugs

that require prereview by the medical director, the plan's clinical pharmacists, or the plan's pharmacy and therapeutics committee. These usually fall into three categories. First are drugs that have utility for treating both actual disease states as well as utility for cosmetic or lifestyle reasons. Second is the off-label use of drugs for a condition that the drug was not certified for by the federal Food and Drug Administration. Third is specialty pharmacy in which highly expensive injectable drugs must meet certain clinical indicators for coverage to apply.

Linkage of Claims Payment to Authorizations

A managed care health plan does not exist as an absolute dictator, preventing a member from accessing services. The only recourse a plan has is to deny full payment for services that have not been authorized. This pertains equally to services obtained from nonparticipating providers (professionals or institutions) and to services obtained without required prior authorization. The counterargument to this concept is that refusal to pay equates to a member's inability to access that service at all. Although this argument has little merit for routine types of services that are affordable even in the absence of insurance, it carries more weight when the services are costly.

In an HMO, payment can be completely denied for services that were not authorized. Point of service (POS) is unique and is discussed later. In most PPOs, CDHPs, and indemnity plans, if a service is not authorized or precertified but is considered a covered benefit, payment may not always be denied, but the amount paid may be significantly reduced. For example, a plan pays 80% of charges for authorized services but only 50% of charges for nonauthorized services or perhaps imposes a flat dollar amount penalty for failure to obtain authorization. Even in such plans, though, certain services such as immunizations may not be covered if not provided by a contracted provider.

In some cases, a plan may deny any payment for a portion of the bill but will pay the rest. For example, if a patient is held over the weekend in the hospital because a clinical service was not available, the plan may not pay the charges related to the extra days even though the inpatient stay was authorized.

In an HMO or a PPO where a contractual relationship exists between the provider and the plan, depending on circumstances, the penalty may fall solely on the provider who may not balance-bill the member for the amount of the penalty. In the case of an indemnity plan (or a PPO in which the member received services from a nonparticipating provider), the penalty falls on the member, who must then pay more out-of-pocket.

Point of Service

POS benefits designs in an HMO are a special challenge for authorization systems and claims management (a thorough discussion of claims management is found in Chapter 18). It is necessary to define what is covered as an authorized service and what is not because services that are not authorized will still be paid, albeit at the lower out-of-network level of benefits. Because POS is sold by HMOs (or mandated on HMOs in certain states) with the expressed intent that members will use out-of-network services, it is not always clear how a service was or was not authorized. Common examples of this issue are illustrated as follows.

If a PCP makes a referral to a specialist for one visit and the member returns for a follow-up, was that authorized? If a PCP authorizes three visits but the member goes four times, does the fourth visit cascade out to an out-of-network level of benefits? If a PCP refers to a specialist and the specialist determines that admission is necessary but the member is admitted to a nonparticipating hospital, is that authorized? What if the member is admitted to a participating hospital but is cared for by a mix of participating and nonparticipating physicians? What if a member is referred to a participating specialist who performs laboratory and radiology testing (even though the plan has capitated for such services); is the visit authorized but not the testing? What if the member claims that he or she had no choice in the matter?

Many other examples of these types of policy questions can be found, and the list of "what ifs" is a long one. Most plans strive to identify an episode of care (*eg,* a hospitalization or a referral) and to remain consistent within that episode. For example, the testing by the specialist referenced earlier may be denied payment and the specialist prohibited from balance billing, or an entire hospitalization would be considered either in-network or out-of-network. In any case, the plan must develop policies and procedures for defining when a service is to be considered authorized (and when it is considered in-network in the case of hospital services that require precertification in any event) and when it is not.

A special problem bedevils POS plans: sometimes the claim arrives before the authorization. This can easily occur in any plan that has a high rate of electronic claims submission, but that depends on a paper-based authorization system. In a typical HMO in which only authorized, in-network benefits are available, this situation usually results in the HMO's claims system "pending" (*ie,* holding) the claim to wait and see if the authorization comes in. But POS is specifically designed to allow for out-of-network, so a claim that does not have an associated authorization immediately cascades down to be processed as an out-of-network or nonauthorized service with lesser benefits, and in some cases then the authorization arrives. When that happens, the member and/or provider complains, the plan has to rework the claim, and the overall cost of rework, to say nothing of the high level of irritation by the member and provider, is a negative event.

Electronic standards for many transactions, including authorizations (both sending and receiving), are mandated under the Health Insurance Portability and Accountability Act (HIPAA) and have been in place since 2002. Unfortunately, the use of electronic authorizations lags the use of electronic claims. As the full HIPAA transaction set comes into use, verification of eligibility will occur at the time of authorization, the authorization will arrive before the claim, and this problem will be lessened. But at this point, it will remain a steady irritant to POS plans, though less of an irritant to the health care market as a whole as a result of the dwindling popularity of POS.

Categories of Authorization

Authorizations may be classified into six types:

- Prospective
- Concurrent
- Retrospective
- Pended (for review)
- Denial (no authorization)
- Subauthorization

For tightly managed MCOs, there is value in categorizing authorization types. By examining how authorizations are actually generated in the plan, management will be able to identify areas of weakness in the system. For example, if all elective admissions are being classified as having prospective authorization but it turns out that in fact most are being authorized either concurrently, or worse yet, retrospectively, medical management will be unable to intervene effectively in managing hospital cases as a result of not knowing about them in a timely manner. A brief description of the authorization categories follows.

Prospective

Prospective means the authorization is issued before any service is rendered. This is commonly used in plans that require prior authorization for elective services. Hospital precertification is the most common form of prospective authorization. The more prospec-

tive the authorization, the more time the medical management has to intervene if necessary, the greater the ability to direct care to the most appropriate setting or provider and the more current the MCO's knowledge regarding utilization trends.

Inexperienced plan managers tend to believe that all authorizations and precertifications are prospective. That naive belief can lead to a real shock when the manager of a troubled plan learns that most claims are actually being paid on the basis of other types of authorizations that were not correctly categorized. This is discussed further later.

Concurrent

A concurrent authorization is generated at the time the service is rendered. For example, the UM nurse discovers that a patient is being admitted to the hospital that day. An authorization is generated by the nurse and not by the PCP. Another example is an urgent service that cannot wait for review, such as setting a broken leg. In that case, the PCP may contact the plan, but the referral or authorization is made at the same time.

Concurrent authorizations allow for timely data gathering and the potential for affecting the outcome, but they do not allow the plan medical managers to intervene in the initial decision to render services. This may result in care being inappropriately delivered or delivered in a setting that is not cost-effective, but it also may result in the plan's being able to alter the course of care in a more cost-effective direction even though care has already commenced. This is especially true when large case management is appropriate as discussed in Chapter 11.

Retrospective

As the term indicates, retrospective authorizations take place after the fact. For example, a patient is admitted, has surgery, and is discharged, and only then does the plan find out. On the surface, it appears that any service rendered without authorization would have payment denied or reduced, but there will be circumstances when the plan will genuinely agree to authorize services after the fact. For example, if a member is involved in a serious automobile accident or has a heart attack while traveling in another state, there is a clear need for care and the plan could not deny that need.

Inexperienced managers often believe not only that most authorizations are prospective but that, except for emergency cases, there are few retrospective authorizations. Unfortunately, there are circumstances when there may be a significant volume of retrospective authorizations. This commonly occurs in HMOs when the PCPs or participating providers fail to cooperate with the authorization system. A claim comes in cold (ie, without an authorization), and the plan must create one after the fact if it finds out that the service was really meant to be authorized. The plan cannot punish the member because it was really the fault of the PCP, so that claim gets paid.

Most plans have a no balance billing clause in their provider contracts (see Chapter 30) and may elect not to pay claims that have not been prospectively authorized, forcing the noncompliance providers to write-off the expense. This is more likely to happen in an HMO than any other type of health plan. Refusal to pay will certainly get a provider's attention, but it comes at some cost in provider relations. Even so, sometimes it becomes necessary if discussions and education attempts fail.

If an HMO's systems allow an authorization to be classified as prospective or concurrent regardless of when it is created relative to the delivery of the service, it is a sure thing that retrospective authorizations will occur but not be labeled retrospective; for example, the physician will say, "I really meant to authorize that," or "It's in the mail," and call the authorization concurrent. Another possibility is that claims clerks may be creating retrospective authorizations on the basis of the belief that a claim was linked to another authorized claim (see discussion later).

When HMOs were relatively small, the ability to create a retrospective authorization

was strictly limited to the medical director or utilization management department, but as they became large, the ability to manage this problem required a loosening of that policy. Even then, most tightly managed plans restrict the ability to create prospective authorizations once the service has actually been rendered, and concurrent authorizations cannot be created after 24 hours have passed since the service was rendered.

Pended (For Review)

Pended is a claims term that refers to a state of authorization purgatory. In this situation, it is not known whether an authorization will be issued, and the case has been pended for review. This refers to medical review (for medical necessity such as an emergency department claim or for medical policy review to determine if the service is covered under the schedule of benefits) or to administrative review. The treatment of pended claims is addressed in Chapter 18.

Denial

Denial refers to the certainty that there will be no authorization forthcoming. As has been discussed, not every claim coming into the plan without an associated authorization will be denied because there are reasons that an unauthorized claim may be paid. In an HMO, denial means no payment is forthcoming; in a POS, PPO, or CDHP, denial usually (but not always) means that payment may be made but at a lesser level of coverage if the service is still considered medically necessary. Payment may be denied in full even by those types of plans if the service is not considered medically necessary or is not a covered benefit. Denial may also occur for some highly restricted services (*eg,* preventive services) that are not received from approved providers regardless of whether they were ordered by the PCP.

Subauthorization

This is a special category that allows one authorization to hitchhike on another. This is most common for hospital-based professional services. For example, a single authorization may be issued for a hospitalization, and that authorization is used to cover anesthesia, pathology, radiology, or even a surgeon's or consultant's fees.

In some HMOs, an authorization to a referral specialist may be used to authorize diagnostic and therapeutic services ordered by that specialist. For example, a referral to an orthopedist automatically allows for authorized payment for radiological services, a referral to a cardiologist allows for electrocardiograms, and so forth.

In the absence of a clear policy, the phenomenon of linking can occur. This refers to the claims system or claims clerks linking unauthorized services to authorized ones and creating subauthorizations to do so. For example, a referral to a specialist is authorized, and a claim is received not only for the specialist's fees but for some expensive procedure or test as well or a bill is received for 10 visits even though the PCP intended to authorize only 1. Fully automated claims systems have algorithms in place to determine payment for real or imputed subauthorizations, and exceptions are pended and require manual review.

The ability of a specialist (or a PCP for that matter) to be reimbursed automatically for tests and procedures must be constrained through one means or another. For example, if a physician has an expensive piece of diagnostic equipment in the office, there may be a subtle pressure to use it to make it pay for itself. One widely cited study looking at physician ownership of radiology equipment documented a fourfold increase in imaging examinations as well as significant increases in charges among physicians who used their own equipment, compared with physicians who referred such studies to radiologists.[56] Similar results have been reported for laboratory services[57] and a wide variety of ancillary services.[58]

The issue of physician-owned diagnostic and therapeutic equipment or services is a difficult one to address and one that has been coming under significant pressure from government regulations, especially in Medicare[59] where there are strict rules applied regarding a physician's ability to bill for nonprofessional services in which the physician has a financial interest. In addition to requiring precertification for selected expensive testing procedures, the best method for dealing with this issue is simply to prohibit or markedly restrict the use of such services. Most managed care plans contract with a limited number of vendors for such ancillary services and may limit referral to only those vendors as discussed in Chapter 7.

Last, as regards subauthorizations, many HMOs prohibit secondary referrals by specialists. This means that a specialist cannot authorize other referrals for a member. In other words, if a specialist feels that a patient needs to see another specialist, then that judgment must be communicated back to the PCP who is the only one able to issue an authorization for services.

Common Data Elements for Authorization Systems

An authorization system operates through the use of data. Standards now exist for these transactions, though even in the absence of a standardized electronic transaction, certain data elements remain commonly used.

Electronic Standards

As noted earlier and as described in Chapter 32, HIPAA has mandated standards for the electronic transmission of authorization data (among other types of electronic transactions): specifically the Prior Authorization Request and Response Transaction (ANSI X12 standard 278) is used to request and receive a response for referrals, certification, and authorization of the following:

- Health care services
- Health care admission
- Extend certification
- Certification appeal

The field descriptions and data requirements of the 278 transaction standard are more complex than those found in a paper-based system as described later. Use of this electronic transaction occurs when many of those data fields are populated by the system itself such as a practice management support system or a hospital information system. The electronic standard is also used in Web-based portals where physicians and hospitals can request an authorization or query the MCO to see if an authorization exists and provide or obtain necessary nonclinical information; in that case, the MCO's system populates many of the fields.

Manual or Nonelectronic Data Elements

As electronic authorization systems continue to come into use, there are still those providers that rely on paper-based communications that are either mailed or (more commonly) faxed to the MCO. Telephonic request and response is also used. Telephonic intake is more cumbersome and may be done either by live intake personnel or by an automated system referred to as interactive voice response (IVR). IVR is more often used when a specialist or hospital is checking on the existence or status of an authorization, though live contact remains common.

What follows is a brief description of the common data elements used in nonelectronic authorization systems. These are illustrated in Table 9-5.

Although most authorization requests would be automatically approved, MCOs may have clinical requirements for authorization or precertification of expensive interventions that are subject to overuse. For example, certain types of cardiac testing, certain types of imaging procedures, bariatric surgery, and so forth. Sometimes this type of precertification review can be automated, but most often it is done by clinical personnel in the UM department. In the event the requesting physician disagrees with an MCO's decision not to provide coverage and fails to convince the medical director of its necessity, external review of the case may also be required, as noted earlier.

It becomes less common for a plan to deny authorization based on medical necessity as the plan matures and the participating physicians become more conversant in definitions of medical necessity, however, the other values of the authorization system remain important. As the use of the EMR and EHR becomes more common, it may be possible for the precertification activity of the MCO to access the clinical information in digital form, easing the burden on physicians to provide required clinical documentation.

Last, when an authorization is made, the system also must be able to generate and link an authorization number or identifier to the data, so that every authorization is unique. In tightly managed plans, any claim for services that are not allowed on a self-referral basis must be accompanied by that unique authorization number to be processed.

PHYSICIAN SERVICES

There is a very practical reason why MCOs encourage or even require members to access PCPs for routine services, whether through the use of differential copays or through the use of a PCP gatekeeper model. In most managed health care plans, the costs associated with nonprimary-care professional services are substantially greater than the cost of primary care services, often between 1.5 and 2.0 times as high. This difference arises from the increased fees associated with specialty services and to the hospital- and procedure-intensive nature of those services; in other words, more than half the costs of specialty services may be associated with hospitalization or procedures, and these associated utilization costs generated by specialists are often overlooked. Not only the fees of the specialists themselves add to the cost of care but also the cost of services ordered by specialists, such as diagnostic studies, facility charges for procedures, and so forth. These costs are not routinely

Table 9–5 Data Elements Commonly Captured in an Authorization System

Member's name _____

Member's birth date _____

Member's plan identification (ID) number _____

Eligibility status _____

Commercial group number or public sector (*ie,* Medicare and Medicaid) group identifier

Line of business (*eg,* HMO, POS, PPO, Medicare, Medicaid, conversion, private, or self-pay)

Benefits code for particular service (*eg,* noncovered, partial coverage, limited benefit, full coverage)

For Specialty Referral Authorization in HMOs

- Primary care physician (PCP)
- Referral provider
- Name
- Specialty
- Outpatient data elements
- Referral or service date
- Diagnosis (*International Classification of Disease* 9th Edition, Clinical Modification [ICD-9-CM], free text)
- Number of visits authorized
- Specific procedures authorized (*Current Procedural Terminology* 4th Edition [CPT-4], free text)
- Inpatient data elements
- Name of institution
- Admitting physician
- Admission or service date
- Diagnosis (ICD-9-CM, diagnosis-related group, free text)
- Planned discharge date
- Subauthorizations (if allowed or required)
- Hospital-based professionals
- Other specialists
- Other procedures or studies
- Free text to be transmitted to the claims processing department

added to the cost of specialist services when data are compiled, but management of specialist services will often lead to management of these outside services as well.

Studies examining the ability of PCP model HMOs to lower costs and maintain quality were most often done in the late 1980s or early 1990s.[60–64] Even in a more recent study, though, the savings generated by managing specialty physician services was actually twice the amount generated from hospital utilization management (adjusted for severity and case mix),[65] and significant reductions of the use of specialty services in Medicare and Medicaid managed care plans have also been documented.[66,67]

In addition, PCPs are often able to deliver many of the same services as a specialist, but at considerable savings and in a more appropriate setting. Even in nonmanaged care systems, PCPs can manage a substantial proportion of their patients' care.[68] On the other hand, some PCPs report feeling uncomfortable about providing some services, with one large survey reporting that nearly one in four HMO PCPs felt that the scope of care they were expected to provide was greater than it should be.[69]

Though specialty referral rates are lower in PCP model HMOs than in other types of health plans, a review of data for referrals to specialists suggests that authorization denial rates have also been relatively low. A study of 2,000 physicians revealed a denial rate of 3% for eight categories of referrals; these rates are measured after appeals, however, with initial denial rates slightly higher. Other denial rates in this study were 1% for hospitalization, 2.6% for specialist referrals, 1.25% for surgical procedures, 0.7% for cardiac catheterizations, and 3.0% for mental health referrals.[70]

There has been some level of controversy, particularly by consumers, about the value of the PCP gatekeeper role in managed care and how the interaction between the PCP model and the reimbursement or financial incentive systems has affected utilization.[71] Physician attitudes also have been variable over recent years, and one study serves as an illustration. In that study, physicians reported that a PCP gatekeeper model was effective in controlling costs and other aspects of care, but those physicians had complaints about the imposition of administrative requirements as well as issues of access to specialists, testing, and other measures. Although decidedly a mixed group of opinions, overall 72% of physicians still thought that the gatekeeper model was better than or comparable to traditional care arrangements.[72]

A PCP-focused model is not a panacea, however. Some studies conclude that a specialist is better at treating a specific condition than is a generalist,[73] and other examples indicate when a specialist will be better at managing the care of chronic and complex diseases such as severe diabetes,[74] chronic rheumatic and musculoskeletal diseases,[75] or debilitating congestive heart failure.[76] For patients with severe chronic conditions who are also involved in an MCO's disease management (DM) program (see Chapter 10), a specialist will almost always be more appropriate than a PCP is in managing that patient's care. In these cases, the appropriate specialist

should have the same level of authorization power as a PCP in an HMO, and in non-HMO plans, the DM program may want to lower any economic barriers to allow access to the specialist. In general, however, PCP-centric approaches are superior for the general population of members.

MANAGEMENT OF INSTITUTIONAL UTILIZATION

Utilization of hospital (or more accurately institutional) services may account for between 35% and 40% of the total expenses in an MCO. That amount can be even greater when utilization is excessive. Management of these expenses is therefore prominent among most health plans' priorities.

The expense of any medical service is a product of the price of that service times the volume of services delivered. Pricing for institutional services is discussed in Chapter 7 and will not be repeated here except as necessary. Volume of services applies to both inpatient care and to ambulatory procedures. UM processes for inpatient care are deployed to manage the inpatient expense, facilitate appropriate discharge services, prevent readmissions, and trigger additional care management programs such as DM and case management. A similar approach is taken to ambulatory procedures but with far greater emphasis on appropriateness of care and where the procedures are performed.

Simple reduction of bed days is of value but can lull the inexperienced manager into a sense of complacency. Management of institutional utilization is therefore to be understood in context with management of other areas of utilization as well. It is possible to reduce inpatient utilization and actually experience a rise in cost, as is discussed later in this chapter.

Management of institutional utilization may be best presented by discussing the key categories for managing the process: prospective, concurrent, and retrospective review, and large (ie, catastrophic) case management

(LCM or CM; see also Chapter 11 for a detailed discussion of case management of hospitalized patients). Prospective review means review of a case before it even happens, *concurrent review* means review occurs while the case is active, and *retrospective review* occurs after the case is finished. Case management refers to managing cases that are expected to result in very large costs so as to provide coordination of care that results in both proper care and cost savings.

Effect of Disease Management

As discussed in detail in Chapter 10, effective DM programs achieve improved outcomes: both clinical and financial. The combination of those outcomes makes perfect sense when it is understood that both are related to preventing visits to the ED and admission to the hospital. By better managing serious chronic conditions, the patient is less likely to require emergency care or hospital admission. The easiest utilization to manage is that which does not occur.

Prospective Review and Precertification

As discussed earlier, precertification refers to a requirement on the part of the admitting physician to notify or obtain authorization from the MCO before a member is admitted for inpatient care or an outpatient procedure.* There is also a requirement for hospitals that contract with the MCO to check for such precertification prior to a nonemergency admission. There is a widespread and rather erroneous belief that the primary role of precertification is to prevent unnecessary admissions from occurring. Although that may occasionally happen (particularly in

workers' compensation cases), it is not the chief reason for precertification and has not been so for a long time.

There are three primary reasons for precertification. The first is to notify the medical management system that a case will be occurring. In most plans, this refers to the software decision support systems that specialize in medical management, creating substantial leverage for the case managers, UM nurses, and the medical director. Precertification also enables UM to prepare discharge planning ahead of time as well as look for the case during concurrent review rounds. In some instances, the LCM function may be notified if the admission diagnosis raises the probability that the case will be expensive (*eg,* a bone marrow transplant).

The second major reason for precertification is to ensure that care takes place in the most appropriate setting or level of care. Perhaps an inpatient case is diverted to the outpatient department or a freestanding ambulatory facility. Another example would be a case that is diverted from a nonparticipating hospital to a participating one or to a facility that has been designated as a center of excellence for a selected procedure.

The third reason is to capture data for financial accruals. Although it is unlikely that a plan can capture every case before or while it is taking place, a mature plan that is running well can capture the great majority of cases, perhaps 90% to 95%. By knowing the number and nature of hospital cases as well as potential or existing catastrophic cases, the plan may more accurately accrue for expenses rather than have to wait for claims to come in. It enables financial managers to take action early so as to avoid nasty financial surprises. Accrual methodology is discussed in Chapter 24.

In any case, for inpatient cases the plan usually assigns a length of stay guideline at the time the admission is certified based on industry standard criteria (*eg,* Milliman* or

---

*The benefit design may actually place the financial penalty, and thus the responsibility, on the member, but as a practical matter, even then it is most likely that it will be the physician or the physician's office staff that make the request.

*See http://www.milliman.com/.

InterQual*), as is discussed shortly. The plan will also use the precertification process to verify the member's eligibility for coverage and to communicate that to the provider, although most plans have a disclaimer stating that ultimate eligibility for coverage will be determined at the time the claim is processed. Eligibility determination through electronic transactions between the providers and the MCO is another example of a defined data set under HIPAA, but will not be further described here.

In the case of an emergency or urgent admission, it is obviously not possible to obtain precertification. In that event, there is usually a contractual requirement in the provider contracts to notify the plan by the next business day or within 24 hours if the plan has UM staffing 24 hours per day. Most plans have contractual language with both physicians and hospitals whereby financial penalties are imposed (eg, a percentage of their fee or a flat penalty) for failure to obtain certification.

In plans that allow members to seek care from noncontracted providers (eg, in PPO and POS plans), the responsibility to contact the plan for precertification rests with members if they choose not to access care through the in-network system. In CDHPs, the responsibility to obtain precertification always lies with the member. In these cases, most plans impose benefits penalties (eg, a higher co-insurance or a flat penalty rate) on members who fail to obtain proper precertification.

Preadmission Testing and Same-Day Surgery

An easy and ubiquitous method for cost control is preadmission testing and same-day surgery for inpatient procedures. A member who is going to be hospitalized on an elective basis has routine preoperative tests done as an outpatient and then is admitted the same day as the surgery is to be performed. Both these policies are confirmed at the time of

precertification. For example, if a member has elective gallbladder surgery scheduled for 10:00am on Thursday, then on Tuesday the member goes to the hospital for preoperative tests. The results are made available to the admitting physician who performs the admission history and physical for the member as an outpatient and either delivers the results to the hospital or calls in the results to the hospital's transcription department. The member arrives at the hospital at 6:00am on Thursday, is admitted, and has the surgery as scheduled.

In many health plans, the plan arranges for laboratory work to be done with a contracted laboratory at reduced rates or has in-house capabilities to perform the laboratory work. Occasionally, a hospital will refuse to accept the results of these laboratories. If the laboratory is accredited and licensed, the hospital has little grounds to require use of its laboratory, electrocardiography, and radiology services for preoperative admission testing. In these cases, it falls to the plan's management team to discuss this issue with the hospital administrator and negotiate an agreement for the hospital to accept laboratory work or to agree to perform the work at equivalent costs. If the hospital refuses to cooperate, the medical director needs to decide whether to direct the elective cases to another, more cooperative hospital.

Mandatory Outpatient Surgery

It has become standard for MCOs to require that certain procedures be done on an outpatient basis unless clinically contraindicated; for example, tonsillectomy or carpal tunnel release. As medical science and technique progress, procedures migrate from inpatient to outpatient; for example, cardiac catheterization is now routinely done on an outpatient basis, but that was not the case 10 years ago. Hospitals themselves, facing inpatient capacity problems combined with their own investments in ambulatory procedure facilities, will often refuse to admit a patient for an inpatient stay for these types

---

*See http://www.interqual.com/IQSite/.

of procedures unless the admitting physician can clinically substantiate the need for admission; hospitals often use the very same guidelines as MCOs in making such determinations.

As mentioned earlier in this chapter as well as in Chapter 7, it is important to ensure that the desired savings are actually achievable from outpatient surgery. In many cases, hospitals or freestanding outpatient surgery facilities have charges that are equal to or greater than those for an inpatient day. In other cases, the facility charge may be lower, but the unbundled charges for anesthesia, recovery, supplies, and so on can drive the costs higher than anticipated. Because of competitive pressures, there may also be substantial differences between what it costs to do the same procedure in a hospital ambulatory facility as compared to a privately-owned freestanding site. When that happens, the MCO works to direct the care to the lower cost facility. When the MCO does not have the ability to do so based on benefits design, it may elect to provide a bonus to physicians for using a lower cost site, as discussed in Chapter 7.

Concurrent Review

MCOs that rely on prospective payment such as diagnosis-related groups (DRGs), case rates, and capitation, as well as loosely managed plans such as CDHPs and some PPOs, may not aggressively manage inpatient utilization once the member is in the hospital. The simple reason is that the hospital has financial responsibility once the patient is admitted, and therefore it is the hospital that will manage the case. Even when this is the case, the MCO needs to stay apprised of what is happening so as to be aware of circumstances that might require activation of DM or LCM or that may trigger additional payments caused by significant cost overruns. MCOs that reimburse hospitals using any charge-based system such as per diems or discounts on charges are more likely to manage inpatient stays aggressively. Although the

focus of this section is from the perspective of MCOs, in either case it is concurrent review that is used. Management of inpatient utilization by the hospital itself is also discussed in Chapter 11.

Concurrent review means managing utilization during the course of a hospitalization (as opposed to an outpatient procedure). Concurrent review results in more effective management of inpatient utilization than does retrospective review.[77] Common techniques for concurrent review involve assignment and tracking of length of stay, review and rounding by UM nurses, and discharge planning. As described later in this section, MCOs typically support concurrent review with on-site nurses at high-volume facilities and then perform the process telephonically for low- and moderate-volume facilities. Loosely managed MCOs do not do any routine concurrent rounding but rather rely on the hospital to notify them when a case exceeds the designated length of stay and only then get involved.

Maximum Length of Stay

As noted earlier, a common approach to hospital utilization management is the assignment of a maximum allowable length of stay (LOS) that sometimes appears in the guise of an estimated length of stay, or ELOS. The plan assigns the LOS on the basis of the admission diagnosis and/or planned procedure, usually the *International Classification of Diseases,* 9th Revision, Clinical Modification (ICD-9-CM) codes. Selecting a norm for the assigned LOS is not always easy given the regional variations. Most MCOs purchase LOS guidelines from commercial third parties but may modify them as required for local variations. The assigned LOS for that stay is all the plan will authorize for payment; for example, an admission for a particular surgical procedure may be assigned 3 days. If the hospital is being paid under prospective payment, it will have its own LOS values. Any costs for days beyond the assigned LOS are not covered unless clinical circumstances support the additional stay. In those plans that cannot or will not restrict payment, the assigned LOS is used only to trigger greater involvement by the medical director. It is worth noting that reduced inpatient utilization is now more a result of management of length of stay than it is of reductions in admission rates.

The advantages of using assigned LOS designations are threefold. First, it allows the plan to cover a relatively large geographic area with few personnel. Second, widely accepted third-party LOS values have the power of legitimacy and do not require continual negotiation. Third, it is a relatively mechanical technique and requires less training of plan personnel and may in fact be automated by the MCO using management support software.

The problems with using assigned LOS designations also are threefold. First, it is easy to get complacent. By choosing certain values for assigned LOS designations, medical managers may fail to evaluate continually whether those are in fact the correct values. Second, designated time becomes free time. In other words, there is less incentive to evaluate critically every day in the hospital for appropriateness and alternatives if plan personnel and the physician feel that there is still time on the meter. Third, using such a mechanical system often achieves less than optimal results. Management of inpatient utilization by the UM nurses and the medical director should produce a reduction in length of stay.

An assigned LOS also may not adequately take into account concurrent or comorbid conditions. There is no one assigned LOS that is applicable to all patients for any given reason for admission. This is not to say that the presence of comorbidity should automatically result in longer inpatient stays but rather that this must be taken into account as part of inpatient UM. The consequences of exceeding the assigned LOS must be defined. Usually, exceeding the assigned LOS results in either a denial or a reduction of payment for services rendered after the assigned LOS has been exceeded.

Role of the Utilization Management Nurse

The one individual who is crucial to the success of a managed care program is the UM nurse. It is the UM nurse who is the eyes and ears of the health plan's medical management department, who is able to apply clinical knowledge to cases, who will coordinate the discharge planning, and who will facilitate all the activities of utilization management.

Staffing levels for UM nurses and others involved in concurrent review vary depending on the size of the geographic area, the number of hospitals, the size of the plan, and the intensity with which UM is performed (eg, by on-site hospital rounding). The advent of advanced clinical management support systems has substantially increased the efficiencies of this function, in some cases nearly doubling the case load that the UM nurse can handle. Last, as MCOs have consolidated (see Chapter 1), there has been a move to centralize much of this function in regional call centers, doing local on-site rounding done by exception rather than routine.

The scope of responsibilities of the UM nurse varies depending on the plan and the personalities and skills of the other members of the medical management team. In some plans, the role simply involves telephone information gathering. Other plans require a more proactive role, including active hospital rounding; frequent communication with attending physicians, the medical director, the hospitals, and the hospitalized members, and their families, as well as discharge planning and facilitation. Some of these activities are briefly described here.

Because of variability in approach to concurrent review, there is widespread variability in staffing levels, even in large MCOs. In the earlier era of HMOs, having one rounding UM nurse for every 6,000 to 8,000 members was the norm,* but such intensity is now more the exception than the rule. Table 9-6 il-

---

*From personal records of the author.

Table 9–6 Staffing Ratios for UM in Large MCOs, 2002

Staffing Ratio for UM Personnel as FTEs* per 100,000 Members	25th Percentile	Mean	75th Percentile
FTEs dedicated to all UM functions	7.1	10.8	13.0
FTEs dedicated to hospital precertification and concurrent UM	2.5	4.4	6.4
FTEs dedicated to case management	2.7	3.6	4.1
FTEs dedicated to referral authorization	0.0	0.3	0.3
FTEs dedicated to ambulatory diagnostic testing and procedure authorization	0.0	1.0	1.5
Percentage of UM FTEs who are RNs	63%	68%	76%

*FTE, full-time equivalent.
Source: Courtesy of Accenture. Used with permission.

lustrates this using data from a proprietary 2002 benchmarking study of large MCOs.

Information Gathering

The one fundamental function of the UM nurse is information gathering. Information about hospital cases must be obtained in an accurate and timely fashion. It falls to the UM nurse to be the focal point of this information collection effort and to ensure that it is obtained and communicated to the necessary individuals in medical management and the claims department. Necessary information includes admission date and diagnosis, the type of hospital service to which the patient was admitted (*eg*, medical, surgical, maternity, and so forth), the admitting physician, specialists, planned procedures (type and timing), expected discharge date, needed discharge planning, and any other pertinent information the plan managers may need. Typically, this information is documented in a core care management software application at the health plan.

Telephone Rounding

In some plans, information gathering is done strictly by telephone. Telephone rounding is used first to check with the admitting office to determine whether any plan members were admitted and then to check with the hospital's own UM department to obtain any further information. Telephone rounding by HMOs is usually done in locations where there is too much geographic area to cover and the plan cannot yet justify adding more UM nurses. It also may be done in those rare instances when a hospital refuses to give the HMO's UM nurse rounding privileges on hospitalized plan members. Telephone rounding also is used when tight controls on utilization do not exist and by many non-HMO MCOs. Telephone rounding generally looks for clear outliers rather than attempting to achieve optimal utilization management.

Hospital Rounding

Rounding in person is far superior to telephone rounding, though it is both more costly and less common than telephone rounding. When hospital rounds are conducted daily by a UM nurse on every hospitalized member, the medical director will obtain the most accurate and timely information and will also have information that might not otherwise be obtainable. For example, in a good quality management program (Chapter 15), the rounding UM nurse can watch for quality problems or significant events that would trigger a quality assurance audit. The rounding nurse is also in the best position to identify "never events," which are events that should never happen in a hospital (*eg,* a serious medication error leading to complications). As discussed in Chapter 7, many MCOs will not pay a hospital for costs associated with never events.

A rounding nurse can pick up information about a patient's condition that may affect discharge planning—information that the attending physician may have failed to communicate (*eg,* home durable medical equipment that must be ordered). The UM nurse also can detect practice behavior that increases utilization simply for the convenience of the physician or the hospital. For example, a patient may be ready for discharge but the physician may have missed making rounds that morning and will not be back until the next day or the hospital may have rescheduled surgery for its own reasons and the patient will have to stay an extra, unnecessary day. In situations such as these, the UM nurse must not be put into an adversarial position but rather should refer such matters to the medical director.

Personal rounding by the UM nurse can have the added advantage of increasing member satisfaction. Many people feel uncomfortable talking to physicians and welcome the chance to express their fears or feelings to the UM nurse. In other cases, inquiring about how members are feeling can let them know that the plan cares about them as people and is not only interested in getting them out as fast as possible. If the UM nurse is seen as trying to "kick the patient out," however, member satisfaction will be decreased, emphasizing the need for good communications skills.

Occasionally, hospitals will refuse to grant rounding privileges to a UM nurse, the typical excuse being that the hospital already has a UM department. The hospital UM department may be inadequate for the needs of an MCO that truly manages care, however, and also does not address the specific member satisfaction and quality assurance needs of the plan. Another frequent excuse is the need to protect the confidentiality of patients. That excuse does not hold if the plan's UM nurse is only rounding on plan members and is properly performing utilization and quality management; even the privacy requirements under HIPAA (see Chapter 32) recognize the need for these functions and allow access to protected medical information to qualified personnel. If a hospital refuses to cooperate on allowing the plan's UM nurse to round, then the plan must seriously question its willingness to do business with that hospital. Fortunately, most hospitals and MCOs are able to accommodate this activity without difficulty.

Review Against Criteria

An important feature of concurrent review is the evaluation of each hospital case against established criteria. Most plans use published or commercially available criteria for such reviews to facilitate evaluation by UM nurses, often with some modification based on regional variation. Experienced nurses use such criteria as an aid in managing utilization, but they do not blindly depend on them. It is possible to keep a patient in the hospital for less than adequate reasons but still meet criteria; the seasoned UM nurse is able to evaluate each case on its own merits. The UM nurse should only approve initial and additional length of stay requests. If at any time, the UM nurse questions the appropriateness of a length of stay, he or she should consult with the health plan medical director or physician advisor.

Most MCOs have automated this function to improve the efficiency of the UM nurse. Software enables the assigned LOS to be generated automatically from the admission diagnosis or procedure. Member and benefit eligibility are checked, diagnostic and procedure codes are generated from entered text, review criteria are automatically displayed for both admission and concurrent review, unlimited text may be entered to allow tracking, census reports are produced, statistics are generated, and so forth. It is commonly done not only at the MCO but also at remote locations using laptop computers that exchange information with the main system through secure Internet connections. UM software also links to the claims and enrollment systems so that claims can be properly processed and also take into consideration any special instructions from the nurses.

Discharge Planning and Follow-up

Discharge planning is an ongoing effort beginning with admission or preadmission screening. Discharge planning includes an estimate of how long the patient will be in the hospital, what the expected outcome will be, whether there will be any special requirements on discharge, and what needs to be facilitated early on. For example, if a patient is admitted with a fractured hip, it is known from the outset that many weeks of rehabilitation will be necessary. It is therefore helpful to contact the rehabilitation facility well prior to discharge to ensure that a bed will be available at the time of transfer. If it is known that a patient will need durable medical equipment, the equipment should be ordered early so that the patient does not spend extra days in the hospital waiting for it to arrive.

Case management as applied to inpatient cases is discussed in detail in Chapter 11. It is an integral aspect of managing utilization of large, complex, and expensive inpatient cases. It is related to discharge planning because many aspects of case management are driven by looking for alternatives to acute care hospitalization, alternatives that are discussed later in this chapter.

An aspect of discharge planning that is often overlooked is informing the patient and family well in advance of actual discharge. Otherwise, they may be upset when the physician tells them that the patient is being discharged because they may have different expectations. Informing the patient and family from the start about when they can expect discharge, how the patient will be feeling,

what they might need to prepare for at home, and how follow-up will occur helps to smooth things considerably.

In the case of short-stay obstetrics, the government has mandated that the minimum length of stay is 2 days, though subsequent studies have demonstrated that there has been no significant effect on the health outcomes of newborns brought about by this policy.[78] From a clinical standpoint, a 1-day LOS for obstetrics is still acceptable if the patient, the physician, and the plan all agree. In the case of short-stay obstetrics, the patient and family must be prepared for the homecoming. Active discharge planning for short-stay obstetrics patients is crucial. Plans must offer home health visits to mothers who are discharged after a short-stay delivery.

In addition to making sure that all goes smoothly to effect a smooth and proper discharge from the hospital, the UM nurse can follow up with the member by telephone after discharge to ensure that all is well. Adverse events occur frequently in the immediate postdischarge period, and many can potentially have been prevented or ameliorated with simple strategies.[79] Many health plans have instituted formal "Welcome Home Call" programs for conditions that have a trend of higher volume of readmissions. The call allows the health plan to educate, coach, and confirm with the member/caregiver that the treatment plan for post-acute care is clear and being followed. Health plans and hospitals have seen a decrease in readmission rates for these conditions, demonstrating both value and improved outcomes; for example, a follow-up phone call by a pharmacist involved in the hospital care of patients was associated with increased patient satisfaction, resolution of medication-related problems, and fewer return visits to the emergency department.[80]

Role of the Physician

As managed care has matured, attention to providing care in the most appropriate setting has matured as well. Two decades ago, many cases that are now managed on an out-patient basis were instead admitted to the hospital. Since then, as inpatient admission rates and lengths of stay have dropped, result-ing in a notably lower rate of bed days per thousand, patients who are admitted tend to be sicker or require more intense services. At the same time, financial pressures on PCPs led many to conclude that caring for hospital-ized patients is not an economically efficient use of their time, leading them essentially to abandon inpatient care as a routine aspect of their practice. PCP management of hospital cases has fallen from 40% of their time to just 10% in a single generation.[81]

If the role of the PCP managing most inpa-tient cases has decreased for multiple rea-sons, it is certainly not completely gone. Straightforward problems that still require admission—diabetic ketoacidosis or a deep venous thrombosis, for example—are often managed by PCPs, particularly when the PCP is a board-certified internist. But even in HMOs it is no longer the case that the major-ity of inpatient stays are routinely managed by PCPs. It is now far more common for in-patient care to be provided by a specialist or, in a growing trend, by a designated rounding physician or "hospitalist." The roles of PCPs, specialists, and hospitalists are briefly de-scribed in the following subsections.

Primary Care Physician Model

In HMOs that emphasize the PCP model, PCPs are encouraged to be involved in and, if appropriate, even manage the hospital care of their patients. In this model, the most im-portant functions of the member's PCP are also the most obvious: to make rounds every day and to coordinate the patient's care. In non-HMO MCOs, the PCP may also be in-volved in the care of patients of course, but this section addresses PCP model HMOs be-cause the approach to UM in such a model often incorporates PCP involvement as a matter of policy. Such PCP involvement is certainly less common now than it was 10 to 20 years ago, but it remains a very effective adjunct to managing inpatient utilization.

Even as patients are now usually hos-pitalized for care delivered primarily by specialists—for example, for surgery, for severe medical conditions (eg, a myocardial infarction), or for prolonged courses of treat-ment (eg, recovery from a stroke)—it is bene-ficial for the PCP to round daily for a number of reasons. First, it helps ensure continuity of care while the patient is in the hospital (ie, the PCP may be able to add pertinent clinical information as needed). Second, it provides a comforting presence for the patient, a pres-ence that results not only in better bonding between physician and patient but also in providing emotional support. Third, it allows for continuity after discharge because the PCP is aware of the clinical course and dis-charge planning.

The PCP also is able to communicate effec-tively with the specialist in the event that the specialist failed to see the patient on rounds. For example, if a busy surgeon misses a pa-tient on rounds because the patient was in the bathroom, the surgeon, because of a heavy operating room schedule, may not make it back to see that patient until late at night. If the patient is actually ready for discharge, the PCP can communicate with the surgeon that morning and arrange for discharge.

In any HMO, however, there are situations in which the PCP is unable to make rounds in person regardless of his or her desire to do so. This happens most frequently when a mem-ber is admitted to a tertiary hospital where the PCP does not have privileges. For example, certain types of cardiac surgery may be done at a teaching hospital with a closed medical staff. In these situations, it is important for the PCP to be in telephone contact with the at-tending physician to keep up with develop-ments and to aid in the discharge planning process. For example, the PCP may be com-fortable in accepting the patient back in trans-fer during the recovery period or may be able to suggest home nursing care. In addition to managing utilization, this helps ensure conti-nuity of care, and the attending physician will almost always remark to the patient how at-tentive the PCP has been.

As a corollary to such involvement, a PCP should be confident and assertive about his or her own abilities. It is an unfortunate by-product of the highly specialized nature of medicine that there are times when a PCP is looked down upon by a specialist. Certainly, a specialist who depends on the PCP for referrals will not knowingly exhibit behavior that the PCP can find offensive, but there remains an unspoken agreement that the specialist calls the shots once the patient is admitted. But in a well-managed UM system, to say nothing of well-managed medical practice, it is the role and responsibility of the PCP to follow the care of the patient and to be aware of the medical issues involved. Furthermore, with the well-documented problem of serious medical errors occurring in hospitalized patients,[82] having an observant PCP may well help to prevent some serious complications, particularly as regards medication errors.

There is the possibility that the PCP will view questioning as confrontational and will be unwilling to appear to question the competence of the specialist. It is important to point out that the PCP is not questioning the specialist's competence (assuming that the specialist is indeed competent) but rather is discussing the case and asking the specialist his or her opinion about alternatives. The fear of such confrontations is far greater than the reality. The PCP has nothing to be shy about. PCPs are trained physicians specializing in primary care, and the specialist is helping care for the PCP's patient, not vice versa. The simple act of asking the specialist questions about care is appropriate and useful and frequently results in improved understanding by all parties as well as improved utilization management.

Specialty Care Physician Model

As a practical matter regardless of MCO type, most inpatient cases are managed totally by a specialist, with no real involvement by the PCP. Unlike the hospitalist model described next, in this model the managing specialist may be any specialist,

in the network or not, depending on the MCO's benefit design.

As noted earlier, in PCP-centric HMOs, the interaction between specialist and PCP remains highly important to good medical management and should be encouraged in all cases. Beyond that, the UM personnel and the medical director work directly with the managing specialist. For example, in one older study that focused on intensive care units—where little discretion would be expected in treatment decisions—HMOs had 30% to 40% lower utilization (measured by length of stay, charges, and use of ventilators) when compared to fee-for-service even when adjusted for case mix.[83] This finding points out once again that specialists, and particularly specialists in a managed care environment, have considerable effect on resource use.

In a loosely managed plan, there are fewer expectations of the specialist than in a tightly managed one. As has been mentioned numerous times, the better the management of utilization, the more one must deal with practice patterns and physician behavior. Specialists are able to add significantly to the cost of care not only from their own fees but also from additional fees generated by extra days in the hospital and through tests, procedures, and secondary referrals to other specialists. Even in non-HMOs, if the MCO's data analytic capabilities are sufficiently robust, it may even categorize specialists into different tiers by outcomes and/or use of resources, providing incentives to members to use those specialists in the more cost-effective tier (see also Chapter 5).

Hospitalist Model

In the hospitalist model, sometimes called the *designated admitting physician* or *rounding physician model,* one physician is designated to care for all admissions of a group or health plan to a given hospital or hospital service (*eg,* to a medical service). Hospitalist is a relatively new term that was coined in the mid-1990s by Wachter and Goldman in an article in the *New England Journal of Medicine* in which they described a "new breed of physicians we call 'hospitalists'—specialists in inpatient medicine—who will be responsible for managing the care of hospitalized patients in the same way that primary care physicians are responsible for managing the care of outpatients."[84] The primary feature of this model is that the PCP or specialist who was providing care in the outpatient setting relinquishes responsibility for the admission, and the hospitalist assumes it.

This model is found in many group and staff model HMOs, large organized private medical groups, and has also appeared in some open-panel HMOs. The hospitalist model is also increasing substantially in hospitals, regardless of payer type, with almost all major teaching hospitals employing it.[85] In fact, there are now more than 8,000 hospitalists, projected to grow to 20,000.[81]

Shy of a fully implemented hospitalist model, a rounding or designated physician model may be in place. In this case, the rounding physician may be on-site on a full-time basis or may simply carry a lighter outpatient load and can devote greater time to rounding on hospitalized patients. In the large closed panels and medical groups, as well as the open-panel plans that have adopted this system, it is more common for the designated physician to be full time on-site at the hospital. In this setting, the responsibility is rotated among members of the medical group, but the group may also use a hospitalist who practices only in the hospital. On a secondary note, large groups find that the use of a hospitalist increases the group's overall efficiency because this model avoids many physicians going into the hospital for just one or two visits.

Some large organized medical groups have gone so far as to create entire hospital care groups that include not only a hospitalist physician, but also a physician's assistant or clinical nurse practitioner, a dedicated rounding nurse, and other clinical team members (*eg,* a clinical pharmacist and a social worker). This may best be described as a hospitalist team and is most suited for medical groups or hospitals that provide care for a high number of patients with serious and complex conditions. Such teams are also commonly used in teaching hospitals, regardless of payer considerations.

The reasoning behind the hospitalist model is that a dedicated, on-site physician is closer to the care that the patient is receiving, is in a better position to coordinate needed services, and is able to monitor care for quality and appropriateness. A dedicated hospitalist is also better able to obtain diagnostic study reports, consultations, and so forth in a timely manner. A hospitalist is available all day (though not necessarily 24 hours per day), rather than once or twice per day that is the norm when private practice physicians care for inpatients. Of course, there will be many clinical conditions for which the hospitalist is not at all in a primary caregiver situation (*eg,* during chemotherapy, for obstetrics, for surgical procedures, and so forth). Even in these cases, however, a hospitalist may follow the case in a fashion similar to that described for the PCP.

The impact of the hospitalist model on both cost and quality is positive. In a review of published results of the movement to a hospitalist model, most studies found that implementation of hospitalist programs was associated with significant reductions in resource use, usually measured as hospital costs (average decrease, 13.4%) or average length of stay (average decrease, 16.6%).[85] A voluntary hospitalist service at a community-based teaching hospital produced reductions in length of stay and costs that became statistically significant in the second year of use, and a mortality benefit extending beyond hospitalization was noted in both years.[86] And in another study in an academic hospital, hospitalist care was also associated with lower costs and lower short-term mortality in the second but not the first year of hospitalists' experience; that study also focused on disease-specific physician experience as an important determinant of the effectiveness of hospitalists.[87]

The hospitalist model works well in a capitation environment (see Chapter 6) in which the medical group and the hospitalist all share in the same capitation payment. Alternatively, if a hospital system is receiving capitation for services, it may wish to employ the hospitalist to manage and monitor cases, even when the outside medical group has no direct financial stake in the cost of institutional services. Teaching hospitals, both academic and community, have been struggling with the financial pressures around the use of hospitalists in a noncapitated environment, however, because cognitive services are always reimbursed at lower rates than procedural ones are. Many MCOs, recognizing the value of hospitalists, have been finding ways to provide financial subsidies for their use.

Medical Director's Responsibilities

In addition to monitoring all the elements discussed in this chapter, medical directors working in UM should perform a few specific functions. The first of these is communication. The medical director should be involved in the most difficult cases from a management standpoint. The difficulty is not necessarily medical but rather may be a problem with a physician, a hospital, a member, or a member's family. Even when dealing with uncooperative individuals, the medical director should take a compassionate, caring, but firm stance when appropriate. Often it is easiest simply to give in, but that can be done only so many times before it becomes a habit that damages the plan's effectiveness. The ability to empathize and sympathize with someone's point of view and to recognize what the real issues are in a dispute is not the same as acquiescing. Although there are indeed times when the medical director will want to loosen the reins, it is important for the medical director to remain firm, refer to evidence-based medicine and industry standards when the situation is clear, and back up his or her subordinates (and the PCPs when they are involved in their patient's admission) when they are right.

If the medical director is heard from only when there is a problem, his or her effectiveness will be diminished. It is important for the medical director to be in direct contact with the attending physician in complex cases where there may be alternatives available or when the UM nurse is unable to obtain adequate information. By asking thoughtful questions in a nonthreatening manner, and by constantly stimulating thought regarding cost-effective clinical management, the medical director may slowly reinforce appropriate patterns of care. The most successful outcome of such contacts occurs when physicians begin asking themselves the questions the medical director would ask and begin improving their practice patterns on that basis.

For optimal management of utilization, a medical director should review the hospital log daily. This task may seem onerous—and it can be—but it is the only way a medical director can consistently spot problems in time to do something about them. As a practical matter, in all but the most tightly managed HMOs and in globally capitated medical groups, review of active inpatient cases is usually done by exception, focusing only on those cases where the UM nurse wishes the medical director to become involved or at least offer advice or an opinion. But for utterly optimal control, daily review of each case is most effective. If possible, it is even better for the medical director to review the hospital log with the UM nurse early in the day because early review enables meaningful action to be taken before noon, the time when many hospitals automatically charge for another day.

Retrospective Review

Retrospective review is done after the case is finished and the patient is discharged and takes two primary forms: claims review and pattern review.

Claims review refers to examining individual claims for improprieties or mistakes. All MCOs use software to screen for and identify claims that are incorrect, misleading, or falsified (see Chapter 18). The most common problems are the result of coding errors by providers, such as diagnosis-procedure mismatch. Other common problems include "upcoding" (ie, submitting a claim using the code for a procedure or diagnosis that is more complex than what was actually the case but will result in higher reimbursement) and "unbundling" (ie, submitting multiple claims by separating out various components and charging for each). Some MCOs have taken this process one step further and use software to automatically change claims that are determined to be problematic; for example, rebundling unbundled claims and paying only the appropriate reimbursement. A more forceful step is to use the software to downcode claims automatically based on statistical norms; in other words, reduce the payment by reducing the type of code, based on how often those types of codes appear under normal circumstances. This last activity has resulted in legal class action by physicians, with some major health plans settling out of court while others continue to defend the practice. While still used by many MCOs, using automated systems to adjust claims downward is now somewhat less broadly applied, and the information about the specifics leading to the adjustment is usually now more readily available to the physicians.

It is routine for plans to review large claims to verify whether services were actually delivered, or whether mistakes were made in collating the claims data. In such large cases, the plan may actually send a representative on-site to the hospital to review the medical record against the claims record. In most cases, this results in some level of payment reduction when information supporting the charges cannot be found.

Review of specific claims will also take place when fraud or abuse is detected, usually through pattern review as discussed next. When MCOs use software to look for patterns of fraud and abuse, thresholds are set so as to focus only on cases or patterns that represent significant financial value. Fraud refers to deliberate criminal activity to submit fraudulent claims, while abuse refers to billing practices that, while not specifically fraudulent, represent attempts to obtain reimbursement far above what is appropriate. When detected, a specialized department in the MCO undertakes detailed scrutiny of submitted claims and supporting documentation (or lack thereof), on-site reviews as necessary and/or possible, and then attempts to recover the money either through direct payment or through offsets to future reimbursement. In other cases, such review takes place before the claims are actually paid. Law enforcement is also brought in when appropriate; reporting fraud and abuse to the federal government for Medicare and Medicaid services is required by law.

Pattern review refers to examining patterns of utilization to determine where action must be taken. This is used not only to detect claims errors or falsifications as discussed earlier, but also refers to detecting patterns of services and utilization that may allow for improvements in cost or quality of care. For example, if three hospitals in the area perform coronary artery bypass surgery, the plan may look to see which one has the best clinical outcomes, the shortest lengths of stay, and the lowest charges. The plan may then preferentially send all such cases to that hospital. Pattern review also allows the plan to focus UM efforts primarily on those areas needing greater attention (ie, Sutton's Law: Go where the money is!). The use of pattern review is complex, requiring attention to case mix, comorbidities, and other factors as discussed in Chapter 16.

One other use of pattern review is to provide feedback to providers. Although not as powerful as active UM by the plan's own department, feedback sometimes can have an effect in and of itself. When combined with other management functions and financial incentives, meaningful and actionable feedback to providers is a useful management tool.[88–90]

EMERGENCY DEPARTMENT

The ED, which used to be more commonly known as the emergency room (ER), is both a source of utilization and expense in its own right and a gateway to inpatient admission. Patients show up in the ED in several ways. They may self-refer based on their perceived need to receive care (*eg,* they may be having chest or abdominal pains or may have cut themselves), they may be transported there by emergency services (*eg,* after a motor vehicle accident), or they may be directed there by their physician (*eg,* after calling their PCP to complain about chest pain). As noted also in Chapter 7, the reported percent distribution of emergency department visits (not specific to managed care) by immediacy with which patient should be seen in 2004 was as follows:

• Urgent: 37.8%
• Semiurgent: 21.8%
• No triage or unknown: 15.1%
• Emergent: 12.9%
• Nonurgent: 12.5% [91]

As regards self-referral by the member, MCOs now usually do not attempt to deny coverage for any but the most egregious misuse of the ED. In the past, some HMOs required EDs to obtain authorization to see the patient, but in 1986 the federal government passed the Emergency Medical Treatment and Active Labor Act (EMTALA) to prevent transfer or "dumping" of uninsured patients by private hospitals to public hospitals.[92] EMTALA requires that all patients presenting to any hospital ED must have a medical screening exam performed by qualified personnel, usually the emergency physician. The medical screening exam cannot be delayed for insurance reasons: either to obtain insurance information or to obtain preauthorization for examination. Although theoretically an MCO could deny payment even though the ED was required by law to provide services, hospitals rightly refused to agree to those terms and MCOs abandoned precertification

for basic ED services as a means to manage utilization (though precertification for admission or for extensive nonemergency services may still be required).

Instead, MCOs have substantially increased the levels of copayment or co-insurance that the member must pay for basic ED services, using financial barriers to cause the member to think twice about whether or not to go to the ED. A 1985 study on the effects of cost sharing was conclusive that cost sharing decreased inappropriate use of the ED without having a negative impact on appropriate use.[93] This was affirmed in studies in 1989 and 1996 involving modest ($25.00 to $35.00) copays.[94,95] Another study looking specifically at the effect of ED copayments of between $25 and $100 on patients with an acute myocardial infarction (heart attack) found that there was no associated delay in treatment.[96] On the other hand, only one-third of adults seem to actually know what their copayment requirement is for ED services.[97]

Regardless of the means by which the member ended up in the ED, what happens next is definitely a focus of UM, particularly as it applies to the ED's function as a gateway to admission to the hospital. In the case of trauma or other obvious significant medical conditions, the role of UM is the same as for any other type of inpatient case. For many other common medical conditions, most EDs have created standardized protocols that improve efficiency and outcomes. But because of concerns about legal liability, many EDs have established chest pain protocols that result either in an admission to the cardiac care unit or in an observation stay, regardless of how serious the patient's condition appears to be or whether there are diagnostic data to support the existence of a serious and acute heart problem. This results in substantially increased costs to the plan as well as to the member if the member has co-insurance. Some plans have addressed this problem by negotiating special rates for such admissions when there is no subsequent evidence of a heart attack. Other plans actually contract with specialty management companies to assume responsibility for the evaluation and disposition of these cases at each hospital's ED, as discussed in Chapter 5.

ALTERNATIVES TO ACUTE-CARE HOSPITALIZATION

There are many instances in which patients are ill or disabled but not to the extent that they need to be in an acute care hospital. Yet, an acute care hospital is where they may stay for a variety of reasons. In some cases, the patient initially needed the services of an acute care hospital (*eg,* the patient had surgery, but the recovery phase requires far fewer resources than the hospital offers). In other cases, there is simply no place for the patient to go (*eg,* a patient is recovering from a broken femur but lives alone). Although now uncommon, there are also times when the patient is kept in the hospital by a physician simply because that's the way they want to do it.

Subacute Care: Skilled or Intermediate Nursing Facilities

One alternative to acute care hospitalization is the skilled or intermediate nursing facility, or subacute facility. This is most suited for prolonged convalescence or recovery cases. For example, if a patient with a broken femur requires more traction than can be provided safely at home and requires many months to recover, the cost for a bed day in a subacute facility will be much less than in an acute care hospital. The same goes for rehabilitation cases such as stroke or trauma to the brain when the damage is too extensive for the patient to go home immediately.

Over the past several years, the subacute care industry has focused on making its facilities a practical alternative to an acute care hospital for a larger variety of medical cases. For example, some subacute care facilities provide a cost-effective location for the administration of chemotherapy that requires close supervision. In some cases, the treatment of certain medical conditions such as acute pneumonia or osteomyelitis when a patient is too sick to be cared for at home may be done in a subacute facility. In other cases, a patient may be able to be cared for at home, but it is still more cost-effective to deliver the therapy in the subacute facility because of more favorable pricing achievable through economies of scale. For a subacute facility to vie effectively for this type of business, it must transform itself into something other than a nursing home.

The main problem with the use of subacute facilities is objection from the patient or the family to the use of a "nursing home," particularly in the case of young patients. A stigma is attached to nursing homes, even if they are renamed subacute facilities. Some people associate them with warehouses for the infirm elderly. To overcome this stigma, a proactive approach is required.

As discussed in Chapter 7, an MCO should contract only with those subacute facilities that meet the plan's (and implicitly the plan's members') needs for pleasant surroundings, and a good subacute facility will be interested in working with the plan to make this option acceptable. For example, the facility might ensure that the plan's members are given a private room (a private room in a subacute facility is still less costly than a semiprivate bed in an acute care hospital) or are placed in a room with a patient with a similar functional status.

Second, discuss the alternative with the patient and the family well in advance of the actual move. Nothing is as distressing as suddenly finding out that you will be shipped out in the morning to a nursing home. If possible, have the family visit the subacute facility to meet the staff and see the environment before the patient is transferred.

Last, do not abandon the patient. In other words, have someone such as the UM nurse and/or a clinical social worker visit the patient on a regular basis. It is easy to rationalize that because the patient is in the subacute facility for long-term care, there is no need to visit often. Although that may be true from a medical standpoint, it is not true from a human relations standpoint.

How the use of subacute facilities is handled has an impact on sales and marketing. If it is perceived that people are coldly shunted into a subacute facility simply to save money, the plan will rapidly get a reputation for placing its financial needs over those of the members. Members will complain to their benefits managers or to other potential members, and growth will be affected. If, however, this option is handled with compassion, taking the time to alleviate the emotional distress that may be caused, most people will be quite understanding and accepting of this alternative.

The other issue to consider in the use of subacute facilities is monitoring the case in regard to the plan's benefit structure. It is easy for a case to go from prolonged recovery to permanent placement or custodial care. Facing the end of coverage benefits can be an emotionally wrenching experience both for the member's family and for the medical managers involved. The problem of who will pay for long-term custodial care is a national dilemma, but it becomes profoundly personal when a family is faced with high costs because the benefits the plan provides do not continue indefinitely. If it is possible or likely that benefits will end, it is wise to make the benefits structure clear to the family early on. This notification does not have to be done in a cold and calculating manner but rather in a way that lays out all the possibilities so that the family can begin early planning.

Step-Down Units

A step-down unit is a ward or section of a ward in an acute-care hospital that is used in much the same way as a skilled nursing facility. A patient who requires less care and monitoring, such as someone recovering from a hip replacement (after all the drains have been removed), may need only bed rest, traction, and minimal nursing care. In recognition of the lesser resource needs, the charge per day is less.

The step-down unit has the advantage of being convenient for the physician and UM nurse and is more acceptable to the patient and family. It also does not require transfer outside the facility. Although the cost per day is sometimes slightly higher than that of a subacute facility, the difference may be worth it in terms of member acceptability.

Outpatient Procedure Units

As discussed earlier in this chapter, a great number of procedures that once required hospitalization are now done on an outpatient basis. Those procedures may be done in the ambulatory facility of an acute-care hospital or at a freestanding facility, may be affiliated with a hospital or may be independent. As discussed in Chapter 7, it is possible for care to shift from inpatient to outpatient and end up costing more, not less, as a result of contractual reimbursement terms that provide for greater remuneration for outpatient procedures. This is an area where MCOs should be directing care to the most cost-effective locations, not simply settling for a shift to outpatient.

Hospice Care

Hospice care is that care given to terminally ill patients. It tends to be care that is supportive to the patient and the family. Much hospice care is outpatient or home-care based, but inpatient forms of hospice are also available and are used most often when such care cannot be given in the home. Statistically speaking, most hospice patients are covered under Medicare. In commercial managed care, it is now a routine benefit, though it once was not. In fact, many MCOs will not cover acute-care hospitalization for purely palliative care for terminally ill patients, requiring the use of hospice for such care. Care of the terminally ill patient has not been a focus of most medical management programs, even though it should be considered a form of case management.

Home Health Care

Home health care is a frequent alternative to acute inpatient care and has become common in MCOs. Services that are particularly amenable to home health care include nursing care for routine reasons (*eg,* checking on a newborn, changing dressings, and the like), home intravenous treatment (*eg,* for osteomyelitis, certain forms of chemotherapy, or home intravenous nutrition), home physical therapy, respiratory therapy, and rehabilitation care.

There should be little trouble negotiating and contracting with home health agencies for services. It is also common for hospitals to have home health care services to aid with caring for patients discharged from their facilities, and those services may be negotiated with the overall contract. Furthermore, as Medicare continues to tighten down on payments for home care, many agencies are looking for alternative sources of revenue. As with hospitals or any other providers of care, home health and high-technology home care agencies need to be evaluated for more than simple pricing breaks. An active quality management program, the presence of a medical director, and evidence of attention to the changes that are constantly occurring in the field are all requisites for contracting.

A warning about home health services is in order. Because the physician and UM nurse seldom visit the patient receiving home health care, it often defaults to the home health nurse to determine how often and how long the patient should receive services, and this practice can lead to some surprising costs. It is advisable to have a firm policy regarding the number of home health visits covered under a single authorization and a requirement for physician review for continued authorization.

Case Management

Case management (also referred to as large or catastrophic case management) refers to specialized techniques for identifying and managing cases that are disproportionately high in cost. This subject is covered in detail in Chapter 11, so is discussed only briefly here within the context of overall management of basic medical-surgical utilization.

Identification of potentially high-dollar cases may be straightforward because patients are hospitalized the first time they are identified, as in the case of trauma. Considerable improvements in outcome and cost are achieved in these programs.[7,98] Other cases may be identified before the patient is hospitalized through the use of predictive modeling as discussed in Chapters 10 and 16. For example, examining the claims system for use of dialysis services may identify an end-stage renal disease patient. In addition to those conditions most commonly managed by the MCO's DM function (*eg,* diabetes, cardiac disease, and so forth), proactively contacting patients with potentially catastrophic illnesses not considered under the DM program not only can save the plan considerable expense by managing the care cost-effectively, but also can result in better medical care because the services are coordinated.

Prenatal care is a specialized form of CM because active coordination occurs before the newborn is delivered. Prenatal CM involves identification of high-risk pregnancies early enough to intervene to improve the chances of a good outcome. With the staggering costs of neonatal intensive care, it only takes a few improved outcomes to yield dramatic savings. Methods for identifying cases include sending out information about pregnancy to all members, reviewing the claims system for pregnancy-related claims, asking (or requiring) PCPs and obstetricians to notify the plan when a delivery is expected, and so forth. After the UM department is informed of the case, the member may be proactively contacted and an assessment undertaken to identify risk factors (*eg,* very young maternal age, diabetes, smoking, alcohol or drug use, other medical problems, poor nutrition, and so forth). If risk factors are noted, then the plan can coordinate prenatal care in a very proactive manner. Although it is impossible to force a member to seek care and to follow-up on problems, it is possible to increase the amount and quality of prenatal care that is delivered. When the pregnant patient is also abusing drugs or alcohol, close coordination with the substance abuse program must then occur.

The degree to which the plan can become involved in CM is in part a function of the benefits structure. In a tightly run managed health care plan, it is common for the UM department to be proactive in CM; in simple PPOs, CM is often voluntary on the part of the member (in other words, if the member chooses not to cooperate, there is little impact on benefits). Even in situations requiring strictly voluntary cooperation by the members and physicians, it is common for CM to be highly effective, though.

Upon acceptance into a CM program, an assessment is typically completed that identifies problems, goals, and applicable interventions for the case. In addition to the standard methods of managing utilization, CM often involves two other techniques. First is the use of community resources. Some catastrophic cases require support structures to help the member function or even return home. Examples of such support include family members, social service agencies, churches, special foundations, and so forth.

The other common technique is to go beyond the contractual benefits to manage the case. For example, if the benefits structure of the group has only limited coverage for durable medical equipment, it may still be in the plan's financial interest as well as the member's interest to cover such expenses to get the patient home and out of the hospital. In self-funded groups, the group administrator may actually be willing to fund extracontractual benefits simply as a benefit for an employee or dependent that is experiencing a terrible medical problem.

In all events, the hallmark of CM is longitudinal management of the case by a single UM nurse or department. Management spans hospital care, rehabilitation, outpatient care, professional services, home care, ancillary services, and so forth. It is in the active coordination of care that both quality and cost-effectiveness are maintained.

CONCLUSION

The provision of basic medical-surgical services involves a broad continuum of care. Managing utilization of these services must focus on managing basic demand, referral and specialty services, and institutional services. The tools and technology utilized by health plans to perform these types of utilization management services have evolved to support multiple channels and provide a more sophisticated level of analytics and business rules to improve efficiency and effectiveness of the programs, as well as acknowledging the longitudinal member record that includes key information regarding health risks, wellness programs, and condition management program participation.

The management of referral and specialty services affects not only professional expenses but also costs associated with tests and procedures, including hospitalizations that may be generated by the specialist. The ability to select only those consultants and referral specialists who practice cost-effectively can yield cost savings, but optimal management depends on an authorization system. The lack of such a system diminishes a plan's abilities to decrease utilization over the long term. At the least, the alternative of using financial incentives as part of the benefit design may create support for the use of primary care versus specialty care.

The management of hospital or institutional utilization is one of the most important aspects of managing overall health care costs. The methods used to manage hospital utilization vary from relatively weak and mechanical to tightly managed, longitudinally integrated, and highly labor intensive. The management of hospital utilization is a function that must be attended to every day to achieve optimal results, and special attention must be paid to CM to produce the greatest savings. Avoidance of hospitalization through prevention, good DM, and access to alternatives to acute hospital care are also important to achieving good results.

References

1. Pilote L, Califf RM, Sapp S, *et al.* Regional variation across the United States in the management of acute myocardial infarction. *N Engl J Med.* 1995, 333(9):567–572.

2. Centers for Medicare and Medicaid Services. National Health Expenditure Data, Overview. Available at: http://www.cms.hhs.gov/National HealthExpendData/. Accessed July 31, 2006.

3. Citrome L. Practice protocols, parameters, pathways, and guidelines: A review. *Adm Policy Ment Health.* 1998, 25(3):257–269.

4. Van Horn RL, Burns LR, Wholey DR. The impact of physician involvement in managed care on efficient use of hospital resources. *Med Care.* 1997, 35:873–889.

5. Wickizer TM. The effects of utilization review on hospital use and expenditures: A covariance analysis. *Health Serv Res.* April 1992, 27(1):103–121.

6. Huggins D, Lehman K. Reducing costs through case management. *Nurs Management.* December 1997, 34–36.

7. Warren BH, Puls T, Fogelstrom-Dezeeuw P. Cost effectiveness of case management experiences of a university managed health care organization. *Am J Med Quality.* Winter 1996, 11(4):173–178.

8. Wickizer TM. Controlling outpatient medical equipment costs through utilization management. *Med Care,* 1995, 33(4):383–391.

9. Plocher DW, Brody RS. Disease management and return on investment. In: Kongstvedt PR, Plocher DW, eds. *Best Practices in Medical Management.* Gaithersburg, Md: Aspen Publishing, 1998.

10. High start-up costs of disease management programs offset by improved outcomes, lower utilization, reduced costs. *Managed Care Week.* June 21, 1999:6–7.

11. Robinson JC, Yegian JM. Medical management after managed care. *Health Affairs.* May 19, 2004. Web Exclusive. W4–269–280.

12. Mays GP, Claxton G, White J. Managed care rebound? Recent changes in health plans' cost containment strategies. *Health Affairs.* August 2004. Web Exclusive. W4–427–436. Accessed August 1, 2006. Available at: http://content.healthaffairs.org/cgi/reprint/hlthaff.w4.427v1. Accessed August 14, 2006.

13. National Committee for Quality Assurance. New NCQA accreditation standards for managed care plans highlight member engagement, wellness, care management. July 31, 2006. Press release. Available at: http://www.ncqa.org/Communications/News/Accred_2007.htm. Accessed August 6, 2006.

14. Vickery DM, Kalmer H, Lowry D. Effect of a self-care education program on medical visits. *JAMA.* 1983, 250:2952–2956.

15. Elsenhans VD, Marquardt C, Bledsoe T. Use of self-care manual shifts utilization pattern. *HMO Pract.* June 1995, 9(2):88–90.

16. Robinson JS, Schwartz ML, Magwene KS, *et al.* The impact of fever health education on clinic utilization. *Am J Dis Children.* June 1989, 143(6):698–704.

17. O'Connor AM, Llewellyn-Thomas HA, Flood AB. Modifying unwarranted variations in health care: shared decision making using patient decision aids. *Health Affairs.* Web Exclusive. October 7, 2004. Available at: http://content.healthaffairs.org/cgi/reprint/hlthaff.var.63v1. Accessed August 12, 2006.

18. Sepucha KR, Fowler FJ Jr, Mulley AG Jr. Policy support for patient-centered care: The need for measurable improvements in decision quality. *Health Affairs.* Web Exclusive. October 7, 2004. Available at: http://content.healthaffairs.org/cgi/reprint/hlthaff.var.54v1. Accessed August 9, 2006.

19. Weinstein JN, Bronner KK, Morgan TS, Wennberg J. Trends and geographic variations in major surgery for degenerative diseases of the hip, knee, and spine. *Health Affairs.* Web

Exclusive. October 7, 2004. Available at: http:// content.healthaffairs.org/cgi/reprint/hlthaff. var.81v1. Accessed August 3, 2006.

20. O'Connor AM, Stacey D, Entwistle V, *et al.* Decision aids for people facing health treatment or screening decisions. *Cochrane Database Syst Review.* 2003, (2):CD001431.

21. Billings J. Promoting the dissemination of decision aids: An odyssey in a dysfunctional health care financing system. *Health Affairs.* Web Exclusive. VAR-128-132, October 7, 2004. Available at: http://content.healthaffairs. org/cgi/reprint/hlthaff.var.128v1. Accessed August 4, 2006.

22. Burton WN, Hoy DA. First Chicago's integrated health data management computer system. *Managed Care Q.* 1993, 1(3):18–23.

23. Pronk NP, Goodman MJ, O'Connor PJ, Martinson BC. Relationship between modifiable health risks and short-term health care charges. *JAMA.* 1999, 282:2235–2239.

24. Elias WS. Introduction to health risk appraisals. In: Kongstvedt PK, Plocher DW, eds. *Best Practices in Medical Management.* Gaithersburg, Md: Aspen Publishers, 1998.

25. Ringle M. Implementing health status measurements. *Health Care Leadership Rev.* February 1998:12.

26. Study proves $6,500 saved per patient thanks to risk assessment program. In: National Health Information LLC, eds. *Medical Management under Medicare Risk.* Marietta, Ga: National Health Information, 1998:22–23.

27. Wennberg JE, Gittelsohn A. Variations in medical care among small areas. *Sci Am.* 1982, 246(4):120–134.

28. Wennberg J, Caper P. Medical practice: why does it vary so much? *Hospitals.* March 1, 1985, 59(5):89.

29. Wennberg JE, Freeman JL, Culp WJ. Are hospital services rationed in New Haven or overutilized in Boston? *Lancet.* 1987, 1:1185–1189.

30. Fisher ES, Wennberg JE, Stukel TA, Sharp SM. Hospital readmission rates for cohorts of Medicare beneficiaries in Boston and New Haven. *N Engl J Med.* 1994, 331:989–995.

31. Restuccia J, Shwartz M, Ash A, Payne S. High hospital rates and inappropriate care. *Health Affairs* (Millwood). 1996, 15(4):156–163.

32. Graves EJ. National hospital discharge survey: annual summary, 1993. *Vital and Health Statistics,* Series 13, No. 121. Washington, DC:

Government Printing Office, 1995. U.S. Dept of Health and Human Services publication PHS 95-1782.

33. Bindman AB, Grumbach K, Osmond D, *et al.* Preventable hospitalizations and access to health care. *JAMA.* 1995, 274:305–311.

34. Weissman JS, Gatsonis C, Epstein AM. Rates of avoidable hospitalization by insurance status in Massachusetts and Maryland. *JAMA.* 1992, 268:2388–2394.

35. Kahan JP, Bernstein SJ, Leape LL. Measuring the necessity of medical procedures. *Med Care.* 1994, 32(4):357–365.

36. Chassin MR. Explaining geographic variations: the enthusiasm hypothesis. *Med Care.* 1993, 31(5, suppl):YS37–YS44.

37. Wennber J, Cooper M, Birkmeyer J, *et al. The Dartmouth Atlas of Health Care.* Chicago, Ill: American Hospital Publishing, 1998.

38. Moore JD. Market pressures say what? *Mod Healthcare.* June 29, 1998, 28(26):150, 156, 168.

39. Asthon CM, Petersen NJ, Souchek J, *et al.* Geographic variations in utilization rates at Veterans Affairs hospitals and clinics. *N Engl J Med.* 1999, 340(1):32–39.

40. Pappas G, Hadden WC, Kozak LJ, *et al.* Potentially avoidable hospitalizations: Inequalities in rates between U.S. socioeconomic groups. *Am J Public Health.* May 1997, 87(5): 811–816.

41. Wennberg JE, Fisher ES, Stukel TA, Shart SM. Use of Medicare claims data to monitor provider-specific performance among patients with severe chronic illness. *Health Affairs.* Web Exclusive. October 2004. Available at: http://content.healthaffairs.org/cgi/ content/full/hlthaff.var.5/DC3. Accessed August 1, 2006.

42. Fisher ES, Wennberg DE, Stukel TA, Gottliev DJ. Variations in the longitudinal efficiency of academic medical centers. *Health Affairs.* Web Exclusive. October 2004. Available at: http:// content.healthaffairs.org/cgi/content/full/ hlthaff.var.19/DC3. Accessed August 1, 2006.

43. Meehan TP, Fine MJ, Krumholz HM, *et al.* Quality of care, process, and outcomes in elderly patients with pneumonia. *JAMA.* 1997, 278(23):2080–2084.

44. Phelps C. The methodologic foundations of studies of the appropriateness of medical care. *N Engl J Med.* 1993, 329(17):1241–1245.

45. Eddy DM. Balancing cost and quality in fee-for-service versus managed care. *Health Affairs* (Millwood). 1997, 16(3):162–173.

46. Chassin MR, Kosecoff J, Park RE, *et al*. Does inappropriate use explain geographic variations in the use of health care services? A study of three procedures. *JAMA*. 1987, 258: 2533–2537.

47. Kahn K, Chassin MR, Flynn MT, *et al*. Measuring the clinical appropriateness of the use of a procedure. Can we do it? *Med Care*. April 1998, 26(4):415–422.

48. Brook RH, Park RE, Chassin MR, *et al*. Predicting the appropriate use of carotid endarterectomy, upper gastrointestinal endoscopy and coronary angiography. *N Engl J Med*. 1990, 323(17):1173–1177.

49. Leape L, Park RE, Soloman DH, *et al*. Relation between surgeons' practice volumes and geographic variation in the rate of carotid endarterectomy. *N Engl J Med*. 1989, 321(10): 653–657.

50. Guadagnoli E, Hauptman PJ, Ayanian JZ, *et al*. Variation in the use of cardiac procedures after acute myocardial infarction. *N Engl J Med*. 1995, 333(9):573–578.

51. O'Connor GT, Quinton HB, Traven ND. Geographic variation in the treatment of acute myocardial infarction. *JAMA*. 1999, 281(7): 627–633.

52. Gaus CR, Clancy CM. Research at the interface of primary and specialty care, adapted from the Agency for Health Care Policy and Research. *JAMA*. 1995, 274(18):1419.

53. Bryce CL, Cline KE. The supply and use of selected medical technologies. *Health Affairs* (Millwood). 1998, 17(1):213–224.

54. HealthCore. *An Economic Evaluation of Use of Payer-Based Electronic Health Record within an Emergency Department*. July 24, 2006. Available at: http://www.healthcore.com.

55. Wynia MK, Cummins DS, VanGeest JB, Wilson IB. Physician manipulation of reimbursement rules for patients: Between a rock and a hard place. *JAMA*. 2000, 283:1858–1865.

56. Hillman BJ, Joseph CA, Mabry MR, *et al*. Frequency and costs of diagnostic imaging in office practice—A comparison of self-referring and radiologist-referring physicians. *N Engl J Med*. 1990, 323:1604–1608.

57. Office of the Inspector General. *Financial Arrangements between Physicians and Health Care Businesses: Report to Congress*. Washington, DC: U.S. Department of Health and Human Services, 1989. U.S. Department of Health and Human Services publication OAI-12-88-01410.

58. State of Florida Health Care Cost Containment Board. *Joint Ventures among Health Care Providers in Florida*. Tallahassee, Fla: State of Florida, 1991:2.

59. The Ethics in Patient Referrals Act—Omnibus Budget Reconciliation Act of 1989.

60. Ware JE, Brook RH, Rogers WH, *et al*. Comparison of health outcomes at a health maintenance organization with those of fee-for-service care. *Lancet*. May 3, 1986, 1(8488): 1017–1022.

61. Udvarhelyi IS, Jennison K, Phillips RS. Comparison of the quality of ambulatory care for fee-for-service and prepaid patients. *Ann Intern Med*. 1991, 115:394–400.

62. Sloss EM, Keeler EB, Brook RH, *et al*. Effect of a health maintenance organization on physiologic health. *Ann Intern Med*. 1987, 106: 130–138.

63. Clancy CM, Hillner BE. Physicians as gatekeepers—The impact of financial incentives. *Arch Intern Med*. 1989, 149:917–920.

64. Martin DP, Diehr P, Price KF, Richardson WC. Effect of a gatekeeper plan on health services use and charges: A randomized trial. *Am J Public Health*. 1989, 79(12):1628–1632.

65. Flood AB, Fremont AM, Jin KB, *et al*. How do HMOs achieve savings? The effectiveness of one organization's strategies. *Health Serv Res*. April 1998, 33(1):79–99.

66. Hurley RE, Freund DA, Gage BJ, *et al*. Gatekeeper effects of patterns of physician use. *J Fam Pract*. 1991, 32(2):167–174.

67. Forrest CB, Reid RJ. Passing the baton: HMOs' influence on referrals to specialty care. *Health Affairs* (Millwood). 1997, 16(6):157–162.

68. Dietrich AJ, Nelson EC, Kirk JW, *et al*. Do primary physicians actually manage their patients' fee-for-service care? *JAMA*. 1988, 259: 3145–3149.

69. St. Peter RF, Reed MC, Kemper P, Blumenthal D. Changes in the scope of care provided by primary care physicians. *N Engl J Med*. 1999, 341:1980–1985.

70. Remler DK, Donelan K, Blendon RJ, *et al*. What do managed care plans do to affect care? *Inquiry*. 1997, 34(3):196–204.

71. Gallagher TH, St. Peter RF, Chesney M, Lo B. Patients' attitudes toward cost containment bonuses for managed care physicians. *Health Affairs*. 2001, 20(2):186-192.

72. Halm EA, Causine N, Blumenthal D. Is gatekeeping better than traditional care? *JAMA*. 1997, 278:1677-1681.

73. Cram P, Ettinger WH. Generalists or specialists—Who does it better? *Physician Executive*. January–February 1998:40-45.

74. Quickel KE. *Managed Care and Diabetes, with Special Attention to the Issue of Who Should Provide Care*. Transactions of the American Clinical and Climatological Association. 1997, 108:184-199.

75. Committee of the American College of Rheumatology Council on Health Care Research. Role of specialty care for chronic diseases: a report from an ad hoc committee of the American College of Rheumatology. *Mayo Clin Proc*. 1996, 71:1179-1181.

76. Bello D, Shah NG, Edep ME, *et al*. Self-reported differences between cardiologists and heart failure specialists in the management of chronic heart failure. *Am Heart J*. 1999, 138:100-107.

77. Santos-Eggimann B, Sidler M, Schopfer D, Blanc T. Comparing results of concurrent and retrospective designs in a hospital utilization review. *Int J Qual Health Care*. April 1997, 9(2):115-120.

78. Madden JM, Soumerai SB, Lieu TA, *et al*. Effects of a law against early postpartum discharge on newborn follow-up, adverse events, and HMO expenditures. *N Engl J Med*. 2002, 347:2031-2039.

79. Forster AJ, Murff HJ, Peterson JF, *et al*. The incidence and severity of adverse events affecting patients after discharge from the hospital. *Ann Intern Med*. 2003, 138(3):161-167.

80. Dudas V, Bookwalter T, Kerr KM, Pantilat SZ. The impact of follow-up telephone calls to patients after hospitalization. *Am J Med*. 2001, 111(9B):26S-30S.

81. Wachter RM. Hospitalists in the United States—Mission accomplished or work in progress? *N Engl J Med*. 2004, 350(19):1935-1936.

82. Kohn LT, Corrigan J, Donaldson MS, eds. *To Err Is Human: Building a Safer Health System*. Washington, DC: National Academies Press, 2000.

83. Rapoport J, Gehlbach S, Lemeshow S, Teres D. Resource utilization among intensive care patients: Managed care vs. traditional insurance. *Arch Intern Med*. 1992, 152:2207-2212.

84. Wachter RM, Goldman L. The emerging role of "hospitalists" in the American health care system. *N Engl J Med*. 1996, 335(7):514-517.

85. Wachter RM, Goldman L. The hospitalist movement 5 years later. *JAMA*. 2002, 287(4):487-494.

86. Auerbach AD, Wachter RM, Katz P, *et al*. Implementation of a voluntary hospitalist service at a community teaching hospital: improved clinical efficiency and patient outcomes. *Ann Intern Med*. 2002, 137(11):859-865.

87. Meltzer D, Manning WG, Morrison J, *et al*. Effects of physician experience on costs and outcomes on an academic general medicine service: results of a trial of hospitalists. *Ann Intern Med*. 2002, 137(11):866-874.

88. Billi JE, Hejna GF, Wolf FM, *et al*. The effects of a cost-education program on hospital charges. *J Gen Intern Med*. 1987, 2:306-311.

89. Kiefe CI, Allison JJ, Williams OD, *et al*. Improving quality improvement using achievable benchmarks for physician feedback: A randomized controlled trial. *JAMA*. 2001, 285(22):2871-2879.

90. Bordley WC, Chelminski A, Margolis PA, Kraus R, Szilagyi PG, Vann JJ. The effect of audit and feedback on immunization delivery. *Am J Prev Med*. May 2000, 18(4):343-350.

91. McCaig LF, Nawar EN. National Hospital Ambulatory Medical Care Survey: 2004 emergency department summary. Advance data from vital and health statistics, no 372. Hyattsville, Md: National Center for Health Statistics, 2006. Available at: http://www.cdc.gov/nchs/data/ad/ad372.pdf. Accessed July 16, 2006.

92. 42, USC 1395 dd (1986) Pub. L. No. 99-272.

93. Grady KF, Mannng WG, Newhouse JP, Brook RH. The impact of cost sharing on emergency department use. *N Engl J Med*. 1985, 313(8):484-490.

94. Selby JV, Fireman BH, Swain BE. Effect of a copayment on use of the emergency department in a health maintenance organization. *N Engl J Med*. 1996, 334:635-641.

95. Shapiro MF, Hayward RA, Freeman HE, Sudman S, Corey CR. Out-of-pocket pay-

ments and use of care for serious and minor symptoms. *Arch Intern Med.* 1989, 149: 1645–1648.

96. Magid DJ, Koepsell TD, Every NT, *et al.* Absence of association between insurance co-payments and delays in seeking emergency care among patients with myocardial infarction. *N Engl J Med.* 1997, 336:1722–1729.

97. Hsu J, Reed M, Brand R, *et al.* Cost sharing: patient knowledge and effects on seeking emergency department care. *Medical Care.* March 2004, 42(3):290–296.

98. Huggins D, Lehman K. Reducing costs through case management. *Nurs Manage.* December 1997, 28(12):34–37.

10

FUNDAMENTALS AND CORE COMPETENCIES OF DISEASE MANAGEMENT

David W. Plocher

Study Objectives

- Understand the meaning of disease management (DM) and be able to explain what is unique about the term.
- Understand how conventional case management differs from disease management.
- Understand the most important characteristics of a disease that make it appropriate for this model.
- Understand why disease management is not enough with regard to the entire spectrum of care management.
- Understand where DM operates.
- Understand the pros and cons of building vs outsourcing DM.
- Understand difficulties in measuring DM ROI.

Discussion Topics

1. Discuss what is unique about disease management.
2. Discuss the key differences between conventional case management and disease management.
3. Describe some characteristics of a disease that would make it appropriate for this model.
4. Discuss how disease management falls short, with regard to the entire spectrum of care management.
5. Discuss how information technology can make disease management programs more successful.

INTRODUCTION

This chapter highlights current and anticipated developments in disease management (DM) at the time of publication. Of the two primary delivery options, built/in-house programs versus those outsourced to a vendor, the emphasis will be on the latter. This is based on observations by the author of multiple installations around the United States showing market segment size much larger in the outsourced mode. Furthermore, in-house programs are especially unique to local circumstances and contents have been proprietary, rarely in the public domain.

There is a specialized form of DM, behavioral health and substance abuse services, that is discussed fully in Chapter 13 and is not the subject of this chapter. Related in many ways to DM and with some overlap, case management (CM) is discussed in Chapter 11 and is noted in this chapter only as it relates to DM activities.

CHRONIC CONDITIONS

The Problem

The largest portion of the U.S. population represented by chronic conditions is composed of more than 40 million Medicare-eligible beneficiaries (see also Chapter 26). The Centers for Medicare and Medicaid Services (CMS) says patients with five or more chronic conditions account for 23% of its beneficiaries but 68% of its spending. Those conditions are primarily heart disease, diabetes, glaucoma, asthma, chronic obstructive pulmonary disease, and cancer.[1] Just below the senior threshold are baby boomers who, by 2020, will raise the level to 25% of Americans having multiple chronic conditions, and the associated care costs are projected to total $1.07 trillion.

Attempts by individual physicians to influence the course of chronic illness have been hampered by reimbursement methods primarily rewarding treatment of acute illness and performance of procedures. Physicians are financially dissuaded from investing time and effort in preventing illness or preventing complications. Unfortunately, it is more remunerative for them to treat complications.

During the 1980s and early 1990s, experiments with full risk capitation of large medical groups intended to remedy this disconnect (see Chapters 2 and 6). However, the labor shortages of the 1990s and associated managed care backlash (see Chapter 1) all but extinguished such efforts. Furthermore, the office visit with a primary care physician is becoming uncomfortably similar to a 5-minute speed bump. Busy physicians, according to Rand research, use the best evidence-based guidelines for care only about half the time.[2] Compounding this problem, patients adhere to their prescription regimens at roughly the same rate.[3]

Response

To address these problems, there arose in the market the DM vendor. Affordable at a scale that can only be accomplished using staffing ratios achievable at large regional call centers, these companies check in on patients *between* physician visits. They review the treatment plan for evidence-based medicine concordance, and if the ordering physician appears to have overlooked something, he or she is contacted. More often, the patients are coached and counseled on adherence to their complex medical regimens. A lot can happen—or not happen—during that 3- to 4-month interval between routine physician visits.

DEFINITION OF DISEASE MANAGEMENT

According to the Disease Management Association of America (DMAA),[4] disease management is a system of coordinated health care interventions and communications for populations with conditions in which patient self-care efforts are significant. Disease management:

- Supports the physician or practitioner–patient relationship and plan of care.
- Emphasizes prevention of exacerbations and complications utilizing evidence-based practice guidelines and patient empowerment strategies.
- Evaluates clinical, humanistic, and economic outcomes on an ongoing basis with the goal of improving overall health.

Disease management components include the following*:

- Population identification processes
- Evidence-based practice guidelines[†]
- Collaborative practice models to include physician and support-service providers
- Patient self-management education (may include primary prevention, behavior modification programs, and compliance/surveillance)
- Process and outcomes measurement, evaluation, and management[5]
- Routine reporting/feedback loop (may include communication with patient, physician, health plan and ancillary providers, and practice profiling)

DISEASE MANAGEMENT COMPANIES

The typical DM company, whether publicly traded or privately held, is primarily call center based, especially for the commercial sector. For the upper age bands in the commercial sector and more commonly with seniors, home-monitoring technology is added for transmission of weight and multiple vital

---

*Full-service disease management programs must include all six components. Programs consisting of fewer components are disease management support services.

[†]Guidelines are updated at least annually as the peer-reviewed medical literature evolves and often are deployed in metric form as reflected in the Health Plan and Employer Data and Information Set (HEDIS) developed by the National Committee for Quality Assurance (NCQA), discussed in Chapter 23.

signs, usually over the Internet to the call centers.

The Medicaid market (see also Chapter 27) requires other layers of intervention, including interaction with participants at community centers, with county public health nurses, with home care agencies, as well as specialized programs such as free (restricted use) cell phones for convenient call center contact and pushing reminders to participants, and even training neighborhood peers to serve as coaches.

Individual companies vary by preferred purchaser. The majority contract with a health plan. Several are interested in working with CMS, as companies have recently contracted for Medicare Health Support projects, in which their fees are at risk for achievement of 5% savings. Fewer have the inclination to bypass the health plan and contract directly with the large, self-insured employer (potentially risky because neither partner is replete with health plan infrastructure). Similarly, few have invested in the specialized programs required for the Medicaid population. Regardless of customer focus, there is less variation in the end-user focus for these companies: The majority are member centered. Very few companies have developed a physician-centered program.

ESSENTIAL ELEMENTS COMMON TO MOST PROGRAMS

The following components represent key components found in disease management programs.

Condition Prioritization

The payer's claims analysis forms the basis for condition selection, and this begins with understanding which major diagnostic categories are the largest drivers of claim trend (see also Chapter 16). Within these, study of disease prevalence versus benchmarks will advance the cause. Then, comparison of the disease per member per month claim cost or annual episode claim cost versus benchmarks will complete calculation of the financial opportunity.

Next is the feasibility analysis. The foundation for treatment decisions should be widely agreed upon evidence-based guidelines. The patients themselves should be symptomatic, motivating them to change behaviors. Preferably, the circumstances will allow incentives to be applied to both patients and physicians; the health plan has a responsibility in such motivation, for example, rewards for enrollment or waiving copays on generic drugs and supplies used to treat these conditions. In aggregate, the condition selected must have a resource-consumption course that can be modified using the disease management arsenal, beginning with the call center. This modification of behavior must be accomplished at an acceptable overhead cost, or the program evaluation will show an unfavorable cost/benefit ratio.

Participant Identification

Most DM companies apply algorithms with condition-definition rules to the payer's claim experience. This is usually a straightforward diagnosis-finding method. In addition, disease management companies apply predictive modeling tools that are beyond diagnosis code dependency. They scan claims experience using artificial intelligence and neural net modeling to discover candidates projected to become high cost. The resulting candidates are screened by CM (see Chapter 11) or DM intake specialists to determine whether CM, DM, or another program is applicable. Figure 10-1 summarizes these case-finding techniques.

Once a candidate for DM is found, the next layer of predictive modeling or stratification becomes condition-specific to plan for intensity of outreach resources. In some settings, the most morbid DM participants may require at least temporary management by CM for stabilization and benefits modeling.

During the past few years, a further layer of data mining has evolved. Claim pattern recognition software is applied to scan for gaps in care. Beyond conventional drug interaction software, these few vendors can determine whether a patient with a key diagnosis is not on recommended prescriptions, not seeing the physician at a minimum frequency, not being immunized, or not having

Population Triage

Case Finding Data Supplied to a Single Call Center

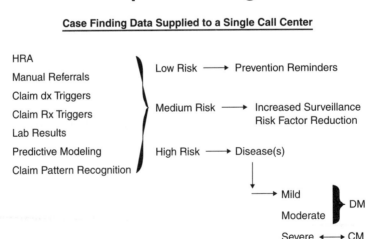

Figure 10–1 Population Triage

Source: Adapted from *Best Practices in Medical Management*, Aspen Publishing, 1998.

a recommended screening test, and so forth. Such services have evolved, in part, in response to the requirement that claims analysis and reporting must produce information that is *actionable*. Typical actions include outreach by mail or phone to the patient, patient's physician, or both.

Recruitment and Engagement

Historic attempts using the opt-in model, whereby the candidate must initiate an enrollment process, have yielded, at most, 30% participation rates. The opt-out method, in which the candidate is automatically enrolled based on passing tests in the rule-based, case-finding algorithm, averages 70% participation rates. The 30% nonparticipation is the sum of true opting out (10%), bad phone numbers (18%), and false positives (2%).* There is rapid evolution in the industry around these activities, to be discussed later in this chapter.

Interaction and Management

Here resides the most important activity of the disease manager. The call center nurse is dynamically interviewing the patients, motivating them to adhere to their complex medical regimens. This is not simply traditional case management, and Table 10-1 summarizes the key activity differences between disease management and case management.

Ten years ago, patients with asthma received much of the attention. Adolescents relying on albuterol for rescue and failing to use steroid inhalers for prevention were vigorously prompted to reverse course. The next most dramatic improvements were made for patients with chronic heart failure, who were offered guidance on low-sodium diets, weight change parameters, diuretic dose adjustments, initiation of angiotensin converting enzyme inhibitors (or, more recently, angiotensin receptor blockers) followed by more recent institution of beta blockers.

_____
*Source: Author's research.

Subsequently, the majority of attention was given to patients with diabetes for blood sugar control, in concert with patients with coronary artery disease, both groups requiring reinforcement of blood pressure and cholesterol management.

Outbound Calls to Participant

Initial welcome call: Orientation to program; administration of health risk appraisal (general) or condition-specific risk assessment; determination of readiness to change; establishing participant's baseline understanding of condition; agreement on preferred language and mode of subsequent communications (phone with desired time of day, mail, Internet, Interactive-Voice Response [IVR]); review of care plan; discussion of methods for closing gaps in adherence; referral to ancillary programs, (*eg* smoking cessation).

Subsequent care calls: Establish progress toward achieving care plan goals and optimal regimen adherence; measure improvement in participant's understanding of condition; coaching on questions to ask during next physician visit.

Reminder calls: Incidental prompts regarding necessary modalities (*eg*, flu shots).

Mailings to Participants

The welcome packet: Complete documentation of program, education about condition, and a symptom checklist (when to call for help).

Periodic updates: Reminders about periodic services needed for condition; updates in educational materials based on medical advances.

Inbound Calls from Participants

Any participant can access the call center to discuss changes in symptoms or other questions about the condition or care plan.

Outbound Calls to Physician

These are rarely needed, unless the member has contacted the call center with a particularly urgent problem, or the claim pattern

Table 10–1 Differences Between CM and DM

Traditional/Catastrophic Case Management	Disease Management
Emphasis is on single patient	Emphasis is on population with a chronic illness
Early identification of people with acute catastrophic conditions (known high cost or known diagnoses that lead to high cost in the near term)	Early identification of all people with targeted chronic diseases (20–40) whether mild, moderate, or severe
Acuity level of catastrophic cases is high, acuity level of traditional cases is high to moderate	Acuity level is moderate
Applies to 0.5–1% of commercial membership	Applies to 15–25% of commercial membership
Value relies heavily on price negotiations and benefit flexing	Value is result of member and provider behavior change that results in improved health status
Requires plan design manipulation	Requires no need to change plan design
Primary objective is to arrange for care using the least restrictive, clinically appropriate alternatives	Primary objective is to avoid hospitalization *and* modify risk factors, lifestyle, medication adherence to improve health status
Episode is 60–90 days	Intervention is 365 days for most conditions
Site of interaction primarily hospital, hospice, subacute facility, or home health care	Site of interaction includes work, school, home
Driven by need for arrangement of support services, community resources, transportation	Driven by nonadherence to medical regimens
Outcome metrics are single-admit length of stay and cost per case	Outcome metrics are annual cost per diseased member and disease-specific functional status

Source: Author.

recognition software has discovered a gap in care requiring prompt attention.

Mailings to Physician

Program orientation: These are informational for the physician, containing confirmation that the program is simply an adjunct to his/her care. Baseline set of practice guidelines pertinent to participant's condition. List of patients in physician panel who have the index condition.

Periodic guideline updates: As the literature advances over time, certain contents of evidence-based guidelines may change.

Periodic participant update: When timing is ideal, these occur just before an electively scheduled office visit. They contain information on the participant's recent contacts with the call center, recent emergency room (ER) visits, and any necessary reminders about tests due or other gaps in care.

Inbound Calls from Physicians

These are very rare and usually consist of questions to aid understanding of the program.

Home Telemonitoring

Participants in the highest risk group with chronic heart failure, chronic obstructive pulmonary disease, and so forth, are equipped with home devices connected (usually) to the Internet so that call centers can monitor real-time results. The most common biometrics transmitted are weight, respiratory rate, blood pressure, heart rate, and oxygen saturation.

Medication Adherence Technology

Still in early-stage trials at the time of publication, several vendors have deployed technology to provide prompts and reminders for participants on complex medication regimens. These take the form of electronic pill boxes, beepers, and specially equipped cell phones.

Documentation

On intake, each new participant's risk stratification is documented. This is usually done informally by each disease management company, though the criteria to establish each stratification level, such as 1 through 4 (low severity to high severity) are objective. Alternatively, there is early use of specialized predictive modeling software designed to be used *not* for the entire population but only for a cohort of participants with a particular condition, again ranking them by levels of severity. The practical purpose is for establishing necessary outbound call frequencies.

Similarly, it is essential to document all baseline inventory obtained during the welcome call, such as scoring and risk stratifying a completed health risk appraisal, readiness to change, and participant's comprehension of their condition. Periodic care call content is also documented, as are occurrences of preventive care reminder calls and mailings.

Information Technology Support

Leading DM companies have invested millions of dollars in the technology providing decision support, automated connections with other programs, and reports. Information technology (IT) is discussed more broadly and at greater length in Chapter 17.

Examples of a few leading practices in the application of IT to DM include the following:

- Automated creation of care plans
- Automated routing of new participant's care plan to the correct disease manager

- Disease manager's ability to view past 12 to 18 months of claim history of the participant
- Disease manager's ability to view the participant's electronic medical record (EMR) at primary care clinic (most advanced practice)

Reporting

Later in this chapter, clinical and economic reporting is addressed. However, for the highest volume of reporting, disease management companies produce fulfillment (activity and participation) reports. These contain the following information:

- Call frequencies, in- and outbound
- Mailing frequencies
- Participants by condition by stratification level
- Participants receiving mail-only versus calls
- Opt-outs
- Bad phone numbers
- False positives
- Complaints and satisfaction survey results for:
    - Participants
    - Physicians

MEASURING EFFECTIVENESS

Methods and metrics used for DM program evaluation have recently been summarized.[6] This continues to be a source of rapid evolution in this industry. At the time of publication, the DMAA is conducting a survey of multiple options in use in an attempt to gain consensus.

The most common method uses the pre-post study. Because many metrics are HEDIS-like, reflecting guidelines used for process measures based on testing required in a year, a requirement of 12 months' continuous enrollment is common. The usual metrics include percentage of diabetes participants with a hemoglobin A1C (HbA1C) test or low-density lipoprotein (LDL) cholesterol test per year, percentage of coronary artery disease

(CAD) participants with LDL cholesterol test per year, percentage of heart failure participants on an angiotensin converting enzyme inhibitor (ACEI), or percentage of CAD (or post myocardial infarction) participants on a beta blocker.

The preceding process measures have clear advantages over outcome measures because of the following reasons:

- Severity adjustment is not needed.
- Sample sizes can be much smaller than those used in outcome data.
- Physicians see process measures as reflecting activity within their more immediate control, whereas there are many other contributors to an unfavorable outcome.

Although measures of process or outcome can be organized from a pre and post study, customers are often interested in using a concurrent control group. This method needs to find a cohort of participants using the same condition—finding algorithms but not being managed by the call center of a DM company (i.e., DM is not available). The most difficult challenge associated with this method is assurance that the two cohorts are actually comparable. Adjustments needed to make them comparable usually include geography, demographics, age, gender, illness burden, provider networks, provider contracts, plan design, and rigor of other medical management programs.

Trusting that such adjustments can be made, the outcome metrics of greatest interest have been as follows:

- Financial:
  ○ Per member per month (PMPM) cost
  ○ Annual episode of care cost
- Utilization (the key savings drivers):
  ○ Acute hospital admits and days per 1,000
  ○ Emergency department (ED or ER) visits per 1,000

Return on Investment

Return on investment (ROI) has been the single largest controversy in the DM industry,

hence the current DMAA survey to obtain an updated consensus. The traditional method establishes baseline participant PMPM cost and projects the following year's expected cost using various trend assumptions such as the following:

- Nondisease trend
- Disease trend
- Overall trend

Such analysis typically excludes outliers, using definitions conventionally above 2 standard deviations beyond the mean. There are other total exclusions, such as acquired immune deficiency syndrome (AIDS), cancer, transplants, trauma, burns, and others. The actual observed following year's cost is then compared with cost that had been projected. Trusting that the observed cost is less than projected, the difference is gross savings, from which program administrative/overhead costs are subtracted to produce net savings. This benefit-to-cost ratio, or ROI, is generally positive and varies by condition.

There are certainly weaknesses in this method. For example, there is no agreement on which trend assumption to use. The largest objection is that this method is influenced by regression to the mean. Hence, there are several new methods in development at the time of publication that attempt to mitigate the error introduced by disease migration, which is the natural progression and regression of various disease care costs over time. Early indications suggest that these methods still usually produce a positive ROI, but less positive than the traditional method. Note that nearly all of the work to date on DM ROI has been done within the population-oriented opt-out engagement model. For those using the opt-in model, methodology revision may be needed.

CHALLENGES USING CURRENT ENGAGEMENT MODEL

Several valuable lessons have recently been learned after years of operating with the current opt out engagement model.

Privacy

The Health Insurance Portability and Accountability Act (HIPAA; see also Chapter 32) has influenced DM companies recently with regard to protected health information (PHI). This risk occurs in the setting of the opt-out engagement model. That is, on its surface, one at least can question HIPAA compliance when PHI is being exchanged around a patient who may not even be aware of his or her automatic enrollment in the DM program, and, if aware, might object. The wording of the final rule around PHI does appear to provide for the use of the opt-out model, but if there is any question, a health plan should rely on proper legal counsel, especially in light of some state-based differences.

Meaningful Engagement

Other recruitment and engagement approaches may be considered. Although the opt-in model has inherent weakness regarding recruitment success, perhaps the opt-out model is the other extreme. For example, opt-out participants might only be receiving but not reading their mail, may not be aware of their participation status, or may have other potential barriers to higher success for the DM program. The near future will likely see a new recruitment model that consolidates the participants into a subset who are confirmed to be engaged.

Physician Integration

As discussed earlier, most DM activity is member-centered. As physicians find out more about DM, there is understandable resentment based on the notion that "Treating diseases is why I went to medical school." Because of this, over the past few years there have been fledgling efforts to involve physicians. Physicians have become progressively more vocal about their concern over being bypassed, or worse, suggesting that the DM company interferes with the doctor–patient relationship. Ironically, it was originally the intent of most DM companies to "not bother" busy physicians.

Resolving such a dilemma may require a series of compromises. However, in the end it remains likely that physicians will not exert a direct role in DM as defined here, nor will they likely obtain a revenue stream from DM. The main reasons are as follows.

As the industry learned during the decade of integrated delivery system development (see Chapter 2), the owner of DM has to be the owner of full financial risk. Today, that owner is the health plan, the employer, CMS, or the state Medicaid department. The physician owns only the office visit component of treatment delivery on a fee-for-service basis, and in some cases, the professional component of an ED visit and/or hospitalization. Therefore, the success of DM, which reduces most of these categories of utilization, would reduce the physician's fee-for-service revenue. As noted in Chapters 1 and 2, attempts to administer full risk capitation to physician groups have receded, though not disappeared from the managed care landscape.

The typical practicing physician's office is not staffed to (and the physician is unaware of how to) provide the required vigilance over the patient at home between visits. Those who have attempted cannot operate at the affordability scale of the DM companies' large call centers. That is, for health plans to yield and create separate reimbursement schemes for individual medical offices to reach out to patients between visits would be grossly inefficient in an environment characterized by enormous pressure on health plans to reduce overhead.

HEALTH PLAN DECISION TO BUILD VERSUS BUY

The debate on having an in-house versus outsourced program is summarized in Table 10-2.

Recent developments find the outsourced mode under pressure. When DM began around a decade ago, health plans had little expertise for delivery. Today, after climbing

Table 10–2 Outsourcing Debate Summary

Build	Buy
Medical management is our core competency.	Lack of internal skills and time to manage rare or complex diseases.
Large organization with existing IT and managerial skills to perform DM.	Speed to market—would take more than 18 months to build.
Tried outsourcing—disagreed on metrics to determine risk-based fee refund.	Revised metrics and contract terms to place vendor at risk.
Tried outsourcing—vendor failed to affect claim cost; or advertised ROI is "too good to be true."	After years of reliable service, transitioned to FFS contract to reduce overhead—no need for risk contract.
Tried outsourcing—vendor used nonclinicians in call center.	Local region has too few RNs with right capabilities to staff call center.
Need control and flexibility.	Require vendor to test guidelines with providers.
Too few dollars at stake for prenatal care and asthma.	Use broad, multicondition DM program.
Tried outsourcing—our members with multiple comorbidities received multiple calls from DM, CM, and UM.	Use single vendor for horizontal contact center.
Integration costs are more than the savings from an outsourced vendor.	Require vendor to use plan identity during communications.

Source: Multiple health plan chief medical officer interviews conducted by author.

the learning curve, health plans are taking a hard look at vendor fees and new integration demands. The nursing shortage notwithstanding, there may be experiments with in-house programs in the near future.

OUTSOURCING CONTRACT FINANCIAL RISKS

The early years featured risk-sharing terms based on a variety of required milestones around service, satisfaction, and achievement of various process and outcome results, including ROI.

The ROI terms are the most rapidly evolving. For example, there is controversy on how to measure in years 3–5 of the program: to use original baseline or update the baseline year. Other controversies arise over what happens to people continuously enrolled over 3 to 5 years. If ROI results become more conservative over time, though proof of concept seems no longer in doubt, it seems logical to waive formal financial ROI risk and related reconciliation overhead. In fact, selected self-insured employers have begun to elect that option, usually in exchange for a reduced program fee and consideration to substitute nonfinancial items, such as adherence to evidence-based process of care measures.

LINKS TO OTHER HEALTH CARE PROGRAMS

In addition to current, conventional hand-offs to and from the health plan's other medical management programs as discussed in Chapters 9, 11, and 13 (*eg*, case management, nurse line, prenatal care, smoking cessation, behavioral health), new linkages are developing for the following types of programs.

Consumer-Directed Health Plans

Consumer-directed health plans (CDHPs) are discussed in both Chapters 1 and 20. Although now in their fourth to fifth year, we are beginning to see early CDHP lessons. For example, it is especially important to allow first-dollar coverage for preventive services and follow with careful measures of HEDIS and other metrics to ensure underutilization of necessary care is not occurring.

Recent experience suggests CDHP enrollees, at least those that enroll in a CDHP on a voluntary basis (*ie*, they can choose between a CDHP and a more traditional type of health plan such as a PPO or HMO), are healthier than non-CDHP enrollees are.* To attract individuals with chronic illnesses, attempts should be made to lower or waive copays for medicines (at least generics) and supplies used for these conditions. There is great interest in avoiding adverse selection, whereby the non-CDH products retain the majority of enrollees with chronic diseases. Perhaps arrangements for a larger risk-adjusted contribution to the Health Savings Account will be an option to accommodate those with chronic illnesses.

Participant Incentives

Several experiments are under way to motivate enrollees, such as immediate reward of cash or gift certificates for agreeing to enroll in DM or additional cash award for completion of a health risk assessment. Because these programs are relatively new, there are no data on overall or long-term effectiveness.

Physician Incentives

Recent initiatives around pay-for-performance (P4P) have linked metrics described earlier to

*Source: Author's analysis.

bonus calculations for physicians. Beyond such clinical measures, other P4P experiments are adding to the bonus calculation the agreement by the physician to adopt an electronic medical record (EMR) and participate in e-prescribing. The interfaces between EMR and DM are multiple, such as electronically checking lab test results, medication lists, and so forth. Performance-based compensation for both physicians and hospitals is discussed more fully in Chapter 8.

Personal Health Records, Regional Health Information Organizations, and Health Information Networks

The newest adjuncts to DM in technology are still to be proven. Personal health records (PHRs), which are populated primarily with data from health plans, may enable more real-time entry and retrieval of participants' health status information. Whether participants will agree on the data entry or physicians will retrieve is being tested. Similarly, regional health information organizations (RHIOs) and state- or federal-sponsored health information networks (HINs) have the promise in DM of assisting with the capture of longitudinal episodes of care (gathering data from all sites of care) as well as transmission of EMR content from provider to provider. As with PHR, both funding and adoption are being tested. PHRs, EMRs, RHIOs, and HINs are discussed in Chapter 17.

INTERNATIONAL DISEASE MANAGEMENT

United States–based DM companies have begun spreading to other countries. Most of the early adopters, primarily Germany followed by Japan, the United Kingdom, and Australia, have presented the implementation challenges of a socialized system. These environments feature largely unregulated physicians and, in some cases, far more use of complementary and alternative medicine modalities.

POTENTIAL FUTURE APPLICATIONS OF DISEASE MANAGEMENT

Disease management programs continue to be market-driven, and are rapidly evolving. Some older approaches have failed, while others evolve and new ones emerge. Integration of different types of programs and activities has also become more common.

New Approaches

An area for intervention that is currently addressed primarily only by prevention and wellness programs (see Chapter 14) is the premorbid population. In the conventional approach to DM, the occurrence of a discharge from the hospital for a myocardial infarction triggers enrollment in the coronary artery disease (CAD) DM program. Can a DM program move upstream and still make the DM program affordable?

Using the findings of asymptomatic hypertension and cholesterol elevation as examples, various experiments are under way to improve upon the older versions of step therapy and the conventional DM call center programs. This draws upon two observations from health care ecology:

- The most frequent health care professional interaction for a patient is with the pharmacist.
- Nonphysician practitioners appear to be "a better buy" for certain routine services (compared to physicians).

Anticipate new delivery models incorporating pharmacists, nurses and health educators, into the care of individuals whose cases are not extremely complex but who have major modifiable risk factors. This should allow tolerance for the multiyear window needed to find impact from risk-factor reduction.[6–8]

Failed Diseases and Failed Approaches

To use resources most effectively, each DM company or program must exert rigorous program evaluation techniques upon each disease in its roster. In the spirit of continuous improvement, the mix should change over time as the low-yield conditions are retired. In addition, greater sophistication will occur as to what interventions fade in effectiveness over time and under what circumstances interventions should be reduced or eliminated, not just changed.

Integration

Medical management strategists have recently proposed a single point of contact for the member, allowing convenient triage to specialized services. The member is to be treated to customized "push" messages at correct intervals. Lavish coaching and counsel that assist the member in navigating the health care system to achieve optimal value are required. This appears to be an outgrowth of the current leading approach to addressing patients with multiple chronic conditions in which a single point of contact is used for managing all conditions.

CONCLUSION

Disease management is a continually evolving but highly effective approach to managing both the cost and quality of care for those members with the most expensive chronic conditions. Predicated on preventing avoidable complications leading to expensive care in the hospital setting, DM is a necessary component of any high-performing care management program.

References

1. Landro L. Eliminating conflicts in medical treatment. *Wall Street Journal*. February 8, 2006:D5.
2. McGlynn EA, Asch SM, Adams J, *et al*. The quality of healthcare delivered to adults in the United States. *N Eng J Med*. Jun 26, 2003:348 (26), 2635–2645.
3. Osterberg L, Blaschke T. Adherence to medication. *N Eng J Med*. August 4, 2005:353(5), 487–497.
4. Disease Management Association of America. DMAA definition of disease management. Available at: http://www.dmaa.org/definition.html. Accessed September 18, 2006.
5. Fitzner K, Sidorov J, Fetterolf D, *et al*. Principles for assessing disease management outcomes. *Dis Management*. 2004:7(3), 191–201.
6. Christianson JB, Pietz L, Taylor R, Woolley A, Knutson D. Implementing programs for chronic illness management: The case of hypertension services. *J Qual Improvement*.1997: 23, 593–601.
7. DiTusa L, Luzier A, Brady G, Reinhardt M, Snyder B. A pharmacy-based approach to cholesterol management. *Am J Manage Care*. October 2001:7(10), 973–979.
8. Menerich J, Lousberg T, Brennan S, Calonge N. Optimizing treatment for dyslipidemia in patients with coronary artery disease in the managed-care environment (The Rocky Mountain Kaiser Permanente experience). *Am J Cardiol*. February 2000:85(3A), 36A–42A.

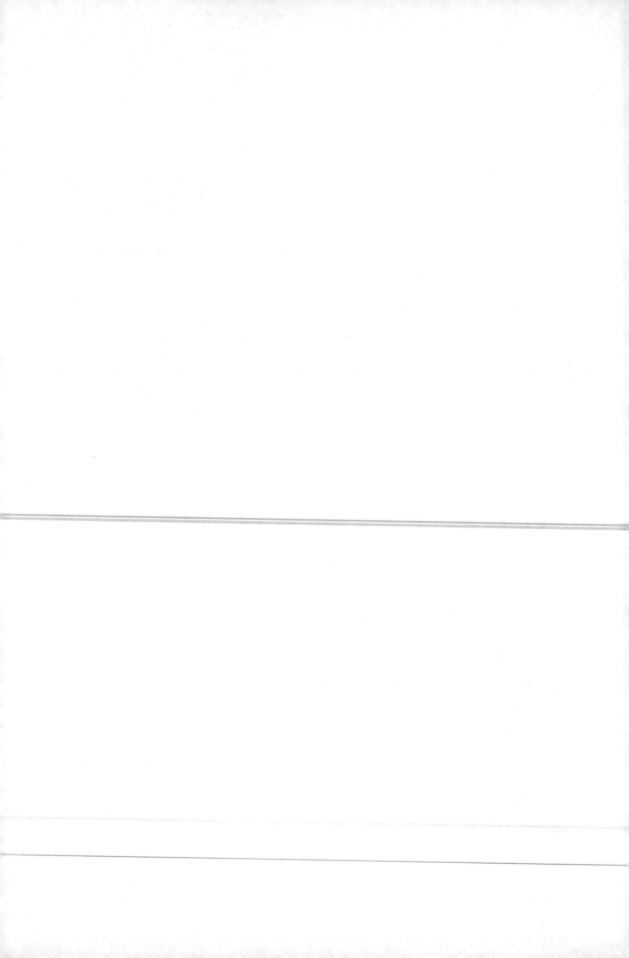

11

CASE MANAGEMENT

Patricia Metzger

Study Objectives

- Understand the basic objectives of case management.
- Understand the distinctions between case management and utilization management, including basic medical/surgical utilization management, as well as disease management.
- Understand the unique contributions case managers make to care and risk/cost management.
- Understand the types of patients who will benefit most from case management.
- Understand several of the indicators that identify a need for case management.
- Understand the basic activities of case management.

Discussion Topics

1. Discuss the purpose of case management.
2. Discuss the differences between case management and utilization management.
3. Discuss how case managers help manage care and risk.
4. Describe the type of patient who will benefit most from case management.
5. Identify several of the key indicators that signify a need for case management.
6. Discuss the role of the case manager, including a case manager's major activities.

CASE MANAGEMENT DEFINED

There are as many definitions of case management as there are theorists about the topic, but for purposes of this chapter we use the definition recognized by the Commission for Case Manager Certification: "Case management is a collaborative process that assesses, plans, implements, coordinates, monitors, and evaluates the options and services required to meet an individual's health needs, using communication and available resources to promote quality, cost effective outcomes."[1] The overall goal of case management is to manage individuals at their maximum level of comfort, functionality, and independence while at the lowest level of intensity of service. As Karen Zander and the staff at the Center for Case Management so aptly put it, case management must address a plan for the following:

- The day—What am I doing today to facilitate the care of this patient along the continuum?
- The stay (on a unit or in a facility)—Is this patient in the right level of care?
- The pay—How will the care be funded and/or who will pay?
- The way (the episode of care)—What are the plans for managing the ongoing care needs of this patient?[2]

No matter how case management is defined, the pivotal role that drives success is that of the case manager. The case manager is the individual who looks at the patient in a fully integrated way and is prepared to address the full spectrum of services required to meet the patient's needs both during the acute phase of illness as well as at discharge. Case managers serve as coordinators, intermediaries, and advocates in securing service, and as the hub of communication for the care team and the individuals who consider the fiscal reasonableness of what is being proposed to manage care.

Case managers work in a variety of venues on the provider side of the equation, including hospitals, clinics, home health agencies, and provider-sponsored disease management programs. They also work in the health plan environment, performing similar functions to the provider-based case managers, while managing the fiduciary obligations of the health plan. Regardless of the setting, the skill set and preparation of the case manager are critical to success. The case manager is consistently challenged with managing fiscal constraints with patient expectations in light of orders and expectations articulated by the care team. This requires a highly skilled individual, certainly not a job for the faint of heart.

In the book *Nursing Case Management: A Practical Guide to Success in Managed Care*,[3] Suzanne Powell lists the characteristics required of a case manager as follows:

- Commitment and desire to be a case manager
- Strong interpersonal communication skills
- Ability to prioritize
- Excellent assessment skills
- Clinical expertise and critical thinking
- Attention to detail
- Organizational skills
- Management skills
- Good follow-through
- Knowledge of community resources
- Respect and trust of peers
- Resourcefulness
- Team player
- Knowledge of legal and quality issues and standards of practice
- Self-esteem and confidence
- Competency and adaptability
- Self-directed and assertive
- Diplomacy
- And last but not least the ability to read poor penmanship

Many of the characteristics outlined by Powell can be captured under three major headings:

- Strong clinical expertise and critical thinking skills
- Strong interpersonal communication skills

- A collaborative relationship with physicians and colleagues, born out of mutual trust and respect

Strong Clinical Expertise and Critical Thinking Skills

The case manager must be the individual to whom the physician or the health plan is willing to entrust oversight of the care of the patient. Case managers have to be capable of discussing the clinical implications of a course of action with the care team in a way that demonstrates their awareness and understanding of the disease process as well as the financial implications of the choices. There is an implied obligation, when assuming the role of case manager, that the individual will maintain clinical expertise and consistently pair that clinical expertise with an understanding of the regulatory and health plan requirements. Additionally, the case manager must be able to prioritize the impact of clinical decisions and financial constraints to arrive at the most reasonable approach to care for the patient. Individuals who have not kept current in their field, or who have not had sufficient experience in caring for patients, may not be well-suited for the case manager's role.

Strong Communication Skills

The case manager has to be capable of communicating up to senior leadership in the organization as well as be able to communicate the plan, both clinical and financial, in such a way that it prompts the entire team to action. The patient interactions facing case managers each day, both from the provider and health plan perspective, vary from the most sophisticated discussions about care to the most basic explanations of the plans of care and the benefits and services available to the patient and family. The ability to listen and understand the other's point of view, be it clinical or personal, is critical to the success of the role. Those individu-

als who are not comfortable with active listening, negotiating, debate, disagreement, controversy, and money, and who cannot manage their own reactions when faced with difficult situations are not likely candidates for the job.

In addition, the case manager must be prepared to communicate information about patterns and trends of clinical and financial performance to leadership in the organization and to physicians. The ability to provide this type of feedback in a factual, nonthreatening way that prompts improvement in performance is an acquired skill. This is an important element in the case manager's job and requires practice and the willingness to take risks because communication of the information may not be well received. A key consideration when evaluating an individual for the case manager role is to determine whether the individual can adapt his or her communication style to the audience with whom the individual is interacting.

Collaborative Relationships

Although no one of these major elements is more important than another, absent good working relationships the case manager is likely to struggle in gaining the cooperation necessary to do the job. An individual who has a strong clinical background and good communication skills but who has not learned to work well with others will not be successful. It is imperative that individuals selected for the role have earned the respect of the medical staff and the care team. Change is difficult and clinical change that affects patients and practitioners carries a higher degree of difficulty. To have the kinds of discussions that often surround clinical practice change, the individual broaching the discussion must be one who has earned both personal and professional respect. If the physicians and other members of the team perceive that they are not being considered as integral to the case management process, the level of cooperation goes down incrementally.

A case manager is not born. Preparation of the individual to assume the role of case manager needs to be undertaken in a very systematic and structured way. The candidate must demonstrate a willingness to invest in the requisite training and education to prepare him- or herself for the job. Nothing replaces the benefits of real-time coaching and mentoring with case managers who are skilled and effective in their positions. The skill set needed by a strong case manager requires preparation from the clinical, financial, and regulatory environments, coupled with interpersonal and self-awareness mentoring.

WHY DO CASE MANAGEMENT?

Case management lives at the junction where, in an organization, margin meets mission. It is the balancing act of managing the patient and the resources one test/procedure/service at a time. Regardless of the venue in which a case manager functions, the crafting of the role and the development of a strong case management program are driven by patient need and organizational expectations. Each organization that puts a case management program into play needs to ask the following questions:

- What do I hope to achieve through this program?
- Am I developing this program in response to some organizational or financial pressure?
- Have all the key stakeholders agreed on the desired outcomes and the metrics that will be used to demonstrate success?
- Is the organization prepared to back the case management effort?
- Have the goals been clearly articulated throughout the organization so that the entire care team is engaged and pulling in the same direction?

Role definition for case management in an organization begins at the leadership level. Without clear definition about the role, case managers can be continuously stressed by the constant reprioritization of work with minimal chance of success. Absent the support of leadership and a strong foundation built on the commitment of time and resources to case management efforts, it is unlikely that any program will achieve the lofty goals most organizations articulate they wish to realize through case management.

THE PATIENT POPULATION

The top three issues confronting hospitals, reported in 2005 by the American College of Healthcare Executives (ACHE), include (1) financial challenges (67%); (2) personnel shortages (36%); and (3) care for the uninsured (35%).[4] As reimbursement strategies change, and the numbers of uninsured or underinsured patients increase, the debate becomes even more heated. According to the Kaiser Family Foundation and Health Research and Educational Trust, the proportion of Americans covered by employment-based health plans dropped to 60% in 2005, down from 69% in 2000.[5] Small businesses claim to no longer be able to afford the hefty health care premiums demanded by insurers. Families with annual incomes of $50,000 or more, who would previously not have considered going without health care insurance, find themselves in positions of having to make choices between health care premiums and day-to-day living with day-to-day living not strictly being defined as survival.

Families are choosing to avail themselves of more spendable income, rather than use that spendable income to "insure" the availability of resources to cover an unplanned illness or hospitalization. As the Generation Xers mature, their choices are based on lifestyle, and these individuals are willing to gamble that they will stay well rather than spend money for "insurance" they may never use. More than 45 million Americans were without health insurance for 12 months or more in 2004,[6] and perhaps twice that many were without health insurance for less than a full year. These figures do not even take into account the undocumented aliens who use hospital emergency rooms as their primary source of health care.

More than half of the care provided in the United States is covered by Medicare and Medicaid. By 2010, the number of Medicare beneficiaries is projected to hit 40.2 million, and by 2030 the number is projected to reach 71.5 million.[7] For the traditional Medicare and Medicaid patients, there have been no expectations that admissions be preauthorized and that ongoing patient stays be reviewed to determine medical necessity and clinical appropriateness. This responsibility to manage patients in these traditional plans has fallen to the providers, some of whom have managed the process effectively, but a far greater number of whom have not managed the process well. Medicare and Medicaid are the provider's risk to manage, and unfortunately these patient populations tend to fall to the bottom of the case manager's work list, given the demands, be they real or perceived, of the payer environment. With no external pressure to address the appropriateness of the admission or the medical necessity of the continued stay, these patients are often the last to be addressed and the least managed. In fact, if providers do not learn how to manage these populations successfully, their organizations are on the fast road to economic failure.

Based on some of the information outlined earlier, the question of whether all patients in the organization or health plan should be case managed comes into play. There are different schools of thought regarding the answer to this question, particularly in the provider arena. Some organizations, and typically most health plans, feel the need to manage only the high-cost, high-risk, complex patient populations. These populations include patients with diagnoses such as HIV/AIDS, cancer, transplant, burn, and spinal cord injuries, to name a few. Other organizations feel that each patient should at least be evaluated to determine if a case management need exists. Although some patients

may not appear to require case management intervention, early involvement by a case manager or a health plan's disease management system (see Chapter 10), particularly on some of the more chronic diagnoses, such as congestive heart failure (CHF), diabetes, and chronic obstructive pulmonary disease (COPD), can oftentimes limit the frequency with which a patient is hospitalized. Still others believe that a case manager should be assigned to each patient in the inpatient environment. There is no one correct answer to the question and each organization must decide, based on needs and strategy and local market, what population of patients it will choose to have managed. Regardless of the decision made, investment in a case management program must produce a return on the investment.

RESOURCES AT A PREMIUM

Organizational development literature is clear that the more task oriented and functionally siloed an organization becomes, the less efficient and effective it becomes because the employees lose sight of the integration points that allow processes to flow smoothly.

According to the U.S. Department of Labor and Statistics, more than 1 million nurses will be needed to meet the growing demands for care by the year 2012.[8] Unfilled positions in nursing, pharmacy, lab, and radiology all translate into potential delays in care. Surgeries will be postponed, capacities reduced, and the efforts of trying to contain cost and promote efficiency will seem impossible. All of the key areas affected by the labor shortage are the areas on which case management relies to help facilitate care and movement of patients through the system.

As staff becomes scarcer and increasingly more stressed with managing the workload of day-to-day expectations for a patient population, it has become apparent that they are focused primarily on their individual work and spend less time looking at the patient from a holistic point of view. The providers and health plans continue to vie for the same pool of dollars, each convinced that it has done all it can to manage the expenditures and improve its performance, while looking only at the point of convergence, the patient. Within the provider and health plan framework, each department or unit works under the same set of assumptions: They have managed their resources effectively, they are working as hard as they can, and they are unique in meeting the needs of the patients they serve.

In the acute-care setting, for example, it is not uncommon to find radiology special procedures closing at 3:00 pm each afternoon, with no availability of weekend hours because of staffing constraints, be they budgetary or the availability of personnel. The impact that the closure has on facilitating care is dramatic. The patient is delayed in getting the testing completed by at least 1 day. Results are returned within 24 hours, adding at least another day to the length of stay. The physician might have already rounded by the time the results are available on the chart, and because nurse staffing is at a premium, the nurse might be too busy to notify the physician that the results are available, adding another 24 hours to the delay in care.

In the health plan environment, the scarcity of personnel has limited the hours of operation and the availability of personnel to interact with providers and patients. Health plans have moved to automated systems and Internet access to answer questions about benefits, coverage, and authorization. Faced with financial constraints on administrative costs, some health plans that previously had staff available at provider sites to interact with patients, families, and provider staff are moving to more telephonic interaction. For the courageous, navigating the process of "press 1 for . . . ," "press 2 for . . .," or being on terminal "hold" can be an exercise in endurance.

It is about cost, resource utilization, and it is about survival of the fittest, but most of all it's about the patient. With that in mind, the remainder of this chapter addresses how case management can positively or negatively affect the patient experience.

ACUTE CARE

Case management in acute care refers to the management of cases that enter the health care system under acute conditions, and then progress through treatment and disposition. This section will describe the basic elements of such care.

Points of Entry

Case management begins at the point of entry to an acute care facility, and there are multiple points of entry. Each point of entry needs to have processes in place that support managing and facilitating care. Health plans have forced providers to evaluate patient information and clinical presentation, couple that with available and authorized resources, and do this prior to rendering care. Health plans have limited the indiscriminate use of precious health care resources and prompted a more clinically systematic approach to decision making.[9]

For most hospitals, one of the primary points of entry is the emergency department (ED). As more and more of the patient population falls into the category of under- or uninsured and increasingly use the ED as the primary means of securing care, managing this access point will become critical to survival. Overlay this challenge with compliance issues specific to rules and regulations under the Emergency Medical Treatment and Active Labor Act of 1986 (EMTALA; see also Chapter 9),[10] and the need for case management in this area becomes critical. Proactive organizations will put aggressive triage processes in place and will establish their own "clinic-like" environments to which the nonacutely ill patient can be referred for follow-up and potential enrollment in an outpatient case management program for the chronically ill to minimize the use of the ED as a primary care clinic.

Once the patient has been triaged in the ED and the determination is made that some level of hospital care is warranted, the critical first step is determining what level of care best suits the patient's needs. A number of clinical criteria sets can be used in helping to make this determination. The criteria are clinically driven, based on physiologic condition, and also provide guidance about the most appropriate level of care, based on the patient's clinical presentation (*ie,* ICU, telemetry, observation status).

Some facilities have chosen to place case management staff in the ED to assist in the application of criteria and the screening of patients for referral to the clinic setting. Others have chosen to manage this telephonically. Still another option is to have the criteria sets available for the ED physicians and nursing staff and to train the ED team to use the criteria when making a determination about the appropriate level of care. In a few instances, health plans have contracted with specialty management companies (see Chapter 5) that focus on ED care to provide for evaluation and disposition of the plan's members that present to the ED and may require admission. Regardless of how the initial screening is accomplished, it is essential that patients presenting to the ED be evaluated to determine the need for services and the level of care in which those services can best be provided.

A good screening process through the admissions area on elective and unscheduled admissions is also essential. This screening process should include both clinical and financial screening that allows the organization to communicate and collaborate with the health plan, the patient, and the physician to obtain the appropriate authorizations for admission or for an alternate care delivery setting; in other words, effective application of a criteria set that drives the placement of the patient in the most clinically appropriate setting. If the services are not a covered benefit, or the services need to be provided in a setting other than the acute care hospital setting, this determination can be made in advance and discussed with the patient prior to the initiation of service. The patient may choose to opt out of receiving the service, or may choose to pay privately for the services to be rendered. The proactive screening process limits the exposure of both the provider and the health plan in addressing both clinical and financial risk.

The tool that is used to initiate this discussion is called an Advance Beneficiary Notice (ABN). It is used by hospitals, many health plans, as well as federally funded programs to inform patients when services may not be covered. The ABN model provided by Medicare is the one typically used and is available as a free download.[11]

Admission and Treatment

Once the patient is admitted, success from both the health plan and provider perspectives begins with optimal discharge planning. A strong working relationship needs to exist among the provider and health plan case management teams. If both provider and health plan case managers understand the rules of engagement, care facilitation proceeds like a well-oiled machine.

Managing resource utilization during the treatment phase of care is critical in controlling costs for both health plan and provider. Unfortunately, perhaps this more than any another aspect of the case manager's role creates the most controversy because it tries to balance the conflicting interests of health care technology, patient and family expectations, physician practice patterns, and reimbursement. The ability to function as both a patient advocate and a fiduciary agent in managing the available resources is challenging and a critical competency for the case manager. Case managers from both the health plan and provider perspectives are uniquely positioned to balance sound clinical decision making with available dollars and resources to achieve the best possible clinical outcomes. Decisions about the course of hospitalization, the course of treatment, the tests and services being provided, and the post acute services that will be required must all be balanced in relationship to the primary admitting diagnosis and the secondary diagnoses related to the primary diagnosis. Too often, the case manager sees secondary workups not related to the primary diagnosis being done for convenience or at patient request. This drives up cost, and in the case of reimbursement under diagnosis-related groups (DRGs; see Chapter 7) yields no additional reimbursement. This requires increased surveillance and vigilance on the part of the case manager and an increased level of understanding by the members of the health care team.

The foundation to manage resource utilization is the application of clinical criteria to determine that the services and treatments that are ordered match the clinical needs of the patient. Early identification of whether the patient has responded more rapidly to treatment or has deteriorated and requires additional intervention is fundamental to effective resource utilization. It is the case manager working in concert with the clinical care team who can identify and respond to clinical condition changes and manage resource utilization effectively. By developing good, strong relationships with the clinical team, and in particular the physicians, the case managers, both from the health plan and provider sides, can establish a climate where patient care needs are center point and where medical necessity and clinical determinations are evaluated using evidence-based leading practice without threat to clinical autonomy. This, however, requires vigilance and engagement of the entire care team.

DRG Payment is the Provider's Risk to Manage

In the case of acute care delivered to the Medicare and Medicaid populations and the DRG-based commercial health plans, resource utilization is the provider case manager's risk to manage. For the DRG-based

health plans, once the initial authorization is given for treatment and the patient is placed in the inpatient setting, any resource consumption is rolled into the DRG reimbursement. Provider case managers need to be very familiar with the insurance rules and payment methodologies for each of their health plans to manage resource consumption most effectively. Based on the reimbursement methodology under the DRG payment system, there is no additional reimbursement for tests and procedures done for a patient that are not related to the primary diagnosis.

In the case of the unfunded patient population, the provider case manager is faced with an even greater challenge in managing resource utilization. Unfunded patients typically present with multiple comorbidities, usually as a result of not having seen a health care provider in a long period of time, not having resources to secure follow-up care, and/or not having good support systems to help with the overall plan of care. The tendency of health care providers has historically been to "tune up everything while we have the patient here," recognizing it is unlikely that the patient will seek follow-up care for issues that are more appropriately managed in the outpatient setting.

The environment in which we live is very litigious. Physicians, in particular, are concerned about their liability should a patient leave the hospital, experience an unplanned complication, and attribute the complication to the physician's "failure to provide me with the care I needed." Case managers recognize that the standard of care must be consistent across all health plan classes. It is important that the case manager be well-versed in leading practice treatment plans when managing this patient population to ensure comprehensive, cost-effective treatment, consistent with standards of care.

It is also imperative that the case manager be familiar with community resources to which these patients can be referred for follow-up care, medication, and post acute services. There may be the case of an un-funded patient who is homeless. Discharge back to the street may be the only plan with which this patient is willing to cooperate. It is the case manager's responsibility to ensure that the discharge plan is the safest possible plan given the circumstances. Involvement of the financial team in trying to secure cover-age alternatives for this patient population is an intrinsic part of the case manager's job.

Discharge planning begins at the time of, or even prior to, admission. Each patient needs to have a clearly identified discharge date in mind. Determination of the date be-gins by identifying the admission diagnosis or "working DRG." The anticipated discharge date needs to be broadcast to all members of the care team, and each care team member should be prepared to manage his or her workflow and processes with the end game in mind. Case management cannot be the only role that is involved in working toward the anticipated discharge date.

Considerations for the patient and the care team as discharge planning begins include such factors as follow:

- **Copayment:** This is an established fee for which the patient/member is respon-sible based on the terms of the plan the patient/member purchased.
- **Deductible:** This is a dollar amount that the patient/member must pay on an an-nual basis for services rendered.
- **In-network offerings:** These are pro-viders, services, facilities, agencies that have accepted a health plan's predeter-mined financial arrangement and from whom the patient/member can select services without financial penalty.
- **Covered benefits:** This is the array of health care services that are paid for fully or partially by the health plan.
- **Secondary coverage:** This is additional health care insurance coverage in addi-tion to the primary insurance coverage carried by the patient/member, for which the patient/member has likely paid an

additional premium, and which may af-ford the patient/member a broader range of services.
- **Patient choice:** This is a requirement, of Medicare in particular, that necessitates providers offer a patient the choice of ser-vice providers within the limitations of their benefit plan and insurance coverage.
- **Referral:** This may be required by some health plans for the patient to receive services from other providers.

Discharge planning requires the orchestra-tion of services and benefits and coupling that with a reality-based clinical and financial plan will allow the patient to receive maxi-mum benefit from the services provided. Discharge planning by its very nature must be multifaceted, and the case manager can-not simply have one plan in mind. There must be a Plan 1 and a Plan 2 in play at all times. Plan 1 is likely to be the preferred op-tion of the patient and family, but Plan 2 is the fallback plan if one or more factors change during the course of the stay. Health plans and providers, when presented with sound clinical information and an array of al-ternatives, are oftentimes very willing to ne-gotiate rates or alternatives for care if it is in the best interests of the patient and fiscally more cost-effective. Each day the case man-ager needs to challenge patient progress by asking four key questions:

1. Is this patient in the correct level of care?
2. If not, what am I doing about it?
3. What is it about this patient's condition today that is preventing him or her from being discharged?
4. What am I doing about it?

Provider and health plan case managers, when working with their patients, are fitting together the pieces of a very complex, not easily navigated health care puzzle. Each case manager assesses from his or her van-tage point the following:

- The patient's and or family's level of un-derstanding of the illness

- The readiness of all involved to participate in the plan of care
- The financial resources available to the patient to manage the disease process
- The support resources available to manage the emotional response to the disease process
- The educational needs of the patient in managing the disease process

Patient Family Understanding

Typically, patients and families who are faced with a newly diagnosed injury or illness necessitating case management intervention are angry, confused, unable to make timely decisions, and unable to deal with the realities of life-altering, role-changing experiences. They are overwhelmed and looking for guidance and direction. A case manager attuned to the life-changing effects a diagnosis can have on an entire family can serve as the conduit to good, sound decision making about choices and alternatives. There will be times when the case manager serves as the intermediary among family members or among family members and physicians. There may be times when the case manager has to challenge the values and culture of a family to discuss life-altering decisions, and this is never easy. There may be times when the case manager is the sole support for the patient and family in a sea of confusion. The readiness of the case manager in being prepared to fill these multiple roles is testimony to the skill set required to function as a case manager.

Readiness to Participate

Depending on the level of understanding of both patient and family and the group dynamics, the case manager must evaluate the readiness of the family to participate in decision making about the plan of care. Obviously, there are legal considerations about who may or may not speak on behalf of the patient, if the patient is unable to speak for himself or herself. The next of kin may or may not be available or able to speak on the patient's behalf. In large families, consensus is not always easily reached. The presence of a medical power of attorney is certainly a consideration. The case manager must be familiar with the law and capable of managing conflict when these circumstances arise.

As one might expect, in cases where the patient and family have no financial resources to manage follow-up care, the readiness to participate in the discharge planning process becomes stalled. Families feel that their loved ones have found a safe place in which to receive care and are unwilling and sometimes unable to manage the implications for follow-up care. It is not uncommon to hear patients and family members say that their loved one will remain in the acute care setting until the family member has reached his or her functional status prior to hospitalization. Case managers need to recognize the stall tactics employed by families and significant others and, while being sensitive to patient/family need, progress confidently down the discharge planning path.

Although not generally a health plan issue, for hospitals in some locations in the country, the number of undocumented aliens that reside in local communities further compounds the readiness of families to participate. There is a tremendous fear that family members will be reported to authorities and deported. Many families "disappear" when faced with imminent discharge plans. There are limitations to what a case manager can do without consent from the family/significant other to proceed. Knowing the legal means available to a case manager to pursue placement, guardianship, and even deportation is an essential element of the case management tool kit.

Financial Resources

From the health plan perspective, case management is more frequently than not done telephonically. As discussed in Chapter 10, some health plans contract with disease management companies to provide case management support to a specific patient population, such as the cardiac disease or oncology patient population. This is particularly effective when dealing with issues of prevention and screening, emotional support, or for follow-up to make certain that the required services are being provided as planned. Telephonic intervention, however, requires a highly skilled, highly sensitive individual who is capable of picking up the subtleties or silences in a conversation that indicate what is really occurring with the patient/member.

The telephonic interventions, even while the patient is in the inpatient environment, will include an assessment of the patient's physical and emotional state, an understanding of the injury or illness, and the confirmation that the course of treatment being provided is consistent with industry standards. For patients admitted to the hospital, based on the information submitted by the patient and/or provider, ongoing care and continued hospitalization will be approved or denied. Provider case managers will often enlist the help of the health plan case managers when addressing discharge plans, and in particular, when difficult situations arise that require consensus building on the part of the care team, patient, family, and health plan.

As discussed in Chapter 9, there are also times when a health plan may elect to bring a case manager on site to the hospital. This may be driven by patient volume, patient complexity, patient noncompliance with the plan and goals of treatment, or concerns on the part of the plan that the care being provided is inconsistent with industry standards. Regardless of the reason, the provider should view this individual as another set of eyes and ears in helping to make the best decisions about the care needs of the patient.

Support Resources and Education

Case managers have a wide variety of resources at their disposal to assist patients and families in coping with the adaptation to illness. Social workers are a vital resource in helping families and patients come to terms with a new diagnosis, or a change in body image, or a terminal diagnosis. Social workers are trained to know the resources available in the community to provide assistance at the level required by the patient and family. Case managers also need to be comfortable in recognizing the need for spiritual support that can be provided through chaplaincy services or local churches.

Health plans often contract with outside agencies to provide support to patients and families with specific diagnoses through specialty management programs (*eg,* oncology or neonatology) or disease management companies (*eg,* COPD or CHF). These programs include not only an ongoing evaluation of the clinical status of the patient but educational materials geared to the specific disease processes and educational readiness level of the patient. Federally funded programs have seen the merit in this type of support and have developed demonstration projects that measure outcomes, both clinical and financial, for patients with specific diseases, such as CHF and diabetes.

Alternative Levels of Care

This chapter has addressed the discharge planning initiatives that must begin at the time of admission to the hospital. Now it is important to discuss how essential it is for the health plan and provider case managers to plan the transition of the patient from the inpatient setting to an alternative level of care.

The first step in transition planning is a solid familiarity with the criteria that drive the selection of post acute services that may be required at the time of discharge. The most desirable setting from the case management vantage point for any patient is a safe transition home. Support services can be provided by home health to the patient upon discharge and can generally be negotiated between the health plan and provider case managers if home care coverage is included in the benefit menu. For federally funded programs, the services that are financially covered for home care are fairly prescriptive. The range of services in the home can include, but is not limited to, the following:

Skilled nursing: These services include care and evaluation by a registered nurse. Frequency of skilled visits is governed by patient need, but generally do not exceed three visits per week.

Rehabilitation services: These services include physical, occupational, and speech therapy. Frequency of these visits is governed by patient need and patient progress toward functional status improvement.

Oxygen support: This service is driven by patient need and is generally provided when the patient's O_2 saturations are less than 85%.

Ventilator support: This service is a very expensive service in the home but can still prove to be more cost-effective than managing the patient in an inpatient setting. Some reimbursement is available to manage the ventilator-dependent patient in the home, but there must also be strong support systems to provide 24-hour per day care.

Wound care: These services can range from providing dressing changes to managing wound vacs.

Homemaker services: These services can be provided in the home, but they are generally an out-of-pocket expense for the patient and family.

Dialysis: This service can be made available in the home and can range from peritoneal dialysis to hemodialysis.

Home infusion: This service is available in the home, but generally is limited to one to two visits per day, and the patient and family must be able to demonstrate some proficiency in self-administration if the frequency is greater than one to two times per day.

No matter what services are provided, the case manager needs to determine that support is available to assist the patient during the time that services are not being provided. If the support structure is not present, discharge to home is not likely to be the best alternative.

Other alternative levels of care include:

Assisted living: This is the setting that most closely mirrors the home environment. It combines housing, supportive services, personalized assistance, and health care. The assisted living environment allows residents to function fairly independently, but provides some level of meal service and some general supervision and assistance with medication administration. The cost for assisted living is absorbed totally by the resident and/or family.

Personal care home: This setting offers meals, accommodation, laundry service, and assistance and/or supervision with personal care. These types of homes are privately owned and independently operated. The minimum requirements for this type of home includes 24-hour supervision; laundry; supervision with grooming, bathing, dressing, and nail care; transportation arrangements; safeguarding medications; and home-based social and recreational activities. The cost of this type of setting can be paid by the resident and/or family or can be subsidized by some federally funded programs.

Custodial care: This setting provides nonmedical care to help individuals with activities of daily living, preparation of special diets, and self-administration of medication, not requiring the constant attention of medical personnel. Most public long-term care programs such as Medicaid will cover the cost of custodial care as long as it is provided within a nursing facility. Custodial care at home can be covered by long-term care insurance but will not be covered by Medicaid.

Skilled nursing care: This type of care is given when the patient needs the services of skilled professionals such as nurses and therapies to manage, observe, and evaluate the care being provided to determine the patient's response. It is provided in the inpatient setting to improve the condition of the patient or prevent the condition from worsening. The costs for these services are covered by most health plans, including Medicare and Medicaid.

Inpatient rehabilitation care: This type of care is provided to coordinate and integrate medical and rehabilitation services 24 hours per day and endorses the active participation and choice of patients. The typical patient populations admitted to inpatient rehabilitation care include but are not limited to cases such as stroke, spinal cord injury, amputation, major trauma, brain injury, polyarthritis, and neurological disorders. Patients must be able to tolerate approximately 3 hours of active therapy and must demonstrate the potential to improve their overall ability to function. The costs for these services are covered by most health plans, including Medicare and Medicaid.

Long-term acute care: The level of care expected in this setting is consistent with that of short-term acute care but for patients who require a longer length of stay than that typically experienced in the short-term acute care setting. The average expected length of stay is 25 days or more for acutely ill/medically complex patients. The long-term acute setting may either be free-standing or a "hospital within a hospital." This level of service is covered by most health plans, including Medicare, but is not covered under most traditional Medicaid plans.

Home health care: This level of care covers a broad range of services, including high-tech services such as IV infusion, home uterine monitoring, ventilator management, chemotherapy, skilled professional (nursing and therapies) and paraprofessional services (home health aides, personal care assistants), durable medical equipment (artificial limbs, orthotics, beds, canes, wheelchairs, oxygen), and custodial care provided and delivered in the home. For these services to be covered, they must be ordered by a physician, medically necessary, and intended to improve the health condition. Home health visits are usually provided on a per-visit rather than an hourly basis. The cost of these services is generally covered by most insurance plans (based on the benefit package selected by the employer or member), including Medicare and Medicaid.

Understanding the payment mechanisms, availability of coverage, and expenditures that may be required of the patient and family are key considerations in determining where best to place the patient to meet the patient's needs. For example, the long-term acute care setting utilizes the same benefit period bank of days for Medicare patients as the short-term acute hospital. In each benefit period, the Medicare recipient has 90 days. To renew a benefit period the Medicare recipient must not have received any type of skilled services for a period of 60 days. If the Medicare recipient has been in the short-term acute care setting for 10 days, transitioned to a long-term acute care setting for 30 days, and is then discharged from long-term acute care, the Medicare recipient has only 50 remaining days in the benefit period. Should the patient require hospitalization again, prior to 60 days without receiving any skilled services have passed, the patient will have only 50 days of hospitalization available. It is essential that the case manager and the care team understand the levels of care and the services provided at each level when working to identify how best to transition the patient.

END OF LIFE

Managing care that involves decisions about end of life is among the most challenging for case managers. Most Americans (63%) die in hospitals and another 17% die in institutional settings.[12] Expenditures at the end of life seem disproportionately large. Payments for dying patients increase exponentially as death approaches, and payments during the last month of life constitute 40% of the payments during the last year of life.[13] Hospice care is now used by about 50% of dying Medicare cancer patients and 19% of dying Medicare patients overall.[14]

Basic Challenges in End of Life Care

Physicians often find discussions about end of life uncomfortable, even though there is general recognition of the importance of addressing this topic.[15] Patients and families want to know how long a person can be expected to live. They expect candid discussion about options and want to be offered alternatives that will allow the family members dignity and respect, with sensitivity to culture and faith.

Conflict for case managers arises when dealing with end-of-life issues because of the highly volatile, complex dynamics of the working environment and the subjectivity that is inherent in managing care and making decisions that affect patient outcomes and organizational performance around this issue. Failure to address the conflict will delay decision making and progress toward the goal.

The challenge of bringing together the wants and needs of patients, families, physicians, and the organization in which the case manager works defines the role of the case manager. The wants and desires of the patient and family may be diametrically opposed to the clinical and financial health of the organization. The ability of the case manager to remain objective and facilitate discussion and decision making around highly emotionally charged issues is tantamount to realizing the best possible outcomes for all concerned. Ineffectively managed conflict will generate dysfunctional behaviors among all involved, and the interested parties will retreat into narrowly marked "safety zones" that allow for minimal negotiation and almost no conflict resolution.

The case manager, in approaching the highly charged discussions around end of life, needs to enter into the discussion with a clearly defined game plan and approach to resolution. The case manager needs to have determined whether there is any room for compromise, or whether consensus has to be reached before all parties involved can proceed. There are distinct differences between the two situations, and it is critical for the case manager to bring the end-of-life discussions to a beneficial and accepted outcome for all concerned.

Palliative Care and Hospice Care

Palliative care and *hospice care* are terms that are sometimes used interchangeably, but in fact mean different things. Both palliative care and hospice care are geared to meeting not only the needs of the patient but also the psychosocial needs of the family and significant others.

Palliative care is comfort care and is primarily directed at providing relief to a terminally ill person through symptom management and pain management. The goal is not to cure but to provide comfort and maintain the highest quality of life for as long as life remains. Well-rounded palliative care programs address mental health and spiritual needs. It is well-suited to a team model that supports the whole person.

Patients who enter palliative care programs are not necessarily facing imminent end-of-life decisions. They may have chronic disease, which may be incapacitating, and participation in palliative care enables these patients to maintain an independence and increased quality of life through symptom management and pain control. Palliative care services are not a distinct benefit election, may not be a covered benefit in health plans, and Medicare and Medicaid do not provide reimbursement for palliative care services in the ambulatory setting. However, a patient can receive palliative care services, although not as a distinct benefit, while inpatient if the patient meets criteria for acute care hospitalization.

Hospice care is a distinct benefit election. Hospice focuses on relieving symptoms and supporting patients with a life expectancy of months, not years. It emphasizes caring not curing, and in most cases hospice care is provided in the home. Patients can receive inpatient hospice care services for short periods of time while symptom control is being achieved or while the patient is actively dying. Hospice is paid for by most private insurers and is a distinct benefit election of Medicare and Medicaid.

It is important that a case manager be able to recognize the distinction of the two services to support patients and families in realizing the maximum level of support available to them when faced with incapacitating illness and pain.

CATASTROPHIC CASES

One of the most challenging situations for any case manager is the management of the catastrophic case. Generally, this type of case presents as the result of some unexpected, personally devastating illness or injury and neither the patient or the family is prepared for the decisions that must be made regarding care, and aftercare should the patient survive. The types of cases referred to here might include the traumatic burn victim, the patient suddenly devastated by a fall or accident who is now a paraplegic or quadriplegic, or the traumatic brain injury patient. Hospitalizations for these types of patients are not measured in days, but rather in weeks or months. Rapidly changing clinical conditions can make anticipatory planning the exception rather than the norm. It takes a highly skilled, clinically solid case manager who understands the pathophysiology of the illness to be able to translate for family and patient alike what to expect and what alternative plans for care might be. The challenges are equally difficult from both the health plan and provider perspectives.

The provider case manager will focus on managing the immediate clinical issues but must be working with the patient and family to make determinations about potential discharge to alternative levels of care. Depending on the nature of the case, and the resources available beyond the acute care setting, this discharge planning process can move smoothly or become intricately complicated. Post acute care decisions and choices will be driven by multiple factors, including but not limited to coverage issues, family financial resources, family dynamics, availability of appropriate alternative levels of care, psychological stresses on the patient and family, and more.

PATHWAYS AND PROTOCOLS

The overall goal for any case manager is to help the patient achieve optimal recovery in the least amount of time while making effective use of clinical resources. The best way to achieve this goal is to utilize a pathway that helps all the members of the team track progress toward the goal. Pathways have been called a variety of names: clinical pathway, protocol, guideline, clinical algorithm, or progress map. Regardless of the name used, pathways help reduce the variation in care, are based on evidence-based medicine to the extent possible, and provide for an efficient use of clinical resources. Not all diagnoses or patients lend themselves to the use of pathways, though, nor will all patients, because of comorbid conditions, be able to be placed on pathways. Where reasonable and appropriate, pathways serve as an excellent guide to cue the care team regarding all aspects of care.

Health plan case managers have been utilizing guidelines for years, when evaluating the appropriateness of the services being rendered to the member population. The most commonly used set of guidelines by health plans is the *Milliman Care Guidelines*,* though others are also used. These are a set of optimal recovery guidelines that demonstrate leading clinical practice benchmarks

---

*Available at http://www.milliman.com.

for treating common conditions. They outline the activities that the case manager should expect to occur during the course of hospitalization and provide an anticipated length of stay for each diagnosis. The intent of these guidelines is not to limit care but rather to minimize waste and inefficiency.

Pathways are an excellent way of achieving the measurable goals of the Institute for Healthcare Improvement (IHI) to "improve the lives of patients, reduce variation and ensure patient safety with no needless deaths."[16] Whether provider or health plan based,* case managers must be very much in tune with the clinical care needs of the patients they serve and work toward the goals so clearly articulated by IHI. Case managers must be able to identify clearly those five to six key elements in the plan of care that, if addressed, will expedite progress of the patient toward the desired outcome, reduce variation, and work with the care team to ensure that those elements are addressed.

Pathway development from the provider perspective can be challenging. The resistance to pathways as "cookbook medicine" has decreased somewhat over the years, but physician individuality and personal preference still weigh in heavily on the ability to use pathways in an organization. Some organizations have been successful at mandating use and have demonstrated both positive clinical and financial outcomes. Other organizations struggle with their cultures and the readiness of the physicians to embrace some form of "standardization." If providers are to maintain viability and achieve good clinical outcomes, they need to be willing to invest the time and risk into the development and implementation of evidence-based pathways that help drive consistency in care.

HOSPITALISTS AND INTENSIVISTS

Twenty years ago 40% to 50% of a primary care physician's time was spent in the hospi-tal seeing 10 to 12 patients, but now only 10% of a typical primary care physician's time is spent in the hospital.[17] Thirty years ago the average length of stay for hospitalized patients was 10 to 12 days; now under managed care, average length of stay has fallen to 3.7 days for non-Medicare and 5.7 for managed Medicare patients.[18] Patients are sicker now when they are admitted than they once were and are now sicker when discharged as well.

As discussed in Chapter 9, the use of hospitalists is on the rise. Perhaps the most important of the many forces promoting the hospitalist movement is the assumption that inpatient care provided by a small, select group of physicians who practice in the hospital most of the time and are available throughout their shifts is less costly, of higher quality, and less variable than the care provided by many primary care physicians who see their patients only briefly once a day. Data has shown that with the implementation of a hospitalist program an organization can expect (1) a 10% to 25% decrease in the length of a hospital stay; (2) no measurable decrease (and possible improvements) in clinical outcomes such as mortality and readmission rates; and (3) no measurable decrease in patient satisfaction.[19]

Hospitalists, working closely with case managers, will continue to have a profound impact on resource utilization and patient transition to the appropriate level of care. Hospitalists are becoming increasingly more involved in decision making about the use of the correct level of care at the time a patient presents in the emergency department. They will make determinations about the use of observation status, intensive care units (ICUs), or telemetry. Because of the accessibility of a hospitalist to the case manager, more timely decision making occurs, test results are validated and acted upon with increased timeliness, and discharge planning discussions occur on a daily basis when the hospitalist and case manager round on the patients under the care of the hospitalist.

*Available at http://www.milliman.com.

Hospitals are beginning to see movement similar to the hospitalist movement in the intensivist model used to manage the care of the critically ill patients usually in an intensive care unit. Similar in philosophy to the hospitalist model, the intensivist model supports the assumption that care of critically ill patients provided by a small, select group of physicians whose practice focuses on critical care medicine and who are available throughout their shifts is less costly, of higher quality, and less variable than the care provided by many physicians who see their patients only briefly once a day. The majority of studies report significant reductions in both costs and in hospital mortality (ranging from 2–17%) when a patient is managed by a hospitalist or an intensivist.[20,21] Intensive care provided by critical care specialists also results in more patients appropriately discharged from the ICU to other hospital wards in fewer days.

The intensivist appears to use resources in the ICU more judiciously, admit fewer patients who are marginally critically ill, use fewer resources for nonsurvivors and more for survivors, and tend to discharge more expediently patients who are no longer critically ill. These efforts, coupled with those of the case manager, available to help the intensivist find the appropriate resources for patient transition to the next level of care or offer support during end-of-life decision making, all serve to demonstrate both the desired clinical and financial outcomes being pursued by organizations today.

COMMUNITY CASE MANAGEMENT

As patients are discharged from the acute care setting, the ability to provide a mechanism for follow-up, particularly for those patients with chronic disease, is an important element in managing the overall care of the patient. The purpose of a community case management program is to assist patients in gaining access to medical, social, financial, educational, and other services to meet the basic needs of living day to day in the community. The services generally consist of five core functions:

- A community-based comprehensive assessment
- Individualized care planning with the patient
- Linkage to and coordination of services in the community
- Ensuring service accountability
- Providing for continued support and advocacy

The goal of a community case management program is to restore each patient's capacity to live independently and achieve a satisfying quality of life while managing a chronic problem. The acute care case managers need to research early and be very familiar with the services offered through community case management programs to enable their patients the best chance of success as they return to the home community environment.

LEGAL ISSUES

A significant aspect of U.S. society is that we are litigious, at least when compared to most other nations. When individuals feel that their rights have been violated, or in some cases if an outcome is not the desired one, litigation ensues. Because case managers work with patients whose illnesses generally have a greater than normal level of complexity, and because the case managers work for organizations, both health plans and providers that are viewed as having "deep pockets," not only will the organization be involved in litigation, but the case manager may be involved as well. With that in mind, it is essential that the case manager be prepared with a working knowledge of standards of care for the region and community and of regulatory requirements.

The purpose of standards of care is to protect and safeguard not only patients but also health care professionals. Standards of care help patients avoid substandard care and describe the minimal requirements that define an acceptable level of care to ensure that no harm comes to the patient. These standards are generally well-founded in evidence-based medicine, which assists physicians in making conscientious, judicious, and individual decisions about the care being provided to patients.

One of the best tools in managing the litigious environment in which we live is concise and accurate documentation of the care being outlined and provided to the patient. Documentation is an essential component of assessment, planning, communication, and evaluation. From a legal standpoint, documentation is oftentimes the deciding factor in whether a case will be won or lost. The old adage "If it's not written, it's not done" still remains valid to this day.

In 1997, President Bill Clinton established the Advisory Commission on Consumer Protection and Quality in Healthcare.[22] This commission's findings led to several key issues for both health plans and providers:

- **Information disclosure:** The rights of the consumer to receive accurate information with which to make informed decisions about care.
- **Choice of providers:** The right of the patient to have a choice of health care providers.
- **Access to emergency services:** The rights of the consumer to receive emergency care when the need arises.
- **Participation in treatment decisions:** The rights of the consumer to participate in decisions about care.
- **Respect and nondiscrimination:** The rights of the consumer to considerate, respectful care at all times and under all circumstances.
- **Confidentiality of health information:** The right to communicate with health care providers in confidence and to have that confidentiality maintained.
- **Complaints and appeals:** The rights of the consumer to have a fair and efficient process to resolve disputes.

The findings of this commission place a substantial burden on the case manager to ensure that the rights of each patient with whom the case manager comes in contact are protected. The case manager needs to consider the wishes of the patient and the family and match those wishes with the resources available to manage the patient's condition.

TECHNOLOGY AND HIPAA

The ability to communicate with other providers about the condition of the patient has become exceedingly more complicated with the introduction of the Health Insurance Portability and Accountability Act (HIPAA; see Chapter 32). Confusion still exists to some extent about this law and how it is strategically implemented in organizations. The law provides for release of information without authorization for treatment, payment, and health care operations.

Treatment is defined as the provision, coordination, or management of health services among health care providers, or by a health care provider with a third party.

Payment encompasses the various activities of health care providers to obtain reimbursement for their services and of a health plan to obtain premiums or to provide reimbursement for services rendered.

Health care operations are those administrative, financial, legal, and quality activities of a covered entity that are necessary to run its business and to support treatment or payment. The activities include quality improvement activities, reviewing the competence or qualifications of health care professionals to provide service, underwriting, and other activities relating to health insurance or health benefits, conducting or arranging medical review, legal and auditing services, business planning and development and business management, and administrative services such as customer service, and grievance resolution.

All other inquiries and provision of information require a signed authorization from the patient.

If the patient is competent, provider and health plan case managers must be cognizant of their responsibility to protect the privacy of the patient and to release information only for specified purposes. When discharge plans are being discussed with the patient and others are present, it is important to secure permission of the patient to discuss care and discharge planning in the presence of others. When the patient is incapable of making health care decisions, the case manager is empowered to discuss protected health information with the immediate next of kin or the individual who has been designated as the patient's legally authorized representative, to determine issues specific to discharge planning and care facilitation.

A legally authorized representative can include one of the following*:

- A parent or legal guardian, if the patient is a minor
- A legal guardian who shows proof of guardianship
- An agent of the patient who is authorized under a valid medical power of attorney
- An attorney ad litem appointed by the courts
- A personal representative such as the administrator of the patient's estate or the executor of the patient's will
- An attorney at law who has been retained by or authorized by the patient to act on the patient's behalf

Special precautions should be taken with photocopying or printing protected health information. The copying should be done only in compliance with the privacy policies of the organization in which the case manager works.

*This information is provided solely for educational purposes. Appropriate and competent legal counsel should be sought for a definitive opinion, if required.

The same precautions apply for the electronic transmission of information. The case manager should be cognizant of the following question, "How completely does an electronic system protect individual health information and protect the information from unauthorized access?"

With advancements in the use of technology, the ability of case managers to communicate should be dramatically enhanced. Case managers can now share information via their automated programs and can provide for enhanced continuity of care. Electronic systems offer a more comprehensive and timely method of communication between the health plan and provider case managers. They allow for a more even distribution of workload, facilitated by the ability to move a patient from one work list to another, guidelines and criteria sets available online that allow the case manager to query information much more rapidly, incorporation of prompts or reminders so that reviews and communication do not go unattended, the creation of a permanent file document that allows for tracking of activities and reviews and that is available for anyone with whom the patient needs to interact, and retention of information to allow for data aggregation, auditing, and response to denials and appeals.

As electronic systems become more sophisticated, patients will interact with their health care providers, including their case managers in a variety of "virtual connections." The connections will assist patients in navigating their way through the very complex maze of health care. Organizations that are slow to adopt the use of electronic connectivity will ultimately need to evaluate their survivability in the times ahead.

CONCLUSION

Facilitating care and managing resource utilization are challenging and rewarding, and it requires a strong skill set, coupled with a solid clinical base to respond to the ever-changing environment of health care today.

Regardless of the venue, the individuals who choose case management as their vocation sign up for work that is often breakneck in speed, with rapid-fire multitasking taking place on a daily basis. The ideal day for any case manager would be to have the time to review patient records and progress, review quality issues, take time to create the multidisciplinary environment critical to make progress, visit one on one with all the patients assigned to the case manager, and have unlimited time to talk with patients and family members about the plan of care. In reality, the days are often riddled with activity, compounded by complications with scheduling, testing, authorizations, and constant reprioritization of a work list of "to-do" items that will need to be followed up on the following day. Major changes in demographics, funding, and reimbursement will always serve as the ongoing challenge in meeting the needs of the patient population. These are exciting times for case management, and the outcomes that can be expected should reap benefits for those who follow.

References

1. Commission for Case Manager Certification. Glossary of terms. 2005. Available at: http://www.ccmcertification.org. Accessed August 6, 2006.
2. Zander K. Planning for the day, the pay, the stay and the way. *New Definition*. Summer: 2003, 18(2).
3. Powell SP. *Nursing Case Management: A Practical Guide to Success in Managed Care*. Philadelphia, Lippincott, 2000.
4. American College of Healthcare Executives. Top issues confronting hospitals: 2005. Available at: http://www.ache.org/pubs/research/ceoissues.cfm. Accessed August 6, 2006.
5. Kaiser Family Foundation. Employer health benefits 2005 annual survey. Available at: http://www.kff.org/insurance/7315.cfm. Accessed June 28, 2006.
6. Kaiser Commission on Medicaid and the Uninsured. The uninsured: A primer. January 2006. Available at: http://www.kff.org/uninsured/upload/7451.pdf. Accessed August 6, 2006.
7. Administration on Aging. Available at: http://www.aoa.gov/press/fact/pdf/ss_stat_profile.pdf. Accessed August 4, 2006.
8. Bureau of Labor Statistics. Table 3d: The 10 occupations with the largest job growth, 2004–14. Available at: http://www.bls.gov/news.release/ecopro.t06.htm. Accessed August 6, 2006.
9. DW Plocher and PL Metzger, eds. 318 pages. Gaithersburg, MD: Aspen, 2001.
10. 42, USC 1395 dd (1986) Pub. L. No. 99-272.
11. Centers for Medicare and Medicaid Services. Letter 1—model hospital-issued notice of noncoverage/HINN—admission or preadmission. Available at: http://www.cms.hhs.gov/BNI/Downloads/HINNs1to10.pdf. Accessed August 6, 2006.
12. Foley KM. Pain, physician assisted dying and euthanasia. *Pain.* 1995:4, 163–178.
13. Isaacs SL and Knickman JR. *To Improve Heath and Health Care.* San Francisco: Jossey-Bass, 1997.
14. Altman D. How to save Medicare? Die sooner? *New York Times* Feb. 27, 2005. Available at: http://select.nytimes.com/search/restricted/article?res = F70F15FC3F590C748EDDAB 0894DD404482. Accessed August 12, 2006.
15. Field MJ, Cassel CK. *Approaching Death: Improving Care at the End of Life.* Institute of Medicine report. Washington, DC: National Academy Press, 1997.
16. Institute for Healthcare Improvement. Improvement methods. Available at: http://www.ihi.org/IHI/Topics/Improvement/Improvement Methods/.
17. Wachter RM. Hospitalists in the United States—Mission accomplished or work in progress? *N Engl J Med.* 2004:350(19), 1935–1936.
18. Sanofi-Aventis. HMO-PPO/Medicare-Medicaid. Managed Care Digest Series. Digest 2005. Available at: http://www.managedcaredigest.com. Accessed July 28, 2006.

19. Wachter RM. The hospitalist movement: Ten issues to consider. *Hosp Pract (Off Ed).* 1999: 34, 95–98,104–106, 111.

20. Wachter RM and Goldman L. The hospitalist movement 5 years later. *JAMA.* 2002:287(4), 487–494.

21. Auerbach AD, Wachter RM, Katz P, *et al.* Implementation of a voluntary hospitalist service at a community teaching hospital: Improved clinical efficiency and patient outcomes. *Ann Intern Med.* 2002:137(11), 859–865.

22. President's Advisory Commission on Consumer Protection and Quality in Health Care. Advisory's Commission's final report. 1998. Available at: http://www.hcqualitycommission. gov. Accessed August 6, 2006.

12

PRESCRIPTION DRUG BENEFITS IN MANAGED HEALTH CARE

Robert P. Navarro and Rusty Hailey

Study Objectives

- Understand why health plans began to manage pharmacy program costs in the early 1980s.
- Understand the factors that contribute to pharmacy program costs.
- Understand trends in pharmacy program costs and utilization rates.
- Understand the metrics commonly used to measure and compare pharmacy program performance.
- Understand the basic components of a pharmacy benefit management information system.
- Understand the advantages and disadvantages of using a PBM for pharmacy program management.
- Understand how the Certificate of Coverage effects pharmacy benefit design.
- Understand the basic components of a pharmacy benefit management program.
- Understand factors involved in the legal basis of pharmacy benefit management.
- Understand the components in a managed care pharmacy distribution network.
- Understand the essential elements of a pharmacy provider contract, including the administrative requirements surrounding the dispensing process.
- Understand the role of the drug formulary in pharmacy benefit management.
- Understand the potential impact of drug formularies on drug access and utilization.
- Understand the influence of prescription drug patient copayments on program costs, drug access, and utilization.

Discussion Topics

1. Discuss the market forces, trends, and changes in the drug benefit over the past 15 years.
2. Discuss the essential elements of a managed care pharmacy benefit management program.
3. Identify the components of pharmacy program costs and discuss the implications of each.
4. Discuss the advantages and disadvantages for a managed care plan in using a PBM to manage its pharmacy services.
5. Discuss the impact of prescription copayments, cost-sharing, and formulary tiering on pharmacy program costs, drug access, and utilization.

INTRODUCTION AND BACKGROUND

A prescription drug program is a vital component of comprehensive health care benefits offered by managed care organizations. Virtually all managed care organizations offer pharmacy benefits, and more than 92% of commercial managed care customers purchase pharmacy benefits for their employees.[1] In addition to commercial health plans, Medicaid programs include a pharmacy benefit (see also Chapter 27), and as of 2006, Medicare Part D offers an outpatient prescription drug benefit to the 41 million Medicare beneficiaries, as discussed in Chapter 26. Therefore, other than the uninsured, the vast majority—approximately 80%—of the U.S. population may obtain prescription coverage through a private or public third-party managed pharmacy benefit program.

Correspondingly, as a result of the Medicare Part D drug benefit, the Center for Medicare and Medicaid Services (CMS) projects that by 2008, 80% of prescription drug expenditures will be paid by a public or private third-party prescription program.[2] The 2004 to 2008 change in prescription drug expenditures by payer source is illustrated in Figure 12-1.

Prescription drug benefits are a highly coveted and a highly utilized benefit by payers as well as members. Payers should understand that offering all health plan members comprehensive pharmacy benefits makes clinical as well as economic sense. Clearly, prescription drugs are a management linchpin of many high-cost and high-prevalence medical conditions, including hypertension, outpatient infections, hyperlipidemia, congestive heart failure, diabetes, cancer, seizure disorders, migraine headache, asthma, allergic rhinitis, depression, psychosis, gastroesophageal reflux disease (GERD), seizure disorders, and many others. Effective outpatient treatment with a pharmaceutical may obviate the need for more expensive and less benign medical resources, such as hospitalization and surgery.

GOALS OF PHARMACY BENEFIT MANAGEMENT

Health care in the United States is a highly competitive market-driven business. Public (Medicaid and Medicare) and private (employer groups) entities have many competitive alternative sources for prescription drug benefits. As a result, providers of pharmacy benefits must understand and anticipate the varied expectations and demands of purchasers, who are quite willing to switch to another pharmacy benefit provider on an annual basis if they are dissatisfied with their current provider. Generally, payers are interested in pharmacy benefit providers who are able to manage program costs, provide reasonable access to necessary medications, and provide excellent customer support pro-

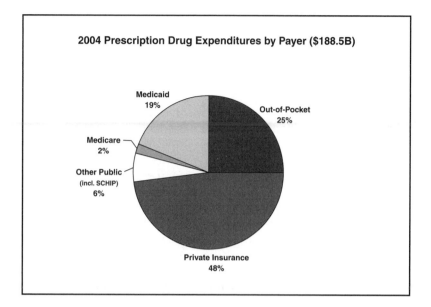

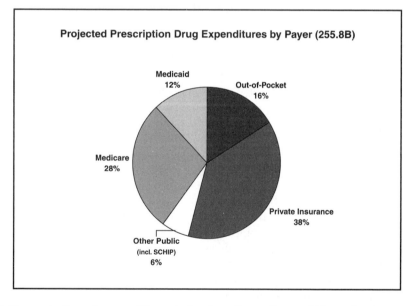

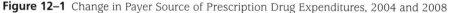

Figure 12–1 Change in Payer Source of Prescription Drug Expenditures, 2004 and 2008

Source: Created by RP Navarro from data obtained from National Health Care Expenditure Projections: 2005–2015. Prescription Drug Expenditures (Table 11). Available at: http://www.cms.hhs.gov/NationalHealthExpendData/downloads/proj2005.pdf. Accessed May 8, 2006.

grams. However, payers are different in their demands, and whereas one payer may place greater importance on cost containment and accept very limited benefits, another group, such as a union trust, may desire a broad range of drug coverage with very low copayments, and still another employer may be more interested in providing greater drug coverage supported by disease management programs. Pharmacy program providers counsel their clients on how they may achieve their desired outcomes by crafting their own customized pharmacy benefit management program.

Pharmacy directors attempt to manage the *supply cost* as well as the *utilization demand* of pharmaceuticals. This is accomplished by influencing the behavior of all individuals and entities that can control the supply and demand of pharmaceuticals by sharing with them the program financial risk. From a pharmacy benefit perspective, managed care implements supply-side contracts with pharmaceutical manufacturers and dispensing pharmacies that essentially extract discounts on the drug ingredient cost (through manufacturer rebates and pharmacy reimbursement discounts) and a discounted pharmacy dispensing fee. Demand-side controls involve member prescription copayments or co-insurances paid by patients/members when they access and obtain pharmacy services. Member cost sharing is designed to encourage use of the most cost-effective products. As noted in Chapter 6, some managed care organizations also share a portion of the pharmacy benefit financial risk with prescribing physicians. The theory behind this strategy is that physicians will prescribe more cost-efficiently if they share in the cost of the drugs they prescribe. Despite the fact that this practice has been criticized for appearing to pay physicians for prescribing certain drugs, physicians with shared financial risk generally prefer generic or less expensive brand products, which also benefits patients through a lower copayment. In summary, pharmacy program managers attempt to obtain discounts on the drug ingredient cost as well as encourage the use of the least expensive yet therapeutically effective products to optimize pharmacy budget expenditures, which benefits payers as well as members.

As a result, pharmacy benefit managers (PBMs) must offer a broad range of program benefit design options to meet varied payer desires, while involving all stakeholders financially to achieve program objectives for each unique customer. The relationships and the flow of money among various stakeholders involved in medical and pharmacy benefits are shown in Figure 12-2. A general rule in identifying entities that may influence supply and demand is to "follow the money" trail. This model includes a managed care organization (MCO) that contracts with a PBM for certain pharmacy benefit services (*eg,* pharmacy distribution network and to contract with pharmaceutical manufacturers). However, large MCOs can provide complete pharmacy benefits directly without using a PBM or by using a PBM that is wholly owned and managed by the large MCO.

MCOs, both public and private, continue to manage pharmacy benefits aggressively in an attempt to promote the appropriate level of prescription utilization rate as well as optimize the drug expenditure. This focus on pharmacy benefit management may seem antithetical to the cost-effectiveness value of pharmaceuticals. However, health care in the United States is a market-driven business. Since the inception of managed health care concepts in the early part of the twentieth century, purchasers of care have demanded cost containment as well as a broad spectrum of health care benefits. As managed care has managed all health care products and services, pharmaceutical benefits continue to be managed aggressively for three primary reasons:

1. Although pharmacy benefits are the third largest health care benefit expenditure of managed care plans (after hospital and outpatient medical benefits), the annual trend rate of prescription drug benefits has historically risen faster than the other two major benefits for many years. At the time of publication, this trend seems to have begun slowing a bit since 2005 and may be reduced more by the loss of patent protection of a number of important high-cost and high-utilization drugs over the next 3 years.

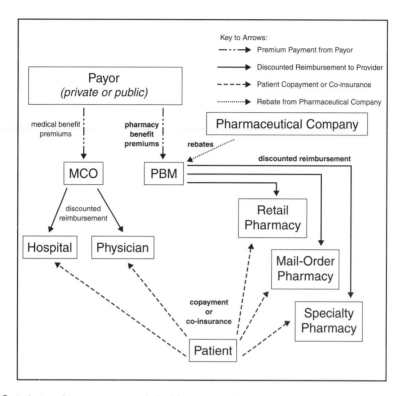

Figure 12–2 Relationships Among Stakeholders in Managed Prescription Drug Benefits (PBM model; deemphasized)

Source: RP Navarro, 2006.

2. Pharmacy benefits are highly visible to government and private payers and are accessed more than hospital or outpatient medical benefits. The average commercial MCO member uses approximately *8 to 11* prescriptions per year, and the average Medicare Part D member uses approximately *17 to 23* prescriptions per year, whereas the average commercial member consults a physician *5 to 6* times per year, and many of those encounters are pediatric visits.

3. Pharmacy benefits *can* be managed. The recipe for managing prescription drug costs and utilization is well-known and can be implemented within months with adequate resources if payers and members are willing to accept benefit limitations. The management strategies

used today were initiated almost 25 years ago and have been used by every pharmacy benefit manager to manage pharmacy benefits. However, although the strategies are well-known, successful implementation is challenging.

Rather than severely restrict or eliminate pharmacy benefits, MCOs and PBMs attempt to counsel their customers to purchase a cost-effective benefit. That is, intelligently managed pharmacy benefits will provide easy access to necessary drugs, even encourage the appropriate use of cost-effective pharmaceuticals, and guard against inappropriate use of unnecessary, ineffective, or overly expensive drugs.

Pharmacy benefit management has been successful in reducing pharmacy benefit costs by 25% to 45%, compared to unmanaged drug costs, depending upon the aggressiveness of the managed program. As pharmacy benefits evolve, and outcomes data demonstrate the comparative value of competitive pharmaceuticals, pharmacy benefits managers and purchases of health care will be in a better position to develop and implement an intelligent pharmacy benefit that optimizes the appropriate use of the most cost-effective pharmaceuticals to achieve the best clinical, economic, and humanistic outcomes.

Pharmacists managing prescription drug benefits must provide high-quality pharmacy benefits while managing program costs. The quest to *manage* costs, rather than merely *minimize* costs, remains the challenge. If pharmacy program costs continue to escalate at an annual trend rate of approximately 10% to 15%, it is tempting to merely restrict expensive drugs, require the use of only generic drugs, and to significantly increase the patient copayment tier amounts. However, simply focusing on cost minimization may be myopic and ultimately cost-ineffective in several therapeutic categories. High-cost drugs *may* produce superior clinical and economic outcomes compared with less expensive alternatives. Also, very high member copayments may be a barrier to drug utilization and adherence and can result in drug failure, which may require more expensive medical treatment. Compliance with an appropriate medication regimen is in fact a fundamental aspect of disease management, as discussed in Chapter 11. Thus, pharmacy directors must consider the cost as well as outcomes associated with competing drug products when developing and managing their pharmacy benefit.

Health plan administrators, as well as commercial and government payers, often consider pharmacy benefits only as a cost center and do not appreciate the value that a well-managed pharmacy benefit can bring to clinical, economic, and humanistic outcomes. In fact, a successfully managed pharmacy benefit should be considered an *investment* in cost-effective health care rather than only a necessary expense. Health outcomes research in health plans, addressed later, provides the linkage between appropriate use of cost-effective drugs and positive outcomes, and helps administrators and payers migrate from cost minimization to optimizing value. To achieve this goal, pharmacy benefit managers attempt to select the most cost-effective drugs for formulary inclusion, implement programs to promote appropriate use and adherence, and document value by measuring outcomes. These goals are no different from those of hospital pharmacists but are more difficult to control because the MCO pharmacy director is often managing prescription benefits for hundreds of thousands or even millions of patients, from pediatric patients to Medicare beneficiaries, with literally every known disease for a prolonged period of time.

NOVEL CHALLENGES AND EFFECTIVE MANAGEMENT STRATEGIES

Pharmacy benefit management has evolved over the past 25 years to meet and, if possible, anticipate the clinical and financial market challenges threatening effective prescription drug benefit management. The events of the years leading up to 2010 and beyond provide some unique market trends not seen in the past two decades. The three most important concerns and challenges managed care pharmacy directors face include the following:

- Successful implementation of the Medicare Modernization Act Part D Medicare pharmacy benefit (see Chapter 26). Although some health plans have had experience in Medicare health benefits, very few have offered a comprehensive pharmacy benefit. Medicare Advantage plans (formerly Medicare + Choice) will hold financial risk for medical as well as pharmacy benefits in this population subgroup with 40 million elderly beneficiaries, who typically have more diseases, comorbidities, and consume more medications.

- Management of injectable biological medications, which are generally extremely expensive and often used in severe or life-threatening medical conditions (*eg,* rheumatoid arthritis and other autoimmune disorders, HIV/AIDS, Crohn's disease, end stage renal disease, certain metabolic diseases, and a variety of cancers). Many health plans and PBMs are using specialty pharmacies to provide and manage injectable biologicals because these products require specialized distribution systems and patient management strategies. Injectable products may not be a component of the pharmacy budget and are often part of the medical budget.* However, even if injectables are not a financial responsibility of the pharmacy budget, often the pharmacy department is involved in managing injectable drug selection and utilization.

- Successfully implementing consumer-driven health care plan (CDHP; see also Chapters 2 and 20) initiatives that include Health Savings Accounts (HSAs) or Health Reimbursement Accounts (HRAs), and higher and more complicated copayments and co-insurance schemes. CDHP initiatives should motivate and reward the consumer for self-management and include financial incentives and cost sharing, without the unintended consequence of inadvertently building in financial disincentives to delay preventive care.[3]

In addition to these novel challenges, health plans and PBMs continue to face the daily challenge of developing and implementing cost-effective pharmacy benefit programs customized for each of their customers. To meet the long-term and unique pharmacy benefit management challenges, pharmacy and medical directors routinely consider the following strategies as most effective (these strategies are discussed in depth later in this chapter):

1. **Increasing the use of generic drugs.** Health plans and PBMs frequently report that 50% to 60% of the prescriptions they reimburse are dispensed with lower-priced generic alternatives. Some closed model plans estimate they may be able to increase this rate to 70% or even 80%, especially in upcoming years when some important high-cost and highly utilized drugs lose patent protection (*eg,* statins, calcium channel blockers, antidepressants, inhaled and nasal corticosteroids).

2. **Raising patient prescription copayments and co-insurance amounts.** Health plans and PBMs continue to increase copayments and co-insurance levels to encourage the use of lower-cost preferred formulary products and to share the cost of medications with members who use them. The impact of copayments is discussed later in the section titled "Drug Formulary Development and Management."

3. **Limiting access to particular drugs.** Health plans and PBMs will more aggressively limit open access to the use of certain expensive drugs, or drugs with a misuse or abuse potential, through the use of prior authorization (physician and/or pharmacist must obtain approval to prescribe or dispense certain drugs), step-care edits (a lower-priced drug must be used before a similar expensive drug is reimbursed), and other limits (*eg,* quantity of units dispensed at one time and the duration of use).

4. **Use of closed drug formularies.** Health plans and PBMs may again promote more closed drug formularies. Closed formularies (a limited number of drugs

---

*In other words, the cost and coverage for these injectable medicines are not part of a drug benefit "rider" to the main insurance or coverage policy, but rather part of the main policy itself. This may vary from state to state and may vary as well in the case of self-insured employers (see also Chapter 31 regarding regulations about self-insured employer benefits programs).

are reimbursed) were more common in the late 1980s and early 1990s, but formularies became more open (increased number of drugs reimbursed using expanded tiered copayments) by the late 1990s. However, with increasing drug program costs, and demands from payers for greater cost containment, pharmacy directors may again encourage the use of closed formularies. This reoccurring trend may be reinforced by the recent implementation of Medicare Part D formularies, which were generally more restrictive and generally closed.[1]

Pharmacy directors will continue to use these and other strategies in the future, but will use them more aggressively and with more therapeutic categories. The following sections discuss important information systems and commonly used prescription drug program management strategies in greater depth and detail.

PHARMACY INFORMATION SYSTEMS AND HEALTH INFORMATICS

Similar to other health care delivery components, pharmacy benefit administration is critically dependent on efficient data and information systems. The basic information systems involved in pharmacy benefit management include the following:

- Internal health plan administrative data systems that include member eligibility files, group benefit claims adjudication files, provider files, and drug files that are used for accurate claims adjudication.
- In-pharmacy point-of-service (POS) third-party claims adjudication systems that dispensing pharmacists use to verify member, provider, and drug eligibility and obtain copayment and reimbursement information in an online, real-time environment.
- Health plan or PBM pharmacy administrative claims file, used for drug

utilization review, pharmacy program performance analysis, research, patient and physician intervention programs, and financial report generation. Drug files are often merged with medical files to generate an integrated claims database suitable for research.

The presence of a universally accepted electronic data interchange standard for pharmacy claims transmission and adjudication has accelerated the adoption of pharmacy e-commerce. This standard, maintained by the National Council for Prescription Drug Programs (NCPDP), "creates and promotes standards for the transfer of data to and from the pharmacy services sector of the healthcare industry."[4] This universal standard has allowed the pharmacy claims systems to be suitable for electronic commerce.

Pharmacy Claims Adjudication

Observation of the NCPDP data standards allows 99% of all managed care prescription claims to be processed electronically online and usually in real time. Pharmacists rely on the third-party prescription drug program benefit design and coverage information provided to them through the in-pharmacy POS system. Pharmacy benefits programs, even within a single MCO or PBM, may be highly variable, may change frequently, and may have complex benefit design elements, and dispensing pharmacists simply must rely on electronic messaging to process prescriptions efficiently.

When a pharmacist fills a managed care prescription, the required patient, drug, and prescriber data are input into the pharmacy POS system. Within seconds, the pharmacist is informed whether the patient and drug are eligible for coverage, is apprised of the copayment to be collected, and is provided any pertinent clinical information (*eg,* drug interactions or clinical edits). If correct, the pharmacist completes the transaction, and within seconds the claim is adjudicated online, informing the pharmacist of the reimbursement amount. The online pharmacy management systems provide patient-specific information at the point of dispensing that identifies adherence problems, drug interactions, dispensing errors, and prints a patient information document. Pharmacy claims data are also used to identify members who may benefit from disease or case management, such as patients who appear to be misusing or abusing redundant prescriptions from multiple providers or displaying other inappropriate or excessive drug use patterns.

Pharmacy and Medical Claims Integration and Clinical Program Support

Over the past decade, health care information system standards have allowed easier integration of medical, administrative, and pharmacy claims datasets. Merging of these databases is accomplished through linking the common shared dimensions, such as identifiers for member, physician, and employer group benefit level. Health plans and PBMs compete on price as well as quality of care and services. Thus, health plans in particular are interested in measuring clinical and economic outcomes and use comparative health plan data for marketing to potential payer customers. For example, a population of case-mix-adjusted patients with a specific medical condition can be stratified according to severity, age, comorbidities, and other characteristics to compare the clinical and economic outcomes of each cohort. Similarly, physician drug-prescribing patterns may also be evaluated and compared. A well-constructed, merged database may be used to identify clinical "best practices" that are associated with the most cost-effective outcomes. Chapter 16 provides further discussion of clinical data usage.

Most health plans participate in the National Commission for Quality Assurance (NCQA; see also Chapter 23) accreditation process and allow their performance metrics to be compared against competitive plans using the NCQA Health Plan Report Card.[5] The NCQA has also established many "effectiveness of care" indicators through its Health Plan Employer Data and Information Set (HEDIS) program. The NCQA HEDIS is a list of almost 70 measures (at the time of this writing) designed to collect data about the quality of care and services provided by the health plans.[6] Approximately one-half of these measures relate to appropriate pharmaceutical or immunization use and can be used to measure pharmacy benefit contributions at a high level. Health plan quality initiatives are addressed specifically in Chapter 15.

Electronic Prescribing

The rapid expansion of information technology applications in health care presents novel opportunities and challenges for pharmacists. Although electronic prescribing (e-prescribing) is not universal, many MCOs are experimenting with real-time electronic data transfer of prescription-related information among trading partners: the health plan, physician, and pharmacy. *E-prescribing* refers to the use of computing devices to enter, modify, review, and output or communicate drug prescriptions. In inpatient care, electronic medication ordering increases prescribing accuracy and dispensing efficiency, and reduces the number of adverse drug events and redundant medications. A number of outpatient pilot projects and initiatives in e-prescribing are proliferating within managed care organizations to achieve the same goals and also provide medication history, drug formulary options, drug hypersensitivities, and other clinically relevant data to the prescriber at the point of prescribing.

E-prescribing is an electronic data interchange application that provides electronic connectivity among all trading partners involved in prescription generation, adjudication, and analysis. E-prescribing links the health plan or PBM with the physician and pharmacy. E-prescribing allows the physician, using a desktop or handheld device, to access a patient's medication history, drug allergies, pharmacy benefits, and drug formulary drugs covered and transmits a "clean" prescription to the patient's preferred pharmacy—all online and in real time. Figure 12-3 illustrates the electronic connectivity among trading partners.

E-prescribing offers several potential financial and patient care advantages to the physician, health plan, pharmacy, and patient. Point-of-prescribing medication information helps enforce drug formulary conformance, informs the physician of the member copayment impact of selected drugs, and prevents rejected prescriptions at the pharmacy. Prior authorization or step-care protocols may be enforced through e-prescribing, and the system can alert physicians of any drug interac-

tions, history of adverse events, redundant prescriptions from other physicians, and incorrect dosages before the patient leaves the physician's office. The potential cost savings from e-prescribing result from reduced administrative costs and less physician and pharmacist time involved in the prescription process, reduction in drug interactions and adverse effects, improved safety and reduced medication errors, and improved medication compliance.

In the ambulatory environment, recent research shows that adverse events are common and can be serious. The Center for Information Technology Leadership reports that more than 8.8 million adverse drug events occur each year in ambulatory care, of which more than 3 million are preventable, many resulting in deaths. In addition to reducing adverse drug effects, e-prescribing can improve quality, efficiency, and reduce costs through other benefits, including the following:

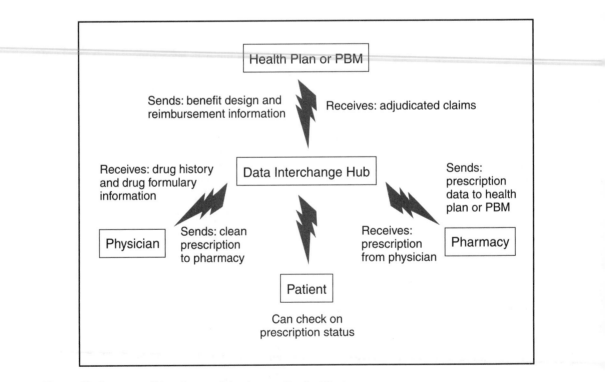

Figure 12–3 E-prescribing Connectivity Among Trading Partners

Source: RP Navarro, 2006.

- Actively promoting appropriate prescription use and adherence
- Providing information about formulary options and copay information
- Improving dispensing efficiency and accuracy by providing instant electronic connectivity between the physician, pharmacy, health plans, and PBMs[7]

More than 3 billion prescriptions are written annually.[8] Given this volume, even a small improvement in quality attributable to e-prescribing would translate into significant health care cost and safety benefits if e-prescribing is broadly adopted. Studies suggest that the national savings from universal adoption of e-prescribing systems could be as high as $27 billion, including $4 billion per-member-per-year (PMPY) savings from reducing preventable adverse drug events, and $35 to $70 PMPY savings from more appropriate use of medications, for a total savings of $39 to $74 PMPY.[7] Electronic prescribing has significant benefits for pharmacists as well. The Institute for Safe Medication Practices estimates that pharmacists spend a significant amount of their time each day on clarifying prescription orders and make 150 million phone calls to physicians annually on prescription accuracy–related issues.[9]

RxHub provides a universal portal that supports prescription electronic data interchange among trading partners. Originally formed in 2001 by three PBMs, the enterprise now enjoys participation of PBMs, health plans, and numerous e-prescribing solution venders, for the following purpose:

> Creating a single point of communication for all participants in the prescription creation and delivery process, the founders formed a neutral organization whose primary mission is to accelerate the adoption of electronic prescribing resulting in better medicine and lower administrative costs.[10]

All advantages of e-prescribing can lead to improved clinical, economic, and quality-of-life outcomes. E-prescribing will unquestionably increase, especially as it is an eventual requirement in the Medicare Modernization Act.

COMPONENTS OF A MANAGED PRESCRIPTION DRUG BENEFIT

Prescription drug benefits are provided through an internal pharmacy department within an MCO* or by a standalone PBM. Regardless of the source (*eg,* MCO or PBM), there is great consistency in the management strategies used to develop and manage a prescription drug program. Pharmacists operating health plan pharmacy benefits have borrowed many management strategies from hospital pharmacy programs, including the pharmacy and therapeutics (P & T) committee, the drug formulary, pharmaceutical company contracting, physician academic counterdetailing, utilization review, and health outcomes research. However, MCOs have had to include additional capabilities, such as development of a pharmacy distribution network, innovative pharmacy benefit design, member copayment schemes, member communication and education, and massive computer systems to process millions of claims in a real-time environment. This section lists and illustrates the components of a successful managed care prescription drug benefit program.

Legal Basis for Pharmacy Benefit Programs

All states have regulatory bodies that control health-related benefit plans as well as licens-

---

*The term *managed care organization* refers to health maintenance organizations (HMOs), preferred provider organizations (PPOs), POS plans, and other health plans, Medicaid programs, and Medicare Part D plans.

ing boards that control the practice of specific health care providers. The Employee Retirement Income Security Act of 1974 (ERISA) is a federal law that sets minimum standards for most voluntarily established pension and health plans in private industry to provide protection for individuals. ERISA is discussed in detail in Chapter 31.

The ERISA act has been supplemented by two important amendments. The Consolidated Omnibus Budget Reconciliation Act (COBRA) provides workers and their families the ability to continue their health coverage after loss of employment, and the Health Insurance Portability and Accountability Act (HIPAA; see also Chapter 32) that provides protection for patients from discrimination related to preexisting medical conditions, as well as enhanced confidentiality of medical information.[11]

MCOs and PBMs, as corporate entities, do not practice medicine or pharmacy and do not claim to provide any and all desired pharmacy products and services. Rather, they arrange for defined medical and pharmacy benefits to be provided by licensed health care professionals within a defined structure and process. Health care professionals participating with an MCO or PBM provide pharmacy benefits that are specified and defined in a state-regulated contract (*eg,* Certificate of Coverage or other similar legal document) between the MCO or PBM and the purchaser of pharmacy benefits. Physicians and pharmacists agree to participate according to policies outlined in their respective provider manuals and contracts, which are generally filed with a state regulatory agency (see Chapter 30 for a full discussion of legal issues in contracting with providers). The contract defines included and excluded benefits, as well as the access rules through which members must obtain benefits. Drugs eligible for reimbursement are normally those included in the drug formulary (a list of reimbursed drugs) that is reviewed and updated from time to time. Drugs typically excluded from reimbursement include the following:

- Experimental or investigational drugs (drugs not approved by the U.S. Food and Drug Administration for commercial sale in the United States).
- FDA-approved drugs when prescribed for unapproved indications ("off-label" indications). This is generally unenforceable through community pharmacies because pharmacists are generally unaware of the prescribed indication or medical diagnosis for most prescriptions dispensed. The approved indication may be enforced if the pharmacist must obtain a prior authorization from the MCO or PBM before receiving reimbursement for the drug product.
- Drugs used for cosmetic purposes (*eg,* Botox™ [botulinum toxin] for wrinkles) or possibly life enhancement drugs (*eg,* phosphodiesterase type 5 [PDE-5] inhibitors used to treat erectile dysfunction).
- A brand-name drug for which there is an identical generic equivalent that is subject to mandatory generic substitution (*eg,* drugs subject to a maximum allowable cost [MAC] reimbursement).
- Drugs available without a prescription (or over-the-counter [OTC] drugs), including brand-name drugs for which there is an identical OTC equivalent. Insulin is an exception because it is a nonprescription drug in most states, but remains covered by health plan pharmacy benefits.

It is important to note that all health plans and PBMs allow for medical exceptions to defined benefits. That is, a physician may appeal to a health plan or PBM for coverage and reimbursement for a noncovered benefit based upon an individual patient's medical needs. Additionally, patients have the ability to purchase directly any noncovered benefit outside of the pharmacy benefit, on a cash basis, with a physician's prescription. Pharmacy benefit design does not limit what a physician may prescribe; benefit design only limits what an MCO or PBM will reimburse.

Changes in Pharmacy Benefit Design

Two principal changes are occurring in benefit design. The first is greater use of formulary prescription copayment and co-insurance tiers, as well as higher copayment tier dollar and co-insurance percentage amounts, especially for nonpreferred and injectable medications. The second major benefit design change is the growth of high-deductible health plans (HDHPs) or CDHPs with HSAs or HRAs (see Chapter 2), encouraged by state and federal regulatory agencies, as well as employer groups and health plans.[12,13] HDHPs and CDHPs usually have lower monthly premiums as well as higher annual deductibles and give members more latitude and freedom in using HSA/HRA funds for health-related expenditures. A potential downside is that HDHP/CDHP members, accustomed to near first-dollar coverage for medical and pharmacy benefits, now have to spend (for example) $2,500 or more in out-of-pocket deductible expenses before benefits are covered 100% by the health plan. Early experiences of a few employer groups have found some members are reluctant to spend their own out-of-pocket money and may delay preventive care, thus resulting in a need for delayed and more expensive acute medical treatment.[14] As discussed in Chapter 20, such types of plans are most effectively used by informed members who are educated and motivated to optimize their health care and who are given appropriate information to make intelligent health care access decisions. HSA members are important targets for pharmaceutical companies with direct-to-consumer advertising for both prescription and over-the-counter medications.

Distribution Channels for Outpatient Pharmaceuticals

MCOs and PBMs must develop a pharmaceutical distribution system that meets member needs for easy access to prescription services as well as controlling drug ingredient and dispensing costs. Closed model health plans (*eg,* staff or group model health maintenance organizations [HMOs] or integrated delivery systems; see Chapter 2) or large employer groups may have in-house, owned pharmacies for member convenience, supplemented with community pharmacies, often with mail service. Open model plans (*eg,* independent practice association [IPAs], network HMOs, or preferred provider organizations [PPOs]) will use a community-based pharmacy network, including chain pharmacies, independent pharmacies, and often mail-service pharmacies. Today, a pure MCO rarely exists, and even most staff and group model plans offer a hybrid distribution network consisting of in-house pharmacists supplemented by community and mail-service pharmacies.

Generally 80% to 90% of third-party outpatient prescriptions are dispensed through community pharmacies (pharmacy chains, independent pharmacies, supermarkets, mass merchandize stores [*eg,* WalMart, Target]). Most of the remaining prescriptions are dispensed through mail-service pharmacies, often owned or associated with PBMs or chain pharmacies. A small percentage of prescriptions, mostly generic drugs and often in rural areas, are dispensed in physician offices, and these may not be reimbursed by third-party payers. Of the $221 billion spent on outpatient prescription drugs in 2004, the National Association of Chain Drug Stores (NACDS) reports that 42.2% were dispensed through chain pharmacies, 18.7% through independent community pharmacies, 18.3% through mail-service pharmacies, 12.2% through supermarkets, and 9.6% through mass merchandize stores.[15] As a result, the basis of a managed care outpatient prescription network is often chain pharmacies, supplemented by other types of pharmacies. However, the NACDS reports that the largest annual growth in prescription sales from 2002 to 2003 occurred in mail-service pharmacies, which grew by almost 18%, in contrast with all other pharmacy types, which grew between 5% and 8%.

Pharmacies participating in the pharmacy provider network agree, by contract, to dispense drugs prescribed by participating physicians to eligible members according to the drug formulary and other benefit design requirements. Open access plans such as point-of-service (POS; see Chapter 2), PPO, or other types of non-HMO plans may reimburse prescriptions from any licensed physician. Pharmacists participate in many different managed pharmacy programs, and by contract must use an online, real-time point-of-service (POS—not to be confused with a POS type of health plan as described in Chapter 2) computer system to verify coverage information (eligible drug, member, and physician), learn any dispensing limitations or requirements (*eg,* quantity limits, step-care protocols), obtain copayment information, and know the level of reimbursement from the health plan or PBM. Busy pharmacists dispensing 200 prescriptions per day simply must rely on an accurate and efficient online system to verify and adjudicate claims.

All participating pharmacies are bound by a provider agreement that stipulates they will provide approved prescriptions dispensed to their members in accordance with drug benefit and coverage policies and for a specified discounted reimbursement. These policies are usually detailed in a participating pharmacy policy and procedure manual that is updated from time to time by the MCO or PBM. Participating pharmacies agree to follow the drug formulary and dispensing requirements, use the POS system to adjudicate claims online and in real time whenever possible, promote the use of generics, discourage the use of "dispense as written" prescriptions that encourage the use of brand-name drugs, and agree to participate in on-site audits of third-party prescription records.

Pharmacists receive a discounted ingredient cost reimbursement based upon a discount off the drug average wholesale price (AWP) plus a discounted dispensing fee. The elements and calculations involved in determining pharmacy reimbursement of a brand-name drug in formulary copayment Tier II (brand preferred) is illustrated by the example in Table 12-1.

The drug AWP is generally used to determine drug ingredient reimbursement. In the example illustrated in Table 12-1, the AWP is discounted by 15%. This level of discount is used to approximate the actual acquisition price (AAC) by the pharmacy. It is actually quite difficult to positively identify the AAC for a particular prescription because the pharmacy inventory is based upon volume discounts, special offers, and early payment discounts. Thus, rather than burden pharmacies with the requirement to identify the exact AAC of a prescription, MCOs and PBMs approximate this amount using a discounted AWP. Brand-name drug AWP discounts may be 15% to 18%, and generic drug discounts are often in the range of AWP less 40% to 60%. Other payments may exist, such as for special incentives for generic substitution or member clinical consultation, such as medication therapy management program (MTMP) activities, as mandated by the Medicare Part D regulations.

Table 12–1 Example of Calculations Involved in Determining Pharmacy Reimbursement from a Managed Care Plan

	Preferred Brand Tier II
Average wholesale price (AWP)	$100.00
Drug reimbursement (AWP – 15% discount)	$ 85.00
Dispensing fee (+)	$ 2.50
Subtotal	$ 87.50
Member Tier II copayment (−)	$ 25.00
MCO reimbursement to pharmacy	$ 62.50

Source: RP Navarro, 2006.

Specialty Pharmacy Distribution

The increasing use of high-cost injectable biological products is identified as the greatest threat to pharmacy benefit management. However, despite the challenge in managing cost and utilization of expensive products, injectable biologicals present unique, advanced therapy for many severely debilitating and life-threatening illnesses. Thus, as much as health plans welcome the launch of life-saving drugs, they are faced with the reality that uncontrolled utilization may place a plan in financial peril. Health plans support the use of evidence-based treatment guidelines and protocols and usually implement prior authorization edits on expensive biological injectables to encourage appropriate use for FDA-approved indications. By way of example, in 2006 a large Blue Cross and Blue Shield plan found that 37% of injectable expenses were for oncology and related products, 11% were for inflammatory diseases of the colon, 9% were for leukocyte stimulants, and 2% was spent on anti-inflammatory and anti-arthritis injectable products.[16]

The unique distribution, storage, and utilization considerations of injectables have caused the development of carve-out specialty pharmacy distributors (SPDs). Specialty pharmacy services may also be offered internally through PBMs and health plans. Specialty pharmacies manage the distribution and use of self- and physician-administered injectable products. SPDs may send injectables directly to a physician office or infusion center specifically for a patient appointment, or self-injectable drugs may be mailed directly to a member's home. Volume purchasing by SPDs introduces cost efficiencies into the system that are passed on to payers and members. SPDs also use rebates, formulary-style product steerage, copayments and coinsurance, and provider discounts as other methods of controlling injectable drug costs.

Health plans may also use SPDs to buy and store inventory on behalf of physicians, which prevents physicians from stocking and storing expensive medications and removes physicians from the flow of dollars. In this scheme, the SPD bills the health plan and/or member directly, and the physician is paid an infusion and/or administration fee by the health plan. The growing availability of biotechnology pharmaceuticals will likely increase the role and importance of SPDs in the future. Traditional discounted reimbursement of injectable products as a Part B Medicare benefit will be altered through the use of a CMS average selling price (ASP) plus 6% method. Many plans are adopting this Medicare-style cost-plus reimbursement for injectables in their commercial plans as well. The implementation of the CMS Competitive Acquisition Program (CAP) for injectables has been delayed, and the impact of the CAP is unknown at the time of this writing.

Internet Pharmacy Access

Internet pharmacies developed in the late 1990s and were thought to be a future threat to community and mail-service pharmacies. However, this has not occurred, and although some Internet pharmacies remain in existence at the time of publication (*eg,* www.drugstore.com), others have ceased doing business. In reality, Internet pharmacies were simply an online method to access traditional pharmacy services with mail delivery. Internet pharmacy access enables patients to refill prescriptions and purchase nonprescription drugs, vitamins, and other health products online. However, rather than Internet pharmacies threatening mail-service pharmacies, chain and mail-service pharmacies have developed patient-friendly Internet portals and have developed their own Internet pharmacy capabilities. Managed care supports Internet access to pharmacy services of U.S.-licensed participating pharmacies because Internet access increases the use of the mail-service pharmacy component, which is considered a growing source of pharmacy budget savings.

Although Internet access to licensed U.S. chain and mail-service pharmacies is a patient convenience, there remains a safety concern about unregulated Internet pharmacies outside of the United States. Counterfeit and inert drugs from international sources have been distributed through Internet pharmacies, and international commerce through the Internet is impossible to control.

In response, the National Association of Boards of Pharmacy (NABP) developed the Verified Internet Pharmacy Practice Sites (VIPPS) program in 1999. To be VIPPS certified, a pharmacy must comply with the licensing and inspection requirements of each state in which they dispense pharmaceuticals. In addition, pharmacies displaying the VIPPS seal have demonstrated to NABP compliance with VIPPS criteria.[17] According to the NABP Web site, 12 Internet pharmacies have satisfied VIPPS criteria,[18] including the mail-service pharmacies of PBMs (eg, Caremark, Medco Health Solutions, Prescription Solutions), health plans (eg, Anthem, CIGNA), pharmacy chains (eg, Hooks SuperRx/CVA, Walgreens), and Internet pharmacies (eg, Familymeds.com, Drugstore.com).

Physician Dispensing

Some health plans may reimburse physicians for dispensing drugs directly from their office, but this is an uncommon practice and most often occurs only in rural areas that lack adequate coverage by community pharmacies. Health plans often do not reimburse physicians for dispensing drugs unless the physician's office agrees to accept the same level of reimbursement as is paid to pharmacies and the physician's office submits pharmacy claims through a POS terminal. Physician dispensing units often contain a limited amount of acute-care drugs and generally promote the use of generics. Some applications link in-office physician dispensing units for acute care drugs with mail order for chronic care medications. The American Academy of Family Practice supports the right of physicians to dispense,[19] but thus far most medical groups have not focused on developing in-house dispensing activities, other than through a colocated and usually independent community pharmacy (state law may allow the medical group to own the pharmacy space and obtain rent, but may prevent the medical group from owning the licensed pharmacy practice itself).

Pharmacy and Therapeutics Committee Management

Managed care has borrowed the P & T committee concept from hospitals as a source for formulary development and drug coverage decisions. In addition to the clinical drug review, the committee must make recommendations on drug formulary coverage and copayment tier and other dispensing limitations or restrictions. Managed care P & T committees typically consist of 10 to 15 physicians and pharmacists who meet quarterly. Clinical pharmacists with the health plan or PBM conduct a review of available data and information and prepare a drug monograph for distribution to members of the P & T committee that contains a recommendation for formulary inclusion or exclusion.

The data and information reviewed by clinical pharmacists typically includes the following:

- Peer-reviewed published clinical efficacy and effectiveness studies
- Safety and toxicity data
- Published health outcomes and economic data
- Data on file and economic models submitted by the pharmaceutical manufacturer usually organized according to the Academy of Managed Care Pharmacy *Format for Formulary Submissions*[20]
- Plan-specific expected utilization patterns
- The positioning and impact on other formulary drugs
- Manufacturer contracts

Because of concerns about drug safety and utilization patterns, new drugs are usually not formally reviewed for formulary consideration for at least 3 to 6 months post launch. During that time, the drug may be available for reimbursement as a nonformulary or nonpreferred drug, usually in the co-payment Tier III. The Medicare Part D regulations require that a drug be reviewed within 90 days, and a formulary decision must be made within 180 days. Medicare Part D regulations also require a separate Medicare P & T committee and members appropriate to evaluate drugs for the elderly. Many health plans share members between commercial and Part D P & T committees and often hold their meetings sequentially.

Clinical data (efficacy, effectiveness, and safety) are the two primary formulary decision criteria, but net cost ranks high as a decision consideration as well. Increasingly, credible health outcomes and economic data are available and considered by managed care P & T committees, and formulary decisions are becoming more based upon clinical and economic outcomes rather than solely on pharmacy budget cost minimization. Humanistic or quality-of-life outcomes remain less important for most drugs, but quality-of-life data are used subjectively when appropriate and convincing. The Academy of Managed Care Pharmacy *Format for Formulary Submissions* has made a significant and positive impact on improving the quality and quantity of data available for reviews as well as the ability of clinical pharmacists to review the body of existing data.

Drug Formulary Development and Management

Health plans and PBMs have used drug formularies for the same reasons they are used in hospitals: to identify and promote the most cost-effective pharmaceuticals in the most appropriate manner. A drug formulary is a preferred list of medications developed by the health plan or PBM P & T committee to guide physician prescribing and pharmacy dispensing. Formularies are not novel but have been used for decades by hospitals, health plans, and other health care institutions as a method of inventory control and to promote the use of the most cost-effective products.[21]

Early formularies in the United States were primarily compilations of formulas and recipes used to prepare medicines. The first hospital formulary, the Lititz Pharmacopoeia (1778), attempted to standardize compounding and dispensing of medicines in military hospitals that were set up during the Revolutionary War.[22] A formulary system is the method and process used that continually updates the formulary's content of prescription medications. The formulary system is a uniquely dynamic system that represents the current body of pharmaceutical knowledge and medical community practice standards resident in the health care setting it serves.

The benefit design is enforced through the formulary, which is the basis for the drug and reimbursement information used by the pharmacist to process eligible claims using the POS system. Formulary booklets are mailed to participating physicians, and often abridged formulary documents are provided to members. However, paper documents are often discarded, and many plans and PBMs provide pharmacy benefit and formulary information for physicians and members online. This allows for more frequent changes and efficiency in communicating formulary matters to providers and members.

Some formularies are "open," signifying that most drugs are eligible for reimbursement although the level of member copayment varies with formulary position. Some drugs are "on formulary" but available only if the patient satisfies certain prior authorization (PA) criteria. Drugs may be subject to a PA based upon cost or safety issues, to attempt to control use for labeled indications only, or to limit use for certain types of patients.

Other formularies may be "closed," indicating a select number of drugs are eligible for reimbursement, while others are not. Closed formularies do not allow for reimbursement of nonformulary products, and if one is prescribed, the pharmacist must contact the prescribing physician to request a change to a formulary product, or the patient must pay cash for a nonformulary product. The open and closed nature of formularies is cyclical. Since the mid-1990s, formularies more often were open and inclusive, with nonpreferred or even nonformulary products covered on Tier III. However, because of rising costs, and also because of the recent development of Medicare formularies, many MCOs are returning to more restrictive, closed formularies as well as including higher and tiered copayments.

Physician and member formulary conformance may be enforced using different mechanisms depending upon whether the formulary is inclusive or exclusive. Closed and open formularies both use a tiered copayment structure, described later, to encourage physician prescribing and member use of generic or preferred formulary products. Some health plans and PBMs use pharmacists to "academically detail" directly to physicians who continuously disregard the formulary. Many health plans and PBMs provide physicians "formulary conformance report cards" and indicate opportunities for prescribing changes that favor formulary products. Some plans and PBMs offer financial incentives to physicians for high levels of formulary conformance.

Formulary Copayment Tiers

MCOs and PBMs often use tiered formulary copayments as an integral component of their pharmacy benefit design. Two copayment tier plans have been in existence for more than 20 years, but in the last decade more plans are adopting three or more copayment tiers benefit plans. The purposes of tiered copayments are as follows:

1. Share some of the prescription costs with the utilizing member and help re-

duce some of the pharmacy program costs to the payer.
2. Encourage physicians to prescribe, and patients to accept, lower-cost drugs, which usually have a lower patient copayment.

Through a copayment system, members pay a flat dollar payment per prescription (ie, $12 or $30), whereas with co-insurance, a patient pays a percentage of the total prescription cost (eg, 50%), sometimes up to a maximum cap amount.

Drugs are placed into copayment tiers generally based upon their value to the plan and payer. A drug's value is based upon its clinical benefits as well as the net cost. Generic drugs are generally less expensive than brand-name alternatives are, and as a result, generic drugs are found on the lowest copayment tier, Tier I. Preferred formulary brand drugs are placed into copayment Tier II, and nonpreferred or nonformulary drugs are found in Tier III. Three-tier formularies are the most common tiered formulary structure, although some programs, notably union trust groups, may still have two-tier formulary copayments (generics in Tier I and all brands in Tier II).

Some large MCOs and PBMs offer greater copayment tier options for their customers and may include four- and five-tiered formularies. Tier IV may include unessential, lifestyle, or cosmetic drugs, and Tier V may contain self-injectable drugs. Copayments are more common today, but co-insurance payments are becoming more popular with self-injectable biologicals and expensive nonessential drugs in higher copayment tiers. An example of average three-tier open formulary structure copayment amounts is found in Table 12-2.

Copayments continue to increase in dollar amount, especially for Tier III nonpreferred products. Many large health plans and PBMs have announced options for Tier III copayments over $60 for clients who desire such cost-containment measures. A summary of average copayment amounts from a number of large health plans over the past 5 years is shown in Figure 12-4.

Table 12–2 Example of Average Three-Tier Drug Formulary Structure Copayments

Tier I	Tier II	Tier III
Generic drugs	Preferred formulary brand drugs	Nonpreferred or nonformulary brand drugs
Copayment $13	Copayment $31	Copayment $53

Source: RP Navarro, 2006.

An example of a formulary and copayment tiers used to encourage the use of lower-priced medications is found in Table 12-3. This table shows possible entries for the HMG Co-A reductase inhibitor therapeutic category (*eg,* statins), a high-cost and high-utilization category, for 2006 and for 2008 (before and after simvastatin and pravastatin lose patent protection). The number of dollar signs ($) is a graphic indication of the relative price of the products within the therapeutic category.

The 2006 statin formulary category includes one generic statin in Tier I, two preferred formulary brand drugs in Tier II, and two nonpreferred brand drugs in Tier III. The 2008 formulary includes three generic statins in Tier I, one high-potency statin in Tier II, one nonpreferred brand statin in Tier III, and the two remaining nonpreferred statins are not reimbursed. This copayment structure will encourage physicians to prescribe, and members to prefer, generic statins first, and, if necessary, Lipitor™ on Tier II, before the nonpreferred Tier III statins, while not providing reimbursement coverage for two brand statins that have acceptable alternatives.

The formulary position of a drug, and the resulting prescription copayment, can have a significant impact on the cost of the drug to a health plan and the member. Table 12-4 illus-

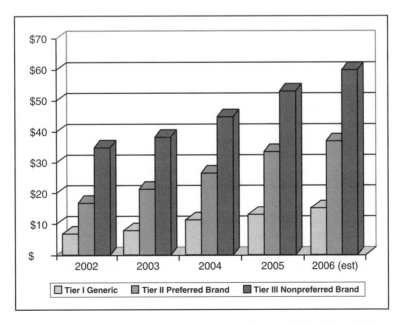

Figure 12–4 Examples of Average Copayment Amounts for Various Tiers, 2002—2006

Source: RP Navarro, 2006. Average health plan copayments compiled from a variety of research projects and personal communications with pharmacy and medical directors, 2002—2006.

Table 12–3 Example of Potential HMG Co-A Reductase Inhibitor Therapeutic Category Drugs (Statins) in a Commercial Formulary in 2006 and 2008

HMG Co-Reductase Inhibitor Formulary (single-entity statins)—2006		
	Tier I	**Tier II**	**Tier III**
Type of Drugs	Generic	Preferred formulary brand	Nonpreferred or nonformulary brand
Drugs Included	$ lovastatin	$$$ Pravachol™ (pravastatin)	$$$$$ Crestor® (resuvastatin)
		$$$ Lipitor (atorvastaton)	$$$$$ Zocor™ (simvastatin)
Copayment Amount	$12	$25	$45

HMG Co-Reductase Inhibitor Formulary (single-entity statins)—2007		
	Tier I	**Tier II**	**Tier III**
Type of Drugs	Generic	Preferred formulary brand	Nonpreferred or nonformulary brand
Drugs Included	$ lovastatin $ simvastatin $ pravastatin	$$$ Lipitor (atorvastaton)	$$$$$ Crestor® (resuvastatin)
Copayment Amount	$18	$35	$65
Nonreimbursed drugs: Pravachol™ (pravastatin) and Zocor™ (simvastatin)		

Source: RP Navarro, 2006.

trates the impact of a Tier II and Tier III copayment on the health plan payment to a pharmacy as well as to the member. The wholesale acquisition cost (WAC) is a realistic price that approximates the actual acquisition cost of a drug. The average wholesale price (AWP) is an artificial, calculated number, somewhat archaic, that often is used in pharmacy reimbursement calculations.

In this example, drugs with identical AWPs ($100) are put in Tier II and Tier III. In Tier II, the patient pays a $25 prescription copayment, and the MCO payment to the pharmacy is $62.50. In the Tier III example, the patient pays a greater portion of the drug cost ($45 copayment), and as a result, the payment from the MCO to the pharmacy is less ($42.50). This illustrates how a health plan or PBM can reduce costs, which are passed on to the payer, by increasing the member copayment cost. When the drug is on Tier II, the MCO pays approximately 60% of the AWP to the pharmacy, whereas in Tier III, the MCO pays approximately 40% of the AWP to the pharmacy, more than a 30% savings, although the patient must pay a copayment that is 180% of the Tier II copayment.

Generic drugs are one of the most important cost-containment components of an effective drug formulary. Members are well accepting of generics and most often ask for a generic drug. Generic drugs generally cost

Table 12–4 Impact of Tier II and Tier III Copayments on the Cost of a Drug to a Health Plan and Member

		Preferred Brand Tier II	Non-Preferred Brand Tier III
Average wholesale price (AWP)		$100.00	$100.00
Drug reimbursement (AWP – 15%)		$ 85.00	$ 85.00
Dispensing fee (+)		$ 2.50	$ 2.50
	Subtotal	$ 87.50	$ 87.50
Member Tier II copayment (−)		$ 25.00	$ 45.00
MCO reimbursement to pharmacy		$ 62.50	$ 42.50

Source: RP Navarro, 2006.

a fraction of the brand costs, and AB-rated products (considered to be bioequivalent and generically substitutable), are increasing in importance because several high-cost and high-utilization drugs will soon lose their patent protection. In addition to encouraging the use of generics through lower copayments, health plans and PBMs also have a mandatory generic reimbursement program, often referred to as a maximum allowable cost (MAC) program.

Through a mandatory generic program, the generic form of a drug is assigned an MAC, which is the upper level of pharmacy reimbursement by the MCO or PBM. This means that if a pharmacist dispenses a brand-name equivalent for a drug with an MAC, the pharmacist will only be reimbursed at the MAC level, which approximates the acquisition cost of the generic. This almost guarantees a generic drug will be dispensed if the drug is subject to an MAC, unless the patient is willing to pay cash for the brand drug or the physician demands the brand drug through a "dispense as written" order. Pharmacists are advised of drugs subject to an MAC as well as the MAC level of reimbursement through the POS pharmacy claims adjudication system.

Health plans and PBMs often develop their own proprietary MAC programs and list of drugs subject to an MAC, and the mechanism they use to establish an MAC level may vary. However, in general, a product is assigned an MAC if there are three or more generic products available from reputable generic manufacturers, and the actual acquisition cost (AAC) is significantly lower than the AAC or WAC of brand drugs. The level of significance varies with different health plans and PBMs, but generally if the AAC of a generic product if more than 50% less than the AAC or WAC of a brand drug, and the generic AAC has stabilized, an MAC will be assigned.

The use and impact of high-tiered copayments on pharmacy program costs and prescription adherence are controversial topics. Certainly, copayments can reduce the cost of drugs by 20% to 40% or more, depending upon the copayment amount. However, critics of high-dollar copayments claim the high copayment amounts are financial deterrents to members obtaining, and remaining on, prescribed drugs, and high copayments results in poor adherence and failed outcomes. Such negative outcomes may occur, but critics must also realize that lack of adherence is caused by a number of other factors, such as lack of member understanding, forgetfulness, belief that mediations are unnecessary, adverse effects or fear of adverse effects, and cultural barriers to medication use.[23-26] Some employer groups have adopted novel copayment structures and have reduced the copayment for chronic medications for several high-cost and high-prevalence medical conditions, such as diabetes, asthma, and hypercholesterolemia.[27,28]

Pharmaceutical Manufacturers Rebate Contracts

Rebates from pharmaceutical manufacturers to health plans began when the first contract was executed in April 1984 between United HealthCare and Abbott Laboratories. Borrowed from hospitals and other industries, health plans sought, and received, a financial incentive (rebate) to more favorably position contracted drug products. It is important to note that the price or rebate is not the most important driver in formulary positioning; clinical efficacy and safety appropriately remain the most important decision criteria. However, in the absence of statistically and clinically significant differentiation among similar drugs, the net cost (which may be reduced by a rebate) can have an important impact on ultimate formulary positioning. This is especially true in crowded, relatively undifferentiated therapeutic categories, such as ACE inhibitors, ARBs, and proton pump inhibitors, as well as expensive, competitive categories with clinical product differentiation, such as antidepressants, statins, and inhaled corticosteroids.

However, a rebate may make a drug more attractive by making it less expensive than competitors, and a rebate may result in a preferred formulary position *if* the clinical features and benefits of the rebated drug are somewhat similar to nonrebated, more expensive alternatives. The rebate savings obtained reduce the net price of contracted drugs, which, in turn, reduces the overall prescription drug program expenses. A reduced net price will result in a more favorable cost-effectiveness ratio and may result in more positive economic outcomes. These savings are passed on to payers through lower premiums (or lower than would be without re-

bates) and to patients through a lower prescription copayment (rebated products are usually in Tier II, which has a lower prescription copayment than Tier III does).

The effect of rebates is similar to discounts. Health plans and PBMs that contract with community pharmacies and do not take possession of drug products are usually offered rebates. In contrast, health plans with in-house, owned pharmacies that take possession of drug products may qualify for a discount (often a wholesale chargeback). The net result is similar, although the administration and flow of money of rebates and discounts are dissimilar.

Rebate contract terms are varied and somewhat complex. However, in simplest terms, rebates provide health plans with incentives to position contracted products in a favorable position because rebates reduce the net cost of the product. The favorable formulary position helps pharmaceutical manufacturers because physicians and members generally prefer drugs with lower copayments, such as found in Tier II. Rebate contracts often contain two components, an access rebate as well as a performance component.

A flat, access rebate (*eg,* 3%–6%) is offered for a Tier II preferred formulary status. The value of the access rebate may vary based upon the number of competitive products sharing Tier II. For example, if a product has an exclusive Tier II position, the access rebate may be higher, but if the product shares Tier II with one or more other products, the access rebate may be lower. Traditionally, with three-tier open formularies, rebates were not offered for Tier III positioning. However, with closed formularies, commonly seen in Medicare Part D, rebates are offered for Tier III status because, if a product is not covered on Tier I, II, or III, it is not reimbursed in a closed formulary. Thus, manufacturers pay for access to Tier III, which is preferable to their product not being reimbursed at all.

The performance rebate component may be based upon market share (in plan or national), volume growth, or other similar metric. Although a rebate contract may allow a health plan or PBM to include more than one product on a formulary tier, there is a better chance of achieving performance tiers if there are a limited number of products in a tier.

Rebates are additive and highly variable based on the therapeutic category, number of similar products, competitive nature of the category, and the clinical and safety differentiation among products. Products in crowded and undifferentiated therapeutic categories may be associated with total rebate potential of 20% to 30% or more. Conversely, unique, highly differentiated products may have no rebate offered or a very low rebate (*eg,* 5% total rebate). Products and categories associated with no or very low rebates include many unique injectable biological products, HIV/AIDS drugs, and atypical antipsychotics.

Health plans and PBMs are, in general, relatively transparent regarding sharing rebates with their clients, although the exact terms of rebate contracts remain confidential. Rebates are generally passed on to clients or are used to reduce pharmacy program costs.

An example of how a rebate may reduce the net cost of a contracted drug is shown in Table 12-5. In the illustration, the drugs of the same wholesale acquisition cost (WAC) have significantly different net costs based upon formulary tier, member copayment, and rebate (paid for Tier II positioning). As stated earlier, WAC is a realistic price that approximates the actual acquisition cost of a drug. AWP is an artificial, calculated number that is often approximately 20% higher than the WAC, is somewhat archaic, but often is used in pharmacy reimbursement calculations. Rebate calculations are usually based on the WAC.

In this example, the net cost of two drugs with identical WACs is shown. The drug on the preferred Tier II position is associated with a 20% rebate off the WAC. The rebate value is $25.60, which results in a net cost $5.60 less than the Tier III product, despite the higher member copayment associated with the Tier III drug. Rebates will remain an important cost-containment strategy to manage the net cost of brand drugs.

Table 12–5 Impact of Copayment and Rebate on Drug Net Cost to an MCO or PBM

	Preferred Brand Tier II	Nonpreferred Brand Tier III
WAC	$128.00	$128.00
AWP	$160.00	$160.00
Drug reimbursement (AWP – 15%)	$136.00	$136.00
Dispensing fee (+)	$ 2.50	$ 2.50
Subtotal	$138.50	$138.50
Member copayment (–)	$ 25.00	$ 45.00
MCO reimbursement to pharmacy	$113.50	$ 93.50
Rebate (15% of WAC)	20%	0%
Rebate amount (–)	$ 25.60	$ —
Net MCO cost	$ 87.90	$ 93.50

Source: RP Navarro, 2006.

Although the regulation is somewhat more complex, an important result of the Omnibus Budget Reconciliation Act of 1990 (OBRA 1990) was to require pharmaceutical manufacturers to extend commercial drug rebates 15.1% or more to state Medicaid programs. As a result, the rebate on many drugs would not exceed this percentage, although in competitive therapeutic categories, rebates could reach the 20% to 45% range, which is extended to Medicaid programs. Additionally, some state Medicaid programs mandate payment of a "supplementary rebate" to assist in reducing program costs. Other novel rebate contracts, including outcomes-based rebates, adherence-based rebates, and drug expense guarantees, are interesting but often difficult to administer.

Clinical Pharmacy and Disease Management Services

Health plans and PBMs offer an array of clinical pharmacy services, many of which are online and real-time edits provided to the dispensing pharmacist. Others include prospective or retrospective utilization monitoring, adherence intervention, and disease management program support.

Online, real-time point-of-dispensing edits provide commonly used guidance regarding drug interactions, early refill prevention, duplicate medications, age and gender edits, and step-care edits. Health plans and PBMs also provide computerized DUR, screening for drug misuse and abuse, polypharmacy, nonadherence, and other dangerous or inappropriate drug use patterns. Interventions may include patient and/or physician communications requesting clarification of the potential dangerous pattern.

Health plans may offer disease-specific management programs to augment health care services provided by plan physicians that may include general disease education, diagnostic screening events, and case management. Diseases most commonly included in clinical programs are diabetes, asthma,

cardiovascular disease (hypertension and lipid disorders), chronic obstructive pulmonary disease (COPD), congestive heart failure (CHF), and behavioral health (see Chapter 13). Disease management programs in managed care are addressed in Chapter 10.

MCO pharmacy departments and PBMs often play a supportive role in health plan and employer disease management programs. Pharmacy program drug utilization data are often used to identify patients with poorly controlled medical conditions (identified by the number and type of medications used) or those who have drug adherence problems (through inconsistent prescription refill records). Pharmacy departments may obtain resource support from pharmaceutical manufacturers that often provide unbranded disease management resources (*eg,* physician or patient education materials or educational grants) to supplement health plan efforts. Disease management offerings from pharmaceutical manufacturers will not influence formulary decisions, and in fact the reverse influence exists. That is, health plans and MCOs may seek clinical program support from manufacturers whose drugs have been previously selected for preferred formulary positions.

Clinical pharmacy programs are important in supporting health plan quality of care initiatives, such as NCQA accreditation and improvement of NCQA HEDIS measures. This was discussed earlier in the section titled "Pharmacy and Medical Claims Integration and Clinical Program Support."

• Pharmacy Benefit Managers (PBMs)

PBMs, such as Medco Health Solutions, Caremark, Express Scripts, Prime Therapeutics, MedImpact, WellPoint Pharmacy Management, and many others, are stand-alone companies that specialize in all aspects of pharmacy benefit management. They sell their services to private or public purchasers, including MCOs, self-insured employers, Medicaid programs, Medicare Advantage Part D plans, as well as directly to Medicare members and other purchasers of pharmacy benefits. Table 12-6 provides a list of the largest PBMs at the time of publication.

PBMs have evolved as specialized experts in pharmacy benefit management. Many large health plans, such as Aetna, Humana, and CIGNA, manage their pharmacy benefit programs through an internal "captive" PBM. Although many large MCOs manage their pharmacy benefit through an internal pharmacy department, they may use a PBM for claims processing, pharmaceutical manufacturer contracting, and other back-end commodity services. Other small MCOs, large self-insured employers, and state Medicaid agencies may use a PBM for full-service, turnkey prescription drug benefits.

Although PBMs do not offer any services a health plan could not develop through an internal pharmacy department, PBMs manage many millions of lives and offer economies of scale to MCOs regarding computer services, patient call centers, contracting with pharmacies and pharmaceutical manufacturers, and other services. The PBM may offer such services less expensively than could be developed by an MCO.

The amount of PBM services purchased by MCOs, Medicare or Medicaid plans, and self-insured employers, depends entirely on the needs of the PBMs' customer. Some of the offered services include the following:

- Pharmacy distribution network (community, mail, and possibly specialty products)
- Drug formulary development and management
- P & T committee support services
- Pharmaceutical manufacturer contracting
- Physician and member communications
- Member service help line support
- Health plan pharmacy benefit Web site development and maintenance
- Clinical pharmacy services (utilization review, adherence monitoring, clinical edit development) and disease management program support
- Claims processing and report generation

The PBM market is very competitive, and most large PBMs offer similar services. Decisions on PBM selection usually come down to aligned interests (*eg,* cost containment, member services, and clinical programs), transparency, quality of service, and cost.

Measuring Pharmacy Benefit Management Program Performance

The competitive managed care environment requires that health plan and PBM pharmacy programs are effectively managed to achieve desired clinical, economic, and qualify-of-life objectives. Health plans have been criticized for managing pharmacy costs separate from medical costs, when the use of resources—and outcomes—of both may be inextricably linked for many medical conditions. As discussed earlier, appropriate use of cost-effective pharmaceuticals may result in higher pharmacy program costs, but may prevent use of more expensive medical resources, such as hospitalizations and emergency department visits.

Despite the awareness that the pharmacy program must be managed to optimize the drug spend, the pharmacy director must focus on pharmacy program performance met-

Table 12–6 Membership of Largest U.S. PBMs

PBM	Number of Members (millions)
Caremark	103
Medco Health Solutions	71
Express Scripts, Inc.	51
WellPoint Pharmacy Management	36
MedImpact	21
Prime Therapeutics	8

Source: Compiled by RP Navarro from PBM Web sites and marketing material, April 2006.

rics as well. The pharmacy program director will monitor specific performance metrics on a monthly basis and attempt to modify controllable factors if performance measures suggest costs are rising more than forecast, member satisfaction is declining, drug-related clinical outcomes are not being achieved, or other markers of poor pharmacy program performance are indicated.

Some of the basic performance benchmarks monitored (monthly, quarterly, or annually) usually include the following financial and quality-of-care metrics:

- Total prescription program costs as well as costs and trends of selected therapeutic categories and specific high-cost and/or highly utilized drugs
- Monthly per member per month (PMPM) and annual PMPY program costs—PMPM and PMPY for high-cost therapeutic categories, as well as cost trends
- Prescription utilization (PMPM and PMPY) overall and for selected highly utilized therapeutic categories
- Administrative and claims processing fees (overall and per prescription)
- Prescription discount or rebate (total amount, per prescription, PMPM, and PMPY)
- Generic dispensing rate (overall, by pharmacy, by group, by therapeutic class, and by physician) and missed generic substitution opportunities
- Drug formulary conformance rate (overall, by physician, and by pharmacy)
- Patient satisfaction and member complaints related to the pharmacy program
- Number of drug formulary prior authorization exception requests and approvals, and review of authorization trend

- NCQA HEDIS measure scores related to pharmacy (*eg,* percentage of post-MI patients receiving a beta blocker)
- Trend of all the preceding performance measurements measured monthly, quarterly, or annually

There are many more performance measurements pharmacy directors routinely monitor, especially with more sophisticated programs that may include drug formulary conversion, compliance, and persistence activities. However, with the preceding basic performance measurements, a pharmacy director can evaluate the effectiveness of his or her prescription drug management program.

CONCLUSION

Pharmacy benefits are an important component in comprehensive health care benefits, and when optimized, can contribute to clinical, economic, and quality-of-life outcomes of benefit to payers as well as members. Purchasers of pharmacy benefits have many options to obtain a customized pharmacy program and must identify their objectives clearly to their pharmacy benefit provider to make certain the benefit is appropriately designed. Primary future challenges will be control of expensive biologicals and implementing a successful consumer-driven health care benefit, such as through a Health Savings Account.

Pharmacy directors see increased use of generics and higher member copayments as two important methods of helping to contain costs. However, the pharmacy benefit must be integrated into the broad medical benefit to demonstrate the contribution of appropriately used, cost-effective pharmaceuticals.

References

1. Navarro RP. Unpublished primary managed care research. 2004–2006.

2. Centers for Medicare and Medicaid Services. Prescription Drug Expenditures (Table 11). In: *National health care expenditure projections: 2005–2015*. Available at: http://www.cms.hhs.gov/NationalHealthExpendData/downloads/proj2005.pdf. Accessed May 8, 2006.

3. RP Navarro. Personal communication with pharmacy and medical directors. 2005–2006.

4. NCPDP. Available at: http://www.ncpdp.org/frame_about.htm. Accessed May 13, 2006.

5. National Committee for Quality Assurance. Health plan report card. Available at: http://hprc.ncqa.org/. Accessed May 13, 2006.

6. National Committee for Quality Assurance. The Health Plan Employer Data and Information Set (HEDIS). Available at: http://www.ncqa.org/programs/hedis/. Accessed May 31, 2006.

7. eHealth Initiative. Electronic prescribing: Toward maximum value and rapid adoption. Recommendations for optimal design and implementation to improve care, increase efficiency and reduce costs in ambulatory care. 2004:11. Available at: http://www.ehealthinitiative.org/initiatives/erx/document.aspx?Category = 249&Document = 270. Accessed April 5, 2005.

8. Agency for Healthcare Research and Quality. MEPS highlights #11: Distribution of health care expenses. 1999. Available at: http://www.meps.ahrq.gov/mepsweb/data_files/publications/ hl11/hl11. shtml.

9. Institute for Safe Medication Practices. A call to action: Eliminate hand-written prescriptions within 3 years. 2000. Available at: http://www.ismp.org/msaarticles/whitepaper.html. Accessed April 5, 2005.

10. RxHub. Available at: http://www.rxhub.net/about.html. Accessed May 31, 2006.

11. U.S. Department of Labor. Health plans and benefits: Employee Retirement Income Security Act—ERISA. Available at: http://www.dol.gov/dol/topic/health-plans/erisa.htm. Accessed April 18, 2006.

12. California Healthline. States consider encouraging increased use of HSAs. February 13, 2006. Available at: http://www.californiahealthline.org/index.cfm?Action = dspItem&itemID = 118692. Accessed June 2, 2006.

13. Consumer Driver Health Care Institute. Our mission. Available at: http://www.cdhci.org/. Accessed June 2, 2006.

14. RP Navarro. Personal communication with benefit consultants and employer health benefit officers. 2006.

15. National Association of Chain Drug Stores. 2004 community pharmacy results. Available at: http://www.nacds.org/user-assets/PDF_files/2004results.PD. Accessed June 2, 2006.

16. Minnesota Blues injectable drug cost July 2003–June 2004. *Specialty Pharmacy News*. January 2006:3(1), 11.

17. National Association of Boards of Pharmacy. VIPPS information and verification. Available at: http://www.nabp.net/. Accessed June 3, 2006.

18. National Association of Boards of Pharmacy. VIPPS database search results. Available at: http://www.nabp.net/vipps/consumer/listall.asp. Accessed June 3, 2006.

19. American Academy of Family Physicians (AAFP). Available at: http://www.aafp.org/online/en/home/policy/policies/d/drugs.html. Accessed June 3, 2006.

20. Academy of Managed Care Pharmacy. AMCP format for formulary submissions Version 2.1. Available at: http://www.amcp.org/amcp.ark?c = pr&sc = link. Accessed June 2, 2006.

21. Goldberg RB. Managing the pharmacy benefit: The formulary system. *J Manag Care*. 1997: 3(5), 565–573.

22. Sax MJ and Emigh R. Managed care formularies in the United States. *Journal of Managed Care Pharmacy*. Vol 5, No. 4 July/August: 289–295. Available at: http://www.aafp.org/online/en/home/policy/policies/d/drugs.html. Accessed June 3, 2006.

23. Rector TS, Finch MD, Danzon PM, *et al*. Effect of tiered prescription copayments on the use of preferred brand medications. *Medical Care*. March 2003:41(3), 398–406.

24. Sokol MC, McGuigan KA, Verbrugge RR, Epstein RS. Impact of medication adherence on hospitalization risk and healthcare cost. *Medical Care*. June 2005:43(6), 521–530.

25. Landsman PB, Yu W, Liu X, Teutsch SM, Berger ML. Impact of 3-tier pharmacy benefit design and increased consumer cost-sharing on drug utilization. *Am J Manag Care*. 2005:11, 621–628.

26. Gibson TB, Ozminkowsk RJ, Goetzel RZ. The effects of prescription drug cost sharing: A review of the evidence. *Am J Manag Care.* 2005:11, 730–740.

27. Rand Corporation. Cutting drug copayments for sicker patients can cut hospitalizations and save money. January 11, 2006. Available at: http://www.rand.org/news/press.06/01.11. html. Accessed June 2, 2006.

28. PR Newswire. Total value/total return tells the Pitney Bowes experience: Healthier employees translate into a healthier bottom line. April 17, 2006. Available at: http://media. prnewswire.com/en/jsp/tradeshows/events.jsp ?option = tradeshow&beat = BEAT_ALL& eventid = 1001951&view = LATEST& resourceid = 3187226. Accessed June 2, 2006.

13

Introduction to Managed Behavioral Health Care Organizations

Joann Albright, Deborah Heggie, Anthony M. Kotin,
Lawrence Nardozzi, and Fred Waxenberg

Study Objectives

- Understand the differences between behavioral health managed care and medical-surgical managed care.
- Understand the different forms of managed care treatment in behavioral managed care.
- Understand how behavioral managed health care is integrated into the larger health system.
- Understand the different approaches a behavioral health management organization might take for different HMOs or non-HMO health plans.

Discussion Topics

1. Discuss the unique factors that present special challenges to behavioral health management as compared to medical-surgical management.
2. Discuss which types of behavioral health treatment methods form the backbone of managed care service.
3. Discuss the advantages and disadvantages of a managed care plan using an external vendor versus managing behavioral health services using internal resources.

INTRODUCTION

The management of mental health benefits has undergone substantial changes over the past two decades. These changes result from a confluence of circumstances, environmental as well as structural. The call for change was hastened when, in February of 2001, President George W. Bush announced his New Freedom Initiative and, subsequently, the New Freedom Commission on Mental Health. The commission established six goals for a "transformed mental health system" that could overcome barriers preventing Americans from receiving appropriate health care for mental health and substance use disorders. The transformed mental health system would have the following characteristics:

1. Recognize that mental health is essential to physical health.
2. Provide mental health care that is consumer- and family-driven.
3. Eliminate disparities in coverage.
4. Make mental health screening, assessment, and referral standard practice.
5. Deliver excellent mental health care and accelerate research.
6. Use technology to increase access to mental health care and information.

We have a long way to go.

In the early days of managed care, mental health utilization was managed by medical directors who were trained in predominantly nonpsychiatric disciplines. Services use was driven by benefit plan designs that were clearly distinct from those used for health benefits. These designs typically included annual "day limits" that rapidly became the average for inpatient days and outpatient services. To the health care system at large, mental health benefits were easily defined, difficult to manage, and consumed 10% of the medical costs.

As the managed care industry matured, payers became increasingly aware that mental health benefits should be managed by mental health specialists. Thus, the managed behavioral health industry emerged. The growth of this new specialty industry was fostered by the emergence of safe, highly effective medications for the treatment of major mental illnesses such as depression and psychosis. Drug spending for mental illnesses grew from $2.7 billion in 1987 to $17.8 billion in 2001.[1] The new drugs made nonpsychiatrists feel comfortable treating patients who presented with symptoms of depression and other mental health disorders and shifted the venue of service from the inpatient to the ambulatory setting. At the same time, the stigma of mental illness began to diminish, primarily because of celebrities publicly revealing their struggles with mental health disorders.

As managed behavioral health care began its ascendance, the seeds were being sown for its diffusion and absorption back into mainstream medical care. According to data recently collected by Magellan Health Services, 75% to 80% of prescriptions for behavioral health medications were written by nonpsychiatrists. The reasons for reabsorption are twofold. First, although stigma in general was reduced, among health care clinicians there remained a hesitation to render a mental health diagnosis for an individual presenting to general medical settings. The second—and perhaps most potent—issue was that most health plans would not pay nonpsychiatrists for treatment of mental health diagnoses. Thus, although 25% of the population was being treated for mental health, only 5%, or the average penetration of the membership covered by a managed behavioral health organization (MBHO) was being appropriately accounted for through accurate diagnosis and service coding. As a result, in 2006 the MBHO calculated share of the total health care expense was 1.5 to 2 cents on the dollar. This is an historic low because between 1971 and 2001 the calculated share of behavioral health relative to national health expenditures fell from 11.1% to 5.9%.[2]

Although inpatient confinements have been reduced substantially and outpatient services have become more effectively managed, when all behavioral health services are accounted for, the actual impact of mental health very well could be greater than the 10% of health care expenditures seen in the early days of managed care.

THE NATURE AND UNIQUENESS OF BEHAVIORAL HEALTH

Although marginalized and misunderstood, mental health is not a minor issue. As Table 13-1 shows, depressive and anxiety disorders affect large numbers of people.

Despite their widespread occurrence, psychiatric conditions remain poorly understood by the general public and incompletely understood by many clinicians outside of psychiatry. This extends to substance-related disorders. Franklin and colleagues note that "stigma associated with the term *alcoholism* frequently inhibits physicians and patients from exploring the connection between [substance] abuse and bio-psychosocial consequences."[3] They further note that "psychiatrists participating in a hospital survey positively identified alcohol

abuse two-thirds of the time, whereas physicians treating gynecology patients diagnosed the disorder only 10% of the time."[3,4]

As understanding of brain chemistry has evolved, there has been a concomitant and significant impact on the treatment of behavioral health conditions. Schatzberg and colleagues summarize this view when they argue that over the past 30 years, psychiatry's "move from a largely psychoanalytic orientation toward a more biological stance radically changed not only its basic approaches to patients but also the professional identities of psychiatrists."[5]

At its core, behavioral health attempts to interpret neurophysiology as manifested by behavior. This is by no means a simple task and proves daunting for even the most talented professionals. Behavior can reasonably be interpreted as the consequence of activities in the mind and the mind as a state of being both influenced by and influencing brain chemistry. Yet psychiatric nosology (*ie*, the systematic classification of diseases) partly ignores this paradigm by its shift from imputed motivation in certain conditions to a phenomenological approach that relies solely on the observation of behavior or a patient's self-report.

Nothing, for example, in the American Psychiatric Association's (APA's) description of a major depressive episode[6] implies a psychological antecedent to depression. The description relies solely on the patient's report, and/or observation by the clinician or others, of a depressed mood, markedly diminished interest in or pleasure from activities, significant weight loss or decreased or increased appetite, insomnia or hypersomnia, psychomotor agitation or retardation, fatigue or loss of energy, feelings of worthlessness or excessive/inappropriate guilt, diminished ability to think or concentrate, and recurrent thoughts of death or suicidal ideation.

Given the plethora of theories and schools of thought about the psychology of human beings, the emphasis on observation of behavior and patient self-report is necessary for

Table 13–1 Prevalence of Depressive and Anxiety Disorders in Adults

Disorder	Estimated Prevalence
Dysthymic disorder	10,900,000
Major depressive disorder	9,900,000
Social phobia	5,300,000
Post-traumatic stress disorder	5,200,000
Generalized anxiety disorder	4,000,000
Obsessive-compulsive disorder	3,300,000
Agoraphobia	3,200,000
Panic disorder	2,400,000
Bipolar disorder	2,300,000

Source: National Institutes of Mental Health, 2004.

the creation of an empirical system that is manageable and easily validated. Although such a system serves the health care industry well, it is necessarily circumscribed and unable to match the complexity of the human condition, especially in regard to an individual's motivation, which may be a key to effecting therapeutic change.

Although the APA's catalog of symptoms, as presented earlier, makes the diagnosis of depression a relatively straightforward task for a psychiatrist or behavioral health clinician, even such a basic task is complicated by differential diagnosis. For example, the symptoms of a major depressive episode occur within the context of major depressive disorder, or they may constitute the depressive phase of Bipolar Disorder, depression secondary to a medical condition, depression as related to substance use or withdrawal, depression as manifested in Premenstrual Dysphoric Disorder, depression as related to bereavement or complicated bereavement, or depression as associated with Cyclothymic Disorder. It is small wonder, then, that diagnosis of behavioral health disorders poses many challenges to clinicians and patients alike. It is no small consideration whether expecting acute care, general medical clinicians to understand the nuances of behavioral diagnosis under the structural and process pressures inherent in general practice settings is realistic or in the public interest.

Another emerging facet of the field of behavioral health is the growing evidence for and understanding of the connection between the body and the mind. Psychosomatic medicine, which is rooted in consultation-liaison psychiatry and has grown from modest beginnings in U.S. medicine in the 1930s, remains a valuable subspecialty. With an emphasis on the mind-body connection, psychosomatic medicine remains a vital force in opposition to the split—predominantly an artifact of having made a distinction between mind and body—that too readily occurs between physical and mental approaches to diagnosis and treatment. Mainstream psychi-

atry acknowledges the mind-body connection by its elimination of "functional" (being emotional or psychological in nature) and "organic" (being physiologic or anatomic in nature—a concept in previous editions of the *Diagnostic and Statistical Manual of Mental Disorders*).

Proper diagnosis is, of course, of paramount importance in any medical specialty. It is no less so in behavioral health. Treatment plans can be effective only if based on proper diagnosis because the diagnosis determines not only the treatments offered (*eg*, medication and/or psychotherapy), but also risk factors and prognosis. Yet, as the example of depression demonstrates, a clear diagnosis is not always evident to even the most skilled clinician, especially on initial evaluation. Accuracy of diagnosis and appropriateness of treatment planning have ramifications for an individual's morbidity, productivity, and sense of well-being, as well as for the cost of effective treatment. Furthermore, because many behavioral health disorders are chronic, and chronicity may become evident only after adequate time in treatment, incorrect diagnosis and inappropriate treatment planning can foster noncompliance, relapse, and excessive costs for treatment. Risks for noncompliance, relapse, and excessive cost may not be as pronounced for general medical conditions (*eg*, hypertension, hyperlipidemia, or diabetes) where laboratory or physical tests to identify and monitor these conditions are readily available.

In response to these challenges, managed behavioral health care organizations have gone beyond the traditional gatekeeper function of utilization management. Prevention and disease management programs identify members at risk because of behavioral health and/or medical conditions and provide education and outreach to reduce morbidity and enhance well-being. Intensive care management programs meet the needs of members with more serious or long-term care needs. Alongside these initiatives are outcome measurement protocols that measure effectiveness in terms of reduction in morbidity and increase in productivity—key issues for the health plans and employers that typically cover the costs of care.

THE PUBLIC SECTOR

If individuals with mental health and substance use disorders pose special challenges for health care systems, individuals that receive care through Medicaid benefits present additional, complex problems. Medicaid-managed care is also discussed in Chapter 27.

Medicaid populations have a much higher incidence of debilitating psychiatric illness, such as schizophrenia and bipolar disorder, than the general population does. Medicaid beneficiaries by definition lack resources to access the private health care system easily, and the serious and persistent nature of their behavioral disorders makes them less likely to comply with treatment or maintain routine follow-up care. Reduced or absent access to routine and preventive care, cultural and linguistic factors, lack of family and social supports, and lack of community resources conspire to make effective participation in behavioral health treatment much less likely. Managed behavioral health care systems have been able to address the unique needs of Medicaid populations through innovative, evidence-based programs that provide solutions to the complex, myriad barriers that reduce participation in behavioral health care.

NETWORKS

As discussed in Chapter 5 regarding the physician network, one of the defining features of managed care in general, and managed behavioral health care in particular, is the establishment and use of a credentialed clinical network. The philosophy of behavioral health network management has changed over the past few decades. Originally, behavioral health care companies developed small, contained networks, contracting with facilities and providers at discounted rates in return for increased referral streams to these pre-

ferred providers. The modest size of these networks allowed behavioral health care companies to track utilization and quality indicators and helped control the cost of care.

As the managed care industry matured, consumers opted for less restrictive products with more choice of providers than in traditional health maintenance organizations (HMOs). Managed behavioral health care companies responded by expanding their networks to include a larger selection of providers to allow greater consumer choice and clinical specialization. Companies created mechanisms to decrease barriers to access and enabled members to search for providers using Internet and telephone technologies. The downside to the development of broader and larger networks was reduced opportunity to collect and interpret meaningful quality data on credentialed providers. Recently, managed behavioral health care companies have responded to this challenge by implementing new strategies designed to collect outcomes and/or quality data regardless of network size and composition.

PAYMENT MECHANISMS

In the last two decades, behavioral health care financing strategies mirrored to a large extent those developed in the medical arena as discussed in Chapter 6. As HMOs developed and matured, there was a movement to share financial risk with large provider groups and delivery systems through capitation contracts. Subcapitated groups were paid set rates regardless of the number of patients served. Contracts varied as to the levels of care and services covered. By the year 2000, however, the popularity of capitation as a risk-sharing strategy ebbed as a result of the well-publicized collapse of a number of large provider groups.

More recently, different financing strategies have developed based on whether a mental health and substance abuse provider operates at the inpatient or outpatient level. Outpatient providers have been contracted with and paid using fee-for-service (FFS) compensation arrangements, with compensation varying based on specific, negotiated fee schedules. Fee-for-service rate schedules depend on provider type (*eg*, psychiatrist, psychologist, social worker), current procedural terminology (CPT) codes, and state(s) in which services are rendered.

Inpatient providers more recently have been compensated using per diem schedules specific to the type of service and program (*eg*, hospital inpatient, intermediate care, residential treatment, partial hospitalization, day treatment, and intensive outpatient). The rates depend on a number of variables, including the facility's retail rates, location, availability of comparable services in the same area, and prevailing market rates.

ACCESS AND DENSITY STANDARDS

As managed behavioral health care organizations grew national in scope, they began to review their clinical networks using access and density standards. Such review was necessary because of variation in the number and availability of mental health and substance use providers across regions and in rural versus urban settings.

A number of factors are considered in reviewing access and density. *Access* is defined as the availability of a provider within a certain geographical distance of the population. Access standards vary depending upon whether an area is considered urban, suburban, or rural as determined by U.S. Census data in conjunction with the latest U.S. Postal Service ZIP code updates.

- Urban = Population of 3,000 or more per square mile
- Suburban = Population of 1,000 to 2,999 per square mile
- Rural = Population of fewer than 1,000 per square mile

Table 13-2 illustrates access standards for urban, suburban, and rural areas.

Density refers to the type and number of professionals per covered member. Psychiatrists are broken out from the other classes of therapists because of the specialized services they provide. Table 13-3 illustrates density standards for psychiatrists and nonpsychiatrists.

Behavioral health care organizations typically use commercially developed computer programs to determine the adequacy of their networks in relation to the characteristics of the population they are serving.

Behavioral health as a discipline is served by a variety of licensed professionals, including psychiatrists, psychologists, social workers, licensed professional counselors, marriage and family therapists, and clinical nurse specialists. Managed behavioral health care companies create their own requirements for acceptance of these provider classes because states vary greatly on their requirements for licensure and the degree of professional autonomy associated with specific licenses.

CREDENTIALING

Providers undergo a standard credentialing and contracting process before they are in-

Table 13–2 Network Provider Access Standards

MHSA	Urban Areas	Suburban Areas	Rural Areas
One psychiatrist and one other behavioral professional	90% within 10 miles	90% within 25 miles	90% within 40 miles
One organizational provider (facility)	90% within 25 miles	90% within 40 miles	90% within 60 miles

Table 13–3 Network Provider Density Standards

Psychiatrist	Nonpsychiatrist	Total	Number of Covered Lives
2	8	10	10,000

cluded in a network. National accrediting bodies such as the National Committee for Quality Assurance (NCQA), the Joint Commission for the Accreditation of Health Care Organizations (JCAHO), and Utilization Review Accreditation Commission (URAC) have established standards for the types of information that must be collected and verified in the credentialing process. External accreditation is discussed in detail in Chapter 23.

Because of the nature of behavioral health services, credentialing processes include review of information on providers' clinical specialty, language, and ethnicity. Providers identify their subspecialties and evidence for them. Some of the more commonly recognized subspecialties are the following:

- Marriage/family
- Child/adolescent
- Substance use disorders
- Eating disorders
- Lesbian/gay issues
- HIV/AIDS
- Anxiety
- Faith-based counseling (provider is asked to identify religion)
- Workplace/career issues

Network providers typically are recredentialed every 3 years. Some states and customers may require recredentialing more frequently. As part of the recredentialing process, essential elements of the provider's application are reviewed again. The credentialing department performs primary source verification for licensure, liability claims history, Medicare/Medicaid sanctions, and history of criminal activity.

A clinical review is performed once the administrative aspects of the recredentialing process are completed. This includes a review of any new malpractice or action against licensure information, presence of complaints, and outcome and patient satisfaction data (if available). The clinical reviewers make the final decision as to whether to recredential the provider.

TYPES OF SERVICES DELIVERED BY BEHAVIORAL NETWORKS

Behavioral health care networks allow for the provision of an extensive array of services and levels of care. The typical commercial delivery system classification includes the following:

- *Inpatient services.* Inpatient services are the highest level of skilled psychiatric and substance abuse services and usually are provided in a hospital facility involving 24-hour medical and nursing care, such as a freestanding psychiatric facility, a general hospital, or a detoxification unit in a hospital.
- *Residential treatment.* Residential treatment services are rendered in a facility that offers 24-hour care and provides patients with severe mental disorders or substance-related disorders a continuum of therapeutic services. Licensure requirements vary by state, but settings that are eligible for this level of care are licensed at the residential intermediate level or as an intermediate care facility.
- *Partial hospitalization.* Partial hospitalization programs provide structured mental health or substance abuse therapeutic services for at least 4 hours per day and at least 3 days per week. Services are delivered by a multidisciplinary team.
- *Intensive outpatient program.* Intensive outpatient programs provide structured therapeutic services for at least 2 hours per day and at least 3 days per week. Services are composed of coordinated

and integrated multidisciplinary services such as individual, family or multifamily group therapy, psychoeducational services, and medical monitoring.

Outpatient treatment. Traditional outpatient therapy includes individual, family, or group treatment rendered by a licensed professional for a specified duration of time. This includes medication evaluation and monitoring by a professional licensed to provide that service (typically psychiatrists or clinical nurse specialists).

Employment assistance programs (EAPs). EAP professionals deliver short-term, problem-focused services for employees and their families. Services are delivered in an outpatient setting and focus on finding solutions for work and personal problems. Services are free to the user and delivered within a 3-, 5-, or 7-session model.

NETWORKS IN THE PUBLIC SECTOR

Public sector networks frequently encompass a greater range of services and delivery systems because myriad services are needed by the public sector population. Consequently, these networks often include nontraditional provider and organization types, such as the following, which usually are provided under the supervision of a community mental health center.

Supervised living. Supervised living includes community-based residential detoxification programs, community-based residential rehabilitation in halfway or quarter-way houses, specialized foster care homes, and group homes. Services include a combination of outpatient therapy and assistance in managing basic day-to-day living activities.

Programs for assertive community treatment (PACT/ACT teams). In PACT/ACT units, multidisciplinary teams deliver services directly in the community to members who demonstrate a pattern of recidi-

vism and symptom chronicity and severity. The structure of the teams and delivery system are highly standardized.

Peer support. In peer support programs, consumers who have attained a high level of recovery work under the supervision of a behavioral health provider and assist patients in building confidence and in improving life skills.

Continuous treatment teams (CTT). Continuous treatment teams are multidisciplinary and provide a range of intensive integrated case management, treatment, and rehabilitative services in an effort to prevent a child's removal from the home to a more restrictive level of care. The team uses a community-based family strengths model and philosophy.

Community case management. Community case management workers coordinate care and social services delivered within the community. They collaborate with the systems and providers rendering the care.

QUALITY MANAGEMENT OF NETWORKS

As with all aspects of managed behavioral health care, quality is a prime concern. Organizations manage the quality of the services delivered by their network providers and facilities through a variety of means, including treatment record audits, satisfaction data, and the tracking of complaints, adverse incidents, and quality of care concerns. Increasingly, managed behavioral health care organizations are expanding their quality measurement efforts to include patient safety considerations, evidence-based guidelines, treatment outcomes data, and objective measures, such as the Health Plan Employer Data Information Set (HEDIS) measures from NCQA for ambulatory follow-up and antidepressant medication management.

Two emerging trends are provider/facility profiles based on clinical, outcomes, and utilization data, and pay-for-performance initiatives. Behavioral health care organizations have lagged behind the medical arena in the development and implementation of these activities, primarily because of the lack of available and widely accepted objective behavioral health measures. Unlike in general medicine, easily identified and accepted tests that indicate improvement in a patient's mental health and well-being are not available. The stigma associated with mental health diagnoses may be another factor in the slow adoption of these trends.[7] Despite these challenges, it is likely that managed behavioral health care companies will move forward in this direction.[8]

Successful pay-for-performance initiatives as described in Chapter 8 are characterized by involvement of the provider community in the program design, adoption of nationally recognized and reliable measurements that are viewed as clinically relevant, a financial incentive that is of a size and structure that is meaningful to the provider, and a compensation methodology that is easy to understand and calculate.[9,10] Under the direction and leadership of the Centers for Medicaid and Medicare Services (CMS), the public sector has been one of the leaders in the adoption and rollout of pay-for-performance initiatives. A summary document prepared by the Center for Health Care Strategies summarizes the different pay-for-performance initiatives that are being tracked across states. Several of the initiatives relate specifically to behavioral health populations,[11] including adolescent readmissions to residential facilities, ambulatory follow-up visits within 30 days post discharge, and community tenure. On the commercial side, there hasn't been consensus yet about the metrics or program structure best suited for a pay for performance program. Different managed behavioral health companies have implemented initiatives targeting different provider populations and financially rewarded the adoption of targeted metrics. There is a strong likelihood that behavioral health-based pay-for-performance programs will continue to expand in the coming years.

USE OF STANDARDIZED ASSESSMENT TOOLS

In recent years, the managed behavioral health care industry has begun using standardized assessment tools in day-to-day clinical operations. This represents a major shift in the industry. The major focus of behavioral health managed care in the 1970s and 1980s was cost containment achieved through the determination of what was medically necessary and what was not, and managing benefits accordingly. Increasingly, employers and other health care purchasers are requiring a focus on clinical outcomes in addition to cost containment.

In response, managed behavioral health care organizations found that the majority of the costs in behavioral health were associated with a minority of chronic patients who required repeated interventions over time. The reason is that once a condition becomes full blown, it often requires very intensive and high-cost services to manage, often with limited success. To conserve resources and achieve optimal return with an ever-growing demand for services, MBHOs began focusing on how to identify and manage this chronic population proactively by intervening in early phases of illness when relatively less intense and less costly treatments could be effective. Increasingly, MBHOs are demonstrating that accurate behavioral diagnosis and attention to medical, neurological, and substance abuse issues reduce repeat hospitalizations and excessive ambulatory visits, with reductions in attendant costs of care and burden of illness.

A growing aspect of the trend toward proactive identification and intervention is an emphasis on high-prevalence mental disorders, such as depressive and anxiety disorders, that frequently coexist with medical disorders, such as heart disease, diabetes, and cancer. This emphasis is based on the belief that medical costs can be significantly lowered if coexisting mental disorders are aggressively managed, such that patients are more engaged in and compliant with medical treatment. This belief is borne out by a growing body of data suggesting that the course and prognosis for at least some medical conditions are affected or mediated by mental disorders. For example, the link between recovery after a coronary event and the presence or absence of depression is now well-established. MBHOs have become more directly involved with general medical patients in activities that provide added value to the efforts of the medical providers to reduce impact, course, and severity of medical disorders.

The prime example of such involvement is the explosion in growth in the last 10 years of disease management programs (see also Chapter 10). These programs have been designed to meet two objectives: (1) to help patients successfully manage chronic behavioral disorders and (2) to identify and mitigate the effects of mental disorders that may reduce treatment effectiveness and increase costs of care for physical illnesses, such as diabetes. In the service of motivating medical patients to engage in self-care and treatments that address their coexisting mental disorders, MBHOs have embraced the technique of motivational coaching. Coaching is offered to patients directly by the MBHO, providing education, encouragement, and other assistance to enhance motivation for and engagement in treatment, assist in the coordination of care with multiple providers, and support the patient during the therapeutic process. Disease management and coaching activities are indications of a major paradigm shift in which MBHOs work directly with patients and not solely with providers. Because these are new and innovative approaches, their clinical and financial effectiveness has not been proved. To demonstrate the return on investment, MBHOs have embedded ongoing outcomes measurement, using standard assessment instruments to establish baseline status and improvement during treatment, into program design.

At present, most MBHOs are using internally developed health risk assessments, which assess a range of behavioral and physical conditions to target areas for assistance. Other widely used general assessment tools include QualityMetric's SF-36 and the SF-12, which often are used in conjunction with tools for assessment for specific conditions, such as the PHQ-9 and Beck Depression Inventory for depression, and the CAGE and AUDIT for substance use disorders.

UTILIZATION MANAGEMENT

For most managed care companies, utilization management is conducted telephonically by licensed mental health professionals, referred to as care managers, who review cases with provider, facility, or program personnel. Reviews may also be conducted with other members of the treatment team as needed. The care managers use evidence-based medical necessity criteria addressing intensity of services and severity of need to determine the most appropriate level of care. The care managers have access to licensed clinical supervisors, board certified psychiatrists, and addictionologists to assist in clinical decision making.

Utilization review occurs when treatment is requested and is reviewed at intervals thereafter to assess treatment issues, screen for potential quality of care issues, and arrange for discharge and aftercare planning.

OUTPATIENT MANAGEMENT

Trends in MBHOs' management of outpatient services have varied during the past few decades. Initially, MBHOs used precertification and concurrent review to manage outpatient care. Typically, 3 to 10 sessions were authorized at the start of treatment. If the clinician required additional sessions, she or he submitted a request that included clinical information on which a clinical reviewer could determine case severity, progress to date, and necessity of additional treatment. Over time, MBHOs reduced the amount of information needed for reviewing care and introduced technologies, such as telephonic and Web-enabled forms, to reduce the administrative burden for clinicians. Currently, MBHOs serving commercial populations vary in the use of precertification and concurrent review for the management of outpatient care. These activities increasingly are being combined with data-driven strategies tailored to members' specific, identified health care needs.

MANAGEMENT OF INPATIENT AND INTERMEDIATE LEVELS OF CARE

Initially, inpatient and intermediate level of care management efforts focused on containment strategies, such as primary care gatekeepers, benefit limitations, discounted provider fees, and restrictions on coverage of certain types of conditions. When MBHOs arrived on the scene, the focus shifted to promoting the delivery of clinically effective specialty care and services in the least restrictive setting that was safe and effective for a given patient.

As MBHOs evolve, utilization management strategies have begun to emphasize the following:

- Addressing the psychosocial precipitants to admission to high levels of care to get early treatment response and avert the need for admission.
- Increasing ambulatory follow-up to help prevent unnecessary readmission to high levels of care.
- Reducing readmission through intensive interventions for at-risk patients.
- Measuring and tracking clinical performance with a focus on outcomes and efficiency.
- Reducing relapse through effective aftercare planning and use of community and social supports.
- Coordinating services among multiple agencies and providers.

- Emphasizing the quality of services provided through supervision, clinical rounds, live call and documentation audits, analysis of complaints, patient and provider satisfaction surveying, in-service staff training, and outcomes tracking.

Two other factors have had a role in utilization management of inpatient and other high levels of care. Employee assistance programs have reduced utilization because EAP counselors assist people in handling social, vocational, and behavioral issues and problems before they reach crisis levels that may require higher levels of care. The use of networks with specialty care clinicians also has reduced high-level utilization through accurate matching of patients with providers who specialize in the presenting issues. Such matching can increase the likelihood that behavioral health needs will be addressed adequately and will not escalate such that higher levels of care will be needed.

RECENT TRENDS IN UTILIZATION MANAGEMENT

The absolute cost of behavioral health services relative to medical costs has historically been, and remains, a relatively small proportion. Thus, the intensity of management resources applied to a large number of members must be carefully managed because the savings opportunity per each contact is far less than it is for members with a medical condition.

This has resulted in a shift of focus from case by case to targeted, data-driven efforts and increased partnerships with providers. For example:

- Through the management of patient and provider data gathered over many years, MBHOs have developed national and regional norms, by diagnosis, for higher levels of care. Routine decisions can be based on these norms with review resources used for complicated cases at high risk for readmission based on past history.

- Reviews increasingly focus on how providers can improve the quality and/or efficiency of treatment and how the MBHO can assist through specialized services, such as intensive care management.
- Field care management programs, in which MBHO staff work with patients in the community, have been found effective in maintaining patient stability while reducing use of higher levels of care.
- Provider education and communication, based on outcomes monitoring, have become the norm.
- Partnerships between MBHOs and facilities or programs with similar values has reduced front-end utilization management and increased joint management by outcomes.

Although utilization management will remain a basic function of MBHOs, current trends suggest that utilization increasingly will be addressed through cooperative efforts with providers on how to increase the quality and efficiency of the care and boost provider self-management through education and data management. Continued innovative efforts, such as field care management aimed at the chronic high-risk population, also will be an ongoing focus.

SPECIALIZED SERVICES

Managed behavioral health companies increasingly are using health risk assessment questionnaires, claims, and pharmacy data to link members proactively to services appropriate to the severity of their condition. Members are assigned to a defined risk level based on their questionnaire responses, diagnosis, and historical utilization pattern. Care management services are then provided based on the associated risk level. This continuum typically ranges from prevention and psychoeducational interventions to intensive care management (ICM) involving direct contact with both members and providers.

INTENSIVE CARE MANAGEMENT

ICM services have a long history in the public behavioral health delivery system. These services emerged out of utilization research showing that a small percentage of patients repeatedly used costly inpatient services. In the late 1970s, Stein and Test implemented an ICM program in Wisconsin characterized by assertive outreach to individuals with frequent psychiatric hospitalization, "hands-on" intensive case management by care managers, and ongoing involvement with patients across service setting.[12] Consistently, such hands-on ICM services have been found effective in reducing inpatient services in the public sector.[13-15]

By the early 2000s, many commercial behavioral health organizations had implemented telephonically based ICM services for their members. Like their public sector counterparts, internal studies by these MBHOs found that a small percentage of members utilized a disproportional amount of treatment services. This research found that age, diagnosis, and comorbidity of diagnoses were factors that contributed to a higher risk of readmission or greater overall cost. Not only was this costly to the MBHOs, but the quality of care was considered less optimal as best illustrated by the pain and disruption in the members' and families' lives that resulted from repeated psychiatric admissions. One large managed behavioral health care company found that of those members who utilized behavioral health services, 5% accounted for 53% of total costs, as illustrated in Figure 13-1.

In companies with such programs, ICM candidates are typically identified by either claims data, notification of an inpatient admission, or by care managers from the managed behavioral health care entity or the health plan partner. Once identified, ICM care managers contact members to explain the program and obtain consent to participate. The ICM care managers then work directly with the members to develop per-

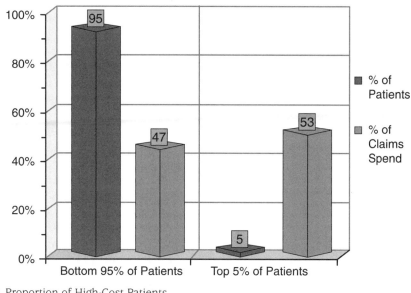

Figure 13–1 Proportion of High-Cost Patients

Source: Magellan Health Services. Used with permission.

sonalized treatment plans that address their clinical needs and then coordinate care delivery with the members and their behavioral health providers across service settings.

Over the past few years the philosophy of ICM programs has expanded to include components of the Chronic Care Model[16] (Wagner, Chronic Care Model,) such as the promotion of self-management skills and integration with evidence-based decision support tools. These concepts associated with the management of chronic illnesses have been adopted by the behavioral health community to address the severity and chronicity of certain mental illnesses such as bipolar disorder, schizophrenia, major depression, and substance abuse. Self-management support involves patient education, problem solving, and collaborative decision making.[17] Care managers use these strategies to support the goals of self-efficacy and behavior change. This requires ICM care managers to use different skill sets such as motivational interviewing, promotion of recovery-based concepts, and resiliency as they work collab-

oratively with members and providers during the delivery of care.

Managed behavioral health companies have begun to use clinical outcomes and return on investment (ROI) measures to evaluate the efficacy and impact of their ICM programs.[18] One such program resulted in decreased admissions, lengths of stay, and overall care costs. These results are promising although yet to be confirmed by other studies.

QUALITY MANAGEMENT

Quality management in behavioral health care encompasses both quality assurance and quality improvement. Early origins of quality management in behavioral health care can be traced to the American College of Surgeons who, in the interest of understanding the variability of patient outcomes, published in 1913 the first set of quality standards for hospitals.[19] In the 1980s and 1990s, the health care industry and behavioral health care began applying principles of Total Quality Management (TQM) and Continuous Quality Improvement (CQI) built on the theories of Walter Shewhart, W. Edwards Deming, Joseph M. Juran, Philip Crosby, and Donald Berwick. These systems and processes were designed to measure process variability and methods for reducing variability to acceptable levels. This method has come to be known as the Plan, Do, Check, Act (PDCA) cycle:

- *Plan:* Identify opportunity for improvement.
- *Do.* Implement interventions.
- *Check.* Measure effect of interventions.
- *Act.* Adjust interventions/change interventions.[20]

Recently, MBHOs have favored quality improvement, a more forward-looking model which includes analysis of system-wide data describing routine care and outcomes, over quality assurance models.[21] With an increased focus on system-wide data, methods and practices to reduce wide variation in quality of care have come under intensified scrutiny. Variations within the field of behavioral health exist in such areas as use of risk assessment protocols, screening for substance abuse, use of evidence-based practices, clinical record keeping, use of electronic treatment records, diagnostic coding, utilization review procedures, performance measures, and quality improvement procedures.

QUALITY OF CARE

Quality of care, as defined by the Institute of Medicine (IOM), is "the degree to which health services for individuals and populations increase the likelihood of desired health outcomes and are consistent with current professional knowledge."[22] Six aims for high-quality care were identified in the IOM's seminal reports, *Crossing the Quality Chasm: A New Health System for the 21st Century*[23] and *Improving the Quality of Health Care for Mental and Substance-Use Conditions.*[24] These aims define care that has the following characteristics:

- *Safe.* Avoiding injuries to patients from the care that is intended to help them.
- *Effective.* Providing services based on scientific knowledge to all who could benefit and refraining from providing services to those not likely to benefit (avoiding underuse and overuse, respectively).
- *Patient centered.* Providing care that is respectful of and responsive to individual patient preferences, needs, and values and ensuring that patient values guide all clinical decisions.
- *Timely.* Reducing waits and sometimes harmful delays for both those who receive and those who give care.
- *Efficient.* Reducing waste, including waste of equipment, supplies, ideas, and energy.
- *Equitable.* Providing care that does not vary in quality because of personal characteristics such as gender, ethnicity, geographical location, and socioeconomic status.

COMPONENTS OF QUALITY MANAGEMENT PROGRAMS

Quality management program components frequently are grouped into structures, processes, and outcomes based on a framework proposed by Donabedian.[25] *Structures* are the components of behavioral health care's quality improvement program. *Processes* represent the behavioral health services provided to or on behalf of a patient. *Outcomes* are the results of the services and care provided to patients. The quality of behavioral health care is measured, monitored, and improved over time using performance measures.

Quality programs in MBHOs vary in size and scope based on the complexity of the organization, the type of products provided, the size of the provider network, and the characteristics of the population served or managed. Another factor affecting the complexity of an MBHO's quality program is its participation in programs that accredit or certify quality processes, such as NCQA or URAC.

Most MBHOs have a quality program with a quality committee and/or team, policies outlining quality and safety standards and procedures, performance measures that define process and outcomes measures, and a system for analysis of barriers and root causes that may cause undue variation in quality or utilization. Formal systems for assessing quality improvement initiatives have been developed. For example, NCQA has developed standards for Quality Improvement Activities (QIAs), and URAC has developed standards for Quality Improvement Projects (QIPs).

ACCREDITATION

The major accreditation organizations used by MBHOs are JCAHO, NCQA, and URAC (see Chapter 23). Less widely used is the Council on Accreditation, which accredits employee assistance programs. Accreditation by these organizations is voluntary and designed to provide external validation of a behavioral health care company's quality program with assurance of quality for consumers and purchasers of services. Increasingly, states require MBHOs to meet accreditation requirements to obtain a utilization review license and/or to deliver services within their state.

In the absence of state-mandated accreditation, MBHOs historically have sought to distinguish themselves on the basis of accreditations. An important factor in voluntary accreditations is that medical managed care organizations that contract with MBHOs in a carve-out arrangement frequently require them to be externally accredited and set monetary guarantees and penalties based on accreditation performance. Although accreditation standards for behavioral health care vary by agency, they include constructs such as those shown in Table 13-4.

MBHOs seeking NCQA accreditation must demonstrate that they have identified opportunities for improvement in service and clinical areas, with targeted interventions and measurement of the effectiveness of interventions. Examples of clinical improvement activities in behavioral health care include increasing the rate of members who attend an ambulatory follow-up visit in the 7 days following hospitalization, improving the rate of provider identification of comorbidities, and strengthening coordination of care between behavioral and primary care clinicians.

With the maturation of MBHO quality programs and increasing numbers of companies obtaining accreditation, a shift is occurring from an emphasis on structures and processes to performance-based measurement and demonstrable outcomes.

PERFORMANCE MEASUREMENT AND OUTCOMES

The purposes of performance measurement include accountability, quality improvement, and research.[26] Performance measurement

---

Table 13–4 Common Constructs in Behavioral Health Care Accreditation Standards

Quality program and improvement activities	Patient safety
Enrollee and provider satisfaction	Performance measures and outcomes
Utilization review program components	Member rights and responsibilities
Medical necessity criteria	Preventive behavioral health
Appeals and complaints	Clinical practice guidelines
Credentialing of providers and organizations	Stakeholder input
Confidentiality and HIPAA compliance	Staff training and management

program components are categorized similarly to quality program components. *Structural* measures are features of a behavioral health care organization relevant to its capacity to provide services and care. *Process* measures are usually expressed as a rate and assess a health care service. *Outcome* measures are the "effects of interventions (or lack of interventions) on primary and secondary consumers."[27] Outcomes-based measures of quality reflect the cumulative impact of multiple processes of care.[28]

Hundreds of measures have been developed to assess behavioral health care. The National Quality Measures Clearinghouse (NQMC), operated by the Agency for Healthcare Research and Quality, includes measures for mental health and substance abuse,[29] as does the National Inventory of Mental Health Quality Measures. Richard Hermann provides an extensive list of applicable measures.[21] A partial list of measures is provided in Table 13-5.

The challenge for behavioral health care is not a lack of measures but difficulties arising from the quality and availability of data and the complexity in computation. A wide array of data sources is used to collect performance metrics in behavioral health care, as illustrated in Figure 13-2.

Administrative data include claims, eligibility information, and various coding sets. Treatment records contain detailed clinical information. Survey data are obtained from providers and consumers and measure experiences and satisfaction with care and services. Access data are gathered from telephone systems and reviews of provider appointment availability. Clinical assessments involve consumer self-report and provider and caretaker observations. Utilization management data include requests for care, nonauthorizations, and appeals. Risk management data include adverse events, medication errors, and rates of seclusion, and restraints. Predictive modeling data are derived from utilization data and population risk adjustment formulas.

Data challenges are significant within behavioral health care. Behavioral health is difficult to measure because there are few laboratory tests with relevance for program monitoring. Use of self-report and provider observations result in wide variation and expensive capture mechanisms. Providers' use of electronic technology is limited for claims submission and treatment records. Code sets and definitions vary widely across the continuum of care resulting in data interface issues. Calculation problems arise as a result of the

Table 13–5 Measures Applicable in Behavioral Health Care Quality Improvement

Developer	Measurement Set
American College of Mental Health Administration	Indicators for Behavioral Health
Child and Adolescent Residential Psychiatric Programs (CHARPP)	CHARPP Improvement Measurement Program
Joint Commission on Accreditation of Healthcare Organizations	National Library of Healthcare Indicators
National Committee for Health Quality Assurance	Health Plan Employer Data and Information Set (HEDIS)
Mental Health Statistics Improvement Program (MHSIP)	Process measures derived from MHSIP consumer survey items
Washington Circle Group	Washington Circle Group Performance Measures

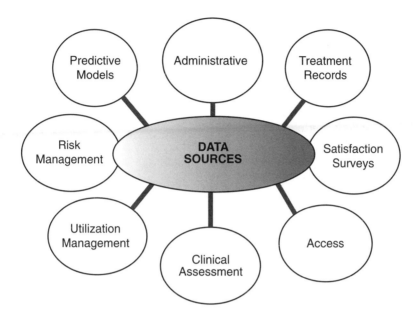

Figure 13–2 Data Sources for Behavioral Health Care Quality Improvement

many variations in data capture and coding systems.

MEASUREMENT SELECTION

Drawing on the available data sources, behavioral health care companies select performance measures based on internal and external needs. The most widely used measurement set in health care is HEDIS, developed by NCQA. Although HEDIS measures are reported by managed care organizations (MCOs), as subcontractors to MCOs, MBHOs share in the collection of data. HEDIS includes behavioral health measures with established thresholds for utilization and effectiveness. Annually, NCQA publishes MCOs' HEDIS results; employers use the results to select among managed care plans and set benchmarks for performance. A sample of performance measures used for quality improvement and accountability by one behavioral health company is presented in Table 13-6.

OUTCOMES

Clinical outcomes measurement is an essential function for MBHOs and serves multiple stakeholders. Purchasers of behavioral health care want demonstrated return on investment and maximum clinical improvement for minimal premium dollars. At the patient or consumer level, outcomes allow for comparison with a standard and/or with consumers using similar services. At the aggregate level, population health and well-being can be assessed, as well as program effectiveness and efficacy. Another purpose, gaining momentum in health care, is that of linking outcome and performance measurement data with incentives to improve quality.[30-32]

Most MBHOs use clinical assessment systems that monitor members' response to treatment and progress over time. The modalities used by MBHOs vary, with some requiring providers to complete assessments and others relying on member self-report. The focus of clinical assessment is broaden-

Table 13–6 Performance Measures Used for Quality Improvement

Domain	Measure	Data Source
Structure	QI and UM program descriptions	Quality data
	Medical necessity criteria	Clinical data
Process	Timeliness of telephone access	Admin data
	Readmission rates	Utilization data
	Appeals overturn rate	Admin data
	Intensive care management enrollment	Admin data
	Adverse events	Clinical data
Outcome	Patient experience of care	Patient survey
	Symptom and function improvement of members	Patient self-report

ing from solely behavioral health to incorporate physical health, recovery and resilience, and productivity.

Patients are increasingly recognized as valid judges of the quality of their health care experience.[33] With the shift to patient-centered care, clinical outcomes reported from the patient perspective are being used by patients and clinicians for treatment planning and monitoring. "Ultimately, the most important questions in assessing quality of care are whether symptoms remit, functioning and quality of life improve, adverse events are avoided and consumers are satisfied."[21]

INCENTIVES TO DRIVE QUALITY

An additional function of clinical outcomes data is in support of incentive programs. Provider profiles and scorecards increasingly are used to aid consumers in choice and selection of providers. As discussed in Chapter 20, there is a trend to publish provider quality data on Web sites for consumers' use. Pay-for-performance programs, with financial incentives, reward high performers for demonstrated quality. Nonfinancial incentives include recognition programs, administrative burden reduction, and preferred provider status. Tying provider incentive payments to investment in technology and using variable copayments to encourage consumers to choose providers with better quality profiles also have been proposed.[34]

The jury is still out on which incentive programs work best and how much they improve quality of care and access to services. The development of a set of principles to guide pay-for-performance systems by JCAHO and the IOM's charge for use and measurement of evidence-based practices suggest that incentives to improve quality will grow with greater use and scrutiny in the years to come. Groups such as Leapfrog, an employer-based group, and the National Quality Forum play a significant role in setting quality standards, use of performance measurement, and reviewing incentives to drive quality.

The behavioral health industry is at a critical juncture in its use of performance measurement to improve quality and measure outcomes. Stakeholders, including purchasers, health plans, provider groups, clinicians, patients, and researchers, need to engage in the process of effectively using measures to drive quality improvement.[35,36]

CONCLUSION

The managed behavioral health care industry is in flux and will likely remain so for the foreseeable future. Significant tension exists among managed care organizations regarding whether the behavioral management function should be in-sourced or outsourced.

The illusion that the percentage of the medical spend allocated to behavioral health is now so small relative to the overall medical spend may suggest that it does not merit a carve-out management approach. Added to this is the growing acknowledgment that there is a significant intersection between behavioral health issues and physical health, leading MCOs to the conclusion that coordinated management under one roof is the preferred way to proceed.

These arguments are counterbalanced with the reality that managing patients who are suffering from emotional distress require a different set of skills, a broader network of provider types, and specialized claims processing standards.

These dynamics will continue to play out with strong advocates on each side of the equation. Most of the large national carriers have built or bought the capability, but the regional and local players will continue to assess their strategic direction on a regular basis.

References

1. Frank RG, Conti RM, Goldman HH. Mental health policy and psychotropic drugs. *Milbank Quarterly. June* 2005:83(2), 271–298.
2. Frank RG and Glied S. Changes in mental health financing since 1971: Implications for Policymakers and patients. *Health Affairs.* May-June 2006:25(3), 601–613.
3. Franklin JE, Levenson JL, McCance-Katz EF. *Substance-related disorders: textbook of psychosomatic medicine.* Washington, DC: American Psychiatric Publishing, 2005.
4. Moore RD, Bone LR, Geller G, et al. Prevalence, detection and treatment of alcoholism in hospitalized patients. *JAMA.* 1989:261, 403–407.
5. Schatzberg AF, Cole JO, DeBattista C. *Manual of Clinical Psychopharmacology,* 5th ed. Washington, DC: American Psychiatric Publishing, 2005.
6. American Psychiatric Association. *Diagnostic and Statistical Manual of Mental Disorders DSM-IV-TR.* Washington, DC: American Psychiatric Association, 2000.
7. Pomerantz JM. *Pay-for-performance could better align incentives in behavioral health care. Drug Benefit Trends.* 2005: 17(3).
8. Patel KK, Butler B, Wells KB. What is necessary to transform the quality of mental health care. *Health Affairs.* 2006:25(3), 681–693.
9. Young G, White B, Burgess J, Berlowitz D, Meterko M, Guldin M, Bokhour B. Conceptual issues in the design and implementation of pay-for-quality programs. *American Journal of Medical Quality.* 2005:20, 144–150.
10. Endsley S, Kirkegaard M, Baker G, Murcko A. Getting rewards for your results: pay-for-performance programs. *Family Practice Mgmt.* 2004:11(3), 45–50.
11. Bailit Health Purchasing. Performance incentive model options. Center for Health Care Strategies. December 2005.
12. Stein LI and Test MA. Alternative to mental hospital treatment 1: Conceptual model, treatment program, clinical evaluation. *Arch of Gen Psychiatry.* 1980:37, 392–397.
13. Bond GR, Miller LD, Krumwied RD, Ward RS. Assertive case management in three CMHCs: A Controlled Study. *Hospital and Community Psychiatry.* 1988:39, 411–418.
14. Tibbo P, Chue P, Wright E. *Hospital outcome measures following assertive community treatment in Edmonton, Alberta,* Can J. Psychiatr. 1999;44:3, 276–279.
15. Ziguras SJ, Stuart GW. A meta-analysis of the effectiveness of mental health case management over 20 years. *Psychiatric Services.* 2000:51, 11, 1410–1421.
16. Wagner. Chronic care model, in Solberg, LI, Crain, AL, Sperl-Hillen, JM, Hroscikoski, MC, Engebretson, KI, O'Connor, PJ. Challenges of change: A qualitative study of chronic care model implementation. *Annals of Family Medicine.* July–August 2006.
17. *Patient Self-Management Tools: An Overview.* California Healthcare Foundation, 2005. Quality Chasm Series. National Academy of Sciences, 2006. California Healthcare Foundation, 2005.
18. Taylor EC, LoPiccolo CJ, Eisdorfer C, Clemcence C. Best practices: Reducing rehospitalization with telephonic targeted care management in a managed health care plan. *Psychiatric Services.* 2005:56(6), 652–654.
19. Ruetsch C, Wadell D, Dewan N. Improving quality and accountability through informa-

tion systems. In Dewan NA, Lorenzi NM, Riley RT, eds. *Behavioral Health Informatics*. New York: Springer-Verlag, 2001.

20. Brassard M, Ritter D. *The Memory Jogger II. A Pocket Guide of Tools for Continuous Improvement and Effective Planning*. Methuen, MA: GOAL/QPC, 1994.

21. Hermann RC. *Improving Mental Healthcare: A Guide to Measurement-Based Quality Improvement*. Washington, DC: American Psychiatric Publishing, 2005.

22. Lohr KN, ed. *Medicare: A Strategy for Quality Assurance*. Washington, DC: National Academy Press, 1990.

23. Institute of Medicine. *Crossing the Quality Chasm: A New Health System for the 21st Century*. Washington, DC: National Academy Press, 2001.

24. Institute of Medicine. *Improving the Quality of Health Care for Mental and Substance-Use Conditions*. Washington, DC: National Academy Press, 2006.

25. Donabedian A. *Exploration in Quality Assessment and Monitoring: The Definition of Quality and Approaches to Its Assessment*. Ann Arbor, MI: Health Administration Press, 1980.

26. Solberg LI, Mosser G, McDonald S. The three faces of performance measurement: Improvement, accountability, and research. *Jt Comm J Qual Improv*. 1997:23(3), 135–147.

27. Decision Support 2000+ Outcomes Measurement Process, Project Overview and Deliberation of Steering Committee, 2003.

28. AcademyHealth. Health Outcomes Core Library Project. Washington, DC: National Information Center on Health Services Research and Health Care Technology, National Library of Medicine, 2004. (No. Order No. P.O. 467-MZ-301222).

29. Agency for Healthcare Research and Quality. National Quality Measures Clearinghouse. 2004. Available at: http://www.qualitymeasures. ahrq.gov/resources/measure_use.aspx# attributes. Accessed September 20, 2004.

30. Dudley R, Frolish A, Robinowitz D, Talavera JA, Broadhead P, Luft HS. Strategies to support quality-based purchasing: A review of the evidence. Rockville, Md: Agency for Healthcare Research and Quality, 2004. Summary, Technical Review Number 10. Available at: http:// www.ahrq.gov/clinic/epcsums/qpurchsum.htm. Accessed November 8, 2006.

31. Rosenthal MB, Fernandopulle HRS, Landon B. Paying for quality: Provider incentives for quality improvement. *Health Affairs*. 2004:23 (2), 127–141.

32. Bachman J. (2004). Pay for performance in the behavioral healthcare arena. Available at: http://www.wpic.pitt.edu/dppc/journalwatch_ 2004_11.htm. Accessed December 19, 2004.

33. Iezzoni L. Assessing quality using administrative data. *Ann Intern Med*. 1997:127, 666–674.

34. Steinberg EP. Improving the quality of care—Can we practice what we preach? *N Eng J Med*. 2003:348(26), 2681–2683.

35. Horgan C, McCorry F, W, GD. Creating policy relevant information: The case of Washington Circle. Presented at: AcademyHealth Annual Meeting, 2003, Nashville, TN.

36. Pincus H, Pechura C, Degruy F. Depression in primary care: Linking clinical and system strategies. Presented at: Robert Wood Johnson Foundation Depression in Primary Care (DPC) Annual Grantee Meeting, 2004, Huntington Beach, CA.

Suggested Reading

Joint Commission on Accreditation of Healthcare Organizations. Facts about ORYX for hospitals. Available at: http://www.jcaho.org/ accredited + organizations/hospitals/oryx/oryx + facts.htm. Accessed June 8, 2006.

National Inventory of Mental Health Quality Measures.

National Committee for Quality Assurance (NCQA). Available at: http://www.ncqa.org. Accessed June 2006.

National Institutes of Mental Health. 2004.

14

DISEASE PREVENTION AND HEALTH PLANS

Marc Manley

Study Objectives

- Understand the role of health plans in prevention.
- Understand the different approaches a managed care plan can use in preventing disease.
- Understand the economic value of prevention.

Discussion Topics

1. Discuss the value of disease prevention; use concrete examples and measures.
2. Discuss the barriers and enablers for health plans to promote prevention.
3. Discuss the role of the individual versus the role of a health plan as regards prevention.
4. Discuss how a health plan might implement, monitor, and modify a prevention program.

INTRODUCTION

The prevention of disease has always been an integral component of the practice of medicine. Hippocrates, the most famous physician of the ancient Greeks, proclaimed, "The function of protecting and developing health must rank even above that of restoring it when it is impaired."[1] Disease prevention strategies have produced major improvements in human longevity, the quality of our lives, and the capability of entire societies. Safe drinking water, polio vaccination, and screening for breast cancer are but three examples of the powerful impact prevention can have on a community's health.

Yet in the twenty-first century, the role of prevention in U.S. health care is far from prominent. The U.S. Department of Health and Human Services projected the nation's medical care costs to be nearly $2.2 trillion in 2006.[2] Former U.S. Surgeon General David Satcher estimated that less than 2% of the nation's expenditure on health care is spent on population-based prevention.[3] In contrast, more than 75% of the nation's health care expenditures is devoted to treating people with chronic diseases.[4]

Prevention has often been regarded as an essential element of managed care. Indeed, the expansion of health maintenance organizations (HMOs) and other managed care organizations (MCOs) in the 1970s and 1980s was expected to result in a greater emphasis on prevention and therefore improved health and control of health care costs (see also Chapter 1). This chapter presents the rationale behind prevention and then reviews the current practices MCOs use to prevent illness, including benefit selection, member services, provider contracting, and influencing public policy. The discussion focuses largely on the prevention of common chronic diseases in adults.

In the context of health and health care, *prevention* can be defined as "action taken to decrease the chance of getting a disease or condition."[5] Three levels of prevention are commonly recognized. *Primary prevention* is the prevention of disease before it starts. For example, individuals who smoke can help avoid lung cancer by quitting smoking before any neoplasm has begun. *Secondary prevention* is the detection of disease before it becomes symptomatic, which allows for earlier and more successful treatment. Mammography is an example of secondary prevention, in which breast cancer is detected before a patient is aware of its existence, and the cancer is treated before it has metastasized. *Tertiary prevention* is the prevention of complications of a chronic disease after diagnosis. MCOs address tertiary prevention through case management and (very specifically) disease management programs as discussed in Chapters 11 and 10, respectively. The focus of this chapter, therefore, is on the need for and practice of primary and secondary prevention strategies.

THE CASE FOR PREVENTION: A COST-EFFECTIVE SOLUTION FOR SAVING LIVES

In the early twenty-first century, noninfectious diseases have replaced infectious diseases as the leading causes of death, illness, and health care costs. Heart disease and cancer lead this list, together causing an estimated 1,242,000 deaths each year.[6] Chronic diseases cause about 70% of all U.S. deaths each year, and five chronic diseases—heart disease, cancer, stroke, chronic obstructive pulmonary disease, and diabetes—are responsible for more than two-thirds of these deaths.[1]

Health care costs are a growing burden on our economy. Heart disease, cancer, and stroke—the top three causes of death in the United States—cost an estimated $523.4 billion each year in direct medical costs and lost productivity.[1] Table 14-1 shows the diseases that cause the most deaths in the United States and the health care costs attributed to these diseases.

Table 14-1 conveys the toll—in human and economic terms—of chronic diseases. But it does not convey one fundamental fact: most

Table 14–1 Mortality Figures and Health Care Costs of the Leading Chronic Diseases

Chronic Disease*	Number of Deaths*	Health Care Costs in Millions**
Heart disease	685,089	$56,678.6
Cancer	556,902	$38,901.8
Stroke	157,689	$14,938.8
Chronic lower respiratory diseases	126,382	$36,476.5
Diabetes	74,219	$18,287.9

Source:
*Hoyert DL, Heron MP, Murphy SL, Kung HC. Deaths: Final data for 2003. *National Vital Statistics Report*. April 19, 2006:54(13), 1–43.
**Thorpe KE, Florence CS, Joski P. Which medical conditions account for the rise in health care spending? *Health Affairs*. Web Exclusive. August 25, 2004: W4, 437–445.

chronic diseases (and thus, the associated mortality and health care costs) are partially or even entirely preventable. At least one-third of all deaths in the United States can be attributed to three very modifiable behaviors—tobacco use, lack of physical activity, and poor eating habits.[1(p5)] Table 14-2 shows the actual causes of death in the United States identified not by disease but by the risk factors that lead to chronic diseases.

Similarly, the costs associated with these avoidable causes of chronic disease are immense. Tobacco use alone is responsible for $75 billion in annual health care costs, with an additional $80 billion per year in lost productivity.[1] Obesity is estimated to cost the nation's health care system $61 billion annually, with an additional $56 billion per year in lost productivity.[1]

Numerous studies have shown the remarkable results that preventive measures can achieve:

- Patients at risk for diabetes could reduce their risk by 58% simply by walking an average of 30 minutes a day, 5 days a week, and by lowering their intake of fat and calories.[1]
- Cervical cancer screening programs can reduce cervical cancer mortality rates by 20% to 60%.[7]

- Treatment for high blood pressure can reduce heart attacks by 21% and strokes by 37%.[8]

By using existing technologies and evidence-based practices known today, we have the potential to reduce chronic disease to nearly the

Table 14–2 Actual Causes of Death in the United States in 2000

Actual Cause of Death	Number (%)* of Deaths in 2000
Tobacco	435,000 (18.1)
Poor diet and physical inactivity	365,000 (15.2)
Alcohol consumption	**85,000 (3.5)**
Microbial agents	75,000 (3.1)
Toxic agents	55,000 (2.3)
Motor vehicle	43,000 (1.8)
Firearms	29,000 (1.2)
Sexual behavior	20,000 (0.8)
Illicit drug use	17,000 (0.7)

*The percentages are for all deaths.
Source: Adapted from Mokdad AH, Marks JS, Stroup DF, et al. Actual causes of death in the United States, 2000. *JAMA*. March 10, 2004:291 (10), 1238–1245.

same extent that immunization reduced infectious disease in the 19th and 20th centuries.

Return on Investment

For a society, the health and financial benefits of preventing disease are obvious. Full implementation of disease prevention programs could produce major reductions in morbidity and mortality caused by chronic disease. Prevention has the potential to produce financial savings for individuals, employers, health plans, governments, and entire societies. Several factors impair the willingness or ability of managed care plans to implement successful primary prevention efforts.

- The time it takes to realize financial gains from prevention is highly variable, depending on the disease that is being prevented, the type of prevention program employed, and the point of view of the return on investment calculation.
- The benefits of member-focused interventions may not be realized by the health plan or employer. (The people who start exercising and lose weight now, employees of Company A and members of Health Plan B, may avoid heart disease and diabetes 10 years from now, but at that point they may well work for a different employer and be covered by a different health plan.)
- For purchasers and even some health plans, the benefits of primary prevention tend to be abstract and distant, whereas the up-front costs are tangible and immediate; they must come out of this year's already-tight budget.

Adding to the complexity, the financial benefits of different prevention programs and services have been calculated and described in many different ways. Thus, it has not always been easy to associate programs with clear, short-term financial returns on investment (ROI).

However, well-designed studies have documented a positive ROI for many health improvement programs. One literature review found an average cost-benefit ratio of 3.48 in these studies.[9] A review of worksite health promotion and disease prevention programs conducted by the U.S. Department of Health and Human Services found that for every dollar companies spend, the median benefit-to-cost ratio is $3.14.[10] Programs to reduce smoking have been studied frequently and found to produce positive returns. One study that examined the relationship between modifiable health risks and short-term health care charges in a health plan population ages 40 years and older found that current tobacco use was related to 18% higher health care charges over an 18-month period.[11] Such results provide evidence that reducing these health risks may offer health plans relatively short-term returns on investments for persons in this age group.

Another analysis, based on a worksite simulation analysis, suggests that for a health plan with a 10% annual turnover rate, a smoking cessation program would more than pay for itself based exclusively on savings in health care costs.[12] A related article suggests that such a program would reach the "break-even" point for a firm implementing it in just over 3 years. The worksite simulation included not just medical care costs but also related costs such as productivity, absenteeism, and life insurance.[13]

A COMPLETE PREVENTION PROGRAM

The fact that preventable chronic disease is so common means that prevention efforts are not reaching their full potential. Effective primary prevention programs are often complex, multifaceted efforts that take years to produce intended results. They are sometimes opposed by powerful organizations; for example, tobacco companies opposed effective strategies to reduce tobacco use such as strong smoke-free workplace laws and ordinances.[14,15] The clinical services that are under the control of MCOs may not be maximally effective in the absence of broader, community-based programs. For example, MCOs can promote regular physical activity, but if members lack safe, accessible places to exercise and the social support to make that behavior change, those efforts are unlikely to succeed. Finally, as recognized earlier, organizations that are asked to pay for prevention programs may not always realize the full return on their investments. Nevertheless, prevention is too important to the future health and economic viability of our communities to ignore or to implement at a minimal level.

Organized and strategic interventions are required to achieve the successful implementation and maintenance of preventive strategies. MCOs have a large arsenal of prevention interventions at their disposal. To have the maximum impact on health and health care costs, MCOs need to use the entire set of prevention tools available to them. Health plans need to offer the right member benefits, provide the right member services, contract effectively with providers, and—perhaps most important—support and implement the right public policies. Table 14-3 shows examples of each of these four basic strategies. Each is described in more detail in the following subsections.

Member Benefits

MCOs typically offer three general types of clinical preventive services: immunizations, screening services, and counseling services. *Immunizations*, once a routine part of pediatric care only, are now used for the prevention of influenza and pneumonia in adults as well. The role of immunizations in adult preventive care is likely to increase. In June 2006, the Food and Drug Administration approved a vaccine for girls and women ages 9 to 26 for the prevention of cancer of the cervix.[16] Immunizations that prevent cancer in other sites may be used in the future. *Screening services* are most often performed to prevent cancer and heart disease in adults, but also include screening of newborns and children for a variety of illnesses. Screening may be accomplished through laboratory tests (*eg,* cholesterol levels), imaging studies (*eg,* mammography), or a clinical examination (*eg,* a skin exam to detect cancer). *Counseling* helps people change their behavior to avoid disease. Counseling to help people quit smoking or lose excess weight results in the prevention of cancer and heart disease.

One challenge for all MCOs is choosing the correct list of preventive services to provide as

Table 14–3 Components of a Strong MCO Prevention Program

Components of a Strong Prevention Program	Examples
Member benefits	• Immunization and screening included in benefit sets • No copayments for preventive services or products • Coverage for nicotine cessation medications and weight loss drugs • Payments to providers for counseling visits
Services for members	• Health risk assessments • Behavior change programs • Discounts for memberships at fitness centers or in weight loss programs
Contracts with providers	• Pay for performance programs • Performance feedback
Public policies	• Increases in taxes on tobacco products • Clean indoor air laws

benefits for their members. Plan leaders understand the importance of providing benefits for services that are proven to prevent disease, but the science of prevention does not always provide complete information. Hence, there is frequent disagreement among health plans about which clinical preventive services to offer as benefits. Respected scientific organizations sometimes disagree about the value of certain services for different age groups. For example, prostate specific antigen (PSA) is a marker for prostate cancer that may detect the disease before it becomes symptomatic. However, because of the nature of prostate cancer, it is less clear whether this early detection leads to longer life spans on average. Until there are well-designed studies of this issue, uncertainty—as well as disagreement—will remain among experts.[17]

Most health plans choose to adopt the recommendations of a single organization, relying on the expertise of this body for these difficult judgments. Since the U.S. Preventive Services Task Force (USPSTF) first published the *Guide to Clinical Preventive Services* in 1989, that guide has become the primary resource for health plans as they design their health maintenance programs and benefit packages.[18] Table 14-4 presents a copy of the USPSTF's recommendations as they stand in 2005.

A recent report issued by the National Commission on Prevention Priorities—a panel of key representatives from health plans, employer groups, academia, clinical practice, and governmental health agencies—ranked preventive services according to two measures: the clinically preventable burden of disease and the cost-effectiveness of the service.[19] The combined score of these two measures provides a rough measure of the value of each service. Each service received a score of 1 to 5 on each of the two measures for a total score possible of 10. Table 14-5 shows the ranking.

Of all preventive services with evidence of effectiveness, the three that ranked highest were aspirin use in high-risk adults, childhood immunization series, and tobacco use screening and brief intervention. This same study ranked the preventive services that would provide the most health benefits if 90% of patients received the service. Tobacco use screening and brief intervention, colorectal cancer screening, and influenza vaccine for adults were the three highest-ranking services.[19]

In addition to scientific evidence and expert opinion, other forces may affect the selection of preventive services. Some benefits may be required by regulators or accreditors, mandated by state laws, or requested by customers. The National Committee for Quality Accreditation (NCQA) assesses the prevention efforts of health plans, including whether the plan has guidelines for doctors about the need to provide immunizations and screening tests to plan members. NCQA evaluates how the plans educate providers and patients about preventive measures and assesses the percentage of eligible patients who receive appropriate services.[20] Accreditation, including examples of these types of measures, is discussed fully in Chapter 23.

Coverage for cancer screening in particular has become a political issue in several states. Many states have mandated some form of cancer screening, but the screening services covered varies from state to state. As of the end of 2005, 46 states required health insurers to provide coverage for mammograms.[21] Many states also require coverage for cervical and colorectal cancer screenings. Twenty-three states use the American Cancer Society's recommendations, while no states used the recommendations of the USPSTF when determining which screening cancer services to mandate.[22] Table 14-6 shows cancer prevention benefits currently mandated by state laws.

Finally, employers and other purchasers may require—or decline to pay for—specific preventive services. Many large employers self-insure, which means that they, not the MCO, decide which benefits to cover. For example, an MCO may recommend coverage for influenza vaccination or smoking cessation or fitness center discounts, but the self-insured purchaser chooses which benefits it

Table 14–4 Preventive Services Recommended by the U.S. Preventive Services Task Force—2005

Recommendations	Adult Men	Adult Women	Pregnant Women	Children
Alcohol misuse, screening and behavioral counseling interventions	X	X	X	
Aspirin for the primary prevention of cardiovascular events	**X**	**X**		
Bacteriuria, screening for asymptomatic			X	
Breast cancer, chemoprevention		X		
Breast cancer, screening		X		
Breastfeeding, behavioral interventions to promote		X	X	
Cervical cancer, screening		X		
Chlamydial infection, screening		X	X	
Colorectal cancer, screening	X	X		
Dental caries in preschool children, prevention				X
Depression, screening	X	X		
Diabetes mellitus in adults, screening for Type 2	X	X		
Diet, behavioral counseling in primary care to promote a healthy weight	X	X		
Hepatitis B virus infection, screening			X	
High blood pressure, screening	X	X		
Lipid disorders, screening	X	X		
Obesity in adults, screening	X	X		
Osteoporosis in postmenopausal women, screening		X		
Rh (D) incompatibility, screening			X	
Syphilis infection, screening	X	X	X	
Tobacco use and tobacco-caused disease, counseling to prevent	X	X	X	
Visual impairment in children younger than age 5 years, screening				X

Note: This table does not include recommendations for immunizations, which are revised frequently.
Source: Reprinted with permission from U.S. Department of Health and Human Services, Agency for Healthcare Research and Quality. Guide to clinical preventive services 2005: table of recommended prevented services (2005). Available at: http://www.ahrq.gov/clinic/pocketgd/gcpstab1.htm.

is willing to cover. As discussed more fully in Chapter 31, under federal law (the Employee Retirement Income and Security Act—ERISA), self-insured employers are also not subject to providing state-mandated benefits such as those listed in Table 14-6. On the other hand, the employer may push the MCO to expand coverage for a preventive service it regards

Table 14–5 National Commission on Prevention Priorities' Rankings of Effective and Cost-Effective Clinical Preventive Services

Preventive Services	Score for Clinically Preventable Burden	Score for Cost-Effectiveness	Total Score
Aspirin chemoprophylaxis	5	5	10
Childhood immunization series	5	5	10
Tobacco use screening and brief intervention	5	5	10
Colorectal cancer screening	4	4	8
Hypertension screening	5	3	8
Influenza immunization	4	4	8
Pneumococcal immunization	3	5	8
Problem drinking screening and brief counseling	4	4	8
Vision screening—adults	3	5	8
Cervical cancer screening	4	3	7
Cholesterol screening	5	2	7
Breast cancer screening	4	2	6
Chlamydia screening	2	4	6
Calcium chemoprophylaxis	3	3	6
Vision screening—children	2	4	6
Folic acid chemoprophylaxis	2	3	5
Obesity screening	3	2	5
Depression screening	3	1	4
Hearing screening	2	2	4
Injury prevention counseling	1	3	4
Osteoporosis screening	2	2	4
Cholesterol screening—high risk	1	1	2
Diabetes screening	1	1	2
Diet counseling	1	1	2
Tetanus-diphtheria booster	1	1	2

Source: Reprinted with permission from Maciosek MV, Coffield AB, Edwards NM, et al. Priorities among effective preventive services: Results of a systematic review and analysis. *Am J Prev Med.* July 2006:31(1), 52–61.

Table 14–6 State Laws Mandating Coverage by Private Insurers for Cancer Screening

State	Breast Cancer Screening*	Prostate Cancer Screening†	Colorectal Cancer Screening‡	Cervical Cancer Screening§
Alabama	X		Y	
Alaska	X	X		X
Arizona	X			X
Arkansas	Y		X	
California	X	X	X	X
Colorado	X	X		
Connecticut	X	X	X	
Delaware	X	X	X	X
District of Columbia	X	X	X	X
Florida	X			
Georgia	X	X	X	X
Hawaii	X			
Idaho	X			
Illinois	X	X	X	X
Indiana	X	X	X, Y	
Iowa	X			
Kansas	X	X		X
Kentucky	X			
Louisiana	X	X	X	X
Maine	X	X		X
Maryland	X	X	X	
Massachusetts	X			X
Michigan	Y			
Minnesota	X	X		X
Mississippi	Y			
Missouri	X	X	X	X
Montana	X			
Nebraska	X			
Nevada	X	X	X	X
New Hampshire	X			
New Jersey	X	X	X	X, Y

continues

Table 14–6 State Laws Mandating Coverage by Private Insurers for Cancer Screening—continued

State	Breast Cancer Screening*	Prostate Cancer Screening†	Colorectal Cancer Screening‡	Cervical Cancer Screening§
New Mexico	X			X
New York	X	X		X
North Carolina	X	X	X	X
North Dakota	X	X		
Ohio	X, Y			X, Y
Oklahoma	X		Y	
Oregon	X	X	X	X
Pennsylvania	X			X
Rhode Island	X	X	X	X
South Carolina	X	X		X
South Dakota	X	X		
Tennessee	X	X	Y	
Texas	X	X	X	
Utah				
Vermont	X			
Virginia	X	X	X	X
Washington	X	X		
West Virginia	X		X	X
Wisconsin	X			
Wyoming	X	X	X	X
Total (of 51)	**50**	**29**	**23**	**26**

X indicates mandatory coverage. Y indicates a requirement to offer coverage.
Source: Adapted with permission from:
*National Cancer Institute, State Legislative Database Program. *Fact Sheet: Breast Cancer.* Bethesda, Md: National Cancer Institute, 2006.
†National Cancer Institute, State Legislative Database Program. *Fact Sheet: Prostrate Cancer Screening.* Bethesda, Md: National Cancer Institute, 2006.
‡National Cancer Institute, State Legislative Database Program. *Fact Sheet: Colorectal Cancer.* Bethesda, Md: National Cancer Institute, 2006.
§National Cancer Institute, State Legislative Database Program. *Fact Sheet: Cervical Cancer.* Bethesda, Md: National Cancer Institute, 2004.

as pertinent to its employee population or may cover such a service separately. As an example, some employers cover weight management programs or exercise programs for all employees, regardless of their health care coverage.

In addition to defining the set of prevention benefits that members receive, MCOs also define the copayments, deductibles, and other disincentives that may be applied to these benefits. These payments by members decrease the use of at least some preventive services. Some health plans eliminate copayments for appropriate preventive services, often those recommended by a trusted national or state organization, such as the USPSTF or the Institute for Clinical Systems Improvement. This practice is especially common for consumer-directed health plans (CDHPs; see also Chapters 2 and 20).[23] By providing appropriate prevention services at no cost to these members, the MCO is encouraging people to manage their own health as well as their own care. Early experience with CDHPs found that CDHP plan members were significantly more likely than members of traditional health plans to participate in health-promoting and preventive behaviors, including joining a wellness program and receiving regular checkups from a physician.[24]

Medicare requires no copayment for screening of certain chronic conditions, such as diabetes screening or colorectal cancer screening, or for certain vaccines, such as the flu vaccine.[25] Based on evidence that reducing patient expense increases the number of smokers who use smoking cessation interventions, as well as the number of smokers who subsequently quit, the Task Force on Community Preventive Services (TFCPS) recommends coverage or reimbursement to patients for expenses incurred for proven smoking cessation interventions.[26] Increasingly, health plans provide coverage for first-line pharmocotherapies and telephone counseling to help smokers quit successfully.[27]

Services for Members

In addition to defined benefits, MCOs can provide a wide variety of other services to help members stay healthy and improve their health. MCOs typically offer some or all of four types of prevention-oriented services: information, assessments of members' risks, programs to change behaviors, and financial incentives to improve health.

Information

MCOs have been providing information about prevention to patients for decades. Printed materials such as brochures and newsletters contain screening recommendations, encouragement for healthy behaviors, and reminders about the use of appropriate immunizations. Many regulators and accreditors expect or require these communications. There is very little evidence that these materials alone change knowledge or behavior.[28] However, the best prevention programs are only useful if people know about them. Especially in the context of broader educational efforts that include other forms of communications plus financial incentives and public policy, distribution of printed information can probably be justified.

MCOs have increasingly turned to the Internet to supply prevention information to their members. Health plans have developed or purchased voluminous Web-based information on prevention and other health issues. Again, the impact of this information on the health behaviors of health plan members is not well documented. It is known that the Internet is a popular resource for health information for the U.S. public: 59% of American adults have access to the Internet, and of these, 79% have searched for health-related information.[29]

Assessment of Members' Health Risks

A major challenge of supplying useful information to patients is the need to tailor information to each person. A nonsmoker, for example, may get no benefit from a brochure promoting a smoking cessation program. Health risk assessments (HRAs) were developed, in part, to address this issue. HRAs are questionnaires about an individual's health behaviors, health status, screening, and immunization history. Algorithms allow the individual's responses to trigger a tailored plan that addresses the specific risks and needs of that individual. Pencil and paper HRAs still exist, but HRAs are more commonly administered and scored electronically.

HRAs are an effective tool for collecting information about a population. That cumulative information can then drive decisions about appropriate interventions. In large populations, the most significant challenge can be encouraging or requiring people to complete the HRA. Employers and some health plans have increased use of HRAs by offering financial or other incentives to individuals who complete them.

Programs to Change Behavior

HRAs require follow-up. When a person is identified with a prevention issue (such as, smoking or obesity), services must be offered to address that issue. Such services can be delivered through e-mail or the Internet, through mailed materials, by telephone, and through face-to-face counseling. Many health plans offer or sell these services to their members through vendors or internal programs. Most commonly, health plans offer members different "modules" to help them with a particular health issue that is identified by the individual's HRA results. Often the modules are Internet-based programs that provide information and e-mail reminders. Common modules cover diet, physical activity, tobacco use, and stress.

HRAs may also be used to direct members to formal counseling programs that help individuals change behavior. Because tobacco use and obesity are the first and second causes of premature death, programs to address these issues are commonly provided to members.[27,30] Tobacco cessation counseling over the telephone is effective and widely available through vendors, state health departments, and health plans. Of all counseling methods, telephone counseling is the most widely covered by health plans.[27] The TFCPS found ample evidence to strongly recommend telephone cessation counseling, especially when used in conjunction with other cessation methods, such as tobacco cessation medications.[26] Several other studies have found telephone counseling to be highly effective in helping patients to modify behaviors and improve health.[31–33]

There is less evidence that Internet programs help smokers quit successfully, but those studies that have been conducted have found promising results. One study of an Internet-based cessation program resulted in one-third of participants quitting or reducing the number of cigarettes they smoked by half. Almost half of the participants made a serious effort to quit. More impressively, 78% of participants reported in a follow-up survey that the Internet program had strengthened their desire to quit.[34]

Group and individual face-to-face counseling is effective, but those methods are utilized by a very small fraction of people trying to quit. A study conducted on the cost-effectiveness of counseling intervention options found group intensive counseling to be the most cost-effective, yet only 5% of smokers were interested in participating in this intervention option.[35]

Programs to treat obesity come in many different formats. There are promising Internet- and telephone-based programs, but their effectiveness is not firmly established. An overview of studies on Internet-based programs found that individuals who participated in Web-based interventions acquired wider knowledge and understanding of chronic conditions and achieved greater health-promoting behavioral modifications.[36] Many studies have found that Internet-based weight loss programs are more effective when they include an interactive behavioral counseling component, such as personalized feedback from trained weight loss counselors via e-mail.[37,38] One study found that a therapist-led, structured Internet-based behavioral program helped participants to lose an average of more than twice as much weight as those who used a basic, commercial Internet-based program.[39] A study on the effectiveness of telephone counseling for treating obesity found that patients who received individualized, telephone-based behavioral counseling from trained professionals achieved weight loss comparable to patients who attend face-to-face behavioral programs.[33]

At least one group support program (Weight Watchers®) has been shown to help people lose weight.[40] There are also more intensive group and individualized programs, some requiring medical management of severe caloric restrictions.

Incentives for Participation

Health plans also promote prevention by providing discounted prices for specific services offered by their own vendors or in the community. For example, discounts may be offered for participation in fitness centers. Such discounts frequently are paid only when a member uses the fitness center a minimum number of times per month (*eg,* eight times per month). Discounts may also be offered for weight management programs, such as Weight Watchers®. Here again, a smart incentive program will pay the discount only for those members who attend the program regularly. It is important to select those programs that can reach large numbers of people, can expect to affect their health, have been studied adequately, and can be reasonably expected to provide a return on investment.

Contracting with Health Care Providers

Managed care organizations can also use the power of the purse to influence physicians and their delivery of preventive services. Health plans' contracts with provider organizations are potentially important tools for promoting good preventive care. For many years, health plans paid clinics to institute quality improvement programs that were designed to make "systems changes" in the care of patients. Payment was often tied to completing the quality improvement project, not necessarily to improving actual care. In recent years, "pay-for-performance" programs have attempted to provide financial incentives for providers to deliver documented improvement in patient outcomes. Many of these programs have strengthened the delivery of preventive services, such as cancer screening or tobacco counseling. Rigorous studies have not yet confirmed the effectiveness of pay-for-performance programs,[41–43]

but many plans are using this technique, which is discussed fully in Chapter 8.

Another approach to promote the delivery of appropriate preventive services is the use of performance feedback for health care providers. Using administrative claims data, health plans have provided information to provider groups and individual practitioners about their patients' use of preventive and other services. Information about an individual provider's performance improves the delivery of preventive services.[44,45] Information that compares a practitioner's or provider's performance to other peers can be particularly compelling because it invites "how did they do that?" questions and leads to system improvements.

In addition to performance feedback, MCOs have also provided reminders to providers about specific patients' needs for services. Using administrative data, health plans have notified clinics about patients who may be overdue for specific screening tests or immunizations. The use of provider reminders to promote screening and immunization has been shown to be effective as a way to increase rates of both immunization and screenings. However, this information may not always be useful to clinics, especially when they lack electronic medical records. A list of patients needing services is difficult to link to a specific medical record at the time of an individual patient's visit. Computer-based medical record systems that create computer-generated reminders have been found to increase the frequency of follow-up visits,[46] to increase the likelihood that practitioners provide preventive care,[47] and to allow clinics to easily provide individualized outreach and services to patients.[48]

The work of prevention requires information that isn't commonly found in an MCO's administrative claims data sets, such as tobacco use, body mass index (BMI), and dates of immunizations. It also requires information that isn't commonly found in a patient's medical record, such as benefits coverage and HRA results. In the future, HRA results may augment health plans' data sets and provide information that can guide programs and monitor progress. Similarly, as electronic medical records become more common, we should expect major improvements in the ability of MCOs and health care providers to use their collective information for tailored interventions.

Public Policy and Prevention

Managed care organizations have both financial and ethical reasons to prevent disease and promote health. Their traditional sphere of influence lies within their membership, their benefits and services, and their provider contracts. Recent decades have seen some notable public health improvements (for example, in immunization rates and smoking rates), but these improvements have not been accomplished through clinical interventions alone. Major improvements in public health come about through multifaceted intervention programs that may include clinical tactics but rely most heavily on public policy. Public policies influence people every day and can provide encouragement, incentives, and (at times) requirements to change behavior in a positive way.

Childhood immunizations provide a good example of the effects of public policy. Vaccination is a clinical intervention, but high rates of childhood immunization were not achieved by clinical means alone. The most powerful intervention for increasing immunization rates has been the public policy that requires children to be vaccinated before they can attend school. All 50 states now require proof of current immunization to enter school, although the specific immunization requirements vary from state to state.[49] This "no shots, no school" policy has made immunization almost universal among school-aged children. A review of immunization interventions concluded that the enforcement of immunization laws requiring proof of vaccination for school attendance resulted in more than 95% of school-age children receiving the proper vaccinations.[50] Although most states allow exemptions for medical, religious, or philosophical reasons, less than 1% of school-age children are exempted.[51]

Adult immunizations are not as widely utilized as childhood immunizations. Vaccines to prevent influenza and pneumococcal pneumonia are both effective and cost-effective, but no public policies require their use. Instead, health departments and health plans invest in programs to encourage voluntary vaccination, and achieve much lower immunization rates. Immunization has the potential to save tens of thousands of adults who die each year from diseases that can be prevented, including 36,000 who die from influenza[52] and 4,000 to 5,000 who die from hepatitis B.[53] Yet, less than half of the 188 million Americans the Centers for Disease Control and Prevention (CDC) estimates should be vaccinated against influenza are vaccinated each year.[54]

Another example of effective public policy is tobacco control. There are effective clinical treatments for nicotine addiction, but large-scale reductions in the prevalence of tobacco use require a multifaceted approach that goes far beyond clinical interventions. Changes in public policy have much larger impact on smoking rates. Two public policies make a big difference: (1) increases in the excise tax (and therefore the price) on tobacco and (2) strong clean indoor air laws that prohibit smoking in all public workplaces, including restaurants and bars. States that have enacted a comprehensive tobacco control program, including public policy and a variety of options to help smokers quit, have seen notable decreases in smoking rates.[55]

Changes in public policies are far more cost-effective methods for improving health than any clinical intervention. A study that compared the cost-effectiveness of cigarette tax increases, nicotine replacement therapies, and "nonprice interventions," including smoking bans, bans on advertising, and public education campaigns, found that tax increases are both the most effective and the most cost-effective intervention. All of the interventions were shown to be cost-effective when compared with the cost in lives and preventable medical expenses, but policy interventions are more cost-efficient because they incur only administrative and enforcement costs as opposed to nicotine replacement therapies, which have the added cost of the pharmacological product.[56]

Health plans that lead or contribute to lobbying efforts for effective primary and secondary prevention strategies demonstrate visible public leadership and active concern for their members' health. Public policy advocacy is a relatively new role for MCOs but one that may gain traction as MCOs, purchasers, and other community leaders realize the cost-effectiveness of this approach.

CONCLUSION

Prevention saves money, saves lives, and improves health. It is an effective and cost-effective strategy. In fact, the health and financial case for prevention has never been stronger as concerns about rising health care costs grow. MCOs have a wide array of tools to promote primary and secondary prevention, including member benefits, member services, provider contracts, and the promotion of public policies. MCOs should work to educate both purchasers and members about effective prevention methods. The policy arena clearly holds the most promise for major future gains. MCOs can expand their roles by becoming catalysts for collaborative efforts among other health plans, purchasers, and other community stakeholders.

References

1. U.S. Centers for Disease Control and Prevention (CDC). *The Power of Prevention: Reducing the Health and Economic Burden of Chronic Disease.* Atlanta, Ga: U.S. Department of Health and Human Services, 2003. Available at: http://www.cdc.gov/NCCdphp/publications/PowerOfPrevention/pdfs/power_of_prevention.pdf. Accessed June 16, 2006.
2. Centers for Medicare and Medicaid Services. National health care expenditures projections: 2005–2015. U.S. Department of Health and Human Services. Available at: http://www.cms.hhs.gov/NationalHealthExpendData/downloads/proj2005.pdf. Accessed July 5, 2006.
3. Satcher D. U.S. Department of Health and Human Services. Keynote address. Presented at the American College Health Association 2000 Annual Meeting, May 31, 2000. Available at: http://www.surgeongeneral.gov/library/history/satcherarchive/speeches/acha_fn.htm. Accessed July 5, 2006.
4. Dartmouth Atlas Project. The care of patients with severe chronic illness: A report on the Medicare program by the Dartmouth Atlas Project. Executive Summary. Center for the Evaluative Clinical Sciences. Available at: http://www.dartmouthatlas.org/atlases/2006_Atlas_Exec_Summary.pdf. Accessed July 6, 2006.
5. National Cancer Institute and U.S. National Institutes of Health. *Dictionary of Cancer Terms.* Available at: http://www.nci.nih.gov/dictionary/. Accessed June 16, 2006.
6. Hoyert DL, Heron MP, Murphy SL, Kung HC. Deaths: Final data for 2003. *Natl Vital Stat Rep.* 2006:54(13), 1–43.
7. U.S. Preventive Services Task Force. *Guide to Clinical Preventive Services*, 2nd ed. Washington, DC: U.S. Department of Health and Human Services, Office of Disease Prevention and Health Promotion, 1996. Available at: http://odphp.osophs.dhhs.gov/pubs/guidecps/. Accessed June 15, 2006.

8. U.S. Centers for Disease Control and Prevention (CDC). *Division for Heart Disease and Stroke Prevention: At a Glance 2006*. Available at: http://www.cdc.gov/nccdphp/publications/aag/cvh.htm. Accessed June 15, 2006.

9. Aldana SG. Financial impact of health promotion programs: A comprehensive review of the literature. *Am J Health Prom*. 2001:15(5), 296–320.

10. U.S. Department of Health and Human Services. *Prevention Makes Common "Cents."* September 2003:2. Available at: http://aspe.hhs.gov/health/prevention/prevention.pdf. Accessed June 29, 2006.

11. Pronk NP, Goodman MJ, O'Connor PJ, Martinson BC. Relationship between modifiable health risks and short-term health care charges. *JAMA*. 1999:282(23), 2235–2239.

12. Warner KE. Smoking out the incentives for tobacco control in managed care settings. *Tobac Contr*. 1998:7(suppl), S50–S54. Available at: http://tc.bmjjournals.com/cgi/content/full/7/suppl_1/S50. Accessed June 19, 2006.

13. Warner KE, Smith RJ, Smith DG, Fries BE. Health and economic implications of a worksite smoking cessation program: A simulation analysis. *J Occ Envir Med*. 1996:38(10), 981–992.

14. Drope J, Chapman S. Tobacco industry efforts at discrediting scientific knowledge of environmental tobacco smoke: A review of internal industry documents. *J Epidemiol Community Health*. 2001:55, 588–594.

15. Tsoukalas T, Glantz SA. The Duluth clean indoor air ordinance: Problems and success in fighting the tobacco industry at the local level in the 21st century. *Am J Public Health*. 2003: 93, 1214–1221.

16. U.S. Food and Drug Administration. FDA licenses new vaccine for prevention of cervical cancer and other diseases in females caused by human papillomavirus. *FDA News*. June 8, 2006. Available at: http://www.fda.gov/bbs/topics/NEWS/2006/NEW01385.html. Accessed June 12, 2006.

17. Collins MM, Fowler FJ Jr, Roberts RG, Oesterling JE, An GJ. Medical malpractice implications of PSA testing for early detection of prostate cancer. *J Law, Med Ethics*. 1997:24(4).

18. Woolf SH, Atkins D. The evolving role of prevention in health care: Contributions of the U.S. Preventive Services Task Force. *Am J Prev Med*. 2001:20(3S), 13–20. Available at: http://www.elsevier.com/locate/ajpmonline. Accessed June 9, 2006.

19. Maciosek MV, Coffield AB, Edwards NM, Flottenmesch TJ, Goodman MJ, Solberg LI. Priorities among effective preventive services: Results of a systematic review and analysis. *Am J Prev Med*. 2006:1–10.

20. National Committee for Quality Assurance. What NCQA looks for in a health plan: Staying healthy. Available at: http://hprc.ncqa.org/stayinghealthy.asp. Accessed June 9, 2006.

21. National Cancer Institute, State Legislative Database Program. *Fact Sheet: Breast Cancer*. Bethesda, MD: National Cancer Institute, 2006.

22. Rathore SS, McGreevey JD, Schulman KA, Atkins D. Mandated coverage for cancer-screening services: Whose guidelines do states follow? *Am J Prev Med*. August 2000:19 (2), 136–137.

23. RAND. *"Consumer Directed" Health Plans: Implications for Health Care Quality and Cost*. Oakland, CA: California Healthcare Foundation. 2005:9. Available at: http://www.chcf.org/documents/insurance/ConsumerDirHealthPlansQualityCost.pdf. Accessed June 22, 2006.

24. Agrawal V, Ehrbeck T, Packard KO, Mango P. *Consumer-Directed Health Plan Report—Early Evidence Is Promising: Insights from Primary Consumer Research*. Pittsburgh, PA: McKinsey & Company, 2005. Available at: http://www.mckinsey.com/clientservice/payorprovider/Health_Plan_Report.pdf. Accessed June 22, 2006.

25. Centers for Medicare and Medicaid Services. Quick reference information: Medicare Preventive Services. U.S. Department of Health and Human Services. March 2006. Available at: http://www.cms.hhs.gov/MLNProducts/downloads/qr_prevent_serv.pdf. Accessed June 29, 2006.

26. Task Force on Community Preventive Services. Recommendations regarding interventions to reduce tobacco use and exposure to environmental tobacco use. *Am J Prev Med*. 2001:20(2S), 14.

27. McPhillips-Tangum C, Bocchino C, Carreon R, Erceg C, Rehm B. Addressing tobacco in managed care: Results of the 2002 survey. *Prev Chron Dis*. October 2004:1(4). Available at: http://www.cdc.gov/pcd/issues/2004/oct/oct/04_0021.htm. Accessed June 9, 2006.

28. Lancaster T, Stead LF. Self-help interventions for smoking cessation. *Cochrane Libr*. 2006:2.

29. Pew Internet and American Life Project. *Health Information Online*. May 17, 2005:i–iv,1–17. Available at: http://www. pewinternet.org/pdfs/PIP_Healthtopics_May05.pdf. Accessed June 20, 2006.

30. National Institute for Health Care Management. Health plans emerging as pragmatic partners in fight against obesity. April 2005. Available at: http://www.nihcm.org/finalweb/ObesityReport.pdf. Accessed June 14, 2006.

31. Zhu SH, Anderson CM, Tedeschi GJ, et al. Evidence of real-world effectiveness of a telephone quitline for smokers. *N Engl J Med*. October 3, 2002:347(14), 1087–1093.

32. Lichtenstein E, Glasgow RE, Lando HA, Ossip-Klein DJ, Boles SM. Telephone counseling for smoking cessation: Rationales and meta-analytic review of evidence. *Health Ed Res*. 1996:11(2), 243–257.

33. Boucher JL, Schaumann JD, Pronk NP, Priest B, Ett T, Gray CM. The effectiveness of telephone-based counseling for weight management. *Diabetes Spectrum*. 1999:12(2), 121–123. Available at: http://journal.diabetes.org/diabetesspectrum/99v12n2/pg121.htm. Accessed June 14, 2006.

34. Lenert L, Muñoz RF, Stoddard J, et al. Design and pilot evaluation of an Internet smoking cessation program. *J Am Med Inform Assoc*. January–February 2003:10(1), 16–20.

35. Cromwell J, Bartosch WJ, Fiore MC, Hasselblad V, Baker T. Cost-effectiveness of the clinical practice recommendations in the AHCPR Guideline for Smoking Cessation. Agency for Health Care Policy and Research. *JAMA*. December 3, 1997:278(21), 1759–1766.

36. Wantland DJ, Portillo CJ, Holzemer WL, Slaughter R, McGhee EM. The effectiveness of Web-based vs. non-Web-based interventions: A meta-analysis of behavioral change outcomes. *J Med Internet Res*. 2004:6(4). Available at: http://www.jmir.org/2004/4/e40/. Accessed June 14, 2006.

37. Rothert K, Strecher VJ, Doyle LA, et al. Web-based weight management programs in an integrated health care setting: A randomized, controlled trial. *Obesity*. 2006:14, 266–272.

38. Tate DF, Jackvony EH, Wing RR. Effects of Internet behavioral counseling on weight loss in adults at risk for type 2 diabetes: A randomized trial. *JAMA*. 2003:289, 1833–1836.

39. Gold BC, Burke S, Buzzell P, Pintauro S, Harvey-Berino J. Weight loss on the Web: A pilot study comparing a commercial website to a structured behavioral intervention. Health e-Technologies Initiative. Available at: http://www.hetinitiative.org/sub-resources/ea-abstract_weightlossweb.html. Accessed June 14, 2006.

40. Tsai AG, Wadden TA. Systematic review: An evaluation of major commercial weight loss programs in the United States. *Ann Intern Med*. 2005:142, 56–66.

41. Dudley RA. Pay-for-performance research: How to learn what clinicians and policy makers need to know. *JAMA*. 2005:294(14), 1821–1823.

42. Rosenthal MB, Frank RG. What is the empirical basis for paying for quality in health care? *Med Care Res Rev*. 2006:63(2), 135–157.

43. Rosenthal MB, Frank RG, Li Z, Epstein AM. Early experience with pay-for-performance: from concept to practice. *JAMA*. 2005:294, 1788–1793.

44. Bordley WC, Chelminski A, Margolis PA, Kraus R, Szilagyi PG, Vann JJ. The effect of audit and feedback on immunization delivery. *Am J Prev Med*. May 2000:18(4), 343–350.

45. Kiefe CI, Allison JJ, Williams OD, Person SD, Weaver MT, Weissman NW. Improving quality improvement using achievable benchmarks for physician feedback. *JAMA*. June 13, 2001: 285(22).

46. Barnett GO, Winickoff RN, Morgan MM, Zielstorff RD. A computer-based monitoring system for follow-up of elevated blood pressure. *Med Care*. April 1983:21(4), 400–409.

47. McDonald CJ, Hui SL, Smith DM, *et al*. Reminders to physicians from an introspective computer medical record: A two-year randomized trial. *Ann Intern Med*. January 1984: 100(1), 130–138.

48. Kleschen MZ, Holbrook J, Rothbaum AK, Stringer RA, McInerney MJ, Helgerson SD. Improving the pneumococcal immunization rate for patients with diabetes in a managed care population: A simple intervention with a rapid effect. *Joint Commiss J Qual Patient Safety*. September 2000:26(9), 538–546.

49. National Network for Immunization Information. Common questions about school immunization laws. March 2004. Available at: http://www.immunizationinfo.org/assets/files/pdfs/4_SCH.pdf. Accessed June 20, 2006.

50. Briss PA, Rodewald LE, Hinman AR, et al. Reviews of evidence regarding interventions to improve vaccination coverage in children,

adolescents, and adults. *Am J Prev Med.* January 2000:18(1).

51. Orenstein WA, Hinman AR. The immunization system in the United States—The role of school immunization laws. *Vaccine.* October 29, 1999:17(suppl 3), S19–S24.

52. U.S. Centers for Disease Control and Prevention (CDC). Influenza: Clinical description and diagnosis. Available at: http://www.cdc.gov/flu/professionals/diagnosis/. Accessed June 9, 2006.

53. U.S. Centers for Disease Control and Prevention (CDC). Achievements in public health: Hepatitis B vaccination—United States, 1982–2002. *MMWR.* June 28, 2002:51 (25), 549–552.

54. Orenstein WA. Testimony of Walter A Orenstein, MD. *Hearing Before House Committee on Government Reform: Averting Future Influenza Vaccine Shortages: Hearing on U.S. Influenza Vaccine Supply.* 109 Cong, 1 Sess. February 10, 2005. Available at: http://a257.g.akamaitech.net/7/257/2422/07apr20051200/www.access.gpo.gov/congress/house/pdf/109hrg/99512.pdf. Accessed June 9, 2006.

55. U.S. Centers for Disease Control and Prevention (CDC). Targeting tobacco use: The nation's leading cause of death. *At a Glance 2006.* Available at: http://www.cdc.gov/NCCdphp/ publications/aag/osh.htm. Accessed June 8, 2006.

56. Ranson K, Jha P, Chaloupka FJ, Nguyen S. The effectiveness and cost-effectiveness of price increases and other tobacco control policies. In: Jha P, Chaloupka FJ, eds. *Tobacco Control in Developing Countries.* New York: Oxford University Press, 2000:427–447. Available at: http://tigger.uic.edu/ ~ fjc/Presentations/Scans/Final % 20PDFs/tc427to448.pdf. Accessed June 8, 2006.

15

QUALITY MANAGEMENT IN MANAGED CARE

Pamela B. Siren

Study Objectives

- Understand the components of a traditional quality assurance program.
- Understand the differences between traditional quality assurance and quality management.
- Identify customers of managed care.
- Understand managed care processes and outcomes and how they meet customer need.
- Understand the key measures used to assess performance of managed care processes.

Discussion Topics

1. Describe and discuss the three criteria Donabedian developed to assess quality and identify circumstances in which they can be applied.
2. Discuss the key components of a quality management program and what features distinguish a quality management program from traditional quality assurance.
3. Discuss how the quality management model can be applied to the development of a new program in preventions, such as one to reduce teen smoking.
4. Describe and discuss the strategies an MCO can use to involve physicians in managed care processes.

INTRODUCTION

The new millennium was marked by two significant publications from the Institute of Medicine (IOM) that took direct aim at quality in our health care system. *To Err is Human: Building a Safer Health System* (1999) and *Crossing the Quality Chasm* (2001) were outputs of the Committee on the Quality of Health Care in America, which was charged with identifying strategies for achieving substantial improvement in the quality of health care delivered to Americans. The findings from the committee's work have influenced purchasers, employers, and government agencies in making decisions regarding health care benefits for their constituents. Managed care, through its design and reimbursement of provider networks and independent medical management approaches, plays a crucial role in the overall strategy of quality improvement. The committee proposed six aims for improvement in our health care system:

- *Safe:* Avoiding injuries to patients from the care that is intended to help them.
- *Effective*: Provision of services basic on scientific knowledge to all who could benefit and refraining from providing services to those not likely to benefit (avoiding overuse and underuse, respectively).
- *Patient-centered*: Providing care that is respectful of and responsive to patient preferences, needs, values and ensuring patient values guide clinical decisions.
- *Timely*: Reducing waits and sometimes harmful delays for both those who receive and those who give care.
- *Efficient*: Avoiding waste, including waste of equipment, supplies, ideas, and energy
- *Equitable*: Providing care that does not vary in quality because of personal characteristics such as gender, ethnicity, geographic location, and socioeconomic status.[1]

The versions of this chapter in prior editions of *The Managed Health Care Handbook* series provided a primer for a managed care quality management program. Considering the changes in the marketplace, those core concepts are still important today and will be repeated, but the concepts also employ the principles of measurement, customer focus, and statistically based decision making and will be enhanced to address the issues of day.

TRADITIONAL QUALITY ASSURANCE

Advocacy for performance assessment in health care can be traced to E. A. Codman, a surgeon who practiced at Massachusetts General Hospital in the early 1900s. He was among the first advocates of systematic performance assessment in health care. His efforts included evaluation of the care provided to his own patients.

In the 1960s and 1970s, the introduction of computers and large administrative datasets (used initially to support Medicare claims processing) permitted investigators to use powerful epidemiological methods in their analyses of practice variations and related phenomena. In this period, Avedias Donabedian developed three criteria for the assessment of quality that are still used today: structure, process, and outcome.[2] His approach to quality assessment of care has stood the test of time and remains useful in managed care settings.

Structure Criteria

Structural measures of health care performance focus on the context in which care and services are provided. These measures provide inferences about the managed care organization's (MCO's) capability to provide the services it proposes to offer. Examples of structural measures include board certification of physicians, licensure of facilities, compliance with safety codes, record keeping, and physician network appointments. Many such requirements are delineated in federal, state, and local regulations that govern licensing or accreditation (see Chapter 23) and mandate periodic review and reporting mechanisms.

Accreditation and regulatory bodies have traditionally emphasized structural criteria because of their ease of documentation. Purchasers support this tradition by requesting such information in their contract negotiations with MCOs. The role of the MCO's leadership in improving performance is increasing and is evaluated by accrediting agencies through assessment of committee function. MCO leadership, executive and governance, needs a complete understanding of the role it plays in ensuring quality of care and service.

Integrated delivery systems' criteria for structural quality are more complex. The regulations and standards that may govern MCOs, such as those of the National Committee for Quality Assurance (NCQA; see Chapter 23), may be different from the standards to which member hospitals are held accountable, such as those of the Joint Commission on Accreditation of Healthcare Organizations (JCAHO) or to those public health licensing requirements for which the primary care practice sites are held responsible. Reconciliation of at least the minimal and widely accepted standards within the MCO and across an integrated delivery system is the first step to developing structural measures and evaluating structural performance and its impact on the quality and cost of health care delivery.

Structural measures generally do not offer adequate specificity to differentiate the capabilities of providers or organizations beyond meeting minimum standards. In addition, the relationship between structure and other measures of performance, such as outcomes, must be clarified to ensure that enforcing structural standards leads to better results.[3]

In an era of increasing demand by consumers and increasing costs, MCOs must manage their structural resources strategically while being mindful of the IOM aims for improvement. For example, some states, in collaboration with MCOs, are streamlining the provider credentialing process through centralization using an intermediary. In Massachusetts, for example, MCOs purchase provider credentialing information for a subscription fee. The efficiency achieved is two-fold: Providers have a single application to complete for all of the state's MCOs, and MCOs can reduce resources associated with their credentialing function without compromising the integrity of the process. From a quality perspective, required credentialing criteria can be consistently met in a timely fashion with a minimum of variation and error. This approach is discussed further in Chapter 5.

Process Criteria

The second traditional criterion for health care quality assessment is process. Langley and Nolan describe a *process* as a set of causes and conditions that repeatedly come together in a series of steps to transfer inputs into outcomes.[4] Processes of care measures evaluate the way in which care is provided. The IOM aims for improvement in process measures focus on safe, effective, timely, patient-centered, efficient, and equitable health care. Examples of care process measures for MCOs include the number of referrals made out-of-network, preventive health screening rates (*eg,* mammography and cholesterol screening), follow-up rates for abnormal diagnostic results, and assessment of adherence to clinical algorithms for different conditions. Such measures are frequently evaluated against national criteria or benchmarks. Process of service measures are also frequently used; for example, appointment waiting times and membership application processing times. As with structural measures, it is important to link process measures to outcomes. Although the field of outcomes research continues to grow, the link between many health care processes and key outcomes has not always been clearly defined.

Freedom of choice and ease of access to specialty care are often common themes in patient-centered approaches to quality improvement. For example, a number of health maintenance organizations (HMOs) have been experimenting with referral-less or open access specialty networks. They are doing so because if processing a referral is not embraced as an opportunity for care management, there may be little value and added administrative expense for requiring one. Evaluation of both the cost and clinical value for specialty referrals as well as designing networks with some flexibility of choice should therefore be considered.

Outcome Criteria

The third traditional category of quality assessment is the outcome of care or service. Examples of traditional outcomes measurements include infection rates, morbidity, and mortality. Relatively poor outcomes performance generally mandates careful review. Unfortunately, although outcomes measures are purported to reflect the performance of the entire system of care and service processes, they often offer little insight into the causes of poor performance.

Despite the limitations of current outcomes assessment, most MCOs have systems in place to assess for adverse events. These screening criteria are often evaluated during the utilization review process to detect sentinel events. Some of these same measures are being applied to the peer review process within the MCO.

Peer Review and Appropriateness Evaluation

In addition to Donabedian's three quality criteria, peer review and appropriateness review have been key components of the traditional quality assurance model. Peer review and appropriateness of care are central to the managed care debate, and they are discussed here.

▪ Peer Review

Peer review involves a comparison of an individual provider's practice either by the provider's peers or against an acceptable standard of care. These standards, or practice guidelines, may be developed within the MCO, be described by national professional associations (eg, the American Academy of Pediatrics), or be created or compiled by a regulatory or legislative agency (eg, the Agency for Healthcare Research and Quality). Practice guidelines are discussed further in a later section of this chapter as well as in Chapter 8.

Cases for peer review are identified either as outliers to specific indicators, perceived deviations from a norm, or through audits of medical records. Peer review has traditionally been used as an informal yet effective educational tool. It is typified by morbidity and mortality conferences currently in existence within medical groups. Within an MCO, peer review frequently occurs following a sentinel or "never event"[5] such as a member suicide during the course of receiving behavioral health treatment or the wrong body part being operated on. These never events are called that because they should never occur, and they are discussed as well in Chapter 7.

Peer review has its limitations. First, opportunities for improvement may be missed by a paradigm that rests on conformance with standards. Deming emphasized that merely meeting specifications does not result in constant improvement but rather ensures the status quo.[6] Second, peer review is limited by the scope of the indicators or processes under review and is traditionally driven by sentinel events.

In today's MCO, more emphasis is being placed on the what, the how, and the who of making clinical decisions to approve or deny coverage. An integral component of a modern quality management program is the evaluation of consistency of decision making by both MCO physicians and case managers. Interrater reliability audits are useful tools to be added to an MCO's internal peer review process to monitor consistency of decision making and application of criteria.

▪ Appropriateness Evaluation

Appropriateness evaluation reviews the extent to which the MCO provides timely and necessary care at the right level of service to those who are likely to benefit. Appropriateness review frequently occurs before an elective clinical event (admission or procedure) as part of a precertification process (see Chapter 9). Procedures or admissions most frequently selected for appropriateness review include those for which there is a wide variation of opinion as to their usefulness or effectiveness and those that have been notably expensive. Examples of procedures frequently selected for appropriateness review include hysterectomy, coronary artery bypass surgery, and laminectomy. The proposed indication for the event is compared with a list of approved indications obtained from a professional society, a specialty vendor or commercial source, or designed by the MCO itself. Appropriateness review is intended to identify and minimize areas of overutilization. Optimal care management systems are applying appropriateness criteria to assess the potential for underutilization of needed services or responding to the IOM improvement aim of ensuring effective care.

BUILDING ON TRADITION: ADDITIONAL COMPONENTS

Donabedian's three criteria for quality assessment provide the essential tools to design a quality management program. The traditional quality assurance model can be improved, however, with an infusion of systems thinking, customer focus, and knowledge for improvement.

Systems Thinking

Systems thinking recognizes that processes are interrelated. Systems thinking offers a method for structural design, assessment, and management of performance with a clear aim and shared purpose. A shared aim permits payers and providers to form a connected, efficient network. Generally, a disconnected network will eventually engage in contradictory and inefficient behaviors. Organizational goals can be achieved first by identifying customer needs of an organiza-

tion, unifying the purpose within the organization, and expanding the shared purpose across the integrated delivery system. Shared purpose and a shared financial risk between MCO and provider groups offers the potential to promote the quality of care delivered through the reduction of inappropriate care/service denials and improved coordination of care.

Customer Focus

Customer focus is the cornerstone of a modern quality management program. An organization that embraces this philosophy as part of its strategic vision is well suited to address the needs associated with increasing consumerism, as discussed in Chapter 20. The modern quality management program identifies key customers, anticipates customer needs, measures how effectively customer needs are met, and improves processes to meet those needs.

Knowledge for Improvement

Finally, an enhancement of the traditional quality assurance model is knowledge for improvement. Improvement involves the methods of measurement and change management. According to Moen and Nolan, three fundamental questions can be used as guides for improvement efforts:

1. What are you trying to accomplish? Information gained from understanding customer needs, the current process and outcome performance, and expected performance will assist the MCO in answering this question.
2. How will you know that a change is an improvement? Establishing performance expectations before implementing an improvement activity assists the MCO in understanding whether a change is an improvement and minimizes any potential confusion between measures of utilization and indicators of quality.

3. What changes can be made that will result in an improvement?[7]

To develop tests and implement changes, the plan-do-study-act (PDSA) cycle is used as a framework for an efficient trial and learning model. The term *study* is used in the third cycle to emphasize this phase's primary purpose: to gain knowledge. Increased knowledge leads to a better prediction of whether a change in a given process will result in an improvement.[4] According to Langley and Nolan, to be considered a PDSA cycle, the following aspects of the activity should be identifiable. First, the activity must be planned, including a strategy to collect data. Second, the plan must be attempted. Third, time must be set aside to analyze the data and study the results. Finally, action must be rationally based on what was learned. For example, an MCO experimenting with the most effective means to ensure an adequate response rate on a member self-reported health risk assessment (see Chapter 9) might deploy two strategies. One strategy includes a telephone call to the member; in the other strategy, a written survey is mailed. Response rates are collected for both methods to determine which yields the most favorable rates. If findings identify that telephone calls yield a higher response rate, then this is the strategy to be deployed. In all events, improvement strategies do not necessarily have to be broad, sweeping changes. Rather, small, incremental improvements offer sustainability over time.

CONTINUOUS IMPROVEMENT PROCESS MODEL

The remainder of this chapter discusses the key steps in developing a modern quality management program that is based on the fundamentals of quality assurance, incorporates the improvement aims of the Institute of Medicine, and is responsive to the changing marketplace. Figure 15-1 illustrates the components of this model.

Understand Customer Need

Understanding customer need is the basis of all quality management programs. Juran and Gryna described a customer as anyone who

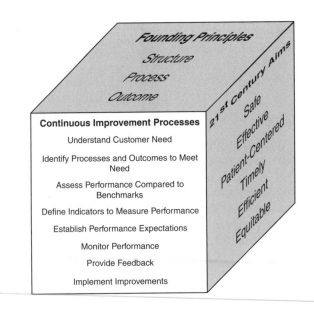

Figure 15–1 Quality Management Cube

is affected by a product or process.[8] Three categories of customers are external customers, internal customers, and suppliers. External customers of an MCO include members or beneficiaries, providers, and purchasers. Internal customers include the departments and services within the MCO, such as claims processing and member education, as well as the MCO's health care professionals themselves. Customer needs may be clear or disguised, rational or less than rational. These needs must be discovered and served.[8] Negotiating and balancing the needs of these diverse and sometimes conflicting customer groups represent a challenge for MCOs, as they do for any organization.

Methods to understand customer need are as diverse as the customer groups. Reactive understanding of customer needs usually comes in the form of complaints. Customer complaints are a usual signal of a quality problem. Low levels of complaints, however, do not necessarily mean high satisfaction. Frequently, dissatisfied customers will purchase services elsewhere without ever registering a complaint. Most MCOs have a formal process to survey their membership for satisfaction with care or services. Member surveys often use a common format as described in Chapter 23 on accreditation. Member complaints and grievances are also categorized and discussed in Chapter 19 on member services.

MCOs need to carefully examine their internal policies and processes that have a direct impact on members. Evaluation of front-end member services to assess the ease of access to care and services and responsiveness to meet member needs is essential. Medical management operations must evaluate the appropriateness and consistency of care decisions, particularly denials, and the degree to which care is coordinated. Analysis of member appeals should focus both on the reason for the care denial but should inform the process of negotiating; balancing the diverse groups of customer needs can represent a challenge. Juran and Gryna state that it is important to recognize that some cus-

tomers are more important than others. It is typical that 80% of the total sales volume comes from about 20% of the customers; these are the vital few customers who command priority.[8] Within these key customer groups, there is a distribution of individual customers that may also have a hierarchy of importance, such as a government agency, a gold card purchaser account, or an academic teaching center. Explicit understanding of the needs of all the MCO customer groups will minimize situations in which one customer's needs are met to the exclusion of another's.

Two key customer needs have moved to the forefront of quality management: patient safety and equitable access. The IOM Quality of Health Care in America Committee reported that as many as 98,000 people die in any given year from medical errors that occur in hospitals.[9] Medication errors alone, occurring in or out of the hospital, are estimated to account for more than 7,000 deaths annually.[10] In addition to the responsibility the MCO has to provide a safe network of providers, MCOs must seek remedy for medical errors. Remedies may come in the form of refusing to reimburse for continuing care associated with medical errors such as an extended hospital stay related to an error or a surgical procedure on the wrong organ or limb, as discussed in Chapter 7. MCOs also have the ability to influence and direct their membership to high-quality hospitals. For example, the Leapfrog Group, an organization of purchasers, asks hospitals if they adhere to three quality and safety practices because significant scientific evidence shows that these practices reduce unnecessary deaths and injuries:

1. Computerized physician order entry.
2. Intensive care unit (ICU) staffing with health care providers who have special training in critical care.
3. High-risk treatments—the process of selecting a hospital with extensive experience and results for specific procedures, surgeries, or conditions is known as evidence-based hospital referral.[11]

The customer need for patient safety is largely being expressed by purchasers and employer groups who are diligently working to inform their constituents.

Equitable health care, that is, providing care that does not vary in quality because of personal characteristics such as gender, ethnicity, geographic location, and socioeconomic status, is a growing customer need. The Institute of Medicine found that racial and ethnic groups receive lower quality of care and needed services than nonminorities do even when factors related to access to care are controlled.[12] The Commonwealth Fund also has demonstrated how race, ethnicity, and English language proficiency can affect access to quality health care.[13] Understanding who your customers are and how the quality of care they receive may vary according to those differences is essential to a modern quality management program.

Identify Processes and Outcomes That Meet Customer Need

Identification of processes and outcomes that meet customer need is the next step of the continuous improvement process. How do customers view the MCO's quality? To begin with, they want to know whether the MCO meets their expectations. MCOs are expected to treat members who are ill and to maintain the health and functional capabilities of those who are not. To treat sick patients, MCOs first have to make it easy for them to access services, and second must provide them with appropriate care. Purchasers and members value access and appropriateness.[14] Purchasers also value assessments of disease screening activities, service quality, and encounter outcomes to the extent that they support or embellish information about access and appropriateness. Similarly, purchasers know that to maintain health and functional capacity, MCOs must support prevention of illness and management of health status. These types of activities are discussed further in the other chapters in Part III of this book.

Assess Performance Compared with Professional or "Best-of-Class" Standards

The third step of the continuous improvement process is assessing the MCO's performance compared with a professional or "best-of-class" standard. This concept of comparison was discussed earlier. Performance can be assessed through appropriateness and peer review, benchmarking, and outcomes assessment.

▪ Appropriateness Review

As discussed for the traditional quality assurance model, appropriateness indicators evaluate the extent to which the MCO provides necessary care and does not provide unnecessary care in the service location best suited for quality and cost efficiencies. Purchasers understand that they cannot obtain good value from an MCO unless it provides appropriate services, so that these indicators are as important as those for accessibility.

Unfortunately, improving the assessment of appropriateness has been dogged by methodological problems, such as adjusting the data for case mix (discussed later) and the surprising lack of data from controlled trials that would define appropriate care in the first place. This issue affects the evaluation of both overutilization and underutilization of services.

In response to these challenges, the MCO can do two things. First, the MCO can identify minimum performance standards for high-cost diagnoses and use them to select processes having excess utilization. Second, the MCO can demonstrate evidence of consistent success and/or an improvement trend in clinical appropriateness indicators. If these two approaches are employed, purchasers seem inclined to offer MCOs some flexibility in the short run even if some isolated indicators suggest that there may be quality problems.

▪ Peer Review

As discussed previously, peer review involves a comparison of an individual provider's practice against an accepted standard of care. A key difference between peer review in a traditional quality assurance model and that in a modern quality management model is the topic of comparison.

▪ Benchmarking

A third method of assessing and comparing an MCO's performance is benchmarking. Robert Camp of Xerox Corporation popularized benchmarking over the last 20 years. Camp and Tweet define *benchmarking* as "the continuous process of measuring products, services, and practices against the company's toughest competitors or those companies renowned as industry leaders."[15] Two types of benchmarking may be used by MCOs. First, internal benchmarking identifies internal functions to serve as pilot sites for comparison. This type of benchmarking is particularly useful in newly integrated delivery systems with multiple, diverse component entities.[15] The second type of benchmarking is external or competitive benchmarking. Competitive benchmarking is the comparison of work processes with those of the best competitor and reveals which performance measure levels can be surpassed.[15] The benchmarking process can be applied to service and clinical processes for knowledge of current performance. Managed care organizations are sometimes reluctant to experiment in benchmarking outside of health care or insurance. Much can be learned from the airline industry (*eg,* scheduling and call center statistics), the banking industry (*eg,* privacy and replacement of lost cards), and the manufacturing industry (*eg,* processing claims).

▪ Outcomes Assessment

An MCO also assesses performance through outcomes assessment. An outcomes assessment may be performed on the MCO's 10 high-volume or high-cost diagnoses or procedure groups. An outcomes assessment permits the MCO to assess its own performance over time and to identify variation within the MCO. Davies and others have out-lined three core activities for an outcomes assessment:

1. Outcomes measurements are "point-in-time" observations.
2. Outcomes monitoring includes the process of repeated measurements over time, which permits causal inferences to be drawn about the observed outcomes.
3. Outcomes management is the application of the information and knowledge gained from outcome assessment to achieve optimal outcomes through improved decision making and delivery.[16]

The purpose of an outcomes assessment is to provide a quantitative comparison among treatment programs, to map the typical course of a chronic disease across a continuum, or to identify variations in the outcome of care as potential markers of process variation.[16]

Define Indicators to Measure Performance

Defining indicators to measure performance is the fourth step of the continuous improvement process. The MCO may apply the quality criteria (structure, process, and outcome) as discussed for the traditional quality assurance model. In addition, it is useful for MCOs to evaluate their process and outcomes by populations of customers served. A key issue faced by MCOs in indicator definition and analysis is case-mix adjustment.

Case-mix adjustment is the process of correcting data for variations in illness or wellness in patient populations. It is a statistical model that takes into account specific attributes of a patient population (*eg,* age, sex, severity of illness, chronic health status) that are beyond the control of the MCO or health provider.[17] This adjustment is particularly important in comparative analyses between providers or among MCOs.

Case-mix adjustment permits fair comparisons among same-population groups because it accounts for preexisting phenomena that may affect the outcome of care. Potentially required variables in a broadly useful risk adjustment system include the following:

- Demographic factors
- Diagnostic information
- Patient-derived health status
- Claims-derived health status
- Prior use of all services
- Prior use of nonelective hospitalization
- Prior use of medical procedures
- Prior or current use of pharmaceuticals[18]

Issues of case mix affect the analysis of both inpatient and outpatient care. The problem, however, is more serious for some performance measures than for others. Case mix is important for clinically oriented indicators such as appropriateness and encounter outcomes. It also has a significant impact on assessments of health status, resource use, and member satisfaction. Case mix is not nearly as important for measures of access and prevention, and thus these measures should be considered more appropriate for physician profiles and report cards. The topic of case-mix adjustment exceeds the scope of this chapter. Chapter 16 provides further discussion of this topic.

The National Committee for Quality Assurance (NCQA; see Chapter 23) has been a leader in indicator development for managed care. The indicator set developed by NCQA, the Health Plan Employer Information Data Set (HEDIS), had its origins in preventive health screenings and procedures such as pediatric immunizations and cancer screenings. With recognition that the population of persons living with chronic conditions and the science of measurement have improved, new HEDIS measures have increasingly focused on care of chronic conditions and proper use of medications. NCQA is moving away from creating new measures that require review of medical records and is advancing toward more measures that utilize administrative data. For example, chronic disease treatment measures now include chronic obstructive pulmonary disease (COPD) and rheumatoid arthritis. Medication monitoring measures a number of treatment do-

mains, including antibiotics, psychoactive medications (for depression and attention deficit hyperactivity disorder—ADHD), and persistent-use medications for chronic conditions such as asthma and hypercholesterolemia. Rates for the new measures are calculated using a combination of claims and pharmacy data.[19] The full HEDIS measurement set for 2006 is illustrated in Table 23-1 in Chapter 23.

Establish Performance Expectations

Establishing performance expectations is the fifth step of the continuous improvement process. Performance expectations are defined by understanding customer needs (step 1), evaluating the performance of the processes and outcomes designed to meet those needs (step 2), and comparing performance against "best-of-class" standards either internal or external to the MCO (step 3). Many MCOs submit the results of their indicators to NCQA's Quality Compass each year. Quality Compass is a valuable source for MCOs to benchmark from and establish stretch goals for performance improvement.

Monitor Performance and Compare with Expectations

Following established expectations, the sixth step is the actual monitoring of performance and comparison with expectations. The frequency of monitoring is determined by the indicators the MCO has selected to measure performance. An MCO can compare its performance against its own over time and against other MCOs if the same indicator definitions are used.

Provide Feedback to Providers and Customers

The seventh step of the continuous improvement process is providing feedback. Two methods of feedback are discussed here: profiling, which assesses the performance of individual providers and report cards, which assess overall MCO performance. Feedback through profiling and/or report cards is also a component of pay-for-performance (P4P) programs, which is discussed in detail in Chapter 8.

▪ Profiling

Profiling focuses on the patterns of an individual provider's care rather than that provider's specific clinical decisions. The practice pattern of an individual provider hospital or physician is expressed as a rate or a measure of resource use during a defined period and for a defined population.[20] The resulting profile can then be compared against a peer group or a standard. MCOs are using profiling to measure provider performance, to guide quality improvement efforts, and to select providers for managed care networks.[21] Examples of measures used in provider profiling include average wait time to schedule a routine physical, number of hospital admissions, number of referrals out-of-network, number of emergency department visits, member satisfaction, percentage compliance with the MCO's clinical practice guidelines, and, if applicable, the percentage of children receiving appropriate immunizations and the Cesarean section rate. Chapter 16 discusses the approach to and uses of profiling in more detail.

▪ Report Cards

Report cards have become a popular method of conveying performance within an individual MCO with multiple geographic sites or across many diverse MCOs. The purpose of a report card is to provide customers (purchasers and consumers) with comparable quality and cost information in a common language for the purpose of selecting a health plan. In 2005, the popular magazine *U.S. News & World Report* published a report card on "America's Best Health Plans," focusing on NCQA accreditation and HEDIS. A similar type of report card has long been used by the publication to report on "America's Best Hospitals."

The benefits of the report card movement (sometimes referred to as *data transparency*) include the stimulus for MCOs to build the capacity to produce performance information and strengthen data quality. Public disclosure of performance information, as illustrated in the *U.S. News & World Report* publication, also lends itself to plan, provider, and hospital accountability. Such public report cards should aim to include the issues of patient safety and equity.

A limitation of the report card movement continues to be measurement. Although the NCQA and HEDIS have made moves to standardize measurement, there continues to be variation in measurement, coding, and clinical classification. Additionally, there is variation in the administrative source datasets that plans use to obtain their measurements. Risk adjustment and a broader clinical focus are opportunities for improvement. Finally, no conclusion can be drawn about processes or outcomes that are not assessed by the report card measurements.

Implement Improvements

The eighth step of the continuous improvement process is implementation of improvements. The PDSA cycle described earlier is a vehicle for learning and acting. According to Langley and Nolan, PDSA can be used to build knowledge about a process, to test a change, or to implement a change. Current strategies employed by MCOs as tools to improve health care delivery processes and outcomes are practice guidelines, improvement teams, and consumer education.

▪ Practice Guidelines

Clinical practice guidelines are systematically developed statements to assist practitioners and patients in making decisions about appropriate health care for specific clinical circumstances. Clinical guidelines may inform a disease management program (see Chapter 10) or be applied separately. Clinical guidelines for selected, high-impact conditions are also incorporated into P4P programs as discussed in Chapter 8.

Guidelines offer an opportunity to improve health care delivery processes by reducing unwanted variation and can also be viewed as restrictive when applied to care or service denials. An appointed committee of the Institute of Medicine recommended the following attributes of guideline design:

- *Validity:* Practice guidelines are deemed valid if they lead to the health and cost outcomes projected for them.
- *Reliability/reproducibility:* If given the same evidence and development methods, another set of experts would come up with the same recommendations, and the guidelines are interpreted and applied consistently across providers.
- *Clinical applicability:* Guidelines should apply to a clearly defined patient population.
- *Clinical flexibility:* Guidelines should recognize the generally anticipated exceptions to the recommendations proposed.
- *Multidisciplinary process:* Representatives of key disciplines involved in the process of care should participate in the guideline development process.
- *Scheduled review:* Guideline evaluation should be planned in advance and occur at a frequency that reflects the evolution of clinical evidence for the guideline topic.
- *Documentation:* Detailed summaries of the guideline development process that reflect the procedures followed, the participants involved, the evidence and analytical methods employed, and the assumptions and rationales accepted should be maintained .[22]

Guidelines can't be effective without a successful implementation process. The first step in designing an implementation strategy for clinical guidelines is to identify the forces driving and restraining clinical practice change.[23] Thus, an MCO may want to convene a group of local content experts along with its own medical leadership to initiate guideline planning and adoption. An effective implementation team strengthens the driving forces for the guideline and weakens the restraining forces for a given clinical practice change. To implement guidelines as an improvement

strategy, performance must be measured on two levels. First, the gap between prior and optimal practice is measured to assess the degree of implementation. Actionable feedback must also be given to providers to reinforce the change in clinical practice.[24]

▪ Consumer Education

The effectiveness of consumer education must also be a part of an MCO's quality plan. Consumer education is targeted at beneficiaries so that they can become effective health care consumers and participate in meeting the aforementioned needs of treating disease and managing health. Examples of consumer education utilized by MCOs include telephone resource lines, health risk appraisals, worksite-based consumer education programs, and consumer health education materials. Many MCOs have developed and provide members with self-care guidelines for preventing illness and treating common complaints at the time of enrollment. These topics are also discussed briefly in Chapter 9 and extensively in Chapter 14.

▪ Setting the Improvement Agenda

Finally, the MCO must evaluate whether improvements actually made a change and met customer need. If not, the cycle begins again with step 1. If improvements did occur and customer needs were met, the cycle can begin again for new or unaddressed customer needs.

How can an MCO design such a cycle? MCOs have limited resources with which to assess and improve performance, and strategic decisions must be made to target resources effectively. An MCO's leadership group may begin the cycle of improvement by applying the following criteria:

1. Identify which customer need is being addressed by the proposed project.
2. Evaluate the strength of the evidence for the need to improve.
3. Assess the probability that there will be a measurable impact.
4. Determine the likelihood of success.

5. Identify the immediacy of impact in meeting the customer's need.

CONCLUSION

Double-digit rate inflation annually for health care premiums in an environment of excessive medical errors and concerns that minorities are not receiving equal care and treatment suggests an opportunity for MCO quality managers to design effective and comprehensive quality programs. Tools to affect such a program are the foundations of quality assurance from Donabedian, addressing the IOM improvement aims for the twenty-first century, and using a planned and deliberate process performance improvement process based on data.

Institute of Medicine. *To Err Is Human: Building a Safer Health Care System.* Washington, DC: National Academy Press; 2000.

Suggested Reading

Institute of Medicine. *To Err Is Human: Building a Safer Health Care System.* Washington, DC: National Academy Press, 2000.

Institute of Medicine. *Crossing the Quality Chasm. A New Health System for the 21st Century.* Washington, DC: National Academy Press, 2001.

Juran JM, Gryna FM. *Quality Planning and Analysis.* New York: McGraw-Hill, 1993.

Langley GJ, Nolan KM, *et al. The Improvement Guide: A Practical Approach to Enhancing Organizational Performance.* San Francisco: Jossey-Bass, 1996.

Senge P. *The Fifth Discipline: The Art and Practice of the Learning Organization.* New York: Currency Doubleday, 1993.

Walton M. *The Deming Management Method.* New York: Putnam, 1986.

References

1. Institute of Medicine. *Crossing the Quality Chasm.* Washington, DC: National Academy Press, 2001: 5–6.
2. Donabedian A. *Exploration in Quality Assessment and Monitoring: The Definition of Quality and Approaches to Its Assessment.* Vol. 1. Ann Arbor: Health Administration Press, 1980.
3. Shortell SM, LoGerfo JP. Hospital medical staff organization and quality of care: Results from myocardial infarction and appendectomy. *Med Care.* 1981:19, 1041–1056.
4. Langley GJ, Nolan KM, Nolan TW. 1994. The foundation of improvement. *Quality Progress, ASQC.* June 1994: 81–86.
5. National Quality Forum. 2002. Available at: http://www.qualityforum.org. Accessed October 2006.
6. Walton M. Improve constantly and forever the system of production and service. In: Walton M. *The Deming Management Method.* New York: Putnam, 1986: 66–67.
7. Moen D, Nolan TW. Process improvement. *Quality Progress.* 1987:9, 62–68.
8. Juran J, Gryna F. Understanding customer need. In: Juran J, Gryna F. *Quality Planning and Analysis.* 3rd ed. New York: McGraw-Hill, 1993: 240–252.
9. Institute of Medicine. *To Err Is Human: Building a Safer Health System.* Washington, DC: National Academy Press, 2000.
10. Phillips DP, Christenfeld N, Glynn LM. Increase in U.S. medication error deaths between 1983–1993. *Lancet.* 1998: 351, 643–644.
11. Leapfrog Group. For hospitals. Available at: http://www.leapfroggroup.org/for_hospitals. Accessed August 11, 2006.
12. Smedley BD, Stith AY, Nelson AR, eds. *Unequal Treatment: Confronting Racial and Ethnic Disparities in Health Care.* Washington, DC: Institute of Medicine, National Academies Press, 2002.

13. Nerenz DR, *et al. Developing a Health Plan Report Card on Quality Care for Minority Populations*. New York: Commonwealth Fund, 2002.

14. Health Care Advisory Board. *Next Generation of Outcomes Tracking*. Washington, DC: Health Care Advisory Board. 1994: 1–57.

15. Camp RL, Tweet AG. Benchmarking applied to health care. *JT Commiss J Qual Improvement*. 1994:20, 229–238.

16. Davies AR, *et al*. Outcomes assessment in clinical settings: a consensus statement on principles and best practices in project management. *JT Commiss J Qual Improvement*. 1994:20, 6–16.

17. Pine M, Harper DL. Designing and using case mix indices. *Manage Care Q*. 1994:2:1–11.

18. Goldfield N. Case mix, risk adjustment, reinsurance, and health reform. *Manage Care Q*. 1994:2, iv.

19. National Committee for Quality Assurance. *HEDIS 2007 Technical Specifications*. Vol. 2. Washington, DC: National Committee for Quality Assurance, July 2006 revision.

20. Lee PR, *et al*. Managed care: provider profiling. *J Ins Med*. 1992:24, 179–181.

21. Walker LM. Can a computer tell how good a doctor you are? *Med Econ*. 1994:71, 136–147.

22. Institute of Medicine, Committee to Advise the Public Health Service on Clinical Practice Guidelines. *Clinical Practice Guidelines: Directions for a New Program*. Washington, DC: National Academies Press, 1990.

23. Handley MR, *et al*. An evidence-based approach to evaluating and improving clinical practice: implementing practice guidelines. *HMO Practice*. 1994:8, 75–83.

24. Kiefe CI, Allison JJ, Williams OD, *et al*. Improving quality improvement using achievable benchmarks for physician feedback: a randomized controlled trial. *JAMA*. 2001:285, 2871–2879.

16

DATA ANALYSIS AND PROVIDER PROFILING IN HEALTH PLANS

David W. Plocher and Nancy Garrett

Study Objectives

- Understand general requirements for using data in medical management.
- Understand basic report format requirements.
- Understand basic types of reports and data for inpatient, outpatient, and ambulatory utilization.
- Understand basic concepts of profiling, and the problems of profiling, and approaches to dealing with those problems.
- Understand the uses of data and the strengths and weaknesses of different approaches to using data to manage medical care.
- Understand the general advantages and pitfalls of case mix/risk adjustment systems.
- Understand the trends in profiling and medical informatics.
- Understand the use of case mix/ risk adjustment measures for quality of care and for utilization/cost.

Discussion Topics

1. Discuss the principles of using data to manage health care delivery systems.
2. List and discuss the most important utilization and cost reports a medical director would need by model type, and describe the key elements in those reports.
3. Discuss the most common technical, clinical, and organizational problems medical directors face in using data to manage utilization and what steps might be taken to deal with those problems.

4. Discuss the most important principles in provider profiling.
5. Discuss the most common problems with profiling and how might a plan address those problems.
6. Identify and discuss how common sources of data are accessed in producing data for medical management and how problems with each of these data sources cause problems with the others.
7. Discuss the types of case mix measures available for each type of health care encounter and the strengths and weaknesses of each type.
8. Discuss HIPAA requirements regarding privacy and protected health information.
9. Discuss the challenges of public versus confidential disclosure of provider information.
10. Discuss some of the questions to ask when considering a case mix/risk adjustment system and/or profiling vendor.

INTRODUCTION

As employers face health care cost increases at least two to three times the consumer price index, they are increasingly turning to analysis of financial and clinical data for insights. In response, health plans are putting more resources into development of reporting and analyses that will help plans provide better medical management and employers better understand where they are spending their excess health care dollars. Additionally, large employers often work with third-party consulting firms that specialize in data analysis and who are able to provide summarized data from many employers for comparison.

A 2004 survey of the National Account Decision Makers found that reporting and analytical capabilities are key criteria employers use in choosing a health insurance carrier. "Providing information to better understand costs" is one of the key drivers of account relationship management, according to the same survey conducted in 2005.[1] Thus, the ability of health plans to use data and information intelligently to explain and manage costs has become a key success factor for sales and marketing efforts.

Because of the importance of analytics to the health plans' relationships with employer groups, this chapter focuses on reporting and analysis from the employer perspective. Other users of health plan data include medical managers in health plans, providers, consumers, and the community. However, all health plan analytic activities can ultimately be linked to their use in providing the best possible service to health plans' primary customers: employers.

By necessity, the focus of these analytics is on administrative claims data. Claims are a type of universal language in the health plan business. Because of government standardization in the way health plan claims are submitted* and increasing sophistication by health plans, consulting firms, and health services researchers in applying uniform rules and definitions to claims data, measures based on administrative data can be compared across employer groups, plans, and regions of the country. Using claims data for analysis is affordable because the data are already collected for the purposes of claims payment and is based on common rules and definitions. Although use of administrative data has many limits and nuances that we

---

*The mandate for standardization of electronic claims and other administrative transactions is a result of the Health Insurance Portability and Accountability Act (HIPAA) as discussed in Chapter 32.

discuss further, it forms the backbone of health plans' analytic services.

The latter part of this chapter focuses on a specific analytic activity: provider profiling. *Profiling* means the identification, collection, collation, and analysis of data to develop provider-specific characterization of their performance. As used in this chapter, providers can be any type of provider of health services, including physicians, clinics, and hospitals. Provider profiling represents an important application of analytics to efforts to improve quality and reduce costs for employer groups.

ADMINISTRATIVE CLAIMS DATA

Claims data are used by health plans to pay the providers of care. These providers include hospitals, pharmacies, group physician practices, and individual physicians. Because the purpose of the data is for payment of claims, a basic operational purpose of health plans, the data must be standardized and stored to be useful for reporting and analysis.

Data Warehousing

The setting in which a health service takes place helps to determine the kind of claims that are submitted to the health plan. For example, claims from a health care facility are often submitted using an electronic standard, the ANSI X12N 837 (required under Health Insurance Portability and Accountability Act [HIPAA] for electronic claims submissions; see Chapters 5, 17, and 31), or rarely now using a paper standard developed by the federal government, the CMS-1450 (previously called the HCFA Uniform Bill-92, or UB-92). Pharmacy claims are submitted in a different format maintained by the National Council for Prescription Drug Programs (NCPDP), often through a pharmacy benefit manager (PBM), a company that specializes in processing pharmacy claims as discussed in Chapter 12.

Other types of administrative data used for health plan payment include membership information, demographic information about the health plan members and the benefits they have; and provider information, demographic and practice information about providers. Because the sources of the data are unique, plans often have separate software systems to process each type of data for claims payment.

To capture and integrate these diverse data sources for clinical reporting and analysis, plans have developed data warehouses. A *data warehouse* is a collection of a broad set of data spanning a significant period of time, as well as a repository of information derived from those data. Standard rules and definitions are applied to reduce data errors and make the data as consistent as possible. This process of applying uniform rules is challenging, given the many different systems that can exist within the same health plan and the differences in how individual providers of care code similar events.

Building a data warehouse also requires agreement within a plan on how business rules apply to claims data. For example, one business unit such as underwriting may use a different definition of what makes up a managed care product compared to another unit, such as marketing. Therefore, creating a useful warehouse requires the collaboration of people throughout an organization.

Data warehouses are also built to maximize efficiency in reporting so that queries can be quickly returned even when accessing files with millions of claim lines. As the speed of the servers that store data and the software that queries against it improves, plans will be able to devote less time to pulling data out of the warehouse and more time to analyzing what it means.

As an example of the types of data that would be available for analysis in a data warehouse, for provider profiling purposes the following data elements are generally necessary:

- Unique patient identifier (scrambled for patient confidentiality).
- Diagnostic information—typically provided using codes from the *International*

Classification of Diseases, 9th ed., Clinical Modification (ICD-9-CM).*

- Procedural information—derived from Volume III of ICD-9-CM, current procedure terminology (CPT), and HCFA Common Procedure Coding System (HCPCS) codes. In addition, identifying information relative to the name of the pharmaceutical used is often present.
- Level of service information—such as that provided by evaluation and management CPT codes.
- Paid dollar amounts from services ordered by the physician or health care facility.
- Unique provider identifier. Universal Provider Identification Numbers (UPINs) codes for physicians, as used by the Center for Medicare and Medicaid Services (CMS), are not necessarily unique. The UPIN code is being replaced by a new numbering convention, the National Provider Identifier (NPI), in 2007. The NPI is discussed in Chapters 5 and 31.

Data warehouses are also being built across multiple health plans by national data consolidators. These consolidators, often private consulting and actuarial firms, specialize in cleansing data and applying uniform rules so that use of health care services can be analyzed for large populations. The consolidators use the national data warehouses for several purposes, including providing data comparing health plans on cost and utilization to large employers; calculating benchmarks of use and cost of health care services that plans can use to compare their performance to others; and conducting studies of postmarket drug reactions. The work of the consolidators in helping large employers interpret and compare their health care patterns is putting pressure on individual health plans to provide more analytical services to their clients.

Validity and Reliability

One issue in using claims data for reporting and analysis is validity, or the extent to which they actually mean what you think they mean. Even when there is great attention to diagnostic coding, the reason for a visit may or may not be related to everything that gets done (for example, a patient is seen with the diagnosis of hypertension but also gets a hearing test), or the diagnostic code may not be the same as the underlying disease (for example, a patient is seen for an upper respiratory infection, but the relevant diagnosis is emphysema). In addition to coding validity, it is important to validate data against other potential sources of the same data. For example, physician identification data may be kept in two separate databases, which may not match. At the time of publication, it is also common for providers to have different identifiers depending on what office they are practicing in, what group they are with, and so forth. For example, a physician may work with a medical group on certain days, but have a solo practice on other days. The problem of providers having different identifiers will eventually be resolved through the introduction of the NPI, which requires that a provider have one single and unique identifier for use in all circumstances.

The measures built using claims data must also be meaningful. It is of no value (other than academic) to measure things that have no real impact on the plan's ability to manage the system or a physician's ability to practice effectively. Even worse, there is potential harm in producing reports that purport to mean one thing but really mean another.

Another important consideration is the reliability of claims data or the extent to which data are consistent and mean the same thing from provider to provider. For exam-

---

*At some point in the future, ICD-9 is expected to be replaced with a new and more complex version, ICD-10. When that will occur is unknown at the time of publication.

ple, one provider may code differently from other providers for the same procedures, and a hospital may code an event differently from the attending physician. Diagnostic coding is particularly problematic when analyzing data from physician outpatient reports. Because diagnostic coding is not as important as procedural information in determining what a physician is paid, there is a great deal of laxity in diagnostic coding for office visits. Procedure coding tends to be more accurate because there is a direct relationship between what a provider codes as having been performed and what the provider gets paid. Accuracy, however, does not rule out creative coding or even fraud, resulting in deliberate coding inconsistencies. For example, one surgeon may bill for a total hysterectomy, whereas another surgeon performing the same procedure may bill for an exploratory laparotomy, removal of the uterus, removal of the ovaries, and lysis of adhesions, all of which generate a fee. The need for consistency may mean having to change or otherwise modify data to force conformance of meaning in the construction of a data warehouse.

Use of Claims Data for Analysis and Reporting

Despite the challenges with reliability and validity of administrative claims data, they are the closest type of information we have to a universal language in the health plan business. Because there is no need for additional data collection efforts such as clinical chart abstraction, using claims data is relatively cost-effective. In the future, clinical data may become more available to health plans as clinics begin using electronic medical records (EMRs; see also Chapter 17), which will allow for more complete and in-depth analysis of the outcomes of medical care.

Claims data are used to produce reports that monitor the utilization patterns and cost of health care, often on a per member per month (PMPM) basis, so that health plan actu-aries can monitor changes in the population-wide cost of specific services. Reports provide a picture of utilization patterns from a clinical perspective, showing the types of treatment that members receive. By tracking the services used by members with particular conditions, plans can produce process measures of the quality of care delivered. Claims also provide a basis for ad hoc investigation into specific clinical questions.

Inpatient claims data, in particular, have often been used for physician and institutional profiling.[2] There are several advantages to the use of inpatient claims data for quality improvement and utilization management purposes:

- With the implementation of diagnosis-related groups (DRGs), there is an extended period of experience with inpatient coding.[3]
- Because there are significant financial issues at stake for the hospital, there typically is a considerable effort to code as accurately as possible.[4]
- For enrollees with a chronic illness—individuals with the highest likelihood of interaction with the health care system—information pertaining to the quality of hospital care is likely to be important. This has become all the more important with the recent decision by CMS to use inpatient diagnoses as the initial risk adjuster for capitation payment rates to Medicare-managed care plans (see Chapter 26).
- Most simplistically, a significant portion of a managed care plan's expenditures comes from a relatively small number of enrollees.
- For at least one important aspect of quality within a hospital, mortality, the information is reliably coded and is of great importance to all consumers interested in physician profiles. Mortality, though, represents a very small set of events, and morbidity must also be measured.

- For many physicians, there are insufficient numbers of patients for whom one can examine issues pertaining to either quality and/or utilization.[5] When that is not possible, there are statistical methods to aggregate clinically dissimilar patients into categories, which have been adjusted for complexity.

Although still sometimes criticized, claims-based data have been widely used for quality improvement purposes.[2] For example, the Maine Medical Assessment Project has extensively utilized inpatient claims data for the purpose of developing physician-specific profiles.[6] These profiles are then released directly to the physician. This project has had a significant impact on medical practice, not only because of the rigorous scientific nature of data elements used within the physician profiles, but, just as important, the release process of the profiles. That is, the physician profiles are not only released for internal purposes, but senior physicians have provided extensive follow-up to the physicians involved in this profile effort.

Controversy still exists with respect to the validity of using claims-based data for quality improvement purposes. Recently published literature has begun to address this controversy, which has until now consisted more of noise than understanding. Chen and colleagues at Yale University determined that at least one methodology—that used in the creation of the *U.S. News and World Report Quality Ranking*—correlated with outcomes and processes of care for the one condition examined, acute myocardial infarction (AMI, or "heart attack").[7] On the other hand, Iezzoni and colleagues determined that complication rates derived from claims data do not correlate with quality of care information abstracted from the medical record.[8] Several entities, such as the state of California, are working to improve the validity of claims data by collecting data that indicate whether a secondary diagnosis was present at admission. In all events, health plans should be cognizant of the inadequacy of hospital complication rates that rely on claims data.

Visit-based ambulatory care claims data can also be used to provide comparative information pertaining to utilization of services across providers (provided that procedures are not a significant part of the case-mix adjustment that is used to account for differences in illness severity of the patient).[9] So long as the objective is clearly specified, profiling can also provide information pertaining to quality of care provided to enrollees. Thus, the following types of information obtained from visit-based ambulatory claims data are useful for physician profiles for quality monitoring purposes:

- Presence or absence of a particular procedure (such as vaccination or mammogram for preventive services or a retinal examination for a diabetic patient), the performance of which typically indicates that quality care has been provided for that particular condition.
- Utilization of inappropriate sites of care (such as the emergency department for an asthmatic), which, if repeated continuously, may indicate an opportunity for improvement.

As summarized in a review of claims data used for physician report cards published in 1998: "Despite the imperfections, claims data can be extremely useful probes to improve utilization, target continuing medical education, help manage complex patients, identify underserved patients and detect misprescribing, as well as fraud and abuse."[10]

THE NEED TO ADJUST FOR RISK

When comparing populations on outcomes related to the quality or cost of care, an important step is to adjust for differences in the illness burden between them. A useful definition of risk adjustment is: "Risk adjustment (RA) consists of a series of techniques that account for the health status of patients when predicting or explaining costs of health care for defined populations or for evaluating retrospectively the performance of providers who care for them."[II] Without rigorous risk adjustment techniques, comparisons of outcomes between populations may be a result of the demographic and health characteristics of each group rather than the care provided.

The terms *risk adjustment*, *severity adjustment*, and *case-mix adjustment* are often used interchangeably. Sometimes, however, *case-mix adjustment* is used specifically to adjust inpatient hospital episodes, as opposed to a population-wide approach to controlling for differences in health status across patients. Until the industry arrives at more standardization of this terminology, it is important to be clear about the definitions used in any particular situation.

Because risk adjustment techniques aim to separate the effect of treatment from characteristics inherent to the members, they need to be based on diagnosis rather than procedure codes. For example, a diagnosis code of diabetes indicates that a person is in a higher risk category for health care utilization compared to someone without diabetes. However, two people with the diagnosis of diabetes may have very different treatment patterns, and these treatment patterns should not influence the risk category because they are part of the outcome of interest.

Traditionally, age and sex served as a proxy for severity and case-mix adjustments, as was discussed in Chapter 6 regarding capitation payments to physicians. The basic and valid argument is that utilization is predictable based on age and sex, using actuarial tables. However, age and sex account for only a portion of risk, and more sophisticated models take into account population morbidity or other factors as well. Risk adjustment systems such as adjusted clinical groups (ACGs, formerly known as ambulatory care groups) explain about 30% of the variance in outcomes. Other unmeasured population differences that influence health include socioeconomic status and psychosocial characteristics.

Risk adjustment requires different tools and approaches depending on the focus of analysis. Approaches for ambulatory visits, inpatient episodes, diagnosis-based risk adjustment, and nursing home care are discussed later.

Ambulatory Visits

Two classification systems were developed and are used in the profiling of individual ambulatory visits or encounters: ambulatory patient groups (APGs) and ambulatory payment classifications (APCs). APGs were developed as a forerunner and are quite similar to APCs. Both are in the public domain. The APCs are used by CMS for outpatient prospective payment in hospital outpatient departments and ambulatory surgery centers for Medicare patients. APGs are already used by a variety of payers (for example, Medicaid and many Blue Cross Blue Shield plans). A number of companies produce mainframe and desktop versions of software for these classification systems.

Inpatient Episodes

A number of case-mix classification systems are available for profiling of inpatient care. Two such examples are as follows:

- DRGs as used by CMS for prospective payment under Medicare are public domain but are not severity adjusted. One needs to profile at an institutional level using CMS's DRGs to know the overall financial performance. However, the reasons for that performance cannot be ascertained without severity adjustment.
- APR-DRGs (3M/HIS Inc.) are proprietary, use claims data, and are commonly used for inpatient severity adjustment.

A number of intermediary vendors aggregate severity-adjusted data from either their own customers or from public use data tapes to produce comparative data. These include not-for-profit alliances and proprietary companies. A practical issue the user needs to decide is whether to mold and manipulate the data in-house and thus have greater flexibility in creating one's own reports or to send the data to a third party and receive reports from that intermediary. Thus, for example, with respect to the APR-DRGs, users can license a workstation that provides both standard and ad hoc reports, but they still must load in their data, or they can work with a third-party vendor that processes the data and provides canned or, at a higher price, tailored reports. This choice is made based on economic issues, internal capabilities, and the need to manipulate data on a frequent basis.

A health plan or large provider system should understand several theoretical issues. One of the most contentious is the inclusion of complications versus comorbidities in the logic of the risk adjustment. For example, with specific respect to myocardial infarction, many secondary diagnoses present on admission after an AMI likely represents comorbidities or sequelae of the AMI. For example, if a patient develops complete atrioventricular blockage (a complication resulting in the heart's inability to beat properly) on the second day of admission, it is likely that this secondary diagnosis represents a comorbidity of the AMI and not an *avoidable* complication of an AMI. One could extend this analysis to a large number of other secondary diagnoses with specific respect to AMI, and the same issue occurs with many other acute illnesses. The state of California has been a leader in providing a middle ground, by collecting data on whether the secondary diagnosis was present on admission.[12] Such knowledge would allow the calculation of separate indices for all codes rather than only those codes present on admission. This issue extends itself to episodes of illness.

Diagnosis-Based Risk Adjustment

Several systems have been developed that adjust for risk based on combined inpatient, ambulatory, and pharmacy data. These systems involve algorithms that look for patterns of diagnosis codes that are associated with higher population morbidity and resource consumption. They allow for comparison of utilization between populations while holding the overall illness burden constant. Thus, they have been used to determine payments to health plans and providers, as well as for clinical analysis. Two major systems in this category are adjusted clinical groups (ACGs)[13] and diagnostic cost groups (DCGs).[14]

Nursing Home, Rehabilitation Facilities, and Home Care

The numerous proposals and enacted federal legislation to pay for these services on a prospective basis have heightened the importance of case-mix measures. Health plans will increasingly need to become familiar with these case-mix measures as disease management programs begin to use these types of facilities more frequently. Descriptions of the two most commonly used case-mix measures follow.

Resource utilization groups (RUGs) have the least severity adjustment built into the system. They are currently used in the prospective payment for nursing homes.[15] Functional independence measure (FIM) and the Patient Evaluation and Conference System (PECS) are used primarily for rehabilitation facilities. Both have excellent severity adjustment measures built into the system. Recently, function resource groups (FRGs) were developed, using the FIM, for prospective payment. The Outcome and Assessment Information Set (OASIS) has been developed as both a quality of care and payment tool for home care services.

PATIENT DATA CONFIDENTIALITY

There have always been requirements on providers and health plans to protect the confidentiality of patient information. Those requirements have been variable from state to state to some degree. That recently changed somewhat with the effective date of HIPAA on April 21, 2005, which created a stringent minimum set of privacy and security standards, though states remain free to impose even greater stringency (see Chapter 32). In addition to privacy and security standards, as noted earlier, the implementation regulations for electronic business transactions also include detailed technical specifications based on ANSI X.12 N transaction data standards for both the data fields contained in a transaction and for the electronic format for transmitting a transaction, and also mandates the use of standard procedure and diagnostic codes; these are discussed in Chapters 5, 17, and 31.

HIPAA focuses on requirements to maintain the physical security of health information. The legislation applies to any person or organization that maintains or transmits electronic health information. HIPAA outlines standards for maintaining reasonable and appropriate administrative, technical, and physical safeguards. The safeguards aim to protect the physical security and integrity of personal health information from threats, hazards, or unauthorized uses. HIPAA prohibits wrongful disclosures of individually identifiable health information and prescribes penalties for violations. However, unlike the other parts of the administrative simplification title, the confidentiality provisions do not supercede all state laws about privacy of health information; a state may implement stricter, but not less strict, regulations.

HIPAA allows data to be used for medical management, including managing utilization and quality. It also allows for the use of "blinded" data—aggregate data for purposes of producing population-level reports—as long as there is no way for someone to use those data to trace back to an individual patient. Special protections are provided for mental health records. There are also situations where specific permission to use the data must be obtained from the patient (for example, providing that information to an employer or to anyone who is not involved in the provision or direct management of the patient's medical care). HIPAA expressly pro-hibits the sale of patient-identifiable data for any marketing or sales purpose. The complete text of the HIPAA regulation is available at the CMS Web site.[16]

Based on the preceding, it is clear that the use of data for analytic purposes requires a high degree of attention to policy and procedure to protect member confidentiality. Methods to produce reports must take these confidentiality requirements into account. Nevertheless, these confidentiality requirements, while creating high standards, do not prevent health plans from using data.

EMPLOYER REPORTING AND ANALYSIS

The purchaser of health coverage is primarily interested in the data analyst's ability to identify cost drivers, that is, the main causes of claim trend escalation. Such discoveries are expected to lead to customized solutions for reducing health care costs. The goal is trend mitigation, and employers competing in a global economy, trying to price their products and services efficiently, would like to see their claim trend approximate the consumer price index.

The Fundamentals

Each employer wishes to see how its paid claims trend compares to competing employers in the same industry. Next, the portion of employee liability is also of interest. That is, has the employer been too paternalistic in taking on the vast majority of health care costs—or conversely, has the option to cost shift been maximized to the point of contributing to workforce turnover?

For each type of service, the employer wants to see the health plan's accounting of exactly where excesses occur. For acute inpatient hospital services, is it unit cost (reimbursement per confinement) or unit frequency (admits per thousand)? Such analysis continues for outpatient/ambulatory services.

These excesses must be justified using credible benchmarks. As stated earlier, benchmarks should match the industry. There should also be adjustment by region of the country, product (HMO versus PPO), demographic (commercial versus Medicare versus Medicaid), and illness burden (adjustment for severity of illness of the employer's workforce and dependants).

Clinical analysis of where an employer's health care dollars are being spent should initially be constructed using a Pareto chart of clinical categories of care, such as the major diagnostic categories recommended by the Agency for Health Care Research and Quality.[17] For the commercial employed population, the top three categories are often oncology, musculoskeletal, and cardiovascular.

As excesses are explored, microcontributors need to be addressed. For example, high levels of emergency room services or of diagnostic imaging, although less of a contributor to total health plan cost, may represent overutilization that should be addressed. Examples of utilization reports for hospital care and an open access health plan are listed in Table 16-1 and 16-2, respectively.

Program Evaluation

Especially when the health plan charges an added fee for a particular medical management program, the plan analyst is required to show, using rigorous methods and metrics, the benefits to cost ratio for each program. Program evaluation involves both process and outcomes measures. For most employers the ultimate goal of health improvement programs is to save money by improving health, so analysts must determine return on investment (ROI) of each program. This is usually expressed as the ratio of dollars saved for each dollar invested, for example, a 2 to 1 ROI. For the most controversial programs, shared reimbursement of such reconciliation by an independent third party may be required.

Historic program evaluation techniques are centered on changes in direct claim costs, usually driven by utilization improvements. Today's analysts must add estimates of the indirect cost gains for the employer caused

Table 16–1 Sample Data Elements for a Monthly Summary of Hospital Utilization

- Plan statistics
  - Days per 1,000
  - Admissions per 1,000
  - Average length of stay
  - Average per diem cost
  - Average per case (per admission) cost
  - Emergency department visits and average cost
- Hospital- and provider-specific statistics
  - Days per 1,000
  - Admissions per 1,000
  - Average length of stay
  - Average per diem cost
  - Average per case (per admission) cost
  - Emergency department visits and average cost
- Statistics by service type (see Table 16-2)
  - Days per 1,0000
  - Admissions per 1,000
  - Average length of stay
  - Average per diem cost
  - Average per case (per admission) cost
- Retrospective authorizations
- Pended cases for review
- In-network compared to out-of-network statistics
- Number and percentage of denied days

Note: The plan will want to produce these statistics not only for the entire plan but for major lines of business as well (that is, commercial, Medicare, Medicaid, self-insured versus fully insured, and so forth).
Source: Created by author and adapted from an earlier version in *The Managed Health Care Handbook,* 4th ed., Jones and Bartlett, 2000.

by improvements in productivity and "presenteeism." These indirect costs are harder to measure, but are necessary to provide a complete picture of the benefits of health improvement programs. An emerging body of research is helping to provide more tools to make this possible.[18]

Table 16–2 Sample Data for an Open Access Model Plan

Outpatient Services

- Average number of visits per member per year

- Average number of visits per member per year to each specialty

- Diagnostic utilization per visit
  - Laboratory
  - Radiology and imaging
  - Other

- Average cost per visit

- Procedures per 1,000 visits per year (annualized)
  - Aggregate
  - By procedure for top 10, by specialty type
  - By individual specialist

- Average cost per episode (as defined for each sentinel diagnosis) over a defined time period, including charges not directly billed by provider

Inpatient Services

- Average total cost per case, including charges not billed by provider, for hospitalized cases

- Average length of stay for defined procedures

- Average rate of performance of a procedure, such as:
  - Cesarean section rate
  - Hysterectomy rate
  - Transurethral prostatectomy rate
  - Cardiac procedures

- Readmission rate or complication rate

- Use of resources before and after hospitalization

Source: Created by author and adapted from an earlier version in *The Managed Health Care Handbook,* 4th ed., Jones and Bartlett, 2000.

Applied Research Studies

Health plans may also conduct applied health services research studies of topics of interest to employers. For example, a health plan could use its administrative claims data and analytical expertise to conduct a study of the effectiveness of consumer-directed health plans in reducing utilization and cost. These studies help plans provide consultations to employers about effective medical management and motivational plan designs.

PROVIDER PROFILING

Provider or practice profiles have a variety of uses. Examples include producing feedback reports to help the providers modify their own behavior, recruiting providers into the network, and finding which providers are not the right fit with the organization's health care philosophy. Other uses include supporting performance-based reimbursement systems, determining specialists to whom the health plan will send certain types of cases, detecting fraud and abuse, determining how to focus the utilization management program, supporting quality management, and performing financial modeling. More recently, profiling has been used to set up multilevel health plan products that encourage members to go to providers with higher quality and/or lower cost through a benefit differential, referred to as a tiered network.

With respect to quality improvement, there are two types of variables one can profile: those that have a direct relation to costs and those that, although over the long term will possibly lead to decreased costs, have a closer relationship to our traditional understanding of quality. An example of the first type would be the variation in use of coronary artery bypass graft (CABG) for patients with angina, whereas mammography rates represent an example of the second category. From a quality of care perspective, both types of variables are of equal value, and both should be used.

Unfortunately, so many meaningless profiles have been developed that providers have become understandably suspicious of their intent. That is, rather than integrating quality with efficiency, many provider profiles today are simply economic reports. Profile implementation focused on quality improvement is always challenging but is necessary to combine with profiles that focus on economic issues.

Also bear in mind that one cannot simply hand out the profile and expect change to occur. Although there are some reports in the literature stating that simply disseminating profile reports results in change, there is more evidence that profile reports, as important as they are, are but one tool out of several when working with physicians to examine and change practice patterns and habits.

When designing provider profiling reports, the following principles should be kept in mind:

- Identify high-volume and costly clinical areas to profile.
- Involve appropriate internal and external customers in the development and implementation of the profile.
- Involve the providers in the development and implementation of the profile.
- Compare results with published performance (external versus internal norms).
- Report performance using a uniform clinical data set.
- When possible, employ an external data source for independent validation of the provider's data.
- Consider on-site verification of data from the provider's information system.
- Present comparative performance using clinically relevant risk stratification.
- Require measures of statistical significance for comparisons and establish thresholds for minimum sample size.
- Revise performance measurements using formal severity adjustment instruments.

Customers and Users of Provider Profiles

There are many customers or users of provider profiles. Identification of these customers and paying attention to their needs when developing and implementing the profile are important to success. Profiles are not inexpensive in both time and money. Profile customers include the following:

- **Health plans:** All levels (provider relations, medical directors, etc.).
- **Consumers:** Although consumers are a key customer, we are still in the process of developing profiles and approaches to the effective dissemination to health plan members.[19]
- **Employers:** With notable exceptions, most employers are still less interested in quality than they are in cost control. Thus, to get employers interested in quality one must use tools and approaches that integrate cost control with quality.
- **Providers:** Most providers are interested in change if methods to measure performance are well grounded in scientific evidence or professional concensus.[20]

Public versus Internal Disclosure of Provider Profiles

A key flashpoint of debate is internal versus external disclosure of provider profiles. By way of example, there are nearly 20 states that produce publicly available profiles of hospital services. Health plans are beginning to use this information in their feedback loop to hospitals. The report format itself is an important aspect of the development process. For example, the state of Florida, which has released hospital-specific mortality and severity of illness rates for several years, has established wide confidence intervals and designed a format that places a great emphasis on information and deliberately underemphasizes identification of poor or excellent performers. This approach improves the acceptance and utility of the report, while lowering the potential for sensationalism. Pennsylvania has undertaken similar efforts in producing reports on hospitals, taking into account severity adjustments.

The National Committee for Quality Assurance (NCQA) uses the Health Plan Employer

Data Information Set (HEDIS) information to evaluate health plans and make this information available through its *Quality Compass* publication (see Chapter 23 for further discussion around health plan accreditation). The Pacific Business Group on Health has also made an effort to use this HEDIS data set to evaluate medical groups that contract with health plans and plans to release this information to the public.[21] Minnesota Community Measurement is an example of an effort to pool data across health plans to provide quality measures to purchasers and consumers.[22] There are also several Internet Web sites that provide information from multiple sources, ranking health plans, hospitals, and physicians. Two examples are Health Grades[23] and Health Share Technologies (now WebMD Quality Services).[24]

More recently, some health plans and employers have produced and released physician practice quality and service profiles to their members or employees and have reported a shifting in enrollment into practices that were reported as "best practices."[25] This is a significant step forward in the development of physician profiles for external or public release. Its importance derives from the fact that many physicians, particularly on the West Coast, are not solo practitioners or members of small medical groups; they are members of large medical groups that contract with health plans for the entire risk and are the key providers of medical care.

DESIRED CHARACTERISTICS OF PROVIDER PROFILES

Provider profiles should share these characteristics, as discussed here:

- Accurately identify the provider in the profile
- Accurately identify the specialty of the provider
- Help to improve the process and outcome of care, both dollar and quality outcomes

- Have a firm basis in scientific literature and professional consensus
- Meet certain statistical thresholds of validity and reliability
- Compare the provider to a norm
- Cost the minimum amount possible to produce
- Respect patient confidentiality and, if obtaining information from the medical record or using patient-derived information, obtain patient consent

Accurate Identification of the Provider

As noted earlier, the accurate identification of the provider is not always easy or straightforward. Problems of multiple databases, the use of multiple identifiers, inconsistent data, and poor linkages between provider codes and clinical information make this a challenge. The use of the NPI will address this issue beginning in 2007. For periods prior to that, unless a health plan uses a single master provider identification file and has taken great care to ensure nonduplication of provider identification data, it will require a significant amount of attention to address this. In addition, profiling software must employ algorithms to ensure that data about cost, utilization, and quality are linked to the appropriate provider(s).

The level of analysis is also important to consider in provider profiling. Profiling at the individual physician level is often not possible because the number of episodes for each physician is too small. The resulting statistical instability introduces too much error to lead to robust comparative conclusions. Instead, profiling should be done at the clinic/group level. This also has the advantage of taking into account the fact that care is delivered by teams of providers, particularly for complex and chronic diseases.

There are increased efforts to link hospital and physician payment for services provided in the hospital because these data are usually not coming from the same sources. In other words, physician claims or encounters are entered into the system via both claims and medical management, whereas hospital data are likewise entered, but independently from the physician data. And none of these sets of data are automatically linked in most information systems.

In hospital care, accurate identification of the "responsible" provider is not always clear. For example, the physician of record for hospital administrative purposes may not be the same as the physician who actually cares for the patient. In addition, several health plans are now able to provide profiles of hospitalizations for a procedure (CABG, for example) that includes 90 days postdischarge. These are much more valuable profiles from both a cost and quality perspective.

An additional problem concerns providers who behave as though they are in a group but are not legally connected and do not appear as a group in the health plan's provider file. An example would be two physicians who share an office, share after-hours on-call responsibilities, and see each other's patients, but who are actually independent of each other. The reason that this is important in managed care is that, if the health plan contracts with one but not the other, the member may wind up seeing the nonparticipating physician and be subject to balance billing. Even if the physicians agree not to balance bill, the health plan still may not actually want the other physician in the network, even on an occasional basis. Related to the preceding is the ability to detect linkages between practices or ancillary services. Examples include orthopedists who own physical therapy practices or neurologists who have a proprietary interest in a magnetic resonance imaging center.

Accurate Identification of the Specialty Type

The specialty of the physician is not always clear. Most health plans have provider files that indicate what specialty type a physician

has self-indicated, but it is surprising how often that information does not match up with specialty indicators in the claims file. Of course, health plans that perform comprehensive verification of board specialty status as part of the credentialing process (see Chapter 5) will have more accurate data than health plans that depend on self-reporting by physicians.

The problem of provider specialty definition is particularly acute when looking at primary care physicians (PCPs). As discussed in Chapter 5, many board-certified medical specialists actually spend a considerable amount of time performing primary care, whereas others spend the majority of their time practicing true specialty medicine. This has great implications for how a health plan will evaluate performance of specialists as well as PCPs when comparisons to peers are used (a common practice). A related issue is determining which physicians will be considered specialists at all because the health plan may not want to send referrals to a specialist who is not particularly active in his or her designated specialty. Even within a single specialty there will be differences in how specialized a specialist is. For example, a specialist may have a majority of primary care patients or may not care for patients in the intensive care unit (ICU). Therefore, the health plan will want to look at the degree to which a physician is truly a specialist in his or her mix of routine and complex cases.

Even when the issue of specialty definition is resolved, there remains the problem that no two practices are exactly alike. As an example, some general internists perform flexible sigmoidoscopies and some do not. If one looks only at charge patterns, the internist who performs the procedure will look more expensive compared to the internist who does not, but that analysis will fail to pick up the fact that the internist who does not perform flexible sigmoidoscopies instead refers them all to a gastroenterologist who charges more than the first internist (in addition, the first internist could be overutilizing the procedure or the second internist could be failing to provide this common preventive care activity, but those are separate types of analysis). The same problem arises outside of primary care medicine. For example, when neurosurgeons are assumed to be a homogeneous group, accurate profiling cannot be done when one neurosurgeon works only on atrioventricular (AV) malformations, another on brain tumors, and so on. This problem extends to related procedures, such as whether neurosurgeons or vascular surgeons perform carotid endarterectomies or whether neurosurgeons or orthopedists perform various types of spine fusions.

Improve Process and Outcome Using Scientific Criteria

It is important not only to be certain that quality of care variables have relevance for either process or outcomes of care, but also that there is scientific and professional consensus that the variables are worth examining. Generally speaking, this can be done in one of four ways:

- Accrediting organizations, such as NCQA, have increasingly put their screening items through a rigorous evaluation process.
- Several proprietary software packages from reputable developers include guidelines or quality of care criteria.
- Most will use professional literature, including peer-reviewed journals or trusted locations on the Internet, such as the Web site hosted by the Agency for Health Care Policy and Research, http://www.guideline.gov.
- Self-development is always an option, but development of reliable and valid quality of care criteria always takes more time than one expects.

Need for Statistics

Appropriate statistical techniques are required for both quality of care and efficiency criteria. Without their use, one can easily be misled by noise into arriving at a mistaken conclusion. Most stand-alone software packages have statistical tests embedded. If one is obtaining reports from the information technology department, it is important to ask for the addition of statistical tests, especially when faced with decisions pertaining to network determination. Reports should include basic measures of confidence, such as standard deviations or P values.

From a design point of view, it is likely that there will be enough data over time to profile a provider using statistical process control (SPC). "SPC consists of a set of powerful techniques to ensure the continued stability of any process and to detect the presence of sources of instability."[2] One can develop control charts or simpler reports if one is not able to use SPC for a wide variety of independent variables using claims data such as the following:

- Daily hospital log
- Length of stay
- Cost of care (by type of cost; claims forms are divided into approximately 20 departmental categories ranging from pharmaceutical to medical supply to ICUs)

Compare the Provider to a Norm

Practice profiles are of no use unless the results are compared to some type of standard. Certain problems are inherent with comparisons in provider profiling. All these problems are resolvable, but medical managers need to be aware of them before embarking on profiling. Comparison against norms is necessary, but it is fraught with potential difficulties, chief of which is defining the norm. There are, broadly speaking, two types of norms: internal norms (that is, one's own norms if one has enough enrollees or patients) and comparative norms (using external data).

The usual way of comparing profiling results is to provide data for each individual practice in comparison to one or more of the following internal norms discussed earlier:

Total health plan average result. This standard is simply the average for the entire health plan and is the crudest method of comparison.

Independent practice association (IPA) or preferred provider organization (PPO). A variation of health plan average, this compares the practice only to other practices within a set of providers smaller than the entire network. This approach may be combined with multiple other approaches when a health plan contracts through organized provider systems. Another variation on this is geography, even in the absence of organized provider groups.

Specialty specific or peer groups. This compares each practice only to its own specialty (for example, internists are only compared to other internists).

Peer group, adjusted for age, sex, and case-mix/severity of illness. This is the most complicated approach, as noted earlier, but provides the most meaningful comparative data.

Budget. This compares the profile to budgeted utilization and cost, a necessary activity when providers are accepting full or substantial risk for medical expenses.

Advanced and statistically based comparisons. This is coupled with confidence intervals so that a provider will know whether the difference versus the peer group is statistically significant. Examples of comparative norms include the following:

- Hospital charges or costs
- Mortality
- Group practice charges
- Certain outcomes, such as hospital admission rates
- Parameters of greatest interest to health plans, such as utilization rates (for example, prescribing behavior), immunization, mammography, or other HEDIS rates

Some of these norms, such as hospital charges and mortality, may be augmented through public use state data tapes. Occasionally, state data repositories (such as exist in Florida, California, Pennsylvania, and Texas) are adjusted using a reputable severity adjustment tool. More often than not, the state data repository is either not available or, if it is, no risk adjustment is performed. Normative data sets may be internally generated if the health plan is large or part of an alliance that pools similar data. Data sets tailored to the needs of a specific organization are also available for purchase from reputable commercial organizations.

Episodes of Care

Grouping claims data into episodes of care is increasingly becoming a standard approach to efficiency analysis across providers. It provides a complete picture of care delivered across the health care continuum.

Episodes of care are defined as time-related intervals that have meaning to the behavior requiring measurement. Episodes may vary considerably both by clinical condition and by provider type. In the case of obstetrics, obvious measures, such as Caesarian section rate, are important but will not reveal the full picture. Looking at the entire prenatal and postnatal episode may reveal significant differences in the use of ultrasound and other diagnostics, differences in early detection and prevention of complications, or perhaps a great deal of unbundled claims during the prenatal period.

Furthermore, it is possible for patients with multiple medical conditions to have overlapping episodes of care, making it more difficult to sort out which resources are being used for which episode. Several of the proprietary software programs attempt to deal with this issue by, for example, identifying patients with both congestive heart failure (CHF) and diabetes and separating this group of patients from those who only have CHF.

Related to the issue of episode construction is the problem of identifying which provider is actually responsible for the patient's care. As an example, an internist or an endocrinologist may be responsible for the care of a diabetic but may have little responsibility for managing that patient's broken leg, other than to refer the patient to an orthopedist. Identification of the responsible physician is also difficult regarding hospitalized patients; it is not uncommon for the admitting physician not to be the attending physician, especially when surgery is involved.

The hallmark of episode definition is the ability to link all the health resources into a defined event. This may mean diagnostic services (laboratory or imaging), therapeutic services (physical therapy), drugs, consultations, outpatient visits, and inpatient visits. In other words, it must be a patient-based analysis rather than a provider-based one; the analysis of the behavior of providers is a product of examining what happens to their patients. Several vendors have constructed proprietary episode grouping systems, such as Episode Treatment Groups (ETG)[26] and the Medstat Episode Grouper (MEG).[27] However, episodes of care may contain heterogeneous levels of severity and thus require further risk adjustment to use them to compare utilization across populations.

SELECTION OF A PROFILING VENDOR

Unless a health plan has an extraordinary information system, it will be required to purchase or license services from an outside vendor of profiling systems. Broadly speaking, there are three types of products:

- Database or data management tools that allow one to collect information and report that information in useful formats. These are sophisticated (from an informatics perspective) empty shells.
- Tools that interface with data management and provide "clinical logic," which points the health professional toward particular avenues of investigation of either cost or quality.
- Risk adjustment systems that provide the user with the assurance that "apples are being compared with apples." This issue is discussed earlier in detail.

As illustrated in Table 16-3, one looks at several distinguishing features to aid in the selection of a system.

Validated Methodology

Methodologies used for severity adjustment and episode construction are more trusted by new users if they have already been evaluated for predictive validity and reliability by the peer-reviewed literature and multiple installations.

Multiple Products for HMO, Point-of-Service (POS), PPO, Medicare, Medicaid

Although profiling in the "lock-in" or 100:0 plan HMO environment is usually straightforward, point-of-service (POS) and preferred provider organization (PPO) products add complexity. Whether referred by the PCP with or without the health plan's approval or if self-referred by the member, resource consumption out of network and in-service area or out-of-service area, strains the information collection completeness and timeliness. Metrics for Medicare must include, for example, adherence rates for influenza and pneumococcal vaccines, pneumonia and CHF readmissions, and additional items beyond HEDIS requirements. Medicaid populations must build profiles that address maternities with high risk, asthma, HIV/AIDS, care for substance abuse, and care for the elderly, blind, and disabled.

Comprehensible by Average User

Customers for profiling software and services in the past may have settled for shipping a claim tape to the vendor and waiting for a report. However, users now expect to have direct access to the information and be trained to design ad hoc reports for customized circumstances in real time. They prefer the visual relief provided by a graphical user interface and deplore tabular data. They want to be self-managing. Several workstation options provide this facility to the average user.

Carve-Out Accommodated

Because many health plans have separate agreements with subcapitated programs (*eg,*

Table 16–3 Distinguishing Features and Selection Criteria to Use When Evaluating Physician Profiling Vendors

Sound Clinical Methodology

- Independently validated in peer-reviewed literature
- Applicable to primary and specialty care physicians
- Intuitive and easy to explain to practicing providers
- Industry standard "universal language" (for example, standard definitions of episodes)
- Ability to incorporate inpatient and outpatient care into episodes of care
- Sound statistical methodologies

Reporting Comprehensiveness

- All data incorporated (eg, ICD-9, CPT, NDC, HCPCS, local codes, NY DRGs)
- All places of services captured
- Ability to incorporate user-defined fields
- Ability to incorporate external benchmarks

Reporting Flexibility and Presentation

- Ability to report by individual provider, specialty, risk pools, or other user-defined group
- Analysis variability to include billed, paid, allowed amounts, relative value units, rates per 1,000, per member per month
- Ability to complete clinical performance reporting
- Ability to vary reporting period and trend data
- Ability to drill down to claim level detail
- Ability to report by product lines (Medicare, Medicaid, commercial) or aggregate products
- Indicates statistical significance for comparisons
- Ability to severity adjust at patient level
- Ability to integrate with existing legacy systems/programs for reporting flexibility
- Graphic presentation
- Actionable reports
- Summary-level report available with ability to add detail pages

System Platform/Training and Support

- Platform and technical requirement compatibility
- Technical and clinical training and support available
- Data cleansing process

Source: Created by author and adapted from an earlier version in *The Managed Health Care Handbook,* 4th ed., Jones and Bartlett, 2000.

managed behavioral health, chiropractic, pharmaceuticals, lab, and so on), the better profilers are equilibrating their report packages to ensure apples-to-apples comparisons. Although important throughout this chapter, profiling from within any capitated entity (especially physician group; see Chapter 6) will not be possible if encounter CPT-4 data are not submitted, such that health plans have had to develop reward programs for completeness-of-capture for encounter information. Carved-out programs must also provide highly detailed information; for example, pharmaceutical information should get to the level of prescribing physician, drug name, dose, and route of administration.

Prioritization of Services for Focused Review

Briefly mentioned earlier in this chapter, this capability represents an essential management tool for health plan utilization management departments. They do not want to hassle righteous physicians. They want to reduce the overhead attached to operating these oversight activities dedicated to micromanagement. They would prefer not having to do old-fashioned utilization review at all. The better profilers arm them with information to perform this targeting.

HEDIS Production and Other Accreditation Requirements

Profiling vendors vary in their willingness to produce the administrative data portion of HEDIS reports (see Chapter 17 for HEDIS data requirements). Conservative vendors argue that claim data integrity is unknown, such that the electronic production of such a report is unreliable. Other vendors dedicate energy to claim tape edits and cleansing processes, whereby a level of confidence is achieved. The user can learn portions of this track record where a vendor has produced a HEDIS report that was externally audited.

Statistical Packages

Simple averages on colorful pie graphs are not adequate today. Tests of statistical power

expressing significance using P values and confidence intervals using standard deviations are essential.

Easy-to-Use Interfaces

This is critical if a user wants to import data from other sources or to integrate plan data with, for example, software that will help build a clinical guideline.

THE FUTURE OF DATA USE

The primary future use of health plan data and analysis will reside under the umbrella term *transparency*.

For consumers, data will need to be accessed on the Internet to allow easily comprehended comparisons in cost and quality among providers. This will prompt more consumers to "vote with their feet," though the magnitude of market share shifts remains to be seen.

For providers, data and analysis provided by health plans allow them to see a more complete picture of the care they provide. Bolstered by seeing their contributions to longitudinal episodes and seeing their performance within their specialty, compared to matched peers, regional national averages, and gold standards, they will have customized information on which to produce quality/performance improvement programs.

The secondary future use of these data will be for original health services research. By having access to national inventories of claims data, investigators will be in a unique position to find out more quickly "what works." For example, postmarket surveillance of Food and Drug Administrations (FDA)–approved drugs is often a poorly funded ad hoc process. Increasingly, one can use claims data for this purpose, avoiding the expense and time of conducting clinical studies. By isolating a drug code, initiating a downstream search for specific complications (ICD-9 diagnosis code), and comparing the results with those who did not use that particular drug, postmarket drug surveillance can be expanded and improved. Similar analysis can be conducted looking for the unintended consequences of deployment of new medical devices.

Furthermore, research will be accelerated for discovering what kinds of behaviors are prompted by various innovations in benefit design. Ultimately, there will be better answers about the relationship between cost and quality in the delivery of health care services.

References

1. Blue Cross and Blue Shield Association. *National Account Decision Maker Survey.* Washington, DC: Blue Cross and Blue Shield Association, 2005.

2. Goldfield N. *Physician Profiling and Risk Adjustment,* 2nd ed. Gaithersburg, Md: Aspen Publishers, 1999.

3. Coulam RF and Gauler GL. Medicare's Prospective Payment System: A critical appraisal. *Health Care Financing Review.* 1997:(suppl 13), 45–76.

4. Russell LB and Manning CL. The effect of prospective payment on Medicare expenditures. *N Engl J Med.* February 16, 1989:320(7), 439–444.

5. Hofer TP, Hayward RA, Greenfield S, Wagner EH, Kaplan SH, Manning WG. The unreliability of individual physician "report cards" for assessing the costs and quality of care of a chronic disease. *JAMA.* June 9, 1999:281(22), 2098–2105.

6. Schneiter EJ, Keller RB, Wennberg D. Physician partnering in Maine: An update from the Maine Medical Assessment Foundation. *Jt Comm J Qual Improv.* October 1998: 24(10), 579–584.

7. Chen J, Radford MJ, Wang Y, Marciniak TA, Krumholz HM. Do "America's best hospitals" perform better for acute myocardial infarction? *N Engl J Med.* January 28, 1999:340(4), 286–292.

8. Iezzoni LI, Davis RB, Palmer RH, et al. Does the Complications Screening Program flag cases with process of care problems? Using explicit criteria to judge processes. *Int J Qual Health Care.* April 1999:11(2), 107–118.

9. Goldfield N. A quality improvement process for ambulatory prospective payment. *J Ambul Care Manage.* April 1993:16(2), 50–60.

10. Dans PE. Caveat doctor: How to analyze claims-based report cards. *Jt Comm J Qual Improv.* January 1998:24(1), 21–30.

11. Blumenthal D, Weissman JS, Wachterman M, *et al.* The who, what, and why of risk adjustment: A technology on the cusp of adoption. *J Health Polit Policy Law.* June 2005:30(3), 453–473.

12. California Health Care Association. Cal-APR-DRGs working draft, internal memo. Sacramento: California Health Care Association, 1999.

13. Starfield B, Weiner J, Mumford L, Steinwachs D. Ambulatory care groups: A categorization of diagnoses for research and management. *Health Serv Res.* April 1991:26(1), 53–74.

14. Ash A, Porell F, Gruenberg L, Sawitz E, Beiser A. Adjusting Medicare capitation payments using prior hospitalization data. *Health Care Financ Rev.* Summer 1989:10(4), 17–29.

15. MedPAC suggests modifications to SNF PPS system, new RUG III group may be an option. *Natl Rep Subacute Care.* March 10, 1999:7(5), 3–5.

16. U.S. Department of Health and Human Services. Centers for Medicare and Medicaid Services: CMS programs and information. Available at: http://www.cms.hhs.gov/. Accessed May 19, 2006.

17. U.S. Department of Health and Human Services. Agency for Healthcare Research and Quality. Available at: http://www.ahrq.gov/. Accessed May 19, 2006.

18. Goetzel RZ, Long SR, Ozminkowski RJ, Hawkins K, Wang S, Lynch W. Health, absence, disability, and presenteeism cost estimates of certain physical and mental health conditions affecting U.S. employers. *J Occup Environ Med.* April 2004:46(4), 398–412.

19. Goldfield N, Larson C, Roblin D, *et al.* The content of report cards: Do primary care physicians and managed care medical directors know what health plan members think is important? *Jt Comm J Qual Improv.* 1999:25(8), 422–433.

20. Stason WB, Auerbach B, Bloomberg M, *et al. Principles for Profiling Physician Performance.* Walton, MA: Massachusetts Medical Society, 1999.

21. Healthscope. View California health care ratings. 2005. Available at: http://www.healthscope.org. Accessed October 10, 2006.

22. Minnesota Community Measurement. Measure up to better health. 2005. Available at: http://www.mnhealthcare.org/. Accessed March 30, 2006.

23. Health Grades. Homepage. 2006. Available at: http://www.healthgrades.com/. Accessed April 4, 2006.

24. WebMD Quality Services. Why WebMD Quality Services. 2005. Available at: http://www.healthshare.com/hosp_why_hst.asp. Accessed April 4, 2006.

25. Larkin H. Doctors starting to feel report cards' impact. *Am Med News.* July 26, 1999.

26. Symmetry Health Data Systems. Episode Treatment Groups: An illness classification and episode building system. 2004. Available at: http://www.symmetry-health.com/ETGTut_Desc1.htm. Accessed March 30, 2006.

27. Thompson Medstat. Medstat Episode Grouper. Available at: http://www.medstat.com/products/productdetail.aspx?id = 72. Accessed October 10, 2006.

Part 4

OPERATIONAL MANAGEMENT AND MARKETING

We could manage this matter to a T.

—Sterne,
Tristram Shandy, bk. II,
ch. 5 [1760]

17

INFORMATION TECHNOLOGY IN THE HEALTH PLAN ORGANIZATION

Thomas Riley and Kelly Hanratty Butler

Study Objectives

- Understand the role of information services in a managed care organization.
- Understand the basic activities of the information systems area.
- Understand different approaches to delivering services and the advantages and disadvantages of those approaches.
- Understand some of the future initiatives in information systems.

Discussion Topics

1. Describe and discuss the key attributes for the information systems area in an MCO.
2. Discuss the different aspects of technology required by a health plan.
3. Discuss the merits of in-house or owned vs. outsourcing.
4. Describe and discuss the data warehouse and its key attributes.
5. Describe and discuss how IT has evolved and how it might evolve in the future.
6. Discuss the role of IT in providing information to health plan executives, to regulators, to providers, and to consumers.

INTRODUCTION

At its core, insurance is the business of risk. In the health plan world, one party pays a fee on a consistent basis to cover unexpected incidents that may or may not occur in his or her individual future; the other party uses that individual's fee, pooled with others, to pay for the unexpected when it occurs. The assessment and allocation of fees is actuarial-driven, a series of complicated statistical mathematical equations that are constantly evolving as new data are collected.

Although the underlying concepts of insurance are actuarial-driven, the execution of the business and the customer experience are nearly entirely information technology-driven. Technology enables everything from core processes, such as claims adjudication, to consumer touch points, such as Web sites and customer service systems, to internal enablers, such as employee e-mail. Medical management, a key feature in managed health care, is likewise enabled by technology.

To the consumer, insurance is not a simple transfer of risk, but rather a series of interactions that are all technology enabled. For example, a young woman is experiencing lower back pain. She visits her health plan Web site to research her symptoms and look for doctors who can help treat her. At the doctor's office, she hands her identification (ID) card to the office staff member at the front desk who confirms the patient's eligibility by dialing the toll-free number and navigating an interactive voice response (IVR) system. After the visit, the provider submits a claim via a claims clearinghouse to the insurance company. The claims processing system adjudicates the claim according to the patient's current benefits. The young woman receives an explanation of benefits in the mail, but is concerned there is an error. She visits the health plan Web site to look for information related to the claim and places a call to customer service. The customer service call is routed to a customer service representative who then uses interfaces to the health plan's internal membership, claims, and benefits systems to respond to the inquiry, documenting the interaction with the member. This very basic scenario illustrates the pervasive nature of technology for the most routine of interactions.

Management of technology falls to the Information Technology (IT) organization within the health plan, regardless of whether the technology solution serves the internal or external community.

Although the IT organization must continue to deliver core business functionality efficiently such as claims processing, customer inquiry, eligibility maintenance, and bill reconciliation, the organization must also respond quickly to market-driven trends and outside influences. The move toward consumerism discussed in Chapters 1 and 20 shifts the focus of the health plan from a reactive claims processing entity toward an organization proactively contributing to the improvement of the health of its membership. Consumerism has also led to the introduction of financial instruments that give membership more control over their health spending, but it also increases the complexity of the relationship with their health plan, and it increases demand on tools to aid consumers in making decisions related to their health care. The federal government is now pushing for more global and interoperable data sharing between physicians and hospitals and has challenged the standard operations of the health plan, with the effects rippling through every organization, especially in IT.

With the increasing media and government attention on the rising cost of health care in the United States, IT organizations must assist the health plan in reducing controllable costs (most often labeled administrative costs) by delivering core functionality in a more efficient manner. Automation of paper processes, increased throughput, and decreased processing errors can all assist in the quest to deliver a greater number of transactions for a lower cost.

In recent years, the expectation of the IT organization has changed dramatically—from the basic delivery of bits and bytes to a delivery of experience. Customers now bring expectations from nonrelated industries such as retail and financial services. Members expect more personalized information delivered across multiple channels (Web, IVR, phone). Employers, battling rising costs, demand more custom solutions and variable price points. Internal IT customers, such as marketing, sales, and member services look to IT to provide guidance on the delivery of these experiences.

To handle the increasing burden of delivering core functionality more efficiently, reacting quickly to an ever-shifting market and legislative landscape, and delivering high-quality experiences to users of all systems—internal and external—the IT organization also requires the influx of nontraditional skill sets such as marketing and sales.

This chapter covers core IT functions, emerging trends, and changes required within the IT organization.

CRITICAL INTERNAL INFORMATION TECHNOLOGY FUNCTION OVERVIEW

The Information Technology department designs, implements, operates, and maintains systems that perform critical core business processes essential to the day-to-day operation of the health plan organization. These processes must be completed efficiently and accurately on an ongoing basis and new efficiencies must be created to achieve cost reduction opportunities. These core processes (which are described in more detail in other chapters of this book) and their enablement by IT are as follows.

Products

Central to any business, products are the entities that are sold by health plans and bought by consumers. In the health insurance market, there are two main consumer groups: employers who purchase the product and offer it to their employees, and individuals who do not receive insurance benefits from their employer and must purchase insurance products directly.

At the highest level, health insurance products are all the same and are pretty straightforward. A fee is assessed in exchange for a set of benefits that define medical services that the health care consumer can receive at some cost. The cost to the consumer normally includes a premium, a standard flat fee assessed on a (normally) monthly basis, and some type of cost sharing between the patient and the health plan based on the service received and the benefit associated with that service. Customer cost sharing can range from $0 to the full cost of the service, depending on the benefit structure. These fees may take the form of an annual deductible, a per-visit copay, or a percentage of the total bill (co-insurance). It is not uncommon for a claim to feature more than one of these cost sharing elements; that is, a deductible and co-insurance, or a deductible and a copay.

Complicating health insurance products even more is the customization demanded by the various types of consumers. To be viable, a product must offer a set of benefits at a price point where consumers feel they are receiving a "value." *Value* is defined differently by different consumers, and therefore, more products must be offered and supported by the health plan to have a viable business. A healthy, young, new college graduate may be more interested in plans with a lower monthly premium; a mother of three may desire more comprehensive coverage and be willing to pay a higher premium.

The IT organization must support the systems that manage the individual variables for each product—and most health plans have a core set of products, but thousands of variations on those core products. IT solutions must facilitate the input and ultimately store benefit levels, procedure code information, deductible amounts, co-insurance or copay amounts, and other data points that ultimately determine how a member's claim gets paid. This storage system must be packaged with a set of interfaces that allow other systems, such and claims and customer service applications, to access this data for processing and inquiries.

Eligibility

Eligibility systems determine whether an individual is currently enrolled and covered by a health plan product. These systems are queried by providers to determine how a patient should be billed at time of service, and by the claims systems during the adjudication process to determine if or how the health plan should pay the claim. Eligibility systems are also involved in determining how to bill the employer or (in some cases) the member.

When an individual, or group of individuals, first signs up for a particular health insurance product, the enrollment piece of eligibility is completed. In this process, information about each individual (eg, name, address, product) is loaded into the eligibility system. In some systems (usually older, or "legacy" systems), the information is loaded only for the subscriber (ie, the employee of the company through which he or she received health insurance), and it is only the subscriber's information that is used to determine eligibility. In other systems, especially health maintenance organizations (HMOs) that pay providers under capitation, eligibility information is entered for all members—both the subscriber and the subscriber's dependants who are also covered under the subscriber's policy.

This load can be manual or through some type of electronic process. When done manually, paper forms are usually first scanned so as to convert them into an image, then optical character recognition (OCR) is applied, with enrollment data entry clerks reviewing the data and correcting errors, or entering the data manually. Some large commercial health insurance companies outsource some or all of this manual process, but the systems that support the activity are run by the insurance company's IT function. When the function is outsourced, paper is never sent overseas; only imaging is used, and privacy and security policies and procedures are strict, meeting or exceeding the privacy and security standards required under Health Insurance Portability and Accountability Act (HIPAA; see Chapter 32 for a description of those requirements).

Electronic loading may be done by the subscribers entering information through a secure Web site or through a password-protected IVR system. Electronic loading may also occur via tape-to-tape database transfers from the employer to the health plan, or through direct transmission via a secure electronic connection. In some advanced health plans that provide automated tools to sales agents and brokers, the broker may actually enter the demographic information on behalf of the client, which is then transmitted to the health plan.

Once enrolled, an eligible member is likely to experience a change in his or her information during some point in the relationship; for example, an address needs to be updated, a product change is made, or a new dependant(s) (eg, birth or adoption of a child, or new dependants as a result of marriage) needs to be added. At this point, the maintenance phase of the eligibility process is engaged and the individual's information is updated appropriately.

IT managed systems must support both the enrollment and maintenance processes. Many large employers expect these processes to be handled electronically. Often, custom feeds must be designed and established to allow the secure transaction of eligibility data from the employer's personnel system to the health plan. Interfaces must also be built to allow the manual enrollment and maintenance of individual records by customer service personnel and directly by members via a secure Web portal.

Because physicians and hospitals are always concerned about being paid for services delivered, they will almost always confirm that a patient does in fact have insurance and is covered for the particular services in question, prior to providing medical services to the patient. Historically, this was done through a phone call to a provider services unit, but the past decade has seen more use of IVR, and recently much of this activity has been moved to Web-based provider portals. The electronic standards for any eligibility transactions (query and response) between a health plan and providers have been standardized under HIPAA as discussed in Chapter 32 (including a listing of the standards).

Claims Processing

Claims processing covers the chain of events after a medical service is delivered and is described and discussed in great detail in Chapter 18. Only a brief overview to illustrate the role IT plays in the claims function is provided here.

A claim is sent to the health plan, and the information on the claim is reviewed for accuracy. Assuming the information on the claim is validated successfully, the claim is then adjudicated. In the adjudication process, the benefits system is accessed to determine what the correct coverage levels are for the services that were performed as part of the claim. In addition, the provider network systems or databases are queried to determine whether the provider or hospital billing for the services is part of any of the health plan's networks (*eg,* HMO or preferred provider organization [PPO]), and if so, what reimbursement methodology is appropriate; if the provider is not under contract to the health plan, then the reimbursement policies for out-of-network claims are applied (see Chapters 6 and 7 for a full discussion of reimbursement issues). The claims system also may need to look for an authorization or

precertification, as discussed later. Once adjudication is complete, an Explanation of Benefits (EOB) is sent to the patient or subscriber (if the patient is a dependant), and reimbursement is sent to the provider (or in some cases to the subscriber if the subscriber has already paid the provider directly).

Many HMOs use an authorization system for precertifying specialty care systems, and most health plans use a precertification system for inpatient hospital and (some) ambulatory facility services, as described fully in Chapter 9. In either case, the claims system must have access to the authorization or precertification to process the claim correctly. HIPAA-mandated standards exist for these systems (submission, query, and response) as listed in Chapter 32, but the use of electronic transactions in this area lags behind other types of plan–provider interactions, though it is starting to grow as physicians, in particular, begin to adopt more modern practice management software. Still, alternate means of authorization and precertification data entry into the system such as paper, fax, and phone are common.

Claims can be submitted to the health plan via multiple entry points. The most common entry method is electronic, often referred to as EDI (electronic data interchange). The electronic submission of claims allows for a great level of automation, reducing the manual labor costs associated with handling claims on an individual basis.

Large hospital systems may submit claims through a direct connection with the plan. In other cases, a claims clearinghouse establishes the electronic connections between physicians, hospitals, billing services, and health plans, and moves claims and inquiries electronically among the parties. HIPAA-mandated standards exist as well for electronic claims; the standards are different for hospitals, physicians, and dentists, as listed in Chapter 32.

Claims can also be submitted manually via postal mail or fax. Claims received via paper are often scanned into imaging systems for electronic retrieval on the claims processing as well as the use of OCR to enter preliminary data that is then reviewed (and corrected as necessary) by data entry personnel, or data may be entered manually. As discussed in Chapter 18, many large commercial health insurance companies have outsourced manual data checking and entry to off-shore locations, similar to that described earlier regarding enrollment data entry. In the case of claims, when off-shore outsourcing is used, it is more common for the data entry aspect to be off-shore while the adjudication is still performed by the health plan. As with off-shore entry of enrollment data, paper is never sent overseas; only imaging is used, and privacy and security policies and procedures are very strict.

Although claims processing was originally viewed as *the* core function of a health plan, the accurate and timely paying of claims is no longer viewed as a market differentiator; a baseline expectation of customers is that this function will operate with high levels of efficiency. Certainly, it is in the plan's competitive interest to continually improve the level of automation and efficiency, and lower the cost of administration, but it is no longer necessarily the only core function. In recent years, much greater emphasis has been placed on customer service, on providing information to patients to help improve their health and their health care–related decision making, and on enabling better medical management.

Medical Management and Predictive Modeling

As discussed in Chapter 1, historically, health insurance has been a reactive industry. Insurance was only engaged after treatment for an illness or injury was delivered. Health care cost inflation in the 1980s and early to mid-1990s led to the rise of managed care, which certainly helped to rein in unnecessary utilization and costs, but both a change in

practice behavior by providers and a change in the market's desire for managed care led to a reduction in the popularity of HMOs and a rise in PPOs and other less tightly managed products. With health care costs once again rising significantly faster than inflation, though for different reasons than existed two decades ago, pressure is being placed once again on the entire health care industry, including health plans, to identify ways to be more proactive in managing the health of individuals. Medical management and predictive modeling are key components of this effort.

Medical management is discussed in great detail throughout Section Three and will not be reiterated here. All medical management activities are supported and enabled by IT, including decision-support systems, tracking and case management systems, and automated authorization and precertification systems. There are even pilot programs using IT-enabled patient-centric devices and interfaces; for example, a scale that automatically sends a congestive heart failure patient's daily weights to the plan's disease management program, or a diabetic regularly reporting self-measured blood sugar levels via a Web portal. The disease and case management functions of the plan may even have access to the claims system so as to provide benefits waivers (ie, allow the plan to pay for a service at a higher level of coverage) to allow for better management of chronically ill patients, resulting in better outcomes and lower costs.

A plan's IT system will also be responsible for the creation of a so-called personal health record (PHR). The PHR is not a full electronic medical record. Rather, it is a record based on the information that the plan has about a member, such as diagnoses, medications being prescribed, procedures that have been performed, and so forth. Plans are making PHRs available to members on an increasing basis.

Through the routine collection of eligibility, claims, and pharmacy data, health plans have access to a wealth of information about the cause and effect of treatments. Other data sources such as laboratory data or clinical data from other sources are not routinely collected, but eventually will be, particularly as the adoption of the electronic medical record increases. In all cases, it is so-called data mining of these large datasets that helps identify trends in successful prevention and treatment patterns.

As discussed in Chapter 10, in predictive modeling, the health plan attempts to locate individuals who might be at risk for chronic illness. It is known that early intervention in keeping members healthier can result in fewer unnecessary office visits, procedures, and so forth. Identified individuals can be engaged in medical management programs that aim to educate these targeted members on managing their conditions more effectively. Predictive modeling is also a mainstay of disease management programs that focus on a small set of common but expensive chronic conditions (*eg,* diabetes, asthma, and heart disease) to identify when an individual with such a condition requires extra attention from the program or the physician to avoid hospitalization.

To support predictive modeling and medical management, IT must maintain large data warehouses and use sophisticated data mining and informatics tools to transform the raw data into information for use by the medical management systems. It is critical that a data dictionary be established both internal to the system and external to the system's users, to ensure common definitions of data elements are enforced. Systems must be designed so that data gathered can be quickly and easily transformed into actionable information.

Provider Credentialing and Network Maintenance

A key decision factor for consumers when selecting their health plan is whether their chosen doctor is covered by their chosen health plan product. Health plans form relationships with a large number and large variety of providers—primary care physicians, specialists, clinics, hospitals, and others. Because members will have a strong financial incentive to use doctors who are in their health plan's network it is important that they have some assurance that the doctors included in the network are "high quality" not just "low cost."

Provider credentialing, described in detail in Chapter 5, begins with the initial collection of data about a given provider—office locations, billing addresses, specialties, and so forth. It is critical the information be accurate for the reimbursement of claims. These data also feed provider directories, printed and online, used by consumers to make contacts.

The credentialing program collects detailed information about the provider's medical training, certifications, any specialties, any disciplinary actions, and so forth. Credentialing, particularly in HMOs but in many other types of plans as well, also entails a detailed process in which random charts are pulled from the provider's office and reviewed for thoroughness of documentation and adherence to specific proven treatment protocols. Accessing national databases such as the National Practitioner Databank is also a requirement under credentialing. Some plans use a third party to perform some or all credentialing activities, as long as that third party is accredited to do so (see Chapter 23). Other plans conduct credentialing using internal resources.

Maintenance of the provider database (sometimes referred to as the provider file) is a function of network management. It is common for two different departments to exist within network management: hospitals and facilities and professional providers (physicians and nonphysician professionals). Updating data, eliminating duplicate entries, and other basic maintenance functions are necessary for the efficient operation of the health plan. In all cases, the IT organization must design solutions and interfaces that can assist in the collection, use, and maintenance of provider data.

Last, as regards providers and the IT function, with the advent of the new National Provider Identifier (NPI) mandated by HIPAA for implementation in May of 2007 for all health plans and providers (May of 2008 for small health plans), some health plans will face substantial challenges. Because some plans use imbedded intelligence* in the provider identifiers to help drive reimbursement systems or for other reasons, new approaches will be required because the NPI does not contain any imbedded intelligence. Other plans may have other challenges such as the hard coding of identifiers in the system, or a provider ID field type that cannot accommodate the format of the NPI. The IT function will be heavily involved in making the change. The NPI is discussed more fully in Chapters 5 and 32.

Member Service

Member service, discussed in Chapter 19 as well as Chapter 20, continues to be a key market differentiator for health plans. Individuals tend to share both positive and negative service experiences, and studies illustrate these experiences do influence future choice. The current challenge facing member service is customer expectations have increased as common channels, such as call centers and Web portals, have evolved.

Members now demand accurate information, delivered via multiple channels at times convenient to their schedule. Many workers do not want to call and discuss health issues from their cubicle, so e-mail and Web chat have become more prominent. Each mem-

ber has unique needs and demands, and multiple channels must be supported to allow for such variety. In addition, members bring expectations from service interactions from other industries such as financial services, retail, and utilities.

Self-service channels such as online member portals and IVR systems must integrate well with more traditional service channels such as customer service representatives. Customers aggregate interactions from individual channels into a complete experience and expect that transactions within one channel are known by the other channels. A member expects the customer service representative on the phone to understand his or her recent interactions with the IVR system and Web portal.

To increase the success of the call center, tracking and reporting solutions must be deployed. These systems assist in identifying issues, reporting key metrics, such as time to resolution, hold times, and so forth, that can help management tune staffing. Sophisticated load-balancing software can help move calls from location to location to assist in overflow or disaster recovery situations. With the integration of predictive modeling solutions into medical management, member service (via the plan's disease management function) now encompasses outbound calls to reach out and try to influence members' behaviors as well as answering customer calls and questions. New processes and systems must be configured to track this new direction of interaction.

The IT organization must support member service by integrating multiple technologies, many provided by external vendors, into a holistic member service solution. IT must also provide guidance on how to use each of the channels so service personnel can educate members on using each channel effectively.

E-Business

Whether serving employers, members, providers, or brokers, health plans are exploring

---

Imbedded intelligence refers to specific characters in the identifier having specific meaning. For example, the letter *P* to indicate the provider participates in the plan's PPO, or the letters *VA* to indicate the provider is in Virginia and the geographically appropriate fee schedule should be used.

the use of e-business (also referred to as e-commerce) to both cut administrative costs and also provide compelling solutions outside of standard business hours for constituent convenience.

For the employer, portals can enable enrollment and maintenance capabilities. Employers can view and edit employee eligibility information, eliminating the need to submit paperwork manually. They can view and pay bills online. In some cases, employers can enable features to allow their employees to complete initial enrollment online, eliminating paperwork and manual processing.

For the provider, e-business provides a method to verify patient eligibility far more efficiently than a phone call can. Providers can also use Web portals to submit claims or reconcile their outstanding receivables against health plan payments.

For brokers and agents, e-business can provide tools and information to assist in the sales cycle—from educating prospective clients about products to generating quotes and submitting applications online.

For the member, e-business provides a way to deliver self-service capabilities to existing customers and a way to deliver product information and decision-support tools to potential customers.

The IT organization must support e-business initiatives by ensuring Web-based solutions are complementary to other channels and are not developed in a silo. It is critical the delivery and execution of e-business align with offline service channels and marketing goals. E-business solutions must be secure, accurate, and geared toward the appropriate customer. Support measures must be in place to monitor and correct system issues outside of business hours.

Internal Enablers

Although this chapter focuses mainly on IT's role in functions that directly affect external customers, such as claims processing, eligibility, and billing, it is important to note that another primary function of the IT organiza-

tion is to manage, maintain, and service enabling capabilities such as e-mail, telephony, and other communications channels for health plan employees.

DELIVERY ATTRIBUTES

In designing and implementing solutions, several key attributes should be considered to ensure the ultimate success of the deployment. These attributes are discussed as follows.

Visibility

With the advent of the Internet, systems designed, maintained, and operated by the IT organization became more visible to everyone who works with or for today's health plans. The increased transparency in the back-end systems of a health plan organization require increased communication from the IT organization to internal and external customers. If a system is unavailable, account teams and customer service centers must be immediately informed so they can proactively communicate to external constituents. A complex data structure that previously was only visible to internal users now forms the basis for the self-service customer experience. The need to aggressively wring complexity out of the environment is more critical than ever before. And the health plan that is unable to reduce and manage its complexity will struggle to provide a significant level of online service to its customers.

Security and Privacy

Several high-profile security breaches of major financial institutions have raised the security concerns of the general population. Federal laws and regulations such as HIPAA and the Sarbanes-Oxley Act (see Chapter 24), as well as state laws and regulations in some cases, mandate additional constraints on technology and processes to ensure the security and privacy of consumers.

In the IT organization, security and privacy have a large impact. First, design decisions must be made to ensure compliance with regulations. Such compliance can be costly and may require new infrastructure and business processes to support. In addition, the information technology organization must be able to communicate priorities to business owners of applications because these mandates may require shifting of resources away from other projects to ensure compliance.

Second, the IT organization must educate its staff on these government mandates. These individuals need to understand how changes in government initiatives translate into system requirements.

Security audits must be performed, both by internal staff and external auditors to proactively identify vulnerabilities in systems. Security experts should train developers on best practices in developing secure applications and perform code reviews to ensure compliance with those standards.

Usability

In delivering technology solutions, the IT organization must be aware of the ultimate use of the system; in other words, how will the system be accessed? What are the characteristics of the users? This picture of the end user will assist in defining appropriate requirements and designing a usable system. Involving users throughout the software development life cycle helps ensure the end product meets user needs appropriately.

Often users bring expectations from interactions with other systems. For example, if asked to design a word processing program, the designer would be wise to review other word processing software such as Microsoft Word to become familiar with standard conventions the user would expect. IT application designers must research applications used by the target population to identify these conventions.

For external-facing solutions, such as Web sites and portals, usability can help create applications that are more compelling—increase sales, convert users to a lower-cost channel,

increase customer satisfaction, and increase utilization of online tools.

For internal-facing solutions, such as customer service inquiry applications, productivity improvements that come with a well-designed product lead to reduction in administrative costs.

Flexibility

IT is often presented with requirements from business leads contained within a single project unit. IT needs to analyze those requirements to identify similarities with requirements from other units. In addition, IT must anticipate future capacity needs to build a solution that will last.

In addition to the requirements outlined by the various business units, IT analysts must add requirements that allow the system to be quickly modified based on customization requests and legislation.

MARKET TRENDS AND IT

The focus of the health plan business is no longer solely on cost containment through administrative efficiency, but rather on proactively contributing to the health care quality and overall wellness of its membership using approaches beyond what have traditionally been used.

Consumerism

As discussed in Chapter 20, one facet of consumerism is the theory that if individuals carry more of the financial burden of their health care, they will become better consumers of health care. By being more educated, they will make smarter decisions on when to engage health care services and will maintain a healthier lifestyle in hopes of preventing health issues that require longer term or more intensive intervention. This has led to the creation of so-called consumer-directed health plans (CDHPs; see Chapter 2) that combine high-deductible health insurance with pre-tax funding vehicles used to pay for at least some of the deductible.

As consumers become more responsible for allocating their dollars in health care, they demand more information on the quality and cost of services they receive. They expect the health plan will provide the tools to help them compare doctors and hospitals based on the services they want to receive.

A key corollary to consumerism is the proactive management of health and not simply the reactive treatment of a condition. Health plans are investing resources in solutions to assist consumers in becoming healthier, including partnerships with health information articles and interactive tools.

As consumers demand more information about their health care providers, IT must be able to collect and disseminate data. Based on business requirements that data take the form of compliance reports, links to state records, consumer feedback, and so forth, the system built must be flexible enough to accommodate structured and unstructured data.

IT must also support the consumerism movement by identifying ways to educate members on their own health—primarily through online tools and information—and supporting innovative product designs that incorporate new financial instruments and benefit designs.

Last, health plans must justify the theory of consumerism to employer groups by reporting on the success of consumerism products. Data are required to illustrate that when more responsibility is transferred to consumers, they use health care services more intelligently.

Pay-for-Performance

With increasing focus on health care costs, health plans are developing new ways to pay providers for services rendered. In an effort to align payment with quality, the pay-for-performance model has recently emerged, as discussed in detail in Chapter 8. In this model, compensation is tied to compliance with best practices and results achieved, not just on the number or duration of services.

IT must support this model by creating solutions that can collect these data from disparate sources, transform and load data into a repository, and provide access methods for reporting systems and consumers. Because relationships with providers are critical to a plan's success, audits of the solution must illustrate the accuracy of the data collected.

Plan as Financial Institution

The health insurance industry has often looked to the financial service industry as a role model in the evolution of the technology organization. The industries share similar concepts (*eg,* risk) and concerns (*eg,* security). With the introduction of Health Savings Accounts (HSAs) and CDHPs with Health Reimbursement Accounts (HRAs) in recent years, the line between the two industries has blurred and in some cases, financial institutions have become competitors of health plans in delivering products and services. Plans offer these new financial instruments associated with products through alliances with banks or internally.

As mentioned previously, consumers often bring expectations from other industries, including financial services. Financial services is a decade ahead of the health plan industry in terms of delivering high-quality self-service capability to consumers. Financial institutions introduced self-service Web sites and automatic teller machines (ATMs) in the late 1980s and have quickly evolved those offerings based on consumer demands and feedback.

IT organizations need to integrate with various financial institutions, help create the infrastructure to support internal financial products, and use the financial industry as a guideline for success in customer self-service.

Maturation of Health Care IT Vendors

Vendor solutions have improved drastically, often making it more efficient to purchase solutions instead of developing custom solutions. With the evolution of consumerism, vendors have emerged in medical management, and health and wellness, capabilities previously not prominent in health plan organizations.

Though vendors have improved, often one vendor excels in one area while another excels in a different area. Many health plans adapt by creating "best of breed" solutions that integrate with their custom solutions. IT must work with multiple vendors with varying technology standards and platforms, and respond to challenges in delivering a consistent user experience.

As the market has matured, a handful of vendors has emerged as market leaders. The solutions delivered by the market leaders are often selected by multiple health plans, further reducing competitive differentiation. IT must continue to evolve the integration of these vendor tools into a seamless solution to regain some differentiation in the marketplace. IT must also adjust to the shifting balance of vendor solutions over home-grown solutions by implementing flexible architecture that allows specialized applications to plug into the larger suite of systems and by developing employees' integration skills.

PERSONAL AND ELECTRONIC HEALTH RECORDS

During the course of his or her lifetime, an individual's health will be cared for by multiple doctors, hospitals, clinics, and other providers. Individuals will be less likely to establish a deep relationship with a single provider, or even if they do, it is likely that they will receive treatment from other sources because of travel, relocation, or the eventual retirement of the provider. And the unfortunate fact is that most physicians' records are still kept on paper charts stored in file cabinets; it is also the case in too many hospitals as well. In other words, it is difficult to have important information about one's health available when it might be needed.

Currently, individuals themselves are the point of consolidation of the information

about their health. However, consumers do not have easy access to test results, x-rays, laboratory test results, detailed procedural notes, or other health records. Under HIPAA, consumers do have the legal right to such access, and providers all have policies and procedures in place to grant such access. But consolidating all the health records of an individual remains by far the exception, not the norm.

Individual providers and facilities maintain health care records. The introduction of PHRs as described earlier, as well as electronic medical records (EMRs) and/or electronic health records (EHRs) that are more comprehensive in the data they contain, aims to provide easy electronic access to health records using a variety of means. For some, it may even mean consolidating these data into a single record. However, until global data stores are created, health plans are the most likely source of data about an individual's claim history, thus the importance to both health plans and members of the PHR.

Whether it is creating the PHR to be accessed by the member, by a provider, or by another health plan, IT will be challenged to create access to the single data store across networks and software that may or may not be compatible with their own. Interoperability will be a key success factor. Certainly, security will be a focal point—IT will need to create a framework to provide data access to the appropriate people, based on consumer wishes, and create detailed logs of activity for analysis should a breach occur.

The solutions created by IT must also be easy to use by providers under appropriate circumstances to prevent errors, improve care, and facilitate the easy update and maintenance of the data contained within.

BUILDING AN IT ORGANIZATION TODAY

The Information Technology organization of today is less about delivering bits and bytes and more about delivering information, solutions, and services to support overarching business goals. High-performing employees with traditional skills such as development and architectural experience are expected; new skills such as communication, portfolio management, usability and design, and marketing, normally considered more "business" than "IT," have become increasingly more important as the pressure to enable business success falls on IT's shoulders.

Information Technology as a Business

IT has long been considered a necessary (and often large) component of the total administrative cost within health plans. Increasingly, though, IT is being asked not only to justify expense, but deliver and measure the organization's return on investment (ROI). Although most IT organizations certainly have reduction of administrative costs as a stated goal, they are now also being asked to stimulate and support growth.

IT must more efficiently allocate resources based on prioritization of business goals and availability of budget. It is critical for IT to communicate with business representatives on constraints in their organization—whether skills gaps, labor shortage, hardware/software limitations, security, or performance risks are inherited in a given solution. In addition, the IT organization must work with the business to identify opportunities to share solutions among certain business lines, working toward delivering a single (but flexible) enterprise solution versus a set of specifically designed solutions.

Traditional Skills

Employees responsible for maintaining and installing hardware need to understand core architectural concepts—network protocols, vendor equipment, and so forth. Strategic thinking is critical in planning future needs. The IT organization needs to work closely with the business units to identify future requirements and growth estimates to ensure the hardware to support the organization can

be procured, installed, and configured for maximum efficiency.

Certainly, skilled development teams are essential to creating and maintaining custom applications. Developers should be well versed in the syntactic structures of languages, but should also be trained in best practices in writing efficient and secure source code. The IT organization should establish a solid application architecture framework that can be used consistently across many areas. In addition, coding standards and methodologies should be communicated and enforced within the developer community. This foundation of standards helps create a pool of skilled development resources that can be moved from application to application to balance resource levels more effectively based on workload.

The security requirements of HIPAA as described in Chapter 32, as well as emphasis on security as a result of recent high-profile lawsuits and public relations nightmares, require a well-educated security organization. To run effectively, the security organization must maintain a level of objectivity. Internal security audits should be performed often. The individuals performing the audits need to be separate from those who train developers and review code to ensure compliance with security best practices.

Funds should be allocated in keeping employees trained in these traditional skills. New hardware and software standards and methodologies constantly evolve and employees must keep current.

Nontraditional Skills

To run IT successfully as a business, competencies long considered unusual within an IT environment now become important for success. Although core architectural, development, and integration skills still require attention, market demands necessitate a more diverse balance of individuals.

Technology has become a key decision point for many employer groups in selection of health plans, and consumers may look at a health plan's technological prowess as a way to differentiate among payer organizations. Within the organization, IT professionals with communication skills are needed to help develop the "technology story," capturing the internal and external capabilities. In addition, these IT employees need to assist in training the traditional sales organization in delivering this technology story in context with other sales messages.

Delivery of solutions, versus bits and bytes, requires a more intimate knowledge of the "customer," however one defines the term. Usability professionals can assist in this endeavor by profiling target customers and creating user interface designs that best meet user needs and exploit current best practices and conventions.

CONCLUSION

Information technology is at the root of the health plan organization. A key participant in reducing administrative costs, IT is now faced with shifting into a more proactive role in keeping membership healthy. Delivering more compelling external-facing experiences, not simply automating back-end processes, will continue to raise the profile of the IT organization within the plan. To respond to the increased visibility as a key player, the IT organization must transform itself from a storehouse of highly technical employees to a mini-business with a more well-rounded workforce.

18

CLAIMS ADMINISTRATION

Donald L. Fowler Jr. and Elizabeth Pascuzzi

Study Objectives

- Understand the purpose of the claims adjudication process within a managed care organization.
- Understand the factors from other plan areas that contribute to, or hinder, accurate and timely claims processing.
- Understand where claims and benefits administration play a key role in improving a plan's operations or market position.
- Understand implications upon claims work flow of organizational structure of claims within an organization and internal to claims.
- Understand the major components of claims operational management to establish, monitor, and maintain efficient work flow, including pertinent measures for productivity and quality.
- Understand standard accuracy measures, what they mean to an organization's sound fiscal, community relations, and market-competitive standing.
- Understand the interrelationships between claims and other MCO functions.
- Understand how to identify common claims administration problems, their repercussions, and how to identify and rectify them.
- Identify the four core competencies of the modern claims capability as well as the three integrated components common to each competency.

Discussion Topics

1. Discuss the purpose of benefits administration and claims adjudication within a managed care organization.
2. Discuss the process and importance of inventory control.
3. Discuss what information reports support claims management.

4. Discuss the differences between "batch" and "online" adjudication, and the advantages or disadvantages of each.
5. Discuss productivity standards and turnaround times, including those factors that improve or hinder each.
6. Discuss the standard accuracy measures and what reasonable levels of accuracy are within these measures.
7. Discuss the sources for definitive interpretation of benefits in order to determine plan liability when adjudicating a claim.
8. Discuss the factors that combine to contribute to final claim reimbursement amount.
9. Discuss the most common claims and benefits administration problems, their repercussions, and how to identify and rectify them.
10. Discuss the circumstances under which a plan would consider outsourcing their claims adjudication function.
11. Discuss the differences between upstream and downstream quality control and why the claims capability must focus on each.
12. Discuss the value of policies and procedures and staff training and development to the modern claims capability.

INTRODUCTION

The modern claims capability, built on decades of evolving and competing demands, operates on a monumental scale. Nationally, today's claims capability facilitates nearly $2 trillion in claims payments annually (approximately 16% of the U.S. GDP[1]), enough financing to fuel the largest sector of the U.S. economy. As such, it protects millions of citizens from catastrophic loss caused by medical expenses through the health benefit programs it administers. In addition to processing claims, the modern claims capability carries out the following functions:

- Supports disease management and specialized medical management programs for approximately 75 million Americans (25% of the insured population).
- Serves as the safeguard against fraud and abuse.
- Supports large social welfare programs (Medicare and Medicaid).
- Plays a role in tracking national health trends and providing early warning signs for health pandemics and bioterrorism.

Closer to home, the modern claims capability is vital to the health and vitality of its managed care organization (MCO), having a crucial impact on virtually all other departments and on the MCO's bottom line. However, it must rely on a number of other MCO departments for faithful execution of their responsibilities to fulfill its mission: to serve customers, internal and external, via timely and accurate claims adjudication.

This chapter describes the evolution of the modern claims capability, defines the various functions within the claims capability, and examines management issues and core business steps. It concludes with a discussion of major risk areas. Several tables and figures are included to illustrate concepts or provide more detailed information.

EVOLUTION OF THE MODERN CLAIMS CAPABILITY

The modern claims capability has evolved over decades of changes in health care delivery and insurance practices. Changes have been driven by expectations and demands of employer groups, consumers, medical providers, legislators, and regulatory agencies. The Centers for Medicare and Medicaid Services (CMS),* which administers Medicare and Medicaid through various public/private business partnerships, has also influenced the modern claims capability in major ways. Additionally, advances in medical technology on the provider side and in transactional processing systems on the payer side have driven claims operations managers continually to upgrade and redefine the role of the claims capability.

As discussed in Chapter 1, the roots of claims operations can be traced back to the 1920s when many employers began offering health care coverage as a method of attracting and retaining employees. Benefits initially focused on hospitalization, but as the labor force grew and large unions began negotiating improved benefit packages, coverage was extended to include the cost of doctors' fees, allied medical expenses, and prescription drugs. Union negotiated benefit plans influenced both product and benefit design and ultimately the benefit packages offered to salaried and other nonunion employees. This evolution in product and benefit design resulted in more and more variations of health insurance coverage with some employer groups ultimately sponsoring dozens of benefit plans. To finance and administer such programs, employer groups looked to multiline insurance companies with their in-house transaction capabilities and actuarial skills to price, underwrite, assume the financial risk, and process claims. Insurers were the first to introduce the idea of cost sharing (deductibles, co-insurance, and stop-loss features) as well as underwriting principles to guard against adverse selection (*ie*, to ensure that

the insurance company does not cover more sick people than it does nonsick).

At the same time that employer groups were developing programs with insurance carriers, medical providers were exploring other methods of providing and financing health care in the form of prepaid health service plans. As early as 1910, the Western Clinic in Tacoma, Washington provided medical care based on a per member per month (PMPM) premium payment. The origins of Blue Cross coverage are traced to Baylor Hospital, which in 1929 offered a prepaid hospitalization plan to teachers. Starting in 1939, Blue Shield plans were formed by state medical societies to reimburse physicians. Other alternatives to commercial health care coverage underwritten by multiline insurance carriers were established before World War II, including the Kaiser Foundation Health Plans and the Group Health Cooperative of Puget Sound.[2]

While the financing and delivery of health care were evolving, provider billing practices also changed to reflect the ever-increasing complexity in medical care. Initially, payment to providers (even in the form of barter) was expected from patients at the time medical services were rendered. Even if covered under an employer health plan, patients often paid for doctor visits or prescription drugs out of their own pockets and filed claims for reimbursement. Once consumers had the ability to seek reimbursement for medical care from the multiline insurance companies, the modern claim form was born.

Over time, hospitals and physicians began to file claims directly with third-party payers as a service to the patients. When providers began filing claims, they began using more sophisticated methods of creating itemized bills. Itemized bills were submitted in a variety of formats and did not always contain all of the data required by the payer to determine coverage or payment. It wasn't until 1966 that common procedure terminology (CPT) codes were introduced by the American Medical Association to standardize itemized

*Centers for Medicare and Medicaid Services (CMS), initially known as the Health Care Financing Administration, or HCFA, is part of the U.S. Department of Health and Human Services.

charges and provide uniformity in billing practices. Health Care Procedure Coding System (HCPCS) Level II codes for ancillary medical services were introduced in 1983, and revenue codes for hospital services were introduced in 1984. Even today, the medical community tries different submission techniques to streamline claims processing, improve claims turnaround time, and maximize payments.

With the advent of government entitlement programs in 1965, the policies and procedures established for the administration of Medicare began to influence the health insurance industry. Medicare processing standards were ultimately adopted (and continue to be adopted) by most payers, even for non-Medicare benefits. Additionally, the Health Care Financing Administration (HCFA, now known as CMS) pushed for uniformity in billing, and ultimately providers began to use standard claim forms: UB92 claim forms for hospital services (also known as the HCFA 1450) and HCFA 1500 (also known as the CMS 1500) claim forms for professional fees. Uniformity was still an issue at the turn of the twenty-first century when the Health Insurance Portability and Accountability Act (HIPAA) mandated standardization of data for more efficient communication among providers and payers. HIPAA, including the mandated standards for transactions and code sets, is discussed in Chapter 32.

Although standardization of coding helped to simplify claims adjudication during the late 1960s and 1970s, the provider practice of decomposing service codes, referred to as "unbundling," introduced a new element of complexity. Early unbundling largely related to hospital-based physician charges, that is, ungrouped services that had been previously included within the hospital bill. As a result, a single hospital stay began to produce multiple paper claims, including those for the hospital facility charges as well as those for professional fees (emergency room physicians, radiologists, surgeons, anesthesiologists, other specialists, ambulance, durable

medical equipment, prescriptions, etc.). Later, unbundling was also carried out by physicians (including a practice known as upcoding) to maximize payments. This practice in turn led to the development of early programs to detect and prevent fraud and abuse, a topic further explored later in this chapter.

The growth of dual household incomes after 1970 increased the likelihood of dual health benefit coverage for all family members. As a result coordination of benefits (COB) became another element of administrative complexity. Initially, primary coverage for dependent children was associated with the father's health plan. But as society changed, so did benefit determination rules and the "birthday rule" (see Table 18-5 for definition) was established in 1984. Other-party liability (OPL) rules associated with automobile insurance, workers' compensation, and subrogation also evolved. Insurers became increasingly focused on assigning financial responsibility and controlling claim payments.

The growth of managed care organizations in the 1970s and 1980s, spurred by the 1973 federal HMO Act, introduced two new elements to the developing claims capability: medical management and much broader use of provider payment agreements. In terms of medical management, claims adjudicators now had to determine if charges submitted by health care providers were preauthorized and/or met other medical management standards. In terms of provider payment agreements, claims adjudicators also had to ensure that the claims payment matched the appropriate fee schedule for the particular type of service and benefit plan. In addition to fee schedules, other payment options for individual providers, including specific discounts and per diem rates, came into use.

The evolving claims capability had to be adaptable, flexible, and forward looking to keep pace with the growth in complexity (as shown in Figure 18-1) of benefit plans within multiple lines of business (commercial, Medicare, Medicaid, TRICARE, etc.), provider pay-

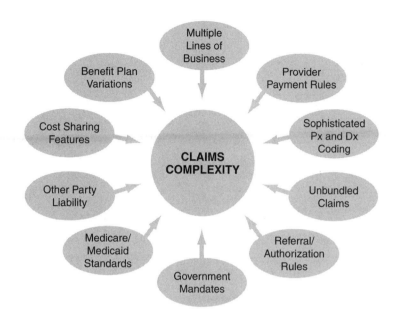

Figure 18–1 Elements of Claims Complexity
Source: Author.

ment rules, increasingly sophisticated procedure and diagnostic coding systems, unbundling practices, multifaceted referral/authorization rules, government mandates; other-party liability rules, and evolving cost sharing features. The claims capability had to be proactive and positioned to respond to changes in the health insurance marketplace, in the practice of medicine, in health care billing practices, and in the payer's own evolving technology needs. While the environment around it became increasingly complex, the claims operations continued to focus on its primary role of transaction processing to ensure the financial integrity of the payer.

As all of the variables shown in Figure 18-1 evolved over the course of the last century and as computer-based transaction processing grew out of its infancy, health insurance payers were required to make greater investment in technology and to continually upgrade both hardware and software. Payers also had to continue to invest in training and development to support evolving medical management practices. For this and a variety of other reasons, many of the multiline insurance carriers that together created the health insurance claims processing industry ultimately opted to divest their health insurance divisions. This divestiture created a new landscape that led to a new breed of organization that shifted the fundamental approach to the delivery and financing of health care from an actuarial point of view to a holistic care management point of view. This new breed of organization evolved during the 1980s and early 1990s into the managed care organizations that dominate the health insurance market today. By the end of the last century mergers and acquisitions had become the norm, with some very large MCOs dominating the industry and subsequently moving the claims capability further along in its development.

DEFINING THE MODERN CLAIMS CAPABILITY

Simply stated, the modern claims capability is the set of operational functions within the MCO that together process claims from receipt to issuance of payment and/or Explanation of Benefits (EOB). The set of operational functions (illustrated in Figure 18-2) includes the following:

- Receipt of paper claims
- Receipt of electronically submitted claims (EDI)
- Initial auto adjudication (first pass)
- Second-attempt auto adjudication following resolution of certain suspension edits
- Manual processing for claims that cannot be auto adjudicated
- Check writing process
- Issuance of Explanation of Benefits (EOB) and/or remittance advice
- Archiving claim records and data

Most often, this collection of functions (described at length on the following pages) is referred to as "claims" by individuals both outside and inside of the MCO. To those outside the MCO, the claims process is often the "face" of the MCO, particularly to the provider community. To MCO business leaders, government agencies, and others within the health insurance industry, claims is the source of information that allows the MCO to gauge and improve its business performance and improve the health care of its members. As the modern claims capability continues to evolve, information management techniques will continue to create a place of greater prominence for the claims capability in the twenty-first century.

In studying the modern claims capability, one quickly concludes that four primary core competencies make up what many of us consider claims. The core competencies include the following:

- Transactional processing
- Quality control
- Service delivery
- Information management

As shown in Figure 18-3, within each of these core competencies are three integrated components: proven business and communication processes, trained and motivated people, and supporting tools and technology. Just as with a three-legged stool, weakness in any

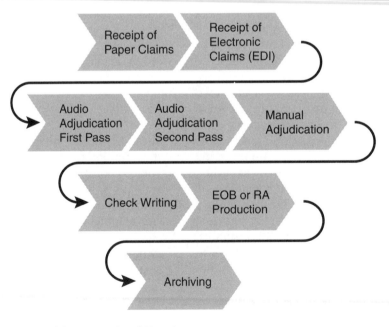

Figure 18–2 Claims Capability Operational Functions

Source: Author.

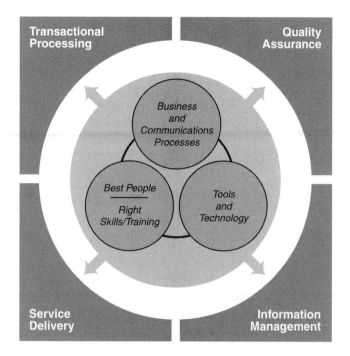

Figure 18–3 Claims Capability Core competencies and Integrated Components

Source: Author.

one integrated component will threaten the entire structure. Each of the core competencies and their integrated components are described in the following subsections.

Core Competency 1: Transactional Processing

Transactional processing is a term that describes the handling and adjudication of health care claims. It is (and always has been) the primary competency of the claims capability. Failure to execute this competency has a profound impact on all of the other core competencies as well as on the MCO as a whole. Successfully executing this competency requires an effective blend of proven business and communication processes, trained and motivated people, and supporting tools and technology.

Business and communication processes should be detailed, transparent, thorough, and integrated. One process should lead to the next in a comprehensive course of events

that allows for all contingencies. The initial business process actually begins with instructions to providers on how to file claims. Over the years, provider instructions have become much more complex yet very specific in terms of standardized claim forms and required data elements.

Two information elements that have undergone the most significant changes in recent years are the member and provider identification (ID) numbers. Regarding member ID numbers, efforts have been made, particularly in response to privacy and security requirements in HIPAA, as discussed in detail in Chapter 32, to discontinue the use of Social Security numbers in favor of an MCO-generated ID number. For provider ID numbers, at the time of publication, efforts are being made by MCOs to convert to the National Provider Identifier (NPI), also required under HIPAA and discussed in Chapters 5 and 31; the NPI is scheduled to be phased in by May 23, 2007 (May 23, 2008, for small health plans).[3] As for other required data elements, virtually all MCOs require the use of standardized place of service, diagnosis, and procedure codes (CPT, HCPCS, revenue, etc.) and have abandoned (for the most part) the use of so-called home-grown or local use codes. Furthermore, the use of the standardized codes is required under HIPAA if the transactions are electronic, thus effectively eliminating the use of local or nonstandard codes.

Personnel outside of the claims capability (often the Provider Relations or Provider Contracting department) generally communicate instructions to providers regarding these and other data elements. Those providers that use modern (*ie*, HIPAA-compliant) practice support or billing Information Technology (IT) systems will already be able to conform. Even then, the claims capability management team is responsible for reviewing and approving claims filing instructions periodically to ensure that new pertinent information is adequately and accurately included.

Within the MCO, specific business processes, discussed in greater detail later in this chapter, govern more detailed policies and procedures for the following:

- Initially handling of submitted claims (paper or electronic)
- Adjudicating claims for payment or denial
- Resolving suspended claims
- Limiting liability by administering other-party liability programs
- Reopening processed claims as a result of errors or appeals

Effective business processes must be well-documented, tested, applied, revised, and reapplied in a quest for continuous process improvement. Business processes must also be coordinated with other MCO departments to ensure that customer concerns are adequately addressed and that the MCO delivers on its key commitments across constituencies.

The claims capability's business architecture, that is, its business and communication processes, defines the tools needed to execute the transaction processing core competency. The key tool is the integrated transactional processing system, a technically advanced software application designed to record data and adjudicate claims according to predetermined rules. This tool must be robust enough to accommodate existing business and membership levels but flexible in its capacity (or scalable) to support membership growth and future complexity. Additional technology tools include scanning solutions for paper claims, applications that enable electronic claims submissions, and a host of special databases to support the management of products, benefit plans, provider contracts, regulatory requirements, and so forth.

To optimize this complex set of tools, (1) functionality (including limitations) should be well understood and communicated, (2) capabilities should be fully exploited to deliver the greatest possible value, and (3) information files should be properly maintained and updated. Optimizing the use of these tools is contingent upon integrating activities and communication within a variety of departments within the MCO (often including functions and/or entities external to the MCO).

When designing and developing products, benefit plans, provider reimbursement terms, and business processes, the MCO should not allow a transactional processing system to dictate its business decisions. However, care should be taken to ensure that benefit plan features and/or provider reimbursement methods are easily configured or programmable in the system and can be supported in such a manner as to avoid manual processing.

Historically, there has been a natural tension between the health insurers' and subsequent MCOs' desire to customize benefit plans and provider contracts in response to marketplace demands, and the MCOs' internal constraints related to business processes and tools. To ensure this natural tension remains in balance, analysis of claims administration costs associated with nonstandard benefits or provider reimbursement schemes is recommended before contracts are signed.

In fact, some MCOs pass the costs of non-standard provisions onto the employer groups and providers who request them. Imbalance within this natural tension will ultimately lead to a decrease in profitable business either through (1) unmanageable internal processes and related cost increases or (2) products that are too out of touch with the marketplace to retain membership.

Just as business processes and technology are important to transaction processing, so are trained and motivated people who perform the tasks required to process claims. Within the transaction processing component of the modern claims capability, these people include the following:

- Clerical personnel who initially prep paper claims
- Technically proficient personnel who support electronic data interchange (EDI) transmissions
- Claims processors who adjudicate claims
- Supervisors and managers who interpret policies and run daily operations
- Directors and vice presidents who strategically manage investments in the claims capability

It is the people who interact with each other, with other MCO departments, and with customers that really put the "face" on the MCO.

Unfortunately, it is the IT component that is often the major focus of attention in many claims capability operations with less and less emphasis placed on personnel. Such an approach is shortsighted, especially when many MCOs still receive large volumes of paper claims, and suspensions of electronic claims are common. Clerical personnel are needed to open, date stamp, sort, and stage claims. They also scan claims or key claims data into the transactional processing system. These front-end procedures are critical to an efficient and accurate process because claims mishandled at this stage bog down the entire workflow and may lead to quality issues such as linking claims to the incorrect

member and benefit plan, or to the incorrect service provider and fee schedule.

Even when claims are submitted via electronic data interchange (EDI), claims personnel are still vital to the front-end process by resolving claims submission problems. The EDI process varies among MCOs depending on the sophistication of their systems and the providers' EDI capabilities. The electronic process also depends on the efforts of the MCO personnel outside of the claims capability who are normally staffed in the MCO's IT department and charged with establishing the electronic links with providers and other third-party invoicing organizations or billers. There must be strong two-way communication between the claims capability and those controlling the EDI process to ensure that all data are received according to established business processes.

The heart and soul of transaction processing is claims adjudication. Today's transactional processing systems auto adjudicate on average 68%[4] of claims that are accepted into the processing system (claims that are not accepted into the processing system are considered "rejected" and never become part of the "record" within the MCO). For the remaining 32% of accepted claims, a suspension occurs during the adjudication process. Suspensions (sometimes called edits) result in manual intervention. Well-trained and experienced claims adjudicators must review suspended claims and judge whether they are paid or denied.

Adjudication not only depends on well-defined business and communication processes, technology and tools as previously described but also on the human element. Within the modern claims capability, it often takes 6 months or more to fully train a claims adjudicator. Although initial training for new employees is vital, ongoing training of tenured staff is also required to remain current in a rapidly changing environment. Claims adjudicators must also be properly motivated, accurately assessed, and suitably rewarded in terms of productivity and quality measures.

Core Competency 2: Quality Control

The second core competency of the modern claims capability is quality control. Quality control focuses on functions and processes from initial intake through preparation/staging and concludes with customer service, appeals, and ultimately renewal of the employer group or government contract. Claims adjudication is where the "rubber meets the road." It is the spot in the MCO where the organization's business processes and system files converge to produce an adjudicated outcome. As such, the claims capability is able to assess quality both "upstream" and "downstream."

Upstream refers to the processes and system files that govern and enable automatic and manual claims adjudication. Those areas and the individuals responsible for these files are usually outside of the traditional claims capability. Some upstream files contain high-level but fundamental information, including data about lines of business, group and sub-group structure, benefit plans, and other "control" data that apply across the board to all transactions. These files do not change much over time. However, other upstream files are continually updated. These include member and provider records, provider reimbursement terms and rates, referral and authorization decisions, and other-party liability details as well as the files that define benefit coding and adjudication rules.

Errors in claims processing can often be traced back to errors in one or more upstream files or records. However, rather than identifying such errors only *after* claims have been erroneously processed (causing customer service issues), the modern claims capability is proactive in monitoring and testing upstream files before providers and members are negatively affected. Just as modern managed health care focuses on preventive medicine (Chapter 14) and quality management (Chapter 15), a tenet of the modern claims capability must be quality assessment through proactive testing, quality reviews, and preventive file maintenance. The people component of this core compe-

tency relies largely on communications with other departments that control upstream processes and files. Interdepartmental relationships must be established, maintained, and nurtured. MCOs without open communication will never be as successful as those that encourage honest dialogue and collaboration.

Downstream refers primarily to the claims capability itself. The claims capability's primary goals are ensuring that claims processing error rates are kept as close to zero as possible while maintaining target production. Claims personnel are the primary focus in most downstream quality and process improvement efforts because downstream quality problems are often traced back to human error. Human error within the claims capability is generally caused by carelessness, unclear policies or procedures, insufficient training, or less than attentive management practices. Preventive measures are also essential to downstream quality assessment in terms of routine claims adjudicator audits, ongoing policy and procedure review and updates, attention to training and retraining, and close daily supervision. Careful attention should also be paid to member and provider complaints and/or appeals as well as to returned checks and other voluntary refunds to discover the root causes of errors and subsequently design corrective measures.

Other downstream factors that affect quality claims adjudication include medical management and many of the third-party programs such as pharmacy benefits management (PBM; see Chapter 12) and mental or behavioral health care programs (see Chapter 13). Tort actions can also be a factor long after claims adjudication. For example, when the MCO is notified by outside attorneys of accidents where automobile insurance, workers' compensation benefits, or subrogation is involved, the claims capability must review processed claims for potential adjustments. In addition to retrospective review of previously paid claims, measures must be taken to avoid future overpayments related to these situations.

Whether errors are considered upstream or downstream, they have a negative impact on the face of the MCO in terms of customer satisfaction. Continuous quality problems have a dampening effect on provider and member retention and could lead to the loss of business, negatively affecting the MCO's bottom line. Even if such customer loss is avoided, quality problems still affect the bottom line in terms of costly rework. Devoting resources to preventing errors is far less expensive than the postadjudication analysis necessary to discover errors or the assets necessary to correct them. Costly rework can quickly change the financial assumptions underlying the MCO's business plan.

Core Competency 3: Service Delivery

A third core competency of the modern claims capability is service delivery to both internal and external customers as described in other chapters in this book. Internal customers include those departments that directly interact with members and providers as well as finance, actuarial and underwriting, product development, sales and marketing, medical management, and internal audit. External customers, including employer groups, brokers, members, and providers, are affected by the claims capability and may have direct contact with the claims capability management team through periodic customer audits and site visits.

Service delivery focused on members or providers can be handled in two ways. One way is to house call centers that respond directly to member and provider claims concerns within the claims capability. The advantage to this approach is that claims adjudicators taking the calls may be able to adjust errors or resolve suspended claims immediately. The disadvantage to this approach is that the caller may have other concerns and must be transferred to a member or provider services representative for resolution. Another disadvantage is that constant interruptions with telephone calls

severely impede claims adjudication productivity and quality if both tasks are assigned to the same person at the same time. Care must be taken to segregate claims adjudication production tasks from call center tasks to ensure appropriate focus. Another issue to consider is whether claims adjudicators assigned to call center duty are trained in customer service skills. Excellent claims adjudicators may not be excellent customer service representatives.

The other way to handle service delivery to members and providers is for the MCO to have a separate call center operation that responds to all member and/or provider inquiries. In this case, customer service representatives (CSRs) must rely on the claims capability to promptly resolve claims problems. The advantage to a centralized call center is that the CSR is trained to respond to all sorts of issues, not just claims-related problems. A disadvantage is that additional extensive training on how claims are adjudicated may be needed to fully prepare CSRs to respond to claims inquiries. Another disadvantage is that adjustments cannot be accomplished as quickly. To address this issue, the claims capability must establish and execute policies and procedures to promptly attend to problem claims identified by the CSRs. Member services, including managing the call center function, are discussed in detail in Chapter 19.

As stated earlier, the claims capability uses technology and sundry tools to support service delivery. The transactional processing systems and other software applications facilitate communication among departments, provide data to research and uncover the root cause of errors, and support the execution of adjustments. Almost as important as the transactional processing system are the business and communication practices that enable an efficient and timely error resolution process. However, well-trained and motivated personnel are the key to delivering the service. The claims capability staff must be reminded that behind every claim is a patient who is ill or injured and is relying on the MCO to deliver on its service commitments. If claims personnel understand the human component, they are more likely to understand their impact on customers and are less likely to think of themselves as just a traditional back-office support operation.

Core Competency 4: Information Management

The fourth core competency of the modern claims capability is information management, that is, the collection and management of data fundamental to the MCO and its customers. Information management plays a major role in data warehousing, security, standard and ad hoc analytics, care and disease management, fraud and abuse detection, other-party liability administration, and financial functions such as forecasting and reporting. As previously noted, the claims capability is the source of much of the data that allows the MCO to operate and improve its business. This fourth core competency relies on the previous three competencies, particularly transactional processing and quality control.

Technology, of course, is vital to information management and is discussed in some detail in Chapter 17. A robust transactional processing system and other technological tools enable the MCO to categorize and house data. MCO personnel can then extract and manipulate key elements. In early processing systems, reporting was limited to so-called canned reports that were hard-coded into the software. Current systems are designed to make virtually all data elements reportable so that MCO analysts can include any number of factors in business and health care improvement models. During the past decade, the science of informatics has grown from infancy to become a robust part of the MCO's business and care delivery model. *Informatics* is defined as "the collection, classification, storage, retrieval, and dissemination of recorded knowledge treated both as a pure and as an applied science."[5]

As informatics has come of age, so have the parallel needs of developing and hiring more personnel with deep analytical skills. To optimize the resources and data collected, well-designed business processes are needed and must be fully coordinated with other operational departments. As such there is a need for two-way communication and understanding between claims personnel and other departments to fully understand and realize the potential of all collected data. For example, administering a profitable other-party liability program usually depends on data collected by personnel outside of the claims capability. If the Enrollment department (or outside vendors) provides other health insurance information on members, it must be cognizant of the specific data elements needed for claims adjudicators to coordinate benefits successfully. Similarly, if utilization nurses identify other insurance potential because of accidental injury, they must be directed to record specific information that can be used to reduce the MCO's liability in favor of automobile or workers' compensation insurance. Data collection and management are ongoing processes that cannot be left unattended. Lags or gaps in maintaining data limits its usability and diminishes its value.

When claims-related information initially became more accessible through software and hardware designs and greater automation, it was mainly used for actuarial purposes to evaluate experience and set rates. Since the 1990s, MCOs have developed more sophisticated means to retrieve data, thus exponentially expanding the use of the information they have collected. Information is now considered a vital asset not only to the MCO but also to employer groups, members, providers, and external parties, including state and federal governments.

For the MCO, and for employer groups as well, claims experience helps to support new product and benefit designs, including the development of consumer-driven health plans (CDHPs; see Chapters 2 and 20). Members have more and more access to data that help them to determine and/or control costs and manage their own health care. Wellness initiatives and disease management programs are evolving to benefit members, providers, and the MCOs in ways not imagined previously. Even the federal government is now realizing that MCOs are a unique aggregator of data that can identify early signs of global health threats or biological terrorism. New community organizations such as regional health information organizations (RHIOs) or public-private state-wide health information networks (HINs) are beginning to leverage this growing information management and informatics experience.

Organization Considerations

The claims capability is typically managed as one consolidated department within the MCO's operations division and reports to a chief operations officer (COO) or a chief financial officer (CFO). In large organizations, the claims capability may report to a senior vice president. Within smaller MCOs, the claims capability often reports to a director of operations. As shown in Figure 18-4, the claims capability is integral to managed care operations and depends upon relationships with virtually all of the other MCO's departments.

Within the claims capability, the organization structure depends on the scope of responsibilities. A large MCO with multiple lines of business may require a separate manager or director for each. An operation focused solely on commercial business may organize around major employer groups especially if each employer group has nonstandard benefit plans that require a certain amount of manual adjudication. MCOs administering entitlement programs (Medicare, Medicaid, and TRICARE, discussed in Chapters 26, 27, and 28, respectively) may organize based on the program guidelines for compliance. Within any of these models, further specialization could be assigned for pharmacy claims, durable medical equip-

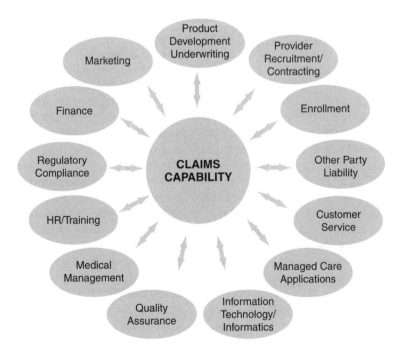

Figure 18–4 Claims Capability Relationships within the MCO

Source: Author.

ment (DME) claims, or claims involving other-party liability (OPL), and so forth.

Additional factors to consider when creating a claims capability organization model involve the transactional processing system in use. Most transactional processing systems are structured by claim type, that is, one set of processing screens and procedures for professional claims, and another set of processing screens and procedures for institutional and ancillary services claims. This structure lends itself to organizing units of claims adjudicators by the types of claims they process. Some MCOs may have one or more legacy transactional processing systems that were developed for health maintenance organization (HMO), preferred provider organization (PPO), or traditional indemnity plans. In some cases, this factor alone may govern how the claims capability organization is structured.

Figure 18-5 shows a claims capability organization chart for a large MCO that incorporates many of these ideas. The organization chart shows several management levels that may or may not conform to specific MCO strategies around organization design. This illustration also shows a claims organization that is rich in varied duties and levels creating a career path vital for employee motivation and retention. Figure 18-5 is not a blueprint but rather an example that suggests options to consider when organizing personnel and business processes by line of business in relation to the available technology.

A single individual should be accountable for the modern claims capability. Whether the individual is a senior vice president, vice president, director, or manager depends on the size of the MCO, the MCO's human resources policies, the number of business lines, annual claims volume, and government protocols if the MCO manages state or federal contracts. The organization chart shows only one supervisor under each manager. However, the number of supervisors (if any) depends on the number of adjudicators needed and the degree of processing special-

ization. Figure 18-5 also shows that quality assessment and training are often separate and shared services across the claims capability organization. These functions should report to the highest management level of the claims capability because they serve the entire claims operation. Placing these functions outside of the claims *production* environment is more likely to ensure (1) fair and equitable quality reviews, (2) an adequate focus on training and cross-training, and (3) the development of comprehensive training materials.

Another organizational issue relates to adjustments defined as those claims that must be corrected or adjusted because of a processing error or a decision reversed upon appeal. Adjustments because of errors include claims that are paid for the wrong patient, paid to the wrong provider, paid an incorrect amount (possibly from the wrong fee schedule), paid for the wrong date of service, paid at the wrong benefit level as well as those denied erroneously. Adjustments also may be caused by decisions reversed upon appeal, including claims denied for no eligibility, ineligible benefit, no authorization, or exhausted benefits. Claims may be reversed upon appeal by a first-time review within the appeals department (often located within claims capability), by medical management or other senior managers, or as the result of provider peer review or legal action. Although there may be some value in returning errors to the original adjudicator for correction, it is usually more efficient to have all adjustments handled by a special unit because the processing steps can be quite complicated. Choosing to staff each unit of the claims capability with adjustors who are familiar with the specific line of business, employer groups, government programs, provider contracts, and so forth is a decision that must be made based on quality, productivity, and training challenges unique to the MCO.

Roles and responsibilities should be coordinated within the organizational model to drive outcomes related to the particular claims capability. Table 18-1 displays a skills

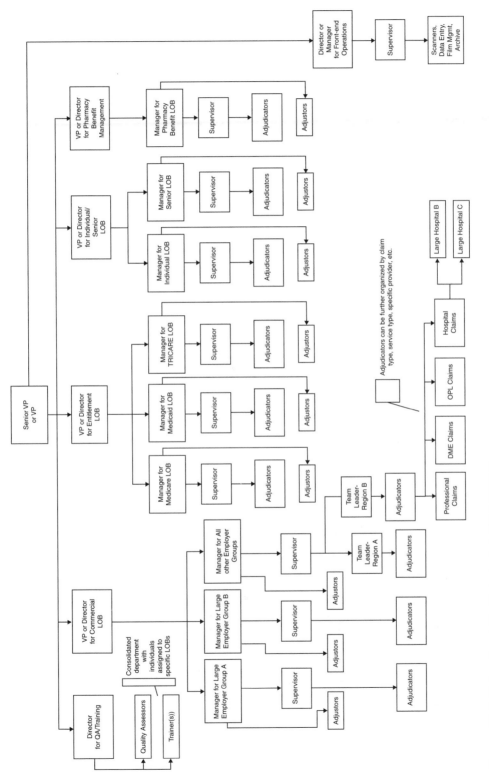

Figure 18–5 Claims Capability Organization Chart Options

Table 18–1 Claims Capability Roles and Responsibilities Matrix

	Sr VP	VP	Dir	Mgr	Sup	Team Lead	Adjudicator	Adjustor	Clerical Staff	Other
Overall responsibility for claims capability (depending on size of operation)	X	X	X	X						
Represents claims capability in management meetings	X	X	X	X						
Represents claims capability with providers and members	X	X	X	X						
Represents claims capability with ASO groups, government, and external auditors	X	X	X	X						
Manages third-party vendors	X	X	X	X						
Security	X	X	X	X						IT
Determines claims capability roles and responsibilities	X	X	X	X						
Determines individual management roles and responsibilities	X	X	X	X						
Determines individual nonmanagement roles and responsibilities			X	X						
Establishes policies and procedures			X	X						
Enforces policies and procedures				X	X	X				
Coordinates policies and procedures with other departments			X	X	X	X				
Coordinates claims adjudication system rules			X	X						
Maintains claims adjudication system rules			X	X	X					IT
Responsible for training and development	X	X	X	X	X					Trainers

Responsibility/role matrix (columns: four staff/role columns unlabeled on this image, plus IT, Quality assessors, Cross-functional team):

Activity					IT	Quality assessors	Cross-functional team
Manages workflow tools			X		X		
Manages work distribution at unit level			X				
Manages work distribution at individual level		X	X				
Quality assessment						X	
Inventory (backlog) management		X	X	X			
Continuous quality improvement		X	X			X	X
Hires, terminates, assesses performance	X	X	X				
Respond to problem resolution calls			X	X			
Special projects			X	X			X
Resolves unadjudicated EDI claims	X						
Adjudicates paper claims	X						
Resolves suspended claims	X						
Adjusts claims caused by processing errors or appeals		X					
Scans or keys claims data into system			X				
Archiving			X				

matrix that can help shape the various roles and responsibilities within the MCO. Some responsibilities are marked for more than one managerial level and should be interpreted to apply to the highest level that exists in a particular MCO. For example, "overall responsibility" is checked for a senior vice president, vice president, and director. However, if all three managerial levels exit, the responsibility resides with the senior vice president.

Claims capability managers often have questions about determining staffing ratios in terms of the number of claims adjudicators, supervisors, or managers needed to respond to the claims volume. There is very little in the way of industry standards to suggest the ideal staffing ratio because there are so many variables to consider. There are also variations in the way claims capability metrics are structured. Some claims operations measure productivity by claims processed per hour; others measure by claims processed per day. The MCO's historical experience can provide a starting point for creating productivity benchmarks if they are not already established. Productivity goals should be set, records kept and analyzed, and ultimately a claims per hour or claims per day (or claim line items per hour or day) quota should be established for staffing determinations as well as performance evaluations. Ultimately, the answer to staffing ratio questions depends on the number needed to meet volume demands, while maintaining quality standards and not relying on overtime hours as a permanent solution.

MANAGING THE CLAIMS CAPABILITY

Shared across the four claims capability core competencies as described earlier are common, enterprise-wide objectives including the following:

- Enabling the MCO to meet contractual obligations to employer groups, government agencies, members, and providers.

- Ensuring timely benefits administration for enrolled members, including the accurate application of cost sharing features, benefit limitations, maximums, and exclusions.
- Administering medical management policies and medical necessity decisions.
- Improving the health care of its members through the development and execution of care management plans.
- Providing prompt and accurate customer service to members, brokers, employer groups, and providers.
- Protecting financial liability by validating eligibility, avoiding duplicate and other inappropriate claims, ensuring accurate processing, administering other-party liability programs, pursuing cost-containment activities related to known or specific financial leakage, and ensuring timely productivity to avoid processing penalties and interest payments.

To achieve these enterprise-wide objectives, the claims capability must be well-managed in terms of the following:

- Inventory control
- Auto Adjudication
- Task allocation and work distribution
- Workflow
- Policies and procedures
- Staff training and development
- Quality assessments
- Reports
- Cost containment
- Use of information technology
- Outsourcing

Each of these management priorities is discussed here in terms of achieving production and quality standards. Refer to Figure 18-6 for a graphic representation of the process steps and functions described in this section.

Inventory Control

Inventory control refers to the management of claims from receipt to final disposition.

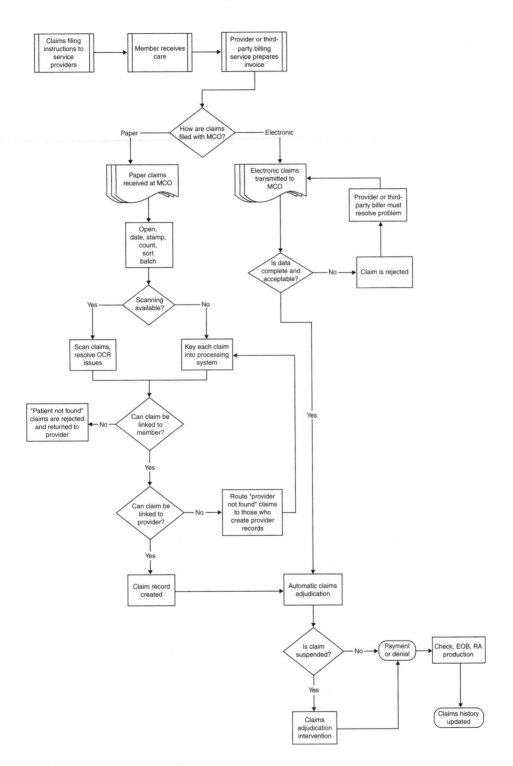

Figure 18–6 Claims Capability Workflow Chart

Ultimately, claims inventory is controlled by the claims capability management team; the claims capability management team should not be controlled by the inventory! Control must be based on accurate claim counts at all stages of the claims adjudication process, as well as on efficient work distribution strategies. Bottlenecks must be quickly recognized, root causes discovered, and action plans formulated and executed to eliminate the problem. The claims capability management team will always be challenged with managing inventory control (production) and quality. A claims capability that does not meet this challenge will suffer from growing inventories or excessive and costly rework.

Inventory control begins with the front-end processes related to receipt and preparation of claims, paper or electronic. Management of the front-end operations should be under the direction of a single director or manager who reports to the most senior claims capability manager as shown in the sample organization chart (Figure 18-5). The front-end process for paper claims is far more clerical in nature than that for electronically submitted claims. In either case, front-end claims-handling procedures are vital to ensure that claims are promptly and accurately prepped for claims adjudication.

Both claim streams, paper and electronic, are dependent on other MCO departments for success. Therefore, it is incumbent upon the claims capability management team to establish and nurture relationships with other MCO functions to ensure coordinated processing. Consider the fact that the front-end process actually begins with instructions to providers as to how to prepare and file claims on behalf of the MCO's members. Claims filing instructions, policies and procedures, and/or guidelines are usually prepared, updated, and distributed by the provider relations or provider contracting personnel. These instructions, which sometimes include certain state and federal government regulations, define what constitutes a valid or "clean" claim. The definition of a clean claim must address the following:

- Required claim forms
- Required data elements
- Additional documentation requirements such as emergency room or operative reports, details of anesthesia units administered, and so forth
- Timely filing rules indicating the number of days from the date of service in which a provider must file a claim

The claims capability management team should review claims filing instructions periodically to ensure that all pertinent information is adequately and accurately included. It is important to remember that claim turnaround rules (defined as the time allowed by government regulation and/or provider contract terms specifying the number of days the claims capability has to process submitted claims for payment or denial) depend on the definition of a clean claim.

Claims Intake for Paper Claims

If claims are filed on paper, the inventory control process begins with initial handling procedures shown in Table 18-2:

- *Open and date stamp:* Remove paper claims from envelopes and date stamp indicating the date the claim is received by the MCO. The date of receipt is vital in measuring claims aging and turnaround time. The date of receipt is also used to apply the timely filing rule. (Claims aging, turnaround time, and timely filing are discussed later in this section.)
- *Sort:* How paper claims are sorted depends entirely on the claims adjudication process and how the claims capability is structured. Sorting categories should enable maximum work distribution efficiency and should be considered a target for change in a continuous process improvement review.

Table 18–2 Initial Handling Procedures for Paper Claims

Open and Date-Stamp	• Allocate secure physical space • Establish detailed procedures to open, date-stamp, count paper claims and other correspondence • Organize and equip mailroom to move the paper through an assembly-line process, ensuring no claims are lost or destroyed • Date-stamp each piece of paper with a date stamp • Avoid marking claims in any way (except for a date stamp and/or document control number) because they are legally binding documents • Ensure that any additional documents submitted with the paper claim (operative or emergency room reports, explanations of benefits from other insurance carriers, letters, etc.) remain with the claim • Discard envelopes except for those showing certified mail information

Sort	• Establish postal mail box numbers for each product or line of business.
	  – Initial sort accomplished by the postal service
	  – Applicable claims filing address can be printed on the member's ID card to ensure compliance
	  – Coordinate with other MCO departments that control the design and production of member ID cards
	• Sort by claim form because most transactional processing systems are designed with two separate processing tracks
	  – HCFA/CMS 1500 for professional services
	  – UB92/HCFA 1450 for hospital services
	• Sort by specialization
	  – Physician charges
	  – Durable medical expense (DME)
	  – Chiropractic and/or physical therapy
	  – Other-party liability (OPL)
	  – Sort by specific providers such as large hospitals or providers with unique contract terms
	CAUTION:
	• Too few categories may adversely affect efficiency of work distribution.
	• Too many categories may be unnecessary and counterproductive.
	• Never carved in stone.

Batch and Count	• Create batches of claims as they are sorted:
	  – 25–50 claims per batch
	  – Rubber-banded
	  – Labeled with a batch control sheet indicating the date of receipt, the number of claims, the type of claims, and any other important data useful to the functional area receiving the work
	• Create batches of equal size to expedite overall claim count and specific claim count per sort category
	• Manual count in smaller operations
	• Automated counting methods in larger operations
	  – Use date-stamping equipment that includes automatic counters.
	  – Use a document control number that is sequentially incremented by one. The document control number not only aids the counting process, it also serves as a link between the source document and the claim recorded in the transactional processing system
	• Execute a thorough physical "hard" count of paper claim forms periodically to ensure accountability and guard against intentional or unintentional misplacement

- *Batch and count:* Batching paper claims helps to secure an accurate claim count, vital in determining overall and specific claims volume per day, per week, per month, and per year. Changes in this volume directly affect budgetary and staffing decisions for the claims capability.

Front-End Systems Procedures for Paper Claims

Once paper claims are sorted, counted and batched, they are ready to be recorded in the transactional processing system: through scanning technologies or through manual keying of data into the system. Scanning has become the preferred method especially in operations that still receive high volumes of paper claims. Scanning technology has progressed from merely creating an electronic image of the paper document to actually populating the claims processing data screens based on optical character recognition (OCR) functionality. Despite these advances, there may be letters or numbers on a particular claim that the scanning application cannot recognize with certainty. Most scanning applications are designed to highlight questionable characters so that the human operator can review the actual claim document (or its scanned image) to make the accurate determination (for example, is the questionable character a "3," an "8," or a "B"?). This process is called resolution.

An alternative to scanning claims is the direct data entry of information from the paper claim into the transactional processing system. Operations that receive a small volume of paper claims may opt for this method rather than investing in scanning technology. Entry-level personnel can perform this task because they will not be making claims adjudication decisions. However, personnel assigned to this task must be well trained and aware of the vital importance of accuracy at this stage. Their work should be closely monitored and assessed for quality to ensure that the claims data submitted on the paper form are the data that is entered into the processing system.

Two critical actions in both the scanning and data entry of claims are linking the claim to the correct member and to the correct service provider. Although outside the control of the claims capability, any critical delays in creating or maintaining member eligibility or provider records in other MCO departments will have a negative impact on the claims capability and will more than likely lead to rework or adjustments to claims later in the process. Specific policies and procedures must be developed to account for missing or questionable data elements and such policies and procedures must be coordinated with other MCO departments.

One problem that has implications beyond the claims capability involves claims for patients who cannot be identified in the processing system. These are often referred to as "member not found" claims. If such claims cannot be linked to processing system member records (even if the member is no longer eligible for benefits), the claims can proceed no further in the process. They are typically returned to the provider of service, indicating that the claim was sent to the wrong MCO. This return process, however, may not work for claims operations administering Medicaid, Medicare, or TRICARE programs. Compliance regulations may require that the "member not found" claims be further researched on other databases to determine if the patient is, in fact, eligible but not yet recorded in the MCO's transactional processing system.

The claims capability must establish precise policies and procedures to answer the following questions:

- Are paper claims routed to another department for research?
- If so, how does the claims capability control the paper and ensure against loss?
- Should paper claims be photocopied?
- If so, how are photocopies coordinated with the originals when the research is complete?
- Can photocopies be kept secure and in compliance with HIPAA regulations?

- Can claims personnel have access to the other eligibility databases?
- How much training is involved?
- Which department is responsible for the transferred claims?
- If claims are sent back to providers, does this create a service issue that another MCO department must resolve?
- Is this issue addressed in member or provider handbooks?

These and a host of other issues must be thoroughly thought through and worked through with cross-functional teams to ensure that inventory control is maintained and members and provider obligations are met.

Similar issues revolve around paper claims where the "provider is not on file." If claims cannot be linked to a processing system provider record, they cannot proceed through claims adjudication. But this time, this problem must be resolved within the MCO. As MCOs convert to using the NPI beginning in 2007 (2008 for small health plans), this problem will eventually diminish as an issue.

Prior to the conversion to using the NPI as well as for some time after (because of lags in billing and to the as-yet unknown ability of all providers to be in compliance with using the NPI by 2007), policies and procedures governing the assignment of provider ID numbers must accommodate the transactional processing system and comply with all regulatory agencies. Most often, primary care physicians and specialists are assigned individual provider ID numbers so that claims can be linked to the individual provider. But there are always exceptions to this rule. For example, professional claims for radiology or anesthesiology can be linked to the group practice or to the individual physician. For behavioral health claims, services provided by social workers can be linked to the overall practice or the individual social worker's tax identification number. Additionally, provider records can be further complicated by turnover within medical practices as well as changes in service providers' statuses within

the MCO. A physician considered as participating or in-network one day, may be nonparticipating and out-of-network the next. Or providers may be participating or in-network for one line of business and nonparticipating and out-of-network for another.

The claims capability management team must have a thorough understanding of how provider records are created in the processing system thus enabling them to design front-end procedures for linking paper claims to the correct provider. As previously noted, claims cannot be returned to service providers because there is no record of the provider in the processing system. Such claims must be worked internally by some combination of claims capability personnel and personnel responsible for creating provider records. Once again the questions about what to do with the paper claim form surface:

- Are paper claims routed to another department for research and resolution?
- If so, how does the claims capability control the paper?
- Should paper claims be photocopied?
- If so, how are photocopies coordinated with the originals when the research is complete?
- Can photocopies be kept secure and in compliance with HIPAA regulations?

Remember, that while these processes occur, the clock continues to tick in terms of claims turnaround commitments. Just as with "member not found" claims, policies and procedures to deal with "provider not found" claims must be thoroughly thought through and documented.

Beyond member and provider issues, there are other data elements that can be missing or illegible on paper claims. How these instances are handled depends on decisions made by the MCO in defining a "clean claim." The claims capability may take a hard line and return all claims with missing or questionable data elements to the submitting provider. However, it is worth considering if making telephone inquiries to clarify questionable data would better serve members, providers, and the MCO. In very large operations, this may not be feasible. But in smaller operations, a few well-placed phone calls may actually be more efficient. After all, service delivery is a core component of the claims capability.

Claims Intake for Electronic Claims

Virtually all of these front-end inventory control issues disappear when claims are submitted electronically through third-party vendors known as clearinghouses. A clearinghouse establishes relationships and electronic connections with both service providers and MCOs to facilitate the immediate delivery of clean claims (those that include all of the required data elements that allow for electronic submission by the provider and receipt by the MCO). "Provider not found" issues are eliminated because each provider must have an identification number already established to submit electronic claims. "Member not found" issues are also eliminated in that the claim will not be accepted (and therefore will be automatically returned to the provider by the clearinghouse) if the patient identification number is not recognized. Claims with other missing data elements are also returned to the provider, thereby ensuring that only clean claims are accepted electronically. Claims that do not meet criteria established by the MCO are considered rejected claims. Data from these claims are never entered into claims history and never become part of MCO reports.

An advantage of working with a clearinghouse (for both providers and MCOs) is that problems are identified and resolved before claims are received by the MCO. Alternatively, some MCOs have established direct electronic links with larger providers to avoid clearinghouse fees. In these situations, the MCO must establish strict policies and procedures to resolve electronic claims issues with the service providers directly.

Claims Intake Metrics

Whether claims are submitted on paper or electronically, inventory receipts must be measured to allocate adequate resources and verify financial assumptions about an insured population. Other measures are also important to track, including the following:

- Timely filing limits.
- Turnaround time based on the date the MCO received the claim.
- "Claims lag," the time elapsed by comparing the date of service to the date of receipt.
- "Incurred but not reported" (IBNR), claims measured by comparing outstanding authorization records ordering care and other unreported encounters to actual claims received. IBNR claims represent rendered but unreported services caused by delays in service providers' submissions. IBNR tracking is very important to effective financial management and is discussed further in Chapter 24.

Turnaround time is probably the most important of these measures because claims capability operations must be structured to ensure that turnaround requirements, governed by provider contracts or government regulations, are met. Shorter turnaround goals may be established for electronically submitted claims. Exceeding the turnaround time limits leads to customer service problems and may also result in interest penalty payments to providers.

To produce accurate and timely reports as well as meet turnaround goals, claims should be recorded in the transactional processing system immediately upon receipt by the MCO. For electronic claims, this process is automatic and, therefore, transparent to the claims capability. For paper claims, however, the front-end operations should be staffed adequately to ensure that all clean claims are initially processed within a day or day and a half of receipt. Volumes will vary each business day with Mondays traditionally being the highest volume day except for weeks that include a Monday holiday. Historical reviews of daily claim receipts should help the management team adjust the staff accordingly and anticipate the need for overtime hours.

Auto Adjudication

The purpose of the front-end process is to record claims data into the transactional processing system so that auto adjudication can be applied. *Auto adjudication* is the process of automatically determining eligibility and correctly applying benefits and payment terms for each claim using predetermined rules without any human intervention. Virtually all transactional processing systems are now capable of auto adjudication, but auto adjudication is based on what seems like a million small decisions and contingencies built into the hundreds of business rule configuration files governing this complex series of automated decision making. MCO employees who build such files (usually a combination of IT and claims personnel) must be knowledgeable about the following topics:

- Both professional and institutional claim types
- How claims are filed
- How charges are reported
- How benefits are expressed in terms of procedure and/or diagnosis codes
- How providers are reimbursed
- How member liability is applied
- How referral and/or authorization rules are applied
- How medical management programs affect claims payment decisions

Typically, there is a hierarchy of decisions that the transactional processing system works through to determine if a claim is payable or if it should be denied or suspended for further attention and human decision making. Indeed, there are three outcomes of auto adjudication once a claim is accepted into the processing system:

- Auto-pay
- Auto-deny
- Suspend

The hierarchy should begin by determining whether the claim meets the timely filing parameter. If the date of service is beyond the timely filing limit, the claim is automatically denied with the appropriate denial reason code before any other data are evaluated. The next decision usually involves the patient's eligibility status. If the patient is not eligible on the date of service, the claim is denied with the appropriate denial reason code before other data are evaluated.

If a claim survives these initial edits, it is then evaluated charge by charge (otherwise referred to as line by line) in terms of benefit coverage and the accepted standards of medical practice. There may be certain types of services that are never covered (autopsy, for example) that are immediately recognized as not covered and denied with the applicable reason code. All other benefits are compared and reviewed in the business rule configuration files in terms of some combination of procedure, diagnosis, place of service, and/or other codes that determine the following:

- If the service is covered under the appropriate benefit plan
- If any cost sharing features (copayments, deductibles, co-insurance) or limitations (maximums or benefit limitations) should be applied and recorded in the member's claim history

At the same time, the system is applying rules specific to the provider of service (whose ID number is coded on the claim) in relation to the member's benefit plan:

- Participating or not
- In-network or not
- Capitated or not
- Payable according to a fee schedule or a different payment calculation, etc.

Claims that do not meet the complex (but relatively clear) criteria for payment or denial are automatically suspended for manual review by a claims adjudicator. Some claims suspend because they "get hung up" in the transactional processing system, thus revealing some problem with the business rule configuration structure. These claims must be attended to immediately so that the problem can be rectified and inventory control, including turnaround time, is not compromised. Other claims suspend precisely because of business configuration rules such as the following:

- Inappropriate combinations of service type, procedure, or diagnosis codes for the patient's age
- Illogical combinations of service type, procedure, or diagnosis codes and the patient's gender
- Services that require specific medical management review
- Procedure codes that must be manually priced
- Missing or inappropriate modifier codes affecting the pricing of surgical claims
- Suspected other-party liability
- Suspicious diagnosis codes related to accidents
- Suspected fraud and abuse

The business rule configuration and auto adjudication process are much more complicated than this brief description implies. Nevertheless, auto adjudication occurs almost instantaneously. The goal of auto adjudication is maximum throughput (the number of claims automatically adjudicated for payment or denial) and is achieved through the knowledge, experience, and tenacity of the personnel assigned to create the rules, tables, and other auto adjudication files. The more complete and precise the business rule configuration files, the higher the throughput.

Some MCOs place the responsibility of maintaining the business rule configuration files within the claims capability; some place it within the IT operation. Other MCOs place it within a separate managed care applications team that includes other specialists who maintain business rule files that govern eligibility, provider contracts and credentialing, medical management, and other fundamental processing functions. If the business rule configuration function is outside of the claims capability, the claims management team must maintain at least a dotted-line connection to the function to ensure accuracy and accountability. Those who create and maintain business rule configuration files must be knowledgeable about the following topics:

- Claim types
- How claims are created and submitted
- How benefits are structured
- How providers are paid
- How referrals and authorizations are applied
- How medical management programs affect claims payments

As part of the MCO's proactive management approach, the claims capability management team must insist on extensive testing of business rule configuration for auto adjudication as well as on prompt fixes to problems discovered through provider and/or member complaints and appeals. Proactive management is challenging because the skill sets and knowledge required to maintain the complex criteria for auto adjudication are often in short supply.

Task Allocation and Work Distribution

As described earlier, claims adjudicators must review suspended claims for final disposition. How suspended claims are assigned to claims adjudicators, however, varies among MCOs. Most large MCOs have linked a workflow software application to their transactional processing system. Workflow software automatically directs suspended claims to claim adjudicator work queues based on any number of factors such as claim type, suspension reason, provider specialty, or dollar threshold. Managers, supervisors, or even team leaders monitor such work distribution to ensure that the claims adjudicators have the training and experience to resolve the suspended claims assigned to their work queues.

For those operations that do not have workflow software, the work distribution is more labor intensive. Managers, supervisors, or team leaders must rely on daily reports generated from the transactional processing system that list suspended claims. The reports are marked up with specific names of assigned adjudicators, photocopied as necessary, and distributed among the staff.

In either case, claims management personnel must constantly monitor claims aging reports to ensure that suspended claims are not left untouched for unnecessary or unacceptable periods of time. They must also identify any bottlenecks in the process especially if other departments must be contacted to resolve suspended claims. Detailed workflow processes as well as policies and procedures with other departments must be established and monitored to ensure that no claim is left behind.

Policies and Procedures

Although several references to policies and procedures have been made throughout this chapter, this topic deserves a section of its own to underscore its importance. Indeed, one cannot overstate the value of thorough, well-written, cross-functional, current, and accessible policies and procedures. They are used to explain the "why" (policy) and the "how" (procedure) of every operational task within the claims capability. Unfortunately, the policies and procedures responsibility is often an orphan. Ideally, the responsibilities for creating and maintaining policies and procedures should be specifically assigned to one or more persons who have claims knowledge and experience as well as analytic and written communication skills. In a large organization, they can be part of the quality assurance (QA)/training function so that there is consistency across the claims capability in style and substance. In a smaller organization, the policies and procedures responsibility may have to be combined with other duties, but care should be taken to ensure that the other duties are subordinate.

Discreet policies and procedures are required for all claims capability tasks. Attri-butes of these policies and procedures are as follows:

- They must be *written* following a well-defined format that identifies who does what, when, and how it is measured or verified. The documents should also show a history of change over time so that an adjudicator or auditor can easily determine the policy or procedure in effect at a specific time.

- They should be *thorough* in that they account for every single step in a process. Thoroughly reviewing and documenting processes helps to reveal inconsistencies or gaps in claims processes that compromise quality and/or efficiency.

- They should be *cross-functional* in that procedures that cross departmental lines should be developed with other departments. For example, if certain suspended claims must be reviewed by medical management personnel, procedures must be developed with the medical management staff so that each department's procedures are clearly defined.

- They must be *current*. Production of policies and procedures is not a one-time event. It is an ongoing process that must reflect changes in the claims capability. Claims personnel must feel confident that the policies and procedures are up-to-date. If found to be unreliable or outdated, personnel will not refer to them.

- They must be *accessible*. Most MCOs have developed intranets to house policies and procedures, which makes searching for applicable information more efficient. This contrasts with the huge "butterfly" policies and procedures manuals that graced claims adjudicators' desks in the past. Search capabilities should be monitored and adjusted as needed based on user feedback.

- They must be *consistent with external information*, that is, internal policies and procedures should correspond to the material that is printed in employer or member marketing vehicles, member handbooks, and provider guides as well as items on the MCO's Web site.

Staff Training and Development

Staff training and development is another discreet function that demands adequate time and resources. Like the development of policies and procedures, training is not a one-time event, but rather a process. It begins with on-boarding new employees with both knowledge and skills related to the position. A major pitfall of current training approaches in many MCOs is that training usually focuses only on the transactional processing system. MCOs often fail to teach new employees the "big picture" concepts of claims processing before teaching processing tactics. When this occurs, employees often do not understand why they should perform steps in a certain order and for specific reasons. They just know how to do the steps. This ultimately limits their abilities to quickly conduct research and analysis on suspensions, errors, adjustments, and so forth. "Systems" training, although vital, must be grounded in knowledge about managed health care in general and the MCO in particular. New employees should understand the MCO's philosophies, organization, lines of business, products, provider networks, and other basic information to provide context and meaning to the systems processing instructions.

Training methods can include classroom training, Web-based and CD-ROM courseware, conference calls, webinars, online simulations, lab-based simulations, job aids, Web pages and/or sites, mentors, chats, and videos. Some organizations are also incorporating newer technologies such as podcasting, vodcasting, and blogging.[6] Blending a number of training delivery methods is also a current trend that allows MCOs to use the most appropriate delivery for the audience and topic. However, various methods must be integrated into an overall training plan aimed at addressing specific performance issues. "A

blended solution doesn't occur when you just bolt on some e-learning modules to an instructor led session. It's only when the pieces fit together logically like finely matched parts of an engine that you create a real blended solution."[7]

To be effective, training must conform to adult learning principles:

- Adults have a need to know why they must learn what is being presented to them.
- Adults approach learning in terms of problem solving.
- Adults must see the relevance of the instruction to their immediate experience.[8]

To provide relevancy, training can be staged over a period of time, so that new hires are instructed on one aspect of claims adjudication (*eg*, laboratory claims), are given time to apply the training with live claims, and are evaluated and advanced to the next level of claims adjudication. In other words, there is not a great deal of value in training all new hires on all aspects of claims adjudication when they are unlikely to be assigned to work with all aspects of claims immediately after formal training. Once new claims adjudicators become proficient with certain types of claims, they can be more easily cross-trained on other types.

Cross-training is actually one type of ongoing staff development that should be part of the claims capability total training strategy. Cross-training is vital in smaller organizations simply because there are fewer individuals to rely on when absenteeism or seasonal increased volume affect productivity. In larger organizations, cross-training is a good motivational tool and keeps staff fresh and more eager to learn and do something new.

Other ongoing staff development that should be part of the total training strategy focuses on updates to policies and procedures or system processing rules. Many MCOs use e-mail to convey new information, but this is not a reliable method to ensure all appropriate parties are informed. It also does not guarantee compliance. Delivering new information requires carefully planned rollouts that could begin with e-mail, but are followed-up with workshops and updated policies and procedures.

Another area of ongoing staff development has to do with softer skills training that may be offered through the MCO's human resource department. Claims capability managers should take responsibility for the development of their personnel to ensure a career path and a more satisfied workforce. Time should be allotted for personnel to pursue internal as well as external training programs relevant to their responsibilities. The management team should be encouraged to attend industry conferences to learn from other organizations and experts in the field. Such external outings should be put to good use, however, with a goal of implementing at least one new idea or process to improve productivity or quality.

Quality Assessments

Earlier in the chapter the core competency of quality control was described in terms of upstream and downstream control. This section focuses on how quality assessment occurs within the claims capability. The quality assessment process is executed by quality assessors who report to a nonproduction manager or director (see Figure 18-5). Quality assessors must have strong analytic and investigative skills as well as a thorough knowledge of the lines of business, products, benefit plan features, provider contracts, and policies and procedures associated with the claims they review. They must also operate with a high level of integrity so that the quality review process is not only fair, but is perceived to be fair by the claims adjudicators.

Typically, quality assessment is conducted on a random sampling of claims selected by the transactional processing system. An equal number (or percentage) of claims are assessed for each adjudicator, and quality scores are calculated based on the number and type of errors uncovered. Some errors are regarded as financial, meaning they directly affect the payment or denial of the claim. Some errors are regarded as statistical in that the payment or denial is not affected, but some data element or aspect of processing is not correct. In the past, statistical errors were considered more of an annoyance or an indication of carelessness. But now that claims data reporting is a factor in new product development, wellness and disease management programs as well as government reporting (as discussed earlier in this chapter), statistical errors take on more significance.

Claims errors discovered via quality assessments must be traced back to determine their origins, system or human, so that steps can be taken to prevent similar errors in the future. "Systems" solutions may include correcting a provider or member record, updating a fee schedule, or adjusting a business rule configuration file. "Human" solutions may include delivering additional training, updating policies and procedures, and/or revising business processes. If the issue is specific to a small group of individuals, the claims capability management team may opt to institute performance monitoring plans for those persons.

Additional errors are also uncovered by reviewing member and provider complaints and/or appeals to discover the root causes of errors. Returned checks and other voluntary refunds are also good resources of such information. This type of research is more likely to be the responsibility of the claims capability management team. But these efforts should be coordinated with the quality assessors so that a broad picture of performance improvement issues can be constructed and attended to.

Reports

Well-designed, useful, and timely reports are vital to the claims capability management team. However, obtaining such reports continues to be a challenge in most MCOs. As previously noted, early transactional processing systems provided so-called canned reports that were hard-coded into the software. These were often of little use, being poorly conceived and having not only too much information, but too much useless information.

Current transactional processing systems are able to produce more customized reports and have evolved to offer a "dashboard" approach so that specific management personnel are able to focus on information of greatest interest to them. While that opportunity exists, there is still a need to design reports that provide the precise detail required for different levels of managers and for different purposes. Over time, MCOs have also implemented specialized reporting databases. Such operational data warehouses enable the flexibility and reporting referenced earlier; these warehouses allow the claims capability to perform analysis, develop statistics and trends, identify incorrectly processed claims, and identify performance improvement opportunities more quickly.

Table 18-3 displays a matrix showing various types of internal and external reports and their recommended utilization. Some reports are financial in nature and are useful to senior management. Other reports facilitate operational decisions. Summary versions of such reports are usually requested by senior claims managers. The detailed versions are used by the claims capability managers, supervisors, and team leaders to monitor and distribute work. They are vital to moving claims through the process and uncovering any bottlenecks. Reports for adjudicators and adjustors are usually limited to those used for work assignments. A special report is produced for the quality assessors listing randomly selected claims for review. Additionally, ad hoc reports can be created for continuous process improvement projects as needed. External reports for employer groups and government regulators must also be produced, including those that address claims capability quality and productivity, group and product experience, OPL savings, and provider-specific reports related to performance and risk

sharing. The data elements included in external reports are often dictated by employer groups and government regulators.

Report design and production is as much art as science. To obtain the needed information in the most useful form, the claims capability management team should develop a good working relationship with report-writing personnel who are often part of the IT operations. If possible, report-writing positions should be staffed within the claims capability to reduce the dependency on nondepartmental resources and produce reports in a more timely fashion. Claims report writers should have the requisite technical skills, but also have claims adjudication knowledge to execute specifications articulated by claims management.

Financial Leakage and Claims Cost Containment

More sophisticated quality review efforts, better analysis, and more flexible reporting have enabled many MCOs to pursue focused but effective claims cost-containment programs designed to curb financial leakage. Some MCOs have created specialized units within the claims capability to identify (prospectively and retrospectively) overpayments caused by complex duplicates, retroactivity, inappropriate dosages, less obvious COB and OPL, inappropriate billing practices, and so forth. These examples are but a few of the hundreds of causes of claims overpayments that directly affect the MCO's bottom line.

To elaborate on one of the examples listed earlier, the term *complex duplicate* primarily refers to services that overlap. One example of the many forms of overlapping services is an emergency department visit that overlaps with a subsequent admission for an inpatient stay. Typically, a separate payment for hospital emergency department charges is not payable if the patient is admitted. The transactional processing system's duplicate logic does not always catch overlapping services, especially if the patient arrives in the emergency department during the afternoon or evening but is not admitted until after mid-

Table 18-3 Reports Matrix

		INTERNAL REPORTS									
		Sr VP	VP	Dir	Mgr	Sup	Team Lead	Adjudicator	Adjustor	Clerical Staff	Other
Executive-level dashboards		X	X								
Financial											
Claims payout		X	X	X							
By LOB, plan, employer group, member											
By day, week, month, quarter, year											
IBNR		X		X							
By LOB, plan, employer group, member											
By day, week, month, quarter, year											
Utilization reports											
By LOB, plan, employer group, member											
By day, week, month, quarter, year											
Overpayment reports	Summary	X	X	X	X						
	Detailed				X	X	X		X		
By LOB, plan, employer group, member											
By day, week, month, quarter, year											
Voluntary refund reports	Summary	X	X	X	X						
	Detailed				X	X	X		X		
By LOB, plan, employer group, member											
By day, week, month, quarter, year											
Productivity/Quality											
Mailroom and EDI receipts	Summary	X	X	X	X						
By LOB, plan, employer group, etc.	Detailed				X	X				X	
By day, week, month, quarter, year											

continues

Table 18-3 Reports Matrix—continued

INTERNAL REPORTS

		Sr VP	VP	Dir	Mgr	Sup	Team Lead	Adjudicator	Adjustor	Clerical Staff	Other
Claims on hand	Summary	X	X	X	X						
By LOB, plan, employer group, etc.	Detailed				X	X					
By status (ready to finalize, suspended)											
Claims processed through auto adjudication	Summary	X	X	X	X						
By LOB, plan, employer group, etc.	Detailed				X	X					
By status (ready to finalize, suspended)											
Suspended claims	Summary	X	X	X	X						
By LOB, plan, employer group, etc.	Detail				X	X	X	X			
By assigned claims adjudicator						X	X				
Claims selected for random quality assessment											Quality Assessors
Ad hoc reports for continuous process improvements											Cross-functional Team

EXTERNAL REPORTS

	Sr VP	VP	Dir	Mgr	Sup Lead	Team	Adjudicator	Adjustor	Clerical Staff	Other
Quality and timeliness reports by customer	X	X	X							
Group experience report	X	X								
Product experience report	X	X								
MTS scores for BCBS plans	X	X								
COB and OPL reports by customer	X	X								
Provider-specific reports related to performance and risk sharing	X	X								

night. The date of service for the emergency department claim will be a day earlier than the date of admission and avoid detection by the business configuration rules.

Another example, retroactivity, refers to members whose termination date is reported by their employers (or government agency) well after the fact. In the interim, thousands of claims may have been paid on behalf of such terminated members. Payment reversals (sometimes known as offsets or clipped payments) can usually be executed within transactional processing systems. However, retroactively terminated members must first be identified and their termination dates verified. Caution must also be exercised to determine how such overpayments can be collected from affected providers. Simply "off-setting" or "clipping" future payments could damage provider relationships.

These examples are intended to be illustrative. Well-managed claims cost-containment functions are constantly looking for new examples of financial leakage. Types of finan-

cial leakage change with new product launches, system conversions, changes to business configuration rules, changes to state or federal legislation, and so forth. Experience also shows that well-managed cost-containment functions continue to find greater quantities of financial leakage year after year.

Information Technology

Much has already been said about transactional processing systems and other technology tools used by the claims capability. This section examines the evolving nature of claims-related IT over the last 50 years (illustrated in Figure 18-7) and how this evolution has affected the management of the modern claims capability.

Generation 1

In the first generation, as depicted in Figure 18-7, claims processing was entirely paper-based with personnel being the vital compo-

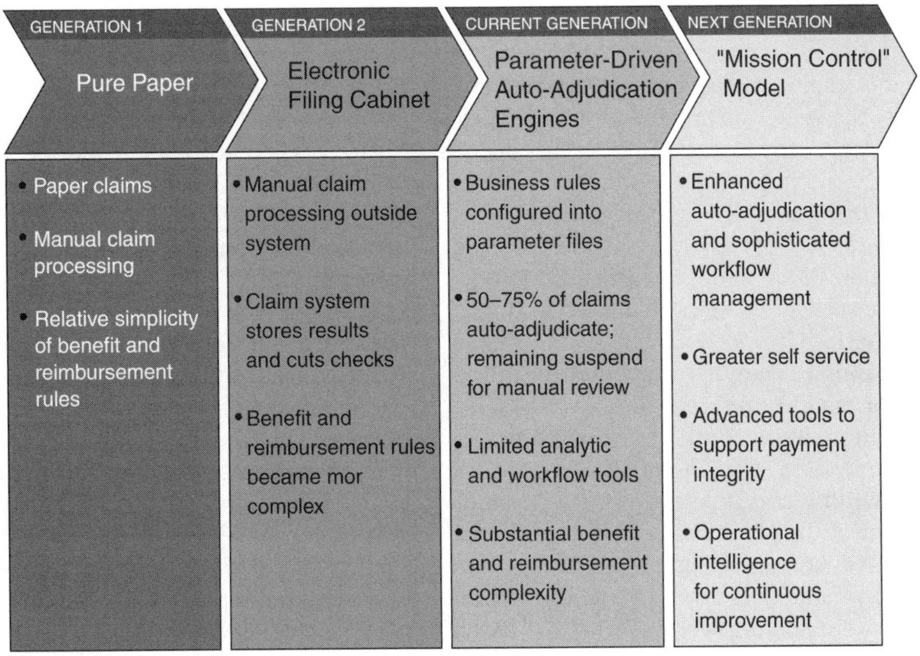

GENERATION 1	GENERATION 2	CURRENT GENERATION	NEXT GENERATION
Pure Paper	**Electronic Filing Cabinet**	**Parameter-Driven Auto-Adjudication Engines**	**"Mission Control" Model**
• Paper claims	• Manual claim processing outside system	• Business rules configured into parameter files	• Enhanced auto-adjudication and sophisticated workflow management
• Manual claim processing	• Claim system stores results and cuts checks	• 50–75% of claims auto-adjudicate; remaining suspend for manual review	• Greater self service
• Relative simplicity of benefit and reimbursement rules	• Benefit and reimbursement rules became mor complex	• Limited analytic and workflow tools	• Advanced tools to support payment integrity
		• Substantial benefit and reimbursement complexity	• Operational intelligence for continuous improvement

Figure 18–7 Evolution of Claims Information Technology

Source: Author.

nent. Paper invoices from doctors, hospitals, and other medical providers, or receipts from patients who were seeking reimbursement were received, date-stamped, and sorted in the mailroom. This paper-based inventory was subsequently placed in staging areas. In the traditional indemnity insurance operations of the 1950s through the 1980s, newly received claims were inserted into file folders created for each insured individual and/or family. Claims adjudicators compared the new claims to the collection of already-processed claims in the folder to prevent duplicate payments. They verified eligibility, coverage, and coordination of benefits status based on information contained in the folder, and then they scanned the new claims for completeness. If data were missing or questionable, a form letter was generated or a phone call was made. If the new claims were cleared for payment, claims adjudicators manually calculated applicable deductibles (individual or family), out-of-pocket expenses, stop-loss amounts, annual and lifetime maximums, and other insurance benefits. Accumulators of various types were maintained on worksheets inside the claims file folder. The process concluded with the completion of a check voucher and the refiling of the patient's folder. The claims capability was an entirely manual process. Even in early managed care claims operations that did not utilize the family file folder system (such as staff or group model HMOs), the process was entirely manual, including the production of an itemized list of claim payments attached to the provider's reimbursement check.

In this first generation, technology (in the form of mainframe computers housed in large temperature-controlled rooms) was in its infancy and was initially used only for check writing and financial reporting. Management of the claims capability focused on personnel. Armies of entry-level clerks were needed to sort, file, and retrieve the paper. Claims adjudicators were the keys to both production and quality. Greater emphasis on production, however, often meant that error

rates would increase. Greater error rates led to higher volumes of costly rework, ultimately producing a negative impact on productivity and financial results of the payer.

Business processes revolved around an assembly-line approach to the movement of claims from mailroom to check production but were often bogged down by sheer volume. In many operations, claims adjudicators not only processed claims, but they also responded to telephone and written inquiries and complaints. Any sudden increase in claims volume easily created claim backlogs, which in turn created larger call volumes—a vicious circle that was difficult to break without the use of costly overtime or temporary help.

Generation 2

The second generation introduced the transactional processing system leading to claims automation and to corresponding improvements in productivity and quality. Claims continued to be submitted on paper and had to be keyed into the transactional processing system. However, the systems could now perform arithmetical calculations for copayments, co-insurance, deductibles, benefit limitations, and even coordination of benefits. Such functionality varied as large insurance carriers and MCOs developed proprietary systems, and software vendors developed and marketed their own applications to meet the needs of specific markets. By the mid-1990s, though, most transactional processing systems could check for duplicates, evaluate eligibility, check for required referral or prior authorization records, and calculate payments based on financial benefit rules (copayments, co-insurance, limitations, etc.) and provider contract terms.

Such automation had an enormous impact on personnel and business processes. There was no longer a need to maintain file folders of claims history once claims data were recorded in the processing systems. In many claims processing operations, tasks performed by entry-level personnel changed from chasing and organizing paper to keying claims into the processing system as they were received and identifying early in the process those claims that could not be processed because of incomplete information. Claims adjudicators were aided in determining payments with the system's financial calculators, thereby reducing errors. Productivity increased in terms of claims processed per hour. However, several challenges continued to bog down productivity, including making benefits determination at the procedure code level, linking referrals/authorizations to claims, and dealing with nonstandard provider contract payment arrangements. Such matters still had to be resolved in a manual process requiring the expertise of experienced claims adjudicators.

Specialization of claims processing became the norm in this generation of claims capability because of the design features of the transactional processing systems. A separate system architecture existed for professional claims (filed with HCFA 1500 claim forms) and hospital claims (filed with UB92 claim forms) to comply with different billing methods for each type of claim. With considerably diverse provider payment schemes, most claims operations divided claims processing duties by claim type. This often resulted in more senior claims adjudicators being assigned to hospital claims processing because many aspects of hospital charges or reimbursement methods were not initially automated. Managing two claim types required two similar but still different sets of business processes, policies and procedures, training curricula, production standards, and quality measures.

Another significant development during this period involved the changing relationship between the claims operation and the other departments within the MCO. For example, most MCOs reassigned the customer service function to call centers that were themselves evolving into higher-performing and specialized operations as described in Chapter 19. The call centers responded to all types of telephone, written inquires, and complaints, including those dealing with claims. Claims production personnel, although freed from these external customer responsibilities, still retained a customer service competency for internal customers.

Additionally, the claims operations became increasingly dependent on other departments to create precise enrollment, provider contracting, and other records to ensure accurate claims processing. Those with claims processing experience were called on to educate those programming the new systems so that all aspects of claims processing would be taken into consideration as processing dictionaries were created. Contrary to some who believed that medical management would become the primary function within the evolving MCO, it soon became apparent that the claims operations would remain the primary functional area within the evolving enterprise.

Current Generation

The last 10 years have ushered in parameter-driven auto adjudication technology currently used by most transactional processing systems. As such, a wide variety of benefit designs can be programmed into the processing software. Rules defined by multiple combinations of various codes sets (procedure, diagnosis, place of service, etc.) along with patient demographics, benefit calculators (copayments, co-insurance, deductibles, limitations, etc.), and provider contract terms allow for automatic claims adjudication. With advances in the filing of electronic claims as well as scanning technologies for the dwindling number of paper claims, most transactions are poised to sail through claims processing without human intervention. Those claims that cannot be finalized automatically are suspended for a claim adjudicator's resolution.

This change has had a profound impact on claims capability personnel. Claims organizations have generally become smaller (fewer headcount) through auto adjudication and electronic receipt of more and more claims. Although total full-time equivalents (FTE) counts are lower, the skill mix is more diverse and robust. Claims adjudicators have become key problem solvers within the MCO and deliver value by resolving the suspension edits that can be numerous and complex. Business processes have also changed dramatically in that workflow, policies and procedures, and training need only focus on the types of claims problems the adjudicators will encounter. Business analysts have taken an increasingly important role in improving production and quality through various quality improvement initiatives and ongoing transactional processing system enhancements.

Technological advances and their corresponding personnel and business policies have evolved to improve accuracy, avoid customer dissatisfaction, and improve the MCO's financial results. Tools that enable early overpayment identification have become increasingly important as health care costs continue to escalate. Many claims capabilities have created cost-containment detection filters and (where possible) prepayment adjustments. Also referred to as forced audits, such final quality checks for a known area of weakness can detect incorrect payments on processed claims that have not yet entered the final check-writing process. Consulting firms and other specialized third-party vendors have helped MCOs save hundreds of millions of dollars through development of specialized programs to detect overpayments.

Future Generation

There is no question that technology will continue to evolve and influence the core competencies of the claims capability. Already common in many MCOs is access to claims records for provider and member self-service inquiries. Many employer groups also now update employee and member eligibility information directly in the MCO's eligibility system. Through the widespread usage of secure, Web-based portals, MCO information is much more readily available to many customers.

Auto-adjudication technology and processes also continue to advance, including real-time adjudication. Workflow management tools are becoming more sophisticated and now typically suspend claims to specific work queues for resolution. As auto-adjudication rates and workflow management tools have improved, the standard work mix directed to claims adjudicators is more complex today than in years past (there simply are not as many "easy" claims that cannot be auto adjudicated). Transactional processing systems continue to become more and more flexible than the legacy transaction systems used into the early 1990s were, thus enabling a broader array of benefit plans and products.

Finally, the analytical and reporting tools that support cost containment and payment integrity have advanced significantly. The most sophisticated MCOs now rely on advanced analytics and even artificial intelligence to identify specific claims and billing patterns that the business configuration rules of the past could not detect.

Outsourcing

The last issue to discuss in terms of managing the claims capability is outsourcing, an option exercised by many large commercial MCOs and more recently by smaller organizations and nonprofits. Outsourcing is occurring across the health care marketplace with both providers and payers participating. For example, many provider organizations are beginning to have X-rays and pathology reports read offshore by U.S.-trained physicians, as well as paperwork completed (including operative report transcriptions and dictation) by well-educated staff in developing nations around the world.

There are many reasons health payers consider outsourcing as a management option with the top reasons focused not only on reduced costs but also on improved service levels. Examples of these reasons include the following:

- Reducing transactions cost
- Improving service levels
- Migrating to new technology

- Focusing management on key aspects of the business, not on routine transactions
- Easier introduction of business process innovations
- Reducing implementation costs and time frames

The functions that have been traditionally outsourced by MCOs have been "non-customer-facing" functions, including, more recently, actual claims adjudication. Although many developments have led to an increased interest and implementation of outsourcing arrangements, the two most significant are (1) the monumental advances in information and communications technologies, and (2) the availability of more sophisticated workforces around the globe that are available to support U.S. business. Just as the modern claims capability has evolved, so have outsourcing options that include the following four models: shared service, onshore, near-shore, and offshore.

The shared service model has been operated for decades by many large regional or national MCOs that have consolidated "back-office" functions into a centralized office while the customer service, medical management, and provider relations and contracting functions remain local. Examples of shared services functions include mail intake, scanning, data entry, ID card and booklet production, and certain types of claims processing. Greater efficiencies and economies of scale can be achieved through a shared services model. In cases in which some claims processing has been centralized, the knowledge and skills of trained, experienced claims adjudicators can be leveraged via cross-training to accommodate spikes in claims volume and serve as a critical component in contingency planning.

As the shared services model matured, many vendors emerged enabling the MCO to migrate shared functions from their own centralized offices to lower-cost third parties. Over time, these lower-cost third-party vendors began to move their own facilities to near-shore and offshore locations to remain competitive. Most of these third-party vendors were able to invest in building their own capabilities outside of the United States by entering into multiyear contracts with MCOs. The rise in third-party administrators (TPAs) during the 1980s and 1990s also bolstered the use of specialized third-party vendors. For example, a relatively young TPA would often outsource its clerical functions (and sometimes certain types of claims processing) to other third-party vendors to keep its own administrative costs low. For a new TPA, it is often more efficient to use the services of an established third-party vendor instead of building and supporting the infrastructure and staff needed for specific functions. This type of outsourcing enables the TPA to focus on product design and services that act as differentiators in the marketplace. Although onshore vendors started with more clerical functions, they now often support core claims processing functions. Their services include not only simple claims resolution tasks, but also highly specialized claims processing for services such as home infusion therapy.

The near-shore model with operations often located in the Caribbean, Canada, or Ireland, was an option developed in the 1980s. This model leveraged English-speaking personnel who were trained to assume some claims capability functions at a lower cost. Lower-level clerical functions such as data entry were often outsourced to the Caribbean whereas higher-level functions were outsourced to Canada and Ireland. Although initially a viable option (from about 1980 to 1995), small labor pools and increasing local labor costs contributed to the migration of outsourcing from these near-shore locations to other parts of the world.

To date, Eastern Europe, India, and the Philippines have been the largest beneficiaries of the labor migration described here. Each of these labor markets includes English-speaking, educated, and highly motivated individuals eager for employment with U.S.-based firms. Even though they are physically located on the other side of the world, many of these operations work during traditional U.S. business hours. Willingness to work U.S. business hours facilitates communication and problem solving and enables outsourced production units to integrate with the MCOs.

In addition to information and communications technology issues, many other matters must be addressed to enable offshore outsourcing. There must be a clear delineation of responsibilities and communication protocols (electronic or telephonic) established between the MCO and the outsourcing operation. This particularly applies to timely and accurate problem resolution. Corresponding policies and procedures and training materials must be designed with both parties in mind, and particular attention must be paid to materials for offshore staff to accommodate language usage and cultural differences.

There are also legal, public relations, financial, and human resource issues to consider when outsourcing. For example, if an MCO is administering Medicare, Medicaid, or TRICARE plans, there may be contractual restrictions on outsourcing, onshore or offshore. Even when administering commercial business, state regulations may restrict out-of-state or off-shore outsourcing. Federal and state government entities, as well as politicians, may also create environments in which the MCO suffers from a public relations perspective if it chooses to outsource even clerical functions; this is particularly the case for non-investor-owned (ie, not-for-profit) health plans. Although many MCOs opt for offshore outsourcing to supplement their current workforce (not replace it), employee relations and human resource issues (often emotionally charged) arise and must be addressed with existing employees, employer groups, providers, and the business community at large.

By 2005, off-shore outsourcing had become a competitive requirement for many large MCOs and will continue to gain traction as a means to curb accelerating health care costs. In addition to the 30% to 50% cost savings that can exist by function, there are many other benefits to outsourcing (applicable to all four models). Creation of an out-sourced claims capability serves as a critical backup for U.S. operations; this backup is particularly useful to mitigating work stoppages caused by facility problems such as electrical outages, natural disasters (such as Hurricane Katrina), and local labor unrest.

Those MCOs that exercise due diligence, carefully plan outsourcing ventures, and more fully integrate the outsourced operations into the parent company ensure a successful outcome. In fact, most MCOs that outsource an initial function continue to take advantage of the better quality results and lower costs associated with outsourcing additional functions. Regardless of political grandstanding and negative stories in the media, outsourcing will continue to have a role for MCOs as it will for other industries.

CORE CLAIMS CAPABILITY BUSINESS STEPS

Regardless of the type of claim or how it is submitted, the same core claims capability business steps apply, including determination of liability, other-party liability, benefits administration, application of provider fee schedules, resubmissions, appeals and adjustments, and fraud and abuse. Each of these is discussed on the following pages.

Determination of liability refers to decisions that establish whether and to what extent the member is eligible for benefits. Liability is directly related to underwriting considerations and premium collection. Other principles related to determining liability pertain to employer-sponsored group health benefits that waive preexisting condition provisions as well as many waiting periods. Additionally, coverage is often broader, including benefits such as alternative medical treatments.

There are several decisions involved with determining liability. The first decision involves the member's eligibility on the date(s) of service. In the auto-adjudication process, the transactional processing system compares the date of service listed on the claim to the span of effective and termination (if any) dates on the member record. Members may have multiple layers of eligibility records if they have been enrolled in various benefit plans over time. The benefit plan in force on the date of service will determine the exact coverage, including any cost sharing features such as copayments, co-insurance, or deductibles as well as any limitations or maximums. See Table 18-4 for details.

The member eligibility record will also indicate the member's provider network and/ or primary care provider (PCP). Whether or not the service provider on a claim is participating in the member's provider network or is the member's PCP will also have an impact on liability. If the member seeks care for certain services outside of the network, the MCO may not be liable for payment or may reduce its payment according to predefined benefit rules.

Other-party liability (OPL) refers to the determination of whether other insurance plans (group health, government health/ entitlement programs, automobile, workers' compensation, etc.) are liable or other individuals are responsible for illness or injury related to specified health care expenses. The claims capability must determine (1) if a member is covered by any other insurance that may be considered liable in whole or in part for specific medical care, and then (2) if the MCO is financially responsible for any part of the care. There are four categories of other-party liability to consider:

- Other group health insurance
- Automobile insurance
- Workers' compensation insurance
- Subrogation

Benefits are *coordinated* with other group health insurance typically based on industry standard coordination of benefit (COB) rules published by the National Association of Insurance Commissioners (NAIC; see also Chapter 33) and defined within the member's subscription agreement. With automobile and workers' compensation, liability is *shifted* from the MCO to another insurance carrier based on state laws or other government regulations. With subrogation, speci-

fied benefit payments are *recovered* from members who have been compensated for incurred health costs via legal action. See Table 18-5 for details.

Ideally, OPL claims are handled by claims specialists who have knowledge of various OPL opportunities and are trained to execute OPL decisions in the transactional processing system. The key to successful OPL efforts is data. The MCO must engage employees in a variety of departments and roles to collect and record other insurance data. Most transactional processing systems provide space on the member record for other group health insurance. Business rule configuration records can be programmed to suspend claims for members who have other coverage so that benefits can be coordinated with the other program. Other group health insurance information must be updated at least once each year, although continuous updating is becoming more common.

Information about accident-related claims can also be captured by personnel outside of the claims capability. Utilization nurses arranging for inpatient stays or durable medical equipment are often able to determine that care is related to an automobile accident or a work-related injury. Such information can be communicated to OPL specialists through an authorization record or a flag attached to the member record to suspend all claims for OPL determination.

Paper claim forms have check boxes and other fields where the service provider can record OPL information. Such claims can be identified in the front-end process and routed immediately to OPL specialists for special handling. The transaction record layouts for electronically submitted claims, standardized under HIPPA (see Chapter 32), also include fields for communication of other-party liability data. Business rule configuration records can be programmed to suspend claims submitted with such data so that benefits can be coordinated with the other program.

Before proceeding with an OPL program, the MCO must make a fundamental decision regarding its approach: "pay and chase" or

Table 18-4 Benefit Plan Cost Sharing Features, Limitations, and Maximums

Feature	Definition	Auto Adjudication	EOB/RA	Balance Billing
Copayment	• Usually a fixed dollar amount • Member must pay out-of-pocket directly to the service provider • Usually applies to office visits, emergency room charges, and prescription drugs	• Automatically calculated and applied • Payment to the provider reduced by copayment amount	• Expressed on the member's EOB and on the provider's remittance advice with an explanatory reason code	• Provider collects copayment at the time services are rendered or by billing the patient directly
Co-insurance	• Usually a percentage such as 20% of the provider payable amount (not the billed charge) • Member must pay out-of-pocket directly to the service provider • Not as common in traditional HMO benefit plans • Usually applies to specified services	• Automatically calculated and applied • Payment to the provider reduced by co-insurance amount	• Expressed on the member's EOB and on the provider's remittance advice with an explanatory reason code	• Provider collects co-insurance by billing the patient directly
Deductible	• A dollar amount that must be paid out-of-pocket directly to the service provider before any benefits are paid by the MCO • Not as common in traditional HMO benefit plans	• Automatically calculated and applied • Payment to the provider reduced by deductible amount Note: If adjustments are made to claims where a deductible has been applied, deductible history must be reset (manually, if necessary).	• Expressed on the member's EOB and on the provider's remittance advice with an explanatory reason code	• Provider collects deductible by billing the patient directly

426

	• A major feature of newer consumer-driven health plan designs with deductibles as high as $5,000 • Usually expressed as an annual amount • Can apply to specific services or globally to all services • Can be designed to apply to an individual or to a family or both			
Limitation	• Usually expressed as the number of services that is allowed for payment during a specified period • Examples include 60 days of physical therapy per course of treatment or 20 outpatient mental health visits per calendar year • Usually applied to specific services	• Automatically calculated and applied • Services exceeding the limitation are denied Note: If adjustments are made to claims where a limitation has been applied, limitation counters must be reset (manually, if necessary).	• Expressed on the member's EOB and on the provider's remittance advice with an explanatory reason code	• Provider collects reimbursement for denied services by billing the patient directly
Maximum	• Usually expressed as a dollar amount limit for specified services or for a lifetime benefit • Examples include $5,000 limit on hospice care or $5M lifetime benefit	• Automatically calculated and applied • Payable amounts exceeding maximums are denied Note: If adjustments are made to claims where maximums have been applied, maximum counters must be reset (manually, if necessary).	• Expressed on the member's EOB and on the provider's remittance advice with an explanatory reason code	• Provider collects reimbursement for denied services by billing the patient directly

Table 18-5 Other-Party Liability

Feature	Definition	Claims Adjudication	EOB/RA	Balance Billing
Coordination of Benefits	• Process by which MCO determines the order of payment when a member is covered under two or more group health insurance programs	• Claims for members whose MCO coverage is considered secondary are suspended for COB specialist review and determination	• Expressed on the member's EOB and on the provider's remittance advice with an explanatory reason code	• Typically no balance exists for the provider because both health plans combined pay 100% of the charges
	• Ensures that providers and/or members are not paid twice for the same care	• Claims may be denied pending receipt of other health plan's EOB		
	• Industry standard rules developed and updated since 1970 by the National Association of Insurance Commissioners (NAIC)	• Payment to the provider reduced by other health plan's payment, if any		
	• COB rules govern which plan is primary (pays first) and which plan is secondary (pays second) and how order is determined			
	• Many rules apply to dependent children when covered under both parents' health plans			
	• Birthday rule most common indicating that parent with the birth date (month, day, not year) earlier in the calendar year is primary for children			
	• MCO must determine calculation method (benefit less benefit or "true" COB)			

Automobile Insurance	• Benefits available under an automobile insurance policy applicable to medical expenses incurred as a result of an automobile accident • Governed by state laws, which vary; some states do not allow coordination • Must determine if auto accident is work-related, creating different liability • MCO utilization management nurses may be alerted to auto benefits potential	• Claims incurred as a result of an automobile-related injury may be autosuspended if associated with accident-related diagnosis or procedure codes • Payment to the provider may be denied until auto insurance liability is established • Once auto insurance liability is confirmed, coverage for the portion of medical care not covered by auto insurance (perhaps to policy dollar limit) is considered for payment	• Expressed on the member's EOB and on the provider's remittance advice with an explanatory reason code	• MCO often made aware of auto insurance settlement if provider refunds claims payments
Workers' Compensation	• Benefits available under a workers' compensation insurance policy applicable to medical expenses incurred as a result of an on-the-job accident or work-related health problems occurring over time • Governed by state laws, which vary • MCO utilization management nurses may be alerted to workers' comp potential	• Claims incurred as a result of a work-related illness/injury may be autosuspended if associated with work-related diagnosis or procedure codes • Payment to the provider may be denied until workers' comp liability is established • Once workers' comp liability is confirmed, coverage for the portion of medical care not related to work-related illness or injury is considered for payment	• Expressed on the member's EOB and on the provider's remittance advice with an explanatory reason code	• MCO often made aware of auto insurance settlement if provider refunds claims payments

continues

Table 18–5 Other-Party Liability—continued

Feature	Definition	Claims Adjudication	EOB/RA	Balance Billing
Subrogation	• The right of the MCO to recover any damages the member may receive from a third party who assumes responsibility for an accidental injury, including those known as "slips and falls" • Usually surfaces after legal action results in a financial settlement to the member • Allows the MCO to seek reimbursement from the member for health care payments made on the member's behalf related to the injury • Must be a subrogation clause in the member's subscription agreement	• Payments of claims related to subrogation settlement may be recovered from member, not provider, unless there is evidence that the provider was paid twice • MCO may agree to engage third-party attorney or specialty vendor to recover funds for a contingency payment	• Expressed on the member's EOB and on the provider's remittance advice with an explanatory reason code	• MCO often made aware of settlement if provider refunds claims payments

"chase and pay." In the "pay and chase" model, the MCO processes claims for payment without coordinating benefits either with other group health plans or with auto carriers or workers' compensation programs. Instead, the OPL program is executed retrospectively (the "chase"). Some MCOs take this approach to limit prompt payment complaints from their provider community especially if interest is calculated on late payments. Recovery, however, is both costly and challenging and may take months to realize OPL savings. Other MCOs follow the "chase and pay" model in that they may suspend or even deny claims until the OPL information is "chased" and a benefit determination is made. This approach conserves claims dollars, but it may generate more customer service issues while claims remain unresolved or denied. Over time, more and more MCOs have moved toward the "chase and pay" model.

Every effort should be made throughout the MCO to identify OPL potential, capture the information, and execute OPL policies and procedures because millions of dollars are at stake. A dedicated OPL unit can pay for itself with upward of a 10:1 return on investment. Financial incentives for the collection of OPL overpayments should also be considered within the context of the MCO's human resources and salary policies. Many MCOs set specific savings targets for OPL personnel, a practice gaining popularity within the industry.

Benefits administration refers to applying the appropriate schedule of benefits during the claims adjudication process. The schedule of benefits consists of covered and noncovered services as well as one or more of the cost-sharing features described in Table 18-4. For MCOs administering a single line of business such as a Medicaid program, the same schedule of benefits usually applies to all members. However, most MCOs now administer (or intend to administer) multiple programs, thus increasing the number of benefit variations. Under earlier (and much diminished but not extinct) traditional indemnity programs, there were separate benefit structures that focused on hospitalization and on physician services. As discussed in Chapter 1, this was the genesis of Blue Cross (hospitalization) and Blue Shield (physician services), respectively, though commercial indemnity insurers followed suit. Traditional indemnity and Blue Cross and Blue Shield plans then added comprehensive benefits structure referred to as Major Medical. HMOs, point-of-service (POS) plans, PPOs, and now CDH benefit programs have been added to the market. To administer benefits accurately, each benefit plan must be assigned a unique code in the transactional processing system, and that benefit code must be attached to the member's eligibility record. As a result, the transactional processing system is able to auto adjudicate claims according to the applicable schedule of benefits.

Every enrolled member receives a benefit booklet or subscription agreement that describes in some detail the services that are covered and subject to copayments, coinsurance, deductibles, limitations, and/or maximums. Also included is a list of exclusions, those items that are not covered under any circumstance. Exclusions can be stated in very specific items such as acupressure or more general items such as services rendered due to civil unrest. Additionally, exclusions may be linked to the provider's status in relation to the member. For example, some preventive care may be excluded if rendered by a physician who is not the member's primary care provider. Other care may be excluded if rendered by out-of-network providers.

MCO personnel must "code" all covered and noncovered benefits into transactional processing system records used to execute auto adjudication, a process referred to as system configuration. This is an enormous and complex undertaking and can result in thousands of business rule configuration files linked together to enable auto adjudication. The heart of benefit coding is the standardized procedure (CPT, HCPCS, revenue, etc.) and diagnosis codes that include tens of thousands of items describing virtually every service a provider can bill and the medical justification underlying the claim.

Making it even more challenging is that procedure and diagnosis codes are continually updated. The American Medical Association updates CPT codes annually. New codes are added as new medical procedures are clinically approved; some procedures are marked as deleted if they are no longer accurate descriptions of current medical practice. Similarly, HCPCS codes are modified, added, or deleted as changes are made to such items as durable medical equipment or injectable drugs. Such changes to HCPCS codes are reported quarterly. Procedure code modifiers can also change over time and are important especially because they further define surgical procedures or differentiate between professional and technical charges. For those claims capability operations that adjudicate prescription drug claims, the U.S. Food and Drug Administration updates its directory of National Drug Codes (NDC) on a quarterly basis.

Changes to diagnosis codes are usually found in the codes beginning with "V" or "E." However, the World Health Organization has been working since 1989 to produce the next generation of the diagnostic coding system designated as ICD-10-CM. Although already in use in other countries as well as the United States to track morbidity, the widespread use of ICD-10-CM diagnosis codes for claims processing purposes will depend on HIPAA implementation standards. There will be a 2-year implementation window once the final notice to implement ICD-10-CM has been published in the *Federal Register*, according to the National Center for Health Statistics.[9]

Those who configure the business rule configuration files must remain vigilant to changes in procedure and diagnosis codes and update the transactional processing system accordingly. If system configuration is poorly or inaccurately executed, thousands of customer service issues will erupt, requiring a massive number of claim adjustments. As stated previously, it is vital for MCOs to test benefit coding thoroughly to ensure accuracy before the effective dates of new or updated benefit plans. However, the claims capability management team must also stay alert to procedure and diagnosis code changes because they may affect policies and procedures and/or training materials.

Application of provider fee schedules refers to automatically determining the payable amount for covered services based on the service provider's fee schedule or other payment methodology. Fee schedules and other payment methods are recorded in the transactional processing system and linked to provider records so that the applicable payment is executed during auto adjudication. Table 18-6 defines the most commonly used payment methodologies and how they are administered. Reimbursement methodologies are discussed in more detail in Chapters 6 and 7.

When a claim is subjected to one or more of these payment methodologies, each line item on the claim (representing each procedure or revenue code billed) is labeled with one or more reason codes that tell the provider how payment was determined. For example, an office visit procedure code of 99201 paid according to a fee schedule and subject to a copayment would most likely have two reason codes attached: (1) one code indicating that the payment was reduced by the copayment amount, which can be collected from the member, and (2) one code indicating that the payment was based on the contracted fee schedule and that the unpaid amount cannot be "balance billed" to the member.

Balance billing rules, when applicable, provide a significant protection for consumers related to paying excessive charges for medical services. *Balance billing* is a billing practice used by some providers to bill the member directly for the amount over and above the provider's contracted rate. Most, if not all, MCOs include a "no balance billing" clause in their provider contracts that prohibits providers from billing the member for any amount other than copayments, co-

Table 18–6 Common Provider Payment Methodologies

Feature	Definition	Auto Adjudication	EOB/RA	Balance Billing
Fee Schedule	• A fixed dollar amount for each procedure code • Most common payment method for physician and most ancillary services • Some procedure codes may be labeled as special consideration and will automatically suspend for manual pricing determination	• Automatically applied based on fee schedule linked to the provider record associated with the member's benefit plan	• Expressed on the member's EOB and on the provider's remittance advice with an explanatory reason code	• May not balance bill the member for amount not paid over the fee schedule amount
Capitation	• A per member/per month reimbursement for rendering specified services to members • A common payment method for primary care providers • Procedure codes associated with capitated services are programmed to result in a zero dollar payment amount (not to be confused with denied services that also result in a zero dollar payment amount)	• Automatically applied based on capitated services linked to the provider record associated with the member's benefit plan	• Expressed on the provider's remittance advice with an explanatory reason code • May or may not be included on the member's EOB	• May not balance bill the member for amount not paid because of capitation
Discount	• A percentage discount off of the billed amount • Biggest disadvantage is that providers can bill any amount • Reasonable and customary language can minimize billing abuse	• Automatically applied based on percentage discount linked to the provider record associated with the member's benefit plan	• Expressed on the member's EOB and on the provider's remittance advice with an explanatory reason code	• May not balance bill the member for amount not paid over the discounted amount

continues

Table 18-6 Common Provider Payment Methodologies—continued

Feature	Definition	Auto Adjudication	EOB/RA	Balance Billing
Per Diem	• Usually applies to hospital charges for inpatient stays • A fixed dollar amount paid per each day of admission regardless of the billed amount • Multiple per diem rates can be established for various types of inpatient stays: medical, surgical, coronary care, maternity, behavioral health, etc. • Multiple per diem rates could apply to the same claim in terms of level of care: semiprivate, intensive care, step-down care, skilled nursing care, etc. • Either the date of admission or the date of discharge should be paid, but not both • If a member changes health plan coverage while admitted, the benefit plan and associated provider agreement effective on the date of admission is applicable (Note: This may be a plan administered by another MCO.)	• Automatically applied based on per diem rates linked to the provider record associated with the member's benefit plan	• Expressed on the member's EOB and on the provider's remittance advice with an explanatory reason code	• May not balance bill the member for amount not paid over the per diem calculation
Case Rate	• Usually applies to hospital charges for inpatient stays • A fixed dollar amount paid per a specific type of admission such as	• Automatically applied based on case rates linked to the provider record associated with the member's benefit plan	• Expressed on the member's EOB and on the provider's remittance advice with an explanatory reason code	• May not balance bill the member for amount not paid over the case rate calculation

	• maternity or cardiac bypass surgery regardless of the number of admitted days or the billed amount • If a member changes health plan coverage while admitted, the benefit plan and associated provider agreement effective on the date of admission is applicable (Note: This may be a plan administered by another MCO.)			
DRG	• Usually applies to hospital charges for inpatient stays • A fixed dollar amount paid per type of admission based on diagnosis-related group • If a member changes health plan coverage while admitted, the benefit plan and associated provider agreement effective on the date of admission is applicable (Note: This may be a plan administered by another MCO.) • DRGs are more common in certain markets	• Automatically applied based on DRG rates linked to the provider record associated with the member's benefit plan	• Expressed on the member's EOB and on the provider's remittance advice with an explanatory reason code	• May not balance bill the member for amount not paid over the DRG calculation
Ambulatory Surgical Codes (ASC)	• Usually applies to hospital charges for out patient surgery • A fixed dollar amount paid per each occurrence of outpatient surgery • ASCs are a newer methodology	• Automatically applied based on ASC rates linked to the provider record associated with the member's benefit plan	• Expressed on the member's EOB and on the provider's remittance advice with an explanatory reason code	• May not balance bill the member for amount not paid over the ASC calculation

insurance, deductibles, and amounts not paid because of limitations, maximums, or exclusions (see Chapter 30). Some states such as California also regulate the practice of balance billing to protect consumers. However, nonparticipating or out-of-network providers are not necessarily subject to balance billing policies. As such, MCOs must determine whether covered charges are to be paid in full (subject to copayments, co-insurance, etc.) when no contract is in force with a provider. Most large MCOs also have a special unit that is dedicated to negotiating with noncontracted providers for significant expenses associated with urgent or emergency out-of-network admissions, and this function is described in Chapters 5 and 7.

An important policy and procedure that must be addressed by the MCO is how to handle claims in the rare occurrence where the billed amount of the service is less than the contracted fee schedule or payment rate. Some MCOs still pay the fee schedule amount; others pay the billed amount. Although this policy may be applied differently to various providers, a consistent policy across the board is preferable for the sake of both auto adjudication and customer service. It must also be determined whether paying the billed amount lower than the contracted rate can be accommodated by the transactional processing system without custom programming (and if such custom programming is worth the cost in the long run).

Another important policy and procedure addresses how to handle claims from providers who are capitated for certain services. As discussed in Chapters 6 and 7, capitation is a fixed PMPM payment to a provider for defined services to members enrolled in the provider's panel. Capitation is used by many HMOs for primary care physicians (PCPs) and is also used to a lesser degree for specialty and hospital services. As regards PCP capitation, decisions must be made at the MCO on how to adjudicate claims for so-called covering PCPs, that is, PCPs who render primary care services to covered members who are not enrolled in their panels. In some cases, a PCP may be considered a specialist depending on the type of service as well as the member's PCP selection and/or benefit plan. These issues are explored further in Chapter 6.

Accurate and timely maintenance of provider payment terms in the transactional processing system are vital to the claims capability's ability to fulfill its obligations to the MCO, the members, and the providers. MCO senior management must recognize that poor quality or untimely maintenance of provider payment records has an enormous negative impact on the claims capability and subsequently on members and providers. Resources must be allocated to MCO personnel assigned to maintaining provider payment records so that fee schedules and other payment methods are error free and recorded before the effective dates of the payment terms. All too often, new or updated provider contracts are applied retroactively, resulting in a large volume of claims adjustments. If this situation arises, the MCO may find that a lump sum financial settlement outside of the transactional processing system may be more advantageous than expending the resources to adjust hundreds or thousands of claims.

Resubmissions refer to those claims submitted for payment by providers (or sometimes members) two or more times. In some cases, providers resubmit claims automatically every 30 days or so until payment or denial is posted to their accounts receivable system. If submitted on paper, resubmitted claims may be stamped as "second" or "third" submissions. If submitted electronically, resubmitted claims will most likely be automatically denied as duplicates even if the original claim is suspended in the transactional processing system.

The claims capability management team must be alert to a high number of resubmitted claims from one or more providers because they signal a problem. The problem could be on the provider side in that payments and/or denials are not being properly or promptly posted. Providers have also been known to resubmit claims toward the end of their fiscal years in hopes that previously denied claims would be paid a second time around. If such trends are noticed, the claims capability managers should enlist the help of provider relations personnel to address these issues. Conversely, the problem could be on the claims capability side, indicating a backlog. This problem is self-perpetuating in that providers will continue to resubmit delayed claims, making the backlog grow even larger. The claims capability management team must keep claims inventory well within contracted turnaround times to help reduce the instances of resubmitted claims.

Appeals and adjustments refer to those claims that are rereviewed based on a formal grievance or appeals process; adjustments are those claims that are "reprocessed" in the transactional processing system as a result of a grievance or appeal. Each MCO establishes and publishes directions for either members or providers to file grievances or appeals (the terms are not necessarily interchangeable). State and federal laws and regulations also place requirements around this process. The appeals and grievance processes (as applied to members) are discussed briefly later and in greater detail in Chapter 19.

There are usually three levels of a grievance or appeal, each level escalating the review process to a higher level of MCO management. The initial level of grievance or appeal brings a problem to the attention of the MCO usually through a telephone call or written correspondence from a member or provider. If a claim was denied in error or an incorrect payment was made, the claim is adjusted in the system. If the original adjudication decision is found to be correct, the member or provider is informed that the grievance or appeal is denied, but the option to provide additional information for further consideration is available.

As such, a second-level grievance or appeal may be submitted, which is usually reviewed by an Appeals Committee. Claims in this cat-egory are often those denied because of no prior authorization or because the service was considered not covered. In some cases, the additional information provided will overturn the original denial, and the claim will be adjusted for payment. For example, if a surgical claim was denied because it was considered cosmetic, the denial may be overturned based on the operative report. However, if the additional information does not result in a reversal, the member and/or provider is again informed that the appeal is denied, but the member and/or provider has the right to provide additional information for further consideration. The member and/or provider may subsequently file a third level of appeal, which is often reviewed by MCO senior management or by an outside party such as a peer review organization. Their decision is usually final.

Requests for adjustments should be expedited by the claims capability especially if the claim was initially adjudicated erroneously. The claims capability management team must monitor aging and turnaround time for adjustments just as they do for new claims. The management team should also analyze the new knowledge gained through the grievance and appeals process and use it as a basis for continuing process improvements.

Fraud and abuse refers to actions taken by internal or external parties that violate security and/or cause a financial loss to the MCO. Fortunately, internal instances of fraud are rare, but the claims capability management team must be ever vigilant over security issues. Employees must be reminded not to share passwords or reveal claims-related information with anyone outside the context of their job responsibilities. External instances of fraud are more the responsibility of the MCO to communicate, especially to the provider community, its intention to investigate and prosecute fraudulent practices. A vulnerable spot within the claims operation occurs when claims are received from providers that are not yet established in the transactional processing system. Before a provider record is created, steps should be taken to verify that the provider is legitimate, especially if it is a high-dollar claim.

Abuse is actually the more common problem and is associated with inflated or inappropriate charges. Whether intentional or not, abuse is best tackled through analysis of claims data, provider payment practices, and anomalies in provider practice patterns within the scope of the claims capability.

15 RISK AREAS AND 40 TIPS

Throughout this chapter, a variety of production and quality issues were described or referenced. To provide a more pointed discussion of claims capability risks, the following is a list of 15 common pitfalls along with suggested resolutions.

1. *Growing backlog:* Claims backlogs do not develop overnight and, therefore, cannot be resolved overnight. Tight control over daily receipts and quick action when production falls behind (with the application of overtime or temporary help) will help prevent a backlog from growing into a monster. Major undertakings such as systems conversions or adding new lines of business require advanced planning to prevent backlogs from taking root.
   - TIP 1: When planning a large new undertaking, make every effort to bring the current claims inventory down to zero, meaning that claims are resolved almost as they are received.
   - TIP 2: When faced with a large backlog, create a "SWAT team," including personnel from other departments experienced in claims adjudication, to focus on the backlog while regular claims personnel focus on current claims.
   - TIP 3: Be on guard for providers who resubmit claims that were previously denied. Enforce the timely filing limits to prevent old dates of service claims

from entering the system again, only to be denied as duplicates.
   - TIP 4: Attempt to reject inappropriate claims from entering the transactional processing system inventory.
   - TIP 5: If still receiving a large volume of paper claims, sort through backlogged claims for old dates of service and investigate if they are duplicates. Some providers or billing services will continue to generate the same invoices until payment or denial is posted. Backlogs can often be reduced substantially simply by weeding out these duplicates.

2. *Inadequate front-end control or "garbage in, garbage out":* EDI procedures must be strictly established to ensure only claims that are complete and with valid data elements are accepted into the system.
   - TIP 6: Enforce claim filing rules with all providers. Work with provider relations personnel to better educate providers on this issue.
   - TIP 7: Make sure that MCO-dictated changes in billing requirements can be accommodated by front-end EDI configuration. For example, if a specific field is required for processing that is not captured by the EDI logic, claims will not be auto adjudicated. EDI configuration may need to be modified to support the modified billing requirements.

3. *Inadequate suspended claims management:* Claims suspended through the auto adjudication process must be strictly followed and quickly resolved.
   - TIP 8: If additional information is required from the provider, deny the claim with the applicable reason code and request the additional information. The burden is placed back on the provider, and the claim is removed from the suspended status. Be sure that providers are informed of all required data, however, so as not to cause a provider relations problem.

- TIP 9: Use reporting to identify aging claims and closely manage those that sit in a suspended status for an extended period of time. These claims are sometimes forgotten or ignored because claims adjudicators do not know how to resolve the problems, or their requests for assistance have not become the priority of others.
- TIP 10: Establish and enforce pended claims procedures and turnaround times with other departments. The claims capability is ultimately responsible for all suspended claims even if awaiting action from other MCO personnel. If turnaround times are not being met, alert senior management.

4. *Inadequate focus on a continuous quality improvement process (CQIP) effort:* Claims capability processes must be considered a work in progress. There is almost always some aspect to improve.

    - TIP 11: Designate specific claims personnel to be responsible for continuous quality improvement. As the name implies, this is not a one-time activity or task.
    - TIP 12: Involve claims adjudicators and other nonmanagement personnel in continuous quality improvement efforts. Those closest to the processes usually have the best ideas.
    - TIP 13: Create rewards or incentives for continuous quality improvement efforts, including gift certificates or time off. Make sure rewards fit within the MCO's human resource guidelines.
    - TIP 14: Consider using specialized outside help to establish and improve CQIP efforts.

5. *Inadequate or ineffective workflow:* Do not allow inadequate or ineffective workflow to create bottlenecks. Claims must be pushed along the process and daily, even hourly; supervisory management is required.

    - TIP 15: Document workflow processes in minute detail using a flowchart software application. Identify every single decision point made by either the transactional processing system or by claims adjudicators. Such detailed examination will reveal opportunities for fine-tuning the workflow.
    - TIP 16: Make sure that management and supervisory staff understand how to utilize the workflow software application. The functionality of this application is not always fully leveraged. Additionally, kept alert to staff members who do not utilize the workflow software and continue to work from paper reports.
    - TIP 17: In the absence of a workflow software application, aggressively manage workflow through daily/weekly reporting.

6. *Poorly maintained claims engine or other operational applications:* The claims capability relies on the transactional processing system and other software applications as its tools. Poor maintenance will compromise both productivity and quality.

    - TIP 18: *Do not* allow poor system maintenance to go unchallenged. Many claims adjudicators often find ways around system problems to meet productivity standards. As a result, system problems are suppressed and worked around rather than identified and resolved.
    - TIP 19: Develop a working relationship with personnel who maintain the transactional processing system and other pertinent software applications. Make detailed reasonable requests for changes. If improvements are not made, enlist the support of senior MCO management to determine priorities.

7. *Inadequate or ineffective data management:* The claims capability relies on other departments' records (member, provider, pricing, authorization, etc.) to adjudicate claims. If other department

files are not timely and accurately up-dated, claims errors will occur.

- TIP 20: Develop working relation-ships with other department heads to catch problems early.
- TIP 21: Analyze quality assessment reports and review the causes of claims adjustments to determine whether poorly maintained records in other departments are the problem. Gather facts and figures to review with other department heads as needed. Avoid confrontation and try a collaborative approach to resolve problems.
- TIP 22: Participate in cross-functional teams to address both upstream and downstream quality and performance issues.

8. *Incorrect benefit setup and group installa-tion:* The claims capability relies on business rule configuration records to process claims. If basic files associated with groups or benefits are incorrectly established, thousands of claims could be at risk. Adjusting large volumes of claims, especially if historical deductible or limitation calculations are affected, can be a nightmare.

- TIP 23: Preventive measures are the key to avoiding this risk. Whenever a new benefit plan is established or a large new group of members is ready to "go live," ask to be part of the final testing phase to ensure that the claim outcomes match the benefit specifi-cations. Test benefit coding through a standard durable and repeatable process.
- TIP 24: Sign off on unique benefit configuration rules to ensure accurate benefit administration within the transactional processing system.

9. *Incorrect provider contract setup and maintenance:* The claims capability relies on all records associated with providers, including contract setup and payment methodologies, to process claims. If provider files, payment methodologies, fee schedules, and so forth are incor-rectly established, thousands of claims could be at risk. Just as in item 8, adjust-ing large volumes of claims, especially if historical deductible or limitation calcu-lations are affected, can be a nightmare.

- TIP 25: It is critical that claims capa-bility personnel be proactive in par-ticipating in the initial and ongoing validation and maintenance of pro-vider contract setups. Staff who process adjustments, in particular, have insight into cases where pro-vider contracts are setup with the wrong reimbursement methodology for a particular service (*eg*, case rate instead of per diem for maternity de-livery inpatient stay) or with the wrong variable value attached to a reimbursement methodology (*eg*, 75% of charges instead of 80% of charges).
- TIP 26: Sign off on unique provider contracts (prior to contract execution if possible) to ensure payment will be processed correctly in the transac-tional processing system.

10. *Inadequate quality and financial controls:* The claims capability must establish and execute a quality control function. It's the flip side of its dual responsibili-ties of production and quality.

- TIP 27: Be sure claims adjudicators and other staff understand and agree to the quality assessment process to ensure that quality review results are accepted.
- TIP 28: Ensure that the quality assess-ment process is "blind" to individual adjudicators so that the process is fair and is *perceived* as fair.

11. *Poor employee recruiting:* Despite the ad-vances in claims adjudication technology, claims adjudicators and other personnel are still vital to the claims capability.

- TIP 29: Organize the claims capability with positions of increasing responsibility and salary grades to create a career path. Talented staff will seek positions outside the claims capability if that is their only path to promotion.

- TIP 30: Be sure to reward good performance, especially exemplary performance. If budgets are tight, consider extra time off, more flexible hours, gift certificates, special award ceremonies, special meals (lunch with the director), and so forth.

12. *Inadequate policy and procedure documentation:* Unwritten and/or unclear policies and procedures lead to inconsistent claims adjudication and low employee morale/motivation.

- TIP 31: Create a space on the MCO's intranet to house policies and procedures. Be sure they are searchable and are kept updated.
- TIP 32: Assign policy and procedure responsibility to a single accountable resource.
- TIP 33: Break the habit of communicating new information via e-mail. Rather, use e-mail to alert staff of updated information posted on the intranet.

13. *Inadequate training:* Training should not be limited to systems processing only. A comprehensive training approach that provides context and background will result in greater retention and transfer to the job.

- TIP 34: Begin training at an industry level and proceed to MCO-specific training topics. Within this context, proceed with unit- and task-level training.
- TIP 35: Employ a variety of means to train and develop staff, including any combination of classroom training, Web-based and CD ROM courseware, conference calls, webinars, online simulations, lab-based simulations, job aids, Web pages and/or sites, mentors, chats, videos, podcasting, vodcasting, and blogging. Be sure to blend various

methods into a cohesive and comprehensive training program.

14. *Inadequate claims management reports:* Reports should aid the management team, not impede them.

- TIP 36: Employ report writers within the claims capability to develop meaningful reports on demand.
- TIP 37: Leverage and expand existing reports; as much as possible avoid report overload.
- TIP 38: Design "dashboard"-type reports to enable various levels of managers to zero in on desired information.

15. *Failure to use the claims capability to identify customer and operational problems early:* The claims capability is the repository of facts, figures, and perceptions that affect performance as well as internal and external customers. Listen to what they have to say!

- TIP 39: Engage claims adjudicators in discussions and/or performance improvement projects. They are the closest to the work at hand and can provide great insight into the inner workings of the MCO when asked.
- TIP 40: Analyze corrections, resubmissions, voluntary refunds, and appeals to reveal root causes of problems and targets for process improvements.

A final risk area that can pervade all the others is cynicism. The claims capability management team must feel that they can rely on senior MCO managers for resources and cooperation especially when thorny problems present themselves. Claims managers must remain positive and lead by example with hard work, a sense of urgency, and a commitment to high quality, integrity, and customer service.

CONCLUSION

The modern claims capability has multiple objectives and multiple constituencies. Its operations directly affect the corporate reputation and bottom line of the MCO. This chapter has attempted to define the modern claims capability, its core competencies, and business steps and how they are managed. It concludes with an examination of the risks that must be confronted as well as tips developed from more than 50 years combined experience of the authors. Ultimately, the claims capability is a service organization. If management and business practices are executed with service to internal and external customers in mind, the claims capability will ensure its own health and vitality as well the financial health of its MCO.

References

1. National Coalition on Health Care. Health insurance cost. 2004. Available at: http://www.nchc.org/facts/cost.shtml. Accessed October 12, 2006.
2. Fox P. An overview of managed care. In: Kongstvedt PR, ed. *The Managed Health Care Handbook.* 3rd ed. Gaithersburg, Md: Aspen; 1996:3–15.
3. *Federal Register.* January 23, 2004;69(15).
4. Center for Policy and Research, America's Health Insurance Plans. An updated survey of health care claims receipt and processing times, May 2006.
5. Merriam Webster Online Dictionary. Information science. Available at: http://www.m-w.com/dictionary/information+science. Accessed October 12, 2006.
6. Higgins J, Mindrum C. New learning technologies for enterprise learning: ready for prime time? Accenture; 2006. Available at: http://www.accenture.com/global/services/by_subject/business_process_outsourcing/accenture_learning/r_and_i/newprimetime.htm. Accessed October 12, 2006.
7. Zenger J, Uehlein C. Why blended will win. *T+D.* 2001;55:54–60.
8. Knolwes M. *Self-Directed Learning: A Guide for Learners and Teachers.* Place: Chicago: Associated Press, 1975.
9. National Center for Health Statistics. About the International Classification of Diseases, Tenth Revision, Clinical Modification (ICD-10-CM). 2006. Available at: http://www.cdc.gov/nchs/about/otheract/icd9/abticd10.htm. Accessed October 12, 2006.

19

Member Services

Kevin Knarr and Peter R. Kongstvedt

Study Objectives

- Understand the basic processes of call center operations.
- Understand how technology supports the member services function.
- Understand the goals of member services in a managed care organization.
- Understand basic staffing and management issues in member services.
- Understand the basics of how a plan addresses member concerns and grievances.
- Understand proactive approaches a plan may take to measuring and maintaining member satisfaction.
- Understand the legal and regulatory aspects of member services.

Discussion Topics

1. Discuss the basic goals of a member services department.
2. Describe the typical types of steps that member services would take to address a member inquiry, problem, a complaint, and a formal grievance.
3. Describe the legal and regulatory milieu affecting member services, and provide hypothetical descriptions of different scenarios to illustrate those effects.
4. Describe actions a plan may take to enhance member satisfaction.
5. Discuss how call center management and technology has evolved and how it may evolve in the future.

INTRODUCTION

Navigating the increasingly complicated world of health care is a daunting task for the average health plan member. Complex benefit structures, confusion surrounding provider networks, the nature of the claims, explanation of benefit (EOB), and billing processes—and the advent of consumer-directed health plans (CDHPs)—all contribute to the increasing need for guidance from the plan itself. That guidance comes most frequently in the form of the member services or, more broadly, the customer services function. The fundamental delivery approach for member services is through a customer interaction center, often referred to interchangeably as a "call center" or "customer contact center." This environment supports inbound inquiries across a broad array of media (though most frequently, inbound telephone calls), blended with outbound contact and outreach transactions.

The customer interaction center enables the member to communicate directly with the insurer, enrolling in the plan, accessing administrative or clinical information, resolving issues, initiating grievances or complaints, and receiving general assistance in procuring care effectively. In turn, the health plan is able to track and report problems encountered, determine the root cause of upstream issues, and help manage the member decision-making process as it relates to accessing care.

Increasingly, plan executives are beginning to understand the rich insight that the center offers the health plan. Whereas the member services function was once considered a cost center, a "necessary evil," more forward-thinking plans realize the immense potential in developing long-term relationships with their membership through a well-designed member services function. This trend is particularly important as one considers the retail nature of the consumer-directed health plan movement (see Chapter 20). In mimicking a consumer products company's approach to managing the customer relationship, plans are more aware than ever of the function's ability to drive member satisfaction, and ultimately, retention, market share, and "wallet share" of the customer as they expand product and service offerings.

THE MEMBER SERVICE ENVIRONMENT

As noted earlier, the bulk of member services activity takes place in the health plan's customer interaction center(s). These centers vary in size between 30 and 400 customer service representatives (CSRs), with the majority of centers falling in the 100 to 200 full-time equivalent (FTE) range. The centers are commonly located with other health plan "back-office" functions, including claims payment, provider services, enrollment and billing, and materials fulfillment. In determining an effective location for their customer interaction center(s), plans will evaluate several criteria:

- Commercial real estate costs (leasing/purchasing)
- Labor wage rates
- Telecommunications and technology infrastructure
- Availability of high school, community college, and (in some cases) college-educated CSR candidates
- Availability of qualified customer interaction center management candidates

Typically, plans locate contact centers in suburban/ex-urban locations, in smaller towns with plentiful availability of "flex-space" or office park real estate; less expensive, educated, and available labor pools with minimal competition for employees; and durable infrastructure. When choosing a location for their customer interaction centers, plans are often able to elicit incentives from the candidate communities because the centers afford stable, long-term job opportunities for their citizens.

Although there is a great degree of variance in the size of health plan customer interaction centers, it is generally understood that plans derive economies of scale from pooling their labor resources into larger centers. However, client demands (such as an employer wishing to have its plan's customer interaction center near its employee base), lack of available labor pools, or structural considerations (*eg*, a state-based Blues plan's requirements to keep customer interaction centers in state) can all affect a plan's ability to scale its centers.

The customer interaction centers themselves present a unique office environment. CSRs are typically housed in cubes with low wall heights to foster teamwork and assistance, sitting with teams varying from 12 to 20, all reporting to a supervisor or team lead, who is normally located with or near the team. These teams may be dedicated to an account (as prescribed during the contracting phase between the plan and an employer group) or may be part of a larger pool of CSRs servicing hundreds of accounts and millions of members.

Aside from the site director and the senior management of the customer interaction center, most employees do not have enclosed offices. This usually results in a very open environment, seen as critical to collaborating to resolve their customers' issues quickly and effectively. This open environment also enables the supervisor to see when a CSR is having difficulty with a member's phone call, and also ensures that CSRs are at their station and available to take incoming calls/correspondence as scheduled. To a person more familiar with a traditional high-rise office environment, a customer interaction center has an unusual appearance.

Special Considerations Regarding the Member Services Environment

Some special issues must be considered in the provision of member services to individual members. The two that are the most important for this discussion are the hours that member services are available to members and the ability to communicate in languages other than English.

Hours of Availability

Availability is the most obvious issue to consider. Although 24 hours per day, 7 days per week (referred to as 24/7) is ideal, it will not be cost justified for all but the largest plans, and not necessarily even then. In fact, one need look no further than the arrival patterns of member calls to see that most members attempt to contact their plan's customer interaction centers between the hours of 7:00am and 6:00pm (in the caller's time zone) on weekdays, with highest call volumes seen on Mondays and lower volumes as the week progresses. The size and geographic distribution of the managed care organization (MCO) play a role in determining the maximum hours that member services will be available. As an example, a state-based Blues plan on the East Coast may choose to stay open from 7:00am to 7:00pm in the eastern time zone on weekdays, with no weekend coverage. However, a large national health insurer may choose to stay open from 7:00am Eastern Standard Time (EST) to 7:00pm Pacific Standard Time (PST) to ensure their entire membership has coverage for their inquiries. To ensure the appropriate level of consumer satisfaction, plans employ several techniques to service their members during "off hours":

- To address the clinical (nonadministrative) call types which come in during off hours, plans may send calls to a 24/7 nurse advice line, where a licensed nurse can help respond to a member's clinical issue or advise the member to call during regular business hours to address administrative issues. It is better for some inappropriate calls to go to the nurse advice line than for a medical problem to go unaddressed. In MCOs that use this approach, it is preferable for the nurse advice line organization (often an outside company with which the MCO has contracted) to have direct access to the

MCO's systems and information, and to be able to input information for action and follow-up by the plan's member services department when it reopens. Nurse advice lines are discussed further in Chapter 9.

- Plans may employ 24/7 electronic media such as the Internet or and Interactive Voice Response (IVR) system (discussed in later sections) that enable members to guide themselves through simple and moderately complex administrative questions.
- Plans may choose to outsource their off-hours call volume to a customer service business process outsourcing (BPO) company, which hires and trains representatives to handle the less-predictable off-hours volume more efficiently than the plan can itself.
- Use of voice mail, once thought to be a good way to handle off-hours calls, has proved to be less effective than planned because iterative games of "phone tag" are carried out between the plan and the member, thus having a negative impact on customer perception. Use of voice mail is typically viewed as a last resort measure for off-hours calls.

For any calls received during periods when the member services department is not open, it is critical that the automated menu a caller hears upon connecting to the closed center makes clear that if the call is in reference to a clinical problem or medical emergency, the member should contact his or her physician or, in the case of a medical emergency, seek medical help directly.

Hours of operation is yet another area where the employer group purchasing the plan may have a direct impact. Some groups demand extended hours of customer interaction center operation, sometimes related to the type of business they operate. For instance, an employer group that is a manufacturing concern with round-the-clock hours may demand the same of its health plan.

Non-English Communications

The ability to communicate with members in languages other than English is becoming increasingly important, particularly in large urban areas with large immigrant populations. In those areas with high concentrations of individuals speaking a particular language other than English (eg, Spanish), the MCO will often employ member services representatives who speak that language. For languages that are not necessarily in high concentration, or in smaller plans, it is common for the multilingual services to be provided through externally contracted interpreter services.

METHODS OF ACCESSING MEMBER SERVICES: INTERACTION MEDIA

A major part of creating an enduring and positive customer experience is giving members a variety of options in terms of how they interact with the health plan; and equally important, ensuring that the plan handles all interaction media effectively and efficiently. The way a member chooses to communicate varies as a result of several factors, most prominently the following:

- Reason that he or she is calling
- Media available to the member at the time of contact
- Level of comfort with electronic media

Generally speaking, there are several major means for the member to contact the interaction center:

- Interactive Voice Response (IVR)
- Inbound telephone calls
- Mail and paper-based communications
- E-mail
- Web chat/text messaging
- Internet/Web self-service

With each interaction medium, plans delivering a good customer experience will employ several integrated and interrelated technologies in routing the transaction to ensure that the CSR is in the best position to handle the inquiry efficiently and with the greatest chance to drive "first contact resolution," that is, completing the transaction such that the member has no need to contact the plan again regarding the issue.

The first of these capabilities is known as Computer Telephony Integration, or CTI. CTI enables the plan to take information the caller provides while in an automated menu (for example, member ID or type of request) or other information (caller's phone number), and access the plan's underlying customer databases to identify the member who is trying to contact the customer interaction center. This is particularly helpful in both routing the contact to the appropriate location and preparing the CSR to process the contact by "popping" the contact information to the CSR's desktop screen.

Second, building on CTI, "intelligent call routing" or "skill-based routing" enables the plan to send the contact to the CSR group best prepared to handle the contact. Criteria for routing may include the severity of the issue, past history of interaction with a specific CSR or set of CSRs, employer group, or other insight/business rules that the plan deems necessary to encourage effective service. These routing mechanisms enable the plan to tailor the customer experience and increase member satisfaction with the outcomes of the contact.

Finally, effective balancing of contact volume is accomplished via the use of an automated call distributor (ACD). This is a device or switch that automatically routes contacts based on programmed distribution instructions. Two levels of ACD may be used in a plan. The first is to serve as the initial automated answering system for inbound calls ("Hello. You have reached the member services department of XYZ Health Care"), which will then send the call on (directly or to an IVR as discussed later), as well as serve to provide wait instructions and background content for those members put on hold. The second function is to distribute all contacts based on CSR availability; in other words,

spread the workload and maximize the level of service provided. Modern ACD systems have the capability of handling all forms of interaction media, but plans typically use the ACD to balance their inbound call volume.

Inbound Telephone Communications Including IVR

The highest volume of interactions between a plan and its members will occur via the telephone, excluding routine mailings such as the issuance of identification cards, member newsletters, and other nonindividualized forms of communications. Several aspects to telephone communications must be looked at by any plan, and these are discussed as follows.

Placing the Call and Initial Navigation

Virtually all plans employ toll-free lines for use by members. In some cases, plans with a high incidence of local membership may opt to also publish local numbers to reduce toll charges. However, with 8nn-number (8nn refers to all toll-free numbers, including 800, 866, 877, etc.) toll charges edging as low as $0.03 per minute, it makes up a very small part of the customer interaction center cost as compared to years past. In some cases, a member's identification card or member handbook lists different numbers for different needs. For example, a plan may have an 8nn number for members to select a new primary care physician (PCP), to access a nurse line, or to resolve a problem. In most instances, plans take the route of having one single member services telephone number, and the member then will be directed via telephone network menus or an IVR. It is critical that these menus (either in the network or in the IVR) be clear, stripped of medical jargon, and simple to navigate. Otherwise, the plan runs the risk of consumer backlash as the service experience fails to satisfy member needs. In a very few cases, the member may be connected immediately to a service representative who will then deal with whatever issue the member has. This is particularly common in situations where the caller might be easily frustrated with IVR menu (*eg*, the senior marketplace), or in the instance of potential high-stress calls (*eg*, behavioral health intake calls). Generally, though, for routing and self-service purposes, the toll-free line will first lead to automated responses.

Ensuring Capacity

It is important for the telephone "trunks" and lines to be adequate in number, and properly automated in function, depending on plan size; for example, automatic call distribution, sequencing, and so forth. These are the functions of the MCO's telephone system, generally referred to as a PBX. For historical reasons, even though this system is actually a specialized computer, it is referred to as a "switch."* It is common for large MCOs to have more than one switch and for some of the switches to be specialized for use by plan functional areas. Because the switch is really a computer that is open to the telephone systems of the entire world, intense and specialized security precautions are required, discussion of which is beyond the scope of this chapter. Suffice it to say that the MCO's telecommunications staff spends a great deal of their time ensuring that capacity exists to handle the volume of inbound calls (with contingency for spikes), that call routing programming is accurate and avoids "misdirected" calls, and that failover plans are in place to ensure uninterrupted member contact response.

Routing the Call to the Right CSR

Call routing requires collaboration of the aforementioned CTI and skill-based routing capabilities, as well as use of the IVR system. The IVR is a system that provides the caller with a menu, or several menus, to choose from to direct the call to the most appropriate department. These menus may be touch-tone in nature, where the caller uses the phone's key pad to interact or may take advantage of the significantly more intuitive and easy to use speech recognition programs, which employ natural language capabilities that almost mimic a live conversation with a CSR.

As an example of an IVR system, the member's call would be answered by the automated system. In a touch-tone or limited speech recognition environment, the member is instructed to "Press or say 1 if your call is about a claim. Press or say 2 if your call is about an identification card. Press or say 3 if your call is about selecting or changing your primary care physician..." and so forth. Some plans nest the menus as well; for example, after the member presses 1 because the call is about a claim, the menu may then instruct the member to "Press or say 1 if your call is about an unpaid claim. Press or say 2 if your call is about an incorrectly paid claim. Press or say 3 if your call is to inquire about the status of a submitted claim . . ." and so forth. The general rule of thumb for best-practice touch-tone environments is to limit the menu structure to a 3×3 matrix; that is, plans should offer no more than three choices at each level and go no more than three levels deep. Also, plans must enable menu repeats and an ability to opt out to a live CSR when the member has exhausted the possibilities within the menu.

The more advanced speech recognition programs have created a paradigm shift for plans in how they employ the IVR. Rather than being beholden to a rigid touch-tone menu structure, the speech recognition IVR might prompt the caller with "Welcome to XYZ Health Care. . . . What is it you are calling about today?" The IVR is programmed for hundreds of permutations of caller responses, so that "I lost my ID card," "I need a new member ID," or "I can't understand why you don't mail my ID to me on time" are all

---

*This is because in the pre-computer days, it actually was a mechanical switch that opened and closed connections. A charming holdover of a term into the computer age.

recognized as a member who is having a problem with an ID card. The IVR might follow up with, "It sounds like you've lost or not received your ID card—is that correct?" When the member answers, "Yes," the call is either forwarded to a CSR who is now prepared to help the member with his or her lost card or else to an automated resolution of the call in a human-like manner.

IVR Self-Service

IVR systems may also provide for member self-service. This refers to providing the member with a form of self-service that does not require the intervention of a member services representative. Examples of these include requesting a new identification card to be mailed, providing fax-back information (*eg*, a listing of all participating PCPs in the member's ZIP code or within 5 miles of the member's ZIP code; or other provider listings), providing a copy of certain plan policies and procedures (*eg*, how the member may receive benefits for alternative medicine), allowing the member to find out the status of a claim in process, determine the status of an authorization for services, or other information.

Self-service IVR may also be used for enrollment purposes.* In this use, the member responds to the IVR questions by entering information via the telephone, not just responding to simple Boolean-type questions. This type of self-service generally requires that the MCO receives a base level of information from the enrolled group (*ie*, the employer) ahead of time, so that the subscriber calling in (*ie*, the member who is the individual actually receiving the benefit from the employer) is able to identify himself or herself by way of an identification number. The enrollment system then collects responses regarding the type of benefit plan the subscriber wants, the PCP each family member wants if enrolling in a health maintenance organization (HMO) by using a directory of PCPs in which numbers are associated with each PCP, and so forth. Additional nonhealth benefits may also be enrolled this way, but often this occurs through a party other than the MCO, such as a benefits consulting firm or outsourced human resources administrator. The advantages of using this type of IVR are obvious: faster data entry, increased accuracy (the IVR simply requires reentry of incorrect data, and also reads back the choices in plain language before asking the subscriber to confirm those choices), and lower costs.

There are two benefits and two limitations to effective IVR self-service usage. From a benefits perspective, the IVR enables the member to get immediate access to answers to inquiries without having to wait on hold for a CSR to answer the call. Additionally, the plan is able to push more call volume to the IVR for self-service, thereby reducing the number of CSRs required to handle calls, optimizing operating costs. Limiting the effectiveness is the fact that when a member calls, she or he is usually calling about issues of health or money, and the sensitive nature of those topics causes them to want to speak to a live CSR, rather than assume that the automated system is really "understanding" their needs. This is the reason for IVR completion rates (member calls satisfied through use of the IVR) have hovered in the high single-digit and low-teen percentages, though speech recognition is having a positive impact here. Second, the Internet is offering a much more intuitive and easy to certify approach to completing transactions. Thus, transactions that were once problematic to complete via the IVR, even with speech recognition, are much better suited to the more visual touch-and-feel nature of the Web.

Delivering the Call to the CSR for Handling

At the point where the plan has exhausted its IVR capabilities for self-service and has

---

*Although enrollment services are not part of the scope of discussion, it is appropriate to discuss this capability here because it is in the context of the overall self-service provision of member services.

picked up enough information from the caller to know who he or she is and have a sense of why the person is reaching out to the plan, the call is routed to a qualified CSR. Also, if the caller opts out of the IVR, the ACD makes a determination as to whom the call should be delivered. CSRs are signed into phone "splits," usually associated with a set of employer groups, a product type, call types, and so forth. The ACD will deliver the call to the split, then assign the call based on predefined parameters, often based on the CSR who has been available the longest.

In MCOs with CTI, the CSR receives the member's (nonmedical) records and other data on his or her terminal screen at the same time the call is coming through. This is done via the switch's ability to recognize the calling number, either via Caller ID or the MCO's own database of numbers, as well as accepting and evaluating information the caller enters into the IVR. Although this provides the member services representative with ability to greet the caller by name, there is no way to ensure that the caller is actually who the system identifies the person to be, and so, to adhere to authentication regulations under the privacy and security requirements of the Health Insurance Portability and Accountability Act (HIPAA; see Chapter 32), the representative must still ask the name of the caller and generally some form of confirmation (eg, the person's address). Once such identification is clear, the representative has the ability to address the caller's needs or questions rapidly because the information is already available, including, of course, notes from prior calls.

The last major type of telephone communications is the outbound, predictive dialer. This is a system in which the call center's switch is programmed to make calls to members on a proactive basis. The most common use for this in an MCO's member services department is outreach to new members, as is discussed later. Another common use of this capability is for follow-up on a member's call; in other words, the MCO representative calls the member to make sure that the member's

issues or needs have been met. The effect on member satisfaction is quite positive. Other uses of outbound predictive dialing exist, particularly in the clinical arena. Examples would include regular follow-up calls to patients with serious chronic diseases (see Chapter 10), or reminders to members to use preventive services (eg, calling women who have no record of a mammogram when they are of an age where screening mammograms are recommended; see Chapter 14).

Mail and Paper-Based Communication

Even though most of the individual-member activity in member services takes place via the telephone (discussed later), mail and paper communication remains highly important and must be managed properly. It is common that inbound mail correspondence will take place in the context of formal complaints or grievances (discussed later in this chapter) as part of a documentation effort by the individual initiating the correspondence, though it can occur in the normal course of communications from those members who simply prefer to use the mail rather than another means of communication.

All inbound correspondence must be logged and tracked, policies and procedures must be in place regarding the routing of correspondence, and master files need to be kept of both incoming and outgoing correspondence. Plans frequently use imaging technology to store the massive amounts of paper documents, the originals of which may then be stored off-site for a number of years. It is important to ensure that paper correspondence receives the same attention that telephone calls do, with time standards for response. In fact, in some of the more sophisticated plans, the paper document is imaged and then routed like a phone call through the ACD to the CSR's desktop for processing.

All MCOs use mail and paper-based correspondence for outbound communications. This is required for any form of communication that takes place on a plan-wide or other large scale (*eg*, to all members of an enrolled group). It is also used by the plan for documentation purposes when communicating important changes or notices to the members, such as a change in the pharmacy network, a change in policy coverage determinations, and so forth.

On an individual member level, outbound mail correspondence will always be used for formal communications and documentation of the complaint or grievance process discussed later in this chapter. Outbound mail is also used to reply to inbound mail from members, though that may serve as a supplement to telephone communications.

E-Mail Communication

E-mail has become ubiquitous in the office environment. Virtually every office worker in the United States relies on an e-mail program to help drive communication and resolve issues. Familiarity with this interaction media has crept into a plan's communication with its membership. On nearly every Web site, and at times on a member's ID card, a plan's customer service e-mail address is available as a means for interaction. Additionally, during the course of a CSR's phone interaction with a member, the CSR may ask the member to e-mail information to him or her to facilitate the closure of the issue.

Plans need to be mindful of the e-mail medium because it can actually be less efficient than live phone interaction is. E-mail intent and content can be open to broad interpretation, such that a CSR's response may not exactly meet the member's needs. This can lead to unnecessary iterations of work. Generally, e-mail interaction should be focused on basic administrative issues with little need for comprehensive evaluation.

Automated e-mail response technologies have been introduced over the last decade and are generally effective when the member request is of a basic administrative nature. Typically, the system will react to keywords in the member's e-mail and at-

tempt to answer the question using standardized responses.

Again, modern-day ACDs enable the processing of e-mails in the same way as they process and deliver inbound phone calls. The e-mail is routed to the CSR (instead of a phone call), and the CSR processes to completion. Once complete, the CSR is then ready to handle another e-mail message, inbound call, or other contact medium.

Interactions between members and plans, including e-mail, are subject to the privacy and security provisions of HIPAA. Therefore, the ability to encrypt data and provide for the assurance that only the member is able to electronically access confidential data about him- or herself is required. This is particularly relevant for both the e-mail medium as well as the next two interaction media, Web chat and Internet self-service.

Web Chat/Text Messaging

Another increasingly common form of communication is a text messaging session, in which the member, usually on the plan's Web site, chooses a "click-to-chat" function. This enables the member to initiate a text session with the CSR, basically a written version of an inbound phone call. More effective than e-mail because of the live nature of the interaction, text chats can be used for a variety of contact reasons. It is not uncommon to see text chats used for more sensitive clinical advice discussions because they give the member just a little more distance between the CSR and him- or herself, enabling a more comfortable "conversation." As with e-mail and imaged paper inquiries, the ACD can be used to deliver text messaging sessions to the appropriate CSR's desktop.

Internet/Web Self-Service

One of the most important developments in the customer interaction center over the past decade has been the meteoric rise of the Web as a means to drive what was once inbound phone volume to the plan's member

Web "portal" to enable self-service. Although the nature of a member's inquiry is often very sensitive, related to health or money, members have shown an increased propensity to use the Internet to retrieve answers to their administrative and clinical questions. Member portals have proved very effective at performing many of the basic administrative activities, including the following:

- Enrollment
- ID card issuance
- Claims status/tracking
- PCP look-up
- Benefits and eligibility look-up

The Web has represented a significant step up from the IVR self-service option of years past, including the breadth and depth of clinical interaction available on the member portal. Treatment decision support, health risk assessments, symptom information, wellness programs, and the like can all be found on a variety of plan Web sites.

As with the IVR, the plan benefits substantially from members completing transactions online because the cost of a Web transaction might be $0.05 to $0.10 versus $7 to $10 for a live interaction.

Accessing Member Services: Summary Points

As discussed on the last few pages, members have many options available to them when they decide to interact with their health plan. Given the proliferation of these interaction media, there are several points to keep in mind when a plan establishes its interaction strategy:

- Not every CSR will be proficient with every transaction medium. Although a CSR may be very skilled in the soft-skill techniques required to be successful on the phone, the person may not have the reading comprehension and letter-writing skills to respond to e-mail. Thus, the human capital aspect of staffing the center needs to be taken into account to ensure

that members are reaching qualified CSRs irrespective of the medium they choose.
- Branding of the various interaction media should be consistent. Members must feel as if they have reached the same member services department, with the same marketing and service "messaging," no matter which medium they have chosen. As a simple example, if the IVR refers to XYZ Health Care as "The Consumer's Choice in Health Plans," that same messaging should be found on the Web site, e-mail footer, and even in the call scripting. The plan should make every effort to appropriately promote its branding and market positioning during the member interaction.
- Issue escalation procedures should be in place for every interaction type. The CSR will not be capable of handling every inbound contact to completion. The member may have a complex question that the CSR cannot answer or may be irate from the outset of the contact. In such instances, more senior personnel must be at the ready to handle escalated issues across all interaction media.
- Plans must be able to manage the workflow of each contact type. Workflow describes the process by which contacts are forwarded throughout the organization to resolve the issue. For instance, a CSR might be required to forward a note to the claims department to review a claim (see also Chapter 18). Workflow must be in place to ensure that the contact is received in claims and that the issue is resolved in a timely manner. Many workflow technologies exist to support such a process.
- All contacts must be tracked and documented through completion, typically using a contact management system found on the CSR's desktop. Many robust technologies exist for such tracking (Oracle, Pega Systems, and SAP are examples of vendors in this space at the time of publication). Perhaps more important, data derived from such transactions must be

used by the plan to drive critical insights about its members, groups, and internal business processes. This insight can be used to drive improved member administrative and clinical outcomes and improved group sales processes and to conduct root-cause analysis to resolve upstream process issues that cause inbound contacts. By its very nature, the customer interaction center is rich with data to enable higher performance on the part of the health plan.

CONTACT TYPES: WHY MEMBERS REACH OUT TO THEIR PLAN

Member services is responsible for helping members use the plan and for disseminating information broadly to the membership. For example, new members commonly have less than complete (or even no) understanding of how the plan operates, how to access care, how to obtain authorization for specialty services (in a PCP case manager type HMO), and so forth. These are services to members as opposed to complaint and concern resolution, which is discussed later. Although the broad *types* of services are generally the same across product lines, plans often find differing levels of need for each of these types of services in the commercial, Medicare, and Medicaid markets; there will also be some differences in *specific* issues depending on whether the plan or product is an HMO, a preferred provider organization (PPO), a point-of-service (POS) plan, or a CDHP (see Chapter 2 for a discussion of different plan types).

Types of Member-Specific Services

Members contact their health plan for a variety of reasons, as illustrated in Table 19-1 later in this chapter. The following are four leading types of issues typically addressed by MCOs:

- Claims issues
- Benefits issues, including appeals and denials of coverage

- Enrollment issues, including ID card issues
- Provider access issues, primarily in HMOs

Claims Issues

Claims-related issues are usually the leading reason members contact the plan. Several aspects to claims may prompt the call, such as denial of payment, incorrect payment, delay of payment, or other errors such as payment to the wrong provider or overpayment. Problems with claims payments will also be a major source of contacts into the provider relations or network management area, and the cost of reworking a claim is grossly higher than is the cost of processing the claim correctly in the first place (see Chapters 9 and 18 for discussions of authorization systems and claims payment systems, respectively). It is no exaggeration to say the incorrectly processed claims account for a disproportionately high amount of administrative cost and dissatisfaction by members and providers.

Claims might be processed incorrectly for myriad reasons. Some of these causes are internal, some external. Examples of internal causes are key entry transpositions (for manually entered claims), incorrect identification of provider, incorrect medical policy application, double payment, and so forth. Examples of external causes include incorrect coding by the provider, illegible paper claims, incorrect identification of the member/patient, failure to actually file the claim, duplicate claims filings that categorize the duplicate as a new claim (*ie*, even paying the first claim leaves the duplicate claim marked as unpaid), and so forth. Causes that include both internal and external include claims being submitted electronically but authorizations being submitted on paper (allowing the claim to be processed immediately as though it were nonauthorized), lack of communication about changes in policy, disputes about the application of medical necessity, inconsistent interpretations of medical policy and benefits policy, and issues surrounding coordination of benefits and other-party liability.

As discussed in Chapter 18, MCOs continue to focus on those processes that will reduce error rates, including increasing the use of electronic claims, to address as many causes for errors as possible. Beyond any required reengineering to eliminate regular causes of claims errors, the member services department is that part of the MCO that must resolve the problem on the member's behalf, while provider or network management may do so on behalf of the provider. Which department is primarily responsible for resolution depends on who initiated the inquiry and where the cause of the problem lies.

For member services to resolve claims problems efficiently, several factors are important to consider. First is the ability of the representative to access information easily and rapidly. MCOs now typically provide CSRs with quick access to claims status screens, demographic information, provider information, medical policy information, and utilization management information. In some older legacy systems, this is done through multiple screens that are reached through menu selection by pressing certain keys. The fewer screens and menus the representative must go through to find necessary information, the better. Those MCOs that are still struggling with multiple systems supporting multiple products will have the most difficult time with this, and in that case, short of replacing the old systems with a single new one, the MCO may need to consider "frontware" that will perform the interface with the old systems, allowing the member services representative to access information more easily. Newer systems generally use a graphics user interface (GUI) that enables the representative to use combinations of the keyboard and mouse to rapidly access information.

It is not enough to access information, though. The CSR must also be able to do something about it. This means that the management of the MCO must set policies about levels of intervention that various types of CSRs may have. For example, all CSRs may be allowed to process enrollment and ID card changes, and to correct informa-

tion that was entered or submitted incorrectly in the first place, enabling the regular processing to then occur. To make a substantial change in a claim payment may require a higher level of CSR—one with more experience and training. For example, the ability of a CSR to override a claim denial based on information the member provides during the course of a telephone call must be available within the member services department, but not necessarily to all CSRs, and clearly not to an unlimited degree. For example, any claims override greater than $500 may need to be approved by the medical management department. In all cases, such overrides must be tracked and patterns analyzed to reduce their occurrence.

In the case of self-funded benefits plans (see Chapter 31), it is not unusual for the client (ie, the company that is self-funded and has contracted with the MCO for benefits administration) to set a general tone of the latitude provided to the member services department. For example, a company may want the CSR to be able to override any claim dispute under $1,000. If this is the case, then as noted earlier, it is reasonable for those CSRs responsible for that company to be organized into a separate unit.

Benefits Issues: Appeals and Denials of Payment

This is a subset of the claims problems discussed earlier. As noted earlier, there is often a level of claim cost that determines whether or not the CSR is able to resolve the issue in an autonomous way; and there may be different levels of override authority for different levels of CSRs based on experience and training. This is not to imply that CSRs can or should override any denied claim just because a member calls in. Rather, this means that good judgment will be applied. For example, a member may be new to an HMO and may make a simple mistake such as going to a nonparticipating provider for an authorized referral, or a new member in a POS plan forgets (or fails) to get a PCP authorization for the referral; in these cases, the member services representative may make the judgment that the goodwill generated by overriding the claim denial (or lower payment, in the case of the POS plan) is worth more in enhanced member satisfaction and retention than the monetary value of denying the claim.

In more serious cases of claim payment disputes, the plan must have a more formal mechanism for the member to appeal the payment denial. This form of appeal or grievance is discussed separately later in this chapter because it is part of the broader discussion of complaints and grievances.

Last in this topic, members may contact the plan proactively to determine whether a particular service is a covered benefit and under what circumstances. This may apply not only to services provided by professionals, but to facility-based services as well as pharmaceutical coverage. MCOs, through proactive member services, try to disseminate this information and make it as easily available as possible, but questions may still arise.

Enrollment Issues and Identification Cards

This is a generally straightforward type of service in which the member needs to correct an enrollment error or make a change to his or her coverage status. Although this chapter does not address the basic issues of entering enrollment information and issuing identification cards, it is inevitable that some members will have problems with their cards, and then member services will need to resolve those problems.

Common reasons for calls include lost cards, cards that were sent to the wrong address, incorrect information on the card, misspelling of the member's (or a dependant's) name, or change of address. Changes in enrollment status may be required because of change of status; for example, adding a new dependant such as a newborn or a newly adopted child, or a change in marital status. In all of these cases, the enrollment information must be updated and a new ID card(s) issued. In many cases, an MCO cannot update

membership information directly, but can only do so when the changes are provided from the employer; the member still contacts the MCO first, but must then be redirected back to the employer's human resources function.

This type of service is increasingly becoming an automated self-service function as described earlier in this chapter.

Primary Care Physician Selection and Network Access

For HMOs that use PCPs to access care, member services will frequently be called on to help members select a PCP. This may occur because the member failed to select a PCP in the first place, particularly in a POS plan in which the member has no intention of using the HMO part of the plan. Even in POS, it is best to require the member to select a PCP because it is not known whether the member will change his or her mind later and because the plan really does want to encourage the member to use the managed care system.

Another reason that an HMO member would need to select a new PCP is if a participating PCP leaves the network for any reason, or if the PCP's practice closes because it is full but that information did not get into the most recent provider directory or even the plan's Web site provider directory, or the member did not realize that a tiny, superscript asterisk meant that the practice was closed. Keeping the provider directory up-to-date is a difficult proposition as discussed in Chapter 5. The Internet provides the most practical solution to this, but not all members (and potential enrollees) have Internet access, particularly in Medicaid and Medicare plans.

OUTREACH

An outreach program can be of great benefit in preventing member complaints and problems, especially in HMOs, Medicare Advantage plans (see Chapter 26), and Medicaid managed care plans (see Chapter 27). An outreach program is one that proactively contacts new members and discusses the way the plan works. By reaching out and letting members know how the authorization system works, how to obtain services, what the benefits are, and so forth, the plan can reduce confusion.

Virtually all MCOs mail some form of an information pack to new members, though as a practical matter it may instead be sent from the employer. This pack typically includes not only the new identification card, but descriptive language about how to use the plan, how to access care, how the authorization or pre-certification system works, information about coordination of benefits (see Chapter 18), how to access urgent or emergency care, in some cases a provider directory (possibly with maps in the case of a closed panel), and a description of how the pharmacy benefit works (see Chapter 12). Some plans may also include a copy of the benefits description, and even possibly the group master contract or legal schedule of benefits. Some plans also include a "Member Bill of Rights" outlining the member's rights and responsibilities. Closed panels, medical groups in open panel plans, and integrated delivery systems (IDSs; see Chapter 2) may also include hours of operation and telephone numbers for their health centers. The various telephone numbers, mailing addresses, and Web site addresses are also provided.

Many plans (particularly HMOs, Medicaid, and Medicare Advantage plans, as noted earlier) accomplish a more aggressive and effective outreach program by conducting a telephone-based outreach program (though some Medicaid recipients may have limited or no regular access to a telephone). A telephonic outreach requires a carefully scripted approach during the contact. Development of scripts enables the plan to use lesser-trained personnel to carry out the program; when questions arise that are not easily answered from the script, or when problems are identified, the member may be transferred to an experienced member services representative. This also gives the member a chance to ask questions about the plan, especially when those questions do not come up until the

member has heard about the plan from the outreach personnel. It is worthwhile to bear in mind that for many members who do not access medical services frequently, this contact may be the most important one; and clearly it is in the plan's interest to retain such members. Outreach is most effective when carried out during both daytime and early evening hours to ensure that contact is made.

Telephone outreach may be especially useful when the plan undergoes a large enrollment surge. The level of problems that members experience with an MCO is generally highest during the initial period of enrollment (because new members are still unfamiliar with the way the plan operates), and outreach can help ameliorate that issue. The sooner the members understand how to access the system, the sooner the burden on the plan to deal with complaints and grievances will diminish.

CUSTOMER INTERACTION SUPPORT ACTIVITIES

Health plan customer interaction centers require several key functions to meet the quality and service levels required by the membership base. Without these functions, questions would be answered insufficiently, CSRs would not feel empowered to do their job, contacts would not be responded to on a timely basis, and there would be no means for recognizing high performance. These activities include the following:

- Training
- Workforce management
- Quality management/performance management

Each of these activities plays a key role in keeping the member service function functioning effectively and efficiently and in keeping member, groups, and plan employees satisfied.

Training

The amount of training required of member services representatives before they are allowed to interact with members varies from plan to plan. It is common for large MCOs to require new representatives to spend at least 30 to 60 working days in training before they begin actually interfacing with members, and even then the first few weeks are monitored by the supervisor. Ongoing training also occurs on a regular basis, particularly if support systems change, as well as training for increasing responsibilities for CSRs, and as a means of increasing employee satisfaction. Timing of training may also be affected by workforce management issues as discussed in the next section.

Workforce Management

The cyclical and variable nature of the inbound customer contact environment make predicting and managing the volume demands a critical part of member services management. Have too few CSRs on hand for the attendant call volume, and contacts will go unanswered, or there will be severe delays in getting to a CSR. Have too many CSRs, and the cost structure of the member services function will be too high. The process of balancing the service level and cost structure falls to the workforce management (WFM) team.

Using an automated set of algorithms in a WFM forecasting and scheduling tool, the WFM team uses historical and projected volume data to forecast the future volume of contacts. Then, based on that projected volume, and taking into account all of the ancillary activities that occur in the center (meetings, training, etc.), the tool creates a schedule to ensure that the right number of people are ready for inbound contacts for every half-hour increment that the member services function is open.

In addition to the static planning function of forecasting and scheduling, which typically occurs every 60 to 90 days, the WFM team manages intraday operations to ensure that call spikes, system outages, and so forth, have little to no impact on the service levels (*eg*, average speed to answer) within the center. The WFM team is also on point to help

plan for such activities as mass mailings and open enrollment periods, ensuring that these cyclical activities are accounted for when planning the staffing need.

Performance Management and Quality Management

Member services are measured on both operational performance, generally focused on hard numbers around answering responsiveness and contact resolution times, as well as more qualitative, soft-skill metrics, such as customer satisfaction and call quality. Each of these measure sets has a direct impact on the member's view of the health plan. Holding member services personnel directly accountable for such metrics helps ensure the member has the best possible perception of the plan's service processes.

Member services departments have responsiveness requirements as part of their performance standards. Such standards generally revolve around a few simple measures, including the following:

- *Average speed to answer (ASA):* Length of time elapsed between the call leaving the IVR and the call being answered by a live CSR (common goal—an average of 30 seconds)
- *Service level percentage:* A specific percentage of calls to be answered within a given timeliness goal (common goal: 75%–80% of all calls handled within 30 seconds)
- *Abandon rates:* Number of calls when the caller hangs up before reaching a live CSR because of lengthy ASA times (common goal: less than 3% of all calls abandoned before a live answer)

Performance standards must be tailored to meet the standards that the *members* would expect, not simply what the plan chooses to measure. For example, a plan may measure ASA by measuring how long it takes a call to be answered by a CSR once the call leaves the IVR; such a measurement would fail to capture the fact that the member had to wade through several menus of an IVR to get there, resulting in 3 minutes of frustration by the member.

Timeliness of response and first contact resolution is also measured against goals. Examples include the percentage of calls that are resolved on the spot (*ie*, no follow-up is required); for example, 90% of calls should require no follow-up. For problems or questions that require follow-up, there are goals for how long that takes; for example, 90% of outstanding inquiries or problems should be resolved within 14 days and 98% within 28 days. Similar standards apply to written correspondence.

CSRs are also measured individually for goals such as the following:

- *Schedule adherence:* Ensuring CSRs are staffed and ready for inbound contacts as scheduled by the WFM team
- *Average handle time:* The length of time each contact takes to complete
- *First call resolution:* Percentage of contacts resolved on the first call

CSRs are usually monitored not just for productivity, but for quality as well. Quality is usually monitored through silent monitoring of the calls themselves. This is usually done through relatively sophisticated systems that enable the quality reviewer to both listen to recorded calls and at the same time view what transpired on the CSR's desktop. These recorded calls can be segmented by call type, CSR name, employer group name, and so forth, to generate rich data for the quality personnel's focused review. The quality reviewer (which may be the CSR's supervisor, but should typically be the responsibility of an objective Quality Management team) will issue a qualitative judgment about how well the service representative handled the call, from both a call process and customer service skills point of view; the answering systems informs the member calling in that the call may be monitored for quality purposes.

It is not enough to take and give information when a member has a problem or complaint; the representative must apply communication techniques developed for customer service to be optimally effective. Some plans routinely send follow-up questionnaires to members after the member services inquiry or complaint is resolved to solicit feedback on the process, as well as reinforce the notion that the member is important.

Other Support Activity

Two other areas that are integral to the success of the member services function are these:

- *Human resources:* The team that recruits and hires the CSR and management professionals, ensuring the function is staffed with qualified resources. Given the potentially stressful environment, the member service function is usually one with high attrition and requires that a steady flow of candidates be evaluated and hired when appropriate.
- *Reporting:* The member services function is heavily reliant on performance and quality data. The dynamic nature of inbound contact volumes require that the customer interaction center management team have the data at their fingertips to make timely decisions to support a member-centric environment. Tools ranging from the WFM system, the call management system, the quality monitoring system, to the HR system are all inputs to the reporting function. This activity is discussed further in the next section.

DATA COLLECTION AND ANALYSIS

The customer interaction center is rich with customer experience information, and the member services department should be responsible for collecting, collating, and analyzing that data. Data may be considered in two broad categories: data regarding general levels of satisfaction and dissatisfaction and data regarding medical and administrative problems.

Satisfaction Data

Satisfaction data may include surveys of current members, disenrollment surveys, telephone response time and waiting time studies (these may be done in conjunction with the quality management department, but they are essentially patient satisfaction studies), and surveys of clients and accounts (although marketing rather than member services may perform many of these studies).

Member surveys are particularly useful when done properly. Even when an MCO is the sole carrier in an account, surveys help the plan evaluate service levels and ascertain what issues are important to the members. Surveys may be focused on a few issues that the plan wants to study, or they may be broad and comprehensive; they may be produced by the MCO, or (more commonly) obtained from an outside source or commercial vendor. The survey activity itself may be conducted by plan personnel, or may be contracted out to an objective third party that specializes in consumer surveys. Of course, any protected health information as defined under HIPAA (see Chapter 32) is subject to HIPAA's privacy requirements.

In an environment where members have multiple choices for their health care coverage, member surveys will be geared toward issues that influence enrollment choices. It is easier and less expensive to retain a member than it is to sell a new one. Of special importance are those members who do not heavily utilize medical services because their premiums pay for the expenses of those members with high medical costs and because such members with low medical costs tend to disenroll more often than members who utilize services heavily. It must be reinforced here, though, that under HIPAA it is not permissible to specifically identify those members by name for purposes of sales, nor may utilization or cost data be made available on a member-identifiable basis to the sales and marketing department.

The Consumer Assessment of Healthcare Providers and Systems (CAHPS), available from the Agency for Health Research and Quality (AHRQ),* was (and still is) focused on health plans, but versions focusing on hospitals and on ambulatory care are being tested at the time of publication. An MCO may be required to perform this standardized member satisfaction survey under several conditions: there is a regulatory requirement or its use in Medicare and Medicaid MCOs, as discussed in Chapters 26 and 27, respectively; and some states require its use as a condition of licensure, as discussed in Chapter 33. The National Committee for Quality Assurance[†] (NCQA; see Chapter 23) also requires use of the CAHPS survey, and it is part of its Health Plan Employer Data Information Set (HEDIS; see also Chapter 23) required for accreditation by that body. In addition to the survey itself, standards exist regarding how often it must be conducted, over what number of members, and under what conditions. Even if an MCO does not face these requirements, many large employers require its use as a condition of offering the plan to their employees.

Satisfaction data are also frequently made available to consumers outside of the auspices of the MCO. Medicare and many states provide Web-based comparative data around member satisfaction to consumers, as do a number of commercial third parties. In addition, data on participating health plans are available for purchase from NCQA under the publication title *Quality Compass*.

Trends Analysis

Problems that are brought to the plan's attention not only require resolution but need to be analyzed to look for trends. If a problem is sporadic or random, there may be little re-

---

*See http://www.cahps.ahrq.gov.
[†]See http://www.ncqa.org.

quired other than helping the individual member as needed. If problems are widespread or stem from something that is likely to cause continual problems, then the plan must act to resolve the problems at the source. Such resolution may mean changing a policy or procedure, improving education materials to the members, dealing with a difficult provider, or any number of other possible actions. The point is that plan management will not know of chronic problems if the data are not analyzed.

Plans automate their member services tracking systems as part of their overall systems support of member services. Such automation not only serves to help member services track and manage individual problems but also serves as a method to collect and collate data. Each member contact with the plan is entered into the computerized tracking system and assigned a category (or multiple categories if necessary); issues involving providers are generally tracked not only by category but by provider as well. Repeat or follow-up contacts are also tracked but usually still count as only one problem or inquiry.

Producing regular reports summarizing frequency of each category, as well as frequency of problems or complaints by provider, enables management to focus attention appropriately. An example of the types of categories that a plan may track is illustrated in Table 19-1. These examples are by no means exhaustive; conversely, it is unlikely that a plan would use all of these categories. In fact, if the plan uses too fine a division of reasons, it may be unable to obtain any statistically significant amounts of data.

Table 19–1 Examples of Categories of Reasons for Member Contacts

Claims Issues

In-network

    Claim denied

    Claim paid at a lower level of benefits

    Unpaid claim

        Provider submitted

        Member submitted

    Received bill from provider

    Coordination of benefits

    Subrogation/other-party liability

Out-of-network

    Claim denied

    Claim paid at a lower level of benefits

    Unpaid claim

        Provider submitted

        Member submitted

    Received bill from provider

    Coordination of benefits

    Subrogation/other-party liability

Benefits Issues

Questions

    Physician services

        Primary care

        Specialty care

    Hospital or institutional services

    Emergency services

    Ancillary services

        Pharmacy

        Other

    Point-of-service benefits questions

Complaints

    Copayment or co-insurance levels

    Limitations on coverage

    Did not know benefits levels

Appeals of denied coverage

Table 19–1 Examples of Categories of Reasons for Member Contacts—continued

Enrollment Issues

ID card(s)
    Never received
    Errors on card
    Change in information
    Lost card
Change in enrollment status
    New dependant
    Delete dependant
    Student of disabled dependant
      verification
Change in address
    Subscriber
    Dependant(s)

Need evidence of coverage or other
    documentation
Need new directory of providers
Selecting a PCP (HMO only)
    Practice closed
    Never selected
    Special needs
Changing PCP (HMO only)
    Dissatisfied with PCP
    PCP no longer participating with plan
    Geographic reasons

Plan Policies and Procedures

Authorization system for specialty care
Precertification system for institutional care
Second opinion procedures
Copayments and co-insurance

Unable to understand printed materials or
    instructions
Formal grievance procedures

Plan Administration

Personnel rude or unhelpful
Incorrect or inappropriate information given
Telephone responsiveness problems
    On hold
    Unanswered calls
    Call not returned

Complaints or grievances not addressed
    satisfactorily

Access to Care

Unable to get an appointment
Too long before appointment scheduled
Office hours not convenient
Waiting time too long in office

Problems accessing care after hours
Too far to travel to get care
No public transportation
Calls not returned

Physician Issues

Unpleasant or rude behavior
Unprofessional or inappropriate behavior
Does not spend adequate time with member
Does not provide adequate information
    Medical
    Financial
    Administrative (eg, referral process)

Lack of compliance with use of plan network
Lack of compliance with authorization policies
Does not speak member's language
Speaks negatively about the plan

continues

Table 19–1 Examples of Categories of Reasons for Member Contacts—continued

Perceived Appropriateness and Quality of Care

Delayed treatment	Incorrect diagnosis or treatment
Inappropriate denial of treatment	Lack of follow-up
Inappropriate denial of referral	Physician visit
Unnecessary treatment	Diagnostic tests

Medical Office Facility Issues

Lack of privacy	Unsafe or ill-equipped
Unclean or unpleasant	Lack of adequate parking

Institutional Care Issues

Perceived poor care in hospital	Facility unclean or unpleasant
Discharged too soon	Facility unsafe or ill-equipped
Hospital or facility staff behavior	Problems with admission or discharge process
Rude or unpleasant behavior	Other administrative errors
Unprofessional or inappropriate behavior	
Spoke negatively about the plan	

PROVISION OF GENERAL INFORMATION

The provision of general information to members is one of the key aspects of member services. This is differentiated from the function of responding to individual inquiries about problems or the need to interact with the plan for some reason (eg, PCP selection, ID card corrections, and so forth). Such information may be broadly disseminated to the entire membership via one or more of the following routes:

- Mass paper-based mailings
- Mass e-mail messages
- Distributed by the employer via its own employee communication modalities
- The plan newsletter
- The MCO's Web site
- Less common modalities such as:
  - Automated outbound telephone calling
  - Group information sessions
  - Electronic kiosks at the work site or other selected areas (eg, an affiliated health club)
  - One-on-one individual sessions

CONSUMERISM AND THE PROACTIVE APPROACH TO MEMBER SERVICES

Most member services departments become complaint departments. When that happens, the plan not only loses a valuable source of member satisfaction but runs the risk of burning out the personnel in the department. It is emotionally draining to listen to complaints all day. Even the satisfaction of successfully resolving the majority of complaints can be inadequate if there is nothing else the plan is doing to address satisfaction. This leads to higher personnel turnover rates in this department than in most other areas of the MCO.

The good news is that the advent of CDH plans and consumerism overall has very positive implications for the member services function; health care consumerism is discussed as well in Chapter 20. Simply stated, the daily monotony of administrative activity is shifting toward one of health coaching, in which the CSR has a greater role and responsibility is assisting a member in navigating the complexity of the new health care environment as well as providing the consumer with information and decision support tools to enhance their ability to participate in health care decision making. The plan is taking a greater stake in developing a longitudinal relationship with the member, to both improve the retention of the member as a customer, and to have a positive effect on the member's overall administrative and clinical well-being.

A number of forces have either required that a CSR take a more proactive approach to member services or have actually enabled that advanced interaction:

- Consumer-directed health plans, with their corresponding savings/investment accounts and debit/credit card solutions, as described in Chapter 2.
- The advent of personal health records (PHR), enabling a longitudinal view of the member's health, as described in Chapter 17.
- Deeper integration of disease management and other health and wellness functions into the health plan (either as plan-owned activities or via relationships with disease management, wellness vendors), as described in Chapters 10 and 14.
- Publicly available provider and facility quality data, evidence-based medicine and outcomes data, and provider/facility unit cost data for procedures, as described in Chapters 8 and 20.
- Easy-to-use decision support tools, enabling the front line to assist members in their treatment choices, as described in Chapter 20.
- Robust customer insight and analytics tools, enabling the identification and segmentation of member populations for targeted interventions.

The member services function is perhaps the most logical arena to execute on a plan's consumerism strategy, given the volume of interaction that takes place between the plan's membership and their CSRs. Given the tools available to them, CSRs will be able to guide a member's decision making throughout the member's health care life cycle.

Many member services departments are now directly responsible for consumer-based, proactive programs. Some examples of such programs are briefly described here.

Member Education Programs

Member education may be clinically oriented or administratively oriented. For the latter topic, that occurs most commonly during new member orientation meetings or seminars. New members are educated on how best to use the health plan, questions are answered, and so forth.

Health education is usually the responsibility of the medical management function of the plan, but it is common for member services to be involved, and in some cases, even be primarily responsible. The two broad categories of health education are general preventive educational services, and disease- or condition-specific education. These programs are often accompanied by medical self-help literature, interactive videos, and other consumer-oriented information.

Examples of general health promotion include smoking cessation, weight control, stress management, and so forth. Examples of health education aimed at specific medical conditions are programs focused on diabetes, congestive heart failure, angina pectoris, pregnancy, and so forth. The actual content of these programs may be provided by the medical department or an outside contractor, but it is member services that organizes the programs and manages communications with the members.

Member Data Transparency and Decision Support Tools

As discussed further in Chapter 20, MCOs are providing more information than ever to members to help them make informed decisions regarding their health care. Although health plans have long made access to self-care information, as well as health risk appraisals, available (see Chapter 9), the provision of information and decision support tools has taken new directions. The initial focus of such efforts was in CDHPs, as described in Chapters 2 and 20, but has now appeared in almost every other type of MCO. Data about actual costs is being made available, as well as automated tools accessed via the Web that will help members with factoring in the financial impact of medical care. Alternatives to various types of clinical services are described, though final decision making ultimately falls to the member and her or his physician.

Member Suggestions and Recommendations

Soliciting member suggestions and recommendations can be valuable. This may be done along with member surveys, or the plan may solicit suggestions through response cards in physicians' offices, in the member newsletter, or via the Internet. There are times when the members will have ways of viewing the plan that provide valuable insight to managers. Although not all the suggestions may be practical, they may at least illuminate trouble spots that need attention of some sort.

Special Services, Affiliations, and Health Promotion Activities

Managed care plans frequently develop affiliations with health clubs and other types of health-related organizations. This usually takes the form of discounts on membership to health clubs, discounts on purchases of health-related products such as safety equipment or home medical equipment, and discounts on medical self-help products such as books or computer programs. This serves to underscore the emphasis on prevention and health maintenance, allows for differentiation with competitors, and provides value-added service to the member. Access to or sponsorship of various health promotion activities (*eg*, support for community smoke-out programs) falls into the same category.

MEMBER COMPLAINTS, GRIEVANCES, AND APPEALS

All health plans seek to prevent or minimize problems that may arise, but no plan can eliminate them entirely. Further, even the correct administration of benefits will occasionally result in a coverage decision that a member does not agree with and wishes to seek a different outcome. Therefore, an essential feature of the member services function is to manage the process of addressing member complaints, grievances, and appeals.

Complaints Compared to Grievances and Appeals

Complaints by members may be generally defined as episodes of dissatisfaction that the member brings to the attention of the plan; they differ from grievances in that grievances are formal complaints, formally demanding resolution by the plan, whereas appeals are a form of formal grievance that is specific to benefits coverage denials. Appeals are by far the most common reason for a formal grievance, as is discussed later in this section.

Complaints differ from routine problems that members encounter (even though those problems certainly may cause dissatisfaction) in that the routine problems are resolved by the member services department as a function of day-to-day operations. MCOs generally categorize something as a complaint if it is not an easily resolvable problem (*eg*, an incorrect ID card, or a small claim problem resolved by member services), or if the attempt at resolution by member services fails to satisfy the member who then continues to express dissatisfaction.

A routine problem can evolve into a complaint if the member continues to follow-up with the plan with the intent of pursuing either a different outcome, or some other action on the part of the plan. Complaints that are not resolved to the satisfaction of the member may evolve into formal grievances. It is clearly in the best interest of the plan to try and re-solve problems and complaints before they become formal grievances because there are greater legal implications and member satis-faction issues involved with grievances.

Resolution of complaints is usually infor-mal, although the plan should have a clear policy for investigating complaints and re-sponding to members. Despite the informal nature of complaint resolution, it is ex-tremely important for the member services department, or in fact any staff member, to document carefully every contact with a member when the member expresses any dissatisfaction. For complaints, the member services representative should keep a log of even casual telephone calls from members as well as notes of any conversations with members while he or she is trying to resolve complaints. Concise and thorough records may prove quite valuable if the complaint turns into a formal grievance. Such documen-tation also helps in data analysis, as dis-cussed earlier in this chapter.

Grievance and appeal resolution is dis-tinctly formal. State and federal regulations, including Medicare Advantage and Medicaid, require health plans to have clearly delineated member grievance and appeal procedures, to inform members of those procedures, and to abide by them. In many instances, mem-bers may be contractually prohibited from fil-ing a lawsuit over benefits denial until they have gone through the plan's grievance proce-dure; however, that requirement has been abolished in some states. If a plan fails to in-form a member of grievance rights or fails to abide by the grievance procedure, the plan has a clear potential for liability. Suggested steps in formal grievance resolution follow later in this chapter.

Benefits Coverage Complaints Compared to Service Complaints

Member complaints fall into two basic cate-gories: benefits coverage complaints and ser-vice complaints. Service complaints fall into two basic categories as well: administrative service and medical service.

Benefits Coverage Complaints

Routine Management of Benefits Coverage Complaints

Benefits coverage complaints generally occur when the member seeks coverage for a ser-vice that is not covered under the schedule of benefits, is not considered medically neces-sary, is from a provider not in an HMO's net-work, or when the member had certain nonurgent services rendered without autho-rization/precertification, leading to denied or reduced coverage. The routine handling of claims problems by member services has been discussed earlier. The focus here is on complaints about benefits coverage denials (either prospective or retrospective) that have not been resolved at the initial contact stage.

In general, the plan will rely on both the schedule of benefits and on determinations of medical necessity by the medical department. In the case of an HMO member seeking cov-erage for services from a nonparticipating provider, the medical department must deter-mine if the same service is available from a participating provider and it is reasonable for the member to use the in-network provider. In the case of denial or reduction in payment of claims already incurred, the issue of plan pol-icy and procedure is also present because this situation usually arises from cold claims re-ceived without prior authorization or precerti-fication (see Chapter 9).

For prospective denial or reduction of cover-age, the plan should respond to the member with the exact contractual language upon which it bases its denial of coverage. A mecha-nism must also be in place for second opinions or external review of the medical director's opinion in those cases where there is a dis-pute over medical necessity. This mechanism for a second opinion may be internal or ex-ternal and is described later. The medical di-rector must be careful not to confuse the issue of medical necessity with that of covered benefits; there may be times when a service can be considered medically necessary but the plan does not cover it under the schedule of benefits. That being said, there are also situations in which the treating physician or the member interprets a medical service as being covered under the schedule of benefits, while the medical director does not; such situations are handled procedurally the same as a disagreement over medical necessity unless the interpretation issue is so obvious that it is more appropriate for it to be handled solely by the plan's legal counsel.

Cases involving denial or reduction in coverage for services already incurred are a bit more complex. The claims department of the plan will receive a claim without an authorization for services. As discussed in detail in Chapter 18, the plan must have clear policies and procedures for processing such claims. In the case of an HMO without any benefits for out-of-network services, the plan may pend or hold the claims to investigate whether an authorization actually does exist (or should have been given). If an authorization for services ultimately is given, the claim is paid; if no authorization is forthcoming, the claim is denied. The plan may occasionally wish to pay the claim even without an authorization in certain circumstances, such as a genuine emergency, an urgent problem out of the area, or a first mistake by a new member, all of which were noted earlier in this chapter.

In POS plans and PPOs, an unauthorized claim is not denied (assuming it is covered under the schedule of benefits), but the coverage is substantially reduced. As discussed in Chapter 9, it is not always clear when a service was actually authorized and when the member chose to self-refer. The plan must have very clear policies to deal with these claims because it is impractical to pend every unauthorized claim because POS plans and PPOs are predicated on a certain level of out-of-network use.

In those instances where, despite the member's complaint about the decision, coverage is ultimately denied or reduced, members need an appeal mechanism. Member services routinely provides information on this process, which is discussed later in this section.

Last, as discussed earlier it is important for plan management to continually analyze the reasons for claims disputes and appeals and to look for patterns. It is common to find certain identifiable causes of these problems. For example, there may be a particular medical group that is not providing adequate after-hours access, or there may be a flaw in the claims processing logic, or there may be a significant change in what is considered accepted and rational medical practice that is not yet reflected in the claims processing logic. When such patterns are identified, remediating the root cause results in lowered disputes and complaints.

External Medical Review of Complaints about Medical Necessity Decisions

As noted earlier, there must be mechanisms in place to obtain a second opinion of a disputed issue of medical necessity in the event that the treating physician and the medical director cannot come to agreement. Of course, if for some reason the denial of coverage has reached the point of dispute and the medical director has not become personally involved, such involvement must occur immediately. Failure of the plan's medical director to be an active participant in this process is unacceptable.

There are both informal and formal approaches to obtaining a second opinion or an external review of a dispute over medical necessity (or the rarer occurrence of a disagreement over the interpretation of what the covered benefit actually is; such situations are often more appropriately managed by the plan's legal department). Formal external review programs are considered part of the formal grievance and appeals process within a health plan and are further discussed later in this chapter.

An informal review process may be as simple as the medical director asking one of the plan's participating physicians in the appropriate specialty to review the case. Such physicians are usually members of a panel of physicians willing to act in this capacity and are appropriately compensated for their time as well as being provided indemnification by the plan for their medical management activities. The opinion of the reviewing physician is not necessarily binding, but rather advisory to the medical director.

Related to the preceding, many HMOs (and some other types of MCOs) have as part of their informal review process a peer review committee that provides advice and counsel to the medical director for such cases rather than occurring ad hoc; however, this committee meets on a regularly scheduled basis and considers multiple cases. Minutes are kept but are subject to confidentiality provisions. The membership of this committee usually spans the spectrum of specialties, with a core group of physicians making up the permanent peer review committee, and a larger group of subspecialists making up an ad hoc group of physicians who participate only when there are cases to review that are appropriate to their specialty. This activity is described further in Chapter 15 as part of a quality management program.

Regardless of state, federal, or accreditation agency requirements as discussed below, many MCOs have developed external appeals programs for sound reasons: this is something that consumers and physicians want, it is a good form of risk-management, it potentially lowers the MCO's exposure to lawsuits, and provides a good and impartial (it is hoped) mechanism for review of the plan's most serious disputes. How often an external appeals process will be used is influenced by many factors, including how well the internal review process works, how well member services is able to communicate with the member, how well members understand the availability of the program and how to access it, and the willingness of an MCO to settle a dispute rather than subject it to the external review program.

Service Complaints

Service complaints include medical services and administrative services. Medical service complaints could include a member's inability to get an appointment, rude treatment, lack of physicians located near where the member lives, difficulty getting a needed referral in an HMO (difficult at least in the opinion of the member), and, most serious, problems with quality of care. Administrative complaints could include incorrect identification cards, not getting a card at all, poor responsiveness to previous inquiries, not answering the telephone, lack of documentation or education materials, and so forth.

When the complaint alleges quality of care problems, the medical director needs to be notified. If investigation reveals a genuine quality of care problem, the matter requires referral to the quality assurance committee or peer review committee (see Chapter 15). Some states require certain types of quality complaints to be reported to a state agency, and Medicare Advantage requires member complaints about quality to be reviewed by a designated quality improvement organization (QIO; formerly called a peer review organization).

Member services personnel need to investigate any type of service complaint and to get a response to the member. Even if most of these are routine problems that are easily resolved as discussed earlier in this chapter, in all cases of service complaints, the key to success is communication. If member services CSRs communicate clearly and promptly to all parties, many problems can be cleared up. Such communication must not be confrontational or accusatory. It is important for member services always to keep in mind that there are at least two ways of looking at any one situation and that there is rarely a clear-cut right or wrong.

FORMAL GRIEVANCE AND APPEAL PROCESS

All MCOs are required to have a formal grievance and appeals process, and the responsibility for implementing it usually falls to the member services department. State regulations for insured plans, federal regulations for Medicare Advantage plans and Medicaid plans, and regulations under the Employee Retirement Income and Security Act (ERISA) for self-funded plans, all contain provisions for this process, as also discussed in Chapters 33, 26, 27, and 31, respectively. The model act used by many states (see Chapter 33) has been revised over the years to more closely align with the federal process described under ERISA. However, variability and overlap can occur between applicable regulations, so most MCOs at the least conduct their grievance and appeals process so as to meet the more stringent timeliness requirements. These various regulations spell out the minimum requirements for the formal procedure, including the following:

- *Timeliness of response:* ERISA requires urgent care claims to be reviewed in 72 hours or less, while some states require 24 hours. ERISA and many states require resolution within 90 days for nonurgent appeals, with an additional 60 days time for resolution of an appeal of the initial decision. Additional time may be allowed under certain circumstances such as the need for additional information.
- *Who will review the grievance or appeal:* The use of external review bodies is required by many states, primarily for external review of medical necessity decisions. That process is discussed further later.
- *Limitations on how long a member has to file a grievance or appeal:* ERISA and many state laws require that a member file an appeal to the initial decision within 180 days of that decision, or else he or she may lose the right under the plan's grievance procedure to file.
- *What recourse a member has:* There are considerable differences in the availability of further recourse to adverse decisions once the grievance and appeals process is exhausted based on whether

the benefits plan is insured, self-funded, or part of a governmental plan.

Filing of Formal Grievance or Appeal

The filing of a formal grievance or appeal is a result of the plan denying coverage for a service or payment of a claim after review by the informal mechanisms discussed earlier in this chapter, and the member choosing to formally appeal that decision, having been provided with a full description of the process, timeliness requirements, and avenues of recourse. This is done with a form specific to that purpose. The member must then fill out a specific form that asks for essential information (*eg*, name, membership number, parties involved, and so forth) and a narrative of the issue and appeal. This begins the formal grievance and appeal process.

Initial Investigation of Grievance or Appeal

Between the time period that begins when the form is filed with the plan and ends when the plan responds, the grievance needs to be investigated. This may include further interviews with the member, interviews with or written responses from other parties, and any other pertinent information that needs to be collected. The information is then reviewed, generally by an officer of the company, a panel of internal or external reviewers, or by an outside reviewer. A qualified physician must be involved in the review process if the claim involves any aspect of clinical judgment. At the end of the review period, the plan responds to the member with its findings and resolution. The response includes the rights and responsibilities for the member to appeal the determination if the resolution is not satisfactory.

Secondary Appeal Process

The formal secondary appeal process occurs as a result of the member exercising his or her right for further review. The member formally requests or files for such an appeal under the required time frames as noted earlier. The secondary appeal review must be undertaken by individuals other than the ones who first made the adverse determination. In the case of a medical necessity issue, this review may occur via the informal medical review process described earlier in this section, or through the more formal process described in the next section. In cases where external medical review is not required or appropriate, the process occurs on an administrative basis. This review may occur solely through the review of pertinent records, including additional material submitted by the member and/or the treating physician. The case is reviewed according to required time frames, and the decision is communicated to the member, along with any additional information about what other options the member has available in the event the decision is still negative (those options may vary, depending on the type of benefits plan the member is covered under).

Some MCOs choose, or may be required, to convene a formal hearing for this type of appeal. The purpose of a formal hearing is to afford the member a chance to present his or her case in person to an unbiased individual or a panel of unbiased individuals, including the opportunity to present any additional pertinent information. The hearing officer or the voting members of the hearing panel should not have participated in the earlier decisions as noted previously. Plan managers who have been involved before will surely participate but not as the hearing officer or as voting members.

It is a poor idea to ask the member's provider to appear at the hearing in those cases where the provider has been involved in the grievance. This carries the potential of disrupting the physician-patient relationship and of placing the provider in a no-win situation, and it can have implications for future legal action against the provider or plan. Any information from the member's provider should be presented by the medical director, accompanied by appropriate documentation.

A resolution of a secondary appeal is rarely given to the member at the close of the hearing. When the hearing is over, the member is told that he or she will be informed of the results within the required time period. After the member and staff have left, the voting members of the panel discuss the case and reach a resolution. That resolution is communicated in writing to the member and any other pertinent parties, along with information that the member has the right of further appeal as appropriate, depending on the benefits plan the member is covered under.

Formal External Medical Review of Appeals of Medical Necessity Decisions

A formal external medical review mechanism is required of MCOs in most states, and such requirements are not preempted under ERISA for self-funded plans. Even if external review is not required by a state, ERISA does incorporate a type of external review for denials based on medical issues as part of a more formal grievance process. External review programs are also required for certification by NCQA (see Chapter 23), and for Medicare Advantage and Medicaid plans. Because there is variability in how external appeal programs operate, what follows are brief descriptions of some of the basic structural and procedural issues that must be addressed.

Determination of Eligibility for the External Medical Review Program

This refers to certain requirements (other than state and federally mandated programs as noted earlier) that must be met for a member to even access the external appeals program. For example, in some state and voluntary (ie, nonmandated) programs, there is a financial threshold that must be met, such as the cost of the disputed service being in excess of $500. The appeals system may also be limited to medical necessity and not to interpretation of covered services. Some plans may require the member to work through the plan's internal appeal process discussed earlier before the member can demand the external review, but that is not uniform from state to state.

Clear Definition of the Time Line for the External Medical Review Process

Similar to the formal grievance procedure discussed later in this chapter, there must be a clear time line for the specific events that occur in the external appeals process. States that require external appeal mechanisms are not uniform in their time requirements. There is usually a time limit on when a member is still able to file for an external review or appeal, and this may vary from 3 months up to a year; ERISA requires a minimum of 180 days. State-mandated time requirements to achieve resolution of nonurgent appeals may vary from 10 to 30 days, with 30 days being required under ERISA.

Clear Communication of the External Medical Review Process

Much like the issue of timelines, it is important to have a formal process in place to ensure that all necessary and appropriate steps are taken, documentation maintained, and requirements met. It is best for a single individual from the MCO to function as the appeals case manager through all steps of the process. If there are managerial "hand-offs" taking place, the likelihood of mistakes occurring or procedures not being followed is high. Plan staff that manage this function, even if they are part of the member services organization, should be dedicated to it and not assigned on an as-needed basis (though because of the low volume of external appeals, that individual will also have other responsibilities). The ability of this individual to gain a deeper understanding of the issues may provide added insight to the medical director before the process proceeds to the final review. Last, most state laws as well as ERISA and Medicare Advantage require that all documentation used in the process be made available to members.

Identification of the External Medical Review Organization

The MCO will have contracts in place with one or more qualified, independent external medical review organizations. The reason for mentioning it here is that there may be different appeal organizations under different circumstances. For example, some formal physician groups or companies have been formed solely to provide this service, and the MCO contracts with that organization. Some states require that the physicians performing the external review be licensed in the state where the member receives services, while other states are silent on this issue and allow for national review organizations to perform this service. Some states require that the review be done only by physicians in the same specialty; others do not address this. Some states require regular certification of the appeals body. Some states mandate that all appeals be reviewed by one single organization and not by an organization selected by the MCO. Most states also provide for immunity from prosecution to the physicians participating in the appeals process, but in those states that do not, either the MCO or the appeals review organization itself must obtain appropriate insurance as well as indemnification from the parties to the appeals process.

Payment for the External Medical Review Process

This refers to who pays what for this service. The MCO generally pays the majority of the cost; this cost is estimated at approximately $500 to $1,000 per review for routine cases, more for complicated cases. Some states require the member to pay a nominal filing fee, such as $25, which is usually refunded if the appeal is successful.

Provision of Information to the External Medical Review Organization

This refers to two structural concepts: the provision of written documentation and the ability of individuals to be physically present to provide information and to argue their case. In all cases, the full medical record needs to be provided to the review organization, as well as all of the MCO's medical management records pertinent to the case at hand. Documentation of plan benefit policies may also be provided, but that may not always be necessary because this process is not one of benefits definition. The member or the member's treating physician may also add material to the medical record, and copies are provided to the plan's medical director. If there is a formal hearing, it must be clear who may attend that session. This is not as obvious an issue as it may first appear. If all parties appear at the same time, the potential for arguments between the parties is high and will significantly impede progress. Whether the member is allowed to have an attorney present is also a major issue because the presence of an attorney transforms the process into one more like a judicial hearing rather than a review of medical necessity and appropriateness. The entire process may take place solely through the review of medical records and written material. However, the appeals organization may want first-hand input, so there may need to be a policy in place that allows for such dialogues to take place, but in a nonconfrontational venue.

Expedited External Medical Review Process for Urgent Cases

An expedited appeals process is required for emergency cases or cases where there is high clinical urgency. For example, ERISA requires a review of a member's appeals of coverage denials or termination of care in urgent situations within 72 hours of the request. For the sake of good clinical decision making as well as risk management, many MCOs have an expedited review process that takes no longer than 24 hours.

Further Recourse

If after exhausting the grievance and appeals process, the member wishes to pursue fur-

ther recourse, there is a variety of means, not all of which may be available. These are briefly described as follows.

Appeal to Government Agencies

In the case of insured products under state regulation, Medicare Advantage and Medicaid plans, if the member is not satisfied with the results of the formal hearing, he or she has the right to appeal to the appropriate government agency.

Further appeal or the filing of a formal grievance with the appropriate state agency is available to members who are in commercial plans that are fully insured. Employees of state or municipal government (regardless if the municipal benefits plan is self-funded or fully insured) are also usually afforded appeal rights to state agencies. For commercially insured members, the state insurance department has jurisdiction. In cases where the grievance involves quality of care, the health department may have jurisdiction. In either case, the state will have a formal process for filing such appeals and grievances, and each MCO must be familiar with these processes and requirements.

Federal employees, or those who are covered under the Office of Personnel Management (OPM), have the right of appeal to OPM. OPM specifically reserves the right in its contract with health plans to resolve and rule on grievances by members who are federal employees. Members who are covered under entitlement programs (Medicare and Medicaid) have the right to appeal to the respective government agency.

Arbitration

In some states, arbitration is allowed for cases involving insured plans. This may occur before or after appeal to the state agency as described earlier. In those states where arbitration is allowed, and if the plan wishes to pursue it (or if it is required), the plan would comply with the regulations regarding arbitration in terms of selection of the arbitrator(s) and form of the hearing.

Lawsuits

Although not a part of a plan's grievance procedure, the last legal remedy for a disgruntled member is legal action. If the plan carefully follows its grievance procedure, the chances of a successful lawsuit against it are small. If the plan fails to follow proper policy and procedure, the chances of successful litigation are high. The right to sue is clear and relatively unfettered for all but self-insured plans, which is much more complicated; see Chapter 31 for a discussion of that issue.

CONCLUSION

Member services are a requirement of any managed care plan. The primary responsibilities of member services are to provide information to the membership in general, help guide members through the system, and help members resolve any problems or questions they may have. Member services must also track and analyze member problems and complaints so that management can act to correct problems at the source. Management of the full range of contacts between members and the health plan requires sophisticated systems support and management processes. Mechanisms to resolve complaints, grievances, and appeals are not only required by law, but make good business sense. Plan management should not be satisfied with a reactive member services function but should take a proactive approach as well.

20

HEALTHCARE CONSUMERISM

Elizabeth Bierbower*

Study Objectives

- Understand the primary drivers of health care consumerism.
- Understand the typical characteristics of today's health care consumer.
- Understand the major implications of consumerism for managed care organizations.
- Understand specific strategies and tactics being used by managed care organizations to address consumerism.
- Understand the role of data transparency in consumerism.

Discussion Topics

1. Discuss the primary drivers of health care consumerism and why each is significant.
2. Describe and discuss today's health care consumer and briefly comment on how these traits affect patients' interactions with the health care system.
3. Discuss the major implications of health care consumerism on managed care organizations. For each, provide a practical example of what an MCO can do to meet this demand.
4. Discuss how data and technology support consumer-driven health care. How might that evolve in the future?
5. Discuss the evolution of benefits design as applied to consumer-driven health care and how those benefits might evolve in the future.

---

*The views expressed in that chapter are those of the author and do not necessarily reflect the views of Humana, Inc., or its customers.

INTRODUCTION

Over the last several years, the term *consumer-driven* or *consumer-directed health plan* (CDHP; see also Chapter 2) has dotted the health insurance industry landscape. These health plans have begun to make their marks with noticeable membership that is expected to continue over the next several years. Although these plans have made an impression, it is important to note that health care consumerism is not simply about benefit plan designs or the much touted cost savings associated with moderated trend increases. Health care consumerism is a much broader concept, one that consists of many moving parts that, when working in unison, can create a powerful change in consumer behavior.

When considering health care consumerism as a broader concept, a look at the analogy of purchasing a car, although admittedly an imperfect comparison, is useful. Most individuals believe they are competent consumers when buying a car. They look at the design of the car; which is likely what attracted them to the car in the first place. A consumer wouldn't be considered savvy if he only considered the car design. An educated consumer also needs to know the price of the car, including not only the purchase price, but also the costs of warranties and even the estimated gas mileage, to determine how much she'll pay for gas each week. Reviewing the car's safety record and reliability, as well as key features such as side impact airbags and alarm systems, are also important. Consumers also want to enjoy the car experience, so features such as the CD and stereo system, the interior design, and other luxury items are assessed.

Most individuals who review all these aspects would be considered good consumers. But how did these individuals become savvy car purchasers? How did they know where to look to find out the safety record or whether the stereo system was state of the art? Consumer magazines and the Internet give individuals access to information that was previously used mostly by car manufacturers and dealerships. Over time, equipped with information, consumers began to ask questions and compare features to determine which vehicle would give the best value, based on an individual's needs and preferences.

Health care consumers are in the early stages of gaining access to information to make informed decisions. Although the Internet has offered a tremendous amount of information, some of which is not trustworthy, by itself the Internet cannot create true health care consumerism. This chapter addresses the key components needed to create and sustain the savvy health care consumer. But first, it is important to understand how the current health care system works against consumerism.

THE HEALTH CARE TRANSACTION

Typically, when purchasing a service, an estimate is provided before the work is performed. The consumer receives an explanation of the issue and an estimate of the cost of the service. In some cases, the consumer may even be provided with some alternatives. Finally, if the work is authorized, the consumer is expected to pay the amount owed in full at the time of service.

Unfortunately, most health care transactions do not work in the same way. If an individual goes to the doctor for an illness, the doctor will likely tell him what is wrong, although he may have to undergo some tests first. The individual probably does not know how much the office visit will cost (a copay is not the true cost of care), and it's doubtful that he knows how much the tests will cost. The individual will leave the doctor's office either paying a copay, if he still has a traditional plan, or pay nothing if he has a plan with a deductible applied first. The individual will go to the hospital to which his doctor has directed him and have the tests. He probably won't price shop to see if he can get the same tests performed less expensively and for equal quality somewhere else. In most cases, he won't even worry about the costs of the tests, assuming that his health plan will cover the amount in full. In fact, with nothing more than a vague understanding, the individual may not even be sure exactly what services will be performed. After the tests are completed, the individual will leave the hospital without paying anything. The individual's actions in the preceding scenario are not reflective of consumerism.

Imagine a customer dining at a restaurant and ordering dinner and drinks from a menu without prices, and then leaving the restaurant without paying. Most businesses using this approach would not be in business very long. The diner may be a frequent, even a favorite customer, but the restaurant is not going to allow her to leave the restaurant without offering a guarantee of payment. Yet the former approach is the approach under which the health care industry has operated for years.

Under the current model, it is difficult for an individual to become a consumer. However, as individuals are introduced to some of the components of consumerism, the current health care model may begin to evolve into one that changes individuals from passive patients into active consumers.

THE PLAN DESIGN

Although the plan design itself is insufficient to create sustainable consumer behavior change, it is nonetheless a very important part of consumerism. One criticism of the health maintenance organization (HMO) benefit design is that the low-cost share, designed to encourage individuals to seek treatment early, masks the true cost of care and creates a sense of entitlement. Office visits "cost" $15, emergency rooms $50, and prescriptions range from $5 to $45. Copays only show the consumer her portion of the bill and not the total cost. As a result, the consumer fails to see the value of the health insurance benefit. In addition, every time the copay increases, the consumer only sees her share of the cost increasing and is not aware of the employer's or health plan's increased costs.

One of the basic concepts behind consumer-driven health plans is that they are designed to expose the consumer to the true cost of health care and to encourage the consumer to take a more active role in his health care. The most prevalent form of plan design associated with consumerism is the high-deductible health plan (HDHP). This type of plan typically eliminates copays and subjects most benefits, including pharmacy, to the deductible. This approach results in the consumer seeing, and paying for, the full cost of the service until the deductible has been met. The ability to understand the true cost of care is often referred to as *transparency*, a concept that is discussed later in this chapter.

In the case of a Health Savings Account (HSA), the HDHP must meet certain requirements to be a qualified plan. The Internal Revenue Service (IRS)* imposes minimum deductibles and maximum out-of-pocket limits for these plans. In addition, the IRS establishes contribution limits each year based on the type of coverage the consumer has (self-only or family). These limits are indexed each year.

HDHPs may be referred to as *catastrophic health plans*. This latter term is used because the deductible is much higher than what many consumers are accustomed to ($1,000 to $1,100 versus a $250 or $500 traditional preferred provider organization deductible). It is important to look past the deductible and at the underlying coverage. Most of these plans provide comprehensive preferred provider organization (PPO) coverage in part or in full once the deductible has been met.

All consumer-driven plans are not high-deductible plans. In fact, any plan that helps the consumer understand the true cost of care might be labeled a consumer-driven plan. In the world of dental insurance, most plans contain a provision known as a *scheduled benefit*, which means the plan agrees to pay a percentage of the bill up to a designated

---

*The IRS has this authority because funds that go into the HSA are considered pre-tax dollars.

amount and the consumer pays the rest. For example, a dental plan may pay 50% of the costs of a crown based on a maximum allowable charge of $700. The consumer understands that if the crown costs $700 or less, his maximum financial exposure is $350. If the cost of the crown exceeds $700, the consumer is responsible for the amount that exceeds $700 in addition to his 50% cost share. Scheduled benefit plans help consumers understand the cost of the service before the service is provided. Some health plans have offered similar medical benefits with limited success. Although these plans do engage the consumer, they often do not provide the "peace of mind protection" associated with other health plan designs in the event of a medical catastrophe.

By way of an example in health insurance, Humana offers its SmartSuite plans as a means to engage consumers in their health care. SmartSuite offers consumers a choice of plan designs, including HMO, PPO, and consumer-driven. These plans are wrapped with decision tools and educational information to help consumers choose their health benefits and then use them throughout the plan year. This approach has yielded SmartSuite customers annualized medical cost trends of 5% to 6%.[1]

Over the years, most plan designs have covered preventive care services in full or with minimal cost share with the thought that consumers would forgo preventive care if forced to pay for these services themselves. Preventive care continues to be an important feature of consumer-driven plan designs. Most CDHPs pay for preventive services prior to the deductible not only to encourage the appropriate behaviors, but also to drive plan adoption.

Some critics believe consumer-driven plan designs will result in nothing more than cost shifting to the consumer and that some consumers may chose to forgo needed treatment. Of particular concern are prescription drugs. A concern is that subjecting these services to a deductible of $1,000 or more will result in less compliance with much-needed medications.

Typically, insurance policies such as homeowners, auto, or life don't cover routine expenses. These insurance plans are designed to cover catastrophic events such as fire, accidents, and even death, leaving the consumer responsible for assuming the cost of routine services. Health plans that want consumers to self-fund a portion of their routine care (preventive and illness-related) must become creative. Consumers will want to understand the trade-off for paying out-of-pocket for routine services. Refer to Figure 20-1 as an example of helping consumers understand the trade-offs between premium and point-of-service costs.

Traditional PPO		High-Deductible Health Plan	
Annual premium		Annual premium	
($100 12 months)	$1,200	($40 12 months)	$480
Deductible	$500	Deductible	$2,500
Office visit copays		Office visit copays	
$305	$150	(part of the deductible)	-$0-
Pharmacy copays		Pharmacy copays	
Avg 2 rx/mo at $20	$480	(part of the deductible)	-$0-
Other out-of-pocket		Other out-of-pocket	
(co-insurance)	$2000	(co-insurance at 100%)	-$0-
Tax savings	-$0-	Tax savings (25%)	$625
Total costs	**$4,330**	**Total costs**	
			$3,625
		Savings	**$705**

Figure 20–1 Understanding Premium and Point-of-Service Costs

Perhaps the benefit is a significantly lower premium or may be the consumer earns credits for obtaining preventive services that can be converted to cash or other rewards. In the short term, health plans have some challenges ahead to reshape consumers' perspective on which services and how much they should self-fund.

Health care is not viewed in the same light as other insurance coverage. Access to health care is viewed as a right by many and, as such, the success of consumer-driven plan designs will be measured in part by access to services. Only time will tell if these plan designs inhibit access to care, and it will be important to monitor compliance for routine care and prescription drugs under consumer-driven plans and traditional HMO and PPO plans.

CONVERGENCE OF HEALTH INSURANCE AND FINANCIAL SERVICES

With the introduction of Health Savings Accounts (HSAs), we have begun to hear about the convergence of health insurance and financial services. Banks and other financial service institutions have begun to partner with health insurers, brokers, and employers to offer Health Savings Accounts and lines of credit. Any discussion of consumerism would be incomplete without addressing these partnerships and services.

Health Care Spending Accounts

The most notable feature of the consumer-driven plan is the HSA or the Health Reimbursement Account (HRA). These accounts are typically attached to an HDHP and are designed to offset a portion of the deductible to ensure that resources are available for routine care. Well before the introduction of the HSA and HRA, the Flexible Spending Account (FSA) was born. In the 1990s, the Archer Medical Savings Account, another form of health care spending account, also became available.

Each of these accounts has its own nuances; however, they are similar in that they are designed primarily for pre-tax contributions (either by the employer, employee, or both) and can be used to offset qualified medical expenses. Some spending accounts are designed exclusively for short-term tax savings and use and others allow consumers to budget or plan for long-term health care expenses.

Regardless of the spending account type, the nature of these accounts engages consumers in paying more attention to how they are spending their health care dollars. Regardless of who makes the contribution under an employer-sponsored plan, proponents of consumerism believe that the employee feels as if she is spending her own money and therefore will be more involved in understanding the costs of her care as well as the treatment alternatives.

Health Savings Accounts

HSAs have filled a void found in other types of spending accounts and present several advantages to consumers. Portability of funds as the consumer moves from one employer to another or into the self-insured pool encourages contribution to the account and overcomes the fear of "use it or lose it" associated with FSAs. HSAs benefit spenders as well as savers. Those who need or choose to use the HSA funds still enjoy the same benefit of tax savings as those individuals who save for retirement. Finally, the HSA can serve as a long-term savings vehicle that becomes increasingly important as employees face retirement without employer-sponsored coverage. Most consumers are not aware of what their out-of-pocket health care expenses might be once they retire and, furthermore, they have not saved enough to cover these costs. In a statement released in March 2006, Fidelity Investments estimates that a 65-year-old couple retiring today without employer-sponsored health insurance will need $200,000 to cover medical costs in retirement.[2] This projection is based on the assumption that the consumer has Medicare.

Employer advantages include lower health insurance premiums, tax savings, and employees that are more engaged in their health. Small employers, who previously have not been able to afford to offer health insurance, may be able to opt back into the insurance pool through CDHPs. All employers benefit from engaging consumers in their health care.

Health Savings Accounts also have detractors. These accounts have been referred to as another tax advantage for the wealthy with concern that lower-income individuals will not be able to afford to fund the account and cover the cost of care. The chronically ill draw additional concerns particularly over whether these individuals will forgo treatment or ever save sufficient funds because their high usage causes them to routinely deplete their account funds. Some consumer satisfaction studies have shown some mixed results with those in these new HDHPs or consumer-driven plans showing less satisfaction than those in a traditional plan. These differences in satisfaction may be linked to lack of education, the newness of the plans, or the fact that the increased upfront cost share creates real concern for consumers.

Spending accounts are a vital part of health care consumerism. Some people believe that, with the introduction of HSAs, the FSA is dead. The FSA continues to have a great deal of potential given that the majority of insureds will not be enrolled in a consumer-driven health plan over the next several years. In addition, coupling an FSA with an HSA for limited purposes or post deductible expenses enables HSA savers to maximize their tax savings. In a very short time, the introduction of the consumer-driven plan design, and in particular the combination of the HDHP and the HSA, is doing very well with significant growth expected to continue over the next 5 years.

Bad Debt

Opponents of consumer-driven health plans believe these plans do nothing more than shift the costs to consumers and force more debt onto their shoulders. Health insurers counter this argument, stating that, with the proper tools and information, consumers can in fact lower their overall health care costs. In the middle are doctors, hospitals, and other health care providers who fear they will be left holding the bag as consumers fail to pay their share of the costs.

New products and services have arisen out of this pending concern of health care debt. For example, Exante Financial Services, a division of UnitedHealth Group, is piloting a line of credit through its subsidiary, Exante Bank. Through this approach, the provider bills the carrier and the bank pays the provider both the health plan's and the member's responsibilities. Members have the opportunity to pay their cost share in full directly to Exante Bank within a designated time frame or to take advantage of the credit option.[3,4]

Other health insurers are offering credit through a more traditional approach, the credit card. These cards may be used for general purposes or they may be limited to health care purchases. Although the approaches vary, what these financial services institutions and health insurers have in common is that they are offering a means for consumers to help bridge the gap between the deductible and the available funds in a health care spending account or to simply fund increasingly higher copayments and deductibles.

Although some may not like the fact that consumers may need to access credit to pay for health care, the reality is that consumers must recognize that health care costs need to be part of their household budgets and have options either through budgeting or credit to pay for these expenses.

Borrowing Technology

Traditionally, health care and insurance systems have been proprietary. Standard transaction sets have been developed over the years to facilitate the exchange of information between health care providers and payers.

Technology from the financial services industry is playing an increasingly important role in the delivery of and payment for health care. The introduction of swipe cards provided consumers with easy access to health care spending account funds and offered providers some minor relief in collections of accounts receivables. Use of these cards has been expanded to verify patients' eligibility for coverage and copay amounts. Smart card technology has been deployed in a limited manner to perform some of the same functions, as well as hold limited personal health records information.

Health plans benefit from these technologies by trading manual transactions for electronic ones. Health care providers receive timely and accurate information that helps minimize bad debt and consumers avoid the hassle of filing manual claims and other paperwork. The challenge that lies ahead is to continue to push health care providers, payers, and the government to adopt lower-cost, open platforms and technologies that have been proven in other industries.

Partnerships

Health insurers have partnered with financial services institutions to bring these various forms of spending accounts to employers and consumers. Although the majority of health plans have formed referral relationships with banks, others have decided to provide HSAs and some other financial transactions as a core competency.

Some health insurers have chartered a bank either on their own or in conjunction with other health plans. The reasons for these moves varies from the desire to own additional pieces in the health care value chain to the desire to provide a lower cost alternative collectively than what a health plan may achieve independently. Those who are choosing to dive deeper into financial services believe that through spending accounts and other services, they can develop strong and lasting employer and consumer relationships.

In the world of 401(k) retirement plans, an employer does not shop for a new plan administrator year after year. The employer desires to maintain a level of stability in managing its employees' funds. Health care spending accounts and lines of credit offer health plans the same opportunity for employer and employee retention. Those plans that can offer seamless medical plan and spending account administration may have an advantage in retaining the employer's and thus the employee's business over a longer period of time.

TRANSPARENCY

Helping consumers gain an effective understanding of health care costs and value requires multiple approaches. Having access to cost, quality, and other relevant information can transform most purchasing processes. The same multifaceted review must apply to health care. Costs alone are inadequate to make a decision on most other treatments or services. When a doctor recommends a prescription, price is certainly a factor. However, consideration should also be given to the drug's possible side effects as well as the frequency and method of consumption of the drug. Understanding each of these factors and collectively assessing whether to proceed with the doctor's treatment plan is all a part of transparency.

Cost

As in other industries, the word *cost* has several meanings in health care. The manufacturer's, retail, and allowable costs all come into play. The retail cost is what is often referred to as "billed charges" and typically includes a substantial profit margin. For a prescription drug, for example, the retail cost would be the price a consumer pays if he or she does not have insurance coverage for drugs (a health plan would pay based on a combination of maximum allowable charge, fill fee, discounts, and rebates as discussed in Chapter 12). Ironically, the uninsured are typically the only individuals subject to the retail cost of health care. Through the effort of consumer advocacy groups, many health care providers and drug manufacturers now offer the uninsured discounts on medical bills for selected services or drugs.

As noted in Chapters 6, 7, and 12, health plans have negotiated to pay providers who are part of the plan's network at less than retail charges. Health insurers are able to negotiate these discounts in exchange for steering a volume of services or consumers to the provider. Like a purchasing club, the health plan buys in bulk, and then passes the savings on to employers and consumers. Most consumers do not realize the significant savings the health plan negotiates on their behalf. Too many individuals believe they are paying more than their fair share of health insurance costs simply because they do not realize what their employer pays toward premiums or what the health plan pays in claims costs.

The consumer's cost is determined based on this allowable amount or is a flat fee or copay. Copays have traditionally been a simple straightforward way for consumers to understand their cost share responsibility. Copay amounts have been increased over the years but have not always kept up with inflation. A concern about the copay is that it masks the cost of care. Individuals only see their cost share and do not see what the health plan pays for the service. As a result, the consumer may believe she is paying a greater portion of the cost share than the health plan or employer. Conversely, if copays are too low, they may drive unnecessary demand for services. For example, a $10 office visit copay could drive increased demand for doctors' services than would a $30 copay (*ie*, the economic barrier is lower at $10 than it is at $30). Sharing information, particularly on retail costs and allowed amounts, will help individuals become more engaged in understanding the cost of care and how they can help become better health care consumers.

In other industries, the cost of the service is determined on a real-time basis or predetermined terminations are made before the service is rendered. A home repair service provides a written estimate, retailers post prices, and even salons and other service-oriented providers provide advance notice of cost. Cost estimates are rare in the health care industry when a third-party payer is involved. Most health plans are unable to provide an estimate for services and procedures. Health plans are not alone; most hospitals and doctors offices can't provide this information either. The inability to get an estimate may have less to do with the uncertainty around the service and procedure and more to do with the fact that health care providers have never been asked for this information and, as a result, have not been equipped to provide price information in a meaningful or useful way.

One reason for not providing estimates may be the uncertainty associated with a procedure. For example, in the case of surgery, complications may arise or a more extensive procedure may be required once the consumer is in the operating room. In addition, a typical outpatient or inpatient procedure involves many different providers, the surgeon, the anesthesiologist, and the hospital. Each of these providers has its own pricing structure and may or may not have an agreement with the health plan. This piecemeal approach to health care makes it challenging for the consumer to understand.

Challenging or not, health plans and providers must begin to share pricing information. Exact figures may not be necessary. Perhaps the consumer can be provided with an estimated range of costs prior to the surgery, a low-end price for no complications, and a high-end price with complications. Some health care providers have begun to take steps to share pricing with consumers. Although still in the early stages, these innovators demonstrate that sharing this information may be a means for creating a competitive advantage and creating differentiation with the competition.

Creative providers will go a step further and alleviate the risk to the consumer. Flat-fee arrangements that factor in that a certain segment of the population will experience complications are standard between provider and payer. Sharing these flat-fee arrangements helps the consumer budget more accurately.

Some health care providers claim that displaying the full cost of care is meaningless because of the health plans' negotiated discounts and the belief that consumers should be concerned only about their own share of the cost. Consumers see the retail price in every other transaction, even when they have the benefit of leveraging a "club" discount. There is no reason to shield the consumer. Information should be provided in a useable format, and consumers should be given the freedom to decide whether and how to use it.

Real-Time Claims Adjudication

Ideally, costs should be shared with the consumer prior to or at the time of service. Health care is the only industry in which a consumer receives a service without understanding the total cost and is not required to pay at the time of service (except for a small copay in the case of most office visits). Consumers don't accept this approach in conducting other transactions but do accept this approach as the norm in health care. The approach to the health care transaction is slowly beginning to change.

Pharmacies have been the exception to the rule. When purchasing a prescription at a pharmacy, the consumer often knows at point-of-sale the retail prescription cost, the allowable amount, what the health plan covers, and her cost share. The consumer can even ask for the cost prior to having the prescription filled and can review lower-cost alternatives. How does the pharmacy give this valuable information on a moment's notice? As discussed in Chapter 12, health plans have contracted with providers called pharmacy benefits managers (PBMs) for years. The PBMs have created real-time claims adjudication systems that enable the pharmacist

to know exactly how much the insurer will pay as well as what to collect from the consumer. The pharmacy is guaranteed payment from the health plan. This process is called real-time claims adjudication, and it is exactly what is needed for health care consumerism to grow. If these PBMs have been able to master the art of real-time claims adjudication for tens of thousands of prescriptions, then why can't health plans and providers do the same?

Some health plans have begun to experiment with this type of real-time processing, even working with competitors to do so. These real-time systems help doctors' offices verify eligibility and process claims on a real-time basis, enabling collection from the consumer at the point of service. Typically, these real-time systems are designed to overlay and extract information from the health insurer's proprietary systems. Investment in real-time technologies is not inexpensive for health plans; however, this technology becomes increasingly more important in a world where copays are being replaced by HDHPs.

Some hospitals and health care professionals don't want to release their costs or negotiated rates for fear that consumers will think they are too expensive and seek services elsewhere. Consumers purchase for a variety of reasons. Some consumers buy almost exclusively on price, whereas others look at the quality of the merchandise, among other features. When it comes to their health, and when armed with the right information, most consumers will consider more than the price when weighing their health care treatment options. Health care providers increasingly will be pressured to share their cost information and demonstrate to consumers the value they offer for the services they provide. The majority of consumers are smart enough to look at multiple factors before making a decision. If one of the results of sharing cost information means that price competition may emerge, the consumer, employer, and the health plan will all benefit.

For example, LASIK* surgery is a procedure that has survived and even thrived in a free-market economy. LASIK is typically a discretionary service, not covered by insurance—and therefore, free of the negative effects of our insurance system. The evolution of the pricing for this procedure demonstrates how price transparency can help drive down health care costs.

When LASIK surgery was introduced in the United States in the early 1990s, few providers performed the service and the cost of the procedure was much higher than it is today. And although prices still vary, overall the average cost of this procedure is much lower today than when the service was first introduced. Consumers who wanted this procedure understood that they were to bear the full cost of the service. Many consumers became early adopters and purchased the service. Some did so for the aesthetic benefits and others had the procedure mostly because they wanted to rid themselves of the hassles and long-term expense associated with eye glasses and contact lenses.

As consumers opted for LASIK surgery, more providers began offering the service and the cost of the procedure decreased. Furthermore, the competition among providers increased, with promotions touting the provider's qualifications, equipment, or relaxed atmosphere becoming the norm. Some providers even used celebrities to promote their capabilities.

LASIK is a discretionary procedure as are many medical services. In many situations, the consumer has the time and the option to gain a second opinion or collect information about his or her condition or proposed treatment plan. Facing increased cost share and armed with the freedom to seek health care from any health care provider, consumers will begin to shop for their health care in a manner similar to how they shop for other goods and services.

---

*Laser-Assisted *In Situ* Keratomileusis (LASIK) is a treatment intended to improve vision.

IT'S NOT JUST ABOUT COST

Cost is clearly an important consideration in health care, but health care consumerism must not be defined as simply knowing the cost of a service or procedure. Consumers want quality goods and services delivered in a convenient manner. They also want to be treated with respect and dignity and to participate in the health care decision-making process. More important, individuals know they have the intelligence and are gaining the confidence to become savvy health care consumers. Other key features that consumers will consider on their path to becoming health care consumers are explored in these next few pages.

Quality

The word *quality* is readily used in health care, but consensus on its meaning has not been reached. In the past, indicators of quality may have included the provider's education or board certification. Some health care providers have touted the volume of procedures as a means to let consumers know their expertise in a certain area. Others have relied on measures such as readmission and mortality rates. No one single measure is an indicator of quality, and nationwide consensus on quality has not been reached. Although the issue of what constitutes quality is not going to be settled in this chapter (the reader is referred to Chapter 15 for a full discussion of quality management by health plans), it does include an overview of some information that is available for consumers to consider when making decisions about their health care.

Credentials are a reasonable place to start, however, many consumers will assume that going to medical school or completing a residency means the doctor is well-qualified to perform the service or procedure needed. Although standards are indeed high, not all medical schools and residency programs are equal in training. Furthermore, board certification in one area does not mean the doctor is qualified to perform any procedure, yet many health plans publish these credentials without providing additional guidance as to how the consumer might use or evaluate this information. Some consumer magazines have published information on doctors and hospitals and display their criteria for assessment. But these assessments are limited in scope and routinely do not help the consumer who is trying to find a family practitioner or an allergist in his neighborhood. What consumers need is access to important information on health care providers and also the ability to search and sort on criteria that are indicative of high performance and are important to the consumer.

Safety is another important aspect of health care consumerism and one that has not been paid the level of attention required by the consumer. Significant progress has been made in the area of safety, in particular by health care coalitions that typically consist of employers who are pushing the health care community on the issues of transparency and safety. Through the efforts of these organizations, health care providers are encouraged to adhere to standards and consumers are provided with useful information about health care safety. Health plans share this information with consumers to help them make choices about where to get their care. The belief is that many quality and safety problems exist in our system; we need transparency to encourage providers to fix them; transparency about performance will create demand pressure as consumers seek out high performers.

Employers have been the most active at promoting transparency and serve in the role of consumer advocates. Through the voices of large employers that are viewed as large purchasers of health care services, providers as well as health plans feel some pressure to participate in developing and adhering to quality and safety guidelines.

Marketing

Marketing and advertising in health care may not be as obvious as they are in other industries. Health care providers freely advertise discretionary services that are not covered by health insurance. Discretionary or self-pay services such as cosmetic surgery, LASIK surgery, or eyeglasses are examples of services that are routinely advertised. Health care professionals who provide these services proudly display the list of services they offer. Beyond noncovered services, more doctors are beginning to advertise their services and promote their competencies. Consumers want to know that their doctors are specialists and whether they specialize in certain areas of need or interest to the consumer. For example, a doctor may advertise herself as a specialist in women's health, thus appealing to a portion of the female population.

Hospitals have been generating direct-to-consumer advertising about their services for years, typically citing the volumes of procedures and perhaps even disclosing some important statistic. Pharmaceutical companies have perhaps been the most effective at marketing their services direct to the consumer. Television and magazine advertisements tout the wonders of the drug (and in fairness the possible list of side effects). Concerns have been raised over direct-to-consumer marketing by drug manufacturers because it is believed to cause some consumers to ask for drugs by name. Brand name recognition will certainly cause a consumer to ask about a particular drug. However, when the consumer also understands the cost of the service as well as availability of lower-cost treatment alternatives, he will use this additional information and not just brand recognition in making a purchasing decision. Knowledge is powerful, and when consumers are provided with useful and actionable information and share in the cost of care, they make better health care decisions.

Show Me the Data

A concern over direct-to-consumer marketing is that the appropriate measures of performance and benchmarks do not exist. Currently, the consumer has limited means of comparing whether the information the provider has shared is meaningful in determining quality or performance. Until meaningful performance information is available, consumers are still at a big disadvantage. Transparency includes coming to agreement about how to measure physician and hospital performance.

Several national initiatives regarding provider performance are under way. For example, the Centers for Medicare and Medicaid Services (CMS) is beginning to invest heavily in measurement development and demonstrations to drive the public availability of information on performance. CMS now publishes hospital data, and other companies provide health plans with hospital information and allow the consumer to compare provider performance. These companies have created tools that use Medicare and limited payer data to show volumes of procedures as well as some quality indicators such as morbidity and mortality rates.

This same level of data sharing has not been applied to health care professionals. With few exceptions, little has been published about the performance of doctors and other health care professionals, yet the performance of these providers is critical to assessing quality. Some insights can be gained by looking at a hospital's performance, but to assume that quality only needs to be monitored in the hospital setting is folly.

Some accreditation organizations publish on their Web sites information geared toward consumers (see Chapter 23). Others are entering into recognition programs that identify physicians that are practicing best-practice medicine. Minor steps have been taken with some health plans engaging in pay-for-performance programs that reward doctors based on efficiency, outcomes, and accreditation for specific diseases such as diabetes (see Chapter 8). Furthermore, some attention is being given to providers who have adopted technology to manage their populations more efficiently.

As noted in Chapter 16, a limited number of health insurers have developed high-performance networks. These networks contain those providers that meet the health plan's criteria for quality or efficiency. Some employers are exploring benefit plan designs such as tiered or high-performance networks to drive employees to cost-efficient or high-quality providers.

These initiatives are a step in the right direction, and these tools provide useful information for consumers. Unfortunately, the use of this information still appears to be low. Without national or uniform standards to measure quality or effectiveness, it is challenging to gain momentum; however, consumers can be a powerful voice and employers can be their proxy at times to push health plans and providers to create standards and release data.

ACCESS

In the past, a consumer may have faced long waiting times in the doctor's office. Some providers were not efficient at managing patient flow, and consumers had lower expectations of appointment timeliness. The days of a consumer waiting patiently well past the appointed time are gone or soon will be. Most consumers highly value their own time, recognizing that they have precious little of it. They resent sitting in a waiting room full of sick individuals because the practice is inefficient.

Some doctors have recognized the need for convenient access to health care that values the consumer's time and allows more time for the doctor-patient interaction. As a result, concierge-style medical practices have been appearing, particularly in areas with a significant retiree or wealthy population. Reactions to these practices have been varied. Some consumers are opposed to the idea of paying an access fee to a physician and then paying for services rendered. Consumers will pay an access fee for a purchasing club membership or access to a country club, and then also pay for the items purchased or the games played but are offended that a doctor's practice would operate under similar principles. This sense of entitlement in health care will begin to shift to a focus on value as the consumer becomes more engaged.

The idea of having access that results in a reduced time for obtaining an appointment, minimal time in the waiting room, and the ability to talk with the physician after hours in the case of an emergency is appealing to some individuals. Those who believe this idea will vanish quickly need to consider the sandwich generation and the baby boomers. Individuals who are raising children and taking care of parents simultaneously are time poor. These individuals may be willing to pay for their parents to have immediate and extended access to a trusted health care provider. The baby boomer generation will change the face of health care. Their consumption of health care services to maintain a healthy and active lifestyle far into their retirement years will drive demand for services, and some boomers with financial means will pay for access to a boutique practice. Not everyone will embrace the idea of concierge services, but enough will that these practices will find a niche market at the very least.

CONVENIENCE

The world today operates on a 24/7 basis. Consumers shop online or telephonically at almost any time of day or night. Automatic teller machines (ATMs) give consumers access to funds not only around the clock, but also around the world. Consumers are busy juggling careers, kids, and households. Consumers are time poor and many are reluctant to take additional time away from work for routine services. And it's not just time, it is location, location, location. Shopping malls have grown over the years because they provide virtually one-stop shopping within the mall or in very close proximity to meet consumers' needs. Consumers want services that are easy to access in a convenient location, and the health care industry is starting to oblige.

A new form of health care provider often referred to as "mini clinics" is appearing in discount retailer and grocery stores. In addition to purchasing groceries, picking up the dry cleaning, renting a DVD, and completing a banking transaction, the consumer can pop into one of these clinics and get basic health care services such as a quick office visit and a strep test. Typically staffed with a physician assistant or a nurse practitioner, these clinics are designed to treat minor illnesses or injuries and issue routine prescriptions that can be filled at the store's in-house pharmacy. Prices are posted so consumers understand what a service will cost. These clinics have typically operated on a cash-only basis, although some are beginning to contract with health insurers. These clinic visits may be lower in cost to the health insurer than a traditional office visit is.

Although some health care providers are concerned that these clinics are in direct competition with family doctors, the companies that manage these clinics beg to differ, stating that they do not treat serious or chronic conditions and urge consumers to establish a relationship with a family doctor. These clinics are filling a niche by providing consumers with low-cost and convenient access to health care services.

These retail-based clinics are not the only type of health care services shifting away from the traditional physician's office or hospital. Freestanding imaging and outpatient surgery centers have been siphoning business away from hospitals for years. They tout extended hours, a more comfortable setting, and convenience. Consumers want to receive routine health services as quickly and painlessly as possible, and these types of facilities meet this need. In many cases, these facilities also meet the cost test. Because many of these facilities are not affiliated with a hospital, their overhead and ultimate cost to the consumer may be lower.

Urgent care centers, which typically provide more comprehensive services than the retail clinic does, have also filled the void of extended physician office hours. Although many physician practices offer some form of extended hours today, in many cases, the number of appointments is severely limited and often confined to urgent situations. In a 24/7 world where the consumer has the freedom to choose any provider, the traditional 9-to-5 model no longer fits. Ironically, hospitals have recognized the need to provide urgent care clinics as a means to reach consumers in their own communities.

But health care providers are not the only entities that need to be more responsive to consumer needs, health plans have opportunities for improvement as well. Many health plans believe that providing access until 8:00pm local time is adequate. Most working families are barely finishing dinner or reviewing homework with the kids by 8:00pm. Consideration has to be given to meeting the consumer's needs for service. Those health care providers and insurers that recognize the value of consumer's time will create loyalty that may lead to retention and higher profits.

INFORMATION AND DECISION SUPPORT TOOLS

Access to information is a major driver of health care consumerism. The Internet has long been regarded as the technology that has transformed access to health information, and one cannot argue that it has had a tremendous impact. The Internet has its issues in that some of the information available is unreliable at best and, in fact, may be untrue. Consumers must have access to trusted sources of information regarding treatment options, costs, and conditions.

Health care content providers have provided useful information on traditional and alternative medicine for consumers. Many health insurers purchase this content and provide it to their members free of charge. Having access to information from an independent third-party resource gives consumers the assurance that the information is not biased by the health insurer and gives the consumer confidence in understanding the condition and various treatment alternatives.

In addition to health content, decision support tools have been developed to assist consumers in choosing and using their health care benefits. When choosing a health plan, consumers often have access to a health plan "wizard" that helps them compare plan features, premiums, and other out-of-pocket expenses. These tools get consumers to think beyond their premium contributions and help them understand the total cost of their health care over the coming year. Using modeling tools, consumers can estimate how many office visits or prescription drugs will be used throughout the year. This use information is factored into the overall costs and the consumer gets a clearer picture of how much he will spend in premium contributions as well as in copayments and deductibles. These budgeting tools also include calculators that help the consumer estimate the amount to put into a flexible spending account or Health Savings Account. Health insurers, consumer advocacy groups, and other independent third parties are making these tools available to consumers as a means to help consumers plan for their health care expenditures.

Although many of these tools are Web based, health insurers have recognized that they must also reach out and engage consumers, rather than relying on the member to come to their Web sites. The use of voice activation technology is one example. Voice activation technology uses a computer-generated voice to generate messages that educate consumers about the need for preventive services or lower-cost drug treatment alternatives. This technology allows consumers the opportunity to ask for additional information via e-mail or snail mail and to leave comments on their experiences with the call. These reach-and-engage strategies have proved to be effective in touching consumers who would otherwise not contact the insurer.

Another emerging means of interacting with consumers is the cell phone. This technology is used by a broad range of consumers, including the very young to the very old. At first used exclusively for talking, cell phones have expanded to text messaging, as well as playing games and capturing information. Imagine a scenario in which a teenage diabetic who has struggled to maintain control of her diet and her health is aided by a cell phone. Through the cell phone, the teenager receives messages that remind her to check her blood glucose level and enter the results into the phone. The information is passed back to a database and can be viewed and monitored by her doctor or her health plan's nurse. Messages reminding the teenager to eat regularly as well as healthy tips are provided as motivation to keep the teen on track.

The use of the cell phone in health care is emerging and it has some predecessor technologies that have laid the foundation. The health care industry has used in-home devices to monitor individuals with diabetes and other conditions, as discussed in Chapter 10. These stationary devices will soon give way to cell phones and other mobile devices to fit with consumer lifestyles. In fact, text messaging has already been used to provide consumers with health information in a limited manner, including information on sexually transmitted diseases and pregnancy. Other mobile technologies are being explored as well. These are a few examples of a growing trend in using widespread technologies to provide health information.

The most common form of contact between a health insurer and a consumer has been the Explanation of Benefits (EOB) statements. Unfortunately, these statements have typically led to confusion. By the time the health insurer has applied its discount and claims administration rules, it's hard to determine exactly what the health insurer paid, and the consumer may be unsure of his cost share. Health plans have followed the lead of financial services and have begun to provide personalized statements to their members. These statements include summary information on the consumer's health care transactions for the quarter or the plan year. They include information on claims, how much the member has spent toward the deductible, as well as tips on saving money on health care services. Health care statements are designed to reach out and engage consumers so they will use their health benefits wisely.

INCENTIVES AND REWARDS

Health isn't only about being sick or accessing information on conditions or treatments. The concept of health involves living and taking care of oneself every day. To foster this interest in health, a plethora of magazines covering healthy lifestyles has blanketed the shelves of retailers, and traditional magazines that cover broader issues routinely include sections on healthy living.

Even though information on healthy living and behaviors is widely available, most consumers don't act on it. They don't loose that extra weight or exercise regularly, and they struggle with portion control. A great advantage of health care consumerism is that it begins to get consumers to think about their health and lifestyles differently. Wellness is back in vogue, but it has a new twist. Once equated with answering a long health questionnaire or attending a smoking cessation class, wellness has graduated to a new level. Consumers are interested in living more active, healthier lifestyles and the idea of sitting on a rocking chair during retirement is dead. Consumers want to look good and feel good at every age, and they now have plenty of choices at their fingertips to help them do so.

This increased interest in healthy living translates to profitable ventures for enterprising individuals. Consumers participate in many forms of lifestyle clubs, including fitness, biking, and walking clubs. They routinely reach into their pockets and pay for exercise videos, yoga mats, workout clothes, and other gear. They spend millions of dollars on home exercise equipment and, increasingly, on body monitoring devices. New players are emerging in the wellness space and some unique partnerships are being formed. Former Internet pioneers are investing in health care. Food companies are partnering in health and well-being companies. Some health insurers have also entered the fray through investment or management arrangements.

Health plans are purchasing services from companies that create incentive and rewards programs designed specifically to motivate consumers to increase their physical activity and improve their health. Consumers earn rewards for routine activities such as walking, running, biking, or going to the gym or for lowering their cholesterol or improving their body mass index. These rewards programs are designed to motivate consumers to get off the couch and live a healthier lifestyle. Recognizing that these measures can lower costs, employers are paying employees to stop smoking or take a health risk assessment similar to covering preventive health services in the past. And when employers do not cover a service, they often provide access at work for weight loss or other programs that can benefit their employees. Whether purchasing a prepackaged program or developing their own customized programs, employers and insurers understand that having employees with healthier lifestyles translates into lower health care costs.

Active employees are not the only individuals who are the target of wellness programs. Health plans that are providing services to the ever-increasing senior population are also interested in keeping seniors active and healthy by offering free fitness club membership with classes that are designed specifically for older adults. Wellness programs coupled with incentives and rewards will continue to grow in importance in health plan or employee benefits offerings not only as a means to lower costs, but also as a means for attracting or retaining employees or members. Wellness and prevention in managed care are discussed in detail in Chapter 14.

THE CONSUMER EXPERIENCE

The fragmented health care system results in a less than optimal consumer experience. If asked to share a positive recent positive experience, a consumer is unlikely to relate a story about receiving health care services. Consumers are often forced to provide redundant information to health care providers year after year or from one location to the next. Their health insurers force them through a series of interactive voice response prompts before they can speak to a representative. The level of customer service in health care has been mediocre at best, but times are changing.

With the rise in health care consumerism, individuals *will* shop for services based on cost, quality, and experience. Increased consumer cost share and access to information will drive this shift. Like the example of LASIK noted earlier, an early sign of the emerging consumer experience can be found in the cosmetic surgery industry. The majority of cosmetic procedures are not covered by insurance; therefore, consumers are looking to minimize expenses and maximize their experience. Because there is no health plan to guide them in-network, the consumer is forced to review the provider's credentials and understand the risks and costs associated with the treatment.

As with other industries, health care providers do not want to be viewed as a commodity. Most want to compete on something other than price. Cosmetic surgery centers are an example of health care providers catering to the consumer's needs and not competing on price. These centers offer state-of-the-art facilities in a relaxing atmosphere that protects the privacy of their clientele. Some facilities arrange for recuperation at a nearby luxury hotel with personal follow-up visits from the center's staff. These extras, atmosphere, privacy, and personal attention equate to value for consumers and profitability for health care providers. Although the majority of cosmetic services are discretionary, it is easy to see how some of these aspects can translate to most any practice or hospital provider, resulting in loyalty, satisfaction, and a source of referrals.

The world of health care has also gone global. Other countries are courting Americans and wealthy individuals from around the world to have heart surgery and other routine procedures performed in their countries. Some foreign nations are offering new and innovative procedures, not yet approved by the U.S. Food and Drug Administration, giving hope and alternatives to consumers who face limited treatment alternatives in their own countries. The term *medical tourism* is used to refer to consumers who receive health care treatments in exotic or foreign locations designed to create an overall lower cost and more pleasant consumer experience. Consumers seek care in other countries for a variety of reasons, including lower costs and to avoid long waiting times. Many of these overseas facilities are state-of-the-art and use U.S.-educated and trained physicians. Whether the service is partly funded by a health plan or paid in full by the consumer, individuals want value for their money. Health care providers and health plans will need to step up and ensure that consumers find this value through their products and services or they risk losing business.

CONCLUSION

Health care consumerism is beginning to take hold. Consumerism is not a fad or fleeting fancy. Faced with increasing health care costs, consumers will take their health care decisions more seriously. Health plans will be forced to provide helpful tools and information as a minimum to compete. Health care providers will be forced to demonstrate their value and quality to consumers. Both parties will begin competing on a platform of transparency.

Health care consumers will demand this information and as they gain knowledge and power will push for more information. Consumers will vote with their feet as well as their pocket books. Employers will no longer make the health plan purchasing decisions solely on cost, and plan designs will play less of a role in health plan selection. The ability to provide consumers with timely and accurate information as well as guidance will be paramount in competing for new and retaining existing members.

Most important, health care consumerism will help create sustainable behavior change rather than the 1-year stop-gap measures typically seen with plan design changes. The consumer is at the table, though some come willingly and others are more reluctant. This transition is to be expected in any industry, with early adopters taking the lead and others following at a little slower pace.

Although predictions about what the future holds vary, most agree that there is no turning back. As consumers gain confidence, health care providers and health plans will be forced to deliver the value consumers expect.

References

1. Health care consumers: Passive or active? A three-year report on Humana's Consumer Solution. June 2005 Penny Hahn.
2. Fidelity.com. Press release. March 6, 2006.
3. Exante Financial Services. Available at: http://www.exantefinancialservices. com. Accessed October 18, 2006.
4. Exante Bank. Exante Bank—Health Savings Accounts. Available at: http://www.exantebankhsa. com. Accessed October 18, 2006.

21

SALES AND MARKETING

Richard F. Birhanzel

Study Objectives

- Understand the basic activities of sales and marketing within a managed care organization.
- Understand how marketing differs from sales.
- Understand compensation of sales and marketing personnel.
- Understand the different segments of the health care market.
- Understand how sales and marketing differ depending on market segments.
- Understand how metrics are used in the sales and marketing processes.

Discussion Topics

1. Discuss how each market segment is unique and how that affects sales and marketing.
2. Discuss how sales and marketing interact with other health plan functions.
3. Discuss how sales and marketing has evolved and how it may evolve in the future.
4. Discuss the different ways that sales and marketing success may be measured and the strengths and weaknesses of each.
5. Discuss how sales and marketing organizational structure may vary by health plan, by market segment, or by regulatory requirements.

INTRODUCTION

Sales and marketing have reemerged as critical capabilities that enable health plans to meet expectations relative to organic growth, which excludes growth through mergers and acquisitions. The historical performance of these capabilities in the managed care market has lagged other industries, notably financial services and retail. However, health plans have prioritized improvements in sales and marketing as key differentiators to fuel the organic growth agenda. This chapter defines health plan sales and marketing, describing fundamentals, as well as providing a view to high performance and a look to the future.

REEMERGENCE OF THE ORGANIC GROWTH AGENDA

After years of unprecedented merger and acquisition activity as the primary driver of growth in the managed care marketplace, several factors are driving renewed interest in organic growth. Inorganic growth may have reached its pinnacle, in terms of fueling managed care growth. Inorganic growth is viewed as having a lower return on investment due to the high acquisition costs per member and the hidden reality of higher-than-expected post-merger integration costs. Anecdotally, some health plans expect organic growth to have a return as much as four times higher than inorganic growth. Further, given the high volume of merger and acquisition activity, the potential future activity is naturally limited as health plans pursue smaller scale, complementary acquisitions or alliances focused on specific geographies, product lines/lines of business, or unique operational capabilities. A shift toward consumerism as discussed in Chapter 20 is another key factor, influenced by the introduction of new consumer-directed products, Medicare reform, and the onset of individual health insurance offerings. Each of these trends demands a deeper understanding of how to influence consumer behavior to drive growth, leading many health plans to look at "retail" disciplines for sales and marketing.

MANAGED CARE MARKETPLACE— DEFINING THE MARKETS

Health plans have typically organized around traditional segmentations of their customer base. These customer segments generally are based on membership size in the commercial space and include individual, small group (typically 2 to 50 member employers), mid-market (51 to approximately 5,000 members), and large case (more than 5,000 members). There is also some designation within each of these segments to reflect the risk arrangement, ranging from fully insured to self-funded administrative services only (ASO),* and the product portfolio purchased, including medical, pharmaceutical, behavioral health, and other ancillary products. In addition, many health plans have organizations and products focused on serving the government-sponsored Medicare and Medicaid markets. In considering health plan sales and marketing, it is important to understand the distinct characteristics and demands of two broader, primary distribution channels: employer-sponsored and direct markets.

The *employer-sponsored* channel is a business-to-business-to-consumer model characterized by heavy reliance on intermediary distribution channels, namely brokers and consultants. In this model, the relationship with the primary buyer, the employer, may be direct or indirect and the relationship with the consumer is typically indirect. The aim of health plan sales and marketing in this model is primarily to influence employer buyers and distribution channel partners, with a secondary focus on consumers. In contrast, the *direct markets* channel, which includes Medicare and individual commercial

---

*The many implications of self-funding under the requirements of the Employee Retirement Income and Security Act (ERISA), in which the employer rather than the health plan is at financial risk for health care costs, are discussed more fully in Chapter 31.

offerings, is characterized by a closer relationship with the consumer. As such, health plan sales and marketing in this model is focused on influencing consumer buyers and the distribution channel partners that service them.

SALES FUNDAMENTALS— EMPLOYER-SPONSORED MODEL

Employer-sponsored health plan sales are typically organized into two groups in each customer segment: new sales and account management for existing customers, focused on renewals. For both new and existing customers, sales activity is heavily reliant on well-established distribution channels, with more than 85% of employer-sponsored business involving an intermediary, typically a broker or consultant. Brokers are typically focused on relatively smaller employers (2–1,000 members) and are compensated based on commissions paid by the health plan (*ie,* some percentage of the premiums paid by the employer to the health plan, though considerable variation exists regarding amounts), whereas consultants are focused on larger employers and receive fee-based compensation paid by the employer.

Given the reliance on distribution partners in driving employer sales and renewals, it has become common among health plans to invest in capabilities that increase the effectiveness of these relationships, particularly the broker relationships. A majority of these investments are focused on driving broker loyalty and improving incentive compensation processes and tools. To drive broker loyalty, health plans have developed databases to gather insight on broker attributes, including performance metrics such as productivity, volume, and profitability. Health plans leverage this insight to tailor relationships with brokers, including commissions and service strategies. The execution of commissions strategies has been significantly improved with the emergence of incentive compensation technology solutions that streamline and drive increased accuracy in commissions payments, which have historically been a trouble spot for health plans.

Health plans are supported by distribution partners through the employer-sponsored sales process. Although this process may vary by health plan, it typically follows several common steps as depicted in Figure 21-1.

- *Lead generation:* The health plan sales process begins with the identification of "leads," prospective employer customers. Leads come from a variety of sources, including brokers and consultants, health plan marketing, and requests for proposals (RFPs) from employers. The basic information about a lead is typically logged in a database, establishing an initial record of the prospective customer.
- *Prospecting:* The health plan salesperson is assigned a lead to qualify through research initial conversations with the

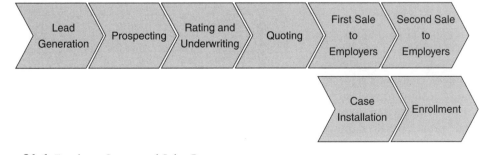

Figure 21–1 Employer-Sponsored Sales Process
Source: Author.

prospective customer, and collaboration with brokers and consultants. If the salesperson interacts directly with the employer, the interaction is likely with benefits coordinators, human resources executives, and potentially c-suite executives. In fact, the involvement of CEOs and CFOs in determining employee health benefits is rapidly increasing because affordability of health insurance is a top priority for many businesses. Successful prospecting will yield enough additional information about a prospective customer to enable rating and underwriting and an initial price quote. This additional information is added to the prospective customer record.

- *Rating and underwriting:* Based on information gathered by brokers and aggregated and submitted by the salesperson, the underwriting organization will evaluate and score the risk to insure the employees of a prospective customer, which drives the initial pricing based on established margin targets. If the prospective customer is interested in ASO, the activity at this stage is focused on underwriting stop-loss insurance coverage and estimating administrative cost, yielding an initial price. Rating and underwriting is discussed more fully in Chapter 25.

- *Quoting:* The next step is for the salesperson or distribution partner to communicate initial pricing to the prospective customer, based on several parameters, including the scope and design of employee benefits and network coverage. There may be several iterations to underwriting and price quoting as parameters are negotiated and adjusted.

- *First Sale (to the employer):* When the employer customer agrees to pricing, benefit design, products, network, and other contract parameters, the salesperson or broker finalizes the contract with the employer and completes the record of the sale in a database that will be used in setting up the customer on the health plan's information systems. In the small group segment, telesales (sometimes referred to as telemarketing) is increasing as an alternative to internal and broker-driven sales.

- *Case installation:* Upon the close of the "first sale," the customer's information, including the details of the services purchased, is entered into the health plan's information systems. Although health plan sales is typically not directly involved in case installation, the quality and completeness of the customer information gathered by the salesperson influences the efficiency and quality of the case installation.

- *Second sale (to the employee):* Although many employers offer insurance from only one health plan, some employers, particularly larger employers, often provide multiple health plan options to their employees. Health plans refer to this as "slice" business because any one insurer will likely service only a portion of the customer's employees. In these situations, there is an open enrollment period for employees to select a health plan. This is referred to as the "second sale," the sale to the employees. During the second sale, the health plan salesperson may be involved in promotions or campaigns to the employees in an effort to influence the selection of the health plan they represent.

- *Enrollment:* When employee selection is complete, the enrolled employees (called subscribers) and dependants (called, along with the subscriber, members) are enrolled in the health plan's systems. Similar to case installation, the salesperson has a limited role in enrollment. However, the salesperson typically follows the status of enrollment to ensure timely completion of fulfillment (*eg,* identification or ID cards to employees) by the employer's effective date. The duration from the first sale to employees' receipt of ID cards is viewed as an important end-to-end measure of a health plan's "front-end" operational efficiency. For small group customers, case installation and enrollment typically occur in one step because both the group and member information is loaded into health plan systems.

Completing the sales process quickly and accurately is a key differentiator from an employer's perspective. An important and increasingly common aid in effective selling is sales force automation (SFA). These applications and databases support the sales process from lead generation through the first sale and become the initial data set for account management to service an employer. SFA tools can also support the gathering of key sales performance metrics. Although specific measures may vary, most health plans evaluate sales based on membership, revenue, and increasingly, profitability; these metrics serve as the basis for compensating sales resources and brokers.

Upon the conclusion of a successful sale, the employer relationship, or "account," is transitioned to an account manager. The account manager's primary responsibilities are to oversee the service provided to the employer and pursue the renewal of the health plan's contract with the employer. Depending on the products and services purchased by the employer, the account manager may interact with the employer on issues related to enrollment, claims, network, care management, and other ancillary services. In providing service to the employer, the account manager is expected to act as a quarterback, owning the customer relationship but able to quickly engage the appropriate health plan expert (*eg,* care management or behavioral health experts) as the issues and opportunities dictate. The volume and complexity of these service-related, transactional issues can diminish the time and focus available for the strategic component of the account man-

ager's responsibilities: renewal and expansion of the customer relationship.

The renewal process begins with a look back at the results from the previous year, leveraging customer reporting that includes metrics demonstrating the service and value delivered. Based on the retrospective view and the anticipated future needs of the customer, the account manager, distribution partner, and employer discuss changes to benefits and other components of the contract. At times, the employer will issue an RFP to evaluate alternatives to the current health plan relationship. Regardless of whether there is an RFP or not, the consideration and negotiation of the renewal often require multiple iterations. Similar to the sales process, changes to the specifics of the benefits, products, network, or other contract components typically require reconsideration by underwriting, as well as updated pricing. Upon the successful conclusion of the renewal, account management follows a process similar to sales, with oversight of updates to case installation, second sales, and updates to enrollment.

Similar to sales, account management is evaluated based on membership, revenue, and profitability. However, account management is also evaluated based on employer satisfaction, employer retention, and member persistency, which is retention at the member level. Account managers and brokers are compensated, in part, on a composite view of these measures.

SALES FUNDAMENTALS— DIRECT MARKETS MODEL

In contrast to the employer-sponsored model, the direct markets of Medicare (see Chapter 26) and individual generally employ a business-to-consumer "campaign" model in influencing consumers to purchase their respective products and services. The exclusion of the employer, however, does not indicate a purely direct consumer relationship. Brokers and other distribution partners remain relevant in this model as a connection to the consumers they serve. Another key distinction of direct markets is that they tend to leverage marketing and customer insight more heavily than the employer-sponsored model does.

In the Medicare market, there exists an array of distribution strategies across and within health plans. Some health plans leverage exclusive relationships with consumer organizations (*eg,* American Association of Retired Persons [AARP]) to sell and provide services to consumers. Others sell and service through brokers who have direct relationships with consumers. Further, most health plans complement internal capabilities with niche vendors in areas such as print fulfillment and telesales. Regardless of distribution relationships and sourcing strategies, Medicare product sales are typically organized around campaigns, and there are a few prevalent go-to-market sales approaches, including the following:

- *Direct mail:* The most common approach is to promote products and services through direct mail to the consumer. The prospective members, or leads, are identified through health plan customer insight and segmentation, broker relationships, consumer purchasing organizations, or Medicare (federal government). Typically, emerging products and services have characteristics that would suit certain consumers better than others. As health plans and their distribution partners apply criteria to prospects, they identify a list of targets for a specific campaign. This list is often delivered to print fulfillment vendors who subsequently distribute campaign materials to consumers.
- *Field sales:* Whether executed by internal sales resources or brokers, field sales involve direct solicitation of prospects at community centers, special events such as health fairs, or at the prospects' homes. By comparison, this is viewed as a high-

touch, high-cost model and is typically reserved for prospects who are unresponsive to other sales approaches.

- *Telesales:* Growing significantly in the Medicare segment, telesales is similar to the direct mail model, with the exception at fulfillment. Instead of sending a list of targeted consumers to a print fulfillment vendor, the targets are delivered to an internal or external call center. Agents in these call centers contact target consumers telephonically, following a specific script intended to promote the sale of a product or service.
- *Web sales:* Emerging in the Medicare segment but more common in the individual segment is Web sales. As the percentage of Web-savvy Medicare-eligible consumers grows, it is expected that Web sales will grow in prominence as a go-to-market approach. Essentially, Web sales involve the steering of consumers to a Web site, where the consumer can evaluate and select insurance coverage.
- *Affinity programs:* In certain cases, Medicare products and services are sold through business relationships outside of the health care space; these relationships are often referred to as *affinity* relationships. As an example, a retailer and health plan may partner to offer the health plan's Medicare products and services in the retailer's stores. In return, the retailer receives a commission and some residual brand enhancement from its involvement in providing health care to retail consumers.

In the individual segment, distribution strategies are even more diverse than in the Medicare space. This is caused, in large part, by the vastly different characteristics of various individual consumer segments, ranging from uninsured to college students to early retirees. As a result, depending on the consumer segment targeted, health plans rely on distribution partners that range from airlines to student loan companies to traditional brokers. A dominant distribution channel does not exist, though traditional and online brokers remain relevant in this segment. Online brokers act as Web-based clearinghouses for Web-savvy consumers seeking individual health insurance. In many cases, online brokers receive a commission for an online referral to the health plan's individual Web site, where the consumer can evaluate insurance options and, in most cases, purchase insurance.

Across the health plans in the individual market, there is significant investment in Web sales capabilities, including the Web site and the functions it supports, such as underwriting and fulfillment. Some health plans intend to mimic the Web sales capabilities of retailers or auto insurers, in terms of the depth and breadth of online functionality. Depending on the targeted segment, Web sales tools may be provided directly to consumers or may be distributed to brokers to be used in selling to consumers. Despite innovation in distribution approaches, sales in the individual segment tend to be influenced by product offerings, pricing, and network coverage.

CHALLENGES TO EFFECTIVE HEALTH PLAN SALES

Although there are common processes and tools, health plan sales organizations face several challenges in acquiring and retaining customers. Examples of these are challenges are as follows.

Employer-Sponsored

- Valuable and usable insight around employers, brokers, and members is limited, by comparison to other industries. Driven by limitations in supporting technology, processes, and customer relationships, this gap tends to limit the ability of sales resources to identify solution needs proactively with targeted value propositions.

The lack of customer insight also naturally limits the quality of the strategic account planning that is critical to growing customer relationships.

- For many health plans, the investment in sales and account management talent has historically been minimized in an effort to reduce operating costs. As health plans increasingly expect this workforce to drive organic growth, there may be a gap in the payroll and training budgets allocated toward expanding the capability of sales and account management.
- The products, networks, and services that health plans sell are becoming commoditized as employers see less differentiation as they consider health plan options. A significant driver of the commoditization is the lack of a demonstrated, quantifiable value story around services aimed at mitigating health care cost.
- Health plan sales and renewals are often complex, given the array of influences on employer buyers. These influences include other brokers, consultants, other employers, providers, employees, and governments. These entities often influence employers in divergent directions and there is a significant challenge for health plans to address the diverse employer concerns emanating from these influencers.
- Most employers purchase health insurance on a calendar year, meaning the coverage period begins on January 1. As a result, both the first sale to the employer and the second sale to the employees have busy periods that resemble the peak volumes accountants face during tax season in the United States, as illustrated in Figure 21-2. In the case of the "second sale" peak that spans from September to December, health plans supplement the sales force with temporary resources to plan and participate in events such as employee benefits fairs. The volume of activity and the inexperience of the team

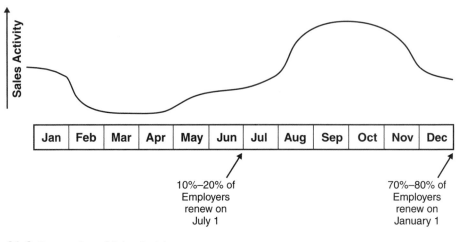

Figure 21–2 Seasonality of Sales Activity

Source: Author.

executing the second sale create a significant challenge.

Direct Markets

- Insight is also critical to direct markets aimed at consumers. Although customer insight is typically more advanced in the Medicare or individual segments, these insight capabilities do not yet enable more advanced "retail" approaches, such as behavioral segmentation.
- Although Web sales is viewed as important to growing both the Medicare and individual segments, health plan capabilities are generally immature in comparison to similar cross-industry capabilities (*eg,* automobile insurance or retail consumer products). As an example, health plans are not currently able to execute the "real-time" underwriting that is common in the automobile insurance Web sales space.
- To a degree exceeding other consumer industries, health plans are burdened by regulatory concerns in their pursuit of organic growth. Federal and state governments have various rules that restrict a pure "retail" model, such as the Health Insurance Portability and Accountability

Act (HIPAA) regulations. As discussed in Chapter 32, that may influence the aggregation and sharing of consumer data. Another example is the limitation on health plans to overtly exclude individual seniors from Medicare offerings. These rules and regulations add an additional layer of complexity to health plan sales efforts in the direct markets.

HIGH PERFORMANCE IN HEALTH PLAN SALES CAPABILITIES

Although many health plans are challenged to execute the fundamentals of sales, some have differentiated certain capabilities in pursuing organic growth and have defined high performance relative to the marketplace. Although no health plan has all of these characteristics, the components of high-performance health plan sales are as follows.

Employer-Sponsored

- *Consultative selling*: Also referred to as "solution selling," this involves a human capital transformation, particularly for account management, from a reactive, transactional, service-focused model to a proactive, consultative, strategic model focused on growth. Several health plans have redefined account management roles, separating the responsibilities for servicing an account from the responsibilities for retaining and growing an account. Another key enabler of this change is a commitment to strategic account planning as a foundation of customer insight. For most health plans, this introduces methods into an area that historically has had minimal structure. In addition, at least modest technology support is needed to enable the creation and refreshing of strategic account plans.

- *Advanced performance measurement:* Increasingly, health plans are moving beyond the fundamental sales metrics, incorporating metrics borrowed from retail paradigms. An example is "share of wallet," which measures both the product penetration and the percentage of eligible members. Another advanced metric is "cost to sell." Although it is not innovative to understand the total cost of the sales force, it is a rather new capability to allocate business development cost to a specific pursuit and, further, to evaluate sales resources based on this metric.

- *Streamlined sales process:* Given the differentiation that comes with a shorter time frame from the time of sale to fulfillment, high-performing health plans are closing process gaps and eliminating redundancies in the sales process. In fact, many have applied Six Sigma methods to examine the end-to-end process and reduce variability. An example of this is providing lead generation and sales force automation tools to brokers to enable involvement earlier in the process and eliminate unnecessary hand-offs.

- *Distribution channel loyalty programs:* Beyond the basics of managing broker and consultant relationships, some health plans have developed approaches to measure distribution partner "loyalty," leveraging deep insight around distribution partner behavior and performance. These health plans are tailoring their financial and service relationships based on this insight, including incentive programs and differentiated broker portal services, based on the membership growth, revenue growth, and data quality.

- *RFP units:* Given the competitive nature of the employer-sponsored market space, RFPs from employers are common and the high-performing plans have developed high-efficiency units focused on supporting the sales force in responding to RFPs. This ensures common and reusable messaging as well as much-needed relief to sales and account management resources.

- *Customer insight and analytics:* Though even high-performing health plans lag other industries in terms of customer insight capabilities, some are investing in gaining a deeper understanding of their current membership. This includes the consideration of new approaches to understand and group brokers, employers, and members, based on behaviors and attitudes rather than the traditional categorizations driven by size, demographics, and claims.

Direct Markets

- *Advanced Web sales:* Particularly in the individual market space, a few health plans have developed Web sales capabilities that emulate the functionality offered by retail or financial services companies. Key capabilities include online product configuration, real-time underwriting, deep online help functions, and telephonic customer service in support of the Web channel.

- *Marketing automation:* In the Medicare segment, several health plans have gained significant efficiencies through investments in campaign automation and marketing resource management tools. These tools enable fast-paced and accurate setup and execution of new campaigns, tracking of campaign results, and management of marketing resources across multiple campaigns.

- *Telesales technology:* Advancements in call center technology have established a platform for improved campaign execution, from the receipt of campaigns to the creation and execution of scripts to the tracking of telesales activity and results. Telesales capability and capacity are viewed as key enablers to health plans dramatically growing direct markets business, particularly in the Medicare segment.

MARKETING FUNDAMENTALS

Health plan marketing has historically been an area of relatively minimal focus when compared to other functions such as claims management or care management. This is changing, given the focus on organic growth. Many health plans have recently invested in acquiring marketing talent from other industries in an effort to infuse cross-industry thinking. Further, the onset of new products, particularly in the consumer-directed and Medicare spaces, has demanded a dramatic increase in marketing spend and improvement in marketing capabilities. Given this rather sudden shift toward a focus on marketing as a key differentiator, many health plans have struggled to advance their capability at a pace necessary to meet the growing demand of the marketplace.

Organizationally, health plans vary relative to a central marketing entity serving all market segments versus allocation of marketing resources to each market segment. In the employer-sponsored segments, sales and marketing are typically distinct organizations, whereas in the direct markets there is very little distinction between sales and the tactical component of marketing. Regardless of structure, most health plan marketing or-

ganizations perform a standard set of functions, including the following:

- *Brand management:* The need to manage brand is a rather recent development in the managed care industry. This process begins with developing a view to the desired market positioning; how does the health plan want be viewed in the eyes of employers, consumers, distribution partners, and providers? For example, is the health plan positioned as a high-touch, premium carrier? Or perhaps the health plan is positioned as a no-frills, low-cost carrier. Whatever the positioning, it is competitively important to clarify the desired market positioning and the key marketplace differentiators aligned with the positioning. Given the strategic importance of brand positioning, health plan c-suite executives are typically involved and health plans often seek assistance from advertising or strategy consulting firms in developing and managing their brand.

- *External communications:* Many health plan marketing organizations own public relations and external communications. This responsibility ranges from managing the content of external Web sites to providing counsel to spokespersons on public comments on specific issues. Marketing is also responsible for ensuring consistency of external communications with the aforementioned brand positioning.

- *Advertising:* Like any other company, health plans utilize a variety of media to advertise their products and services, including television, radio, print, and the Internet. Health plans use advertising firms heavily in determining the mix of advertising channels and in executing broad-based and targeted advertising campaigns. The marketing organization is responsible for setting the overall advertising strategy and objectives, based on the brand positioning, and then providing oversight to the work of the advertising firms. As affinity relationships and go-to-market alliances become more prevalent, marketing organizations are also responsible for representing the health plan in shared branding and advertising.

- *Market research:* Marketing organizations execute basic market research in support of the health plan. Marketing's research scope typically includes marketplace trends, competitive intelligence, and surveying of health plan stakeholders, including employers, distribution partners, members, and providers. For specific needs, health plan marketing purchases specific research from niche vendors.
- *Lead generation:* As market research uncovers opportunities for new markets or customers, marketing provides leads to sales organizations in the various market segments. These leads may be as directional as market intelligence around the attractiveness of a particular industry or as specific as a list of prospective customers.
- *Sales campaign support:* Marketing often provides guidance and support to the sales organizations in the planning and execution of campaigns, particularly around presentations and customer messaging. This support ranges from hands-on edits to proposals to employers to directional advice on key selling messages.

CHALLENGES TO EFFECTIVE HEALTH PLAN MARKETING

Health plan marketing organizations face several challenges in executing the fundamentals, particularly when compared to enablers commonly found in other industries. These challenges are briefly described as follows.

Similar to the challenge faced by the health plan sales force, marketing is severely limited by a lack of customer insight. Although the typical financial services or retail company is armed with advanced customer segmentation based on behaviors and preferences, health plan marketing organizations typically rely on anecdotal data or data that are not specific to the membership base they serve. This customer insight gap limits the ability to tailor marketing campaigns to influence employer or consumer behavior based on behaviors or preferences. Some health plans have mitigated this challenge in the direct markets by purchasing consumer insight from marketing database vendors. However, in the employer-sponsored market, meaningful customer insight around employers or employees has remained elusive.

Historically, health plans have limited investment in the marketing space. Although this has changed over the last few years, the impact of years of underinvestment is manifest in the gaps in human capital and technology assets that reside in many health plan marketing organizations. Only recently, health plans have looked to other industries for marketing talent and started to invest in modernizing supporting marketing technology, such as campaign automation tools.

Targeted marketing in the employer-sponsored space can be very difficult because an employee's purchasing decision may be complex and has many potential influences, including employers, brokers, physicians, unions, other consumers, and media sources. This presents a challenge to health plan marketing organizations as they attempt to design and execute campaigns to establish brand position or promote a product or service.

HIGH PERFORMANCE IN HEALTH PLAN MARKETING CAPABILITIES

There is significant variability in health plans' execution of marketing fundamentals, and health plan marketing generally continues to lag other industries from a capability perspective. Nonetheless, some health plans have achieved marketplace differentiation in certain marketing capabilities, in their pursuit of organic growth. Though not considered exceptional by cross-industry standards, examples of high-performance health plan marketing include the following:

- *Measuring brand value:* Advanced health plan marketing organizations are able to measure the value of the brand they represent. Accomplished through quantitative surveys, this activity provides insight validating brand strategy, measuring the effectiveness of campaigns to adjust brand positioning and quantifying the current value of the brand. Some are also developing an understanding of the brand and customer experience factors that drive conversion through the marketing funnel and yield increased sales and profitability.
- *Marketing portfolio optimization:* Although limited by rudimentary capabilities to measure specific marketing return on investment (MROI), some health plans have started to apply a more scientific approach to the mix of marketing and advertising activities and investments. Health plan marketers currently rely on qualitative, survey-based information and third-party advice in adjusting the mix of their portfolios. Further, they depend on basic information such as "cost per impression," rather than "cost per desired outcome" or quantitative ROI.
- *Consumer segmentation:* Beyond the traditional segmentation of members by age, gender, and claims experience, some health plans are adding qualitative, "life stage" information to their segments. This information is gathered through consumer surveys and clusters members based on the attitudes common to their life stage, a mix of demographics, socioeconomics, lifestyle, and views on health care issues. Some health plans are further advancing their con-

sumer segmentation to include behavioral segmentation, as defined by utilization of health care services, call centers, and portals.
- *Targeted marketing campaigns:* Leveraging advances in consumer segmentation, some health plans have effectively tailored marketing campaigns to support specific objectives, typically around the introduction of new products or services. Examples abound in the consumer-directed product space because health plans have developed intelligence on favorable consumer segments and key selling messages around these products. This intelligence has also been applied to drive advertising content and other marketing campaigns.

A LOOK TO THE FUTURE

Organic growth has returned as a strategic priority for health plans and this is an exciting time for sales and marketing organizations because they are asked to fuel the organic growth engines across managed care. These areas are pressured to mature quickly and drive differentiation in the marketplace at a time when health plan products and services are in danger of becoming commoditized. So, the challenge is great, but those who succeed have a tremendous opportunity to gain competitive advantage and drive significant growth. There are several advanced capabilities that have been demonstrated in other industries but are not yet evident in the health plan space. Although it cannot be known with certainty, the following could be the capabilities that provide real competitive differentiation and growth for health plans.

- *The health plan consumer analytic record:* There is significant and unanticipated value in developing a comprehensive understanding of the health plan consumer. This view begins with basic demographics and claims information.

This information could be complemented with external data from sources such as financial institutions. This expanding consumer record could be further supplemented by qualitative, attitudinal categorization and behavioral data. Behavioral data would include any utilization of health plan services. This can be accomplished, as other industries (*eg,* financial services, retail consumer products) have demonstrated. Further, given the wealth of behavioral data available to health plans, the potential value of the consumer analytic record could be greater than in other industries. The depth of understanding around which combinations of data are indicative of future behaviors could optimize sales, marketing, and service strategies to a degree not previously realized.

- *Closed-loop promotion:* Some industries, notably pharmaceuticals, have made great advances in the integration of sales and marketing. The notion of closed-loop promotion involves a more direct relationship between sales and marketing, with marketing driving specific campaigns to the sales force with specific and tailored selling messages. Sales, then, provides immediate quantitative and qualitative feedback on these messages, allowing real-time and continuous learning for the marketing organization, which they, in turn, incorporate back into the next wave of selling messages. Although some health plans have direct markets that have an integrated sales and marketing team, the employer-sponsored model requires significant transformation to achieve this level of integration.

- *Second sale excellence:* Most health plans scramble to minimally participate in the annual open enrollment peak season. However, the application of fundamental customer relationship management approaches and tools, such as campaign design and diversification of marketing approaches based on customer insight, will create significant competitive advantage for those health plans investing in this space.

- *Sales and marketing outsourcing:* Over the last few years, health plans have reaped significant benefits in outsourcing certain core administrative functions such as enrollment, billing, and claims, often to offshore locations. Although there has been clear savings from the lower labor costs realized, often there have also been efficiency gains in streamlining and standardizing operations as a part of the outsourcing transition. In other industries, companies have outsourced support functions in the sales and marketing space, with some companies outsourcing marketing altogether. In health plans, there remains significant administrative cost in supporting sales and marketing and, although it may not make sense to outsource the customer relationship management or marketing strategy responsibilities, the roles that support these should be considered, in the interests of profitability and efficiency gains.

- *Demonstrated value:* Employers are searching for the health plan that can clearly demonstrate fact-based results for the products and services purchased by the employer, with a particular emphasis on controlling health care cost. Although some niche vendors are able to demonstrate value for specific offerings and most health plans claim to demonstrate value, the mechanics required to demonstrate that a health plan's actions had a direct impact on member behaviors that drive health care cost are missing. Many are pursuing the quantifiable value story and those that can get there first will have a leadership position in the marketplace. What do sales and marketing have to do with this? A deeper understanding of the customer and the customer's health care objectives will lead to better articulation of the value proposition and, retrospectively, the value delivered.

- *Quantitative MROI:* Increased health plan investment in marketing is accompanied by an interest in understanding the facts around the yield from this investment. Many companies have sought and achieved a more structured and quantitative method to measuring the impact of marketing investments. The value of this insight is in better tailoring the go-forward marketing portfolio mix to produce the greatest yield, measured in terms of health plan growth.

- *Internet marketing:* Advances in Internet marketing have been dramatic and dynamic, making it difficult to describe "state of the market." However, advances such as "micromarketing," the steering of targeted Internet users to specific Web sites to provide tailored marketing messages, are growing in importance as the desire to market to consumers or specific employer decision makers expands. Health plans able to master the Internet channel to promote growth have a distinct competitive advantage in the marketplace.

CONCLUSION

This is a challenging but exciting time for health plan sales and marketing organizations. Although there is generally a need to advance sales and marketing quickly to fuel organic growth, indications are that organizational focus and investment are catching up to the ambitious performance expectations in these areas. In the increasingly commoditized employer-sponsored space, sales and marketing are already crucial differentiators in the competition for customers. In the direct markets, the execution of retail sales and marketing approaches will soon be standard for health plans competing for Medicare and individual business. The health plan sales and marketing transformation is under way; the plans that achieve high performance will find the organic growth they seek.

22

THE EMPLOYER'S VIEW OF MANAGED CARE

Michael J. Taylor

Study Objectives

- Understand the managed care trends affecting employers today and how they affect different size employers.
- Understand how employers define value in managed health care.
- Understand that there is no single bullet solution to rising health care costs and increased consumer dissatisfaction with the delivery and administration of health care.
- Understand the drivers of employer business performance that need to be aligned with health care value purchasing.
- Understand how employers want their employees to become more involved with health care decision making.

Discussion Topics

1. Discuss how managed care trends affect large employers. How would trends have different effects on a small employer?
2. Discuss the issue of cost shifting from the government payor to the private employer payor.
3. Discuss different value equation for employer purchasing.
4. Discuss what interventions with the provider community have already been tried and what interventions are new.
5. Discuss how the move towards individual consumerism affects the large employer and the small employer.
6. Discuss the current common defined health care contributions for employees and how that may evolve in the future.

INTRODUCTION

Managed care has almost run its course in the lexicon of U.S. health care. Bold words perhaps, but the gradual decline of what had traditionally been referred to as managed care has gained momentum since the beginning of 2000 when the fourth edition of this book was written. For years, it was felt that it was managed *cost* and not managed *care*. Now, it is all about managing a continuum of costs and care for the individual rather than a group of average employees. Previously, employers focused on purchasing value. Now, employers continue to purchase for value, but value has a different spin to it and involves the employee in several creative ways. This chapter explores current health care trends, and how they affect employers large and small; how managed care evolved into care continuum management and collided with consumerism. The final section of the chapter tries to predict where this employer view will go in the next 5 years.

As described in other chapters in this book, there are a number of key stakeholders involved in the complicated dynamic of health care delivery in the United States. They can be categorized as consumers, employers, providers, health plans, and the government. The needs of these stakeholders are not fully aligned, but they are finally moving closer after years of separate activity.

HEALTH CARE TRENDS THAT AFFECT EMPLOYER STAKEHOLDERS IN 2006

Generally, market forces and government policy shape the U.S. health care delivery dynamic. The employer stakeholder is responsible for providing health care to 160 million people out of the total adult U.S. population of 290 million. This number has been shrinking of late because of the increase in uninsured persons. The issue of rising numbers of uninsureds is a heavy focus for government policy, particularly its impact on state Medicaid budgets, as discussed in Chapter 27.

The following health care trends affect employers:

- *Restructuring*. Restructuring continues throughout the health care delivery system. Merger and acquisition activity is spread across health plans, disease management, pharmacy management, and behavioral health management companies, integrated delivery systems, and provider-owned delivery systems and technology companies. Some new entrants are also experiencing restructuring. These include companies expanding into the content and connectivity space, health and productivity management companies, and consumer health care services, including health account management and debit/credit cards for health care. This restructuring makes the delivery system more complex with more partners so that selecting and evaluating which delivery system makes sense for each employer is getting more difficult rather than less difficult.

- *Competition*. As a result of this restructuring and the growing number of for-profit health care businesses, Wall Street and associated shareholders are becoming more influential with the providers, health plans, and other delivery system stakeholders. The rise in account-based health plans has also attracted many financial services companies. Increased competition forces the delivery system to produce favorable finances both short and long term. Some are arguing that competition is still at the wrong level, namely, at the health plan level when it should be at the provider-patient level.[1] However you define competition, it has a major role in the value shift for employers.

- *Consumerism*. Consumerism is now a full-fledged trend and growing stronger each month. Born out of the backlash against managed care and part of a new deal relationship between employers and employees, consumerism is calling into question the definition of the buyer of health care. As with other aspects of the economy and general purchaser behavior, consumers want more knowledge about health care and the products offered before, during, and after the purchase. In most cases, they also want more control over how health care is delivered and how value is determined. Consumerism is discussed more fully in Chapter 20.

- *Cost increases.* Moderate cost increases are back with severe consequences to employers both large and small.[2] Many factors such as the aging of the population, more educated consumers, advances in treatment modalities and medical technology, and increasing costs (particularly hospital costs) are driving up utilization and cost. As discussed in Chapter 7, providers (again, hospitals in particular) have seized the initiative away from employers and health plans and resist the standard contracting pressures for discounts. The decreased abilities of health plans to control cost and utilization are being addressed in multiple ways. They include more sophisticated employer/employee cost sharing mechanisms, care management, and consumer engagement initiatives.

- *Medicare.* Medicare was not singled out as a trend in the previous edition but now Part D is taking effect. This prescription drug offering for retirees is changing the landscape of health plans and changing the lives of providers and patients; sadly, not always in positive ways. A complicated plan design created to meet budget targets and to satisfy political agendas has lead to a massive implementation in 2005/2006 that is off to a rocky start at the time of publication. Thus, in the short term, the impact of Part D will be on how members are enrolled and use the plan. In the long term, the impact will be on generic substitution rates, drug pricing, and formulary management; it is also possible that the

benefits structure of Part D will change because of political forces. Employers were slow to react to the 2006 enrollment deadline for retiree health plans, and many took the subsidy as an interim step. A more robust strategy involving Medicare Advantage plans, standalone prescription drug plans, and even private fee-for-service will be needed for the long term. More details are provided in Chapter 26.

- *Technology.* Again, in the previous edition, technology was not given its due as a standalone trend in this chapter but has now earned that position. Significant advances in genomics, replacement of organs and structures, and medical device miniaturization are having and will continue to have increased impact on costs and utilization. So will the use of informational tools such as electronic medical records and regional or state-based health information networks. Employers will be forced to come up with a strategy to deal with covering these advances.

- *Quality.* Quality improvement continues its slow development and is still alive and kicking. Several new organizations such as Leapfrog, Bridges to Excellence, and Ambulatory Care Quality Alliance have joined the fray.* Many existing employer coalitions have stepped up their efforts to include this in their health care delivery initiatives. Most stakeholders now realize that collective effort around quality improvement is needed rather than individual efforts. The providers have also responded more strongly than in the past, and several specialty societies and medical organizations have offered to participate with such employer collaborative efforts.

---

*A fuller, though still partial list of these and other organizations, as well as their Web addresses, may be found in Chapter 8.

HOW THESE TRENDS AFFECT EMPLOYERS BOTH LARGE AND SMALL

The type of managed care delivery system and associated plan design and financing provided by employers are still heavily dependent on the size of the employer. There are several reasons for this, but fundamentally it has to do with the amount of resources, financial and human, that is available to make purchase decisions and then to manage the benefit and vendor relationship. However, for the first time a new reason is emerging. This new reason is the relationship that the employer and the business have with the employee. For example, employers with low-wage workers and high turnover have a different view of the labor pool and its employees than does an old-line manufacturer or business that needs experienced, highly educated labor. This relationship of benefits to business and workforce effectiveness continues to unfold as employers create a line of sight through their workforce attraction and retention to products and services and finally to profitability and growth (see Figure 22-1).

Health plans are also changing their approaches to the different size employers for the first time in many years. They are hedging their bets about who will be the prime buyer of health care in the future (employer sponsored or individual consumer).

In terms of changed approach, the large national health plans have created a menu of services in account management, claims and customer service, and now care management that can be put together to meet the different size employer needs. These services are priced separately and are offered in different combinations. Some of this flexibility is the result of more sophisticated technology and some, such as care management, is in response to market demand. Large regional health plans (plans with enrollment of 200,000 to 1 million lives) can also offer some of this flexibility, but it often results in a higher noncompetitive price. Smaller health plans (10,000 to 200,000 lives) have great difficulty in offering such flexibility.

THE LARGE EMPLOYER: 5,000 LIVES PLUS

These employers are commonly multisite and increasingly multinational. Self-funding under the Employee Retirement Income and Security Act (ERISA; see Chapter 31) is very prevalent. In prior years, the employer would be very involved in managing the health plans and might use an outsourced network manager. With increased health plan consolidation and improved reporting, many employers are taking back that responsibility or shifting it back to the health plan. Almost all use benefits consultants to facilitate strategy and purchasing decisions.

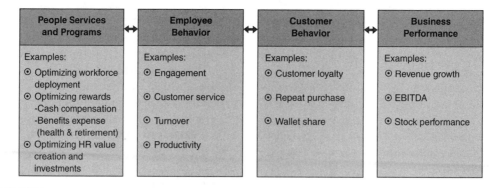

Figure 22–1 Line of Sight from Broad People and Reward Issues to Profitability and Growth
Source: Courtesy of Towers Perrin, New York, NY.

Most large employers are revisiting their health care strategies to combat the cost increases (not necessarily the increase in trend but the absolute cost increase from a higher base) and to align them with their changing business strategies (see Figure 22-2). Most large employers use a 3-year time horizon for strategy, but the rapid changes in the delivery system mentioned earlier have accelerated their review of current strategy in place. Also, improvements in data collection and program measurement have provided employers with more actionable information. Health care strategy and tactics are also being discussed at the CEO/CFO level of most large employers. This is because employee health care costs are often equal to corporate profits.[3]

These new strategies are more likely to be focused on details of health care delivery than on a wider choice of plans. As health maintenance organization (HMO), point-of-service (POS), and preferred provider organization

(PPO) products* have merged together, and as customer service has become automated, attention is being directed toward provider network configuration and care management. Large employers that are self-funded will always negotiate hard on administrative services only (ASO) fees and performance guarantees, but now they include health plan accountability measures around the performance of the network and the care management function.

In response to these demands, health plans have recontracted networks in a variety of ways to reduce cost without harming access or dramatically affecting referral patterns. Many of these networks are referred to as high performance networks or premium designated networks. Other network approaches use the concept of centers of excellence for

*See Chapter 2 for a discussion of these and other health plan and product designs.

	1996	1997	1998	1999	2000	2001	2002	2003	2004	2005	2006
Health Care Plans											
Active employees	4%	3%	4%	7%	10%	12%	13%	15%	12%	8%	7%
Retirees under age 65	4	4	4	6	10	17	13	17	15	9	9
Retirees age 65 and older	3	7	5	10	24	18	19	19	13	9	6
Combined	4	4	4	7	12	13	14	16	12	8	7
Dental Plans											
Active employees	5%	5%	5%	7%	6%	7%	6%	7%	5%	5%	4%
Retirees under age 65	4	5	4	4	6	6	5	6	5	7	7*
Retirees age 65 and older	3	5	3	3	6	4	4	5	6		
Inflation Measures											
Consumer Price Index (CPI)	3%	2%	2%	2.7%	3.4%	1.6%	2.0%	2.3%	3.2%	4.3%**	
Medical care component of CPI	4	3	3	3.7	4.2	4.7	4.8	4.0	4.5	4.1	

*Average cost increase for retirees under and over age 65
**Unadjusted 12 months ended 10/31/05

Figure 22–2A Average Cost Increases: 1996–2006
Source: Courtesy of Towers Perrin, New York, NY.

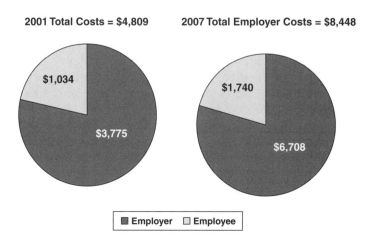

Figure 22-2B Total Health Care Cost Dollar Amount Per Employee
Source: Courtesy of Towers Perrin, New York, NY.

certain low-volume, high-cost procedures. In most cases, the network is a subset of the largest geographic network, and the providers (hospitals and physicians) have been selected based on criteria of cost and quality.

The health plan response to increased scrutiny of care management by employers has been to create targeted care interventions for different types of members and situations. Recognizing that one care management approach cannot fit all situations, this has lead to the development of a care continuum (see Figure 22-3). Different components of care management are directed to different sections of the care continuum; more details on this are provided in section three of this book.

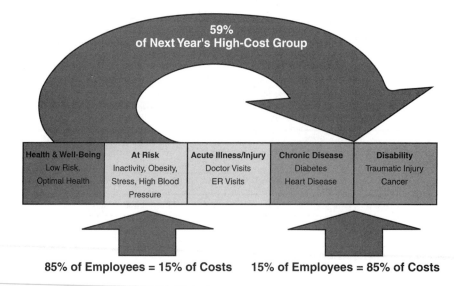

Figure 22–3 The Care Continuum
Source: Courtesy of Towers Perrin, New York, NY.

THE MODERATE GROUP EMPLOYER: 500 TO 5,000 LIVES

These companies continue to be pressured to deliver benefits in a cost-effective way. They have experienced the greatest reduction in benefits staffing. They usually rely on benefits consultants or brokers for purchasing decisions, but some have moved to Web-based purchasing tools or self-service. As business competition within the United States and abroad increases, price sensitivity for health benefits has increased. These employers still value network access and member service but need low cost (see Figure 22-4). Flexibility of plan design and funding are still important. The good news for this group is that health plans are viewing this segment and the next smallest as the growth area, and competition is very healthy.

This group continues to be very demanding in the area of data reporting because they often have to allocate actual employee medical costs to the various divisions within the company.

Consumer-driven health plans (CDHPs; see Chapters 2 and 20) have achieved better penetration in this segment than in the large group segment because of the attractive choices, pricing, data reporting, and self-service.

THE MEDIUM GROUP EMPLOYER: 50 TO 500 LIVES

The economy has produced strong growth in this segment for the first time in many years. The purchasing habits of this group are quite variable. Price sensitivity is very significant, and unfortunately many companies in this segment are not offering health care insurance because it is unaffordable. This has lead to some of the increase in the uninsured population. Most recent estimates put the uninsured population at 41.2 million (see Figure 22-5).

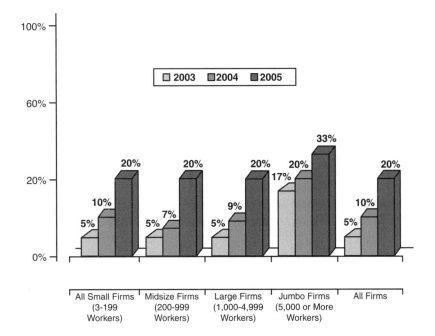

Figure 22–4 Percentage of Firms that Offer Employees a High-Deductible Health Plan by Firm Size, 2003–2005

Source: Kaiser/HRET survey of employer-sponsored health benefits, 2003–2005.

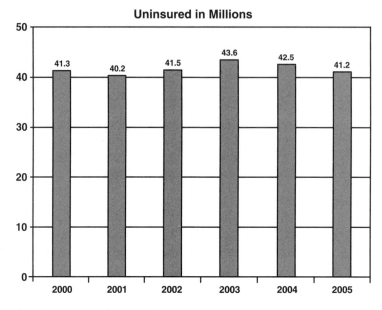

Figure 22–5 Number of Persons without Health Insurance
Source: CDC: Family Core Component of the 1997–2005 NHIS.

The nature of this employer is still local and network composition and access are second in importance after price. However, the dramatic increase in plan merger and acquisition has eliminated many of the local health plans that were the plan of choice for this segment. Consequently, these employers are more likely to be contracting with national plans or the local Blue Cross Blue Shield plan (although the Blue Cross Blue Shield network of plans has itself experienced the greatest amount of consolidation: down from 50 plans to 39 in the last 5 years). The result has been positive in some markets because the national plans can price competitively and leverage scale of technology. In others it has lead to market dominance and a diminished price competition. Generally speaking, though, the days of the high-priced local plan trading on its reputation are almost gone, which is good news for this price-sensitive group.

Brokers remain the primary distribution channel, but there is a significant increase in direct sales by the health plan's own sales force, through health plan self-service portals, or by using Internet aggregators of health in-surance. See also Chapter 21 regarding sales and marketing.

Self-funding is still on the increase for this segment as better data is obtained and underwriting rules are becoming more uniform. Some markets and states are encouraging self-funding through small group cooperatives.

THE SMALL GROUP EMPLOYER: 0 TO 50 LIVES

This group purchases on price. Brokers and agents are the distribution channel. Companies in this group have migrated away from HMOs for cost reasons and are now looking at minimal plan design PPOs. There has been some interest in CDHPs: high-deductible PPOs with either a Health Savings Account (HSA) or Health Reimbursement Account (HRA) as described in Chapters 2 and 20. CDHPs are often priced attractively, but the out-of-pocket or employee share can sometimes be daunting to the consumer, especially to large families.

The small employer group has suffered a great deal from the unaffordability of health insurance. Many of the uninsured actually have some coverage, but it is not enough to handle catastrophic or even chronic care and so they present as uninsured to the providers, (see Figure 22-6). These costs are then borne by the public system under Medicaid or as uncompensated care by providers with attendant cost shifting to the private system, resulting in increased premiums. Families USA has calculated that the increase in average family premium to pay for the health costs of the uninsured is $922 in 2005 and will be $1,502 by 2010.[4]

VALUE FOR THE EMPLOYER CONTINUES TO EVOLVE

In the previous edition of this book, we focused on how employers purchase value in their health benefits. The definition of value changed slightly from the 1980s, 1990s, and into 2000. The 2000 value equation was expressed as a series of interventions affecting cost and quality. The notion of these interventions acting in concert rather than as isolated components was also being tried. Six years later in 2006, the value definition evolves with increased focus on alignment of health care delivery and interventions with an employer's business strategy.

This alignment with business strategy includes broad people and rewards issues. One

people issue that is receiving more attention is employee productivity. The impact of health status on productivity has been extensively studied in recent years, and the results are startling. The cost of disability and absence is the second largest controllable benefit spend of employers. Few employers consider that a significant portion of health care costs (more than 50%) are incurred by disabled employees, and research has shown that a decrease in disability duration drives a 2 to 1 reduction in health care cost. Thus, health and productivity are now part of the employer value definition.

Although value to the employer as described earlier has evolved slightly, value to the employee is rapidly evolving, and for the time being these two are inextricably linked (see Figure 22-7). The evolution and adoption of individual health care consumerism are the catalysts at work here. Individual health care consumerism is covered in Chapter 20, and in the employer world it is all about making employees and to a lesser extent employees' families accountable and responsible for their own health and the associated costs.

For an employer to make its employees accountable and responsible for their own health care, the employer needs to know about its employee population. There has been a significant increase in the amount of analysis of employer populations from a

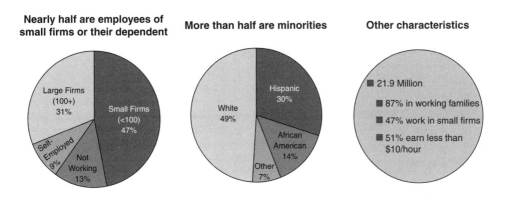

Figure 22–6 Snapshot of Lower-Income Uninsured

Source: Actuarial Research Corporation (ARC) analysis of March 2004 CPS data (CY2003).

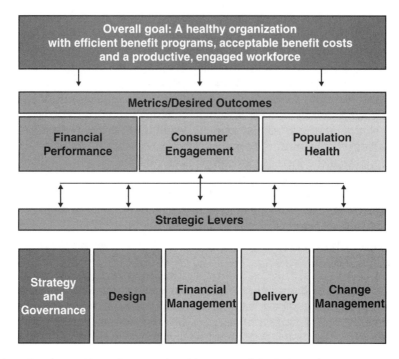

Figure 22–7 How Employers Use a Framework to Measure and Optimize Value

Source: Courtesy of Towers Perrin, New York, NY.

health risk and cost viewpoint. Often this involves the completion of a health risk assessment by the employee and a detailed analysis of medical claims, pharmacy claims, and sometimes disability claims. Once the employer knows where the employees are on the care continuum and what costs are associated with that, the process of employee engagement can begin (see Figure 22-8).

As shown in Figure 22-8, analysis of the cost and risk leads to a number of interventions. Employers are asking their health plans to provide these interventions in an integrated and aligned manner. Health plans have responded positively to this for large self-insured employers, and many have adopted similar responses for their fully insured books of business covering large and small businesses.

However, intervening along the care continuum in an integrated and aligned manner is no easy task. There are many handoffs and data exchanges that need to take place. To

help facilitate this, some health plans and employers have created a layer of resource called a health advocate that sits on top of the various interventions shown in Figure 22-8. These health advocates are usually nurses who are assigned to different employees to help guide them through the care continuum using the resources that the health plan offers within the parameters of the employer health plan benefit design. The health advocates are able to look up information from multiple sources to help make these decisions. Typically, this might involve medical claims information (including pharmacy, diagnostic laboratory), health risk appraisal information, prior history from disease management or case management, employer benefit plan information, prior customer service contacts, community resources, health care content, and so forth. The nurse can then recommend how the employee should proceed, and in some cases, they can make

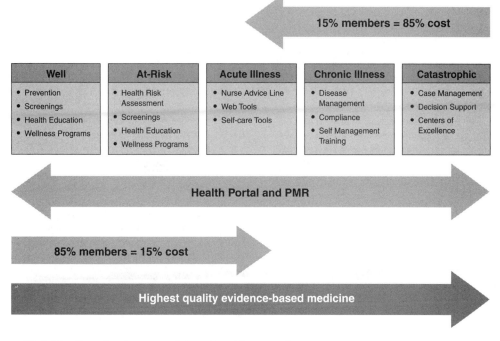

Figure 22–8 The Care Continuum and Associated Interventions

Source: Courtesy of Towers Perrin, New York, NY.

appointments or referrals. These health advocate nurses remain with the employee indefinitely, even if the medical condition has been resolved. Health advocate programs have proved cost effective and have great employee satisfaction. The health advocate concept can also assist in the process of employee engagement.

WHAT IS EMPLOYEE ENGAGEMENT?

Employee engagement is a recognition that one size health care does not fit all and that there are some serious disconnects between what the employer thinks the employee wants and needs and what the employees themselves think (see Figure 22-9).

A number of factors both emotional and rational drive employee behavior. For example, employer commitment and access and use of support tools can affect how employees behave (see Figure 22-10).

Another reason that employee engagement is important is because the more engaged a consumer is, the lower that person's costs (see Figure 22-11).

This collision of consumerism, employee engagement, and care continuum management has spawned the phrase "building a culture of health." The overall goal of a culture of health is a healthy organization. This means an employer will have efficient benefit programs, acceptable costs, and a productive, engaged workforce.

THE FUTURE

Consumerism and technology are the dominant themes that will continue. Health care consumerism is evolving rapidly as better data become available on what drives employee health care behavior. Consumers are accepting some accountability and responsibility but in small doses. At the time of pub-

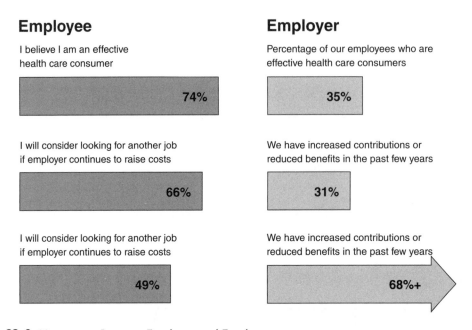

Figure 22–9 Disconnects Between Employee and Employer
Source: Towers Perrin 2005 Health Care Consumerism Survey.

lication, between 5 million and 6 million people were enrolled in a CDHP with an HRA or a high-deductible health plan with or without an HSA.

Technology is benefiting from strong government support of electronic medical records and regional health information networks.

The full power of Medicare Part D will be in effect. The result will be increased government purchasing leverage, increased enrollment in Medicare Advantage plans, and more transparency in pharmacy benefit management.

Prevention is back. No longer shackled by the fuzzy wellness label, prevention is part of the care continuum and has multiple dimensions. Well-designed, engaging, and cost-effective programs for stress reduction, exercise, nutrition counseling, and weight reduction are leading this resurgence. Prevention in managed care is discussed fully in Chapter 14.

Convergence of health and wealth will continue to be a major factor. The major force be-

hind this convergence is the recent U.S. regulatory change that created tax-advantaged HSAs and HRAs that encourage consumers to take more responsibility for their own health care. Many financial services companies are offering savings accounts and investment products to attract HSA assets.

Health insurers not wishing to cede these services have acted to partner with or even charter banks. This convergence is likely to restructure the value chain of the health insurance industry. Cross-industry partnerships will develop and leading companies will invest to build their capabilities. Eventually, traditional insurers and financial firms may combine capabilities and assets to deliver integrated products.[5]

Medical practice is still slow to change. Much progress has been made on reducing variations using tools and technology to support systemization and use of evidence-based guidelines. Several collaborative efforts between medical providers, employers, and researchers are under way. There is general

How Employer Committment Affects Consumer Behavior

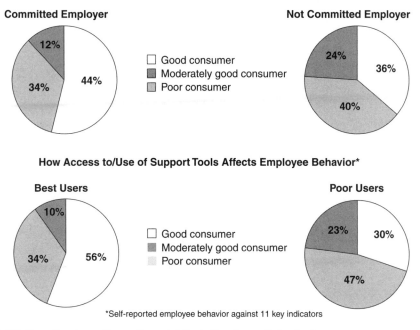

Committed Employer

12%
34%
44%

□ Good consumer
■ Moderately good consumer
□ Poor consumer

Not Committed Employer

24%
36%
40%

How Access to/Use of Support Tools Affects Employee Behavior*

Best Users

10%
34%
56%

□ Good consumer
■ Moderately good consumer
□ Poor consumer

Poor Users

23%
30%
47%

*Self-reported employee behavior against 11 key indicators

Figure 22–10 How Employer Commitment Affects Employee Behavior*

Source: Towers Perrin 2005 Health Care Consumerism Survey.

agreement that greater cooperation is needed to avoid duplication of effort and fragmentation of outcomes.

All of these trends have significant implications for employers. The major implication is the role of the employer in providing health benefits for its employees. As employers look at the people and business drivers and the impact of health benefits on the value of their employees and the effectiveness of their workforce, some may consider getting out of providing health care benefits directly. They may prefer to contribute a defined amount and let the employee decide. They are questioning whether there is adequate business value in continuing to act as the buffer between unhappy health care consumers and unhappy providers. There has been lots of talk about this, but not a lot of employers are exiting the role of sponsoring active health care. However, many employers *are* exiting the retiree medical coverage business.[6]

The more common view is that employers want to stay in the game of providing employee benefits, but they want their employees to be more aware of costs and to be more engaged. Transparency and engagement are the key themes. They are manifested in reduced choice of plan but better designs to match employee segmentation. CDHPs in the form of account-based plans are growing in popularity as one of the remaining choices.

The Bush administration has been very supportive of account-based plans as a way to combat rising costs and to create a medical savings vehicle for retirees that may help Medicare as it runs out of money. Current estimates have Medicare's Hospital Insurance Trust Fund in deficit by 2012.[7]

Some states are looking at universal coverage as a way to reduce the level of uninsureds, which will benefit the private employer-sponsored sector as well as the pub-

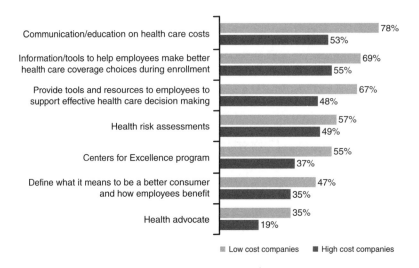

Figure 22–11 A Focus on Consumer Engagement and Health Links to Better Results

Source: Towers Perrin 2006 Health Care Cost Survey.

lic sector. At the time of publication, Massachusetts is trying to implement a health care reform law that will require every resident over 18 years of age to purchase affordable and in some cases subsidized coverage. Vermont and Maryland are considering similar efforts.[8]

CONCLUSION

Much has changed in the 5 years since the previous version of this book, but much has stayed the same. Employers and health plans are hedging their bets about how much health care will be delivered by employer sponsors and how much will be an individual purchase.

The convergence of health and wealth should not be underestimated. The financial sector will have significant impact on the health sector. Adoption of cost-saving and efficient technology will increase; brand loyalty and rewards programs will be introduced; simplified administration may occur; and credit and debit cards will become a major transaction mechanism rather than solely used for claims.

Offsetting these trends are continued upward pressures on health care costs caused by provider costs and charges, advances in medical science, and increasing use of medical services for a variety of reasons. They remain wildcards in this rapidly evolving environment.

Finally, a word should be said about the flattening of the world.[9] As multinational employers in the United States look to increase their workforces in other countries, they should be mindful that many social welfare systems are in dire financial shape. Many countries are looking to revamp their health care systems and shift more cost and responsibility to the private employer sector. Lessons learned here in the United States can be taken abroad. Improving care management, stressing prevention, and engaging employees can be tried in many countries today regardless of the delivery systems and the social welfare funding mechanism.

References

1. Porter M, Teisberg E. Redefining competition in healthcare. *Harvard Bus Rev*. June 2004.
2. Ellis M. GM/UAW deal changes landscape. *Detroit Free Press*. October 18, 2005.
3. How to control health benefit costs. *McKinsey Quarterly*. January 2004.
4. Healthcare for uninsured will add $922 to family insurance premiums in 2005. *Families USA* [press release]. June 8, 2005.
5. The coming convergence of U.S. healthcare and financial services. *McKinsey Quarterly*. June 2005.
6. Employers getting out of retiree healthcare business. *USA Today*. June 28, 2006.
7. Social Security Administration. Status of the Social Security and Medicare programs. *Summary of 2006 Annual Report*. Social Security Administration. May 2, 2006.
8. *2006 Bills on Universal Healthcare Coverage*. National Conference of State Legislatures. June 2006.
9. Friedman T. *The World is Flat*. New York. Farrar, Straus and Giroux, 2005.

Suggested Reading

McKinsey and Company. *An Executive Perspective on Employee Benefits. A McKinsey Survey*. New York: McKinsey and Company, 2006.

Rethinking health reform. *Health Affairs*. November/December. 2005:24(6).

23

ACCREDITATION AND PERFORMANCE MEASUREMENT PROGRAMS FOR MANAGED CARE ORGANIZATIONS

Margaret E. O'Kane

Study Objectives

- Understand rationale for accrediting health care organizations and the intended uses for the information provided by different accreditation/certification programs.
- Understand the differences in approach and intent between the nation's primary accreditors of managed care organizations.
- Understand accreditation of providers within managed care.
- Understand the main elements of each accreditation program.
- Understand which sectors of the health care market are currently accountable for quality and which are not.

Discussion Topics

1. Discuss the main elements of the accreditation process and the importance of each.
2. Discuss how different entities are accredited; for example, HMOs, PPOs, utilization review organizations, and credentialing verification organizations.
3. Discuss how accreditation information is currently used and how such use might evolve in the future.
4. Discuss the difference between accreditation and certification.
5. Discuss why a health plan may or may not participate in a voluntary accreditation program.
6. Discuss how accreditation differs from state or federal licensure.

INTRODUCTION

Since 1991, accreditation and performance measurement have become enduring features in the managed care landscape. Practice patterns, information systems, and key administrative and management functions have all been refined or built from the ground up to promote quality improvement and satisfy the demands of external oversight. Driven by mandates from employers, state and federal government, and consumers, and a desire by health plans to demonstrate quality objectively as market distinction, a majority of the nation's health maintenance organizations (HMOs) and point-of-service (POS) health plans now participate in some form of accreditation.

During this same period, the oversight process has evolved from its initial exclusive focus on HMOs to include accreditation, certification, and performance measurement programs that cover the full spectrum of affiliated health care organizations—managed behavioral health care organizations (MBHOs), credentials verification organizations (CVOs), preferred provider organizations (PPOs), disease management programs, and provider groups. In addition, oversight programs have become more sophisticated and targeted, and are now able, utilizing current information technology, to focus on specific population subsets and disease states.

Growing legislative and market forces continue to advance this trend with accountability applying not just to health plans and related organizations, but also to facilities, Web-based health management, education programs, and individual providers. Consumers, employers, and others need and want to know about the quality of their health care.

Despite the trend, it is notable that accreditation and performance measurement in managed care remain largely voluntary. Current federal legislation requires Medicare health plans to submit performance data (see also Chapter 26), and the Office of Personnel Management recently added a requirement for fee-for-service plans contracting with PPOs as well. At the state level, selected states require health plans to do either accreditation, provide performance measures, or both; sometimes this is a condition of licensure, in other instances it is to gain entry into the state employee market. In place of legislative mandates, however, the market has developed its own mandate. Dozens of the nation's leading corporations will not do business with a health plan that has not earned some form of external accreditation—in particular by the National Committee for Quality Assurance (NCQA), whose seal of approval is now required by several states and more than 30% of the nation's largest firms. An even larger number of employers require their health plan partners to report on their performance, a prerequisite to assessing value.

Three organizations, each of which approaches its oversight role from a different perspective and each of which specializes in a different sector of the market, have developed managed care oversight programs of note:

- NCQA
- URAC
- Accreditation Association for Ambulatory Health Care, also known as the Accreditation Association, or AAAHC

Each of these accredits managed care organizations and each offers related accreditation or certification programs. These organizations and the various oversight programs they offer are described later in this chapter. In addition, NCQA manages and implements the predominant form of performance measurement tool used to evaluate managed care plans—the Health Plan Employer Data and Information Set (HEDIS®), used by more than 90% of all health plans and referred to in several other chapters in this book.

The Joint Commission on Accreditation of Healthcare Organizations (Joint Commission), a major organization for facility-based accreditation and certification, discontinued its network accreditation program (for integrated delivery systems, managed care organizations, managed behavioral health care organizations, and preferred provider organizations), effective January 1, 2006. However, the Joint Commission provides support services and oversight to organizations accredited under this program through the end of each organization's respective accreditation award period.

It is important to note that there are differences among the accreditation programs offered by each organization. These differences reflect the accreditors' varied histories and perspectives for which their programs were designed. Although each of these organizations is discussed in greater detail later in this chapter, a brief description follows.

For NCQA, the major emphasis is on improving the quality of health care by measuring results and providing the market—consumers and employers—with information that will allow for direct comparisons between the organizations on the basis of quality. Hence, NCQA's focus on quality is underscored by the fact that effectiveness of care and member satisfaction performance make up a full 40% of accreditation score. Using the objective, evidence-based HEDIS® measures, NCQA puts emphasis on those mechanisms that the organization has established for continuous improvement in quality. Historically, NCQA focused on evaluating HMO and POS plans, but its agenda has expanded considerably in recent years and now includes behavioral health care organizations, PPOs, CVOs, provider groups, and other health care entities. NCQA believes that by providing the market with this information, it rewards those health plans that are providing excellent care and service, thus giving all health plans a strong incentive to focus on quality.

URAC was formed in 1990 with the backing of a broad range of consumers, employers, regulators, providers, and industry representatives to provide an efficient and effective method for evaluating utilization review (UR) processes. The organization has since branched out beyond UR oversight and into the evaluation of health plans and PPOs, CVOs, disease management programs, health Web sites, and other health care entities. The stated mission of URAC is "to promote continuous improvement in the quality and efficiency of health care management through processes of accreditation and education." Originally, URAC was incorporated under the name "Utilization Review Accreditation Commission." However, that name was shortened to just the acronym URAC in 1996 when URAC began accrediting other types of organizations such as health plans and preferred provider organizations. In addition, URAC sometimes uses a second corporate name or "DBA," which is the "American Accreditation HealthCare Commission, Inc."

The Accreditation Association for Ambulatory Health Care (AAAHC) was formed in 1979 to assist ambulatory health care organizations improve the quality of care provided to patients. AAAHC accredits more than 2,700 health care organizations, including endoscopy centers, ambulatory surgery centers, office-based surgery centers, student health centers, and large medical and dental group practices. The AAAHC also surveys and accredits managed care organizations and independent practice associations (IPAs). The organization's managed care standards are developed with active industry input and include the evaluation of enrollee communications systems, enrollee complaint and grievance resolution systems, utilization management, including enrollee appeal procedures, quality management and improvement, and provider credentialing and recredentialing systems.

OVERSIGHT BY TYPE OF ORGANIZATION

Managed care is a loosely defined term that can be applied to a number of different types of health care organizations, including HMOs, POS plans, PPOs, IPAs, UR firms, and a host of other derivative organizational models as discussed in Chapter 2. Accreditation and performance measurement have not weighed equally on the various systems of care. Historically, only the most tightly managed delivery systems—HMO and POS plans—have been impelled to seek external accreditation. The reasons for the focus on HMO and POS plans were primarily because of responsible employers and leading health plans seeking market distinction volunteering to come forward. No doubt the movement was supported by the extensive media coverage of HMO "horror stories" and the public's general reluctance in the 1990s to accept change in the health care system.

HMOs' participation in accreditation and performance measurement programs over the years has paid an important dividend: improved quality. Since the mid-1990s, the percentage of HMOs earning the highest levels of accreditation, excellent or commendable, from the nation's leading HMO accreditor, NCQA, has steadily risen. At the same time, HEDIS® scores for accredited plans outperform their non-accredited counterparts, evidence that accredited health plans are providing superior care.

Similarly, data collected since 1996 show that most HMOs that publicly report on their performance (using HEDIS®) in such areas as immunization and mammography rates have steadily, and in some cases dramatically, improved their performance. For example, participating HMO and POS plans have gone

from treating just 62% of heart attack patients with beta blockers to treating 96%, an improvement that annually saves thousands of lives. Figure 23-1 illustrates the improvement in other selected clinically important HEDIS® measures over 5 years.

By contrast, there have been few accreditation mechanisms for PPOs and little information available about what proportion of PPOs have quality assurance programs or about the efficacy of those programs. Until recently, the majority of PPOs have not pursued external accreditation by any oversight organization in large part because appropriate oversight programs have not existed. However, this has changed as two of the major oversight organizations—NCQA and URAC—have developed and are implementing accreditation and performance measurement programs for PPOs.

Accreditation and performance measurement tools have become more sophisticated and versatile along with changes in the health care delivery system. Several important organizations have challenged the health care industry to provide better and safer care, and performance measurement is more and more focusing on individual physicians and patients with specific chronic diseases.

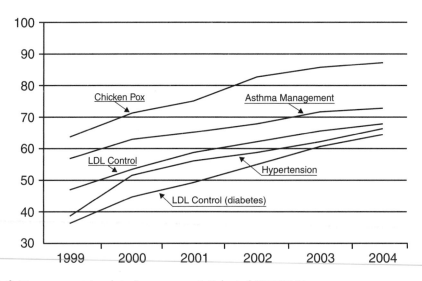

Figure 23–1 Measurement Leads to Improvement: Selected HEDIS® Measures

In fact, a growing number of states are making data about the quality of hospital services available online and consumers, armed with this information, health education materials from the Internet, and health plan report cards from accreditation organizations are making more informed choices, as discussed further in Chapter 20.

As indicated previously, the accreditation programs offered by the three MCOs discussed in this chapter are unique, as are the organizations behind each program. These differences are reflected in the focus of their review process, in the governance of the organizations, and in the actual accreditation process. A review of each of them follows.

NATIONAL COMMITTEE FOR QUALITY ASSURANCE

NCQA is a private, nonprofit organization dedicated to improving health care quality. NCQA accredits and certifies a wide range of health care organizations, including managed care plans (HMOs, POS products, PPOs), managed behavioral health care organizations, physician organizations, and credentials verification organizations. NCQA implements and manages the evolution of HEDIS®, a performance measurement tool used by more than 90% of the nation's health plans. NCQA is committed to providing health care quality information through the Web and the media to help consumers, employers, and others make more informed health care choices.

NCQA is governed by a board of directors of independent experts representing key stakeholders in health quality such as employers, consumers, labor representatives, health plans, quality experts, policymakers, and representatives from organized medicine. Copies of NCQA's accreditation standards, HEDIS® specifications, application materials, and current accreditation status of health plans can be obtained by contacting NCQA, 2000 L Street NW, Suite 500, Washington, DC 20036; (888) 275-7585; or on the Internet: http://www.ncqa.org.

History

NCQA was established in 1979 by the Group Health Association of America and the American Managed Care Review Association, the trade associations at that time for HMOs and IPAs.* Original NCQA governance was by the HMO industry. In 1987, HMO industry leaders, believing that NCQA provided a good base for external quality review, studied a broader role for NCQA and began a process to separate it from the trade associations and make it independent, a recognized prerequisite for its credibility. As part of that process, the board was restructured to empower purchasers and other users.

In 1988, the Robert Wood Johnson Foundation funded a series of meetings to explore interest in the purchaser community in NCQA's potential as an independent external review organization. The group of purchaser representatives, benefits managers from Fortune 500 companies who were at the leading edge of external quality assessment, gave a resounding mandate for NCQA to go forward. In late 1989, the foundation awarded NCQA a grant to support its development as an independent entity. As evidence of industry support, the grant required that matching monies be raised from the managed care industry. Industry contributions demonstrated support, and NCQA was officially launched in March of 1990.

NCQA conducted the first health plan accreditation survey in 1991. During the ensuing 15 years, the organization has conducted thousands of reviews of participating health plans and other health care entities, which currently enroll about 21.5% of all Americans with health care benefits.

---

*These trade associations eventually merged to become the American Association of Health Plans (AAHP), which then later merged with the Health Insurance Association of America (HIAA) to become America's Health Insurance Plans (AHIP). AHIP is the trade association that now represents the managed care and health insurance industries in the United States.

During the 1990s, NCQA took responsibility for the management and further development of the Health Plan Data and Information Set (HEDIS®) and introduced accreditation or certification programs for credentials verification organizations, managed behavioral health care organizations, physician organizations, and preferred provider organizations.

In 2001, NCQA began accreditation and certification of disease management programs and assumed management of the Diabetes Provider Recognition Program. And, in 2004, NCQA introduced *Quality Plus*, an initiative that recognizes health plans that take innovative approaches to ensuring that their members receive high-quality care.

Areas of Health Plan Review

The content of NCQA's accreditation programs is determined by NCQA's Standards Committee, a 15-member group that represents employers, consumers, health plans, and policymakers. NCQA also actively solicits input on all its programs through public review and comment periods.

A health plan's overall accreditation status is determined based on its performance in three areas—clinical performance using HEDIS® measures, member satisfaction using the Consumer Assessment of Health Providers and Systems (CAHPS) survey, and a review of key structures and processes using NCQA Standards and Guidelines. HEDIS® and CAHPS together account for about 40% of a health plan's accreditation results, with performance against standards accounting for the remainder. Using these methods, NCQA evaluates and reports to the public the following:

- *Access and service.* NCQA evaluates how well a health plan provides its members with access to needed care and with good customer service.
- *Qualified providers.* NCQA evaluates how a health plan ensures that each provider is licensed and appropriately trained to practice, and that members are satisfied with their doctors.

- *Staying healthy.* NCQA evaluates health plan activities that help people maintain good health and avoid illness.
- *Getting better.* NCQA evaluates health plan activities that help people recover from illness.
- *Living with illness.* NCQA evaluates health plan activities that help people manage chronic illness.

Compliance with NCQA Standards and Guidelines

Sixty percent of a health plan's accreditation results are based on compliance with NCQA's standards and guidelines, including the scope and function of key operations:

- Quality improvement
- Utilization management
- Credentialing and network development
- Members' rights and responsibilities

Quality Improvement

The first and most rigorous area of NCQA review is a health plan's own internal quality control systems (see also Chapter 15). To meet NCQA standards, an organization must have a well-organized, comprehensive quality improvement (QI) program accountable to the governing body of the organization. The QI program must include a written description of the QI program, which is updated annually and overseen by a QI committee that meets regularly.

The QI program's scope must be comprehensive, covering the full spectrum of services included in the organization's benefit design. The QI program must focus on important aspects of care and services and address clinical issues with major impact on the health status of the enrolled population. These should include the following:

- Accessibility of health care services
- Assistance for people with chronic health conditions
- Continuity and coordination of care
- Coordination between medical and behavioral health care

- Documentation of clinical quality improvement

To ensure practitioner participation in QI activities, contracts with physicians and other health care providers must be explicit about the requirement to cooperate with the health plan's QI program. In addition, the health plan must ensure access to care by creating a provider network that considers the needs of its members. The health plan must also develop and distribute clinical practice guidelines and policies for medical record documentation to its provider network.

If the health plan delegates QI activities to another organization, it must work with the delegated party to develop a mutually agreed-upon document that outlines responsibilities, delegated activities, and monitoring processes.

Most important, a health plan must document program effectiveness in improving its quality of care and service. The plan must measure and demonstrate at least three clinical care improvements, including one in behavioral health. Quality improvement can also be documented comparing successive years' HEDIS® results in the areas in which the health plan has chosen to focus (*eg*, immunization rates, eye exams for diabetics, and so on).

NCQA establishes compliance with its standards by thorough on-site review of a health plan's QI program description and related policies and procedures, quality improvement studies, projects and monitoring activities, QI committee and governing body minutes, interviews with key staff, tracking of issues uncovered by the QI system to ensure resolution, and documented evidence of quality improvement.

Processes for Reviewing and Authorizing Medical Care

Utilization management (UM; see also Chapter 9), one of the foundations of effective managed care, is an important determinant of both the cost and the quality of an MCO. To earn NCQA accreditation, a health plan must meet rigorous utilization management standards designed to ensure that this key function promotes good health care rather than acting as an arbitrary barrier to accessing appropriate services.

NCQA requires that review decisions be made by qualified medical professionals and that the organization has a written description of its program for managing care, which includes clearly documented criteria and procedures for approving and denying care. The UM plan must also address triage and referral for behavioral health care, procedures for drug coverage, access to emergency services without precertification, and the evaluation and coverage of new technology.

NCQA UM standards specify that qualified health professionals oversee all review decisions and that an appropriate practitioner reviews any denial of care based on medical necessity. These standards ensure that if a medical specialist appeals a decision to deny a requested treatment, another similarly trained practitioner will rule on the appeal. This issue is an especially critical consideration for appeals dealing with complex medical questions where simply referring to preexisting medical guidelines may not adequately account for a specific patient's situation.

Health plans must have written policies and procedures for the resolution of member UM appeals. To make sure that UM decisions and appeals are processed in a timely manner, NCQA sets explicit "turnaround time" requirements that specify the maximum allowable time between appeal and determination by the health plan.

Although consumers and others are typically most concerned about overaggressive UM, insufficient UM can be problematic as well, leading to unnecessary care and expense. Thus, NCQA requires that a health plan's UM system monitor for over- as well as underutilization.

Compliance with UM standards is determined during a thorough on-site review of a health plan's written UM program description and related policies and procedures, review determinations, appeals process and determinations, interviews with key staff, tracking of issues uncovered by the UM system, and documented evidence of appropriate oversight.

Delegation

Delegation occurs when the organization gives another entity the authority to carry out a function that it would otherwise perform to meet requirements within NCQA standards. This authority includes the right to decide what to do and how to do it, within the parameters agreed on by the organization and the other entity. When delegation exists, NCQA requires the presence of a mutual agreement between the delegating organization and its delegate that is performing specific functions related to NCQA standards. Although the organization does not directly perform delegated functions, it must oversee them to ensure that the delegate is properly performing the functions. The organization may reclaim the right to carry out its delegated functions at any time.

Subdelegation occurs when the organization's delegate gives a third entity the authority to carry out a delegated function. Subdelegation is acceptable if either the delegate or the organization oversees the work performed by the subdelegate to ensure that it meets NCQA standards. If the delegate oversees the subdelegate, it must report to the organization regarding the subdelegate's performance. NCQA holds the organization ultimately accountable for all NCQA-related activities performed by both the delegate and subdelegate on the organization's behalf.

Quality of Provider Network

To ensure the quality of the health plan's provider network, NCQA's accreditation process includes a thorough review of an organization's credentialing system (see also Chapter 5). In addition to a credentialing process for primary care physicians and medical specialists, the health plan must also confirm that hospitals, home health care agencies, skilled nursing facilities, nursing homes, and behavioral health facilities in its network are in good standing with state and federal agencies and accrediting organizations.

NCQA requires that health plans have a process to identify which types of practitioners must be credentialed, clearly defined and documented procedures for assessing its practitioners' qualifications and practice history, and policies that define practitioner rights to review and correct credentialing information.

Prior to allowing network participation, health plans must verify practitioners' credentials, including a valid license to practice medicine, education and training, malpractice history, and work history. Before making a decision on a practitioner's qualifications, the health plan must receive and review information from third parties, such as information about any disciplinary actions. In addition, the health plan must verify through an on-site visit that primary care practitioners, obstetricians/gynecologists, and high-volume behavioral health care practitioners' offices meet the organization's standards.

An important part of ensuring delivery system integrity is periodic recertification of providers, and NCQA requires that the health plan reevaluate practitioners' qualifications every 36 months. Before reevaluating a practitioner's qualifications, the health plan must receive information from third parties, such as information about disciplinary actions. Between recredentialing cycles, the organization must monitor practitioner member complaints and satisfaction and information from quality improvement activities. NCQA standards require the health plan to monitor sanctions, complaints, and quality issues on a regular basis and take appropriate action when issues are identified.

If the health plan delegates to a third party decisions on evaluating or reevaluating a provider's qualifications, the decision-making process—including the responsibilities of the plan and delegated party—must be clearly documented and the plan must evaluate and approve the delegated party's credentialing process on a regular basis. In 1995, NCQA released standards to certify credentials verification organizations (CVOs), thus eliminating the need for health plans to conduct an annual review of those organizations. This program is described in more detail later in this chapter as well as in Chapter 5.

Compliance with credentialing standards is ascertained by reviewing an organization's credentialing policies and procedures, sampling individual provider files, conducting interviews with relevant staff, reviewing credentialing committee minutes, and tracking issues identified through the complaint system or quality improvement findings.

Member Rights and Responsibilities

To meet NCQA standards, a health plan must have written policies that state its commitment to treating members in a manner that respects their rights as well as delineate the plan's expectations of members' responsibilities. These policies must be distributed to members and participating practitioners.

NCQA requires a health plan to have a system for the timely resolution of member complaints and appeals, to aggregate and analyze complaint appeal data, and to use the information for quality improvement. This activity, often undertaken by the health plan's member services function, is also discussed in Chapter 19.

NCQA standards require written communication to members of certain types of information about how the health plan works, including benefits and charges for which members are responsible, as well as copayments, how to obtain care, how to file a complaint or appeal, and how to choose a new provider when members' practitioners leave the plan's network.

The standards require that member information be written in readable prose and be available in the languages of the major population groups served. Health plans must also have mechanisms ensuring confidentiality and take steps to protect the privacy of members' information and records.

A health plan's marketing materials must describe its procedures for approving or denying coverage, covered benefits, including pharmacy benefits, noncovered services, availability of practitioners and providers, and any applicable restrictions. In addition, the health plan must monitor new members' understanding of its procedures and update its marketing materials accordingly.

Compliance with member rights and responsibility standards is determined by reviewing an organization's written policies and procedures, marketing materials, conducting interviews with relevant staff, and tracking issues identified through the complaint and appeals system.

HEDIS®

As noted earlier, HEDIS® is a performance measurement tool used by more than 90% of the nation's managed care organizations. It is a robust set of standardized measures that specifies how health plans collect, audit, and report on their performance in important areas such as delivery of preventive health services, member satisfaction with care, utilization of services, and treatment efficacy for various illnesses. Measures are reviewed annually and are updated, revised, and even retired through a broad-based process that includes public comment on each proposed new measure or change.

By specifying not only what to measure, but also how to measure it, HEDIS® allows true "apples-to-apples" comparisons between health plans. HEDIS® allows health plans to manage and improve quality and purchasers of health care to make informed choices. Every year, dozens of national news magazines, local newspapers, employers, and others use HEDIS® data to generate health plan "report cards" during open enrollment. All HEDIS® data are independently audited and verified.

HEDIS® consists of more than 60 measures (not including the CAHPS 3.0H survey, which includes dozens of individual questions) that fall into six broad categories or domains:

- Effectiveness of care
- Access/availability of care

- Satisfaction with the experience
- Health plan stability
- Use of services
- Health plan descriptive information

The full 2006 HEDIS® measure set is listed in Table 23-1.

Effectiveness of Care

Measures in this category underlie such oft-reported statistics as childhood immunization rates, cancer screening, appropriate use of antibiotics, management of behavioral health conditions, and common chronic illnesses, including asthma, coronary artery disease, diabetes, and chronic obstructive pulmonary disease (COPD). These and other measures seek to establish whether the health plan is responding to the needs of those who are ill ("Does the health plan make me better when I am sick?") and also to the needs of those who are well ("Does the health plan help me stay healthy when I am well?"). The 2006 HEDIS® Effectiveness of Care measures are listed in Table 23-2.

Access/Availability of Care

Measures in this category assess whether care is available to members in a timely manner when they need it and where they need it. Among others, important measures in this category include adults' access to preventive health care, children and adolescents' access to primary care, and women's access to prenatal and postpartum care.

Satisfaction with the Experience

These measures from the CAHPS Health Plan Adult and Child Surveys provide important information about whether a health plan is able to satisfy the diverse needs of its members. Two different surveys—one for adults, the other related to parents' impressions of the care their children receive—include numerous questions related to many key consumer issues, including getting needed care, getting care quickly, how well doctors communicate, helpfulness of office staff, customer service, claims processing, and overall rating of health plan. The survey of children's care is not required for accreditation.

Health Plan Stability

These measures—practitioner turnover, years in business, and total membership—provide information about the soundness and dependability of a health plan.

Use of Services

How a health plan uses its resources is a signal of how competently care is managed. Measures in this category permit members and other users to understand patterns of service utilization across different health plans. Measures look at important areas such as the frequency of ongoing prenatal care, well child and adolescent visits, frequency of selected procedures, inpatient utilization, maternity care length of stay, and several indicators of mental health utilization.

Health Plan Descriptive Information

Although not technically performance measures, HEDIS® includes several general questions about aspects of a health plan that employers and consumers have found useful when selecting among plans. These include indicators such as board certification of network physicians, enrollment by product line and state, and racial and ethnic diversity of membership.

Significantly, HEDIS® is applicable to both the public and private sectors. The same measurement standards (with some variations for population demographics) are applied to care provided to Medicaid beneficiaries, commercial health plan enrollees, and Medicare populations opting for managed care plans. This not only increases the efficiency of measurement but also allows for performance comparisons across populations and health plan types.

Measures included in HEDIS® typically undergo exhaustive testing and review prior to inclusion and must possess three key attributes:

- *Relevance.* Measures must address health issues of significant concern, and

Table 23–1 2006 HEDIS Measures

Effectiveness of Care Measures
- Childhood Immunization
- Adolescent Immunization
- Appropriate Treatment for Children with Upper Respiratory Infection
- Appropriate Testing for Children with Pharyngitis
- Colorectal Cancer Screening
- Breast Cancer Screening
- Cervical Cancer Screening
- Chlamydia Screening
- Osteoporosis Management in Women
- Controlling High Blood Pressure
- Beta-Blocker Treatment
- Persistence of Beta-Blocker Treatment
- Cholesterol Management
- Comprehensive Diabetes Care
- Use of Appropriate Medication for Asthma
- Follow-up After Hospital, for Mental Illness
- Antidepressant Medication Management
- Glaucoma Screening
- Imaging Studies for Low Back Pain
- Medical Assistance with Smoking Cessation
- Flu Shots, Adults 50–64
- Flu Shots, Older Adults
- Pneumonia Vaccination
- Medicare Health Outcomes Survey
- Management of Urinary Incontinence in Older Adults
- Physical Activity in Older Adults
- Inappropriate Treatment for Adults with Acute Bronchitis
- Use of Spirometry Testing in COPD
- Follow-up Care for Children Prescribed ADHD Medication
- Disease-modifying Antirheumatic Drug Therapy in Rheumatoid Arthritis
- Annual Monitoring for Patients on Persistent Medications
- Drugs to be Avoided in the Elderly

Access and Availability
- Adults' Access to Preventive/Ambulatory Services
- Children/Adolescents' Access to PCPs
- Prenatal and Postpartum Care
- Annual Dental Visit
- Initiation and Engagement: Alcohol and Other Drug Treatment
- Claims Timeliness
- Call Answer Timeliness
- Call Abandonment

Use of Services
- Frequency of Ongoing Prenatal Care
- Well-child Visits/15 Months
- Well-child Visits/3–6 Years
- Adolescent Well-care Visits
- Frequency of Selected Procedures
- Inpatient Use—General Hospital/Acute
- Inpatient Use—Nonacute
- Discharges and ALOS—Maternity
- Births and ALOS—Newborns
- Mental health Use—discharges and ALOS
- Chemical Dependency Use—Discharges and ALOS
- Ambulatory Care
- Mental Health Use—% of Inpatient, Intermediate, and Ambulatory Services
- Identification of Alcohol and Other Drug Services
- Outpatient Drug Use
- Antibiotic Utilization

Health Plan Stability
- Practitioner Turnover
- Years in Business/Total Membership

Satification with the Experience of Care
- HEDIS®/CAHPS 3.0H, Adult
  –Commercial and Medicaid
  –CMS administers CAHPS® 3.0 for Medicare
- HEDIS®/CAHPS 3.0H, Child
  –Information from parents of children with Medicaid or commerical coverage
  –Special section for children with chronic conditions
- ECHOTM 3.0H Survey
  –For MBHOs only
  –Captures enrollee's experiences
    - With Behavioral Health Care
    - Mental and Chemical Dependency Services

Health Plan Descriptive Information
- Board Certification
- Enrollment by Product Line
- Enrollment by State
- Unduplicated Count of Medicaid Members
- Race/Ethnicity Diversity of Medicaid Members
- Language Diversity of Medicaid Members
- Weeks of Pregnancy at Time of Enrollment

Informed Health Care Choices
- Previous Measures Retired
- No Current Measures
- Exploring Future Measures

Cost of Care
- Previous Measures Retired
- No Current Measures
- Exploring Future Measures

Source: NCQA.

Table 23–2 HEDIS Effectiveness of Care Measures

• Prevention
  – Cancer Screening
    • Breast cancer
    • Cervical cancer
    • Colon cancer
  – Immunizations (Children and Adolescents)
  – Chlamydia screen
  – Antibiotic prescribing
  – Elderly care
    • Pneumonia vaccination
    • Influenza vaccination
    • Urinary incontinence
    • Vision screening
    • Advice for physical activity
	• Chronic Care Conditions
	  – Hypertension
	  – Diabetes (6)
	  – Cardiovascular Disease
	    • Cholesterol test and results
	    • Betablocker after AMI
	    • Betablocker long-term compliance
	  – Smoking cessation
	  – Osteoporosis
	  – Arthritis
	  – Asthma
	  – COPD
	  – Depression (3)
	  – Substance Use (3)
	  – Coordination of care psychiatry
	  – ADHD
	  – Low back pain
	  – Safe Medication Management
	    • Never medications
	    • Appropriate testing

Source: NCQA, 2006.

performance on measures should be controllable (at least to some extent) by the health plan. Also, information produced by a given measure should be useful to consumers and employers.

• *Scientific soundness.* Measures must focus on processes of care that are evidence-based. They must also generate reproducible, valid, and accurate results. Measures also must be sensitive enough to detect meaningful differences in performance between health plans.

• *Feasibility.* It should be possible to collect the data required for a measure at a reasonable cost and effort.

As part of the NCQA accreditation process, health plans are required to report on their performance on HEDIS® measures, including a subset from the effectiveness of care category and a subset derived from the CAHPS Health Plan surveys. To ensure that quality and performance are maintained between on-site surveys (which occur at least every 36 months), NCQA requires health plans to submit independently audited HEDIS® results annually. Should these results, or other factors such as regulatory action, suggest a lapse in quality, NCQA may elect to resurvey the health plan sooner. Accreditation status can change as well.

CAHPS Health Plan Survey

Member satisfaction surveys have long been a popular way to assess health plan performance, and such a survey has been featured in HEDIS® since 1996. Previously, information about member satisfaction was gathered using a variety of surveys and instruments developed by the health plans for use with their enrolled population. Because no standardized survey was in broad use, what little member satisfaction data were available could not be used to compare plans because the survey instruments and survey methodology varied from plan to plan.

At the insistence of various constituencies—including health plans, which were often required by their clients to field dozens of different satisfaction surveys annually—satisfaction survey data are now collected in a more rational, efficient manner using a standard tool, the CAHPS Health Plan Survey. This survey was jointly developed by NCQA and the federal Agency for Health Research and Quality (AHRQ).

CAHPS Health Plan surveys are similar to patient satisfaction surveys and include ratings of providers and health plans. But they go beyond this type of question by asking health plan members to report on their experiences with health care services. Reports about care are regarded as more specific, actionable, understandable, and objective than general ratings alone.

Since 1999, NCQA has required CAHPS Health Plan survey results from health plans seeking accreditation and/or submitting data as part of HEDIS®. CAHPS, like HEDIS®, is designed to be applicable to all health plans regardless of the population they serve: Medicare, Medicaid, or commercial. CAHPS consists of several different surveys: one for the adult population, another designed to assess parents' impressions of their children's health care, and a third for use specifically with the Medicare and Medicaid populations. To ensure that CAHPS data are collected using only the approved, standardized methodology, health plans are required to contract with an NCQA-certified third-party vendor to administer the survey.

Although each CAHPS Health Plan survey consists of dozens of questions, the questions are grouped in "composites" to make comparisons between plans easier. The composites provide information on plan performance in the following areas:

- Getting needed care
- Getting care quickly
- How well doctors communicate
- Courteous and helpful office staff
- Customer service

- Claims processing
- Overall rating of health plan

HEDIS® AND CAHPS IN ACCREDITATION

HEDIS® and CAHPS data are an integral part of NCQA accreditation. Together these data comprise 40% of the total accreditation score. This reflects an emphasis on quality performance and customer (member) satisfaction. HEDIS® and CAHPS scores are publicly reported by NCQA on its Web site, the annual State of Health Care Quality report each fall, and most recently as part of the "America's Best Health Plans" program in conjunction with *U.S. News & World Report*.

THE HEDIS® COMPLIANCE AUDIT

HEDIS® has been praised as an important tool for health plan assessment. An integral part of the process is a way to validate data collected and reported by health plans. Despite the clear specifications defined in HEDIS®, data collection and calculation methods employed by health plans may vary, and other errors may taint the results, diminishing the usefulness of HEDIS® data for health plan comparison. NCQA's analysis of HEDIS® data collected as part of a national report card pilot project and experience with numerous state and local projects confirms that these are justifiable concerns.

An independent audit of the HEDIS® collection and reporting processes, as well as an audit of the data that are produced by those processes, is necessary to ensure that HEDIS® specifications are met and that HEDIS® data are valid and reliable. In response to requests from purchasers, regulators, and health plans, NCQA has established and implemented a consistent audit methodology for use by all HEDIS® auditors. The *NCQA HEDIS® Compliance Audit* is a two-part program that consists of an overall information systems capabilities assessment (IS standards) followed by an evaluation of the health plan's ability to comply with HEDIS® specifications. NCQA-certified auditors using standard audit methodologies help purchasers make more reliable "apples-to-apples" comparisons between health plans.

The *NCQA HEDIS® Compliance Audit* indicates whether a managed care organization has adequate and sound capabilities for processing medical, member, and provider information as a foundation for accurate and automated performance measurement, including HEDIS® reporting. The audit standards were designed to complement other verification activities that already occur within health plans. As a result, the standards do not address information audited by other organizations (*eg*, financial/accounting firms or state regulatory agencies), or information based on narrative descriptions of programs that are addressed in the NCQA Accreditation Standards, which are reviewed during accreditation survey visits.

Two different types of Certified HEDIS® compliance audits are offered, partial and full audits. In a partial audit, the health plan, state regulators, or purchaser determines which health plan-reported HEDIS® measures will be audited. Health plans that undergo a partial audit cannot use the NCQA audit seal to market that they have undergone a full NCQA HEDIS® Compliance Audit.

In contrast, in a full audit the certified auditor evaluates a core set of measures across all applicable domains in HEDIS® and then extrapolates the findings from the core set to all measures reported by the MCO. If problem areas are identified, the certified auditor may expand the core set measures. Following a completion of a full audit, the health plan can use NCQA's audit seal to market itself as having undergone a full NCQA HEDIS® Compliance Audit.

Certification of individual auditors and licensing of qualified organizations helps to ensure that standard auditing methodologies are used during all NCQA HEDIS® Compliance Audits. NCQA has developed a qualifying exam with a division of the Educational Testing Service, which individuals must pass before being designated NCQA-Certified HEDIS® Compliance Auditors. The exam con-

sists, in part, of an audit of a hypothetical health plan's HEDIS® processes against NCQA's standards. To maintain certification, auditors must participate in two audits per year, obtain 12 hours of preapproved continuing education credits, and attend the Auditor Update Conference annually. Recertification is required every 2 years.

NCQA also licenses organizations to conduct HEDIS® Compliance Audits. Individuals taking the certification exam must be employed by or contract with an NCQA-licensed organization. NCQA also monitors the quality of an auditor's work through ongoing assessments of audit performances by individual auditors and licensed organizations.

A list of the licensed organizations and certified auditors can be found on NCQA's Web site at http://www.ncqa.org.

QUALITY PLUS

Introduced in 2005, Quality Plus was NCQA's program designed to facilitate the transition to a more flexible generation of measurement and accreditation programs designed with the full range of health care entities—particularly newer models such as consumer-directed plans (CDHPs; see Chapter 2)—in mind. The program was initially voluntary, allowing health plans to earn distinction in each of three content areas:

- *Member connections*. Assesses members' access to interactive information, ability to track claims online, functionality of the plan's Web site, plan's ability to use available technology to provide good service, and provision of online health risk appraisal tools.
- *Care management and health improvement*. Assesses if a plan offers its members specific services based on their own unique health status, how effectively the plan manages chronic conditions and members with complex conditions, and whether the plan works to make all its members healthier.

- *Physician and hospital quality.* Assesses if the plan regularly measures and reports on the performance of network doctors and hospitals, whether physicians are given any incentives for delivering high-quality care, and if members have incentives for selecting a high-quality physician.

More than 130 reviews were scheduled or conducted with health plans seeking distinction. That fact, combined with the growing emphasis on improving members' access to health care information, facilitating early identification and outreach to members at risk for illness, and providing the necessary tools to guide informed decision making, led to NCQA's decision to integrate member connections and care management and health improvement into accreditation beginning in 2007.

NCQA ACCREDITATION REVIEW PROCESS

NCQA uses an Internet-based survey tool for health plan accreditation. The Interactive Survey System (ISS) allows an organization to perform a readiness evaluation at its own pace before submitting data to NCQA. A health plan can assess its programs and operations and estimate its performance against NCQA standards.

The NCQA review process begins with the submission of the survey tool and ends with an on-site survey. When a health plan applies for NCQA accreditation review, a date is set for the electronic submission of the survey tool and a subsequent on-site survey. The review process is separated into two stages:

- The off-site review of a health plan's electronically submitted materials and readiness evaluation
- The on-site survey of an organization's credentialing, denial, and appeal files, as well as a review of the organization's delegation oversight

The on-site survey occurs approximately 8 weeks after the submission of the survey tool. This part of the review process, which typically takes 2 days, consists of a brief opening/introduction, a review of the elements indicated for on-site review, completion of the review of previously submitted documentation, an interview with key personnel, and a closing conference.

During the on-site visit, members of the survey team complete an extensive review of health plan documentation, such as minutes of quality improvement committee and board meetings, policies and procedures relating to various areas of the standards, provider contracts, quality improvement studies, reports, and case files, utilization management review criteria, reports, and files, credentialing files, complaint and grievance files, and member satisfaction and disenrollment surveys.

The survey team also interviews the health plan's chief executive officer, medical director, directors of quality improvement, utilization management, provider relations, and member services, members of the quality improvement committee, a member of the board of directors, and participating physicians.

The survey team checks for evidence of compliance with each of the NCQA standards and presents a summary of its findings at the end of the site visit. A member of the review team prepares a report that is submitted to NCQA. An independent oversight committee analyzes the team's findings and the organization's clinical performance and then assigns an overall accreditation outcome.

Reviewers

NCQA survey teams typically consist of one or two administrative reviewers and two or three physician reviewers. Administrative reviewers are nonphysician clinicians or quality management experts with extensive experience in quality improvement in managed care organizations. Physician reviewers are medical directors, associate medical directors, or directors of quality management from noncompeting health plans.

Accreditation Decisions and Information

Following an on-site survey, NCQA assigns the health plan one of five possible accreditation levels based on the plan's performance:

- *Excellent.* NCQA's highest accreditation outcome is granted only to those plans that demonstrate levels of service and clinical quality that meet or exceed NCQA's rigorous requirements for consumer protection and quality improvement. Plans earning this accreditation level must also achieve HEDIS® results that are in the highest range of national or regional performance.
- *Commendable.* This accreditation outcome is awarded to plans that demonstrate levels of service and clinical quality that meet or exceed NCQA's rigorous requirements for consumer protection and quality improvement.
- *Accredited.* Health plans that earn the accredited outcome must meet most of NCQA's basic requirements for consumer protection and quality improvement.
- *Provisional.* Provisional accreditation indicates that a health plan's service and clinical quality meet some but not all of NCQA's basic requirements for consumer protection and quality improvement.
- *Denied.* Denied is an indication that a health plan did not meet NCQA's requirements during its review.

Accreditation of New Health Plans

NCQA maintains an accreditation program designed for MCOs that otherwise would not be eligible to participate in NCQA accreditation: the Accreditation of New Health Plans Program. The program is designed especially for organizations less than 2 years old, using a core set of standards derived from the *Standards for the Accreditation of Managed Care Organizations (MCOs)*, and applies to health plans that are less than 2 years old, making the program distinct and different from NCQA's Accreditation of MCOs Program. This program for new health plans (NHPs) is fun-damentally similar to NCQA's regular MCO accreditation program, except for three key differences:

- The program contains no requirement that a plan demonstrate improvement over time (an unrealistic expectation given the short history of the plan).
- Results are on a pass or fail basis (to distinguish it from NCQA's main MCO accreditation program).
- New health plans are not required to submit HEDIS® or CAHPS data.

NHP accreditation evaluates how well a plan that has been in operation less than 2 years manages its clinical and administrative systems to continuously improve health care for its members. The accreditation survey results are essentially on a pass or fail basis with plans receiving either NHP accreditation or a denial. Plans may apply for new health plan accreditation only once, and the accreditation period for plans that receive a "pass" designation is 2 years.

NCQA's standards for quality NHPs fall into six categories:

- *Quality improvement.* The NHP must have the appropriate organizational structures and processes in place to monitor and improve the quality of care and service provided to its members and must fully examine the quality of care given to its members.
- *Practitioner credentials.* The NHP must meet the specific NCQA requirements for investigating the training and experience of all practitioners in its network.
- *Members' rights and responsibilities.* The NHP must clearly inform members about how to access health services, how to choose a practitioner or change practitioners, and how to make a complaint.
- *Preventive health services.* The NHP must encourage members to use its preventive health programs and encourage its practitioners to deliver preventive services.
- *Utilization management.* The NHP must use a reasonable and consistent process

when deciding what health services are appropriate for individuals' needs, and when the NHP denies payment for services, it must respond appropriately to member and practitioner appeals.

- *Medical records.* The medical records kept by the NHP's practitioners must consistently meet NCQA standards for quality care.

OTHER NCQA ACCREDITATION PROGRAMS

The managed health care era has given rise to a diverse array of managed systems of care beyond HMOs and POS plans—PPOs, physician-hospital organizations, IPAs, managed behavioral health organizations, and many others—about which quality information historically had been scarce. To help address the need for information about these organizations and to facilitate NCQA's core MCO accreditation program by reducing the oversight burden for health plans, NCQA has implemented a number of other accreditation and certification programs. Taken together, these programs point to one of the trends for the future of quality oversight—targeted accreditation and certification programs suited to particular types of health care delivery systems.

Preferred Provider Organization Accreditation

Preferred provider organizations (PPOs) constitute the largest and fastest growing sector of the health care industry—more than 100 million Americans are enrolled in PPOs. In 1999, NCQA introduced a survey tool—adapted from the CAHPS 2.0H instrument—to assess PPO members' experience with their plans. The survey included questions designed to rate enrollees' experiences with the PPO and addressed specific issues, such as how well appeals procedures work, whether there are any obstacles to getting needed care, claims processing, and customer service.

In 2000, NCQA introduced a PPO accreditation program modeled on NCQA's existing HMO accreditation program. This program features on-site reviews of the core systems and processes that define a PPO—appeal procedures, provider evaluation processes, medical review systems, and quality improvement efforts. NCQA's review of these systems, combined with the PPO's results on the enrollee experiences survey, determines its overall accreditation decision. Some PPOs also report HEDIS® measures.

NCQA's PPO Plan Accreditation program is appropriate for PPO plans, organizations that take responsibility both for providing health benefits-related services to covered individuals, and for managing a practitioner network. NCQA distinguishes PPO plans from PPO *networks*, which are not responsible for the full range of functions included in NCQA's program, but perform one or more of the essential functions that NCQA evaluates. Certification modules allow PPO networks to demonstrate their commitment to quality, alone or as part of an accredited PPO plan. NCQA also offers certification programs that evaluate specific functions performed by PPO networks and plans, including utilization management and credentialing.

NCQA's PPO plan accreditation involves a comprehensive review of the key functions PPO plans perform. Expert surveyors review participating organizations against standards in the following areas:

- *Consumer protection.* Members must be informed about their appeal rights, and medical review decisions must be made quickly and fairly.
- *Customer service.* Member complaints must be resolved appropriately and in a timely manner, and members must receive complete information about benefits and providers.
- *Access to care.* The PPO's provider network must be adequate, and the plan must measure customer satisfaction.
- *Provider credentialing.* The PPO must thoroughly verify practitioners' credentials as well as monitor provider quality, license, and sanction information.

- *Medical group oversight.* The PPO must monitor entities to which responsibility for care and/or service has been delegated.

NCQA assigns PPOs one of four accreditation outcomes:

Full. NCQA's highest accreditation outcome for PPOs is granted to those plans that have excellent programs for quality improvement and consumer protection and that meet or exceed NCQA's standards. Full accreditation is effective for a 3-year period.

One-year. The PPO has well-established programs for quality improvement and consumer protection and meets most NCQA standards. NCQA has given the PPO plan a list of recommendations and will review the organization again after 1 year to determine if it qualifies for full accreditation.

Provisional. The PPO's service and clinical quality meet some but not all of NCQA's basic requirements for consumer protection and quality improvement.

Denied. Indicates that a PPO did not meet NCQA's requirements during its review.

NCQA offers a streamlined process for PPO plans affiliated with an accredited HMO. A health plan may undergo a single review covering its HMO, PPO, and other health plan products. In addition, if the HMO and PPO rely on the same systems (*eg*, credentialing), NCQA reviews that system once. Accredited MCOs also may accredit their PPO products through special add-on surveys. In an effort to provide consumers with comparable data regardless of plan type, NCQA has begun the process of integrating HEDIS® measures into PPO accreditation. Public reporting of PPO HEDIS® data will begin with aggregated data in 2007 and expand to plan by plan results.

Disease Management Accreditation and Certification

NCQA offers a flexible evaluation program, including accreditation for organizations that offer comprehensive disease management (DM) programs with services to patients, practitioners, or both, and certification for organizations that provide specific DM functions. Because they evaluate functions, rather than specific types of organizations, NCQA's DM accreditation and certification programs are available to a wide variety of organizations, including DM organizations, health plans (HMOs and PPOs), pharmaceutical companies, provider organizations, pharmacy benefit management companies, medical groups, and nurse call centers.

NCQA offers six different DM evaluation options—three types of accreditation and three types of certification.

Accreditation Options

1. Patient and Practitioner Accreditation—comprehensive accreditation that includes all standards.
2. Patient-Oriented Accreditation—comprehensive patient-focused accreditation that includes all standards (except select practitioner requirements).
3. Practitioner-Oriented Accreditation—comprehensive practitioner-focused accreditation that includes all standards (except select patient requirements).

Certification Options

1. Program Design Certification—specialized certification for organizations that develop the content for DM programs.
2. Systems Certification—specialized certification for organizations that develop or provide the clinical systems to support DM programs.
3. Contact Certification—specialized certification for organizations that interact with the patients and practitioners in a less comprehensive manner than full DM accreditation (*ie*, no measurement or systems capabilities). Likely organizations include nurse call centers.

Disease Management Standards

NCQA DM standards address the key areas that an organization is required to address for the implementation of disease management. These areas include the following:

- *Program Content* standards include the use of evidence-based guidelines, periodic review of the guidelines, the addition of new information, and the content of interventions for patients and practitioners.
- *Patient Services* standards include the provision of program information, patient participation, interventions, feedback to the patient, and patients' rights and responsibilities.
- *Practitioner Services* standards include the provision of program information, practitioners' rights, and decision support services such as interventions to the practitioner and feedback.
- *Clinical Systems* standards are related to the organization's system capabilities including the coordination of information, the processes for patient identification, stratification and assessment, privacy and confidentiality, and patient safety.
- *Measurement and Quality Improvement* addresses the selection, methodology, analysis, reporting and action related to the organization's clinical quality measures, patient and practitioner feedback, and the evaluation of QI initiatives.
- *Program Operations* of DM include access and service issues, marketing and advertising, staff training, qualifications, and credentialing.

Managed Behavioral Healthcare Organization Accreditation

NCQA's Managed Behavioral Healthcare Organization (MBHO; see also Chapter 13) Accreditation program was launched in 1996 to provide employers and the more than 140 million Americans enrolled in MBHOs with information about the quality of those organizations. Since then, NCQA's health plan and MBHO accreditation programs have become closely aligned, with nearly identical sets of

standards applying to both types of organizations. Both accreditation programs seek to promote access to behavioral health care and coordination between medical and behavioral health professionals, a prerequisite to good quality care.

The NCQA MBHO standards were developed and are updated through a consensus process by a task force composed of representatives of employers, public purchasers, consumers, managed care organizations, MBHOs, and mental health and substance abuse experts. The standards emphasize the importance of access to care and services, coordination of behavioral health services with medical care, and preservation of patient confidentiality.

The MBHO review process consists of both on- and off-site evaluations conducted by teams of behavioral health clinicians (which may include psychologists, psychiatrists, and/or clinical social workers) and managed care experts. A national oversight committee analyzes the team's findings and assigns an accreditation level based on the MBHO's compliance with NCQA's standards.

The standards against which NCQA measures MBHOs are organized into seven categories:

- *Quality improvement.* The MBHO has systems in place to ensure that care and service improve over time.
- *Accessibility of services.* MBHO services must be readily available and accessible, and referral and triage systems must be efficient and effective.
- *Utilization management.* The MBHO is required to make decisions about approving or denying care in a fair, informed, and timely manner with a staff of qualified decision makers.
- *Credentialing.* NCQA reviews how thoroughly the MBHO checks the credentials of its providers.
- *Members' rights and responsibilities.* The MBHO must do a good job of communicating with members and there needs to be evidence that member handbooks

and customer service staff are accessible, and that members understand their rights and how the system works.

- *Preventive behavioral health programs.* The organization is required to take proactive steps to keep members healthy.
- *Treatment records.* Treatment records must be kept confidential and show evidence of coordination between medical and behavioral health providers.

Based on their compliance with NCQA's requirements, MBHOs can earn the following NCQA Accreditation status levels:

Full Accreditation is granted for a period of 3 years to those MBHOs that have excellent programs for continuous quality improvement and meet NCQA's standards.

One-Year Accreditation is granted to MBHOs that have well-established quality improvement programs and meet most NCQA's standards. NCQA provides the MBHOs with a specific list of recommendations and reviews the MBHOs again after 1 year to determine if they have progressed enough to move up to Full Accreditation.

Provisional Accreditation is granted for 1 year to MBHOs that have adequate quality improvement programs and meet some of NCQA's standards.

Denial of Accreditation is given to MBHOs when NCQA's assessment reveals serious flaws in systems for consumer protection and quality improvement.

NCQA has accredited approximately 25% of the nation's major MBHOs.

OTHER NCQA CERTIFICATION PROGRAMS

Credentials Verification Organization (CVO) Certification Program

NCQA's CVO Certification is a quality assessment program designed to assist managed care organizations in assessing credentials verification organizations (CVOs) and other organizations that verify the credentials of physicians (see also Chapter 5). CVOs that are certified have demonstrated that they provide the protections required by NCQA's standards, that they have developed a sound management structure, and that they monitor, and are continually improving, the quality of the services they deliver.

The NCQA CVO survey is a comprehensive on-site evaluation conducted by a team of health care professionals and certified credentialing specialists. A national oversight committee of physicians analyzes the team's findings and determines certification based on the CVO's performance against NCQA standards. These standards were developed and are updated with the assistance of representatives from the credentials verification industry, as well as input from managed care organizations. Certified CVOs must meet these standards, as well as all applicable credentialing standards from NCQA's Standards for the Accreditation of Managed Care Organizations.

For managed care organizations seeking to be accredited by NCQA, CVO Certification takes the place of health plan review of a CVO's structure and performance in verifying provider credentials. Accordingly, health plans that contract for credentials verification with an organization that has been certified by NCQA are exempt from some due diligence oversight requirements specified in NCQA Credentialing Standards.

NCQA's CVO Certification Standards

There are two major components to the CVO Certification Survey:

1. Determination of compliance with the CVO Standards, which includes a review of the following in an organization:
   - Policies and procedures for credentials verification
   - Mechanisms for maintaining credentials data integrity and confidentiality
   - Capabilities for ongoing data collection
   - Internal quality assurance processes
   - Physician application components

- Reporting of physician disciplinary actions
2. An audit of completed credentials files to determine compliance with NCQA's MCO Credentialing Standards.

Certification is awarded to participating organizations on an individual credentials element basis (*eg*, verification of license to practice, DEA registration). CVOs may be certified for all, some, or none of the ten credentials elements addressed in the NCQA Standards. These elements are as follows:

- License to practice
- Drug Enforcement Agency (DEA) registration
- Education and training
- Work history
- Malpractice claims history
- Medical board sanctions
- Medicare/Medicaid sanctions
- Practitioner application processing
- CVO application and attestation content
- Ongoing monitoring

There are no different levels of certification (full, provisional, etc.), and certification is not considered all inclusive; status for all participating CVOs is maintained on an individual credentials element basis and pertains *only* to those elements reviewed as part of NCQA's CVO certification process.

National Association of Medical Staff Services

NCQA partners with the National Association of Medical Staff Services (NAMSS; http://www.namss.org), an international organization for the development of individuals responsible for managing credentialing, privileging, practitioner/provider organizations, and regulatory compliance in the health care industry. All NCQA surveyors conducting CVO surveys must be NAMSS-certified.

Physician Organization Certification (POC)

Physician organizations (POs) such as IPAs, medical groups, and similar organizations have emerged to play an important role as delegated providers of a wide range of administrative and clinical services for HMOs and other health plans. Historically, the more health plan contracts physician organizations held, the more annual audits they faced from plans seeking to satisfy NCQA accreditation requirements. The PO Certification program allows physician organizations to substitute one NCQA survey for the many overlapping annual surveys they may currently face from their health plan partners.

NCQA's PO Certification evaluates how well a physician organization manages its clinical and administrative systems to improve health care continuously for its members. Certification focuses on the PO's role as a delegate, or agent performing a function on behalf of health plans. The POC standards are composed largely of a subset of NCQA's health plan accreditation standards, including quality improvement, physician credentials, preventive health services, and utilization management. Although a few new program-specific standards have been added—requiring open, ongoing communication between the physician organization and the MCO, for example—no significant changes were made to the existing health plan standards to apply them to physician organizations. The survey process for physician organizations is fundamentally similar to that of health plans.

NCQA's Physician Organization Certification is a modular program. Unlike health plans, which must be reviewed on all sections of standards, POs vary in the services they provide relative to standards. Therefore, a PO may choose to be reviewed for certification for any one or more of the four categories.

Utilization Management (UR) and Credentialing (CR) Certification

UR and CR NCQA certification is available to any organization that performs these specified functions and is not eligible for NCQA's accreditation programs for managed care organizations and managed behavioral health care organizations.

The standards have been adapted from the CR and UM sections of NCQA's PPO Plan

Accreditation program to allow PPO networks and other organizations performing these functions the opportunity to demonstrate the quality of their utilization management and credentialing programs. Organizations holding URAC UM accreditation that pursue NCQA UM certification receive credit for the corresponding NCQA requirements.

Organizations can earn one of two possible outcomes—certification or denial of certification—based on their performance against NCQA's standards.

NCQA PHYSICIAN RECOGNITION PROGRAMS

In collaboration with leading experts and consumer-related health care organizations, NCQA has implemented several physician recognition programs. Consumers are able to identify physicians in their area using a search tool available on the NCQA Web site.

Diabetes Physician Recognition Program

The Diabetes Physician Recognition Program, developed by NCQA and the American Diabetes Association, awards recognition to physicians who demonstrate that they provide high-quality care to patients with diabetes. The program assesses key measures that were carefully defined and tested for their relationship to improved care for people with diabetes.

Heart/Stroke Physician Recognition Program

The Heart/Stroke Physician Recognition Program, developed by NCQA and the American Heart Association/American Stroke Association, awards recognition to physicians who demonstrate that they provide high-quality care to patients with cardiac conditions or who have had a stroke.

Physician Practice Connections

Physician Practice Connections, which NCQA developed in collaboration with Bridges to Excellence, a group of large employers, awards

recognition to physician practices that use up-to-date information and systems to enhance patient care.

Some MCOs have also incorporated these recognition programs into their pay-for-performance programs as discussed in Chapter 8. For further information on these programs, visit http://www.ncqa.org.

NCQA REPORT CARDS

Since 1994, NCQA has made the results of all its accreditation and certification surveys available to the public through a set of Health Plan Report Card and Status Lists. These reports are all available online at NCQA's Web site, and they are searched or downloaded by thousands of visitors each month. The following reports are available.

NCQA's Health Plan Report Card

This tool equips consumers with information about the quality of health plans (including HMOs, POS plans, and PPOs) based on their performance in five key areas—access and service, qualified providers, staying healthy, getting better, living with illness—and overall accreditation. Consumers can compare the ratings of various health plans and get detailed information on individual plans.

NCQA's Report Card for Managed Behavioral Healthcare Organizations (MBHOs)

This tool lists all MBHOs currently in the accreditation process, along with detailed information on individual organizations. Employers and health plans can review accreditation information about MBHOs before making critical decisions and consumers can see whether their MBHO is accredited.

NCQA's Status List for New Health Plans

This is a list of NCQA-accredited health plans that have been in operation for less than 3 years and provides information about the status of the plans' accreditation.

Disease Management Accreditation and Certification Status List

This is a list of NCQA-accredited organizations that offer comprehensive disease management programs with services to patients, practitioners, or both, organizations that have achieved NCQA certification for specific disease management functions, and organizations that are scheduled to be reviewed by NCQA for DM accreditation or certification.

NCQA's Certification Status List

This is a list of health care organizations that achieved NCQA certification in specific functions as indicated within the list. Employers and health plans can use this information to ensure that all discrete functions in a delivery system are working together. The Certification Status List covers the following areas:

- Physician Organization Certification
- Credentials Verification Organization Certification
- Credentialing Certification
- Utilization Management Certification

AMERICA'S BEST HEALTH PLANS

NCQA collaborates each year with *U.S. News & World Report* to rank commercial, Medicare, and Medicaid health plans in their annual "America's Best Health Plans" feature. The magazine is published during the open enrollment period in the fall, but the rankings are included on http://www.usnews.com throughout the year. Whereas the magazine includes both ranked lists and "honor rolls" of the top plans in each category, the Web site includes hundreds of plans and enables people to review publicly reported information and compare several plans at once.

URAC

History

URAC is an independent nonprofit organization that was established in December 1990 by the American Managed Care and Review Association (AMCRA), the trade association at that time for UR firms, PPOs, and HMOs. AMCRA's goal was to address provider concerns about the diversity of UR procedures and the growing impact of UR on physicians and hospitals. In addition, at the time of URAC's inception, managed care advocates believed that a number of state legislative initiatives under consideration would severely limit the impact of UR in some instances and make it impossible to conduct UR in others. URAC developed its first set of standards, the Health Utilization Management Standards, as a response to these legislative initiatives.

URAC was originally incorporated under the name "Utilization Review Accreditation Commission." That name was shortened to the acronym "URAC" in 1996 when URAC began accrediting other types of health care entities in addition to UR organizations.

Over the years, URAC has continued to create accreditation programs covering a range of health care processes and organizations. URAC currently offers 16 health care accreditation and certification programs, several of which are relevant for managed care organizations. New accreditation programs, including one for pharmacy benefit management programs, are continually under development.

URAC Accreditation Process

The URAC accreditation process involves four phases. The first phase includes completing the required application forms, gathering supporting documentation (formal policies and procedures, organizational charts, position and program descriptions, etc.), and submitting all materials and an application fee to URAC.

The second phase is a desktop review of the application, performed by a URAC accreditation review team. At the conclusion of the desktop review, the team sends a written request to the applicant for any additional information or documentation needed.

An on-site review represents the third phase. During the visit, the review team interviews managers and staff members, observes the work of the organization, and reviews documents and programs to ensure compliance with URAC standards. Following the visit, the reviewers write a report summarizing the findings of the desktop and on-site reviews.

The fourth phase is a review by two URAC committees consisting of representatives from URAC member organizations and industry experts. The executive summary is reviewed by URAC's Accreditation Committee, which then forwards an accreditation recommendation to URAC's Executive Committee, the group that makes all final accreditation decisions.

Accreditation Status

Full 2-year accreditation is awarded to organizations that meet all requirements. Conditional accreditation may be conferred upon organizations that provide appropriate documentation but have not completely implemented all policies and procedures, while provisional accreditation may be granted to start-up companies; in these circumstances, additional documentation or another on-site review may lead to full accreditation status. Organizations that do not meet URAC requirements may be placed on corrective action status, denied accreditation, or choose to withdraw.

Accredited organizations must continue to remain in compliance with the applicable standards throughout the accreditation cycle. URAC may rescind accreditation status if an accredited company is unable to comply with standards. In addition, URAC may sanction an accredited company with penalties ranging from a letter of reprimand to revocation of accreditation following investigation of complaints made by consumers, providers, or regulators.

The following are summaries of URAC's health utilization management, health network, health plan, disease management,

health provider, credential verification organization, and health Web site standards. Copies of the URAC standards and application materials can be obtained by writing to URAC at 1220 L Street NW, Suite 400, Washington, DC 20005, or calling (202) 216-9010. Summaries of all URAC accreditation standards are available at http://www.urac.org. The summaries provide an overview of the standards.

URAC Core Accreditation

URAC has created a set of core standards that reflect the quality of basic health care functions of an organization. All URAC-accredited programs must meet these core standards in addition to the function-specific requirements set forth by each individual program. Core standards cover the following health care organization functions.

Organizational structure. Requirements include a defined organization structure and oversight responsibility, policies and procedures, job descriptions, current licensure of clinical personnel, a regulatory compliance program, confidentiality and conflict of interest policies, a quality management program, and programs and processes that address consumer protection.

Personnel management. The organization must maintain written job descriptions for all staff members that clearly define qualifications with regard to education, training, professional experience and competencies, licensure and certification, and job responsibilities.

Operations and processes. The organization must maintain communication processes that promote collaboration and coordination, as well as formal processes for information management, business relationships, clinical oversight, regulatory compliance, and incentive programs.

Quality improvement. The organization must maintain a quality management program that promotes objective, systemic monitoring, and evaluation of services. Specific quality management activities may vary across organizations.

Delegation of responsibilities. The organization must maintain oversight and responsibility for functions delegated to other entities, although oversight requirements are less stringent if the other entities are URAC-accredited.

Consumer protection. Communication to consumers must clearly and accurately describe the organization's services and how to obtain them. A grievance process must be in place. A quick-response process must address situations that present an immediate threat to consumer safety or welfare.

Health Utilization Management Standards

URAC's UM standards may be applied to standalone UM organizations or to the UM processes of indemnity insurers, HMOs, or PPOs. The standards ensure that a formal utilization review process is in place, that qualified personnel oversee the process, and that only valid clinical criteria form the basis of medical decisions.

In addition to URAC's core standards, accredited organizations must meet standards related to the following areas:

- Clinical criteria
- The utilization management process
- Staff qualifications
- Confidentiality

Clinical Criteria

The UM process must involve explicit clinical review criteria based on current clinical principles and processes. These criteria must be reviewed and revised periodically and must be disclosed to the patient or treating provider upon request.

Utilization Management Process

Organizations must establish and implement a three-step process to determine medical necessity.

1. *Initial clinical review.* Initial clinical review must be performed by licensed clinical professionals, such as nurses who must have access to licensed physicians or other appropriate clinicians for consultation.
2. *Peer clinical review.* Peer clinical review is implemented if the proposed service cannot be approved during initial clinical review. Peer clinical review is conducted by a physician qualified to render a clinical opinion about the service or by a provider similar to the treating provider if the treating provider is not a physician.
3. *Appeals consideration.* If the proposed service is not approved during peer clinical review, the treating provider and the patient may request an appeal. Appeals must be considered by clinical peers who are board-certified and in a similar specialty as the provider and who were not involved in the initial review. Appropriate time frames for appeals decisions are outlined by the standards.

The standards outline the scope of review information that can be considered during the UM process. The organization must have a formal process to address situations in which information is insufficient to conduct a review. Retrospective and concurrent review time frames are also set by the standards and the organization must have a formal process for communicating certification decisions.

Staff Qualifications

UM staff must be qualified, trained, supervised, and supported by written clinical review criteria.

Confidentiality

Written policies and procedures must ensure that information obtained during the UM process is kept confidential in accordance with the law. That information must be limited to only what is necessary for UM of the services under review, and must be used solely for the purpose of UM, quality management, discharge planning, and case management.

Health Network Standards

URAC's Health Network Accreditation Standards apply to a variety of health care networks, including specialty-specific networks, physician-hospital organizations, and networks related to behavioral health, complementary medicine, skilled nursing, and home care. Both payer- and provider-based models can qualify.

In addition to URAC's core standards, health networks must meet accreditation criteria related to the following areas:

- Network management
- Provider credentialing
- Quality management and improvement
- Consumer protection

Network Management Standards

URAC standards require that networks define, in writing, the scope of the services they offer, including type of service and region served. A network must also establish goals, track performance, and make ongoing improvements regarding access to care and provider availability.

The network must establish provider selection criteria that address care quality, service quality, and organization needs. The network and the participating providers must have written agreements; specified inclusions and exclusions are outlined in the standards. For example, URAC bars "gag clauses" that would restrict providers from discussing available treatment options with eligible persons.

Provider Credentialing

The network must have a formal credentialing program that includes a credentialing committee and defines the senior clinician of the network as overseer of the clinical aspects of the organization.

The network's executive staff must approve a written credentialing plan, which must list the selection criteria for participating providers (including facilities) and the credentialing information to be gathered. The program must verify credentials, and confidentiality of the credentialing process must be ensured.

Providers' continuing compliance with criteria for network participation must be monitored via a formal process. Time frames for credentialing phase-in are set forth in the standards; recredentialing must occur every 3 years. Finally, the network must comply with URAC's core standards for any credentialing functions it delegates to another entity.

Health Plan Standards

URAC's Health Plan Standards apply to health plans such as HMOs and PPOs. In addition to the URAC core standards, health plans must meet standards related to network management, provider credentialing, member relations/consumer protection, utilization management, and quality management. Network management and credentialing standards are similar to those outlined in the Health Network Standards described earlier. Member relations/consumer protection, utilization management, and quality management standards are discussed later.

Member Relations/Consumer Protection

The health plan must implement a mechanism to communicate information effectively and accurately about network services to eligible persons. A communications plan must ensure that particular materials are provided to consumers upon enrollment and an ongoing basis, including provider lists, cost-sharing features, medical management requirements, administrative requirements, consumer satisfaction statistics, coordination of benefits, and descriptions of provider compensation arrangements. The network must implement a mechanism to solicit consumer suggestions and maintain a responsive complaint and grievance policy.

Utilization Management

Organizations seeking health plan accreditation must comply with URAC's Utilization Management Standards. In addition, the health plan must establish a mechanism for consumers to access an independent review process.

Quality Management

In addition to the quality improvement projects required under the core standards, the plan must maintain at least one additional project, and at least two of the three projects must focus on clinical quality.

Disease Management Standards

URAC's Disease Management Standards apply to health plans with DM programs, stand-alone DM organizations, and medical management organizations. The standards, which are not disease-specific, promote evidence-based practice, collaborative relationships with providers, patient education, and shared decision making with consumers.

In addition to the URAC core standards, DM programs must meet standards related to program scope and objectives, administration and staffing, performance measurement and reporting, consumer rights and responsibilities, population management, and program design.

Program Scope and Objectives

A DM program must maintain policies and procedures that address scope of services with regard to each clinical condition it addresses, collaboration with providers to ensure evidence-based care, promotion of patient self-management, and outcomes measurement.

Administration and Staffing

The program must define scope of responsibilities for licensed and nonlicensed staff members as appropriate and maintain a process for coordinating services with the client and with other health care programs.

Performance Measurement and Reporting

The program must develop an outcomes evaluation methodology for measuring both condition-specific and overall program performance. Measurement should be based on reliable data sources and reflect evidence-based standards of care. Clinical processes and outcomes objectives should be established for each condition, and program performance should be compared to outcome goals. Financial outcomes should be reported by condition at least annually. Program member feedback should be solicited at least annually, and feedback should be provided to participating clinicians to promote improvements in care.

Consumer Rights and Responsibilities

Eligible consumers must be informed about the structure and characteristics of the program, including criteria for eligibility and procedures for opting in and out of program participation. Participants must be informed of their rights and responsibilities upon enrollment.

Population Management

The program must maintain a standard, consistent process that includes defined criteria for identification of eligible participants and a process for patient stratification based on clinical evidence that will inform service provision.

Program Design

Clinical decision-support tools used by the program should support evidence-based practice and reflect current specialty knowledge. Tools should be reviewed and updated annually with input from clinical experts. In addition, the program should provide ongoing patient education that addresses self-management, provides educational materials, and encourages use of appropriate resources.

Health Provider Credentialing Standards

URAC established Health Provider Credentialing Standards to ensure that network clinicians maintain appropriate credentials, qualifications, and licensure and that networks have verified the education, training, liability record, and practice history of their providers. Organizations seeking accreditation include HMOs, PPOs, physician-hospital organizations (PHOs), and workers' compensation networks.

In addition to the URAC core standards, organizations must meet standards related to program structure, organization and staffing, and the credentialing process.

Structure, Organization, and Staffing

The organization must maintain a formal program to verify the professional qualifications of all participating providers and facilities that provide services to consumers. The program must have a committee consisting of at least one practicing provider who has no other role in the organization. The committee provides guidance to the organization on credentialing matters and votes on participant applications.

Credentialing Process

All practitioners requesting network participation must submit a written credentialing application with information that can be verified with regard to their qualifications. Primary sources must be used to verify licensure and certification. The organization must monitor providers for compliance and implement response mechanisms in cases of noncompliance. Providers must be recredentialed every 3 years.

Credentials Verification Organizations

URAC's credentials verification organization (CVO) standards pertain to organizations that gather data and verify the credentials of health practitioners, including physicians, who contract with managed care networks. In addition to the URAC core standards, CVOs must meet standards related to scope of services, personnel, the credentialing process, quality improvement, delegation of responsibilities, and confidentiality.

Scope of Services

The CVO must have a written contract with each client that specifies the CVO's responsibilities, including which category of providers the CVO will credential.

CVO Personnel

The CVO must train staff regarding policies and procedures for verification as well as in other responsibilities, including relevant URAC standards.

Credentialing Process

The CVO must document the sources it uses to verify credentials. Applications for credentialing must include comprehensive information that reflects qualifications and professional care quality. Primary sources must be used to verify licensure and certification. The CVO must permit providers to submit information when necessary to correct errors or inconsistencies. On-site reviews of providers' offices must examine patient access, public health policies and procedures, and safety standards for fire, emergency, and equipment maintenance and must be conducted by health care practitioners.

Quality Improvement

A written organization quality improvement plan must exist and should include evidence of routine inspections of data and databases, annual random sampling of staff activities, and improvements when required.

Delegation of Responsibilities

Subcontractors must maintain compliance with URAC standards. The CVO must retain authority over and oversee all subcontracted verification activities. The CVO must perform a comprehensive review of the subcontractor's verification program, perform quarterly reviews, and perform annual random file audits.

Confidentiality

Written policies and procedures must address the integrity of the CVO's databases. All databases should be updated at least annually. Practitioner information may be made public only with the practitioner's consent.

Health Web Site

URAC's Health Web Site accreditation program verifies that health-related Web sites meet certain standards for quality. Topics addressed through the program include privacy and security, health content editorial processes, disclosure of financial relationships, linking policies, consumer complaints, and emerging best practices.

Applicants must complete a formal online application that includes questions related to the standards. The online application is assigned to a reviewer who conducts a desktop review and a telephone interview of corporate officials; then the reviewer presents the application to the URAC committees.

In addition to the URAC core standards, Web sites must meet standards related to operations and processes, quality improvement, privacy and security, and delegation of responsibilities.

Operations/Process

The standards address organizational policies and structures, disclosure, health content, external linking, privacy, security, and accountability. Information that must be disclosed to consumers includes the site's sponsors and financial backers, privacy and advertising policies, and content development method.

The site must maintain an editorial policy that identifies the author and requires that information be evidence-based. Paid advertising and content must be easily distinguishable. A process must govern links to

other sites, which must be periodically reviewed.

Quality Improvement

The organization must have a quality oversight committee to oversee the quality of the site's content; this committee must include the clinicians responsible for content and the individual responsible for the site's privacy practices.

Privacy and Security

The site may not collect personal health information without first requesting user permission and must also notify users if their information is to be sold to third-party entities.

Delegation of Responsibilities

The site must disclose the involvement of third-party entities that have significant interests in the site. The site must also disclose significant relationships between commercial sponsors and health content.

ACCREDITATION ASSOCIATION FOR AMBULATORY HEALTH CARE

History

The Accreditation Association for Ambulatory Health Care, also known as the Accreditation Association or AAAHC, was created in 1979 to assist ambulatory health care organizations improve the quality of care provided to patients. The founding members of the association were the American College Health Association, the American Group Practice Association (now known as the American Group Medical Association), the Federated Ambulatory Surgery Association, the Group Health Association of America (the successor of which is AHIP), the Medical Group Management Association, and the National Association of Community Health Centers. Presently, the AAAHC includes 15 member organizations representing a broad spectrum of ambulatory health care.

The AAAHC currently accredits more than 2,700 health care organizations, including endoscopy centers, ambulatory surgery centers, office-based surgery centers, student health centers, and large medical and dental group practices. In addition, the Accreditation Association surveys and accredits managed care organizations, including HMOs, PPOs, and IPAs.

The AAAHC's managed care standards have been developed with industry input and incorporate the evaluation of functional areas such as member communications systems, member complaint and grievance resolution systems, utilization management, including member appeal procedures, quality management and improvement, and provider credentialing and recredentialing systems. The association's Managed Care Program has received Medicare Advantage Deemed Status from the Centers for Medicare and Medicaid Services.

AAAHC Accreditation Process

An accreditation decision is based on an assessment of a health care organization's compliance with applicable standards and adherence to the policies and procedures of the Accreditation Association. Compliance is assessed by AAAHC through at least one of the following means: documented evidence, answers to detailed questions concerning implementation, or on-site observations and interviews by surveyors.

The Accreditation Association surveyors are physicians, dentists, nurses, and administrators who are selected, to the extent possible, on the basis of their knowledge of and experience with the range of services provided by the organization seeking an accreditation survey. At the close of an on-site survey, the reviewers schedule a summation conference during which they present their findings to representatives of the organization for discussion and clarification. Members of the health care organization's governing body, medical staff, and administration are encouraged to comment on the findings as well as express their perceptions of the survey.

After the on-site survey is completed, association staff members review the survey findings and recommendations, including the survey team's recommendation regarding accreditation, and make a recommendation regarding accreditation to the Accreditation Committee of the AAAHC. Accreditation is awarded to organizations that demonstrate substantial compliance with the AAAHC standards and adhere to the AAAHC accreditation policies. Possible terms of accreditation awarded by the Accreditation Committee include 3-year, 1-year, 6-month, deferred decision, and denial or revocation of accreditation.

AAAHC Accreditation Standards

The AAAHC Accreditation standards are divided into a set of core standards that apply to all organizations seeking accreditation and adjunct standards that apply to organizations based on the specific programs and services they provide.

AAAHC core standards that apply to all organizations include the following:

- Rights of patients
- Governance
- Administration
- Quality of care provided
- Quality management and improvement
- Clinical records and health information
- Facilities and environment

AAAHC adjunct standards that may apply to health plans include the following:

- Managed care organizations
- Health education and wellness

Copies of the AAAHC managed care standards and application materials can be obtained by writing to AAAHC at 5200 Old Orchard Road, Suite 200, Skokie, IL 60077, or calling (847) 853-6060. Information is also available at http://www.aaahc.org.

CONCLUSION

This chapter has presented a summary of three organizations that currently accredit managed care organizations and related health care entities, as well as some details of the oversight programs they offer. Like the organizations they review, the three accreditation organizations vary in their goals and in their approach to external review. Although they vary considerably in their approach, all of these organizations hold the potential for rationalizing and consolidating current external review processes for employers, state, federal, and individual purchasers. These processes are sometimes duplicative or contradictory in their requirements and, in some cases, may have a detrimental impact on managed care programs. Ultimately, however, their effectiveness must be judged in terms of their ability to improve the quality of care and service that health care organizations provide to their customers. And, most important, there is no doubt that these organizations have had a positive impact on the quality of health care in this country.

24

OPERATIONAL FINANCE AND BUDGETING

Dale F. Cook

Study Objectives

- Understand the basic flow of funds in a typical managed care organization.
- Understand the basic types of revenues and expenses.
- Understand some of the key issues involved in statutory accounting.
- Understand basic regulatory requirements as they pertain to financial activities.
- Understand the budgeting process.

Discussion Topics

1. Discuss what regulatory agencies/organizations govern financial reporting and solvency of different types of managed care organizations, and describe the different aspects of their governance.
2. Discuss how profit and loss and forecast information might be segregated and why. Why is it important to analyze the results using PMPM data?
3. Describe and discuss the key elements an HMO finance officer needs to properly set the claims accruals.
4. Discuss what is on a lag report and what completion factors are. What are the strengths and problems associated with completion factors?
5. Discuss how premiums are billed and received.
6. Discuss what a premium deficiency is, why its identification is important, and how this should be reflected in the accounting records.
7. Discuss the more significant issues related to Risk Pool Liabilities.
8. Discuss the minimum capital requirements and risk-based capital requirements under the NAIC Model Act.

> 9. Discuss the key differences between Statutory Accounting Principles and Generally Accepted Accounting Principles. Why is this important to a managed care plan?

INTRODUCTION

To manage successfully a managed care organization (MCO), financial managers' challenge lies in their ability to interact with operational and medical managers, manage changes in the regulatory environment, and gather timely information to facilitate communication of financial results to the organization and its constituencies to react appropriately to sustain or exceed financial goals. Accuracy of the reported financial results is affected by significant accounting estimates that are based on historical trends and results and appropriately adjusted for recent changes affecting such estimates. The interaction between operational managers and financial managers is key to developing timely, accurate financial results.

Overall financial management of an MCO begins with the MCO's product pricing strategies. Strategic pricing is based on an assessment of the competition, targeted profitability, the MCO's estimate of costs incurred for the provision of health care, and the costs to support the operation of the business. Managing and controlling costs and reacting to the medical cost trends as well as the construct of administrative costs are critical to achieving desired results and preserving profitability. Detailed operating budgets are then developed under the same assumptions used in the pricing strategy. Financial managers rely significantly upon information captured and monitored by operational departments to develop the detailed budgets.

Information provided by operational departments is also used as the basis for certain accounting estimates recorded in financial statements. The financial manager's ability to report on actual results, analyze budget variances, and assess the reasonableness of pricing strategies in a timely manner is dependent on the support of operating functions.

In this chapter, through a review of the components of the financial statements of a health maintenance organization (HMO), key information and operational procedures that the financial manager will need and rely upon are discussed. The discussion addresses typical problems that occur in gathering information and provides insight into challenging the integrity of information.

BACKGROUND

Accounting policy for MCOs is set by many regulatory entities. MCOs are primarily regulated at the state level, although certain federal regulations may be imposed if an MCO offers federally regulated products such as Medicare risk contracts. State regulation may be imposed by both the Department of Insurance and the Department of Health. Additionally, there are many publicly held MCOs that are subject to the rules and regulations of the Securities and Exchange Commission (SEC). This more recently includes the Public Company Accounting Oversight Board, which was created when in 2002, as discussed later in this chapter, the Sarbanes-Oxley Act of 2002 was introduced into law.

The state's Department of Insurance is generally concerned with the fiscal solvency of the MCO to ensure that the health benefits of enrollees will be provided. The state's Department of Health (to the extent that it is involved at all) is generally concerned with quality of care issues as well as access to care issues, including the location of providers within specific geographic boundaries and the mix of primary care physicians and specialists to serve the population within these boundaries.

Financial management of MCOs must consider the interests of each of the users of financial information, whether they be senior management, the board of directors, insurance regulators, the SEC, tax authorities, or investors. Balancing the concerns of each interested party represents a challenge for the financial manager. Senior management is concerned with the profitability of products and market segment performance. Management will require internal reporting that focuses on line of business management and also meets regulatory reporting requirements. Regulators are concerned with protecting the insured members and focus on liquidity of the MCO. The SEC is concerned with the protection of investor interests. Balancing conservatism and positive performance with the best return on investment is a difficult task.

The requirements imposed by the state's Department of Insurance and Department of Health can be found in the state laws and regulations, as discussed in Chapter 33. The National Association of Insurance Commissioners (NAIC) is an organization comprising the state commissioners of insurance who set guidelines at a national level. The NAIC has no governing authority over the individual states, however. Generally, states will introduce legislation modeling NAIC guidelines. The NAIC has adopted an annual statement report format that has been adopted by most states. The financial information is prepared in accordance with statutory accounting practices (SAP). Other financial statement users (lenders, the SEC, and investors) require that financial statements be prepared in accordance with generally accepted accounting principles (GAAP). The American Institute of Certified Public Accountants (AICPA) issued an audit and accounting guide for health care providers that provides additional guidance on audit, accounting, and reporting matters for prepaid health plans.

The financial manager should also be aware of the continuous changes taking place in the regulatory arena. For many states, managed care market penetration has historically been minimal, and legislation has not kept pace with recent growth in managed care. Many varieties of MCOs or managed care strategies have emerged, such as physician-hospital organizations (PHOs), integrated delivery systems, management services organizations, direct contracting arrangements among employers and providers, and so forth (see Chapter 2), and there may be little or no legislation governing these non-health plan organizations. For example, many regulators have imposed policy (absent legislative authority) to exercise financial restrictions on PHOs or other provider organizations that contract directly with self-insured plans. Other developments include the NAIC's development of risk-based capital requirements for health insurers, including HMOs, which imposes stricter minimum capital requirements. Also in the past few years, expanded financial disclosure requirements regarding changes in claims reserves have been imposed on health insurers.

FINANCIAL STATEMENT COMPONENTS

Operating Statement

A typical high-level profit and loss statement for an HMO is depicted in Figure 24-1. For internal management reporting purposes, the ability to develop profit and loss reports by product line/market segment is critical to the

Percentage Revenue

> Premiums earned: 95%
> Other income: 5
> Total revenue: 100

Percentage Expenses

> Health care expenses: 84
> General and administrative expenses: 11
> Total expenses: 95

Percentage income or
loss before income taxes: 5

Figure 24–1 Sample profit and loss statement for an MCO-percentage of total revenue.
Source: Author.

financial management process. Assumptions and financial benchmarks may vary widely by product or market segment. For example, medical cost estimates are based on utilization patterns and provider reimbursement strategies that will differ by product and market segment. Likewise, administration of lines of business may be different. For example, the costs associated with supporting a Medicare or Medicaid product will differ from those associated with the commercial population because the customers have unique service needs and because dedicated staff with specific skill sets will be needed to service Medicare and Medicaid enrollees. Pricing is based on the medical cost and administrative cost components; therefore, premium pricing by product will vary consistent with the variations in these cost components. In the following discussion of the components of the financial statement, keep in mind the importance of segregating the reporting by product line or market segment. Analyzing financial results by line of business not only will enhance management's ability to understand the fluctuations from budgeted results but will provide information needed to redirect strategies to preserve the overall success of the operation.

Premium Revenue

Premium revenue is the primary revenue source for HMOs. Premiums are generally received in advance of the coverage period, which is usually monthly. Premium rates are generally effective for a 12-month period. Rates or rating methodologies are usually filed with and must be approved by the state's Department of Insurance. MCOs may file revisions to the rates or methodology, which will also be subject to approval by the Department of Insurance. New rates will not be effective for existing groups until the renewal of the annual contract.

Premiums are determined using actuarial and underwriting techniques, as discussed in Chapter 25. Premiums are intended to cover all medical and administrative expenses as well as to provide a profit margin. Premium rates are therefore directly related to medical expense and administrative expense projections. If the premium rates are not adequate to cover the actual medical expenses and administrative costs, expected profit margins will diminish. If losses for a line of business are anticipated, a premium deficiency exists. Under GAAP accounting, because premium rates are fixed until the end of the coverage period, the aggregate anticipated net loss for the line of business may need to be recorded immediately, not ratably over the remaining coverage period.

Certain premium rates may not be in part or in total controlled by the MCO, such as those for Medicare risk or Medicaid contracts. These rates are subject to review and final determination by the government, as discussed in Chapters 26 (Medicare) and 27 (Medicaid). For example, Medicare premium rates are determined based upon the federal government's review of bids submitted by the MCO. The federal government then evaluates the respective bids and determines the appropriate reimbursement rate to the MCO. It is then the responsibility of the MCO to be able to perform medical management and administrative expense management so that the premium is sufficient to cover costs and yield a profit.

Rating methodologies derive rates based on an evaluation of demographic data (eg, the age and sex mix or geographic location) of the population to insure. Rates may be determined using a community rating methodology or an experience rating methodology. Community rating is often used for small groups (less than 50 subscribers) or individuals, and experience rating is used for large groups. In many states, community rating is mandatory for small groups and individuals. States may also mandate community rating for all groups regardless of size.

Basic community rating entails the application of a standard rate to all groups within the community being underwritten. The standard rate is applied to groups on the basis of the number of rate tiers quoted, the average family size, and the contract mix assumed for the group. Rate tiers are developed based on the age and sex of members as well as the classification of single versus family. Community rating by class considers an adjustment to the basic rate for specific demographics and/or industry classification of the group. Adjusted community rating allows for adjustments to the base rate for group-specific information other than demographics and industry classification.

The experience rating methodology develops a group rate based on a group's actual experience. After determining actual past experience, expenses are trended forward. Experience-rated contracts can be retrospectively rated or prospectively rated. Retrospective rate adjustments allow for an adjustment to the current period premium based on actual experience. The premium adjustment should be accrued in the current financial statement period and may need to be estimated if the settlement date is subsequent to the end of the accounting period. Prospectively rated premiums provide for increases in rates in the next contract period based on the actual experience of the previous period. When premium adjustments are prospectively rated, there are no accounting entries required in the current reporting period.

Revenues are recorded in the financial statements as a function of the underlying billing process. The effectiveness of the billing process is further dependent upon the membership or enrollment process. Membership data must be gathered in sufficient detail from the enrollment forms to allow for the proper classification of the enrollee to ensure that the appropriate rates are charged. Timely updating of enrollment records for changes in membership status not only ensures the accuracy of rates charged but also ensures that medical services are only provided to active enrollees. Furthermore, compliance with billing and enrollment procedures may affect whether the MCO will incur costs for health care services provided to inactive enrollees.

Subscribers, providers, and the MCO each have contractual obligations related to updating and verification of the enrollee's status. Failure to meet contractual obligations to maintain enrollment records properly and accurately could result in additional costs to the MCO. Therefore, the financial manager should have the information needed to ensure that revenue is being billed for all active enrollees and that business processes are functioning in a manner to prevent loss as a result of noncompliance with contract terms.

Premium billing may occur under two methods: self-billing or retroactive billing. The self-billing method permits the subscriber (or the group) to adjust the invoice for changes in enrollment. In this situation, the amount billed and recorded as premium revenue receivable will differ from the actual amounts paid by the group. Differences in the amount billed and received require adjustment to revenue and accounts receivable records. A secondary process should include communication of changes to ensure timely updating of enrollment records and notification of enrollment changes to providers. If processes are not in place to ensure that such differences are reconciled and resolved on a timely basis, revenue and accounts receivable may not be recorded properly in the financial statements, and health care benefits may be provided to individuals who are no longer insured.

The retroactive billing method results in adjustments to be recorded in the next month's billing cycle. Under this method, payments made by the group should equal amounts billed. Any changes in enrollment will be adjusted on the next billing. Any changes in enrollment noted should also be forwarded to the appropriate department to ensure updating of enrollment records.

For either billing method, the financial manager must develop a methodology of estimating adjustments affecting the current accounting period. Because the actual adjustments are not known until payment is received or reported in the next billing cycle, an estimate of expected adjustments should be accrued in the current reporting cycle.

Certain large commercial or government clients remit payment without detailed hard copy explanation of the adjustment. These customers often request electronic data transfer for billing purposes. Financial managers should be aware that significant resources may be needed to service these customers. Information systems personnel will be needed to deal with technical aspects of the electronic data transfer process. Support personnel with specific training will be needed to handle the unique challenges associated with large accounts. The process of reconciling the MCO's records with the customer's records can be time-consuming but is absolutely necessary. The financial manager should monitor the status (timeliness and completeness) of the reconciliations of these accounts to ensure that any potential problems with the reconciliations do not also affect other financial statement components, such as medical expense accruals.

Other Revenue Sources

Fee revenue is typically the largest component of other revenue. Fee revenue is charged to subscribers under administrative services contracts (ASC, also sometimes referred to as administrative services only, or ASO) whereby the subscriber typically selects a managed care product as an access fee for use of the provider network established by the MCO. For example, preferred provider organization (PPO) product fees are generally based on a specified per member per month charge. Fees for PPO products vary depending upon the level of service. There is a base fee for accessing the provider network, but enhanced services such as utilization management or providing a gatekeeper mechanism to manage utilization would increase the PPO access fee charged. Pricing of access fees should consider costs of performing administrative functions related to maintaining the provider network, such as credentialing, contract negotiations, and monitoring physician practice patterns.

Coordination of benefits (COB) recoverable is another source of revenue for the MCO. MCOs must have sufficient procedures in place to identify recoveries of costs under COB. COB usually exists when there is a two-wage earner family and individuals will have insurance coverage under two policies with a different insurer or health plan. Policies and procedures are established by insurance organizations to determine which insurer or health plan will serve as the primary or secondary payer. Procedures need to be in place to ensure that costs that are the responsibility of the other carrier are recovered. The data necessary to perform this procedure are usually gathered during the enrollment and billing process. Again, accuracy and completeness during the enrollment process are key to securing the data necessary to determine the amounts recoverable.

There are two primary methods of recovering COB: pay and pursue and pursue and pay. Under the pay and pursue method, claims are paid, and COB recovery is sought later from the other carrier. Under pursue and pay, the claim net of any COB is paid. To ensure that medical expenses are not recorded net, it is important that gross claim costs and COB recoverable are identifiable by the financial manager. See Chapter 18 for a detailed discussion of COB.

Reinsurance recoverable is another source of income to the MCO. Reinsurance against catastrophic claims or claims in excess of specified dollar limits is often obtained to reduce the risk of individual large losses for the MCO. MCOs may forgo obtaining reinsurance based on the cost versus benefit of the coverage. The financial manager needs to perform a risk assessment to determine whether stop-loss insurance is appropriate. Procedures need to exist to ensure that costs recoverable under reinsurance are identifiable, so that the MCO receives the full benefit to which it is entitled under the reinsurance arrangement. Reinsurance premiums should be recorded as health care costs, and reinsurance recoverable should be shown net of health care costs.

Another source of income for HMOs is interest income. Excess cash is generally invested in short-term instruments to ensure cash availability for the payment of claims.

Medical Expenses

Table 24-1, from Chapter 25 ("Underwriting and Rating Functions," Table 25-2), summarizes the breakdown of medical costs among hospital, physician, and ancillary services. Medical expenses may be incurred on a capitated basis, fee schedule, or per diem arrangement. Another form of reimbursement that is similar to capitation is percentage of premium. Capitation and percentage of premium represent risk transfer arrangements. Risk transfer arrangements place the providers at risk if utilization exceeds expected results. Reimbursement strategies are discussed in more detail in Chapters 6 through 8.

Medical expenses reported in the financial statements should represent paid claims plus accruals for claims reported but unpaid and claims incurred but not reported (IBNR). The development of the accruals for both reported and unreported claims is an accounting estimate whereby the accuracy of the estimate is dependent upon the data captured by operations personnel and communicated to the financial managers. For reported claims, the incidence of claims is known (*eg*, estimated length of stay for inpatient service, number of referred visits for outpatient services), and the type of claim is known (*eg*, inpatient procedure codes, type of outpatient service). The costs related to the claim incident must be estimated. For reported claims there is less unknown, and there can be more accuracy when ultimate costs are projected, although the ultimate disposition of the claims must still be estimated.

For IBNR claims, both the incidence of claims and the type of claims are unknown and must be estimated. IBNR estimates are often developed with the assistance of actuaries. A preferred methodology for estimating IBNR is the development of loss triangles

(Table 24-2). These triangles graphically depict the lag between either the date of service and the payment date or the date of service and the date the claim is reported. From the lag analysis, completion factors are developed to estimate the remaining claims to be reported or paid at each duration. Claim severity, or the estimated average claim costs, is then used to calculate the total projected costs yet to be incurred. The total projected costs are the basis for accruals to be recorded in the financial statements for the IBNR claims.

Loss triangles are often developed separately for hospital and physician claims. Physician claims can also be further analyzed by type of specialty claim where appropriate. Also the IBNR claims analysis should be segregated by line of business. Although greater level of details can assist in a more refined estimate, caution should be used when one is developing estimates from small population sizes. The smaller the base population, the less precise the estimates. It is prudent to limit the level of detail used in the analysis.

As discussed earlier, the adequacy of the estimates for reported claims developed by financial managers is dependent upon the availability of data from the operating areas within the MCO. These data are usually developed from the utilization management program. Inpatient care, excluding nonemergency care, typically requires preauthorization; therefore, if the utilization managers are keeping accurate records of admissions and length of stay statistics, the data needed by the financial managers to estimate admissions and cost of services should be readily available.

For outpatient services and specialist services, referrals are usually required for more services. Again, if the utilization management program is properly monitoring outpatient and specialist utilization and is maintaining accurate records of referrals, the data needed to estimate outpatient and specialist visits should be readily available to the financial manager. To be usable, the authorization information must be carefully controlled so that

Table 24–1 Sample Actuarial Cost Model

Medical Service Category	Medical Service	(1) Annual Utilization per 1,000 Members		(2) Allowed Average Charge Per Service	(3) Per Member Per Month (PMPM) Medical Cost	(4) Copay Frequency	(5) Copay Amount	(6) Net Claim Cost Sharing PMPM	(7) Costs PMPM
Hospital Inpatient	Medical/Surgical	180	Days	$5,100.00	$76.50				$76.50
	Psychiatric/Substance Abuse	45	Days	1,400.00	5.25				5.25
	Skilled Nursing Care	10	Days	950.00	0.79				0.79
	Subtotal	**235**	**Days**	**$4214.89**	**$82.54**				**$82.54**
Hospital Outpatient	Emergency Room	200	Visits	$1,250.00	$20.83	175	$100.00	$1.46	$19.38
	Surgery	75	Visits	3,600.00	22.50				22.50
	Radiology/Pathology	400	Cases	420.00	14.00				14.00
	Other	450	Cases	455.00	17.06				17.06
	Subtotal				**$74.40**			**$1.46**	**$72.92**
Physician	Office and Inpatient Visits	2,800	Visits	$135.00	$31.50	2,400	$25.00	$5.00	$26.50
	Preventative Care	1,200	Services	50.00	5.00	600	10.00	0.50	4.50
	Surgery	525	Procedures	750.00	32.81				32.81
	Radiology/Pathology	2,050	Procedures	120.00	20.50				20.50
	Other	2,350	Services	130.00	25.46				25.46
	Subtotal				**$115.27**			**$5.50**	**$109.77**
Other	Prescription Drugs	8,500	Scripts	$68.00	$48.17	8,000	$15.00	$10.00	$38.17
	Home Health Care	165	Units	350.00	4.81				4.81
	Ambulance	45	Runs	550.00	2.06				2.06
	Durable Medical Equipment	145	Units	390.00	4.71				4.71
	Subtotal				**$59.75**			**$10.00**	**$49.75**
Total Medical Costs PMPM					**$331.96**			**$16.96**	**$315.00**
Retention Load PMPM (10% of the Required Rate)									**$35.00**
Required Rate PMPM									**$350.00**

Source: Milliman U.S.A. as Table 25–2 in Chapter 25. Used with permission.

Table 24–2 Example of Loss Triangles

Inpatient Services

Claims Paid by Month of Receipt

Service Month	Jan	Feb	Mar	Apr	May	Jun	July	Aug	Sep	Oct	Nov	Dec
Jan	10	100	150	50	35	2	1		1		4	1
Feb		7	126	164	44	22	1	1		6	5	1
Mar			24	89	201	33	46	53				
Apr				12	109	177	3	25	2	2	1	
May					1	188	156	45	59	3	4	2
Jun						3	255	189	67	55	4	1
July							9	163	198	84	54	8
Aug								33	127	199	87	62
Sep									27	244	149	88
Oct										17	155	205
Nov											5	104
Dec												12
Total	10	107	300	315	390	425	471	509	481	610	468	484

continues

561

Table 24-2 Example of Loss Triangles—continued

Inpatient Services

Completion Factors by Month of Receipt

Service Month	Cur	+1	+2	+3	+4	+5	+6	+7	+8	+9	+10	+11	Total
Jan	0.03	0.31	0.73	0.88	0.97	0.98	0.98	0.98	0.99	0.99	1.00	1.00	
Feb	0.02	0.36	0.80	0.92	0.98	0.98	0.98	0.98	1.00	1.00	1.00		
Mar	0.05	0.25	0.69	0.77	0.87	0.99	0.99	0.99	1.00	1.00			
Apr	0.04	0.37	0.90	0.91	0.98	0.99	1.00	1.00	1.00				
May	0.00	0.41	0.75	0.85	0.98	0.99	1.00	1.00					
Jun	0.01	0.45	0.78	0.90	0.99	1.00	1.00						
July		0.02	0.33	0.72	0.88	0.98	1.00						
Aug	0.06	0.31	0.71	0.88	1.00								
Sep	0.05	0.53	0.83	1.00									
Oct	0.05	0.46	1.00										
Nov	0.05	1.00											
Dec	1.00												
Jan-Jun	0.02	0.36	0.78	0.87	0.96	0.99	0.99	0.99	1.00	1.00	1.00	1.00	

authorizations unlikely to be used are eliminated before ultimate utilization is estimated. It is extremely important that the utilization managers understand the significance of their responsibilities in that utilization managers not only are vital to controlling overall utilization but also provide necessary information to predict medical costs accurately, prepare reports on financial results, and develop budgets and financial forecasts.

Because the tools used by the financial managers to estimate medical costs also rely heavily on the accuracy of paid claims data, the claims processing department also plays an important role in financial management. The accuracy of claims data and the timely processing of claims will affect the reliability of the data used to develop the loss triangles. The extent of any backlogs in claim processing must be communicated in a timely fashion to the financial manager. See Chapter 18 for a detailed discussion of claims.

Loss triangles represent the most frequently used method to estimate claim costs. Other analyses can also be performed to substantiate further the reasonableness of the estimates for IBNR claims. Analyzing the monthly trends in claims costs or loss ratios by service type (inpatient, outpatient, physician services by specialty, etc.) within product lines and on a per member per month basis provides a basis for determining whether the overall trends in claim costs are consistent with expected results and, where appropriate, industry benchmarks. Factors that may affect the trends include the following:

- Significant changes in enrollment
- Unusual or large claims (isolated occurrences versus changes in utilization/cost patterns)
- Changes in pricing or product design
- Seasonal utilization or reporting patterns
- Claim processing backlogs
- Major changes to the provider network or reimbursement methods

Each of these factors provides a basis for explaining fluctuations when one is preparing trend analyses. It is important to note, however, that significant changes in enrollment also affect the financial manager's ability to determine reasonable estimates used in financial statements. For example, during periods of enrollment growth, it is difficult to estimate medical cost trends because there is little history associated with the current enrollment base and revenue begins on the first day of enrollment but medical costs generally do not; this may lull an inexperienced financial manager into believing that the medical costs ratio is low. In times of significant disenrollment, there is a risk of adverse selection. Adverse selection exists when the characteristics of the remaining population of insureds is weighted toward a high-risk group. Significant disenrollment often occurs when it is generally not an optimal condition for the enrollee to maintain the current coverage. Usually, those insureds with less choice (*eg*, those who are unable to opt for other coverage because of current health status) remain enrolled. Medical cost estimates must be adjusted under these circumstances.

Additionally, as the competitive landscape changes, and pressures to contain premium costs to employers and their members, MCOs need to continuously look to be innovative in product design; for example, consumer-directed health plans as discussed in Chapters 2 and 20. The rising cost of health care, particularly driven by the advancement in medical technology, continue to challenge the ability to market profitable and reasonably priced products. New product initiatives often affect the claims activity and can increase the difficulty in measuring and estimating medical cost trends.

Administrative Expenses

Administrative expenses include salaries as well as sales, marketing, and other operating expenses. Administrative expenses also vary by product and market segment. Administrative expenses can be measured using percentage of premium and per member per month benchmarks. Administrative expenses may also be tracked by functional area (*eg*, finance, sales, underwriting, member services). Administrative expenses will vary with volume as a result of economies of scale. In growth periods, administrative expenses tend to be high as a percentage of premium.

Tracking of administrative expenses by product and market segment enables management to identify whether the appropriate resources are being allocated to product lines. Additionally, if the MCO experience rates certain groups, management needs to track adequately costs associated with a particular group's business to ensure that costs are appropriately allocated to the group and are recovered. The financial manager should also be aware that certain products or market segments, such as government groups and Medicare or Medicaid, place limits on administrative expense allocations to these product lines.

BALANCE SHEET

Cash and Investments

Cash and investments represent a significant balance sheet account for an MCO. The major source of cash is premium revenue. An MCO's investment portfolio usually consists of short-term investments because cash outlays for claims are frequent. Because cash does churn quickly through the MCO, management may benefit from implementing strong cash management practices, such as using lock-box arrangements for premiums. Maximizing the investment in short-term instruments is the main focus of the investment risk.

Premium Receivable

Another significant balance sheet account is premium receivable. Premiums are generally collected monthly; therefore, problems with the aging of accounts will probably arise from many old items that are not reconciled often. Unreconciled differences may occur when billing problems exist or as a result of discrepancies in the enrollment records of the MCO in comparison with customer records.

Timely update of membership records ensures the accuracy of premium billings and further ensures that claims are paid appropriately. Policies and procedures to ensure timely updating of membership records protect the MCO from paying claims for terminated members or ensures the recoverability of amounts paid incorrectly. In general, if membership records are not up-to-date and the MCO bills incorrectly for terminated or inactive members, upon remittance a group will adjust the payment accordingly. If the MCO does not have procedures in place to reconcile remittances to billed amounts, premium receivable records will show amounts outstanding and past due. Because of the large number of individual members within a group and the potentially large number of billings, management must monitor closely the status of premium reconciliation procedures.

The reconciliation process related to premium receivable for government accounts is usually a more complex problem. For example, federal and state employers often remit premium on a cycle that differs from the normal billing cycle of the MCO. The remittances by these institutions are consistent with the institution's payroll cycles. Premium is remitted only for those employees noted as active on the payroll. There are many events that affect the active status of federal and state employees (*eg*, leave of absence, summer recess for educators), but these employees may still be eligible for health benefits. For this reason, the MCO will bill and accrue for premiums that will not be paid until the employee's status on the institution's records is reinstated to active status. Often, MCOs that provide coverage to federal and state groups will have dedicated resources to support the reconciliation process.

The reconciliation process for certain large groups may also be complex. The high enrollment volume or the need to accept enrollment data in compatible electronic format may present a challenge for the MCO.

Other Assets

The significance of other assets of an MCO will vary. Another typical large asset may be fixed assets, for example, an HMO is organized as a staff model HMO that owns and operates physician offices. Because of standards under SAP regarding what may or may not be counted as an asset for purposes of calculating the statutory net worth of the MCO as discussed later in this chapter, it is relatively uncommon for MCOs to own property, however, since it is not considered liquid.

Unearned Premiums

Unearned premiums are premiums received by the MCO that at the close of the financial reporting period have not been earned, principally because the premiums are for the ensuing month and are in actuality premiums received in advance. Because most MCOs bill on a monthly basis, unearned premium is generally not a major accounting issue. If premiums are billed and collected other than monthly (*eg,* quarterly), an unearned premium reserve would be required.

Claims Payable and IBNR

As discussed earlier, the basis for the recording of claim reserves, including IBNR, is dependent upon information provided by other operating areas of the MCO. Claim liabilities are separated between hospital claims and physician claims. In addition to the matters discussed for medical expenses, the financial manager should prepare further analyses of claim reserves and IBNR estimates.

The financial manager should compare the actual claim payments since the close of the accounting period with the original estimates. Significant differences in the actual results compared with estimated results should be investigated. Information obtained from the investigation should be considered when the sufficiency of current estimates is evaluated.

Risk Pool Liabilities

As discussed in Chapters 6 and 7, reimbursement strategies may provide for risk pools, which will require the MCO to maintain accurate records of payment withholds from hospitals and physicians. Amounts payable to the providers from the withhold should be maintained in separate accounts. In addition, shortfalls in the risk pool that must be recovered from the providers need to be evaluated to ensure that the amounts are recoverable, and where necessary the financial manager should consider the need for a provision for unrecoverable amounts. Additionally, any contributions to be made by the MCO for its participation in a risk pool should be appropriately accrued in the financial statements.

Equity

The MCO will need to track its SAP and GAAP basis equity. SAP equity generally differs from GAAP equity as a result of certain assets being nonadmitted and also where permitted certain liabilities being recognized as equity. For example, the statutory balance sheet may permit certain surplus notes to be classified as equity for purposes of determining statutory net worth (issues regarding statutory net worth are discussed later). Surplus notes are obligations to investors that meet certain requirements of the state insurance laws, which are generally subordinated to all obligations of the MCOs. Repayment of surplus notes is subject to the approval of the state's commissioners of insurance. Other transactions affecting equity that are generally subject to the approval of the state's commissioners of insurance include restrictions on the payout of dividends.

REGULATORY REPORTING CONSIDERATIONS

Generally, HMOs and health insurance companies are required to file quarterly financial statements with the state Department of

Insurance, which are due 45 days after the close of the quarter. An annual statement filing is also required. The annual filing is due March 1. Effective with the reporting for calendar year 1998, changes were made to the NAIC annual statement format. The changes to investment reporting (Schedule D to the NAIC annual statement) resulted in HMOs reporting of investment activity which is identical to that reported by other types of insurance organizations (*eg,* life and health insurers and property/casualty insurers). Previously, HMOs were not required to submit such detailed information of their investment activity and holdings at the end of the reporting period. Another important change included the addition of Schedule L to the NAIC annual statement, which reports information and activities with intermediaries, including the concentration of business with intermediaries and whether or not the intermediaries are subject to regulatory oversight, including risk-based capital requirements and provides an indication as to whether the requirements have been met. Schedule L provides the regulators with more up-to-date information on the extent of risk transfer arrangements between the MCO and an intermediary organization that may not in turn be subject to regulatory oversight. This is particularly important to the regulators because when risk is transferred to unregulated entities, there is an increased risk that the assuming entity may not have adequate capital to sustain adverse underwriting risk. In these situations, the funds for the provision of care have already been disbursed by the MCO. If the intermediary is in financial distress, the funds may no longer be available, further increasing the financial risk to the MCO.

The information provided on both Schedules D and L also facilitated the development of the data to be reported in the MCOs risk-based capital filing. There is a direct feed of information from both Schedule D and Schedule L to the risk-based capital filing.

Many states also require the filing of a certification on claims reserves prepared by a licensed actuary. Audited financial statements are also required; the filing deadline may vary by state but is generally June 1. Any differences in the amounts reported in the audited financial statements and the annual filing due on March 1 must be disclosed in the footnotes to the audited financial statements. Depending on the applicable state's requirements, the audited financial statements may be prepared on either an SAP basis or a GAAP basis.

GAAP focuses more on the matching of revenue and expenses in a given reporting period to measure the earnings of an entity. The state insurance departments that have jurisdiction over the MCO are concerned with the MCO's ability to pay claims in the future. For example, certain expenditures (*eg,* capital assets) may benefit future earnings ability and therefore are likely to be capitalized and expensed ratably over future periods for GAAP. However, such costs are expensed immediately in accordance with SAP because moneys expended are no longer available to pay future liabilities.

Many differences between SAP and GAAP accounting are generally based on the premise of the state insurance department's ability to determine liquidity of the MCO. Some of the major differences include the following:

- Treatment of certain assets and investments as nonadmitted under SAP (*eg,* fixed assets other than electronic data processing equipment, past due premium receivables, certain loans and other receivables, and investments not authorized by statute or in excess of statutory limitations)
- Deferred tax accounts
- Carrying value of investments in subsidiaries (which is primarily affected by limitations in the carrying amount and the amortization period of goodwill)

The state Department of Insurance imposes minimum statutory capital requirements for HMOs and insurance companies. The NAIC adopted a model act for HMOs that specified that minimum capital for HMOs should be determined as follows:

- The greater of $1,000,000, or
- 2% of annual premium as reported on the most recent annual financial statement filed with the commissioners of insurance on the first $150 million of premium and 1% of annual premium on premium greater than $150 million, or
- An amount equal to the sum of 3 months' uncovered health care expenditures as reported on the most recent financial statement filed with the commissioners, or
- An amount equal to the sum of:

    1. 8% of annual health care expenditures except those paid on a capitated basis or a managed hospital payment basis as reported on the most recent financial statement filed with the commissioner, and
    2. 4% of annual health care expenditures paid on a managed hospital payment basis as reported on the most recent financial statement filed with the commissioner

Managed hospital basis means agreements wherein the financial risk is primarily related to the degree of utilization rather than to the cost of services. *Uncovered expenditures* means the costs to the HMO for health care services that are the obligation of the HMO, for which an enrollee may also be liable in the event of HMO insolvency and for which no alternative arrangements have been made that are acceptable to the commissioner.

The requirements of each of the states generally call for plans of action when an entity's capital falls within a close range of the minimum requirement.

Although the states' minimum requirements have provided a means to measure the financial viability of an insurance entity, the states' requirements were often a flat minimum and disregarded the size of an entity or the differing degrees of risk to which different entities are exposed. Insurance entities' exposure to risk has become more diverse, and although some are conservative in investment and underwriting practices, others have been more aggressive.

The NAIC began examining existing capital requirements and concluded that consumers should be further protected by having companies that assume a more aggressive, risk-taking approach be subject to higher capital requirements. Risk-based capital (RBC) requirements were first required for life and health insurers and property/casualty insurers. A working group was formed in 1993 to develop a separate risk-based capital formula for health organizations, including traditional health insurers, HMOs, Blue Cross/Blue Shield plans, and health service plans. The working group completed its assignment and now, the Risk-Based Capital (RBC) for Insurers Model Law published by the NAIC* (the Law) covers the RBC requirements for such health organizations. In the final stages of development of the Law, MCOs were required to complete model filings using financial information reported in prior reporting periods. For the calendar year ending 1998, MCOs were required to file electronic and paper filings with the NAIC and to respective state regulators, and beginning with the calendar year 1999, MCOs needed to complete the "RBC Plan" to be submitted as required by the Law in the event the reporting MCO's RBC requirements are not met. Consistent with the deadline for filing the MCO's NAIC annual statement, the RBC filing is due on March 1.

RBC is a method of measuring the minimum amount of capital appropriate for an MCO to support its overall business operations based on its size and degree of risk taken in each of the five major categories of risk: asset risk—affiliates, asset risk—other, underwriting risk, credit risk, and business risk. An MCO's RBC is calculated by applying factors to various asset, premium, and reserve items that result in a charge to the MCO's actual capital and arrives at adjusted capital. The MCO's actual capital is compared to varying levels of the adjusted capital to determine levels of actions, if any, to be taken to improve actual capital. For example, if the

---

*See http://www.naic.org.

MCO's actual capital is greater than 200% of the adjusted capital, no action is required. At 200% of adjusted capital, the MCO is required to develop and submit a plan of action. If actual capital is below 150%, regulatory action is required, unless the actual capital falls to 70% or below, and then mandatory control of the MCO is required.

Of the five categories of risk, underwriting risk results in the largest charge to adjusted capital. The development of this charge was to protect against the risk of fluctuation in underwriting experience. The net charge for underwriting risk is offset by credits that are based to a great extent upon the positive effect that management care arrangements may have on underwriting risk. There is a presumed benefit from certain managed care arrangements that may reduce the uncertainty about future claims payments. For example, capitated fee arrangements with no risk-sharing features are generally fixed costs per member per month (PMPM) that therefore reduce the MCO's risk associated with adverse fluctuations in utilization or intensity, thus providing for a more defined estimate of the cost of the capitated fee arrangement. The impact on an MCO's RBC for the other categories of risk include protection against investments in assets of affiliates, including subsidiary entities with their own RBC requirements, investments in other assets whose value may be subject to fluctuation in market value, credit risk associated with the recoverability of amounts owed to the MCO (ie, premium receivables, recoverables from providers), and business risk including the effect of excessive business growth on the MCO's capital.

The regulatory environment under which MCOs operate is continuously changing to meet market changes, and entities need to prepare themselves in particular to meet the challenges imposed by new or expected legislation.

BUDGETING AND FINANCIAL FORECASTING

The importance of maintaining detailed budgets has been discussed throughout this chapter. Financial forecasts, which project activity and results beyond the current period, are also important management tools. Financial forecasts are often developed several months in advance of the actual reporting period. In developing the forecasts, a balance between complexity and simplicity is sought by the financial manager. Although it is essential to capture much detail to develop the overall forecast, the detail information must roll up to a summary level that will facilitate presentation to senior decision makers within the organization and to provide ease for monitoring variances in actual results. At the early stages of development, if the financial forecast evolves from the appropriate level of detail, the overall summaries discussed by senior management teams will be more meaningful.

At the highest level, membership data priced at blended premium rates must be presented. The development of both the aggregate membership growth and the blended premium rates is based upon input from personnel within sales and marketing, underwriting, and actuarial functions and should have considered specific assumptions for the different array of products offered by the MCO. It is important to verify assumptions with the sales function's expectations and the organizations underwriting policies and pricing strategies.

Because both new and renewal membership and premium rate changes are affected by seasonal patterns, the assumptions should trend from quarterly, if not monthly, baseline data. Developing the overall financial forecasts from this level of detail will assist the financial manager in providing the most accurate report of actual versus budgeted results. Understanding variances in planned to actual premium revenue will support whether expected rate changes or net membership growth assumptions were achieved. Sometimes the rate increase by product and the net membership growth may meet expected targets; however, changes in the membership by product type could still result in the aggregate premium levels not being achieved. The ability of the financial manager to identify the root cause of variances between forecast and actual results is essential to achieving an organization's overall financial goals.

The baseline for the medical expense component of the financial forecast is generally developed from a historical "look back" of the results. At the time that financial forecasts are being developed, there is still some level of estimation in the historical results, which further complicates the development of the baseline estimate of medical expenses. This baseline must then be adjusted for expected changes including but not limited to medical inflation trends, expected changes in regulations (*eg,* new benefit mandates), changes in provider contracting arrangements, enhancements to patient management programs, and introduction of new plan designs. The effects of changes in provider contracts may be dependent upon whether the changes affect a significant portion of the overall membership. Additionally, the effects of patient management programs often require a period of time before the financial impact of the benefit is achieved and/or measurable.

It may also be beneficial, to the extent it is practicable, to segregate average medical costs by types of provider contract arrangements. For example, identifying expected PMPM costs for global contract arrangements, fee-for-service arrangements, specialty capitation, and other ancillary arrangements could provide critical information for monitoring the success of the various types of provider arrangements. If it is difficult to identify expected or actual costs for these arrangements, one may question the appropriateness of the arrangement and the viability of the rate that was negotiated with the provider.

Other key components of forecasting medical expenses include the impact of risk-sharing arrangements with providers and the cost and/or benefit of the historical settlement in additions to regulatory imposed costs, such as interest assessed on late payment of claims or surcharges assessed as subsidies to finance the cost of individual and small employer insurance and care for the uninsured.

Administrative costs need to be forecast. Consideration of the cost to invest in planned growth as well as sustain existing membership volumes is necessary. The most significant component of the administrative costs is typically salary and related expenses.

Whether the financial manager is developing premium revenue, medical expense, or administrative costs, the development of the financial forecast is an iterative process and the financial model must be flexible to facilitate this process while at the same time be responsive and not unreasonably complex.

The financial forecasting process must also include the development of a projected balance sheet. This is particularly important to evaluate the impact of the projected growth in operations on minimum capital requirements. Additionally, the forecasting process should require variations from the baseline projections to determine the risks and exposures if the actual results fall short of the baseline and also to project the impact if actual results are better than expected. Cash flow analyses are also important to ensure that cash will be generated from operations or to determine the extent to which cash reserves will be needed, particularly as new lines of business are pursued.

Sarbanes-Oxley Act of 2002

In July 2002, the Sarbanes-Oxley Act of 2002* was signed into law. The act came in response to a string of corporate scandals, including the collapse of a number of businesses, that negatively affected the confidence of investors in the capital markets of the United States.

---

*Pub. L. No. 107-204, 116 Stat. 745, also known as the Public Company Accounting Reform and Investor Protection Act of 2002 and commonly called SOX or SarbOx.

Focusing primarily on investor-owned companies (not specifically on health insurance), the act contains 11 titles (sections) that range from board responsibilities, to "whistle blower" protections, to penalties. Most important, it created the Public Company Accounting Oversight Board, a quasi-government agency that oversees the audits of public companies, intending to protect the interest of investors and other users of an "issuer's" financial statements. The board, which is subject to SEC oversight, is empowered to establish auditing standards for public company audits, inspect accounting firms that audit public companies, investigate possible rule violations, and sanction violators.

In passing the act, Congress reasoned that the restoration of investors' trust in public companies would depend on demanding that public companies possess strong internal control over financial reporting (ICOFR) and then report on that assessment at the close of its fiscal year. The act also requires a company's external auditor to attest to and report on the assessment made by management.

Specifically pertaining to financial management, Section 404 of the act has two parts:

- Section 404(a) describes management's responsibility for establishing and maintaining an adequate internal control structure and procedures for financial reporting. It also outlines management's responsibility for assessing the effectiveness of internal control over financial reporting.
- Section 404(b) describes the independent auditor's responsibility for attesting to and reporting on management's internal control assessment.

CONCLUSION

Whether the financial manager is developing budgets or financial forecasts or preparing financial statements, he or she must depend on the information prepared and maintained by the operating departments. This information is an integral part of the financial manager's decision-making process. Communication among the various functional areas in the MCO will be key to the successful operation of the entity. Timely financial reporting enhances management's ability to determine performance against anticipated results and redirect its strategies to minimize exposure to loss and preserve a favorable financial performance.

25

Underwriting and Rating Functions

Michael G. Sturm and Troy M. Filipek

Study Objectives

- Understand the development of premium rates in managed care plans.
- Understand the basic issues involved in underwriting.
- Understand the basic elements that go into rate development.
- Understand how per member per month medical costs are calculated.

Discussion Topics

1. Describe and discuss the differences between rating and underwriting.
2. Describe and discuss the basic approach to developing premium rates for MCOs.
3. Describe and discuss the basic elements that go into typical rate development formulas.
4. Describe different times at which underwriting may occur and discuss the importance of underwriting at each time.

INTRODUCTION

Underwriting and rating are two very important functions for any health plan. Successful underwriting and rating strikes a balance among adequacy, competitiveness, and equity of rates. It can be a difficult and delicate balance to achieve. Moving too far in any direction can lead to financial disaster for a health plan.

Adequate rates are high enough to generate sufficient revenue to cover all claims and other plan expenses and to yield an acceptable return on equity. Competitive rates are low enough to sell enough policies and enroll enough members to meet health plan volume and growth targets. Equitable rates will approximate any given group's costs without an unreasonable amount of cross-subsidization among groups. Equitable rates are achieved through applying various rating factors appropriately and result in higher persistency if groups realize they are being charged a fair amount for their insurance.

A health plan should continually assess its success in each of these areas. Although always important, this is particularly true for a newly established plan or product offering. For example, a plan cannot be sure whether a high volume of sales is good or bad until adequacy and equitability are assessed because competitive rates are not necessarily adequate or equitable.

This chapter discusses underwriting and rating functions common to most major health insurance markets. Major markets include private individual, commercial group (both small and large), and government business (Medicare and Medicaid). Several core underwriting and rating functions are common to these markets, which are addressed in this chapter. However, each major market segment also has several components with unique risk characteristics that require different approaches to underwriting and rating. These unique to market topics are outside the scope of this chapter and are not addressed here.

UNDERWRITING

Underwriting involves gathering information about applicants or groups of applicants to determine an adequate, competitive, and equitable rate at which to insure them. The type of underwriting and level of scrutiny depend on many factors, including the time at which the underwriting is done (at issue, during the plan year, or at renewal), the group size (individual, small, or large), and the risk arrangement (fully insured or self-insured).

Underwriting is a function that often is specific to the market being served. For example, individual and small group underwriting generally requires review of individual medical records, whereas large group underwriting does not require this level of depth. As a result, this section provides only a high-level discussion of underwriting techniques and philosophies, without discussing the technical details specific to a particular market.

At Issue

Effective underwriting at issue determines the following information for the individual or group:

- Health status
- Ability to pay the premium
- Availability of other coverage (if any)
- Historical persistency (applies mainly to groups with high start-up costs)

Health Status

Information gathered to determine health status varies. The following types of information might be requested:

- Physical exams and/or attending physician statements (individual)
- Prescription drug histories (individual and small group)
- Individual medical questionnaires (individual and small group)
- An employer disclosure listing major health conditions (large group)

- Medical cost experience (large group)
- No health status information (Medicare and Medicaid risk contracts)

Some carriers use health status information in certain markets (where allowed by law) to apply a preexisting condition limitation or exclusion (*ie,* a temporary or permanent limit on medical payments for existing health conditions). Preexisting condition limitations are often used in conjunction with underwriting to limit antiselection and therefore provide incentive to prospective enrollees to apply for coverage prior to becoming sick. This ensures appropriate risk pooling, which is essential for a successful insurance arrangement.

Other underwriting policies are used to screen for health status at both issue and renewal, such as ensuring a valid employer-employee relationship exists and a minimum percentage of employees participate in the medical plan. These policies, along with others, prevent groups with higher than average morbidity from being issued coverage at average rates (*ie,* adverse selection).

The propensity to purchase coverage is dictated by several factors, including cost concerns, the need to attract and retain employees with health benefits, and whether health insurance premiums are tax-deductible. The chance of adverse selection increases as group size decreases because individual and small group applicants are likely to buy insurance only if they need it. In addition, large groups often submit claims experience, which enables the underwriter to better estimate a specific group's rates. Therefore, underwriting with medical questionnaires to determine health status is common for individuals and small groups and uncommon for large groups.

Other markets, such as Medicaid and Medicare risk, do not allow medical underwriting for rate setting. Risk-adjusted revenue payments from the federal and state governments help address the adverse selection issues in these markets.

Ability to Pay

Information gathered to determine an applicant's premium-paying ability might include income and credit history. Income can be verified through tax returns or audited financial statements. Credit history can be verified through independent credit agencies. Credit history is particularly important for employers in industries facing financial hardship, new employers, or employers first offering medical coverage to employees.

Insurers do not necessarily decline coverage to applicants with poor credit histories. Insurers customarily require groups with a poor credit rating to produce some form of collateral or a letter of credit (for up to 2 months of premium) instead of declining coverage. Insurers nearly always require individual policyholders to pay premiums in advance of the coverage period to ensure their ability to meet premium requirements.

Other Coverage

Insureds are often asked on the application (or are surveyed during the plan year) if they have other health insurance coverage. The presence of other coverage should be noted, such that the claim adjudicator can determine which insurer is responsible for payment of claims based on coordination of benefit rules as discussed in Chapter 18. Coordinating payment for benefits enables insurers to reduce their premium.

Further, it is important to ensure that workers' compensation insurance is in place for commercially insured groups. This insurance provides for coverage in the event of a workplace injury. The coverage enables the medical insurer to subrogate claims it pays initially that occur in a workplace setting. Premium loads of 10% to 20% are common for employers without workers' compensation insurance.

Persistency

Insurers should be cautious when writing groups that frequently change carriers because there can be a significant amount of fixed costs (*eg,* advertising, underwriting, and commissions) to write a new group. The group should appear to be committed to a multiple-year relationship, as demonstrated by a history of persistency with prior carriers. It may be more beneficial not to quote groups with poor persistency in certain cases.

Small groups that frequently change carriers could be placed in the highest rating tier, as allowed by state rating limitations. Large groups with more than two carriers in the past 5 years might not be offered coverage at all.

Carrier actions based on underwriting information include issuing coverage at the standard rate, issuing coverage at a higher rate, excluding certain services, or declining coverage (where allowed by law).

During the Plan Year and at Renewal

Underwriting during the plan year and at renewal varies greatly by major market segment and, therefore, is not discussed in depth here. However, in general, underwriting during the plan year involves a stringent review to prevent adverse selection. At renewal, the underwriter usually has more information on the insureds (possibly including claims experience) and implements rate changes based on this additional information and any projected changes that could affect future experience.

RATING

Rating uses information gathered through underwriting to calculate the premium for a specific individual or group. The premium calculation is generally done using a rate formula, historical experience, predictive underwriting tools, or some combination of these three.

The result of the rate formula is sometimes called the manual or book rate. The manual rate is developed using the experience of all individuals or groups in a specific block or pool (*ie,* a base rate). The starting base rate is adjusted through the rate formula for de-

mographics, area, group size, and other characteristics to arrive at a manual rate specific to a group or individual.

In a group setting, the manual rate might then be blended with group-specific historical experience depending on the group size and credibility of the data. Generally, group sizes of more than 50 are rated at least partially based on experience. State regulation and carrier practices dictate the level of this threshold. Adjusting an individual's rate (whether the individual has individual or group coverage) based on the individual's experience is not allowed by law.

Group-specific experience rating involves varying the manual rate (*ie,* the combination of all the groups' experience) based on a specific group's experience. Experience rating can be thought of as the converse of pooling experience because recognizing a group's experience in its rate calculation reduces the extent to which groups subsidize each other.

The rate formula should recognize all health plan costs, be easy to apply in most situations, and result in an appropriate premium rate. Health plans' costs include medical services, prescription drugs, sales and marketing expenses, administrative expenses, and profit. The rate formula typically expresses rates on a per member per month (PMPM) basis that must be transformed into contract rates for each employee based on the average number of covered members per contract and the contract tiers (*eg,* employee only, employee plus spouse, family).

The rate formula is updated through various analyses that measure carrier experience. These analyses can also be helpful in establishing budgets by medical service category or department, measuring cost and utilization trends, establishing funding for provider-based risk pools, and identifying, quantifying, and prioritizing medical management opportunities within the health plan. Timely analyses will allow the health plan to establish the proper provider-based education and incentives necessary to realize opportunities within the health plan.

Rate Formula

The rate formula provides the mechanism to adjust the base rate to a group-specific premium to quote. The formula adjusts the base rate for demographics, area, group size, and other characteristics to arrive at the manual rate specific to a group or individual. Then, upon adding the retention costs and converting to a per contract rate, the premium quote is determined.

Base Rate Development

Most rate formulas start with a base rate, developed from PMPM incurred medical costs over a historical experience period. The base rate generally reflects the following specific information:

- Population (*eg,* commercial, Medicare, Medicaid, or other population)
- Set of covered services (including service-specific limits)
- Set of cost-sharing provisions
- Set of provider reimbursement arrangements
- Demographic (*ie,* age and gender)
- Average members per contract
- Geographical area
- Occupation/industry
- Health status
- Degree of health care management
- Coverage effective date
- Level of out-of-network usage (if applicable)
- Presence or absence of workers' compensation insurance
- Use of preexisting condition clauses
- Set of underwriting practices
- Set of claim administration practices
- Blend of distribution methods (*eg,* agents, brokers, direct)
- Set of other variables affecting medical costs

The projection period base rate is developed by analyzing historical incurred medical costs for a given time period (*ie,* the base period) and trending it forward to the projec-

tion period, recognizing actual and anticipated changes in the block of business. Historical medical costs are often summarized in 12-month segments of incurred medical costs to provide a credible experience base and to avoid any seasonal variations.

Claims data are generally summarized according to when payments are made. Paid claims data should be converted to an incurred basis, including incurred but not reported (IBNR) reserves, using various estimation techniques (*eg,* claim lag analyses and loss ratio techniques) as discussed in Chapter 24. Incurred claims are then matched with health plan exposure (as generally measured in member months) to develop a base period PMPM medical cost.

Incurred claim estimation techniques should account for a health plan's unique payment arrangements. The actuary should know whether the paid claims data include capitations, withhold payments, stop-loss recoveries, and/or coordination of benefit savings. If these are not included, the actuary should make the necessary adjustments to account for these plan provisions as part of the incurred claims. In addition, the actuary may need to modify incurred claims for any accrued medical incentives, such as provider bonuses.

Projection adjustments should be made to recognize and account for changes in health plan operations between the base period and projection period. Table 25-1 presents elements to consider that may change between the base period and projection period. The elements listed in Table 25-1 may be offsetting. For example, the underlying demand to use more health care services, as the U.S. population ages and technology advances, may be offset by anticipated medical management improvements.

The projection period base rate can be summarized in an actuarial cost model. Table 25-2 displays a sample actuarial cost model. The model contains, by service category, the following information:

- Annual utilization per 1,000 members (column 1)

Table 25–1 Adjustments to Convert a Historical Base Rate to a Projection Period Base Rate

Actual and/or anticipated changes in incurred claims as a result of changes in:

- The underlying demand for medical services
- Medical management
- Provider reimbursement
- Wellness and preventive care programs
- Contractual benefit levels or member cost sharing
- The level of consumer involvement in directing and paying for care
- The average amounts contained in consumer-directed health spending accounts
- The insured population (*eg*, age, gender, Medicare/Medicaid eligibility)
- The geographical area of the insured population
- Claims administration
- Underwriting requirements
- Distribution methods
- The mix of medical services (*eg*, because of new technologies or treatment procedures)
- Intensity (*ie*, the amount of services per day or visit)
- Other variables affecting health care costs

- The allowed average charge per service (column 2)
- Per member per month (PMPM) medical costs (column 3 = (column 1) × (column 2)/12,000); these do not reflect cost-sharing provisions
- Cost-sharing adjustments (columns 4, 5, and 6); these should be composited across the underlying benefit plans offered
- PMPM medical costs net of cost sharing (column 7)

Each service category is defined by a unique set of procedure codes. For example, hospital inpatient services can be grouped by diagnosis-related group (DRG) and physician services can be grouped using current procedural terminology (CPT). Prescription drugs are generally analyzed separately, using the national drug code (NDC).

One major component of the cost model is the rate at which the population is assumed to use medical services (*ie*, utilization). Utilization can vary substantially depending on the efficiency of network providers. Two or more utilization scenarios are often developed to estimate medical costs under current levels of health care management and well-managed levels. Utilization can also vary depending on the benefit designs in place, the level of consumer involvement in directing and paying for care, demographics, and area, among other variables.

The other major cost model component, the average charge per service, is based on the provider reimbursement negotiated and specified in the health plan's provider contracts. The average charge per service can be in the form of discounts from billed charges, per diems, case rates, negotiated fee schedules, capitation payments, or other forms of reimbursement. Reimbursement of providers is discussed in Chapters 6 and 7.

The impact of copays on the cost model depends on the benefit plan design and the plan's policy for copay collection. The PMPM medical cost equals the annual utilization per 1,000 members, multiplied by the average charge per service, divided by 12,000 less the value of cost sharing (*ie*, the copay frequency multiplied by the copay, divided by 12,000). The values in the actuarial cost

Table 25-2 Sample Actuarial Cost Model

Medical Service Category	Medical Service	(1) Annual Utilization per 1,000 Members		(2) Allowed Average Charge Per Service	(3) Per Member Per Month (PMPM) Medical Cost	(4) Copay Frequency	(5) Copay Amount	(6) Net Claim Cost Sharing PMPM	(7) Costs PMPM
Hospital Inpatient	Medical/Surgical Psychiatric/	180	Days	$5,100.00	$76.50				$76.50
	Substance Abuse	45	Days	1,400.00	5.25				5.25
	Skilled Nursing Care	10	Days	950.00	0.79				0.79
	Subtotal	**235**	**Days**	**$4,214.89**	**$82.54**				**$82.54**
Hospital Outpatient	Emergency Room	200	Visits	$1,250.00	$20.83	175	$100.00	$1.46	$19.38
	Surgery	75	Visits	3,600.00	22.50				22.50
	Radiology/Pathology	400	Cases	420.00	14.00				14.00
	Other	450	Cases	455.00	17.06				17.06
	Subtotal				**$74.40**			**$1.46**	**$72.94**
Physician	Office and Inpatient Visits	2,800	Visits	$135.00	$31.50	2,400	$25.00	$5.00	$26.50
	Preventative Care	1,200	Services	50.00	5.00	600	10.00	0.50	4.50
	Surgery	525	Procedures	750.00	32.81				32.81
	Radiology/Pathology	2,050	Procedures	120.00	20.50				20.50
	Other	2,350	Services	130.00	25.46				25.46
	Subtotal				**$115.27**			**$5.50**	**$109.77**
Other	Prescription Drugs	8,500	Scripts	$68.00	$48.17	8,000	$15.00	$10.00	$38.17
	Home Health Care	165	Units	350.00	4.81				4.81
	Ambulance	45	Runs	550.00	2.06				2.06
	Durable Medical Equipment	145	Units	390.00	4.71				4.71
	Subtotal				**$59.75**			**$10.00**	**$49.75**
Total Medical Costs PMPM					**$331.96**			**$16.96**	**$315.00**
Retention Load PMPM (10% of the Required Rate)									**$35.00**
Required Rate PMPM									**$350.00**

Source: Milliman, Inc. Used with permission.

model will differ for each group depending on the group's characteristics.

Rate Determination

Table 25-3 contains a sample rate formula with case-specific adjustments to the base rate. Steps 2 to 5 in the formula adjust the projection period base rate to reflect the specific group and plan characteristics because the projection period base rate assumes that all characteristics of a particular insured individual/group are the same as the block, or group of policies the base rate represents.

The rate formula adjustments should consider relevant, measurable factors that predict medical cost differences among individuals/groups, but the formula should still be easy to measure and apply as well. The adjustments might be additive or multiplicative, depending on the type of adjustment and user's preference. For example, the base rate may need to have costs added to it to reflect additional covered services for mandated benefits in certain states. Conversely, the base rate may need to be multiplied by a factor to reflect lower utilization of services as a result of an efficient health care provider network (*ie,* degree of health care management).

Retention

Retention items are usually built into the rate formula once medical costs are calculated. Retention can include administrative expenses, a buildup of contingency reserves, coordination of benefit savings, and profit. Retention can be combined with medical costs to arrive at the PMPM premium by dividing the medical costs by a target loss ratio (fixed or variable by group size) or adding specific PMPM retention costs.

Retention must be sufficient to cover all functions performed by the carrier, including claims administration, distribution, and underwriting, among others. Retention might only include a subset of a normal carrier's costs if the targets are developed for a physician-hospital organization or other provider-based group that is responsible for only a portion of the administrative duties.

Conversion of Rates from Member to Employee Level

Lastly, the PMPM manual rate must be converted from a member rate to a contract (*ie,* per employee) rate. Individual and some small group contracts covering multiple members are generally rated by adding together the appropriate rates for each member based on their age and gender (*ie,* list bill rating). Conversely, large groups and some small groups are often charged rates according to specific contract tiers without varying rates by age or gender (*ie,* composite rates). Composite rates need to be set such that the total premium generated for the group reflects the average number of members per contract tier in the

---

Table 25–3 Sample Rate Formula

Step 1:	Incurred medical costs PMPM (*ie,* the base rate)
Step 2:	Add or subtract: • Covered services [not] reflected in the base rate • Reinsurance costs
Step 3:	Multiply by: • Benefit plan factor • Geographical area factor • Age/gender factor • Degree of health care management factor • Provider reimbursement factor • Health status factor • Trend factor • Other factors
Step 4:	Retention load (multiply or add) • Administrative expenses • Contingency reserves • Coordination of benefits savings • Profit
Step 5:	Convert the member rate to a contract rate

group. Medicare and Medicaid rates are nearly always stated on a per member (*ie*, individual) basis.

Data Sources

The best data source for any health plan is its own experience because it implicitly recognizes all of the plan-specific characteristics. However, some carriers have trouble collecting their experience in the necessary format. Alternatively, some carriers have recently been established or are expanding into new markets or products. As a result, many health plans look to published data sources or actuarial consulting firms to provide initial medical cost targets, calibrated to be relevant to the situation. The carrier can substitute experience for the estimates with data from their own health plan over time as it becomes available.

Consumer-driven health plans (CDHPs; see Chapters 2 and 20), which are high-deductible health plans using Health Reimbursement Arrangements (HRA), or Health Savings Accounts (HSA), are an example of when historical experience data may not be directly usable for predicting future experience. This new type of coverage pairs a high-deductible health plan with a consumer spending account that can be used to offset member cost sharing or allowed to accumulate over time. Given the uncertainty of consumer behavior with the high-deductible plan and the associated account, a health plan would not want to use traditional plan experience (*ie,* health maintenance organization [HMO] and preferred provider organization [PPO] products without the use of HRA or HSA accounts) to predict utilization behavior under consumer-driven plans.

Managing the Business

The rate formula should be routinely updated. Most health plans review and update the formula at least once per year, with some carriers doing quarterly updates. Updates are done using analyses and data accumulated in various management reports. The management reports might include the following information:

- Financial gain/loss summaries by:
  - Total block of business
  - Line of business (commercial versus Medicare)
  - Product line (HMO versus PPO, traditional versus CDHP)
  - Group size (large group versus small group)
  - Type of business (new versus renewal)
  - Type of medical service (hospital inpatient, hospital outpatient, etc.)
  - Calendar year or quarter
  - Each group individually (usually large group)

- Incurred claim costs by:
  - Total block of business
  - Line of business (commercial versus Medicare)
  - Product line (HMO versus PPO, traditional versus CDHP)
  - Group size (large group versus small group)
  - Type of business (new versus renewal)
  - Funding arrangement (fully insured versus self-insured)
  - Geographical area
  - Policy duration of the individual/small group (not usually applicable to large groups)

- Group-specific reports (applies mostly to large groups), including the following:
  - Earned premium
  - Paid claims
  - Medical loss ratio
  - Large claim information
  - Benefit plan changes
  - Subscriber and membership counts by contract type

- A development of IBNR claims. This report should contain paid claim information, a lag development of incurred claims, a projection development of incurred claims, paid claim lags to monitor the speed of claim processing, and medical cost trends, along with monthly, quarterly, and annual incurred claim estimates. Carriers might produce IBNR reports by:

- ○ Line of business (commercial versus Medicare)
- ○ Product line (HMO versus PPO, traditional versus CDHP)
- ○ Type of medical service (hospital inpatient, hospital outpatient, etc.)

- • Membership by:
  - ○ Line of business (commercial versus Medicare)
  - ○ Product line (HMO versus PPO, traditional versus CDHP)
  - ○ Group size (large group versus small group)
  - ○ Type of business (new versus renewal)
  - ○ Contract tier
  - ○ Geographical area
  - ○ Age and gender

These reports can assist the health plan in analyzing experience and updating the rate formula on a consistent basis.

Most carriers also produce traditional accounting reports such as the income statement, balance sheet, and cash flow statement. These reports help measure health plan success in reaching its financial goals. One measure might be return on equity, a popular and universal measure of the value creation of a business. Return on equity is universal because it enables a business to compare its value to other types of investments, such as investing the carrier's surplus in a money market account, bonds, or the stock market. It is also easily comparable across different companies and industries. Other carriers instead target a percentage of premium and, as a result, might find it difficult measuring the performance of the business versus noninsurance-oriented businesses. Accounting reports are discussed in Chapter 24.

CONCLUSION

The underwriting and rating functions seek to achieve an optimal balance between adequate, competitive, and equitable rates. Underwriting involves gathering information to analyze applicants' risk characteristics. Rating includes using the information gathered through underwriting and management reports to develop a final rate.

Suggested Reading

O'Grady FT. *Individual Health Insurance.* Schaumberg, IL: Society of Actuaries, 1988.

Bluhm WF. *Group Insurance,* 4th ed. Winstead, CT: Actex Publications, 2003.

Pyenson BS. *Managing Risk: A Leader's Guide to Creating a Successful Managed Care Provider Organization.* Atlanta, GA: AHA Press, 1998.

Sutton HL, Sorbo AJ. *Actuarial Issues in the Fee-For-Service/Prepaid Medical Group,* 2nd ed. Englewood, CO: Medical Group Management Association, 1993.

SPECIAL MARKET SEGMENTS

"*We're One*
But we're not the same."

—Bono [1991]

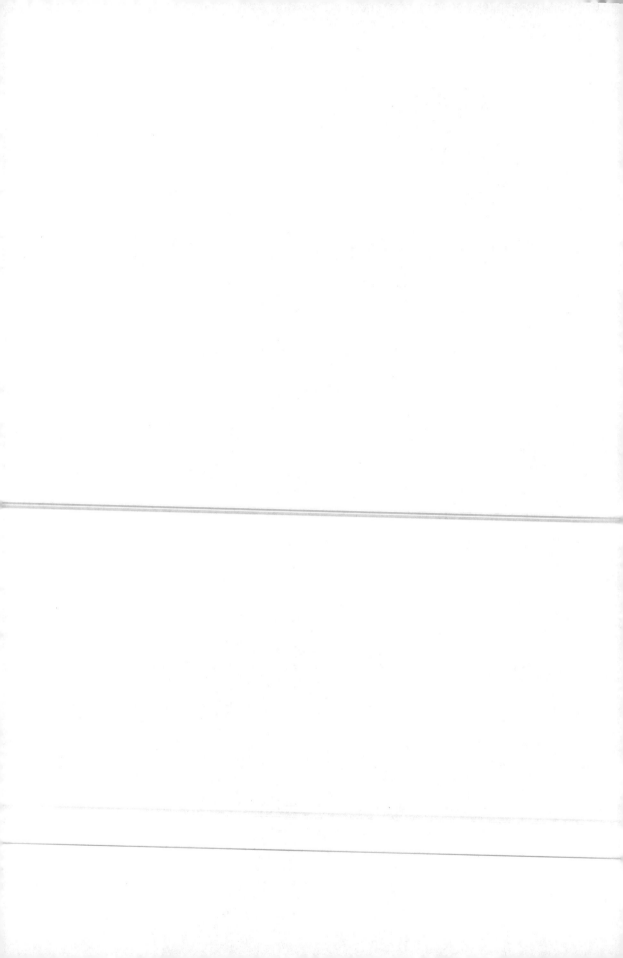

26

HEALTH PLANS AND MEDICARE

Carlos J. Zarabozo and Sidney J. Lindenberg

Study Objectives

- Understand recent changes in the Medicare Modernization Act affecting Medicare managed care contracting and the significance of those changes.
- Understand the different types of Medicare D and Medicare Advantage programs.
- Understand what kinds of organizations can have Medicare Advantage contracts.
- Understand what the ongoing contract requirements are for organizations that have entered into contracts.
- Understand the factors the government uses in determining payments to Medicare Advantage organizations.
- Understand the rights and responsibilities of Medicare enrollees of health plans.
- Understand some of the issues related to how an organization administers a Medicare contract.

Discussion Topics

1. Discuss state licensure requirements that an organization must comply with to become a Medicare Advantage plan, any exceptions to the state licensure requirement, and any cases in which special consideration is given to particular types of entities.
2. Discuss the different types of Medicare Advantage plans, the key differences between them, and why such differences exist.
3. Discuss the impact of the new Medicare D drug benefit and how that benefit affects the market.

4. Discuss the kinds of consumer rights and protections available to enrollees, or prospective enrollees, of Medicare Advantage plans.
5. Discuss how the new reimbursement methodology for payments to Medicare Advantage plans will be applied. How does this differ from prior methodologies?

INTRODUCTION

On the morning of November 22, 2003, the House of Representatives passed a historic bill reforming the Medicare system. This event was historic in many ways. The hour of the morning happened to be 6:00 am or so, with passage of the bill coming after the voting on the floor was left open for a historic record of nearly 3 hours. Also historic was the content of the legislation that the House passed, which the Senate eventually passed and the president signed. The *Medicare Prescription Drug Improvement and Modernization Act of 2003* was heralded as the most significant reform of Medicare in the history of the program because it added drug coverage as a Medicare benefit, nearly 40 years after the beginning of Medicare. Although the headlines of the day were about the drug benefit, the bill that came to be known as the *Medicare Modernization Act* (MMA) also significantly changed the Medicare provisions dealing with private health plans. This chapter provides a summary of Medicare contracting provisions for managed care plans, and other types of plans, as modified by the MMA.

The chapter discusses Medicare private plan contracting from a primarily "operational" viewpoint. After the introductory sections, the sections of the chapter are ordered in a way that roughly matches the decision process of a person or organization deciding whether to enter into a Medicare contract. The chapter explains what kind of organization may enter into a risk contract, how the contractor is paid and what limits there are on the sources and uses of revenue under the contract, what the contractor is required to do, how marketing and information dissemination occurs, how enrollment occurs, and what rights beneficiaries and providers have.

BACKGROUND

With regard to the traditional Medicare program of Part A (hospital) and Part B (medical) benefits (as distinguished from the new drug benefit, Part D, that is described in the next section), one objective of the MMA was to extend the reach of private health plans in Medicare.* This was not a new goal for Congress, which had already tried a number of mechanisms to have health plans made available to more Medicare beneficiaries, and particularly to address the lack of such plans in rural areas, where nearly a quarter of Medicare's 42 million beneficiaries reside. For example, the Balanced Budget Act of 1997 (BBA) introduced a payment "floor" for rural areas, which in some counties doubled the payment rates for Medicare plans operating in those counties. Although the payment floor did not bring more coordinated care plans such as health maintenance organizations (HMOs) and preferred provider organizations (PPOs) to rural areas, the provision did lead to the proliferation of a particular type of plan newly authorized in the BBA, "private fee-for-service" (PFFS) plans (described later in this chapter).

Under the MMA, what had been the Medicare+Choice program became the Medicare Advantage (MA) program. To summarize briefly and succinctly what the MMA did with respect to health plans: it provided more money for health plans in a variety of ways. In addition, the MMA introduced a new approach to plan contracting through the

---

*In the case of the drug benefit, it is administered separately from the traditional Medicare program, and the benefit is available only through private plans, including through Medicare Advantage plans.

regional plan option. The Centers for Medicare and Medicaid Services (CMS), part of the federal Department of Health and Human Services (DHHS), has divided the United States into 26 regions. A regional plan agrees to offer PPO coverage throughout one or more of these regions. In addition to requiring that regional plans be set up as preferred provider organizations offered in every county of a region, payment rules and certain contracting provisions are different for regional plans.

In 2006, 36 states had a regional plan available. Although it was intended that regional plans would be the key to extending access to private plans throughout the country, 88% of Medicare beneficiaries have access to regional plans. This compares to the 80% of beneficiaries who have access to a "local" (nonregional) HMO or PPO (a historic—to use the word *historic* one last time—high in Medicare, exceeding the previous high of 74% in 1998), and the 99% of enrollees who have access to either a local coordinated care plan (HMO or PPO) or a PFFS plan (all of which are defined as local plans even though they may cover an entire region).[1] Thus, the MMA has been successful—one might say wildly successful—in extending the availability of private plans in Medicare.

The MMA created a second type of new MA plan—the Special Needs Plan (SNP). This type of plan may exclusively enroll, or enroll a disproportionate percentage of, special needs Medicare beneficiaries. Individuals with special needs include beneficiaries entitled to both Medicare and Medicaid ("dual eligibles" or "duals"), institutionalized beneficiaries, and individuals with severe or disabling chronic conditions.

THE MEDICARE PART D DRUG BENEFIT IN MEDICARE ADVANTAGE

All Medicare Advantage organizations other than PFFS plans and medical savings account (MSA) plans (both PFFS and MSA plans are described later in this chapter) are required to offer a plan with Medicare Part D drug coverage throughout their service area.

Organizations are free to offer plans that do not include drug coverage for beneficiaries electing to decline drug coverage. PFFS plans can include Part D drug coverage, but MSA plans are not permitted to include Part D coverage as part of the plan.

Overall Design and Financing of the Drug Benefit Program

As noted at the beginning of this chapter, 40 years after its inception, the Medicare program added drug coverage as a voluntary benefit to be administered, it was hoped (and the hope came to fruition), by private entities. The private entities are the "stand-alone" prescription drug plans (PDPs) and Medicare Advantage Prescription Drug (MA-PD) plans.* The benefit is primarily paid for by Federal subsidies, with a portion paid by beneficiaries in the form of premiums and cost sharing, and a portion financed by plans that are partly at risk for the provision of the benefit. Access standards apply to ensure that beneficiaries have convenient access to pharmacies.

A major feature of the benefit is that the drug benefit for dual-eligible (Medicare/Medicaid) beneficiaries (also described later in this chapter) that was previously a Medicaid benefit became a federal benefit, with the states reimbursing the federal government for the cost of the benefit through a mechanism referred to as the "clawback." Some drugs not covered under Part D continue to be provided through state programs. The migration to Part D of this population meant that there was a segment of the population that would be automatically enrolled in the otherwise voluntary Part D program. As explained later, this sometimes resulted in the assignment of this population into particular plans (or their being covered through MA

---

*Residents of long-term care (LTC) facilities obtain drug benefits from the pharmacy selected by the facility. There is a special enrollment period for people who enter, reside in, or leave an LTC facility.

if they were MA enrollees at the time of conversion from the state program to Part D).

Another feature of the program is that, in the interest of maintaining drug coverage for Medicare-eligible retirees through employers and unions—a major source of drug coverage for Medicare beneficiaries before the MMA—employers and unions could elect to continue to provide drug coverage, and they would receive a federal subsidy offsetting a portion of the cost.

There are four sources of federal payment to Part D plans for the benefit: (1) the direct subsidy (*ie*, the subsidization of beneficiary premiums) for all beneficiaries; (2) the low-income subsidy for Medicare/Medicaid dual-eligible beneficiaries and other low-income beneficiaries who apply for assistance under Part D rules (subsidizing premiums and cost sharing, fully or partly); (3) the reinsurance subsidy, whereby Medicare is responsible for the majority of costs at the catastrophic level of coverage; and (4) risk corridor payments, whereby risk is shared with plans around target amounts.

The Benefit Design

The statute specifies the Medicare drug benefit design, but variations in the design are permitted if they are actuarially equivalent to the basic benefit (as specified in law and regulations) or if there is an enhancement of the benefit (for which beneficiaries will pay an additional premium). The benefit is subsidized for all Medicare beneficiaries (as is Medicare Part B coverage), and low-income beneficiaries can receive additional subsidies for premiums and cost sharing.

The benefit is voluntary for beneficiaries, but delayed enrollment in Part D subjects a beneficiary to a premium penalty that the person pays throughout the entire coverage period after late enrollment. A penalty does not apply, however, if the person is not enrolling in Part D because he or she has "creditable coverage," which is drug coverage from another source that is as good as or better

than Part D coverage. Many retirees have such coverage through their former employer and can retain the coverage. If the person loses the coverage—the employer discontinues the coverage—the individual is given the opportunity to enroll in Part D without a premium penalty.

The basic Part D benefit structure (referred to as the "defined standard" benefit) is somewhat complicated and is characterized by a "donut hole," or coverage gap, during which an enrollee who has no low-income subsidy is responsible for 100% of the cost of drugs (albeit at the discounted rate that his or her plan offers). Figure 26-1 is the graphic display that CMS uses to illustrate the defined standard drug benefit (as of 2006).

In the standard benefit for 2006, there was a $250 deductible, after which a beneficiary paid co-insurance of 25% until reaching $2,250 (the "initial coverage limit") in total drug expenditures (including the deductible). On reaching that point—the donut hole—the beneficiary pays 100% of the cost of drugs, as noted, until total expenditures reach $5,100 (representing $3,600 in true out-of-pocket costs for the beneficiary). At that point, catastrophic coverage begins. Under the standard benefit in 2006, catastrophic coverage had the beneficiary paying a 5% co-insurance (unless the person is a low-income beneficiary entitled to a subsidy that would pick up the co-insurance). The dollar amounts of the deductible, initial coverage limits, and catastrophic threshold will change from year to year; this explanation and Figure 26-1 use the 2006 dollar amounts.

Plans have the option of offering a benefit package that is different from the basic benefit. In place of the defined standard benefit, a plan may offer "actuarially equivalent standard coverage," whereby the cost sharing is actuarially equivalent to the 25% level after the initial coverage limit and the 5% level after the catastrophic limit. For example, plans can use this approach to use copayments in lieu of cost sharing or to eliminate cost sharing for generic drugs. The other type of op-

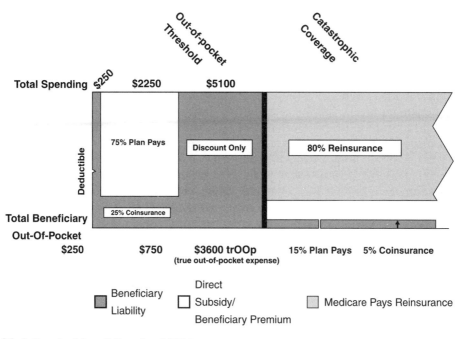

Figure 26–1 Standard Part D Benefit of 2006

Source: CMS.

tion that a plan can offer is an enhanced benefit that, for example, can fill in the deductible and/or the donut hole, but beneficiaries would pay the cost of such coverage through a plan premium, though an MA plan can also use rebate dollars (described later in this chapter) to buy down the Part D premium for any of the Part D options.

In designing a drug benefit, PDPs and MA-PDs may have a formulary, but CMS ensures that there is adequate coverage within classes of drugs and that the formularies used by plans do not discourage enrollment among certain groups of people.* CMS approves formularies in advance of the bidding process for plans to complete their bids. There is also an exception process for bene-

_____

*Formulary review requirements are posted on the CMS Web site at http://www.cms.hhs.gov/ PrescriptionDrugCovContra/03_RxContracting_Fo rmularyGuidance.asp#TopOfPage. This Web address is current at the time of publication, but may be subject to change.

ficiaries to obtain drugs not on a plan's formulary or to obtain the drugs at a lower cost-sharing level.

Payment and Bidding for Part D

Figure 26-1 also illustrates the points at which the government subsidizes the costs, or shares in the cost of the coverage, for all beneficiaries. The government shares risk with health plans for the provision of the Part D benefit after beneficiaries reach the catastrophic level of coverage. (As of 2006, there is also a demonstration project in which plans accept capitation payments in lieu of the reinsurance subsidy.)

The Part D bid of an MA organization is separate from the bid for Medicare A/B benefits, though as noted, A/B rebate dollars can be used to reduce the Part D premium of an MA-PD plan. The bidding process for Medicare A/B benefits by MA plans, including the issue of rebates, is described later in this chapter.

The Part D bid is based on the standard benefit (even for a plan offering an enhanced benefit). The standard benefit excludes beneficiary cost sharing, reinsurance, and low-income cost-sharing subsidies. For a plan offering an enhanced benefit, to arrive at a standard benefit bid the cost associated with induced utilization because of lowered cost sharing must be excluded. This exclusion from the bid is in addition to excluding the cost to the plan of drugs that are not covered in the standard benefit—such as when the enhancement of the plan consists of doing away with the deductible—and excluding as a cost the filling in of cost sharing that would otherwise be the enrollee's responsibility in a standard benefit. The bids are based on the plan's projected enrollment, adjusted by the expected risk factors of the population, to arrive at a standardized bid. CMS has developed risk factors for Part D separate from those for the MA A/B bidding and payment process.

The Part D bids of MA-PD plans and those of standalone PDPs are aggregated and weighted by enrollment in the prior year to arrive at a "national average monthly bid amount."* This bid amount is used to determine the basic beneficiary premium, taking into account the government's direct subsidy of the Part D benefit. The basic beneficiary premium is 25.5% of the national average bid amount (ie, about three-fourths of the premium is subsidized), less projected reinsurance payments the government will make.

The premium at the individual plan level for a PDP or an MA-PD is the basic beneficiary premium, adjusted by the difference between (1) the national average bid amount across all plans and (2) the plan's standardized bid (standardized to a person with average risk, or a risk score of 1.0). That is, there are higher premiums for plans bidding over the national average monthly bid, which the

beneficiary would pay. MA-PD plans may lower the premium (including to zero), using rebate dollars from the Medicare A/B bid, as previously mentioned. As noted earlier, a beneficiary may also be required to pay an additional premium penalty if he or she delayed enrollment in Part D, unless the delay was caused by the loss of creditable coverage benefits from another source.

Once an individual reaches the out-of-pocket threshold (the catastrophic limit—$3,600 in true out-of-pocket [trOOp] in 2006), Medicare will reimburse 80% of allowable individual costs under the reinsurance provisions of the law.* Organizations are permitted to obtain commercial reinsurance for the risk they assume in covering Part D drugs. Plans will receive interim payments for reinsurance, based on their bids, and there is a reconciliation performed after the end of the year.

Risk Corridor Payments and Targets

The government's risk sharing with plans occurs in corridors surrounding a target amount. The target amount is computed as the total direct government subsidy, plus beneficiary premiums, less administrative costs. The administrative costs are based on the percentage administration included in the plan bid. Risk corridor payment adjustments are made on allowed amounts actually incurred by the plan above or below the target amount.

Risk corridor payment adjustments are based on allowed amounts actually incurred by the plan above or below the target. The

---

*Not included are the bids of MA private fee-for-service plans or special needs plans, or the bids of cost-reimbursed plans.

*There are certain rules about what can or cannot be counted as a beneficiary "true" out-of-pocket (OOP) cost. For example, most third-party payments cannot count as a beneficiary out-of-pocket expense. An important point is that a beneficiary's out-of-pocket expenses for drugs that are not on his or her plan's formulary do not count toward true out-of-pocket costs in determining whether the beneficiary has reached the out-of-pocket limit.

adjusted allowable risk corridor costs are composed of (1) the covered Part D drug costs as determined by claims—ingredient cost, dispensing fee, and any sales tax—less (2) cost sharing, low-income subsidy payments, the drug costs and cost sharing of enhanced benefits, the induced utilization of an enhanced benefit, and any rebate dollars applicable to Part D drugs.

For 2006 and 2007, it is anticipated that plans would be at full risk for adjusted allowable risk corridor costs within 2.5% above or below the target. Plans with adjusted allowable costs above the "first threshold" limit of 102.5% of the target, up to the "second threshold" limit of 105% of the target, would be at risk for 25% of those costs. Above 105% of the target, plans would be at risk for 20% of the costs. If plans have savings in relation to the target, they are shared with the government, with plans retaining 25% of the savings and the remainder going to the government.

From 2008 to 2011, the level of risk assumed by plans increases. Plans are at full risk for allowable costs that are 5% above or below the target. Plans would have 50% risk between the first (105% of the target) and second (110% of the target) threshold levels. After the 110% level, plans would be at risk for 20% of the costs. For allowable costs below the target, plans would retain 50% of the savings between 95% and 90% of the target, and 20% of the savings below 90% of the target.

After 2011, the threshold amounts would be determined in such a way as to produce incentives for market entry. However, the first threshold risk percentage has to be 5% or more, and the second threshold percentage has to be 10% or more of the target amount.

Low-Income Subsidy Provisions

Low-income individuals are given financial assistance for their cost sharing and premiums for the Part D benefit. For those with the highest level of subsidy, the full-benefit dual eligibles with Medicaid coverage whose incomes are at or below 100% of the federal poverty level, their only cost-sharing obligation is a nominal copayment ($1 for a generic drug or preferred multiple source, and $3 for any other drug) until the catastrophic limit is reached (the equivalent of $3,600 in out-of-pocket expenses, if the individual had not had a low-income subsidy). For full-benefit duals with income above 100% but below 135% of the federal poverty level who meet an assets test, there is also only nominal cost sharing ($2/$5). For beneficiaries with income below 150% of the federal poverty level and limited resources who apply for assistance, there is premium assistance based on a sliding scale and partial assistance with cost sharing. CMS notifies the plan of a member's eligibility for low-income subsidization.

For a full-benefit dual to have his or her entire Part D premium subsidized, the person must be enrolled in a plan with a premium at or below a certain level in a given region. That is, not all plans would be available to low-income individuals with the premium fully subsidized. The premium subsidy amount for a PDP region is the greater of (1) the low-income benchmark premium (essentially the enrollment-weighted average of all PDP premiums for basic drug coverage [the standard benefit] and the MA-PD drug premiums) or (2) the lowest monthly premium for a plan that offers basic prescription drug coverage. A person may enroll in a higher-cost plan by paying the difference between the computed premium subsidy amount and the actual premium.

BASIC REQUIREMENTS FOR ANY ORGANIZATION TO BE ELIGIBLE FOR A MEDICARE RISK CONTRACT

State Licensure

The most basic requirement for an organization to obtain a Medicare contract is that the organization must be licensed by the appropriate state regulatory authority as a risk-bearing entity under a scope of licensure that permits the organization to assume risk for the comprehensive set of benefits that compose Medicare Parts A and B (as well as Part D). For all organizations, CMS requires that the state provide a certification that the nature of the licensure or authority to offer risk products is, in the opinion of the state, consistent with the requirements for assumption of risk as an MA organization.

Under CMS's regulatory interpretation of the statute, an entity need not be formally licensed by the state regulatory body overseeing HMOs and health insurers, as long as that regulatory body finds the legal status and financial status of the organization to be sufficient to manage the risk entailed by a Medicare risk contract. For example, an organization operating in a state as a "state-defined" Medicaid HMO that was not licensed by the insurance department (as the state regulatory body licensing HMOs in the particular state), but that was instead authorized to operate as a Medicaid plan by the state health department, could have an MA contract as long as the insurance department consented—agreeing, for example, that the state health department's standards for Medicaid contracts were sufficient for the purposes of MA contracting.

For regional plans (regional PPOs) only, the state licensure requirement can be temporarily waived if an organization is licensed in at least one of the states of the CMS-designated region and the organization has applied for licensure in the other state(s) in the region. State licensure requirements and regulatory oversight are discussed further in Chapter 33.

Minimum Enrollment

An organization seeking a Medicare Advantage contract must meet a minimum enrollment requirement of 5,000 "individuals . . . who are receiving health benefits through the organization," or 1,500 such individuals if the organization primarily serves rural areas. However, the requirement may be waived during the first three Medicare contract years.

TYPES OF MEDICARE PLANS

As noted earlier, the MMA introduced the regional plan concept, setting up an important distinction between regional plans (all of which are PPOs serving an entire region) and all other plans—referred to as "local" plans. Even though a local PPO may cover every county in one of the 26 MA regions, such a local plan is not considered a regional plan unless it chooses that designation and adheres to the rules that apply to regional plans.

The Medicare law also makes a distinction between coordinated care plans and other plans. Coordinated care plans include HMOs, PPOs (both regional and local), provider-sponsored organizations that operate like HMOs, and HMOs with point-of-service products. Other types of MA plans include PFFS plans and Medicare medical savings account (MSA) plans. One basis of the difference between the two broad categories is that coordinated care plans can require enrollees to use a network of providers for coverage of Medicare services. Other than in an emergency, a coordinated care plan has no obligation to cover the cost of care if a nonnetwork provider is used, even if the care would have been covered in fee-for-service Medicare. Private fee-for-service plans and MSA plans are not network plans in the sense of being able to limit coverage to a network. Enrollees of such plans have the right to expect the plan to cover the cost of care at any provider willing to accept the individual as a patient, consistent with the rules of the plan regarding coverage (eg, an MSA plan has no coverage before a deductible is met).

There are other differences between the two major categories—coordinated care plans and others—in terms of the statutory provisions that apply. With respect to bidding, while coordinated care plans are subject to a review of actuarial soundness and acceptability of the bids, and there can be negotiation over the bid, the bids of MSA plans and private fee-for-service plans are not subject to that level of review or negotiation.

Another difference between the two major categories is that MSA plans and private fee-for-service plans are not subject to the quality improvement requirements applied to coordinated care plans.

On the assumption that most readers are familiar with the HMO model and HMOs with point-of-service products,* this section describes the features of each of the other types of MA contracting organizations recognized under Medicare law.

Plan versus Organization

Because of certain statutory provisions, CMS makes a distinction between an organization holding an MA contract and the "plans" that organization offers. One organization may offer multiple plans in a given service area or multiple areas (including noncontiguous areas), as long as each plan meets applicable MA standards. The plans may differ slightly (*eg*, point-of-service benefits are or are not included) or they may be significantly different: the same organization offers a PFFS plan and a traditional HMO option. As will be discussed, each plan must have a uniform premium and benefit offering available to all residents of the service area of the plan (except that—to further confuse matters—there can also be "segments" of plans with different premiums). Where one organization has multiple plans, CMS will treat plans as severable if, for example, the need arises to impose a corrective action on a given plan or if a termination or nonrenewal of a particular plan of the organization is deemed appropriate. With regard to the bidding process that is explained later, there is a separate bid required for each plan.

Preferred Provider Organizations and Regional Plans

The Medicare law defines a preferred provider organization, but the definition is provided

only in connection with quality improvement requirements that may or may not apply to the plan. According to the law, a PPO is a "plan that . . . has a network of providers that have agreed to a contractually specified reimbursement for covered benefits with the organization offering the plan; . . . provides for reimbursement for all covered benefits regardless of whether such benefits are provided within such network of providers; and . . . is offered by an organization that is not licensed or organized under state law as a health maintenance organization." Except perhaps for the very last provision, the definition seems to be consistent with most people's opinion of what a PPO is. The definition is placed in the statutory section dealing with the reporting of quality indicators and states that local PPOs will provide data for contracted providers only (and that regional PPOs will have their own rules on quality reporting, established by CMS, but which would not exceed the requirements imposed on local PPOs).

One of the distinctions between regional plans (all of which, again, are PPOs) and local PPOs is that the law specifies that regional plans that wish to impose a deductible must have a single deductible for Part A and Part B services (unlike fee-for-service Medicare). The single deductible may be different for in-network and nonnetwork services, and it may be waived for preventive services or other services. The regional plan is required to have a catastrophic limit on out-of-pocket expenditures for in-network items and services that are Medicare-covered benefits, and a limit for total Medicare-covered expenditures. Although regional PPOs are required to have a network of providers, the access standard can be met by paying for nonnetwork services at Medicare fee-for-service rates. There is also a provision whereby the Medicare program will make payments to an "essential provider," defined as a hospital that is necessary to include in the network but which, after a good faith effort on the part of the plan, does not agree to a contract with

---

*See Chapter 2 for descriptions of these types of models.

payment at Medicare rates. For such cases, Congress has authorized funding of $25 billion to provide additional Medicare payments to an "essential" hospital to have services provided to regional MA plan enrollees.

Private Fee-for-Service Plans

An organization may choose to enter into a contract with CMS to offer a private insurance plan that reimburses providers on a fee-for-service basis and does not limit enrollees to the use of network providers: an MA PFFS plan. As an enrollee of an MA PFFS plan, a Medicare beneficiary may use any Medicare-participating provider who agrees to provide services to the beneficiary, and the organization sponsoring the PFFS plan (*eg*, a private insurer) will make payment for covered services in a manner similar to a traditional indemnity plan operating in the private marketplace. A PFFS plan may not pay its providers on other than a fee-for-service basis, and it may not place providers at financial risk for the utilization of services.

The PFFS plan may have a network of providers who agree to the terms of the plan, but the law also provides for "deemed" participating providers. A provider is deemed to be a participating provider if he or she (or the entity) is aware of the beneficiary's enrollment in the PFFS plan and the provider is aware of, or has been given a reasonable opportunity to be made aware of, the terms and conditions of payment under the plan "in a manner reasonably designed to effect informed agreement" to participate, as stated in the regulations. A noncontracting provider may receive, in total payments (from the PFFS plan and from enrollee cost sharing), only an amount equal to what would have been paid in total under original Medicare. Contracting and deemed providers may also receive additional payments from the enrollee ("balance billing") up to 15% of the PFFS plan payment amount. The PFFS organization is charged with ensuring that providers adhere to the limits on permissible

balance billed amounts; failure to monitor adherence to the requirement can result in CMS's decision not to renew the organization's contract. Enrollees may incur additional liability if the PFFS retrospectively denies coverage (as not Medicare-covered or for non-Medicare-covered benefits not covered under the plan).

As noted in the Conference Report accompanying the BBA of 1997, which introduced PFFS plans, the PFFS option is the first Medicare option that had the structure of a defined contribution. That is, the government contribution toward the cost of the option is limited to the MA payment amount, but there are no limits on what the organization may charge as a member premium for the benefit package. This is now the case for all plans under the MMA, as explained in the section on bidding.

Medical Savings Account Plans

The MA MSA option is a medical savings account combined with a high-deductible plan that is responsible for paying 100% of the cost of covered care after a deductible is met. A portion of the capitation that would otherwise be paid to the MA organization is deposited in an account that the beneficiary can use, on a tax-preferred basis, to finance the cost of medical care, including medical care that is not covered by Medicare. The Medicare payment to the enrollee's account is made at the beginning of the year for use during the year or in subsequent years (*ie*, unused funds roll over). The Medicare contribution may also be used to finance the cost of items or services that the Internal Revenue Service does not define as qualified medical expenses, and in such a case the withdrawal from the account would be taxable. After an enrollee meets the deductible of the high-deductible plan, the MA MSA plan covers 100% of the cost of Medicare-covered services (up to Medicare payment limits). There is no member premium for an MA MSA plan (unless the plan's equivalent of a bid exceeds the benchmark, in which case there is no enrollee deposit possible), and only Medicare services may be included in the plan, though additional benefits can be offered through an optional supplemental package.

The rationale for MSA plans, similar to the rationale discussed in Chapters 1, 2, and 20 regarding consumer-directed health plans (CDHPs), is that they eliminate "first dollar" coverage by a third party and thereby make individuals more prudent purchasers of health care. That is, until the deductible is met, a Medicare beneficiary uses his or her own money—including any money available from the MSA account—to pay for the cost of care. The actual expenses a person must incur out-of-pocket will vary with his or her health care needs, by the size of the deductible (no minimum has been established, but the maximum is $9,500 per year in 2007), and by the level of contribution available from Medicare. In some cases, it may take several years to accumulate a Medicare contribution equal to the deductible.

On choosing this option, a Medicare beneficiary must remain enrolled in the MA MSA plan for at least 1 year (or until the next MA annual coordinated election period if coverage began during a person's initial period of Medicare eligibility during the calendar year). Certain beneficiaries are not eligible to enroll in the MSA option: those on Medicaid and individuals obtaining health care coverage through certain federal programs such as the Federal Employees Health Benefits Program. A person must also reside in the United States at least half the year to be eligible to enroll.

In July 2006, CMS announced the availability of an MSA demonstration project whereby the benefit package would be changed to more closely resemble Health Savings Accounts (HSAs—a type of CDHP introduced by the MMA for the non-Medicare market). In the demonstration, there is a specified minimum deductible ($2,000 in 2007) and a maximum deductible ($9,500, as under the statute for nondemonstration plans), and a plan can provide coverage for preventive services prior to a person's meeting the deductible (as in the case of an HSA). The demonstration also permits plans to impose cost sharing between the deductible and the out-of-pocket limit, and to use differential cost sharing depending on whether the enrollee uses contracted or noncontracted providers. Under the demonstration, the MSA plan can include only service areas comprising an entire state, whereas nondemonstration MSAs can choose in which counties to operate without covering an entire state.

Service Areas and Special Rules for Employer Group Plans

In the early history of the Medicare HMO program, an organization's Medicare service area was required to match its commercial service area, although one would be hard put to find specific statutory language expressing such a requirement. It was assumed that an organization would merely add a Medicare line of business to its products, with much of the remaining structure untouched (service area, provider network, and so forth).

Over time, CMS changed its policy and permitted organizations to operate in a smaller area for Medicare, as long as "county integrity" was maintained. That is, an organization could choose which counties within its authorized service area it wanted to include in the Medicare contract, but a geographical unit smaller than a county could not be designated as the Medicare service area for a given county unless the organization served only that portion of the county in its other lines of business. CMS approved Medicare service area designations requested by applicants on the basis of network adequacy (the ability to provide the full range of services under the contract in the service area), using standards to prevent discrimination or other "gaming" through service area configurations. This is essentially the current policy. However, there is a requirement that a plan's premium and benefits be uniform throughout the service area (or in each "segment" of the plan's service area), which often dictates how an organization wishes to designate the service areas of its plans.

With regard to employer group offerings (discussed later), a health plan may elect to serve a particular county or set of counties only for employer group accounts. That is, although there is an open enrollment requirement for MA plans, a health plan can limit enrollment in a county to only those Medicare beneficiaries enrolling in a plan sponsored by an employer or union for its Medicare retirees.

Other Special Rules for Employer Group Retirees

Although CMS has historically offered health plans wide latitude in their arrangements with employers and unions that offer Medicare coverage to their retirees, the MMA went further by including a very broad waiver provision that encourages the offering of employer- or union-sponsored plans, including the option of having employers or unions directly contract with CMS as Medicare Advantage plans (as opposed to the indirect method of having the employer or union offer benefits through a licensed HMO or other type of health plan operating in the marketplace). To facilitate retiree coverage, among the kinds of waivers CMS has allowed recently are waivers allowing plans to enroll beneficiaries from outside the plan's service area, waivers pertaining to the publication of evidences of coverage and marketing material, and a waiver allowing plans to use Employee Retirement Income Security Act (ERISA) appeals provisions rather than Medicare appeals provisions.[2]

PAYMENT

Payment to plans is based on payment rates established by law and a comparison of these payment rates to plan bids under what is referred to as a competitive bidding system. In many respects the bidding system is similar to the earlier system of plans filing adjusted community rate proposals to determine premiums and benefit packages.

Local MA Plans

The Bid

The bid of a local MA plan for coverage of Medicare A and B services is compared to a benchmark to determine whether there is a premium for Medicare-covered services and to determine the level of savings a plan projects if the plan believes that it can provide the Medicare package for less than the benchmark. For a plan operating in a single county, the benchmark is the county MA payment rate that is published in advance of the calendar year.

To explain the bidding process using the simplest of examples—a one-county plan—the plan would submit a bid for Medicare A and B services for its expected enrollment. That is, the plan would predict the demographic and health status makeup of its expected enrollment using the demographic and health status adjustment factors that form the basis of Medicare payments at the level of the individual enrollee. If, for example, the benchmark in a given county is $1,000, and a plan is bidding at the benchmark, but the plan expects a relatively sicker enrollment averaging 1.1 times sicker (ie, 10% sicker) than the average, the average payment will be $1,100 across the expected membership. If the plan is bidding at the benchmark, it means that the plan projects that its revenue needs would average $1,100 per person to provide the Medicare A and B benefit. If the same plan expected a healthier set of enrollees—at 0.8 the average health status (ie, 20% less sick)—the benchmark would average $800 (ie, the expected actual payments from Medicare), and, all other things being equal, the plan revenue requirements for the A and B benefits would be $800.

For a plan that is bidding above the benchmark, enrollees will have to pay a premium for the Medicare A and B benefit package. This

A/B premium is determined based on a bid-to-benchmark comparison for a beneficiary of average health status (a 1.0 beneficiary)—that is, the bid and benchmark are standardized to determine the member premium for A and B benefits. In the case of a county in which the benchmark is $1,000, where a plan expects an enrollment with exactly average health status (1.0), and the plan bids $1,100 for covering the A/B benefits, Medicare beneficiaries will have to pay $100 for A/B coverage in that plan.

To continue the example, assume instead that the plan had bid $1,210 (1.1 times $1,100) because it was expecting enrollees to be 1.1 times sicker than average. Enrollees of the 1.1 plan would still pay $100 for A/B benefits through the plan because the bid and benchmark comparison is done on a normalized basis (1.0 risk status) for determining the A/B premium. In such a case, what is referred to as the government premium adjustment would result in a payment from CMS for a "1.1 person" of the plan bid ($1,210) less the premium revenue from the enrollee ($100), or $1,110. The $1,110 payment is $10 more than the benchmark payment for a 1.1 person ($1,000 × 1.1 = $1,100). In the case of a plan expecting an enrollment that on average has a 0.8 health status (healthier than average), the beneficiary premium would still be computed on a standardized basis—that is, for a 1.0 person. If this plan's bid for the expected enrollment was $880 (which normalizes to $1,100 for a "1.0 person"), the CMS payment for a "0.8 person" would be $780, in recognition of the $100 revenue received from the member. In this case, the plan receives from CMS $20 less than what the benchmark payment would have been for a "0.8 person" ($800).

The preceding example of the government premium adjustment illustrates how each plan is made whole for its revenue needs through a combination of member premiums and payments for Medicare. The basic approach of the MMA is to pay plans their bids. Beneficiaries are expected to choose among plans based on quality and price. For plans bidding over the benchmark, the government premium adjustment serves to put all plans on an equal footing with regard to price in that both plans in these examples operate at an equal level of efficiency (or inefficiency) in their ability to provide the Medicare A and B benefits. The revenue needs for providing the benefit exceed the benchmark, but the difference in revenue needs between one plan and the other, for their expected enrollment ($1,210 versus $880), is based solely on the risk status of the expected membership, not on the greater efficiency of one plan versus the other.

This example also illustrates a difference between the MMA provisions and pre-MMA law for risk contractors (under Medicare+Choice). The ability to charge a premium for Medicare A and B services because a plan's revenue needs were greater than the Medicare payment in a given county did not exist prior to the MMA, except in the case of private fee-for-service plans. Previously, a plan had to live with the Medicare payment as the maximum revenue for the provision of A and B services, plus revenue representing Medicare's cost sharing, which was also limited to the equivalent of what the beneficiary obligation would have been in fee-for-service Medicare.

A component of expenditures for Medicare A/B services that has to come from individual Medicare beneficiaries (or is paid through supplemental coverage) is Medicare's cost sharing, such as the inpatient hospital (Part A) and Part B deductibles, and the 20% coinsurance for physician and supplier services. These expenditures are not the responsibility of the Medicare program, and therefore would not be included in determining Medicare program expenditures. For Medicare Advantage plans this means, for example, that only the Medicare program's expenditures, and not those of beneficiaries for A/B cost sharing, are included in the benchmark of a county where the benchmark was set at 100% of projected fee-for-service costs.

In implementing the Medicare Advantage program, the MMA changed the approach to computing the value of Medicare cost sharing associated with the A/B benefit package, and the law also changed provisions regarding the amount that could be collected as Medicare cost sharing. Previously, the cost sharing limit, and the assumed revenue from cost sharing a plan would have to collect from members, was—for all plans—equal to the national average actuarial value of A/B cost sharing in fee-for-service Medicare. The MMA takes a different approach. The A/B cost sharing that can be collected from enrollees is computed using a proportional method, varying by geographic area, based on categories of service and the level of cost sharing for such services in fee-for-service Medicare. For example, for skilled nursing facility care, cost sharing in a particular area represents 18.7% of Medicare's skilled nursing expenditures. This percentage is applied to a plan's bid for providing Medicare-covered skilled nursing care for purposes of determining a level of cost sharing that would be actuarially equivalent to that of Medicare (resulting in a computed level of cost sharing that might be less than Medicare fee-for-service if, for example, a plan has the same rate of utilization of skilled nursing care but the services are obtained at a discount off of Medicare rates). The sum of the actuarially equivalent level of cost sharing for each category of service, based on a plan's bid, represents the portion of plan revenue that is expected to be derived from cost sharing for Medicare-covered services.

As noted earlier, another departure from the past is that the proportional factors used to determine cost sharing and the upper limit of cost sharing—which was previously a national figure—are now determined for the specific geographic area(s) in which a plan operates, generally at the level of the Metropolitan Statistical Area (or for all nonmetropolitan areas in a given state). Note that for a regional plan, in determining whether the actuarial limit of cost sharing is exceeded, CMS considers only the catastrophic limit on out-of-pocket expenses for in-network benefits (not out-of-network benefits).

With respect to the upper limit of cost sharing for Medicare A and B benefits, the MMA changed the earlier approach in another way. Under pre-MMA rules, the total of the actuarial value of cost sharing at the point of service, plus any portion of the plan premium charged in lieu of Medicare cost sharing at the point of service, could not exceed the national actuarial value of Medicare's cost sharing (except in the case of PFFS plans). Under the MMA, cost sharing that is charged in the form of a premium rather than beneficiary out-of-pocket cost sharing at the point of service is not included when evaluating whether a plan's cost sharing for Medicare-covered services exceeds the actuarial value for the geographic area in fee-for-service Medicare.

This approach reflects the grand scheme of things in which all plans are paid their bid, and the total revenue a plan needs to provide the A and B services will be received in the form of government payments, member premiums, and cost sharing. Under pre-MMA law, only PFFS plans could charge a premium that would allow them to exceed the then-equivalent of a county benchmark plus allowable cost sharing.

Bids Below the Benchmark and the "Rebate"

The far more common case among MA plans would be a plan bidding below the benchmark because plans bidding above the benchmark may not be particularly attractive to beneficiaries. A plan bidding below the benchmark generates savings, 75% of which are given over to beneficiaries in the form of extra benefits such as cost sharing reductions in A/B, a reduced Part B or Part D (drug) premium, or added benefits not covered by Medicare (such as vision or dental care). The 75% of savings is referred to as the rebate. The 25% retention of savings by the government is a new feature under the MMA.

The amount of savings a plan generates is computed based on its expected enrollment. That is, the bid to benchmark comparison is not on a standardized basis (1.0), but rather it is based on actual expected expenditures compared to actual projected payments from Medicare. As was previously true, such savings have to be returned to beneficiaries in the form of extra benefits, as just noted, though with the advent of the Part D drug benefit, rebate dollars can be used to reduce, fully or partly, any Part D premium. Plans can "mix and match" the benefits they choose to fund with rebate dollars.

The rebate dollars are a fixed revenue stream. That is to say, once the rebate amount has been determined based on the expected enrollment in advance of the contract year, the per capita dollar amount CMS pays for funding rebates remains unchanged. If for example, a plan computed that it could provide a rebate valued at $44 a month (*eg*, it chooses to reduce each enrollee's part B premium by $44), the plan receives $44 per enrollee per month to finance rebates, regardless of the actual risk and demographic status of its enrollees. However, the bid that generated the $44 in savings, which is the basis of CMS's payment to the plan, is subject to risk adjustment (and geographic adjustment, as explained later) at the level of the individual enrollee.

Geographic Adjustment and the Bid

More common than a single-county bid is a bid that covers more than one county. In such a case, the bid takes into account the county of residence of the expected enrollees, and the benchmark is a weighted average of the benchmarks across the counties, based on the expected enrollment from each county (and the demographic and other risk characteristics of the expected enrollment). This is illustrated in Table 26-1, which shows both the effect on the bid of different benchmarks in each county as well as the expected average health status (shown as risk) of the enrollees coming from each county. Note that

the risk-adjusted bid and the risk-adjusted benchmark, as explained earlier, are used to determine the amount of the rebate.

In the example of Table 26-1, because the risk-adjusted bid is below the risk-adjusted benchmark, there is no basic premium for Medicare A and B services. If, for example, the plan described in Table 26-1 had bid $700.50 for the expected population, there would be a premium charged for Medicare services, computed on the basis of a 1.0 benchmark ($792) and a standardized (1.0) bid (equal to $809, rounded). The member basic premium for Parts A and B services would be $17 per month—which is greater than the risk-adjusted bid-to-benchmark difference would be for this over-the-benchmark plan ($700.50 less $690.50, or $10). As explained earlier, the $10 difference is smaller than the $17 premium because the plan is expecting a healthier than average population.

Other Components of the Bid; Use of Rebate Dollars

Also part of the bidding process is the presentation of a bid for non-Medicare-covered services, which can be either mandatory or optional. Optional benefits are financed entirely by member premiums and can be declined by an enrollee. Mandatory benefits cannot be declined. However, non-Medicare benefits can be financed by rebate dollars. In the example of Table 26-1, the $60 rebate can be used to finance the inclusion of $60 worth of non-Medicare benefits for each enrollee.

As noted earlier, the rebate may also be used to reduce Medicare cost sharing, the value of which is determined through the bidding process. In the example of Table 26-1, the plan may have computed Medicare cost sharing as averaging $90 per month. The plan may use its rebate dollars to buy down $60 of cost sharing and charge beneficiaries a premium of $30 per month to finance the Medicare cost-sharing obligation (in which case there could be no cost sharing for Medicare benefits at the point of service; alternatively there could be no

Table 26–1 Example of Local Medicare Advantage Plan Bidding, Below the Benchmark, Multiple Counties

	Local Monthly MA Payment (= Benchmark of One-County Plan)	Expected Number of Enrollees	Computation of Weighted-Average Benchmark If All 1.0 Risk (Each County's Portion of Total Benchmark)	Expected Risk Score of Enrollees in Each County	Revised Weighted Average Benchmark Based on Expected Risk	Projected Plan Revenue on Expected Risk and County of Origin of Enrollees = BID
Big County	$1,000	100	$455	0.9	$409.50	
Medium County	$700	70	$223	0.8	$178.40	
Small County	$500	50	$114	0.9	$102.60	
Total or Average		220	$792		$690.50	$610.50
					Savings (risk-adjusted benchmark less bid)	$80.00
					Rebate (75% of savings)	$60.00

premium, and the plan can have cost sharing charges at the point of service, the actuarial value of which averages $30 per month).

Geographic Adjustment at the Time of Payment

When it comes time to pay plans that have submitted multicounty bids, the payment is the standardized bid (or the standardized benchmark—for plans at or above the benchmark), adjusted for geography and the risk status of individual enrollees. The way in which the geographic adjustment is made is via what is called the intra–service area rate (ISAR) adjustment. This serves to "correct" erroneous projections regarding the county of origin by adjusting the bid based on the relationship among the local MA payment rates of the individual counties that are included in the bid. For example, if a plan was expecting an equal enrollment distribution from two counties, one of which had a benchmark of $1,000 and the other a benchmark of $500, and the plan bid equals the benchmark, the bid and benchmark would equal $750 for the plan for each enrollee. If the enrollee was coming from the $1,000 county, the plan-level benchmark of $750 would have an ISAR adjustment (1 1/3) to arrive at a payment of $1,000. If all enrollees came from the $1,000 county, each enrollee (with a 1.0 risk status) would have a payment of $1,000. (The ISAR adjustment does not apply to the MA MSA plans, and the adjustment can be done differently for regional plans, as explained later.)

As noted earlier, the rebate dollars remain fixed and are not subject to adjustment for geography or for risk status of the actual enrollment.

Regional Plan Benchmarks and Bids

The principle of bidding is the same for regional plans as for local plans, except that there is a different method for determining regional benchmarks, and there is an alternative approach to ISAR adjustment that plans may choose. The plan-level benchmark for regional plans (all of which are of necessity composed of multiple counties) is determined not on the basis of the expected enrollment across counties, but rather through a formula made of two components. One component includes plan bids (the competitive component), and the other component is the statutory component that sets a portion of the benchmark for a region based on the Medicare population distribution in the region. The MMA specified which percentage of the regional benchmark would be composed of each of these two components. The statutory component of the benchmark is the Medicare population-weighted average of all local MA payments in the region, times the percentage of Medicare beneficiaries throughout the nation who are *not* enrolled in MA (ie, are in fee-for-service Medicare). The plan bid component is the enrollment-weighted average of all regional plan bids, based on the plans' expected enrollment, times the percentage of Medicare beneficiaries in the nation enrolled in MA plans.

As noted earlier, the introduction of regional plans was intended to extend the availability of private plans and to make coordinated care plans available in rural areas. The MMA provided a number of advantages to regional plans. Through 2007, regional plans share risk with the government, and through 2007 regional plans, which are structured as PPOs, do not face any competition from new local Medicare Advantage PPOs.

Beginning in 2012 and thereafter, regional plans have access to a stabilization fund of $3.5 billion, plus half of the government share of savings from regional plan bids (the 25 percent of savings that is the government share of savings in the bid-to-benchmark comparison to determine rebate amounts). The stabilization fund is used to subsidize an organization operating as a national plan covering all 26 regions of the nation as a regional MA plan, entitling such an organization to a 3% increase in the benchmark for 1 year. The fund is also used to encourage new entry of regional organizations into regions where no regional plans are available, by increasing the benchmark, and to encourage the retention of a regional MA organization in a particular region if an organization is contemplating exiting the program and fewer than two MA regional plans would be available and the enrollment in regional MA plans in that region is below the national average.

A payment option available to regional plans only is the use of a plan-specified ISAR adjustment. CMS allows regional plans to specify the relative cost (revenue needs) by county for purposes of making the geographic adjustment that applies at the point of payment. That is, when the county-level payment is determined based on the residence of the individual beneficiary, whereas a local plan's bid is adjusted by the relationship between the county's MA payment rate and the rate for other counties in the service area of the plan, the regional plan can specify what the relationship is among county rates.

To repeat the example from the local plan ISAR explanation earlier in this section, if a plan was expecting an equal enrollment distribution from two counties, one of which had a benchmark (ie, local MA county payment rate) of $1,000 and the other a benchmark of $500, and the plan bid equals the benchmark, the bid and benchmark would equal $750 for the plan for each enrollee. If the enrollee was coming from the $1,000 county, the plan-level benchmark of $750 would have an ISAR adjustment ($1\frac{1}{3}$) to arrive at a payment of $1,000. A regional plan could state that the relationship in revenue needs between the two counties was something other than the $1\frac{1}{3}$ applicable to local plans that is based on the county MA payment rates.

Risk Adjustment

An important change in payment policy addresses the issue of selection bias among Medicare risk plans. Previously, the payment adjustment factors were limited to demographic factors such as age and sex. Beginning in the year 2000, on a phased-in basis, CMS payments to health plans are adjusted

at the individual level by demographic factors and health status factors of a plan's individual enrollees, based on diagnostic information submitted by Medicare Advantage plans. The factors are available at the CMS Web site. As of 2004, the demographic factors include age/sex, Medicaid, and previous entitlement to Medicare as a disabled person. There is a separate set of factors for the institutionalized, and there are adjustments made for the "working aged" (beneficiaries who have employment-based health care coverage that is primary in relation to Medicare coverage).

The health status risk adjustment system is known as the CMS-Hierarchical Condition Categories (CMS-HCC) system, which is based on diagnoses made in inpatient and outpatient settings as well as physician settings of care. Beneficiaries are classified by disease group, including a no-disease group. There are different factors within each disease group, and beneficiaries are placed in the most severe category within a specific disease group. The payment adjustment factors become additive when a person is included in more than one disease group.

The diagnostic information for the CMS-HCC adjustments is based on a minimum data set submitted by health plans at least once per quarter. The risk adjustment system is based on the factors as they apply to the entire Medicare population, and therefore Medicare fee-for-service beneficiaries are included when the factors are determined and updated. Payments to health plans are affected by a lag in updating of the factors. At the beginning of the year, payments are based on factors computed for a 12-month period that began 18 months prior to January. In the middle of the year, CMS updates the payment factors and makes retroactive adjustments to payments for the first half of the year. After the end of the contract year, there is a calculation of final reconciliation factors based on diagnostic data for the payment year in question. The final reconciliation occurs in the fall of the following year, and MA plans are allowed one year to correct initial diagnostic data for an individual. A health plan's data submissions are subject to validation and monitoring to ensure the integrity of the risk adjustment system.

There continues to be a phase-in of risk-adjusted payments in that, while (as of 2006) health plans continue to enroll healthier-than-average beneficiaries, Medicare does not fully reduce plan payments to the level that would occur if the system were fully phased in. Instead, MA plans receive a portion of the difference in payment between the fully risk-adjusted level and the level of payment based on an exclusively demographic adjustment system without health status factors. In 2007, health plans received 60% of this difference; in 2008, plans will receive 45% of the difference; in 2009, 30%; and in 2010, the last phase-in year, 15%. The difference is redistributed among health plans based on the relative health status of each plan's enrollees.

User Fees

One more factor affects payments, which is a reduction in payments on the basis of a pro rata user fee collected from all MA organizations for the cost of MA information activities described later in this chapter and for counseling and assistance programs.

Announcement of Rates; Computation of Rates

The announcement of rates for each calendar year occurs early in the year to allow time for development of the informational material necessary for the coordinated open enrollment period. At least 45 days before the announcement of rates, CMS is required to provide advance notice of proposed changes to be made in the methodology and invite comment on those changes and on the actuarial assumptions that form the basis of the following year's payment rates. By the first Monday of April, the rates for the subsequent year are published. This rate book lists, for all U.S. counties, Medicare Part A and Part B base rates for the aged and the disabled (beneficiaries younger than 65 years entitled to Med-

icare because of their disability), together with the demographic and health status adjustment factors that are to be used to adjust the base rates. State-level rates are given for individuals with end-stage renal disease, for whom payment is made on the basis of a separate risk adjustment system. Also announced in the spring are the statutory components of the benchmarks for regional plans.

The Tyranny of the Calendar

The Medicare Advantage program forces organizations to do advance planning revolving around the various deadlines that are imposed. Table 26-2, lifted wholesale from the CMS Web site, shows all the dates of relevance to an MA plan for the 2007 contract year; although specific dates will change each year, Table 26-2 illustrates the relative points in time for specific activities. By March, a newly contracting organization needs to know what its intentions are for the following year, and if the organization is unable to submit a bid by June, it will be another year and a half before the organization will be able to enroll its first Medicare members. Table 26-2 also provides a quick summary of the major steps that a plan has to take in operating a Medicare contract.

Premium Tax Prohibition and Other Preemption of State Laws

The MMA continues the federal law that prohibits states from imposing premium taxes on CMS payments to MA organizations, and the MMA broadened the federal preemption of state law provisions so that all state laws are preempted with respect to Medicare Advantage plans and their Medicare operations, except for state laws governing health plan licensure and solvency standards.

WHAT THE CONTRACT REQUIRES

All MA organizations sign a standard contract; there is no negotiation over the terms of the contract. The contractor must comply with the terms of the contract, federal regula-

Table 26–2 Key Projected Dates in the 2007 Application/Renewal Process for Medicare Health Plan Organizations and Prescription Drug Plans

This calendar outlines key dates in the 2007 individual and employer group market Medicare Advantage (MA), Medicare Advantage-Prescription Drug (MA-PD), Prescription Drug Plan (PDP) application and renewal processes, as well as in the 1833 and 1876 cost plan renewal processes. This calendar is posted on the CMS Web site at www.cms.hhs.gov/PrescriptionDrugCovContra/Downloads/CY2007timeline.pdf. This calendar will be updated and expanded periodically. We encourage you to check the Web site and calendar regularly for changes and to take note of the timelines and deadlines for partcipating in these programs.

2006	
March	March 20—Deadline for submission of ALL 2007 initial Applications MA, MA-PD (including SNPs and Demonstrations), PDP, Direct Contract Employer/Union–Only Group Waiver Plans (EGWPs), and MA Organization, PDP, or Cost Based Plan Sponsor offering EGWPs, and ALL 2007 SAE applications March 22—Issuance of final formulary guidance March 27—Release of Health Plan Management System (HPMS) formulary submissions module March 30—Posting of the final call letters March 31—Transition Guidance Release target date
April	April 3—Issuance of Calendar Year (CY) 2007 Medicare Advantge Payment Rates April 3—2007 Reporting Requirements Comment period ends April 5, 6, 11—Bidders Conference (April 5 MA-PD Sessions, April 6 Actuaries Sessions, April 11 Actuaries Repeat Sessions) April 7—Plan Creation module, Plan Benefit Package, and Bid Pricing Tool available on HPMS April 17—Formulary Submissions Due from all MA-PDs and PDPs (including Direct Contract EGWPs and MA Organizations, PDPs and Cost-PD [for Part D] Sponsors offering EGWPs)
May	May 1—Deadline for CMS to inform currently contracted organizations that CMS has authorized renewal of their contract May 1—Transition Policy Submission target date May 1—Deadline for notifying CMS of organization's intent to stop offering RPPO's in an MA region May 15—End of IEP for Part D and AEP for MA May 19—PBP/BPT upload module available on HPMS
June	June 5—Deadline for submission of bids for all MA, MA-PD, Cost PD and PDP applicants and renewing organizations (including direct contract EGWPs and MA organizations, PDPs and cost based plan sponsors offering EGWPs) June 6—Submission of CY 2007 marketing materials scheduled to begin June 30—End of the MA Open Enrollment Period
July	July 15—Last date by which applicant must receive a determination (as a result of either CMS' initial application review or a favorable redetermination) that it is qualified to enter into a Part D contract for program year 2007
August	August 5—Deadline for cost plans not offering Part D to submit A/B benefit information in order to appear in Medicare Compare and Medicare and You Handbook
September	Early September—CMS signs contract with successful Part C & Part D applicants September 14–15—Plans preview data for the *Medicare and You 2007* handbook (date tentative)

continues

Table 26–2 Key Projected Dates in the 2007 Application/Renewal Process for Medicare Health Plan Organizations and Prescription Drug Plans—continued

October	October 2—Deadline for cost plan information of intent to non-renew for 2007 October 12 (tentatively scheduled)—Medicare Personal Plan Finder and Medicare Personal Drug Plan Finder data goes up on the Web October 30—*Medicare and You 2007* handbooks in mail to beneficiaries
November	November 15—2007 Annual Coordinated Election Period begins
December	December 31—2007 Annual Coordinated Election Period ends

Source: CMS.

tions and statutes governing the contract, and certain other federal laws, as outlined in the standard contract (*eg*, the Civil Rights Act of 1964, the Americans with Disabilities Act, Health Insurance Portability and Accountability Act [HIPAA], among others). However, federal acquisition regulations do not apply to MA contracts.

In contrast to prior regulations, the MA regulations are much more explicit in listing the contracting requirements that an MA organization must comply with and their responsibilities with respect to subcontractors. The standard for administrative and management capability is carried over from prior regulations but now includes a compliance plan to ensure that the MA organization has dedicated and accountable resources to ensure compliance with MA contract requirements.

CMS has also exercised regulatory discretion in certain areas, for example, in departing from the practice of making renewals of contracts automatic in the absence of notice by either party of an intent not to renew. Instead, CMS will make a determination each year as to whether a contract should be renewed. CMS may choose not to renew a contract if the organization has failed to implement quality improvement, has an insufficient level of enrollment, or has committed an action that would subject the organization to a civil money penalty under MA rules.

Due process provisions for contract nonrenewals and terminations are clarified in the regulations. There is also a provision allowing CMS to terminate a contract immediately before the outcome of any appeal of the decision if a situation arises in which the health of enrollees is put at risk because services are not made available.

Some Basic Requirements

An organization must have sufficient administrative ability to carry out the terms of a Medicare contract. Organizations are also required to be able to provide at least the Medicare benefit package to their Medicare enrollees, following Medicare coverage rules.

A contractor must make available all the Medicare services available in fee-for-service Medicare to beneficiaries residing in the service area and must use Medicare-certified providers—hospitals, skilled nursing facilities, and home health agencies. The plan's physicians and suppliers must not be barred from participation in either Medicare or Medicaid because of program abuse or fraud.

For network plans, services must be available through staff providers or providers that are under contract with the organization (with an exception for regional plans, as discussed earlier). Although all plans must follow Medicare coverage guidelines applicable in the geographic area in terms of what services are considered to be "reasonable and necessary" and therefore covered by Medicare, because Medicare's fee-for-service coverage varies by area (*ie*, there are local coverage determinations), a regional MA plan may elect to have any local coverage determination that applies in any part of an MA region apply to all parts of that same MA region. An example of some of these access requirements as they apply to network physicians is provided in Chapter 5.

Organizations are required to provide the benefits in a manner that ensures quality, availability, and accessibility of services. However, some of the requirements vary between network plans (HMOs, PPOs) and non-network plans (PFFS plans and MSA plans).

Under a network plan, an organization must be able to provide 24-hour emergency services and must have provisions for the payment of claims for emergency services within the service area and for out-of-area emergent or urgently needed services. All services that an organization is required to render (including any non-Medicare services in the benefit packages) must be accessible with reasonable promptness, and there must be a record keeping system that ensures continuity of care. The organization is required to maintain the confidentiality of the medical and nonmedical records of its Medicare members.

Quality Standards

Each MA plan (other than PFFS and MSA plans) must have an ongoing quality improvement program through which the organization conducts quality improvement projects that can be expected to have a favorable effect on health outcomes and enrollee satisfaction. The organization must also encourage its providers to participate in CMS and DHHS quality improvement initiatives.

In addition, each plan must have a chronic care improvement program (CCIP). The CCIP identifies enrollees with multiple or sufficiently severe chronic conditions who meet the criteria for participation in the program, and the program must have a mechanism for monitoring enrollees' participation. MA organizations are required to submit annual reports on their CCIP program to CMS.

Other quality requirements include the need to follow written policies and procedures that reflect current standards of medical practice when processing requests for initial or continued authorization of services (see Chapter 9). The plan must have in effect mechanisms to detect both underutilization and overutilization of services. A plan must be able to measure its performance, using the measurement tools required by CMS. Plans will report information on quality and outcomes measures to CMS so that CMS can provide this information to Medicare beneficiaries.

MA plans are responsible for selecting and initiating quality improvement projects on topics relevant to their population, as discussed in more detail in Chapter 15. The quality improvement projects that an organization undertakes are to focus on specified clinical and nonclinical areas and would involve performance measurement, system interventions, performance improvement, and systematic and periodic follow-up on the effect of the interventions. Quality improvement project reports will be submitted as part of a health plan's CMS monitoring visit (occurring every 3 years). Project reports will be collected as part of presite visit preparation and will be sent to a review entity. Results of the project evaluation will be incorporated into the monitoring report, and any corrective action plan requirements will also be fulfilled under ongoing monitoring oversight.

The plan must perform a formal evaluation at least annually of the impact and effectiveness of its program, and all problems that are revealed through internal surveillance, complaints, or other mechanisms must be corrected.

Quality Reports and Surveys

In addition to the reporting and auditing of Health Plan Employer Data Information Set (HEDIS)* data, which is the responsibility of MA organizations, Medicare enrollees

---

*See Chapter 23 for detailed descriptions of HEDIS and CAHPS.

of health plans participate in satisfaction surveys—the annual Consumer Assessment of Health Plans Survey (CAHPS) for enrollees and disenrollees, the quarterly CAHPS Disenrollment Reasons Survey, and the Health Outcomes Survey (HOS). CMS arranges for and pays for administration of the CAHPS survey, whereas MA organizations are responsible for administering the HOS survey. PPOs report on a subset of HEDIS data.

CMS uses the reported data to provide information to Medicare beneficiaries and others. The HEDIS, CAHPS, and Disenrollment summary data are part of the Medicare Personal Plan Finder, the online tool at Medicare.gov that beneficiaries can use to select Medicare health plans. CMS also expects plans to use the data, including HOS data, for internal quality improvement. The data should help plans identify some of the areas where their quality improvement efforts need to be targeted and may be used as the baseline data for quality improvement projects. Additionally, all four data sets may be used for research purposes by public or private entities.

CMS may target areas that warrant further review based on the data. For example, CMS has developed a Performance Assessment System that will array information from the HEDIS, HOS, CAHPS, and Disenrollment data sets in a manner that will permit performance evaluation by CMS. Plans can also view their own information online via secured access to the CMS's Health Plan Management System.

External Review

Coordinated care plans are subject to external review of the quality of care they render. The Quality Improvement Organizations (QIOs, formerly peer review organizations) that are under contract to CMS to review the quality of care of hospitals in fee-for-service Medicare also review the quality of care among MA enrollees. The current approach

to the role of the QIOs moves away from review of individual cases and toward a collaborative approach focusing on patterns of care. QIOs are also authorized to provide technical assistance to plans when they design their quality improvement projects and to evaluate the results of these projects. QIOs also review complaints by MA enrollees about the quality of care in an MA plan. As in fee-for-service Medicare, QIOs process beneficiary requests for review of hospital discharge decisions.

Deemed Compliance with Quality Requirements

MA organizations may meet certain quality standards through accreditation by a private accrediting body (such as the National Committee for Quality Assurance; see Chapter 23). The only requirements that may be deemed as met are quality assessment and performance improvement requirements and confidentiality and accuracy of enrollee records requirements. The accrediting organization must be approved by CMS, with approval subject to notice and comment in the *Federal Register*. Approval of the accrediting body may be withdrawn under certain conditions.

LIMITATIONS ON PHYSICIAN INCENTIVE PLANS

A plan that has a physician incentive plan that places physicians at substantial financial risk, as defined in Medicare regulations, for the care of Medicare or Medicaid enrollees, must provide for continuous monitoring of the potential effects of the incentive plan on access or quality of care. This monitoring should include assessment of the results of surveys of enrollees and former enrollees, and the plan should review utilization data to identify patterns of possible underutilization of services that may be related to the incentive plan. Concerns identified as a result of this monitoring should be considered in development of the organization's focus areas for quality improvement projects. More detail on these limitations is provided in Chapter 5.

CONSUMER PROTECTIONS

MA plans are subject to certain requirements relating to access to services for beneficiaries, information to be provided to enrollees, and appeal rights that must be provided to Medicare members.

Access Standards

With regard to access to care standards, the regulations have a number of requirements, including the following:

- Requiring unrestricted communication between patients and health care professionals through the prohibition of "gag" clauses
- Using the "prudent lay person" definition of what constitutes an emergency, the liability of the MA organization for the cost of such care, and a requirement to cover appropriate maintenance and poststabilization care after an emergency
- Covering out-of-area dialysis during an enrollee's temporary absence from the service area
- Limiting copayments for emergency services to no more than $50
- Specifying that the decision of the examining physician treating the individual enrollee prevails regarding when the enrollee may be considered stabilized for discharge or transfer (codification of existing policy)
- Requiring plans to permit women enrollees to choose direct access to a women's health specialist within the network for women's routine and preventive health
- Requiring that services be provided in a "culturally competent" manner (ie, with sensitivity toward cultural, ethnic, and language differences)

Information on Advance Directives

MA organizations must meet the same requirements applicable to hospitals under Medicare with regard to maintaining written policies and procedures for advance directives.

Member Appeals and Grievances

MA enrollees have the right to an administrative and judicial appeals process for claims and payment issues, and the right to a plan grievance process for other issues. The rules for Medicare appeals (referred to in regulations as organization determinations) pertain to decisions regarding coverage or cost of an item or service included in the Medicare contract (Medicare-covered items and services and additional and supplemental benefits), including payment for out-of-network services received in an emergency.

Appeals

The steps of the appeals process include the following:

- The determination by the organization (or a subcontracted entity)
- Reconsideration by the organization, or, if the organization proposes a reconsideration decision adverse to the beneficiary, review of that decision by an external review entity under contract to CMS
- Review by an administrative law judge (for claims valued at $110 at the time of publication [an indexed amount subject to change each year]) of the external review entity's decision if adverse to the beneficiary (but the MA organization is not entitled to appeal a decision by the external review entity when the decision is in favor of the beneficiary)
- Review of the administrative law judge decision by the Departmental Appeals Board of the US Department of Health and Human Services (a right available to members and to the MA organization)

- Judicial review in federal court for claims valued at $1,090 or more (as of the time of publication—this amount is also indexed)

The first-level determination is to be made by the MA organization within 14 days (or "as expeditiously as the enrollee's health condition requires" but no later than 14 days), and a reconsideration decision (by the organization or the review entity) is to be made within 30 days (with the same requirement for expeditious processing). For expedited appeals, the standard is that a decision must be rendered within 72 hours.

QIOs also review beneficiary complaints, including beneficiary appeals about the appropriateness of a hospital discharge. Expedited time frames similar to those of fee-for-service Medicare apply in such a case.

Grievances

Grievances against a plan, as opposed to Medicare appeals, are subject to different standards. Beneficiaries must currently be afforded a meaningful grievance right when the matter in dispute is an issue other than coverage or cost of an item or service the MA organization is obligated to provide. The statute requires organizations to provide data on the number of grievances and their disposition in the aggregate on an enrollee's request.

PROVIDER PROTECTIONS AND RIGHTS

Medicare contracting health plans are required to afford certain rights to contracting providers, and plans are required to make timely payment on claims from noncontracting providers.

Basic Provider Rights

The MA statute contains provider protections, including the following:

- A provision prohibiting discrimination against particular providers, in selection of providers or payment or indemnification provisions, solely on the basis of the provider's licensure status
- Appeal rights afforded to providers in the event of exclusion from a network
- A requirement that MA organizations consult with plan physicians regarding medical policy, quality, and medical management procedures

The MA statute also permits a health care professional to refuse to provide advice, counseling, or referral for a service that the provider objects to on moral and religious grounds, as long as the MA organization provides notification to enrollees of the applicability of this provision.

Prompt Payment to Noncontracted Providers

MA plans are required to meet the same prompt payment standards that apply to Medicare carriers and intermediaries in fee-for-service Medicare with respect to the timeliness of payments made to noncontracted physicians and other providers. The standards apply to clean claims; that is, claims having no "defect or impropriety" as the law says and not lacking "substantiating documentation" or "requiring special treatment." The standard is that 95% of clean claims must be paid within 30 days.

ENROLLMENT OF MEDICARE BENEFICIARIES INTO MA PLANS

There are specific rules that MA plans must follow with respect to enrollment and disenrollment of Medicare beneficiaries.

Information Dissemination

Until the BBA, marketing and information dissemination regarding private health plan options were primarily functions undertaken by the contracting organizations themselves.

The BBA sought to increase CMS's role in the dissemination of information and also took a number of steps to facilitate MA enrollment in certain cases, such as when a person first becomes eligible for Medicare. Beginning with an information campaign in 1998 and a coordinated open enrollment in 1999, the BBA directed CMS to provide comparative information containing comprehensive, detailed information about health plan choices. As noted, this activity is funded by user fees imposed on participating MA plans. CMS is also required to maintain a toll-free number accessible to beneficiaries residing in areas with MA plans.

The national Medicare education program includes a Medicare handbook with prominent mention of private health plan options and the Internet site at http://www.medicare.gov, which provides comparative information on all plan choices. The outreach and education program also includes a toll-free number (1-800-Medicare or 1-800-633-4227), local health fairs before the annual election period, and other outreach efforts with various partners.

Enrollment and Election Periods

A previous version of this chapter published many years ago began, "TGIF—The Government Is Frightening, unless you know your acronyms." Acronyms continue to abound at CMS, particularly on the subject of enrollment, with the Annual (A), Initial (I), Open (O), and Special (S) Enrollment Periods (EPs). The AEP is what is commonly referred to as an open enrollment period, during which time any eligible Medicare beneficiary may enroll in an MA plan. IEPs and SEPs apply to particular circumstances, with IEPs applicable to individuals newly becoming eligible for Medicare and SEPs applicable to special circumstances.

Who May Enroll

Except in the case of a plan that is not open for enrollment because it has a capacity

waiver, or a plan for which enrollment is limited to special needs individuals or employer group members only, during an election period, any Medicare beneficiary residing in the service area of an MA plan is entitled to enroll in the plan, as long as the person has both Part A (hospital insurance) and Part B (supplementary medical insurance) of Medicare. Medicare beneficiaries who are Medicaid recipients may also enroll.

The only Medicare beneficiaries not entitled to enroll (and to whom a plan must refuse enrollment under the law) are beneficiaries who have end-stage renal disease (ESRD), whether aged, disabled, or entitled to Medicare solely because of their disease. However, enrollees who acquire ESRD after enrollment in the plan may not be disenrolled because they have ESRD, and individuals who were enrolled as non-Medicare members of a plan who have ESRD may be retained as Medicare enrollees on becoming eligible for Medicare. The one exception to the rule is that there can be special needs plans offered to individuals with ESRD, who would not otherwise be entitled to enroll in an MA plan.

The annual election period (AEP) runs from November 15 through December 31, for enrollments effective the following calendar year. This is an election period in the sense that what occurs is an election between traditional fee-for-service Medicare and enrollment in an MA plan, along with the election of drug coverage under traditional Medicare or through MA. After what is referred to as the open enrollment period (OEP), January 1 through March 31, a Medicare beneficiary is locked in to the election he or she has made for the remainder of the calendar year. During the January to March OEP, individuals may make one election in or out of Medicare Advantage, but there can be no change in the person's election of drug coverage. For example, a person who elected a Medicare Advantage plan with drug coverage (an MA-PD [prescription drug] plan) on December 25, 2006, may return to traditional fee-for-service Medicare, but he or she must enroll in a stand-alone prescription drug plan (PDP) because of the election with respect to drug coverage made in the annual election period.

An individual who becomes MA eligible during the year may make one MA "OEP-NEW" election during the period that begins the month the individual is entitled to both Part A and Part B and ends the last day of the third month of entitlement, or on December 31, whichever occurs first. An OEP-NEW election is separate from an OEP election. OEP and OEP-NEW elections are effective on the first of the month following the month the election was made.

During this annual election period, beneficiaries receive comparative information on all of their health care options, including fee-for-service Medicare and its Medigap (supplemental coverage) options. They may elect new coverage and switch back and forth between MA and traditional fee-for-service Medicare, effective the following January. Newly eligible enrollees who do not choose an MA plan are deemed to have chosen the original Medicare fee-for-service option, except that "age-ins" enrolled in a contracting plan may be deemed to have elected the entity's MA plan.

MA plans are also required to be open during special election periods, for example plans must accept beneficiaries when they first become entitled to Medicare, and they must be open when another organization in the service area terminates a Medicare contract. Organizations that have MA contracts are required to offer the option of continued enrollment as Medicare members to current non-Medicare enrollees when they become eligible for Medicare and meet MA eligibility criteria (*eg*, having both Part A and Part B).

Disenrollment and the Lock-In

As noted earlier, beneficiaries may only disenroll from an MA coordinated care plan and choose another plan, leave Medicare fee-for-service to enroll in an MA plan, or return to Medicare fee-for-service one time during the first 3 months of the calendar year. Beneficiaries will be effectively locked in to their MA plan election for the remaining 9 months after this window.

Exceptions to the lock-in period are available for enrollees under the following circumstances: the MA plan contract is terminated, the beneficiary leaves the plan service area, the MA plan fails to provide covered benefits or is found to be improperly marketing the Medicare product, or under other conditions specified by CMS. In the years 2007 and 2008, there is another exception whereby beneficiaries in fee-for-service Medicare have a one-time opportunity to enroll in an MA-only (not MA-PD) plan outside of the open enrollment period. For example, a beneficiary could decide in July of 2007 to enroll in an MA-only plan after having elected fee-for-service Medicare coverage (and a stand-alone PDP plan) during the open enrollment period. The person's Part D election would be unaffected by the MA enrollment. In addition, the lock-in does not apply to institutionalized individuals or to beneficiaries entitled to both Medicare and Medicaid. These categories of individuals may elect fee-for-service Medicare coverage or choose another MA plan at any time during the year.

Involuntary Disenrollment

An MA organization may involuntarily disenroll a Medicare beneficiary if the person leaves the service area permanently (defined by regulations as an absence lasting more than 12 months); if the person has committed fraud in enrolling in a plan or permits others to use his or her enrollment card to obtain care, for failure to pay premiums in a timely manner (including optional supplemental premiums), or because of disruptive or abusive behavior, subject to CMS approval.

Capacity Limits

Although a plan is ordinarily required to be open for enrollment during the election and enrollment periods described previously, a plan may limit or close its enrollment if it does not have the capacity to continue enrollment. In such a case, a plan may discontinue enrollment but may set aside a specified number of vacancies to enroll members who age-in from the plan's commercial product into its Medicare product. Capacity limits may be based on several different reasons and the limit may apply to specific plan benefit packages or counties in different configurations, for example, by plan or by county.

MARKETING RULES

MA provisions include requirements specifying the type of marketing plans are required or permitted to undertake, as well as specifying prohibited marketing activities.

Basic Requirement

The basic marketing requirement is that an organization must market its MA plan or plans throughout the entire service area in a nondiscriminatory manner. Prospective enrollees must be given descriptive material sufficient for them to make an informed choice. One of the required marketing documents is a standardized summary of benefits form that uses standard benefit definitions and a standardized format to allow beneficiaries to make "apples to apples" comparisons among MA offerings and between MA and fee-for-service.

Prohibited Marketing

Prohibited marketing activities include door-to-door solicitation, discriminatory marketing (avoiding low-income areas, for example), and misleading marketing or misrepresentation. These activities are subject to sanctions, including suspension of enrollment, suspension of payment for new enrollees, or civil monetary penalties. MA plans are prohibited from giving monetary incentives as an inducement to enroll and from completing any portion of the enrollment application for a prospective enrollee.

Prior Approval

All marketing and enrollment material (including enrollment forms) an organization proposes to use must have CMS prior approval. CMS has 45 days to review marketing materials. If 45 days pass without CMS comments on the material, it is deemed approved. If an MA plan's marketing materials were approved for one service area, they will be deemed to be approved in all of the plan's service areas, except with regard to area-specific information.

For certain marketing and enrollment documents, CMS has developed model language. Use of the model language reduces the approval time period to 10 days. Under certain circumstances, CMS also allows a "file and use" approach for certain materials, whereby no prior approval is required.

Description of Plan (Evidence of Coverage)

The statute specifies the kind of information an MA member must receive on enrollment and annually thereafter. This includes information on benefits and exclusions; the number, mix, and distribution of plan providers; out-of-network and out-of-area coverage; emergency coverage—how it is defined and how to gain access to emergency care (including use of 911 services); prior authorization or other review requirements; grievances and appeals; and a description of the plan's quality assurance program. On request, the organization must provide information on utilization control practices, the number and disposition of appeals and grievances, and a summary description of physician compensation.

Notifications to Enrollees

Medicare enrollees must be notified at least 30 days in advance of changes in plan membership rules (which must be approved by CMS). However, for the change in benefits occurring from one year to the next, the notice must be sent by October 15 before the coordinated open enrollment period.

THE CONTRACTING PROCESS

The first step in the contracting process is to submit an application in the manner described in the following sections of this chapter. The following are some of the issues addressed in the application:

- Legal and financial structure of the organization
- Types, numbers, and location of providers the plan will use
- Listing of benefits
- Description of the Medicare marketing strategy
- Copies of marketing material to be used
- Evidence of coverage or subscriber agreement listing membership rules, enrollee rights, and plan benefits
- Quality assurance plan
- Enrollment and disenrollment procedures
- Grievance and Medicare appeals procedures

The application review is done jointly by CMS's central and regional offices and will involve a site visit.

CMS uses a highly automated process for plans to submit bid information and plan descriptions that form the basis of the Medicare "personal plan finder" at http://www.medicare. gov. One of the first actions that a new applicant must take is to gain access to this system, the Health Plan Management System (HPMS).

Health Plan Management System

The HPMS system serves many different and crucial functions in CMS for both contractors and the government. Since 2001, HPMS has supported various functions in support of the communication between CMS and contracting organizations, as well as the monitoring of Medicare Advantage organizations. HPMS is also the means by which marketing material is submitted for review, and CMS uses the HPMS system to inform plans of new developments, training opportunities, deadlines, and so forth. Stand-alone prescription drug plans are also supported through HPMS.

At the end of March of each year, the HPMS formulary submission module for MA-PDs and PDPs is released. In early April, the MA plan creation module, the plan benefit package (PBP), and bid pricing tool (BPT) become available to organizations on HPMS. Formulary submissions are due in mid-April from all MA-PDs and PDPs, including direct contract employer group plans, Medicare Advantage organizations, PDPs, and cost-based plan sponsors offering Part D employer group plans.

In mid-May, the PBP/BPT upload module is available on HPMS. The first week of June is the deadline for submission of bids via HPMS for all MA, MA-PD, Cost PD, and PDP applications and renewing contracting organizations. A new MA or PDP applicant with no prior or current access to HPMS must complete and submit a signed hard copy of the form.*

The organization's initial request for CMS systems access should be for HPMS access alone and submitted with its application. MA and PDP applicants and contractors are required to access HPMS to execute a variety of Medicare functions, including the application process, formulary submission, bid submission, ongoing operations of the MA and Part D programs, reporting and oversight activities, and so forth. Failure to have access to HPMS will endanger the timely progress of

---

*This form can be found at http://www.cms. hhs.gov/mdcn/access.pdf. This Web address was current at the time of publication, but may be subject to change.

application review during the critical 8-week time frame. CMS provides MA and PDP applicant organizations with additional technical instructions on how to access HPMS, including the Web site address, once the request for a user ID has been processed.

A new MA or PDP applicant (same legal entity) organization that already has HPMS access for other functions, such as for another MA or PDP plan or product, need not request a new CMS user ID. Once the organization has received its new pending contract number, it can contact CMS and request that the new contract number be assigned to an existing HPMS user ID.

Currently contracting Medicare Advantage organizations complete the HPMS plan crosswalk when uploading their next year contract bids and to designate the relationship between plans they offer in the current year to plans being submitted for the following year. A Medicare Advantage organization is free to change benefits, premiums, and cost sharing under an MA plan or an MA-PD plan from year to year.

Part D sponsors provide notice to CMS of a decision to renew contracts for the following year by submitting a new set of bids in early June. They are required to submit one or more formularies through HPMS in April in accordance with the released Final Formulary Guidance.

The Call Letter and Key Projected Dates Calendar

In April of each year, CMS releases the call letter for the next contract year, which provides instructions and guidance for MA and MA-PD plans. A separate call letter is issued for stand-alone PDPs. The call letter includes both new and clarified policy statements as well as restatements of existing program requirements. It also provides instructions with regard to contract renewal and nonrenewal processes for the next year for currently contracting MA, MA-PD, and cost contract plans (which are described later in this section).

The calendar illustrated in Table 26-2 earlier in this chapter is posted on the CMS Web site early in the year and is updated and expanded periodically. It outlines key dates for application and renewal processes for individual and employer group market MAs, MA-PDPs, and PDPs, as well as cost-based plans.

In February, the draft call letter for the next year's contracts is posted on the Web for public comment, and CMS issues the Advance Notice of Methodological Changes for the next contract year's MA payment rates.

In March, PDP and MA-PD final formulary guidance is released as is the HPMS formulary submissions module (FSM) and the final call letters for MAs, MA-PDs, and PDPs. In April, CMS issues the next year's MA payment rates, holds a bidders' conference, and makes available on HPMS the plan creation module, the plan benefit package, and bid pricing tool.

Early May is the deadline for CMS to inform currently contracted organizations that renewal of their contracts has been authorized. The plan benefit package and bid pricing tool upload module becomes available on HPMS. In early June, all bid submissions are due as are all notifications from currently contracting organizations of their intent to not renew contracts for the following year.

In September, Medicare Advantage organizations can first preview their plan(s) data as they will appear in the *Medicare and You* handbook. In October, Medicare Personal Plan Finder and Medicare Personal Drug Plan Finder data are available on the Medicare Web site, and *Medicare and You* handbooks are mailed to Medicare beneficiaries.

Applying to CMS for a Medicare Advantage Contract

Current year applications for the following MA contract types are posted at http://www.cms.hhs.gov/MedicareAdvantageApps/*:

---

*This Web address was current at the time of publication, but may be subject to change.

- Coordinated Care Plan (CCP)
- Regional Preferred Provider Organization (RPPO)
- Private-Fee-for-Service (PFFS)
- Medical Savings Account (MSA)
- Application for Service Area Expansion (SAE; described later)

Medicare Advantage organizations offering CCP or PFFS plans in the current year that want to expand the existing service areas in the following year use the Service Area Expansion Application (SAE). A date in mid-March is usually the deadline for submission.

There is not a separate application for a MA Special Needs Plan (SNP), which is a type of coordinated care plan.* Organizations that do not hold a current contract with CMS complete the full MA CCP application to apply to offer an SNP. Any contracting MA organization that wants to add an SNP in its contracted service area must complete the SNP section of the MA CCP application. Any contracting MA organization that wants to expand its service area and add an SNP in that expanded service area completes the MA SAE application, including the SNP section of the SAE application. All these applications require submission of a Part D (drug benefit) application as well.

Managed care organizations/sponsors interested in applying for a Medicare Advantage and/or MA-PD contract with CMS for the next contract year are required to submit applications to CMS in March. If an applicant currently has an MA contract, it is nevertheless required to complete a new application to offer one or more different plan types. A current contractor is generally permitted to submit an abbreviated application that focuses only on additional or different information requirements specific to the new plan type(s) that it wants to offer. Organizations

applying to become qualified to enter into an MA contract with CMS for the first time complete the entire application. A Medicare Advantage organization submissions matrix has been posted at the CMS Web site to assist applicants in submitting application-related documents and items.

Medicare Advantage CCPs must offer at least one MA plan that includes Part D prescription drug benefits in each of their service areas. All new or expanding CCP-offering organizations must submit an MA prescription drug plan sponsor application as a condition of approval of the CCP application. The Part D application is found at the CMS Web site. The MMA continues to prohibit new cost-based plans (under section 1876 of the Social Security Act) and precludes any organization from operating a cost-based plan in the same area in which it operates an MA plan; such plans are briefly described later in this section.

CMS also issues guidance and information through HPMS and conducts industry outreach through conference calls and other mechanisms. One or more conference calls are typically scheduled to discuss the MA/MA-PD call letter following its release.

Medicare Advantage organizations submit next contract year marketing materials such as the Summary of Benefits (SB) and Annual Notice of Change (ANOC—the advance notice of new contract year changes provided to current enrollees) after bid submission. All marketing materials are submitted via the HPMS marketing module. Regional office staff will review the materials and approve or disapprove them. After CMS approves the Medicare Advantage organization's bid, any necessary changes to conditionally approved or approved marketing materials must be resubmitted to CMS based on the approved bid. All Medicare Advantage organizations are required to place on all marketing materials the CMS contract number as part of their unique material identification number. Contract number and unique material identification numbers must be printed on the front page of the Summary of Benefits and Evi-

---

*SNP guidance is found at http://www.cms.hhs.gov/SpecialNeedsPlan/. This Web address was current at the time of publication, but may be subject to change.

dence of Coverage. The member identification card must include the contract number and Plan Benefit Package (PBP) number.

As noted previously, CMS regional and central office staff review MA applications. Regional PPO and MSA applications are handled directly by central office staff.

Regional Preferred Provider Organizations

If an applicant wanting to offer an RPPO plan currently has an MA contract with CMS, it is usually permitted to submit an abbreviated application that focuses on additional or differing requirements specific to the RPPO requirements. As previously noted, each RPPO applicant entity must demonstrate state licensure in at least one state in each region for which it is applying and attest that it will apply for or has already been granted licensure in the remaining states in each region prior to September of the year prior to the contract year. Licensure waiver issues with regard to Part D applications must be resolved as well.

Entities that wish to offer an RPPO in multiple regions or to offer multiple RPPO products in one region can submit a single application but must provide full and complete information about each product in each proposed region. As is the case with other MA application types, full documentation of arrangements for health services delivery in the region or regions should be made at the time of application submission.

Private Fee-for-Service Applications

The major difference in the application process for a PFFS plan is the issue of the validation of the claims system, given that PFFS plans are not coordinated care plans and pay noncontracted deemed providers at Medicare fee-for-service rates. An applicant to offer a PFFS plan can validate its claim system in the PFFS application process by one of the following methods:

- Use of a claims system previously tested by CMS (such as a third-party claims administrator previously validated by CMS)
- Use of a CMS-approved claims system for a PFFS plan
- Validation of the applicant's own claims system

In the case of a plan using its own claims system, the applicant must demonstrate that it operates a system that is duly tested and able to properly pay providers at rates that are not less than rates under traditional fee-for-service Medicare. In addition, the applicant must agree to sign an attestation form that it has instituted a reimbursement grid and tested its claims system; that it will submit provider dispute resolution policies and procedures to address written or verbal provider disputes/complaints, particularly with regard to reimbursement amounts. The plan must submit biweekly reports to CMS with regard to provider complaints, verbal and written, for 6 months following receipt of the first PFFS claim, along with data with regard to enrollee appeals/complaints related to claims for the same time period.

Special Needs Plans

As noted earlier, the MMA created a second type of new MA plan, the SNP, which can exclusively enroll or disproportionately enroll special needs Medicare beneficiaries. Those SNPs that elect to enroll a disproportionate percentage of a target population must maintain enrollment in the SNP for that target population as a percentage of total SNP enrollment greater than the proportion that occurs nationally in the Medicare beneficiary population. The three types of beneficiaries that SNPs might serve are as follows:

Special needs plans for dual eligibles. Dual eligibles are divided into different eligibility categories based on income relative to the federal poverty level and assets. Of 7 million dual eligibles as of 2006, about 6 million are full duals who qualify to receive full Medicaid benefits. Beneficiaries with higher income and asset levels are eligible for more limited Medicaid coverage under the categories of the Medicare Savings Program (MSP).

SNPs for dual eligibles are the most common type of SNP plan, and these plans may either accept all dual eligibles or limit enrollment to full benefit duals. The same MA organization can elect to offer two dual-eligible SNPs in the same service area: one for full-benefit duals and another for all duals. However, SNPs cannot limit enrollment solely to the MSP duals. All SNPs apply the same premium and copayments to all members. States may pay Medicare's Part B premium for all dual eligibles and cost sharing for all duals and qualified Medicare beneficiaries (QMBs). States may also pay SNP premiums and/or copayments for certain members or contract with an SNP for some or all Medicaid services.

Special needs plans for institutionalized beneficiaries. Institutional SNPs serve beneficiaries who reside or are expected to reside for 90 days or more in a long-term care facility. They may also elect to enroll beneficiaries living in the community who require an equivalent level of care. CMS has permitted organizations offering these plans to limit enrollment to contracted long-term care facilities within a geographic service area. The SNP must identify in its application to CMS whether it will be facility-based and/or community-based. Community-based enrollees must meet the criteria of the state for nursing home certification (certifiable population).

Special needs plans for beneficiaries with severe or disabling chronic conditions. Chronic care SNPs are designed for beneficiaries with severe chronic diseases and/or conditions. CMS has to date evaluated these proposed SNP applications on a case-by-case basis. That evaluation considers the appropriateness of the tar-

get population, the clinical programs and expertise available, and how the SNP will cover the target population without discrimination against sicker enrollees.

The major characteristic that distinguishes SNPs from other MA plans is their ability to limit enrollment (a statutory provision that expires at the end of 2008, unless extended or made permanent by the Congress). SNPs are paid on the same basis as other MA plans.

SNP applicants must indicate whether they are exclusive to the target population or are disproportionate share plans. The SNP is then restricted to that option through the contract year. A SNP that selects disproportionate share status is required to market to all Medicare beneficiaries.

Dual-eligible and chronic condition SNPs are required to meet all MA requirements for collecting and reporting HEDIS, CAHPS, and HOS at present. Institutional SNPs are not required to report HEDIS measures. CMS will extract the Minimum Data Set (MDS) measures used for nursing homes.

Section 1876 Cost-Based Plans

No new cost-based plan applications under section 1876 are being accepted by CMS (as opposed to cost reimbursement arrangements under section 1833 for employer/union groups). Cost-based plans may continue contracting with CMS through contract year 2007. Cost-based plans have the option of providing Medicare Part D benefits beginning in contract year 2007.

After September 1, 2006, service area expansion applications received from cost-based plans will be accepted only if there are less than two MA plans of the same type meeting minimum enrollment requirements in the area in which the cost-based plan intends to expand. CMS provides cost-based plans with data on competing MA plans in the service areas in which they are offered. Where there is already an existing MA-PD plan or PDP plan in the area in which the cost-based PD plan proposes to expand, no midyear service area expansion will be permitted into that area.

Cost-based plans must be open for enrollment for a period of at least 30 consecutive days. They may offer a Part D plan as an optional supplemental benefit. Enrollment in this optional supplemental benefit must take place during a Part D plan enrollment period. Individuals who disenroll from the cost-based plan are automatically disenrolled from the optional supplemental Part D plan and may enroll in another Part D plan only during established Part D enrollment periods.

Service Area Expansions and New Midyear Plans

An MA organization can apply to CMS to offer a new midyear MA plan or request an SAE of an existing MA plan only if that plan's bid is not included in a competitive benchmark calculation required by the MMA and only if there are no contracting competitors in the geographic area(s) the new plan would serve. The comparison to determine if midyear entry of a new plan or the service area expansion of an existing MA-PD plan will introduce unfair competition is whether there are other Part D competitors: MA-PD plans and standalone PDPs. The comparison to determine whether midyear entry or service area expansion of an MA-only plan will introduce unfair competition is whether or not there are other MA competitors: MA-only and MA-PDs.

In 2006, there was a national PDP plan, which meant that every county had at least one PDP. Consequently, no SNP plan was able to offer a new midyear plan or an SAE during 2006 because each SNP must offer Part D benefits (must be an MA-PD).

Web Sites and the Managed Care Manual

The CMS Web site at http://www.cms.hhs.gov contains an index page at www.cms.hhs.gov/home/medicare.asp that links the user to in-

formation on Medicare topics. Under Health Plans can be found links to topics such as the Benefit Pricing Tool, Bid Form, and Plan Benefit Package, Health Care Prepayment Plans (section 1833 cost-reimbursed contracts for employer-union groups covering only Part B services), Cost Plans, Private Fee-for-Service Plans, and Special Needs Plans. Under Medicare Advantage are MA applications and information on MA-PD contracting.

Also at this Web site is a link to Regulations and Guidance, which includes the manuals, including Chapters 1 to 15 and 17 to 20 of the Medicare *Managed Care Manual*, Publication 100-16, and a link to the Part C Marketing Guidelines for MA organizations.

Other Web sites relating to Medicare Advantage are the following:

- Employer/Union-Only Group Waiver Plans (EGWP) Guidance at http://www.cms.hhs.gov/EmpGrpWaivers/
- Prescription Drug Coverage General information at http://www.cms.hhs.gov/PrescriptionDrugCovGenInfo/
- Medicare Health Plans at http://ww.cms.hhs.gov/Helath PlanGenInfo/
- 2006 Medicare Advantage Payment Rates at http://www.cms.hhs.gov/ MedicareAdvtgSpecRateStats/AD?list.asp#TopOfPage
- MA Applications at http://www.cms.hhs.gov/MedicareAdvantageApps/

All Web site addresses are current at the time of publication, but may be subject to change.

CONTRACTOR MONITORING

Once an organization signs a Medicare contract, CMS maintains ongoing monitoring of the plan. The monitoring is accomplished through self-reporting of financial and other information by the organization on a quarterly basis. If certain criteria are met, the information may be reported on a yearly basis.

Specific to Medicare is a monitoring process that is performed by the CMS central office and, principally, by the 10 regional offices of the CMS. By the end of the first year of contracting, each plan will have a monitoring visit, during which the reviewers will determine whether the health plan is complying with regulatory requirements in such areas as financial arrangements, legal and financial requirements for the entity as a whole, quality of care issues, marketing practices, enrollment/disenrollment, claims payment, and grievance and appeals procedures. The reviewers follow a specific written protocol in conducting the review. After such a monitoring visit, a report is prepared, and if necessary, the organization is required to submit a corrective action plan to correct any deficiencies. Close monitoring of the plan continues until CMS is satisfied that the problems have been resolved. If the initial review goes well, there may not necessarily be a review of the same plan for another 2 years.

CMS must conduct a financial audit of one-third of the plans each year. This means that CMS and its contractors will visit each plan every 3 years to review financial records, including documentation used to develop plan bids, establish administrative costs, and pay providers.

CONCLUSION

The *Federal Register* does not immediately spring to mind as a good source if one is searching for amusing anecdotes in the history of health care policy. However, in volume 69, number 148, of the *Federal Register* of Tuesday, August 3, 2004, page 46,921, there is a little dig at people who presume to make predictions of what the future will bring in health care. That particular *FR* publication—the proposed rules for implementation of the MA provisions of the MMA—noted that when the BBA of 1997 introduced the option of provider-sponsored health plans, it was predicted that provider-based plans would proliferate and take over the world of Medicare managed care. The *FR* of 2004 goes on to point out that the prediction was not even remotely accurate.

So what is one to make of the projections and predictions made in the same August 3,

2004, *FR* publication regarding the Medicare Advantage program—for example, predicting that MA PFFS plans would not be very competitive (page 46,931), or that in 2006 there would be 3 million enrollees of regional MA plans (page 46,928)? What about the fear, as the MMA was being crafted, that no private plans would want to assume even partial risk for providing a drug benefit to Medicare beneficiaries? Given that enrollment in MA private fee-for-service plans was about 750,000 in mid-2006 (compared to about 38,000 in August of 2004), and that regional plans had 83,000 enrollees in mid-2006, and given the number of PDPs and MA-PD plans in 2006, the lesson to be learned is perhaps that predictions are dangerous—something that was stated in the conclusion of the preceding version of this chapter of the *Handbook*, and which seems to hold true to this day. Furthermore, as any student of managed care trends knows, numbers cited today about managed care plans and benefit designs can change drastically in 5 years, up or down.

Instead of making predictions, this chapter concludes with a number of elliptical and possibly cryptic observations about Medicare in general and the MA program. The federal budget has a large deficit. As a federal entitlement program, Medicare contributes to that deficit. The number of Medicare beneficiaries is expected to increase exponentially in the very near future. As indicated by the first two words of its title, the Balanced Budget Act of 1997 sought to address a budget issue by reducing Medicare outlays. A federal budget that has a large deficit is a not a balanced budget. Therefore, to conclude, it seems that something is probably going to happen in the future with regard to Medicare, including the outlays that Medicare makes in payments to providers and health plans and outlays that Medicare makes through the subsidization of beneficiary costs. Of course the prediction that something is going to happen could itself be wrong, in the same way that all those *Federal Register* predictions were wrong. We shall see.

References

1. Data are from Table 9-1 of the Medicare Payment Advisory Commission's "Report to the Congress: Increasing the Value of Medicare," June 2006, p. 206. The section of the report on Medicare Advantage is available at http://www.medpac.gov/publications/congressional_reports/Jun06_Ch09.pdf.

2. At the time of publication, information on waivers can be found at the CMS Web site, at http://www.cms.hhs.gov/EmpGrpWaivers.

27

MEDICAID MANAGED CARE

Robert E. Hurley and Stephen A. Somers

Study Objectives

- Understand why and how managed care emerged as a major Medicaid reform strategy.
- Recognize key similarities and differences between Medicaid and commercial managed care.
- Examine the principal operational features of Medicaid managed care programs.
- Review the major successes and shortfalls associated with implementation of Medicaid managed care across the nation.
- Identify the current and longer term questions and concerns facing Medicaid managed care.

Discussion Topics

1. Discuss the reasons why implementing Medicaid managed care is more complex than developing private sector managed care programs.
2. Discuss the factors that contribute to making capitation rates paid to HMOs so controversial in the Medicaid program.
3. Discuss the evidence that Medicaid agencies are getting better value for their money when they contract with HMOs. Is such evidence convincing? Is there evidence to the contrary?
4. Discuss why or why not a health plan might enter or exit the Medicaid managed care market. Discuss the differences between a Medicaid-only managed care health plan and a managed care plan that also operates in the commercial sector.

5. Discuss the primary care case management (PCCM) program and how that differs from a full Medicaid managed care program.

INTRODUCTION

State Medicaid programs and their beneficiaries have been well-served by managed care arrangements. The implementation of a variety of financing and delivery models has enabled states to achieve a measure of cost control, to promote improved access and quality of care, and to extract more accountability from medical care providers than traditional fee-for-service arrangements permitted. State agencies have been and continue to be resourceful and creative in adapting managed care designs to meet their varied circumstances, needs, and capabilities. Given the success to date, states seem likely to rely further on managed care arrangements to exploit additional flexibility given them by the federal government to try to reform Medicaid. Continued support for managed care bodes well for plans that have chosen to pursue the Medicaid market.

After briefly reviewing why and how Medicaid has embraced managed care, an overview of the current marketplace is presented. The distinctive operational challenges that have led to increasing specialization and focus among plans in this market are detailed with particular attention to how state expectations for health plans are rising along with contract demands. Finally, the roles that managed care arrangements may play in a reformed Medicaid program are discussed, including strategic and structural changes that may be required of health plans that continue to pursue this market.

BACKGROUND AND HISTORY

Despite its image as both a meager provider payer and a state budget buster, Medicaid has consistently met key policy goals for more than 40 years.[1] It is a crucial source of coverage for several vulnerable populations, the largest of which includes low-income mothers and children, individuals with serious chronic illness and disability, and aged persons needing nursing home care who are either impoverished at the time of their admission or become so during their stay. In the course of any recent year, more than 50 million persons will have received coverage from this program that is jointly financed by federal and state tax revenues. Beyond covering individuals, Medicaid also provides major subsidies to safety net hospitals to provide uncompensated care to millions of uninsured persons. Despite dramatic growth in Medicaid coverage during its history, the number of uninsured persons has continued to grow as well. Both factors have intensified the need for the financial resources Medicaid provides.

The financial distress that Medicaid has faced from its earliest days has shaped and, some would say, warped the program in distinct ways.[2] It has persistently paid below-market rates to most providers of services, discouraging providers from participating or encouraging them to limit participation. Consequently, Medicaid beneficiaries encountered difficulties in seeing many types of providers and grew increasingly reliant on hospital emergency departments, health centers, or other community-based providers who because of location or reputation were unable to attract a more favorable payer mix in their practices. Over time, concerns grew that Medicaid agencies could not obtain access to appropriate care from quality providers for their beneficiaries despite the fact that at the same time growth in the number of persons enrolled in Medicaid was creating increasing stress on state budgets, making it difficult to improve payment rates.

In the early 1980s, a few states began to explore whether Medicaid could use selective contracting strategies with subsets of providers or with prepaid health plans (early vintage health maintenance organizations—HMOs; see Chapter 2) to obtain guaranteed access to reputable providers at more predictable and, ideally, more manageable future costs. Led by Arizona and programs in selected counties in California, first-generation Medicaid managed care was born. Additional states soon followed suit, including some such as Utah and Michigan that chose to contract with individual primary care physicians as primary care case managers (PCCMs) because they had few or no willing prepaid health plans. By the end of the 1980s, enrollment in managed care arrangements approached 3 million or about 15% of Medicaid beneficiaries.

Models proliferated and enrollment jumped in the mid-1990s when, after the failure of the Clinton health reform initiatives, states chose, with encouragement from federal authorities, to devise a variety of reform strategies that included combinations of managed care and eligibility expansions.[3] Oregon, Tennessee, Rhode Island, and Hawaii led this new wave of activity, but more than half of all states soon had some managed care initiatives. By 1997, the federal government extended to states the opportunity to routinely require low-income beneficiaries to obtain Medicaid benefits through choice-restricting prepaid health plans or primary care case management programs. This promoted further expansion and by the end of the 1990s nearly 20 million individuals or more than 50% of the Medicaid population were in some kind of managed care arrangement.

During this period, nearly all managed care enrollees were low-income women and children because most states were hesitant to bring the more costly and medically complex people with serious chronic illnesses and/or disabilities into these programs. In the early 2000s, Medicaid enrollment continued to grow with more than 40 states offering some

form of managed care and several beginning to test managed care for disabled and chronically ill beneficiaries. This has been a slow transition, but it remains a key priority because it is this component of the Medicaid population that is the most costly and has the most complex medical management needs. To serve this population new models of care management are being explored and developed beyond the traditional full-risk prepaid health plans that have enrolled the bulk of the Medicaid population to date.

THE LOGIC OF MEDICAID MANAGED CARE

The aims of states in embracing managed care models in Medicaid—revolving around familiar access, cost, and quality concerns—have largely been satisfied, or at least sufficiently met for nearly all states to remain committed to these arrangements.[4] The evidence in support of improved access is the most compelling in large measure because states have been able to obtain guaranteed access to primary care providers through the contractual commitments they received from health plans or from primary care providers in PCCM programs. Obtaining a stable medical home that provides or coordinates care is a nontrivial contribution to beneficiary well-being in its own right and brings other gains such as reduced emergency department use and less "doctor-shopping."

Evidence of sustained cost savings is somewhat more uneven given the analytical complexity of such assessments. However, most states with prepaid arrangements believe rate setting enables them to determine a predetermined rate of increase and to build in savings relative to what they think they would have paid in a fee-for-service environment. Cost savings caused by managed care in Medicaid are constrained by virtue of the fact that payment rates have historically been low and thus price discounting—the source of considerable savings in commercial managed care—is very challenging and of questionable desirability. More significantly, because the least costly Medicaid beneficiaries (low-income women and children) are the ones most likely to be enrolled in prepaid managed care to date, the yield for these arrangements to the overall Medicaid budget has been relatively limited. A recent study estimates only about 15% of the Medicaid budget is currently influenced by prepaid managed care.[5]

The impact of Medicaid managed care on quality reveals both promise and disappointment. The promise lies in the possibility that performance improvement can be systematically measured and monitored through plans. One aspect of the disappointment reflects the unevenness of the more rigorous research done in this realm, which seems to underscore that some states have experienced success in quality enhancement and improvement whereas others have shown little effect at all. Alternatively, national data sets such as the Health Plan Employer Data Information Set (HEDIS; see Chapter 23) that have Medicaid-specific versions, or those maintained in specific states such as New York, have been able to portray evidence of considerable improvement on selected measures of health plan performance, but not necessarily on all measures. Also, many states still have inadequate data collection and analytical capacity to really know how well their plans are performing and how much beneficiaries may be benefiting.

A larger concern lies with the fact that despite important contributions made by managed care, a number of measures in the HEDIS data indicate Medicaid beneficiaries still lag their commercial counterparts quite substantially.[6] Though many of these disparities are caused by social and environmental circumstances and factors often well beyond the capacity of health plans to influence, they continue to suggest to critics of Medicaid managed care that it is still not doing enough to ensure equity in access and quality.

Many Medicaid officials are quick to contend that even without compelling research

evidence of the impact of Medicaid managed care on beneficiaries it remains an appealing strategy because it provides them with a much stronger sense of control and accountability than the traditional fee-for-service program gives them.[4] After a slow and halting start, states have become more detailed and demanding in their contracting with health plans including key requirements such as provider network access standards, customer service requirements, performance data submission, external reviews, and many others. Some states have pushed plans to move into pay-for-performance arrangements and, in a few instances, to extend these models on to network providers. By working through plans and placing performance reporting requirements on them, states can exert more influence on providers than most chose to do when they dealt with them directly. Though many states focused almost exclusively on *managing costs* at the outset, more and more of them are shifting their emphasis to *managing care*, both as a way of improving quality in response to their critics, but also as a way of better controlling long-term costs.

BENEFICIARIES AND PLANS IN THE CURRENT MARKETPLACE

By 2005, Medicaid managed enrollment totaled nearly 30 million beneficiaries or 63% of total population in the program. Approximately 80% of these persons are enrolled in fully capitated health plans (though selected services are carved out in some states),* and the remainder are in PCCM programs. The latter remain popular in rural states and other areas where prepaid managed care has never flourished. In keeping with the way that many states have heightened their contractual demands on their health plans, some of those committed to primary care case

---

*In this context, capitating a health plan is essentially identical to paying an insurance premium to an HMO as discussed in Chapter 24.

management have enhanced their expectations for their PCCM programs, instituting relevant features of managed care into their own administration of these programs.

Also, a number of other arrangements are in place for selected services such as carve-outs and specialized models for behavioral health (see also Chapter 13), special-needs populations (*eg,* foster care, developmentally delayed children), and, in some states, pharmacy benefits carve-outs (see also Chapter 12). As detailed later, several states are now employing disease management and intensive care management (see also Chapter 10) for certain beneficiaries, and a number have entered contracts with Special Needs Plans created under the Medicare Modernization Act for persons with dual eligibility for Medicaid and Medicare (see also Chapter 26).

The composition of the health plans participating in Medicaid has varied over time, revealing both changing perspectives on the relative attractiveness of the market and varied experiences of those plans and plan sponsors who have ventured into the market.[7] The first plans to participate were the classic group practice HMOs that enrolled small numbers of women and children on a voluntary basis. As states began to expand enrollment and some, such as Arizona, pursued mandatory enrollment, they found relatively few existing plans willing and able to accept large numbers of beneficiaries. This meant creating or fostering the creation of new plans, many of which were sponsored by high-volume Medicaid providers. To facilitate market entry, a number of states authorized these plans to participate without securing bona fide HMO licensure. Concerns about states contracting with predominantly Medicaid plans led to federal regulations that made it necessary for Medicaid-participating plans to have a minimum of 25% non-Medicaid membership—the so-called 75/25 rule.

In the early to mid-1990s, as more states converted beneficiaries from fee-for-service to prepaid managed care, Medicaid came to be seen as a major growth market not only for newly formed plans, again including many provider systems, but also for multi-product commercial health insurers seeking to populate new HMO product lines. By 1996, there were more than 330 plans participating in Medicaid, including most of the major national and regional carriers. Enthusiasm among commercial insurance firms proved short lived as the complexities and uncertainties of Medicaid contracting became more apparent. They discovered the rigid nature of Medicaid's administrative policies. They encountered difficulties in adapting commercial networks and operating systems to serving low-income populations, and their profit margins were disappointing or were inferior to what they could obtain in commercial and Medicare lines of business.

Many multiproduct firms left the market abruptly, but states were able to replace them as a new wave of Medicaid-only plans arrived on the scene as the Balanced Budget Act of 1997 removed the 75/25 rule. This rule change opened the way for a new set of market entrants—multistate, investor-owned health plans that focused on the Medicaid product line.[8] A number of these firms subsequently converted from privately held to publicly traded firms with initial stock offerings in the period between 2001 and 2004. A few of the major national, multi-product carriers remained in Medicaid and developed or acquired operating units or subsidiaries that also employed a comparable specialization and focus. Both of these industry segments experienced impressive financial success in terms of profitability and enrollment growth, expanding via organic growth or purchase of existing plans. Their eagerness to grow has enabled a number of states to launch new prepaid programs, to expand the geographic coverage of existing programs, or to extend enrollment to heretofore unenrolled eligibility groups such as persons with disabilities and chronic illnesses. By 2006, about one-quarter of the 220 plans in Medicaid managed care were owned by these types of firms, and they had about one-third of total prepaid health plan enrollment.

OPERATIONAL CHALLENGES FOR MEDICAID HEALTH PLANS

The notable success of Medicaid-focused firms, including both provider-sponsored and publicly traded firms, underscores the specialized nature of the Medicaid managed care market. It is an administratively demanding line of business, requiring plans to serve populations with complex medical and social needs, and forcing them to develop provider networks of considerable diversity—both in terms of service capabilities and cultural competencies. Beyond this, plans still must operate in an uncertain and, at times, politically charged policy environment that is driven to a great extent by state budgetary concerns.

Administrative Demands

Medicaid agencies employ multiple approaches to selecting which plans will be offered to their beneficiaries. Some states set participation qualifications for interested plans—including payment rates—and select all who meet them. Others require periodic bidding and may award a limited number of contracts, often to ensure that winning bidders get sufficient enrollment. More recently, a number of states have created substate regions and set targets for the number of plans selected in each region to promote competition at entry, and, again, to ensure them of relatively large enrollments. Though bidding may be demanding for plans, the prospects of being able to enroll large numbers of beneficiaries on a predetermined date is attractive to them, and when the number of awards is restricted, rapid growth is achievable.

Most states currently mandate enrollment in managed care for low-income women and children, essentially setting enrollment in a choice-restricting environment as a condition of getting Medicaid benefits. A few states do this for other populations, but in most states where disabled or chronically ill persons are eligible for managed care plans, enrollment is voluntary, or, if mandatory, liberal exemptions are permitted. Medicaid agencies carefully regulate marketing by health plans, typically relying on independent enrollment brokers to orchestrate the plan choice process and prohibiting plans from doing direct marketing. For persons who do not make a plan choice, an auto-assignment algorithm is used, with some states experimenting with auto-assignment of additional members who fail to make a plan selection to the highest-performing health plans. This approach evolved in the 1990s in response to marketing scandals that persuaded states to carefully manage customer acquisition by plans. On the positive side for plans, it reduces their marketing expense substantially.

One of the more frustrating and pernicious administrative concerns for Medicaid managed care plans is the high rate of member turnover commonly referred to as "churning."[9] Tying enrollment to Medicaid eligibility means plan members drop in and out based on fluctuations in their income and assets and the diligence with which they remember to reapply for benefits that have periodic recertification requirements. Although many states have in the past addressed this with automatic recertification and guaranteed yearlong enrollment, during periods of budget cutting states are prone to tighten these requirements, which, in turn, intensifies churning. Participating plans contend this drives up their administrative expenses needlessly and, more significantly, undermines efforts to promote preventive services, cultivate appropriate patterns of service use, and better manage the care of those with chronic conditions.

Challenging Populations

In theory, low-income women and children in Medicaid are not unlike much of the commercial population cared for by private health plans. They are typically in good over-all health with the major reason for inpatient care being obstetrics-related admissions and, for outpatient services, prenatal and well child care. However, the low incomes, cultural diversity, language and literacy problems, and social disadvantages of these populations introduce a number of important complications that plans attempting to serve them must address. Transportation services, proactive outreach, attentiveness to physical and social environmental factors, and increasing cultural competency are all areas where plans must develop proficiency to have positive, sustained impacts on their members. The concentration of high-risk pregnancies in this population, as well as persistence of chronic conditions such as asthma, diabetes, depression, and substance abuse, demand well-planned interventions to promote member well-being and make the most cost-effective use of public dollars.

For plans that have ventured into serving disabled and chronically ill beneficiaries, the stakes become much higher. The complex problems that some of these individuals have often mean they are under the care of multiple providers, may be receiving a large number of prescriptions, and may have living situations requiring a number of medical and social supports. When enrolled in prepaid plans, the capitation payments made on behalf of these persons can be as much as 5 to 10 times as high as for a low-income child, creating the potential for sizable financial gains if fragmentation, duplication, or ineffective care can be reduced. But the high payments reflect expected higher costs, and inadequate management or failure to carefully monitor serious chronic conditions can result in financial disasters for plans and serious adverse health consequences for members. It is because of these special complications that many states have yet to mandate enrollment for these high-need/high-cost beneficiaries, and many plans have discouraged states from doing so. As discussed later, this is now beginning to change.

Provider Networks

Some early advocates of managed care in Medicaid suggested or, at least, hoped that this could be a vehicle to achieve access to "mainstream" providers who may not have previously served Medicaid beneficiaries.[2] Commercial plans were expected to use existing networks and employ their leverage with providers to persuade them to see Medicaid as well as privately insured members. These hopes faded as commercial plans pulled away from Medicaid in the late 1990s and Medicaid-focused plans, often built around traditional Medicaid providers, came to dominate the market.

In practice, even commercial plans that stayed in Medicaid found it necessary to expand networks to include these traditional providers for several reasons. Plans lacked the leverage to compel other providers to accept Medicaid members because, they argued, Medicaid payments did not allow them to pay providers the same rates for Medicaid and commercial members. Additionally, many Medicaid beneficiaries preferred to continue with traditional providers of care who were more likely to be located closer to where beneficiaries reside and may be more accommodating and welcoming than providers in more remote locations. In some cases, plans had to include the traditional providers to meet mandated access standards that, for instance, limited the distance or time a beneficiary needed to travel. Finally, states responded to pressures directly from high-volume Medicaid providers or, in the case of federally qualified health centers, indirectly brought to bear on them through federal policies that required plans to include traditional providers in their networks. Not surprisingly, then, aspirations for mainstreaming beneficiaries faded as their medical homes—the places where they obtain routine care—tended to be familiar ones to them.

Because Medicaid payment rates have been notoriously low, especially for physician services, participating plans have had to work hard to meet access and capacity standards. For many plans, this has meant having to pay primary care providers and some specialists such as obstetricians and gynecologists in particular, at rates above Medicaid fee schedules and to finance supplementation through aggressive medical management or reductions in emergency department use. Negotiations with hospitals can be even more challenging, particularly those such as children's hospitals that must be in Medicaid managed care networks because they are so integral to the inpatient and specialty care required for children. Some states allow plans to invoke Medicaid rates for nonparticipating providers when they are unable to come to terms with key providers, but many others do not.

Network composition has another important implication for Medicaid health plans— the selection dynamics of members. Plans that are committed to the market may be strongly motivated to include those providers who have large Medicaid patient panels to enable them to grow quickly and compete against other plans. Some states have even allowed providers to choose the plan or plans to which their current patients will be assigned. But plans can also use network composition to manage their member mix and, in so doing, promote favorable risk selection by excluding those providers who may be a magnet for high-cost beneficiaries. In states where plans do not receive any risk adjustment in average payment levels beyond age, gender, and eligibility category, favorable selection can be an easy but unsavory way to achieve profitability. Accordingly, states have become increasingly sophisticated about scrutinizing plan behavior in this regard.

Uncertain Policy and Payment Environment

As Medicaid enrollment and spending has grown dramatically over the life of the program, Medicaid's impact on state budgets has been profound—approaching or exceeding 20% of total spending in many states.[10] This positions Medicaid to be highly sensitive to state revenue cycles, and when there is a downturn, Medicaid is a common target for serious budget cutting. The high degree of reliance on prepaid health plans creates a conundrum for Medicaid. Rather than being able to reduce payments to providers directly as was typically done in the past, states must consider whether they can reduce payment rates to plans without losing plan participation. If so, plans may then have to renegotiate rates with providers to pass reductions along. In some cases, expenses such as pharmaceuticals may not be amenable to negotiated reductions, and thus prepaid plans can be squeezed between lower capitation rates and rising vendor payments. Despite this potential for disaster, during the recent severe recession of the early 2000s most states were able to maintain healthy participation among health plans, though in a number of cases they did so by freezing rate increases.

States did go through a period in the mid-1990s when a number of them attempted to extract large savings from health plans, relative to fees for services, by reducing their payments or slowing or forgoing rate increases. This resulted in plan departures and destabilized managed care programs in some states, a number of which ultimately backtracked on planned or enacted rate reductions.[7] About this same time, a small number of states began to use risk adjustment schemes to more precisely calibrate their rates to reduce the prospects of overpayment as a result of risk selection, and more states have followed suit. In recent years, federal authorities have imposed an "actuarial soundness" requirement on states that ostensibly ensures that the rates paid to plans are fair and appropriate—to try to build in more stability to the marketplace. Although the impact of this requirement has yet to be clearly demonstrated, most health plans in the Medicaid market have been able to achieve and sustain profitability. In fact, the experience of the investor-owned, multistate firms whose financial performance data are publicly available strongly attests to the surprisingly lucrative nature of this market.

RISING DEMANDS AND EXPECTATIONS

Although continued growth in enrollment bodes well for health plans in the Medicaid market, these opportunities will be accompanied by challenges caused by growing purchaser sophistication and aggressiveness in the Medicaid market.

Pressure to Demonstrate Quality Improvement

Longstanding concerns about the rate of growth in health care costs have been coupled more recently with increasing consternation about the poor quality of care Americans are getting for those expenditures. The Institute of Medicine report *The Quality Chasm* was followed by a series of studies including those of the Rand Corporation documenting care delivery at accepted standard of care only 50% of the time.[11,12] Not surprisingly, some get worse care than others do. Another Institute of Medicine report, *Unequal Treatment*, has led to a series of efforts to examine the socioeconomic, geographic, and demographic reasons why low-income people of certain races and ethnicities in certain parts of the country served by certain kinds of providers tend to have poorer access to care and poorer outcomes than other Americans do.[13] Medicaid finds itself in the middle of many of these discussions.

Making the Business Case for Quality

Medicaid decision makers are also recognizing that short-term fixes—such as cutting rates, benefits, or eligibility—do not constitute long-term solutions. Low-income families left without access to needed services will eventually show up in publicly financed clinics and emergency rooms with serious and costly health care exacerbations that could have been avoided had their problems been addressed earlier. Therefore, policymakers are looking for more enlightened approaches that will give their states sustained value for the public dollars spent. Among the options they are considering are full-risk managed care for people with disabilities; disease management and care management models; special needs plans for beneficiaries eligible for both Medicare and Medicaid; and, more recently, pay-for-performance initiatives comparable to those gaining considerable traction in the Medicare and commercial sectors.

Embedded in all of these approaches is recognition that a small percentage of Medicaid enrollees is responsible for a vast majority of the costs, and many of those costs are predictable because chronic disease is chronic and long-term care is for the long term. Addressing chronic conditions and related care needs with a fragmented fee-for-service system is not fiscally prudent. Assuring that high-need individuals receive coordinated, high-quality services is likely to be what is best for them and for those who pay for their care. A strong business case for quality can be made that recognizes that the state, its contractors, and its beneficiaries are likely to receive superior returns on investments from targeted efforts to identify, stratify, reach out to, and intervene with higher-risk segments of the Medicaid population. Medicaid may be better suited than other health care sectors to demonstrate the business case for quality because of the alignment of financial incentives in capitated managed care and the disproportionate dependence on its services among its highest-risk beneficiaries.[14,15]

Intensified Focus on Special-Needs Populations

Although a few states (Arizona, Maryland, and Texas, for example) have demonstrated that managed care approaches for some special-needs populations can work, the movement to enroll people with disabilities in mandatory, full-risk managed care has been slow. Resistance to it comes from consumers, providers, plans, and, as a consequence, state legislators and bureaucrats, who fear managed care's incentives to underserve and to restrict choice. Even in states such as California, New York, and Wisconsin that have approached their proposed transitions to managed care for recipients of Supplemental Security Income SSI with deliberateness, resistance remains. Despite efforts to involve consumers, ensure a measure of choice, and develop appropriate performance measures, the process of gaining acceptance to full-risk managed care has been frustrating to its champions. As a result, some states have turned to less intense alternatives, including chronic disease management and care management, enhanced primary care case management, and administrative services organizations (ASOs)—all of which are intended to perform the targeting and care coordination functions of managed care for a fee, but without full risk. Although logical and more politically palatable, few of these alternatives have been subjected to rigorous, independent review, either in terms of cost controls or the quality of care that results.

Many of the states experimenting with less comprehensive models of care management may ultimately pursue full-risk options to achieve the budgetary predictability afforded by assigning risk for their most expensive populations to managed care. But they also are aware these expensive beneficiaries are so costly because they have more than one chronic disease and they know that the typical single-disease models will not work well for those with multiple complex, chronic conditions. Treating individuals with comorbidities requires a more comprehensive approach, the kind that full-risk managed care programs with such members are compelled to develop. Often starting with very small, specialized—or "boutique"—plans serving people with severe physical disabilities, AIDS, or other high-cost conditions, the most successful care management approaches involve diverse care teams composed of physicians,

nurses, social workers, and community or peer outreach workers. Indeed, Programs of All-Inclusive Care for the Elderly (PACE) for high-risk dual eligibles, which began in the late 1980s, are among the first of these highly specialized plans.[3] These plans usually need to have innovative financing arrangements with their state Medicaid agencies, including sophisticated risk adjustment and risk-sharing schemes. They may also carve in pharmacy and behavioral health services because so many of these beneficiaries often have serious mental illnesses and substance abuse problems.

In states where people with disabilities are mandatorily enrolled on a full-risk basis, larger managed care organizations—including, in particular, safety-net-based plans as well as the multistate investor-owned plans now prevalent in Medicaid—have developed greater capacity in these areas, employing the techniques available to them in data analysis, predictive modeling, and care management. States, as well, are becoming increasingly sophisticated contractors in terms of assessing risk, adjusting payments, monitoring risk selection, and imposing performance requirements. Still, there are a number of outstanding issues that need to be addressed before consumer advocates and other key stakeholders will become sufficiently comfortable with full-risk approaches to make it the standard way states contract for their care.

NEW FRONTIERS FOR MEDICAID MANAGED CARE

Several major issues requiring further insight and innovation in Medicaid managed care will come to the fore as policymakers refine models of managed care, bring the benefits of managed care to more needy populations, and ultimately attempt to reform more fundamentally the entire Medicaid program.

Aligning Financial Incentives

Aligning financial incentives to promote quality is gaining great attention throughout the health care marketplace. Medicaid managed care is no exception. The most popular form today of financing innovation across the health care marketplace is pay-for-performance, wherein plans, hospitals, physicians, and even consumers are rewarded for participating in quality improvement activities, for investing in health information technology, for implementing evidence-based best practices, and for achieving results in terms of beneficiary outcomes and reduced use of costly and inappropriate care, especially in emergency rooms and inpatient settings. Pay-for-performance is discussed fully in Chapter 8.

A significant number of states have adopted various forms of monetary and non-monetary pay-for-performance approaches for their health plans, including favorable auto-assignment formulae and financial incentives.[16] For example, New York sets aside 3% of premium for this purpose. These states are interested in seeing their health plans institute initiatives to pass incentives through to their physician networks. Other states are working on direct incentive programs for their physicians, particularly in primary care case management programs.

Models for Dual Medicare/Medicaid Beneficiaries

A little-known component of the Medicare Modernization Act (MMA) of 2004 authorizing the creation of Special Needs Plans to serve dual-eligible persons is generating significant federal, state, and health plan commitment to removing the administrative and policy barriers to integrating preventive, acute, behavioral, and long-term care for those dually eligible for Medicare and Medicaid. Many forget that among the "duals" are both low-income and frail seniors as well as younger adults with disabling chronic illnesses and disabilities. As a whole, the 7 million dual-eligible individuals represent about 18% of its 40 million enrollees, but they are nearly twice as expensive as other Medicare beneficiaries. For Medicaid, this 14% of the total 50 million enrollees represents about

40% of expenditures, primarily because of their needs for long-term supports and services. The number of these newly created plans has grown rapidly, but few have yet developed contracts for complete Medicaid services, and even fewer are yet prepared to develop long-term care services. Given the broad stakeholder interest in further integration of care for the duals, many states are likely to seek contracts with special needs plans in the future.

Pursuing Physical/Behavioral Health Integration

Although carve-outs of behavioral health services at both the state and health plan levels remain common, the increasing recognition of physical/behavioral health comorbidities is leading decision makers at both levels to reconsider more comprehensive approaches that promote reintegrating care. Beyond the clinical difficulties associated with managing behavioral health conditions, these efforts are made more challenging by complex intergovernmental and interagency jurisdictional issues. But because large numbers of severely and persistently mentally ill persons qualify for and depend on Medicaid for coverage of their service needs, these organizations that serve this population are highly sensitive to program designs that may put their funding sources at risk.

Identification and Management of Comorbid Condition Clusters in Medicaid

Many persons who qualify for Medicaid because of a significant disability or chronic condition are beset by multiple conditions, making their care management especially challenging. Few programs have been developed to address commonly occurring condition clusters in a systematic manner, in part because of limited information about these clusters. Research sponsored by the Center for Health Care Strategies is attempting to analyze claims and encounter data to identify the most prevalent clusters. Medicaid promises to make it easier for state decision makers and plans interested in enrolling the SSI in managed care to design cost-effective delivery systems for serving these populations in the future.

Exploring Managed Long-Term Care Models

A number of states, led by Wisconsin, New York, Florida, and Texas, have implemented programs to capitate Medicaid-financed long-term services, often including both institutional care and home and community-based waiver services, and contract with specialized managed care entities. Many of the programs rely on traditional county and nonprofit agencies, but increasingly investor-owned health plans are entering this field. In light of the enormous burden that long-term care represents for state Medicaid programs, this area is viewed as one of the most promising opportunities but challenging endeavors for both states and their potential partnering contractors.

Experimenting with Consumer-Directed Designs

Recently, a few states, notably Florida, Kentucky, West Virginia, and South Carolina, have embarked upon controversial efforts to give consumers/beneficiaries incentives for healthy behaviors and making better health care choices. To date, these initiatives have not been fully integrated into managed care models, although aspects of consumer-directed care within a managed care environment are currently being pilot tested in two Florida counties. Although initiatives focused on creating rewards for consumers are not always thought of as part of efforts to align financing to improve performance, they are in fact consistent with the increased focus on using incentives to drive quality. The Deficit Reduction Act of 2005 (DRA) is rife with calls

for consumer responsibility and gives states far greater freedom to experiment in this and other ways that rely on incentives for Medicaid plans and providers to give tax payers the best value for limited public funds. Like the MMA before it, the DRA reveals a heavy reliance on the private sector, including consumers, to achieve these ends.

MOST ROADS LEAD TO MORE MANAGED CARE

The ability of models of managed care to allow Medicaid programs to select their vendors, to extract greater accountability from them, to obtain reasonable cost savings, and to gather promising, albeit uneven, evidence of improvements in access and quality has solidified broad support for this strategy. The new frontiers identified previously lend further support for states to continue to pursue structured arrangements to managing and coordinating care and to seek systematic approaches to establish that Medicaid is getting value commensurate with its investments. Because many of these models are still in embryonic stages of development, states will have to actively nurture them and cultivate collaborative relationships with the innovators who are implementing them.

There are also powerful policy and political reasons why managed care models will continue to be seen as integral features of the Medicaid landscape. Budget pressures for a program with a growth rate that has persistently exceeded state revenue growth will only intensify and compel states to seek new and more effective measures to limit cost growth. The continued devolution of Medicaid policy entrepreneurship to the states is a direct invitation to them to push the envelope, as several of them are now doing with consumer-directed designs and limited benefit offerings. Medicaid managed care is also a vivid example of *privatization* in action—as states shift many programmatic and operational decisions out of their highly constrained domains and onto private contractors who have much more flexibility with which to maneuver. There is little indication that the appetite for privatization among elected officials is waning.

Finally, the success of the investor-owned, multistate firms in Medicaid provides yet another source of momentum for managed care expansion. Investor expectations and burgeoning state opportunities are propelling these plans forward to new states, new populations, and new products. Their desire to grow and diversify their enrollment across multiple states in turn encourages states to raise their expectations about their capacity to find sufficient, competent contractors to facilitate managed care expansion. As strong advocates for the value of managed care models and the embodiment of the asserted virtues of privatization, these plans have found widespread support among many influential policymakers.

CONCLUSION

The evident mutual dependence of Medicaid on managed care evokes imagery of a potentially "lasting marriage" that weathered some stormy early episodes and has now settled into a mature, moderately comfortable, and durable relationship.[4] The sense of joint past accomplishment shared by both states and health plans is an important factor in suggesting they are reasonably well-prepared to address successfully several important challenges that will arise in the years ahead. The sense of partnership that has endured so well in Medicaid contrasts sharply with the far more volatile Medicare managed care experience and the widespread retreat from care management evident in the commercial world.

References

1. Weil A. There's something about Medicaid. *Health Affairs*. January/February 2003:22(1), 13–30.

2. Hurley R, Freund D, Paul J. *Managed Care in Medicaid*. Ann Arbor, MI: Health Administration Press, 1993.

3. Davidson S, Somers S. *Remaking Medicaid: Managed Care for the Public Good*. San Francisco, CA: Jossey-Bass, 1998.

4. Hurley R, Somers S. Medicaid and managed care: A lasting relationship? *Health Affairs*. January/February 2003:22(1), 77–88.

5. Lewin Group. Medicaid capitation expansion's potential costs savings. Presented at Association of Community Affiliated Plans. April 2006, Washington, DC.

6. Thompson JW, Ryan KW, Pinidiya SD, Bost J. Quality of care for children in Medicaid managed care: Are differences between commercial and Medicaid beneficiaries inevitable? *JAMA*. September 2003:290, 1486–1493.

7. McCue M, Hurley R, Draper D, Jurgensen M. Reversal of fortune: Commercial HMOs in the Medicaid market. *Health Affairs*. 1999:18(1), 223–230.

8. Draper D, Hurley R, Short A. Medicaid managed care: Last bastion of the HMO? *Health Affairs*. March/April 2004:23(2), 155–167.

9. Fairbrother G, Dutton M, Bachrach D Newell K, Boozang P, Cooper R. Costs of enrolling children in Medicaid and SCHIP. *Health Affairs*. January/February 2004:23(1), 237–243.

10. Smith V, Ramesh R, Gifford K, Ellis E, Wachino V, O'Malley M. *States Respond to Fiscal Pressure: A 50 State Update of State Medicaid Spending Growth and Cost Containment Actions*. Kaiser Commission Medicaid and the Uninsured. January 2004. Available at: http://www.kff.org/medicaid/7001.cfm. Accessed August 12, 2005.

11. Institute of Medicine. *Crossing the Quality Chasm: A New Health System for the 21st Century*. Washington, DC: National Academy Press, 2001.

12. McGlynn E, Asch S, Adams J, *et al.* The quality of health care delivered to adults in the United

States. *N Engl J Med.* June 26, 2003:348, 2635–2645.

13. Institute of Medicine. *Unequal Treatment: Confronting Racial and Ethnic Disparities in Health.* Washington, DC: National Academy Press, 2002.

14. Leatherman S, Berwick D, Iles D, *et al.* The business case for quality: Case studies and an analysis. *Health Affairs.* March/April 2003:22 (2), 17–30.

15. Somers S. Medicaid can push for quality—Letter to editors. *Health Affairs.* July/August 2003:22(4), 260.

16. Highsmith N, Rothstein J. *Rewarding Performance in Medicaid Managed Care.* Princeton, NJ: Center for Health Care Strategies, March 2006. CHCS Issue Brief.

28

THE MILITARY MANAGED HEALTHCARE SYSTEM

M. Nicholas Coppola, Jeffrey P. Harrison, Bernie Kerr, and Dawn Erckenbrack

Study Objectives

- Understand the difference between direct care and purchased care.
- Understand the importance of readiness in the military health system.
- Understand the governance process in military managed care.
- Understand TRICARE performance metrics.
- Understand the influence of outside stakeholders on military health care policy.
- Understand the history of military performance improvement programs leading to Lean Six-Sigma.
- Understand the relationships and competing priorities of actors within the Managed Care Quaternion.

Discussion Topics

1. Discuss the following statement made by a former Assistant Secretary of Defense for Health Affairs, "The military health system operates the only Health Maintenance Organization (HMO) that goes to war." Why is this statement important in understanding the military health system?
2. Discuss key legislative events in military health care that resulted in the implementation of the current TRICARE program.
3. Discuss key differences and advantages of TRICARE Prime, Extra, and Standard. What other TRICARE programs are available for specific beneficiaries?
4. Discuss the historical events that resulted in "TRICARE for Life" becoming a right for eligible beneficiaries.
5. Discuss strengths and threats to the survival of the military health system.
6. Discuss and describe the Parity of Healthcare.

INTRODUCTION

This chapter discusses the military health system (MHS). The MHS operates a specialized form of managed care called TRICARE and responds to the challenge of maintaining medical combat readiness while providing health services for all eligible beneficiaries. TRICARE brings together the worldwide health resources of the Army, Navy, Air Force, Coast Guard, and commissioned corps of the Public Health Service (often referred to as direct care) and supplements this capability with network and nonnetwork civilian health professionals, hospitals, pharmacies, and suppliers (referred to as purchased care) to provide better access and quality service while maintaining the capability to support military operations.

On the direct care side, the MHS oversees more than 70 military hospitals/medical centers, 411 medical clinics, 417 dental clinics, and more than 100 region-specific *first aid stations* located worldwide. Each service's medical department is headed by a flag officer, or general officer equivalent. By law, the Army, Navy, and Air Force Surgeon General must be a medical doctor. Each military Surgeon General is responsible for the care provided in his or her respective service's military treatment facility (MTF). MTFs are analogous to civilian hospitals, medical centers, and health clinics. In a typical week, the MHS does more than 19,000 inpatient admissions, 1.7 million professional encounters (outpatient), 2,000 births; fills 1.9 million prescriptions; and does more than 400,000 dental procedures.

The MHS managed care plan, TRICARE, offers a range of primary, secondary, and tertiary care benefits to approximately 9.2 million eligible beneficiaries at an annual cost of more than $38.4 billion. Approximately 7.5 million nonactive duty beneficiaries (dependants and retirees) constitute part of the 9.2 million. Active duty service members account for the remaining 1.7 million. In terms of dollars and eligible beneficiaries, TRICARE is the largest single provider of any form of managed care in the United States.

A unique aspect of military managed care is the MHS's readiness mission. *Readiness* is defined as the ability of forces, units, technical systems, and equipment to deliver the output for which they were designed.[1] Readiness is also associated with maintaining the health status of active duty personnel well above the health standing associated with nonmilitary personnel. Furthermore, *readiness* is synonymous with ensuring efficient supplies are available for national disasters and war and ensuring that appropriate processes are in place to support mobilizations. This means that readiness is associated with the ability of certain elements of brick and mortar health care facilities to become mobile and deploy worldwide when necessary. Finally, readiness is concerned with operations management processes and the efficient and effective use associated with the transformation of inputs into outputs. No other managed care plan in the United States—or the world—has a similar focus and responsibility. Former Assistant Secretary of Defense for Health Affairs Dr. Sue Bailey once said that the military health system operates the only health maintenance organization (HMO) that goes to war.[2]

To understand the current structure and process of military managed care it is first necessary to review the seminal events in military managed care evolution. Factors affecting military managed care evolution stem from issues in war, directives from Congress, beneficiary demands, and adoption of civilian best practices over 200 years. In contrast, some civilian managed care practices may have antecedent roots in earlier military health programs. The end result is a civilian managed care system with undeniable ties to military initiatives and a military managed care system that is similar to civilian managed care in many ways while still maintaining distinctiveness in mission and purpose.

BRIEF HISTORY OF THE MILITARY HEALTH SYSTEM

The Revolutionary War through Post World War II

The history of military health care traces its origins to the establishment of the Army Medical Department on July 27, 1775. The Continental Congress also established the fledgling nation's first Director General and Chief Physician. This position eventually evolved into the office of the Surgeon General of the United States, in which such notable figures as Dr. C. Everett Koop and Dr. Richard Carmona have served. During the American Revolution, military health care was delivered in the field and often in churches and barns. After 1777, several fixed facility hospitals were established in various northern states. On March 2, 1799, Congress established An Act to Regulate the Medical Establishment. This legislation gave the Physician General (renamed from the Director General and Chief Physician) the authority and responsibility of overseeing the development of (primarily) Army hospitals. That same year, General George Washington approved the construction of one of the first military hospitals in the Colonies, in Morristown, New Jersey. Although the act did not provide for dependants of one service to be treated in the hospital of another branch of service, both the Army and the Navy routinely took care of members from their sister service.

One of the unique features of the act was a directive to collect prospective payments for health care services. The 1779 act directed the Secretary of the Navy to deduct 20 cents a month from the pay of sailors and marines for their care in civilian treatment facilities. This was necessary because of the lack of access to alternative health care structures for seamen and marines in the military system. The act also suggested structures for remuneration of civilian health personnel and entities. This complicated debit and credit system resulted in the requirement to establish sound accounting systems for the collecting and distribution of funds for health care and may represent the first time in U.S. managed care history that prepayment for prospective health services was established in the health system.

In addition to this new methodology for financing, 1779 also saw innovations in inpatient services by the military. Under the supervision of Dr. James Tilton, the Army built new facilities with isolation wards to segregate the sickest and most critically wounded soldiers. Dr. Tilton's design broke from the traditional one-size-fits-all construction of hospitals. For example, early hospitals were boxlike, and common beds were filled by a diversity of patients from the wounded to the diseased. Dr. Tilton's new hospital design assisted in the prevention and spread of illness—and subsequently promoted recovery rates. In 1813, Dr. Tilton wrote a book titled *Economical Observations on Military Hospitals and the Prevention and Cure of Diseases Incident to an Army*. It was one of the nation's first books on how to improve the performance of hospitals. Dr. Tilton's treatise influenced the design, construction, operation, and administration of all hospitals built in the United States for decades.[3]

From the Revolutionary War through the Civil War, the military attempted to differentiate between care for dependants and active duty access. However, the westward growth of the nation required Army posts to be located in remote areas with no alternative access to health care. As military posts expanded west, families accompanied soldiers. Although departmental regulations prohibited military surgeons from treating civilians, some exceptions were granted. Finally, in 1834, the Adjutant General ruled that military surgeons had permission to treat civilians when it did not interfere with their required military duties.[4] This policy established the benefit—and later entitlement—to free health care for authorized dependants of the military that currently exists. More important, this may also be the first instance in

U.S. health care that nonmonetary benefits (*ie*, health care) were granted by an organization to family members of the employed person. The preponderance of the civilian sector did not adopt a similar provision for providing free health care to an employed person's family on a regular basis until the late 1920s.

CHAMPUS and the Modern Military Health Care Era

In 1956, in an effort to keep up with a growing civilian trend to offer health care benefits and entitlements to retired persons, Congress enacted the Dependants Medical Care Act. This act provided that "medical and dental care in any medical facility of the uniformed services may, under regulations prescribed jointly by the Secretaries of Defense and Health, Education and Welfare, be furnished upon request and subject to the availability of space, facilities, and capabilities of the medical staff, to retired members of uniformed services." The act additionally applied to dependants of uniformed retirees. The significance of the act was that it legitimized standing policies already in widespread application throughout the military health system.[5]

In 1966, Congress created Medicare. One of the original goals of Medicare was to provide health care for retired workers who were no longer covered by a health plan after retirement. However, a problem existed for many military personnel who often retired from a military career in their mid- to late-40s. As a result of the space availability clause of the Dependants Medical Care Act, a problem arose where some military retired members could not gain access to military treatment facilities—and were too young to participate in Medicare. As a result, some service members found themselves paying for medical care in civilian institutions out of pocket.

In an effort to address the inability to gain access to health care for some categories of beneficiaries, Congress amended the Dependants Medical Care Act and created the Civilian Health and Medical Program of the Uniformed Services (CHAMPUS). CHAMPUS was created under Public Law 89-614, the Military Medical Benefits Amendments Act of 1966. Modeled after the Blue Cross/Blue Shield option, CHAMPUS was a fee-for-service benefit that provided for comprehensive medical care when there was not space available in the MTF.[6] For the first time in the history of the military, two different systems existed to provide care to beneficiaries. The resulting composite organization was composed of a direct military care system for active duty personnel that used all available military hospitals and clinics, and a second system monitored through CHAMPUS that acted as a gatekeeper to the civilian care system.[7] Although CHAMPUS did not require a monthly premium like Medicare did, CHAMPUS had an annual deductible and a cost share for care received outside of the MTF.

Through the late 1980s, CHAMPUS benefits remained relatively stable and unchanged. However, spiraling health care costs in the 1980s affecting civilian health care organizations also began affecting CHAMPUS. As a result, the Department of Defense (DOD) began to explore options and alternatives to control costs, monitor access, and maintain health care quality. One option centered on closing inefficient military hospitals. The second option focused on reengineering military health care.

The first option implemented by Congress to control military health care costs was the Base Realignment and Closure (BRAC) initiative. From 1987 through 1997, Congress mandated a 35% reduction of military health care assets.[8] The second option focused on quality and access and resulted in a series of five notable demonstration projects initiated from 1986 through 1993. These demonstration projects were conducted to validate the ability to use defined civilian networks effectively to treat military beneficiaries as well as to conduct a cost benefit analysis between purchased civilian health care services and CHAMPUS expenditures. These demonstrations included the CHAMPUS Reform Initiative (CRI), the New Orleans managed care demonstration, Catchments Area Management (CAM) projects, the Southeast region preferred provider organization (PPO) demonstration, and the Contracted Provider Arrangement (CPA) in Norfolk, Virginia.[9]

THE TRANSFORMATION AND REENGINEERING OF THE MILITARY HEALTH SYSTEM

CHAMPUS Reform Initiative

The CRI demonstration was designed to improve CHAMPUS through competitive selection of financially at-risk contractors to underwrite the delivery of CHAMPUS health care services. The CRI had four primary objectives: to decrease the costs of CHAMPUS and MTF care, to decrease the utilization of civilian health care providers and hospitals, to improve coordination between the military and civilian components of the MHS, and to increase beneficiary satisfaction within the MHS. The CRI was intended to make the military health system more accessible while increasing the program's overall efficiency.[10] The program offered two options. One was an enrollment program similar to an HMO, called CHAMPUS Prime, and the second enrollment program was similar to a PPO, called CHAMPUS Extra. The intent of both options centered on improving cost, access, and quality while maintaining patient satisfaction. The CRI demonstration also experimented with a patient referral system, a health care finder system, and resource-sharing agreements between contractors and military hospitals. A final economic analysis of the CRI demonstration suggested the program could provide marginal benefits to military beneficiaries.[8,11]

New Orleans Demonstration Project

The New Orleans demonstration project was intended to study the effects of using managed care techniques in a geographic area without military MTFs. In June 1991, after a competitive selection process, Foundation Health Federal Services was awarded the contract to provide private-based health services in the region. The design of the service contract was similar in nature to the CRI demonstration: a risk-based contract with a triple option (*ie*, HMO, PPO, and standard CHAMPUS), provider networks, and comprehensive utilization management and quality assurance programs. The New Orleans demonstration likewise met with mixed approbation from government stakeholders. One of the more significant concerns to military leaders was the lack of federal control over the health plan. However, the experiment with a large civilian network for the delivery of care to military beneficiaries proved to be feasible.[9]

Catchments Area Management

The Catchments Area Management (CAM) demonstration project was intended to pursue an alternative management technique to contain MHS costs. The concept was designed around the local MTF commander maintaining responsibility and control over the delivery and financing of health care services for the entire beneficiary population within the MTF's catchment area. The catchment area was defined as the area surrounding the MTF, approximately within a 40-mile radius. By having full autonomy, the hospital commander determined the appropriate means to deliver health care with allocated resources. Although there was only one approved CAM design authorized by the DOD, five demonstration sites were operational across the services. This led to significant operational differences among the CAM sites. However, commonalities among the sites included a health care finder service, enhanced claims management, HMO enrollment requirements, modifications to the standard CHAMPUS benefits package, reduced or eliminated deductibles, discounted inpatient or outpatient service charges, utilization management practices, and quality assurance programs. The CAM projects met with relatively high approval by key military stakeholders because of the advantage of operational control. Elements of the CAM process were eventually adopted in final military managed care models.[9]

Southeast Region PPO

The fourth demonstration project was the Southeast region PPO project. This project introduced a PPO option in the military health system. The goal was to impede CHAMPUS's inflationary growth while simultaneously increasing beneficiary satisfaction by organizing an accessible, cost-effective network of health care providers. The contract was awarded to Wisconsin Physicians Service. The design of the contract was similar in scope to a traditional PPO, requiring no enrollment, more choice of providers, and incentives to use preferred providers. This program also resulted in several successful learning outcomes for key military stakeholders who were experimenting with a managed care PPO option for the first time.[9]

Contracted Provider Arrangement

The final demonstration project was an experiment with managed care carve-outs and was coined the Contracted Provider Arrangement—Norfolk. In this demonstration, services were limited to mental health. This provided the military with an opportunity to experiment with providing care through a civilian contractor for traditional managed care carve-out specialties. Norfolk was selected because of the fact that it had twice the per capita mental health costs compared to the nation. The military anticipated that managed care carve-out techniques and practices would be successful in lowering costs while improving quality and access to care for service members.[9]

As with the former demonstration projects, CPA provided successful outcomes in specific areas of interest to key military stakeholders. As a result, the military has established several carve-out arrangements through specific contractors for specialty care

needs. One of the most notable examples is the Extended Healthcare Option (EHCO) program (discussed later). The EHCO program provides active duty military beneficiaries with very specific and additional options for receiving health care for their dependants when their dependants suffer from specific disabilities. For example, if the active duty service member has an autistic child in need of specialized services, such as applied behavioral analysis (ABA) therapy, those services will be provided through a civilian health care facility identified through a carve-out contract within the military managed care network.

CHAMPUS Demonstration Project Outcomes and the Creation of TRICARE

In 1993, the CHAMPUS demonstration projects suggested a reorganization of military health care was prudent. The demonstrations provided evidence that civilian managed care techniques could help the military contain costs, improve quality, increase access, and advance patient satisfaction. In 1994, Congress enacted the National Defense Authorization Act (NDAA). The NDAA directed the DOD to prescribe and implement a health benefit option for beneficiaries eligible for health care under Chapter 55 of Title 10, United States Code (USC). The NDAA also directed the military health system to implement health programs modeled on managed care plans in the private sector. In response to the DOD and Congress, the military health system developed the military managed care plan called TRICARE. TRICARE's name was coined to represent the three primary military services involved in providing health care to DOD beneficiaries (Army, Navy, and Air Force). The name also represents the three managed care options developed to administer care. The three managed care options are called TRICARE Prime, TRICARE Extra, and TRICARE Standard (Table 28-1). Overall, TRICARE adopted several successful managed care features, such as primary care managers,

Table 28–1 TRICARE Beneficiary Costs

Active Duty Family Members

	TRICARE Prime	TRICARE Extra	TRICARE Standard
Annual deductible	None	$150/individual or $300/family for E-5 and above; $50/$100 for E-4 and below	$150/individual or $300/family for E-5 and above; $50/100 E-4 and below
Annual enrollment fee	None	None	None
Civilian outpatient visit	No cost	15% of negotiated fee	20% of allowed charges for covered service
Civilian inpatient admission	No cost	Greater of $25 or $14.35/day	Greater of $25 or $14.35/day
Civilian inpatient behavioral health	No cost	Greater of $20 per day or $25 per admission	Greater of $20 per day or $25 per admission
Civilian inpatient skilled nursing facility care	$0 per diem charge per admission No separate cost share for separately billed professional charges	$11/day ($25 minimum) charge per admission	$11/day ($25 minimum) charge per admission

Retirees, Their Family Members, and Others

	TRICARE Prime	TRICARE Extra	TRICARE Standard
Annual deductible	None	$150/individual or $300/family	$150/individual or $300/family
Annual enrollment fee	$230/individual $460/family	None	None
Civilian cost shares		20% of negotiated fee	25% of allowed charges for covered service
Outpatient emergency care mental health visit	$12 $30 $25 $17 (group visit)		
Civilian inpatient cost share	Greater of $11 per day or $25 per admission; no separate copayment for separately billed professional charges	Lesser of $250/day or 25% of negotiated charges plus 20% of negotiated professional fees	Lesser of $535/day or 25% of billed charges plus 25% of allowed professional fees
Civilian inpatient skilled nursing facility care	$11/day ($25 minimum) charge per admission	$250 per diem cost share or 20% cost share of total	25% cost share of allowed charges for institutional services,

continues

Table 28–1 TRICARE Beneficiary Costs—continued

Retirees, Their Family Members, and Others

	TRICARE Prime	TRICARE Extra	TRICARE Standard
		charges, whichever is less, for institutional services, plus 20% cost share of separately billed professional charges	plus 25% cost share of allowable for separately billed professional charges
Civilian inpatient behavioral health	$40 per day; no charge for separately billed professional charges	20% of total charge plus, 20% of the allowable charge for separately billed professional services	High-volume hospitals—25% hospital-specific per diem, plus 25% of the allowable charge for separately billed professional services; low-volume hospitals—$175 per day or 25% of the billed charges, whichever is lower, plus 25% of the allowable charge for separately billed services

Source: TRICARE Management Agency, Washington, DC, 2006.

gatekeeper access, enrolled beneficiaries, and empanelled providers. The program also includes capitation budgeting and case, disease, risk, and utilization management principles.

THE TRICARE PROGRAM

TRICARE Eligibility

The TRICARE program is available to uniformed service members, retired military, and their families worldwide. Family members include spouses, unmarried children under age 21, unmarried children under age 23 who are full-time students, and stepchildren adopted by the sponsor. Those who are eligible must be listed in the Defense Depart-

ment's worldwide, computerized database, the Defense Enrollment Eligibility Reporting System (DEERS). The following are not eligible for TRICARE benefits: parents and parents-in-law of active duty service members, or retirees and people who are eligible for health benefits under Civilian Health and Medical Program of the Department of Veterans Affairs (CHAMPVA). Costs for each TRICARE option are provided in Table 28-1.

TRICARE Governance

To implement and administer TRICARE, in 1994, the DOD originally reorganized the military health system into 12 joint-service regions. All 12 regions were subordinate to the TRICARE Management Agency (TMA). The TMA is led by the Assistant Secretary for Defense for Health Affairs who ultimately reports to the president of the United States. The decision to separate contracts for different TRICARE regions was made in an effort to prevent any one contractor from having too much control over the care delivered to DOD beneficiaries.[12] The initial 12-region governance structure proved to be ineffective. As a result, the TMA slowly began to eliminate and reorganize regions.

In 2004, the Assistant Secretary of Defense (Health Affairs) and the services' Surgeons General established a governance structure consisting of three TRICARE regions. The new governance structure is designed to monitor performance and resolve problems at the lowest possible level for managing the military health benefit with force readiness as the first priority followed closely by beneficiary satisfaction. Each of the three TRICARE regions in the United States has a regional contractor to coordinate medical services available at the military treatment facility and the civilian network.[13] The regional contractors work with the TRICARE regional offices (TROs) to manage TRICARE at a regional level. Both the regional contractors

and the TROs receive overall guidance from the TMA. The three TRICARE regions are organized geographically into a North, South, and West region as depicted in Figure 28-1.[14]

Governance of the three TRICARE service regions remains complex. The TRICARE regional offices are responsible for planning, coordinating, and monitoring all health care delivered throughout their region. Additionally, each region establishes contracts with civilian health care organizations to provide medical care to beneficiaries. However, both military commanders and civilian contractors struggle with dual missions to maintain wartime readiness requirements and peacetime beneficiary health care with limited budgets in a not-for-profit environment.

Performance Metrics for TRICARE Contractors

TRICARE contractors are charged with providing or arranging for delivery of quality, timely health care services and have the responsibility of providing the timely and accurate processing of claims received into their custody, whether for network or nonnetwork care. In addition, the contractor must provide courteous, accurate, and timely response to

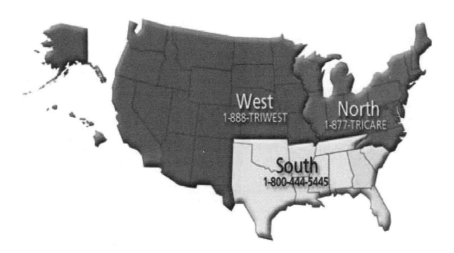

Figure 28–1 TRICARE Regions
Source: Department of Defense.

inquiries from beneficiaries, providers, the TMA, and other legitimately interested parties. TMA has established standards of performance that are monitored by TMA and other government agencies to measure contractor performance. Key performance standards include such measures as preauthorizations/ authorizations, referrals, and claims processing timeliness requirements.

The standard of performance for contractors to issue preauthorizations/authorizations requires the contractor to issue determinations on at least 90% of all requests within 2 working days following receipt of the request and all required information. This requirement also specifies that 100% of such requests be issued determinations within 5 working days following receipt of the request and all required information. For referrals, following the date of receipt of a request for a referral, the contractor shall issue a referral authorization or denial on at least 85% of all requests within 2 workdays and 100% of all requests within 3 workdays. Moreover, 96% of all referrals of beneficiaries residing in TRI-CARE Prime service areas (does not include TRICARE Prime Remote areas) shall be to the MTF or a civilian network provider. (This percentage includes services rendered in network institutions by hospital-based providers even though no formal referral was made to that individual.) Last, the contractors must meet strict guidelines for claims processing timeliness, for example, 95% of retained claims and adjustment claims shall be processed to completion within 30 calendar days from the date of receipt, and 100% of retained claims and adjustment claims shall be processed to completion within 60 calendar days from the date of receipt.

TRICARE Options

TRICARE Prime

TRICARE Prime is the HMO-like plan in which beneficiaries enroll in this benefit option where it is offered. Each enrollee chooses or is assigned a primary care manager (PCM), a health care professional who is responsible for helping the patient manage his or her care, promoting preventive health services (eg, routine exams, immunizations), and arranging for specialty provider services as appropriate. Prime offers enrollees additional benefits such as access standards in terms of maximum allowable waiting times to obtain an appointment, emergency services (24 hours per day, 7 days per week), and waiting times in doctors' offices, as well as preventive and wellness services (eg, routine eye exams, immunizations, hearing tests, mammograms, Pap tests, and prostate examinations). A point-of-service (POS) option permits enrollees to seek care from non-network providers, but with significantly higher cost sharing than under standard care.

Active duty service members must enroll in TRICARE Prime and must receive all health care benefits at military treatment facilities—unless otherwise authorized. All health benefits are free, and there are no out-of-pocket costs to service members. TRICARE Prime is also available to other eligible beneficiaries, such as family members of active duty service members and retirees. If enrolled in TRICARE Prime, dependants must also receive health care at a military treatment facility unless otherwise authorized. Retirees can enroll in TRICARE Prime; however, they must pay an annual enrollment fee and normally enroll for 1 year at a time. TRICARE Prime enrollees must follow well-defined rules and procedures. Failure to follow strict TRICARE Prime guidelines may result in refusal of care, refusal of payment, and costly POS option charges.

In addition to no out-of-pocket costs, an advantage of being enrolled in TRICARE Prime is the policy-directed access to care standards for appointments. Access to care standards differ by the level of care sought. For emergency care, MHS beneficiaries have the right to access emergency health care services when and where the need arises. For urgent (acute) care, the standard is an appointment within 24 hours and within 30 minutes travel time; routine care within 7 calendar days and within 30 minutes drive time; for wellness and specialty care, the appointment must be within 4 weeks and within 30 minutes drive time from the beneficiary's residence. If these access standards cannot be met, TRICARE offers the beneficiary a referral and authorization to seek care in the civilian network. Moreover, TRICARE access standards state that office waiting times in nonemergency circumstances shall not exceed 30 minutes for Prime enrollees.

For service members and their families who do not live near an MTF, TRICARE offers TRICARE Prime Remote (TPR). TPR is specific to certain geographic locations, and eligibility is based on residence and/or work address. To be eligible for TPR, active duty members and their families must live and work more than 50 miles—or approximately 1 hour drive time—from the nearest military treatment facility. The beneficiary must enroll in TPR to be eligible for the TPR option. If specific screening criteria are met, care and benefits at civilian treatment facilities may be authorized for TPR enrollees at the TRICARE Prime option.

TRICARE Standard

TRICARE Standard is the traditional indemnity benefit (also known as fee-for-service or FFS), formerly known as CHAMPUS, open to all eligible Department of Defense beneficiaries, except active duty service members (and, until recently, Medicare eligibles). No enrollment is required to obtain care from civilian providers. TRICARE Standard gives beneficiaries the option to see any provider. Advantages include a wider selection of providers and health care facilities and the option to participate in TRICARE Extra. There is no required annual enrollment, and the option offers comprehensive health care coverage for beneficiaries not enrolled in TRICARE Prime. Standard offers the greatest flexibility in choosing a provider, however, the plan results in the most out-of-pocket expenses for the beneficiary. For example, TRICARE Standard requires that the beneficiary satisfy a yearly deductible before TRICARE cost sharing begins. Furthermore, the plan requires beneficiaries to pay copayments or cost shares for outpatient care, medications, and inpatient care. Another disadvantage is that the patient may also be required to file his or her own claims. Last, the option also does not provide a PCM benefit.

TRICARE Extra

TRICARE Extra is based on a civilian PPO model in which beneficiaries eligible for TRICARE Standard may decide to use preferred civilian network providers on a case-by-case basis (*ie*, they may switch between the Standard and Extra benefits). TRICARE Extra is open to any TRICARE-eligible beneficiary who is not active duty, not otherwise enrolled in Prime, and not eligible for TRICARE for Life (discussed later in this chapter). TRICARE Extra requires no enrollment and there is no enrollment fee. Under this option, beneficiaries can see civilian providers and go to civilian health care organizations that are on an approved list of TRICARE providers called the TRICARE Provider Directory. Extra is essentially an option for TRICARE Standard beneficiaries who want to save on out-of-pocket expenses by making an appointment with a TRICARE Prime network provider. TRICARE Extra requires the same deductible as TRICARE Standard, however, by using network providers, beneficiaries reduce their cost sharing by 5%. An advantage of TRICARE Extra is that the Extra option user can expect that the network provider will file all claims forms—similar to TRICARE Prime. An additional advantage is that the access to the authorized provider may be more geographically convenient to the Extra user. However, disadvantages include extra fees associated with deductibles and copayments, the loss of a PCM, some restrictions on specialty care access, and limited provider choice.

Outcomes of the TRICARE Program

Initial results of the TRICARE reengineering initiative, combined with other improvements within the military health system, suggest that cost containment and quality improvement have been achieved.[15] Quality indicators suggest that military hospitals have higher Joint Commission of Accreditation of Healthcare Organizations (JCAHO) scores than civilian organizations have. Additionally, military report cards suggest that military hospitals have a higher percentage of board-certified doctors, administrators, and allied health personnel than civilian hospitals do. Finally, some studies suggest that care delivered in military treatment facilities is more cost-effective than care delivered outside military treatment facilities is.[3] Congress, the DOD, TMA, and the beneficiary base largely consider TRICARE a success. As a result, in an effort to maintain satisfaction with key stakeholders, the military health system is continually developing process improvement initiatives.

TRICARE Process Improvements

TRICARE continually seeks to enhance the benefit offered to uniformed service members, their families, and retirees and their families. As a result, in addition to the managed care options of Prime, Standard, and Extra, several niche-specific programs and adaptations have evolved to provide benefits to a larger population of beneficiaries. The preponderance of these programs resulted from initiatives in Congress to improve health care access and quality of care. One of the most significant changes to TRICARE came about with the signing of Public Law 106-398 as part of the 2001 National Defense Authorization Act (NDAA). Dr. J. Jarrett Clinton, the acting Assistant Secretary of Defense for Health Affairs in 2001, said, "Collectively, this act represents the most significant change to military healthcare benefits since the implementation of the CHAMPUS in 1966."[16] The 2001 NDAA authorized several key TRICARE improvements, including the following:

1. Established TRICARE as the secondary payer for Medicare-eligible military retirees (MEMR)

2. Established a pharmacy benefit for MEMR called TRICARE Senior Pharmacy Program (TSPP)
3. Established a MEMR Healthcare Trust Fund (HCTF)
4. Eliminated copayments for TRICARE Prime active duty family members
5. Expanded TRICARE Prime Remote
6. Introduced chiropractic care for active duty soldiers
7. Established the Individual Case Management Program (ICMP) for persons with extraordinary conditions
8. Reduced the catastrophic cap from $7,500 to $3,000[14]

Other mentionable benefits included in this act were permanent health benefits for Medal of Honor recipients and their families, extension of medical and dental benefits for survivors of deceased active duty soldiers, and authorization of payment for school physicals. The 2001 NDAA also authorized the DOD to expand TRICARE health benefits to niche-specific programs. The significant programs that were eventually enacted as a result of the original 2001 NDAA—and subsequent amendments—included TRICARE for Life, TRICARE Reserve Select, and the TRICARE Dental Program.

TRICARE for Life

In the early 1990s, military retirees and family members older than 65 years of age slowly lost access to military health benefits. Over the years, agents (recruiters), representing the U.S. government, continued to market "free health care for life" to soldiers. Potential recruits were promised this benefit for themselves and certain family members if they served a proscribed time in uniform.[17] However, in 1956, Public Law 569 changed the century-old, quasi–health care for life entitlement to a benefit. PL 569, Section 301, changed from: "Hospital space *SHALL* be made available;" to "Hospital space *MAY* be made available (*sic*)."[18] Despite the change in law, retirees and family members continued to receive benefits well into the early 1990s. However, in the mid-1990s under congressional and presidential guidance, these beneficiaries were required to use a civilian health care provider, use a civilian organization, and rely on Medicare or other health insurance (OHI) as payers.[19] The Pentagon estimated that approximately 1.5 million personnel, approximately 20% of the beneficiary base, were locked out of the military health system in the late 1990s.[17]

In response to restricted access to health care for military facilities, on July 16, 1996, retired Air Force colonel George E. Day, recipient of the Medal of Honor and an attorney, and others filed a lawsuit in federal court in Pensacola, Florida, on behalf of Medicare-eligible military retirees (MEMRs). More than 250,000 members and a coalition of 30 lobby organizations supported Colonel Day's initiative. The suit alleged breach of contract with military retirees to provide the promised medical care for life. Based partially on the grassroots response, TRICARE for Life (TFL) was passed by Congress and signed into public law (PL 106-398) as part of the 2001 National Defense Authorization Act. TFL replaced earlier demonstration projects conducted to provide MEMRs with some form of health care benefits. These earlier programs were called TRICARE Senior Prime, TRICARE Senior Supplement, and the Federal Employees Health Benefit Plan for MEMRs.

TFL effectively fulfills the promise of lifetime health care made to older retirees for a career in uniform. TFL restores TRICARE coverage for all Medicare-eligible retired beneficiaries who are enrolled in Medicare Parts A and B.[20] Congress established TFL as a "fully funded entitlement program"[21] by means of a new Medicare-Eligible Retiree Health Care Trust Fund. To qualify for TFL, a retiree must have served at least 20 years in the military (including retired members of the National Guard and the reserves). There are no enrollment fees, premiums, or deductibles for TFL. Beneficiaries receive most of their care from civilian providers and Medicare is the first payer, whereas TRICARE (or other health insurance) serves as the secondary payer. TFL makes TRICARE a secondary payer to Medicare at no cost to a retiree.

Another option available to eligible TFL beneficiaries is TRICARE Plus. TRICARE Plus affords beneficiaries the opportunity to receive primary care and specialty care at their local military treatment facility—provided that facility has space available. There are no charges or fees for TRICARE Plus, if offered by the MTF. Basically, TRICARE for Life (benefits received from civilian providers) and TRICARE Plus (care received at MTFs) give beneficiaries more coverage while simultaneously allowing the military health system the ability to control costs. The enactment of TFL represents one of the many military managed care outcomes that can be traced to antecedent activist actions by constituents.

TRICARE Reserve Select

The NDAA of 2005 authorized a new program called TRICARE Reserve Select (TRS). TRS is a premium-based health plan for eligible reserve component members who qualify. TRS offers comprehensive health care coverage similar to TRICARE Standard and TRICARE Extra. TRS members and covered family members can access care by making an appointment with any TRICARE authorized provider, hospital, or pharmacy—TRICARE network or nonnetwork. TRS members may access care at an MTF on a space-available basis only, however, pharmacy services are available from an MTF pharmacy through TRICARE Mail Order Pharmacy and TRICARE network and nonnetwork retail pharmacies. Medical coverage (direct care at the military treatment facility) is available when the member is activated. When ordered to active duty for more than 30 consecutive days, reserve component members and their families have comprehensive health care coverage under TRICARE.[14]

TRICARE Dental Program

The TRICARE Dental Program (TDP) is a voluntary dental insurance program that is available to eligible active duty family members, select reserve component personnel, Individual Ready Reserve (IRR) members, select retirees, and other eligible beneficiaries. This premium-based program has annual costs and deductibles for both family members of active duty personnel as well as other classes of beneficiaries.[14] The plan covers ordinary dental procedures such as annual screenings, preventive care, and standard dental treatments.

Other TRICARE Niche Programs

Other TRICARE niche programs include TRICARE Overseas, Transitional Health Care Benefits such as the Continued Healthcare Benefit Program (CHCBP), and programs for special needs beneficiaries. TRICARE Overseas Prime allows service members and their families who live overseas to get their health care under a TRICARE Prime-like option. Active duty service members must enroll in TRICARE Overseas Prime, however, family members can select between two options: TRICARE Overseas Prime and TRICARE Standard. TRICARE Overseas also extends to military retirees and their families. However, these beneficiaries cannot enroll in TRICARE Prime, but they can use TRICARE Standard.

Individuals who lose TRICARE eligibility or other coverage under the military health system are eligible for transitional health care coverage, such as that offered by the Continued Healthcare Benefit Program (CHCBP). CHCBP is not part of TRICARE but provides similar benefits and operates under most of the rules of TRICARE Standard. To obtain this coverage, the member must enroll in CHCBP within 60 days after separation from active duty or loss of eligibility for military health care.[14]

TRICARE offers three enhancements to the traditional TRICARE program for active duty family members with special needs: TRICARE Extended Care Health Option (ECHO),

ECHO Home Health Care (EHHC), and EHHC Respite Care. ECHO delivers financial assistance and additional benefits, including supplies and services, beyond those available from the basic benefit in TRICARE Prime, Standard, or Extra. The benefit increased from $1,000 (through the Program for Persons with Disabilities) to $2,500 per eligible family member in fiscal year 2004 under ECHO. Additionally, beneficiaries who are homebound may qualify for extended in-home health care through ECHO. ECHO Home Health Care provides medically necessary skilled services to eligible homebound beneficiaries who generally require more than 28 to 35 hours per week of home health services or respite care. This benefit helps eligible beneficiaries stay home rather than having to go to an institutional/acute care facility or skilled nursing home. Similarly, the EHHC Respite Benefit provides temporary relief or a rest period for the primary caregiver to promote well-being for both the caregiver and the homebound beneficiary. This benefit offers 8 hours of respite care, 5 days per calendar week.

Future

TRICARE Next Generation

The military health system is continually adapting the structure of its health care delivery system to meet DOD requirements. In 2004, the DOD began to implement many congressional recommendations through an initiative called the Next Generation of TRICARE Contracts. The goal of the Next Generation of TRICARE Contracts was to implement replacement contracts for administrative services, improve health care delivery, expand education and marketing initiatives, and increase pharmacy access—among other projects. The Next Generation of TRICARE Contracts is currently in operation in all military MTFs. Through these innovative goals, TRICARE seeks to maintain effectiveness to meet future challenges. Some of the key priorities include the following:

1. Support each respective service's readiness and peacetime mission requirements.
2. Maintain beneficiary satisfaction.
3. Improve beneficiaries' health status.
4. Minimize disruptions in care for beneficiaries when military treatment facilities are actively supporting wartime mission requirements.
5. Improve relationships between government stakeholders, contractors, and beneficiaries.
6. Minimize administrative burdens for providers, organizations, and beneficiaries.
7. Increase the use of secondary data for financial planning, medical resource management, clinical management, clinical research, and contract administration.
8. Improve relationships with other federal health care agencies, such as the Department of Veteran Affairs and the Centers for Medicare and Medicaid Services.[22]

Moreover, the 2005 BRAC process afforded the MHS with an opportunity to reorganize its assets to capitalize on the synergies of an increasingly joint service environment and to invest in and modernize facilities supporting these efforts. This initiative gives the MHS a chance to realign resources to better serve the Armed Forces and its beneficiary population. By pursuing the BRAC recommendations, the MHS hopes to further enhance the reputation of its flagship facilities in clinical, research, educational, and training excellence rivaling that found at Johns Hopkins, Mayo Clinic, and other top-rated medical centers. Most important, the MHS will be better positioned to serve its 9.2 million beneficiaries in state-of-the-art health facilities.

Threats to TRICARE

The biggest threat to TRICARE is the cost of the program. According to the Inter Agency Institute for Federal Heath Care Executives, the Department of Defense is experiencing significant increases in the cost of health care. For example, costs have doubled in just 5 years and DOD analysts project steep increases over the next 10 years, to $64 billion in 2015, which represents 12% of the projected defense budget in that year. As DOD has implemented the many enhancements to TRICARE, individuals' cost shares have essentially remained the same since 1995. As a result, TRICARE pays a continually increasing percentage of its beneficiaries' health costs. In 1995, beneficiaries paid approximately 27% of their health care costs; today they pay only 12%. These factors have led some civilian employers and state governments to shift health care costs to the DOD by encouraging their employees who are military retirees to use the very attractive TRICARE health benefit instead of their own health insurance options.

In addition to benefit enhancements, increased use by more beneficiaries, and no cost share increases, the MHS has experienced the same double-digit health care inflation as all health plans in the nation. The MHS implemented a number of management initiatives designed to reduce the costs of delivery and to enhance performance within its health system, but these actions alone will not contain the escalating costs.

Having the enormous responsibility and accountability to be a good steward of tax payers' dollars often makes the MHS a keen concern of Congress. Because the health care industry is the largest service industry in the United States, and health care costs have historically shown a trend of rapid increase, it is little wonder that health care expenditures are a significant issue in terms of the annual military budget and a potential threat to the TRICARE program.

Another concern is loss of stakeholder satisfaction. Issues being addressed through TRICARE leadership include poor claims processing, low reimbursement rates to providers, maintaining access standards in both military health care facilities and the civilian network, access to specialty care, and a perceived lack of plan choices, especially for the retiree population.

Last, fraud is another threat to TRICARE. An escalation in health care fraud emerged in the 1990s because of the money flowing into managed care organizations and the lack of enforcement of antifraud regulations.[23] The need to investigate health care fraud committed by providers in the TRICARE system led to the creation of the TRICARE Management Activity Program Integrity Office (TMA PI), which orchestrates the prevention, detection, and investigation of these increased allegations.

Lean Six-Sigma

From the 1970s through 2006, the MHS adopted and internalized various management paradigms to meet demands of the environment. For example, in the 1970s, the Euclidean concept of management by objectives was a widespread practice in the military health system. In the 1980s, Deming's popular statistical principles of total quality management and continuous quality improvement were required parts of officer training and education in many basic branch courses. In the early 1990s, as the military was drastically downsizing, Hammer and Champy's principles of reengineering and Drucker's ideals of reinvention were widely used to justify cuts in personnel and resources. In the mid-1990s, the military implemented several business-oriented strategies under Vice President Gore's reinventing government ideology. The latter 1990s and early 2000s saw the adoption of Kaplan and Norton's balanced scorecard as a panacea for operationalizing requirements for military health readiness and productivity. As of the writing of this chapter in 2006, and in the present environment of the war on terror, the ideological emphasis is on military efficiency. The military health system is slowly adopting Lean Six-Sigma methodologies to achieve an added benefit from synergizing existing inputs in a process that will (in theory) result in a significant and measurable increase of outputs.

Value Shift

The most significant struggle the military managed care system has grappled with from the inception of TRICARE to the present is the careful balance between elements of Coppola's Managed Care Quaternion (MCQ)[24] and Kissick's Iron Triangle.[25]

The term *Managed Care Quaternion* was coined in the Army-Baylor Graduate Program in Health and Business Administration in 2003. The Army-Baylor Program has been responsible for training and educating the next generation of military health care executives since 1953. The Quaternion has been used for several years to help explain the complex interactions among employers, patients, providers, and payers in regards to partisan and competing views about health care. Moreover, these health care actors also have dissimilar views in reference to Kissick's Iron Triangle. Kissick coined the term *Iron Triangle* in the 1990s to demonstrate the difficulty in selecting priorities for health care as they relate to health care costs, health care quality, and access to health care.

When juxtaposed together, the two models create a new decision-making paradigm Coppola coined, "The Parity of Health Care,"[24] as shown in Figure 28-2. Coppola developed the Parity of Health Care concept and model to assist in explaining to military health care leaders why consensus on any single aspect of health care is difficult.

For example, because each actor in the Quaternion may have different priorities when organizing Kissick's options of cost, quality and access, it is unlikely that any one actor in the Quaternion will organize Kissick's options the same way over a sustained period of time. As a result, actors in Coppola's Quaternion become rivals and antagonists rather than partners and altruistic allies. Figure 28-3 suggests one conceptual priority ranking among actors and demonstrates the complexity of relationships within the Quaternion. Figure 28-3 also assists in explaining why sustained consensus is difficult

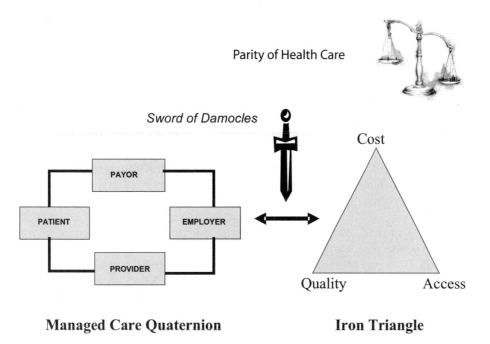

Parity of Health Care

Sword of Damocles

PAYOR

PATIENT

EMPLOYER

PROVIDER

Cost

Quality   Access

Managed Care Quaternion   **Iron Triangle**

Measuring the ineffable balance between healthcare paradigms

Figure 28–2 Parity of Health Care

in developing health policy between Coppola's Quaternion and Kissick's Iron Triangle since each actor persists in setting priorities in a mutually exclusive and competitive manner.

Payor	Patient
Cost-Quality-Access	Access-Cost-Quality
Access-Cost-Quality	Quality-Access-Cost
Quality-Access-Cost	Quality-Cost-Access
Quality-Cost-Access	Access-Quality-Cost
Access-Quality-Cost	Cost-Access-Quality
Cost-Access-Quality	Cost-Quality-Access
Employer	**Provider**
Access-Quality-Cost	Quality-Cost-Access
Cost-Access-Quality	Access-Quality-Cost
Cost-Quality-Access	Cost-Access-Quality
Access-Cost-Quality	Cost-Quality-Access
Quality-Access-Cost	Access-Cost-Quality
Quality-Cost-Access	Quality-Access-Cost

Figure 28–3 Parity of Health Care Competing Priorities

Since each actor must prioritize issues of cost, quality and access in health care decision making, and when one actor's priorities are not in sync with another actor's health care objectives, stress, competition and frailty of relationships is always the outcome.

From a reductionist point of view, consider that a payer may view priorities of "cost, quality, and access" as a primary hierarchy and expectation standard when receiving care. In this regard, the payer seeks to achieve low out-of-pocket costs while simultaneously seeking satisfactory quality outcomes. However, in this scenario, the payer is willing to trade reasonable access priorities to obtain low-cost care and satisfactory quality (since quality outcomes were a secondary issue to costs).

To completely understand this model, it is important to view the complexity of Coppola's Parity of Health Care through the lens of a different Quaternion actor. For example, a payer's goals may be out of sync with the employer's goal if an employer is primarily concerned with the time away from work an individual is forced to take to receive care. In this perspective, the employer—who may be a middle manager or first line supervisor—does not see the advantage of low cost or high quality care. He or she may only be focused on the fact that it took 3 days for a patient to get the appointment—and the final appointment resulted in 3 hours away from the normal work day. In an instance like this, payers and employers have competing views of priorities. In a worst-case scenario, each actor may engage in machination and subterfuge to superimpose individual actor priorities on the other. Such actions rarely result in positive outcomes in regards to efficient and effective delivery of health care.

Compounding the complicated relationship between actors and priorities is the Sword of Damocles. In Greek mythology, the Sword of Damocles represents "ever-present peril." It is also used as a metaphor to suggest a "frailty in existing relationships." For example, in the parity of health care, the Sword of Damocles represents an inability of any one actor to reach sustained consensus reference priorities of cost, quality, and access. With health care priorities constantly changing because of environmental demands, it is no wonder that agreements on health care policy are difficult to reach. However, an understanding of the parity of health care can be helpful in the military health system for strategically forecasting threats to relationships amid actors—and also balancing priorities among actors.

Kissick's Iron Triangle has been used by civilian health care leaders for more than a decade to guide strategic plans, vision, and mission statements. Optimally, it is every health care leader's intent to deliver high-quality care, while increasing access to services and simultaneously lowering costs. However, as health leaders try to make improvements in one area, there is often a trade-off consideration in another area. For instance, increasing access to pharmacy benefits by opening an after-hours pharmacy window might improve access and be seen as a quality initiative, however, it might not generate enough new revenue to pay for itself. As a result, civilian health care leaders must make careful executions with new policy ideas or agendas to maintain an effective balance between health care costs, quality, and access. The same has not always been true in the military health care system.

The military health system operates in a unique cost environment. Military treatment facilities operate in a typical government fiscal bureaucracy. Under this paradigm, health care dollars are allocated to the military treatment facility at the beginning of the fiscal year on October 1. The hospital commander (similar to a civilian hospital CEO) is then encouraged to spend all the allocated monies prior to September 30 of the following year. Typically, hospital commanders attempt to exhaust all allocated dollars by the end of August—and then request more year-end funds. Under this federal bureaucracy and paradigm, military health leaders have little incentive to conserve resources, seek synergies, or save money. All money not used by September 30 of the fiscal year is lost. Ironically, then, commanders and health leaders failing to spend all their allocated dollars may be considered poor financial managers under this paradigm. However, a significant advantage of this philosophy is that military treatment facilities are able to consider aspects of quality and access over costs in many cases.

A similar disconnect exists between the military and civilian perspective of the Managed Care Quaternion. The challenge with civilian health care professionals in regards to employers, patients, providers, and payers is in maintaining high satisfaction with each actor along the continuum of care as they relate to aspects of cost, quality, and access. For example, in regards to quality, a primary care clinic without extended and weekend office hours may be regarded as low quality to the patient and employer but high quality to the payer and by the providers that work in the clinic. However, if employers and patients continue to perceive lack of extended and weekend office hours as low quality, dissatisfaction with the overall health plan may result. A worst-case scenario might result in the termination of the health contract. As a result, civilian health professionals are in a constant struggle to maintain high satisfaction with all elements of the Managed Care Quaternion. Until the terrorist attacks of September 11, 2001 (9/11), the same situation may not have existed in the military health system.

In regards to the military health system, all elements of the Managed Care Quaternion are controlled by a single entity—the Department of Defense. The employer is the military, the patients are all employees or beneficiaries of the military, the provider of care is the military (or a federally contracted agent), and the payer is the federal government. Until 9/11, this placed the military health system in a unique situation where it was able to focus attention and resources on matters of self-interest first rather than key stakeholder and actor priorities. However, since 9/11 and the Global War on Terror, priorities have changed.

Since 9/11, Congress closely monitors military health care budgets and major health care expenditures. Although military treatment facilities still operate on a 12-month exhaustible account, military treatment facility budgets are closely reviewed for superfluous spending. Additionally, under a revised financing initiative, military treatment facilities only are allocated funds based on the number of enrolled beneficiaries and workload produced. Additionally, as the retiree and beneficiary population continues to increase from its current standing of 9.2 million, non-active duty beneficiaries have found they have a voice in Congress and the power to influence military health policy. The recent passing of the TRICARE for Life and the TRICARE Reserve Select options are only two of the examples of stakeholder influence on the modern military health system.

Finally, the local military hospital commander now finds himself in competition with the local TRICARE network. Because certain classifications of beneficiaries have a choice of en-rolling in TRICARE Prime (care at the local military treatment facility) or choosing TRICARE Extra or Standard (care rendered through the civilian network), for every one patient who elects not to enroll (or disenroll) in TRICARE Prime, the local military treatment facility commander loses money. As a result, contrary to the friendly relationship that existed between the TRICARE contractor and the local military treatment facility in the 1990s, both the TRICARE contractor and the military hospital are competing more and more for the same health care dollars that are associated with every one DOD beneficiary.

As a result, if the military health system is to continue to survive, military health leaders must understand the parity of health care. Furthermore, the military health system must, in essence, discontinue thinking "military" and adopt best practices and processes used by civilian peers. Military health leaders must consider aspects of the Managed Care Quaternion when formulating policy. Additionally, federal health care leaders must consider the consequences of cost, quality, and access to Quaternion actors. Failing to consider the complex relationships associated with the parity of health care will affect the efficiency, effectiveness, and survival of military health care in the future.

CONCLUSION

The military health system operates the oldest form of organized health care delivery in the United States. Originally founded in 1775, the military health system has more than 225 years of experience in the effective operation and delivery of military medicine and management. The success of the military health system is caused in part by its ability to adapt to changes in the internal and external environments to maintain effectiveness. Developing initially as colloquial health programs designed to treat specific categories of beneficiaries and active duty service personnel, the military medical system eventually developed comprehensive direct care and purchased care systems. The purchased care system, called CHAMPUS, provided health care to a large standing military throughout the Cold War era. However, in response to changes in the health care environment, the military developed and implemented TRICARE. TRICARE is the DOD's managed care model that delivers health care to more than 9.2 million beneficiaries.

Although it struggled through its initial growing pains during the late 1990s, the TRICARE program has become a viable model of success. Significant advantages of TRICARE include extremely high-quality care and the lowest out-of-pocket costs as compared to civilian managed care models. Threats include costs associated with implementing TRICARE, providing care to an aging retiree population, and the additional mission of providing care to select reserve members. Additional threats include a loss of stakeholder satisfaction and the stretching of scarce military health assets and dollars. Finally, the military health system is grappling to achieve equifinality with Coppola's *Parity of Health Care*. However, if past success predicts future behavior, the military health system will continue to be a relevant and ready health care entity for the rest of the century.

ACKNOWLEDGMENTS

The authors wish to thank the Army-Baylor classes of 2005, 2006 and Army-Baylor Students Eric McClung, Joseph Edger, and Joe Phillips for earlier contributions to this chapter. A portion of this chapter was adapted from Boyer JF, Sobel LS. CHAMPUS and the Department of Defense managed care programs. In: Kongstvedt PR, ed. *The Managed Health Care Handbook*. 3rd ed. Gaithersburg, Md: Aspen Publishers, 1996.

DISCLOSURE

The opinions or assertions contained herein are the private view of the authors and are not to be considered as official policy or position or as reflecting the views of the Department of Defense or the United States government.

References

1. Joint Chiefs of Staff. Policy Memorandum of Policy No. 172. Pentagon, Washington, DC: 1983.

2. Bailey S. Key note address. Presented at: TRICARE Conference. Washington, DC: 1999.

3. Coppola MN. *Correlates of Military Medical Treatment Facility (MTF) Performance: Measuring Technical Efficiency with the Structural Adaptation to Regain Fit (SARFIT) Model and Data Envelopment Analysis (DEA)*. Doctoral dissertation. August 2003. Medical College of Virginia Campus, Virginia Commonwealth University, Richmond, VA.

4. Gillett MC. *The Army Medical Department 1775–1818*. Washington, DC: Government Printing Office, 1981.

5. Military Healthcare Reclamation Group. Detailed history of healthcare issues. White Paper. Military Grass Roots Group Priorities 2003/4 (Tab E); 2002. Available at: http://rebel.212.net/mhcrg/tabe.htm. Accessed February 15, 2004.

6. Burrelli DF. *Report for Congress on Military Healthcare: The Issue of "Promised" Benefits*. 2002. Congressional Research Service Publication No. 98-1006F, Library of Congress, Washington, DC.

7. Government Accountability Office. *DOD's Managed Care Program Continues to Face Challenges*. GAO, Washington, DC: 1995.

8. Zwanziger J, Hart KD, Kravitz RL, Sloss EM. Evaluating large and complex demonstrations: The CHAMPUS reform initiative experience. *Health Serv Res*. 2001:35(6), 1229–1244.

9. Boyer JF, Sobel LS. CHAMPUS and the Department of Defense managed care programs. In: Kongstvedt PR, ed. *The Managed Health Care Handbook*. 3rd ed. Gaithersburg, MD: Aspen, 1996.

10. Sloss EM, Hosek SD, *Beneficiary Access and Satisfaction*. Santa Monica, CA: RAND National Defense Research Institute. 1993. *Evaluation of the CHAMPUS Reform Initiative,* Vol. 2, R-4244/2-HA.

11. RAND National Defense Research Institute. *Evaluation of the CHAMPUS Reform Initiative.* Vols. 3 and 6. Santa Monica, CA: RAND National Defense Research Institute. 1993 and 1994. R-4244/3-HA and R-4244/6-HA.

12. TRICARE Management Activity Policy Memo. TRICARE Management Activity Sky 5, Suite 810, 5111 Leesburg Pike, Falls Church, VA 22041-3206 Washington, DC, 2003.

13. TRICARE Management Activity Policy Memo. TRICARE Management Activity Sky 5, Suite 810, 5111 Leesburg Pike, Falls Church, VA 22041-3206 Washington, DC, 2005.

14. TRICARE Management Activity Policy Memo. TRICARE Management Activity Sky 5, Suite 810, 5111 Leesburg Pike, Falls Church, VA 22041-3206 Washington, DC, 2006.

15. TRICARE Stakeholders' Report. Vol. I. 1999. A report to the people who care about TRICARE. Available at: http://www.tricare.osd.mil/stakeholders/default.cfm. Accessed March 6, 2004.

16. Mientka M. TRICARE for Life in need of supplemental. *US Medicine*, 2021 L Street, #400, Washington, DC April 2001 Available at: http://www.google.de/search?hl = de&q = %22TRICARE + for + Life + in + need + of + supplemental%22&btnG = Google-Suche&meta. Accessed February 22, 2004.

17. Coppola MN, Hudak R, Gidwani P. A theoretical perspective utilizing resource dependency to predict issues with the repatriation of Medicare eligible military beneficiaries back into TRICARE. *Military Medicine*. 2002:167(9), 726–731.

18. Public Law 569, The Dependants Medical Care Act (37 USC, Chapter 7). 1956.

19. The Retired Enlisted Association (TREA). July, 2001. *History of Lost Benefits The Creation of the Military Health Care System.* Unpublished white paper. Legislative Affairs Office, 909 North Washington Avenue, Suite 301A.

20. National Defense Authorization Act of 2001.

21. U.S. Medicine Institute. *TRICARE for Life— Roundtable Forum Addressing the Impact of Provisions of the National Defense Authorization Act for 2001.* Washington, DC: Charles Sumner Museum and Archives. January 16, 2001.

22. TRICARE Management Activity Policy Memo. TRICARE Management Activity Sky 5, Suite 810, 5111 Leesburg Pike, Falls Church, VA 22041-3206 Washington, DC, 2004.

23. Gillette B. Vulnerable system no longer taking chances on claims. *Managed Healthcare Executive*. February 2003:38–39.

24. Coppola MN. *Essay on the Managed Care Quaternion* (unpublished). Fort Sam Houston, San Antonio, Texas, 2004.

25. Kissick WL. *The Past is Prologue in Medicine's Dilemmas: Infinite Needs versus Finite Resources*. New Haven, CT: Yale University Press, 1994.

29

Managed Care in a Global Context

Jonathan P. Weiner, Joanna Case Famadas, Hugh Waters, and Djordje Gikic

Study Objectives

- Understand, compare, and contrast the financing and organization of the U.S. health care system with the health care infrastructures in other selected nations.
- Understand paradigms and typologies useful in framing a global comparative analysis in the managed care arena.
- Understand some of the international experience to date of U.S. managed care companies and U.S. inspired, but locally grown, managed care models.
- Identify and understand some of the promises and pitfalls of U.S. style managed care for other nations in the arenas of financing, organization, and care management.

Discussion Topics

1. Discuss what types of system measures/indicators are used to describe the financing and organization of health care systems. What do these measures tell us about different systems? What other information would you like to have?
2. Discuss some of the aspects of one or more international health care systems of interest to you and discuss how they provide an opportunity or challenge for systems organized using managed care principles.
3. Discuss what some of the biggest challenges are that U.S. MCOs have faced in operating abroad. What are some of the ways that these MCOs have dealt with these challenges?
4. Discuss some of the current opportunities for U.S. MCOs abroad. If you were the CEO of a U.S. MCO that had decided to operate abroad, what type of services would you try to offer? Why?

> **5. Discuss what you think U.S. MCOs and policymakers can learn from other health care systems.**

INTRODUCTION

This is the global century. Although more "local" than other sectors, health care must increasingly be viewed from a global perspective. International boundaries are becoming porous; on a daily basis health-related goods, information, staff, financial capital, services, patients, pathogens, and of course, ideas and innovations are exchanged. The global dimension has implications for U.S. providers of health care and health insurance.

This chapter provides an international context for the readers of this book wishing to learn more about U.S. managed health care. This chapter is relevant to Americans who want to share their knowledge or services with other nations, or who believe they will be affected in one way or another by events in the global health care community. Also, this chapter is designed to facilitate the uptake of this book's many lessons for persons in other nations wishing to learn from the U.S. managed care experience. Perhaps less obvious, but also important, we believe that those leading the U.S. managed care industry have something to gain by stepping back and comparing and contrasting our system to those in other lands.

Cross-national comparative analysis of multiple health care systems is not an easy undertaking. Therefore, the goals of this chapter of necessity must be broad-brush. The specific objectives we have set for this chapter include discussion of the various types of health systems around the globe, the role, or potential role, of managed care in other nations, the experience of U.S. managed care companies abroad, and future opportunities for the cross-national export of managed care methods.

This chapter focuses on issues and frameworks useful in the United States and other developed nations. However, given the rapid economic and health sector development of middle- and lower-income nations as well as the logarithmic growth of the middle class in such places as China and India, we believe aspects of this analysis are relevant in a wide variety of countries.

As described in detail in Chapter 1, managed care organizations (MCOs; see also Chapter 2 for more detailed descriptions of different types of MCOs) were developed in the United States largely as a response to escalating health care costs. Like "traditional" health insurers (such as Blue Cross Blue Shield plans), most MCOs function as third-party payers in the employer-based health system, but unlike traditional insurers, many MCOs, and health maintenance organizations (HMOs) in particular, have legal responsibility for both the financing and delivery of care.[1] The structure of MCOs has evolved and become diverse, but the core functions of managed care include the sharing and management of financial risk, development and management of provider networks, management of service utilization, care management, and—increasingly—the management of information flow as well as quality and outcome measurement; all of these operational issues are described and discussed in detail in other chapters of this book. Although managed care is sometimes considered a uniquely American invention, all public and private health systems around the globe face similar trade-offs between cost, quality, access, and ever increasing consumer needs and demands.

In the United States, we tend to think of an MCO as a private, often investor-owned organization with which employers or governments contract to provide health care to an enrolled population. Among health econ-omists in the United States and internation-ally, much has been written about the potential competition that can ensue when MCOs vie for consumers in a given market.[2,3] Over the years, there has been substantial international interest, at least among market-oriented parties, in the importation of MCO-based American-style competition.[3,4]

Today, witnessing the run-away costs in the United States, less than stellar health out-comes, and strong public sentiments asso-ciated with the "managed care backlash" described in Chapter 1, policymakers and managers in other developed nations are not so keen on adopting U.S. models on a whole-sale basis. Rather, they tend to be interested in the possibility of carefully grafting selected managed care tools onto their existing uni-versal government or social insurance mod-els. Although not without controversy, some policymakers in Canada, Europe, and other high-income nations are calling for the ex-pansion of private health insurance as a way to supplement or complement universally available, publicly provided or coordinated programs. This "topping up" is especially ap-pealing to higher-income members of soci-ety, who may wish to purchase coverage for services beyond the basic levels of care. In emerging markets and middle-income coun-tries with rapidly growing economies, the possibility of using private sector health plans as a vehicle for increasing the middle class's investment in the health sector, while allowing government to focus on care for those with lower incomes, is also gaining some degree of attention.[5] We explore these types of potential cross-national exchange is-sues in this chapter.

A QUICK AROUND-THE-WORLD REVIEW OF HEALTH CARE

Financing and Organization

Before proceeding, we offer a high-level overview of how major nations structure and finance their health care delivery systems.

For selected nations from several continents, Table 29-1 presents some key demographic, economic, and health care cost descriptors, illustrating the diversity of economies and sources and levels of health care system fi-nancing around the world. This table not only summarizes the size of the overall and health care economies, it also offers some basic markers of the health of these nations.

Basic System Structure and Health Levels

The first column of Table 29-1 presents the in-come of each country in gross domestic prod-uct (GDP) per capita in U.S. dollars, measured in purchasing parity units, and the second shows the size of the country's population. Columns 3 and 4 show health outcomes in terms of life expectancy at birth and the rate of child (under age 5) mortality. Column 5 pre-sents total estimated health care expenditure per capita from all sources capita (in U.S. $), and column 6 presents this figure as a per-centage of the nation's GDP. Although low-income countries with low health care outlays tend to have poor health measures, as has of-ten been observed, among higher-income countries there is not always a strong correla-tion between spending on health and health outcomes. For example, the life expectancy and child mortality outcomes of Singapore, Australia, and the United Kingdom are all sig-nificantly better than the U.S. outcomes al-though the resources spent on health care per capita in those countries are from one-third to one-half of what the United States spends (and these countries insure all residents, un-like the United States).

The remaining columns of Table 29-1 focus on the role of government and nongovern-mental sources in financing health care. Column 7 shows the percentage from all non-governmental sources. Column 7 (used as the base) is broken down further in the next two columns into the two major "private" compo-nents: column 8 presents the percentage of total outlays that is paid out-of-pocket from consumers, and column 9 shows the same for prepaid plans. This includes various social in-surance funds (generally sponsored by unions

Table 29-1 Economic and Health Indicators for Selected Countries

	(1)	(2)	(3)	(4)	(5)	(6)	(7)	(8)	(9)	(10)	(11)
Country	GDP per capita, PPP (current int'l $)	Total Population (millions)	Life Expectancy at Birth (years)	Under-5 Mortality Rate (per 1,000)	Health Expenditure per Capita (current US $)	Total Expenditure on Health as proportion of GDP	Private Expenditure on Health as proportion of Total Expenditure on Health	Out-Of-Pocket Expenditure as proportion of Total Expenditure on Health	Private Prepaid Plans as proportion of Total Expenditure on Health	General Government Expenditure Health as proportion of Total Expenditure on Health	% of Population Covered by Government/ Social Insurance (OECD countries)
Argentina	$13,298	38	74.6	18.2	$305	0.089	0.514	0.286	0.196	0.486	—
Australia	$30,331	20	79.9	5.5	$2,519	0.095	0.325	0.220	0.078	0.675	100.0
Austria	$32,276	8	79.2	4.9	$2,358	0.075	0.324	0.192	0.076	0.676	98.0
Canada	$31,263	32	79.8	5.7	$2,669	0.099	0.301	0.149	0.127	0.699	100.0
Chile	$10,874	16	78.0	8.4	$282	0.061	0.512	0.237	0.275	0.488	—
China	$5,896	1,296	71.4	31.0	$61	0.056	0.638	0.559	0.037	0.362	—
Czech Republic	$19,408	10	75.7	4.4	$667	0.075	0.100	0.084	0.003	0.900	100.0
France	$29,300	60	80.2	4.6	$2,981	0.101	0.237	0.100	0.127	0.763	99.9
Germany	$28,303	82	78.5	4.7	$3,204	0.111	0.218	0.104	0.088	0.782	89.8
Hungary	$16,814	10	72.6	8.0	$684	0.084	0.276	0.245	0.006	0.724	100.0
India	$3,139	1,080	63.5	85.2	$27	0.048	0.752	0.729	0.007	0.248	—
Japan	$29,251	128	81.8	3.8	$2,662	0.079	0.190	0.171	0.003	0.810	100.0
Mexico	$9,803	104	75.1	27.6	$372	0.062	0.536	0.505	0.031	0.464	51.0
Netherlands	$31,789	16	78.7	5.6	$3,088	0.098	0.376	0.078	0.172	0.624	76.3
New Zealand	$23,413	4	79.2	6.5	$1,618	0.081	0.217	0.156	0.058	0.783	100.0
Singapore	$28,077	4	79.3	3.3	$964	0.045	0.639	0.620	0.000	0.361	—
South Africa	$11,192	45	44.6	67.0	$295	0.084	0.614	0.105	0.477	0.386	—
Sweden	$29,541	9	80.5	3.7	$3,149	0.094	0.148	0.136	0.003	0.852	100.0
Switzerland	$33,040	7	81.1	5.1	$5,035	0.115	0.415	0.315	0.090	0.585	100.0
United Kingdom	$30,821	60	78.5	5.8	$2,428	0.080	0.143	0.110	0.033	0.857	100.0
United States	$39,676	294	77.4	7.6	$5,711	0.152	0.554	0.135	0.365	0.446	26.6
Uruguay	$9,421	3	75.2	17.0	$323	0.098	0.728	0.182	0.546	0.272	—

Source: Columns 1–5: 2006 World Development Indicators; Columns 6–10: 2006 World Health Report; Column 11: OECD Health Data 2006; data generally from 2002–2005 period.

and other social collectives) as well as private sector health insurance companies and managed care plans that are usually considered distinct from private social insurance funds. (The structure and role of private insurance are discussed in greater detail later in this chapter.) For example, take the first row for Argentina: a bit more than half of all non-governmental outlays (which represent 51.4% of all health care costs in that nation) are made up of direct payments. So, for Argentina, it is estimated that about 29% of all health care outlays are paid for out-of-pocket.

Column 10 presents the approximate percentage that the government-sponsored health care or health insurance represents of the total outlay for health care, and column 11 shows the percentage of the population covered by such programs, where available.

Tables like this one can be used to make broad comparisons between countries. For example, Singapore and New Zealand have similar population sizes and GDP per capita, but New Zealand spends almost twice as much as Singapore on health, in absolute terms. In addition, New Zealand health expenditures are financed primarily by the government, whereas private expenditures compose the bulk of Singapore's health spending. Moreover, Singapore compares quite favorably with New Zealand in terms of life expectancy and under-5 child mortality, two common health indicators. This comparison illustrates that there is no one "right" way to design a health system.

For U.S. readers not familiar with such broad comparisons as outlined in Table 29-1, the difference between the U.S. system and those of other high-income countries on this list is stark. The U.S. spends more than any other nation, both per capita and in terms of percentage of GDP, our health outcome measures are middling, and we are the only high-income nation on the list without universal, or nearly universal, coverage.

The Role of Private Insurance

In this single chapter, it is not feasible to discuss even this limited subset of 22 health care systems along all dimensions. However, it is our objective to add to the reader's understanding of these selected systems by categorizing them along several organizational and functional dimensions relevant to this chapter's discussion on health care delivery, financing, and care management. Table 29-2 extends upon the information presented in Table 29-1 by offering a categorization of the type of health care system financing and management found in each nation as well as the role and estimated market share of private (non-social insurance) health care companies.

Although there are many variations within each category, the first dimension on Table 29-2 (column 1) classifies the system by whether it is primarily government-sponsored, run by independent or quasi-independent social insurance funds, or the private health insurance sector. Each of these types of systems is described in greater detail.

The *government-sponsored systems* include both systems where many or most providers are employees or contractors of a government (or quasi-governmental) entity (for example, the United Kingdom and Sweden), as well as "single" payer models (such as Canada) where national or regional government reimburses independent providers. Most systems of this type have compulsory universal coverage, financed from general government revenues. Health care delivery in these countries is generally organized around distinct geographic administrative units, which have the added value of providing the potential (not always realized) of a population-based orientation, based on place of residence.

In a *social insurance model*, health care is predominantly financed through payroll taxes rather than general taxation. Purchasing social insurance may be mandatory for a designated population, but eligibility is based on payment of a contribution (ie, insurance premium) usually linked to the place of employment. Social insurance is not a right of every citizen, and social insurance programs are financially autonomous and must maintain solvency. Social insurance funds are generally not-for-profit collectives (sometimes

Table 29-2 Summary of System Structure and Role of Private Insurance in Selected Countries

Country	(1) Primary Type of Health System	(2) Main Administrator(s)	(3) Role of Private Insurance	(4) Est. % with Private Primary/Secondary Health Insurance
Argentina	Private sector/government sponsored	Private plans and social insurance funds	Primary/supplementary	NA
Australia	Government sponsored	Regional and national government	Complementary and supplementary	0%/45%
Austria	Social insurance	Regional government	Complementary and supplementary	0.1%/31.8%
Canada	Government sponsored	Regional government	Supplementary	0%/65%
Chile	Social insurance	Private plans and social insurance funds	Primary/supplementary	34%/NA
China	Private sector/government sponsored	None/national government	None	0%/0%
Czech Republic	Social insurance	National government	None	0%/0%
France	Social insurance	Social insurance funds	Complementary and supplementary	0%/92%
Germany	Social insurance	Social insurance funds	Primary/complementary and supplementary	9%/9%
Hungary	Social insurance	National government	None	0%/0%
India	Private sector	None/national government	Primary	NA
Japan	Social insurance	Social insurance funds	None	0%/0%
Mexico	Social insurance/private sector	National government/private plans	Supplementary	NA*/2.8%
Netherlands	Social insurance	Private plans and social insurance funds	Primary/complementary	28%/64%
New Zealand	Government Sponsored	National government/QUANGOs	Complementary/supplementary	0% / 35%
Singapore	Government Sponsored/mixed	National government	Primary/supplementary	NA
South Africa	Government Sponsored/mixed	Government/private plans	Primary/supplementary	NA

Sweden	Government Sponsored	Regional and national government	Complementary and supplementary	0%/1-1.5 %
Switzerland	Social Insurance	Private plans and social insurance funds	Primary/supplementary	0%/80%
United Kingdom	Government Sponsored	QUANGOs/national government	Supplementary	0%/10%
United States	Private sector/government sponsored	Private plans/national and regional government	Primary/supplementary	72%/7%**
Uruguay	Private Sector/government sponsored	Private plans and social insurance funds	Primary/supplementary	NA

Definitions: Government-sponsored, government provides care or is the sole payer for care; social insurance, compulsory participation or contribution in health insurance scheme for designated population; private sector, reliance on individuals and private corporations for the purchase and provision of health insurance; QUANGO, quasi-autonomous nongovernmental organizations; NA, data not available.

*In Mexico, many people choose to pay out-of-pocket for medical care rather than purchase insurance.

**In the United States, supplementary private insurance includes private plans contracting with the government Medicare program for the elderly.

Source: Organisation for Economic Co-operation and Development. *Private Health Insurance in OECD Countries.* Paris, France: OECD, 2004.

known as "sickness funds") often linked to unions or political parties. Under these models, government directly provides care or subsidizes the premiums for those who cannot afford the payments on their own (such as persons who are unemployed, poor, or disabled). Examples of countries with social insurance systems include Germany and Japan. Several other countries, such as France, have "hybrid" health insurance systems that are primarily based on social insurance but also incorporate substantive elements paid through general taxation and private insurance.

Only a few countries in the world have national systems based primarily or heavily on multiple private insurers mixed with government insurance providers. Among high-income countries, a national system based on multiple private insurers exists only in the United States; even in the United States, public sources account for 45% of health expenditures nationwide.[6] Other nations with a substantial private insurance market include Chile, South Africa, and the Philippines.

Although the sources of health care financing are key, so too are the structure and locus of the management of care and resources. Column 2 of Table 29-2 provides a summary of the type of administrative entity that dominates the key policy and management decisions. This has implications for whether and how the various managed care tools described in this book might be applicable. The most common administrators of health benefits include national government, regional government, social insurance funds, private insurers/MCOs, and quasi-autonomous nongovernmental management units, such as locally controlled Primary Care Trusts in the United Kingdom.[7]

Categorizing health systems in this way can be challenging, particularly for countries with no nationalized system. In Mexico, for example, although almost all of the population has access to some basic health services, many Mexicans choose to pay out-of-pocket for health services because of dissatisfaction with the public programs.[8] The system is thus divided among the social security system, the government program for the uninsured, and the private sector, with none having a dominant role.

Even in countries with universal, national systems, private insurance may play a significant role; columns 3 and 4 of Table 29-2 provide a summary of the role and scope of private insurance in this subset of countries. The role of private insurance is classified in one of three ways: (1) "primary" plan or as a *substitute* for the public program (ie, where enrollees opt out of an available public plan); (2) as a *complement* to public programs (ie, where consumer out-of-pocket outlays for the government program's co-insurance is reimbursed); or (3) as a *supplement* to public programs (ie, where excluded services, such as private providers not affiliated with the public system, are covered). The latter two types of secondary coverage are sometimes referred to as "topping-up" above and beyond the publicly available plan.

Column 4 provides an estimate of the percentage of the resident population of each country that relies on private insurance on a primary or secondary basis. Note that nonnationals in the country (such as U.S. expatriates) who may have private insurance as a primary type of coverage are not included in these figures. It is estimated that there are hundreds of thousands of Americans with such coverage. Although difficult to count, individuals working for American companies are increasingly insured by a number of U.S. and global insurance companies in a similar fashion.

The wide variety of approaches to paying and organizing health care provide many opportunities for managed care approaches and organizations. But this also adds significantly to the complexity involved in assessing the scope, appropriateness, and viability of those opportunities around the globe. The diversity also complicates—but does not eliminate—the lessons that we can learn from some of these settings.

EXPORTING MANAGED CARE

There are many opportunities around the globe for the application of managed care models and tools. This section discusses the international experiences of U.S. private health insurers and MCOs and local entities patterned after them. We address challenges, opportunities, and recent history in both middle-income and high-income nations.

Managed Care as a Tool for Development

The most common approach to health financing in lower-income countries is direct out-of-pocket consumer payments to doctors, hospitals, and other providers. Although some level of out-of-pocket payments may be needed in any health system to prevent overutilization (what economists term "moral hazard"), out-of-pocket payments are generally a regressive type of financing and one that leaves the most vulnerable groups particularly susceptible to financial shocks. As a nation's economy progresses (for example, China) public sector insurance schemes are introduced and they generally struggle to find enough resources to provide basic coverage to all of the population. Many believe that the introduction of private insurance in this context allows the public sector to focus on delivering services that benefit the people most in need, while those that can do so (generally the middle class) purchase coverage on their own.[9-12] Thus, in countries with growing middle classes, MCOs can play a complementary role to the public system. These "complementary" plans can be purchased either by employers or the individuals themselves.

An interesting case is the Philippines where unsuccessful attempts were made in 1978 to establish the first HMO. However, a few years later five HMOs were created, a number that has since grown to about 35 companies.[13] This growth occurred without government regulation or promotion, but rather through private sector initiatives. The primary driving force was the need for financial access to quality heath services in the private sector. A mechanism for risk pooling was strongly needed in the private sector, as opposed to the public sector, where free medical care was being dispensed generally to the poor. As in many lower-income countries, the Philippines has limited resources for health care and spends just 3.2% of its GDP on health.[6] With the introduction of managed care, HMO enrollees can now access private providers without risking bankruptcy. In addition, the government was able to reallocate its limited resources and strengthen its programs for the poor.

Although there is great opportunity for private plans to play a role in the expansion of access to affordable care in middle-income developing nations, among some camps there is concern that the problem of limited management capacities in these developing countries will only be exacerbated by the expansion of the private sector and the need to regulate it. For example, managers may leave the public sector to work for these private plans, and some of the remaining ones will need to devote time to regulating the private plans rather than managing care for the poor.

On the flip side, as one managed care company may become an alternative insurer in a developing nation, another may choose to offer its expertise to government to help regulate the growing private sector. Private companies usually have good institutional capacity, well-developed information systems, and skills that can be transferred to the public sector to help in this regulation process to enable them to more effectively manage expanding publicly funded schemes.

Case Study: Managed Care in Chile

The Chilean health system[14] is financed through the public National Health Fund (FONASA) and a group of regulated private insurers (ISAPREs). Since reforms put into place in 1982, employed individuals not otherwise covered are required to contribute 7% of their income to FONASA or to purchase health insurance from an ISAPRE. The ISAPREs currently cover approximately 20% of the population (increased from 2% in 1983); 67% of the population is covered by FONASA. The remainder either lacks health insurance or obtains it through completely private coverage.

The ISAPREs offer subscribers and their dependants a package of health services, subject to copayments, in their own health care facilities or through contracts with other providers. Affiliates pay the obligatory 7% salary deduction and may also make additional payments to improve the coverage of their plan. The ISAPREs also receive a series of public subsidies. One of these is a tax rebate to employers, who contribute an additional 2% of payroll to complement the compulsory 7% salary deduction used to pay ISAPRE premiums for low-income employees. Other subsidies correspond to public health programs—maternity leave payments, free distribution of vaccines, and food supplementation products to ISAPREs' members.

In 1990, the *Superintendencía de las ISAPRES* was created as a regulatory body. The ISAPREs must set premiums at community rates—by age, sex, and family size. Other private insurance companies offer differentiated plans that vary according to the premium paid and the health risk of the insured family. For those covered by FONASA, contributions are calculated based on income. Individuals may move between FONASA and the ISAPREs. The Ministry of Health, which supervises the private insurance system through the *Superintendencía de las ISAPREs*, regulates both subsectors. The ISAPREs offer a wide range of premiums, copayments, and coverage plans; there are many thousands of different coverage plans. As of October 2004, there were 16 active ISAPREs.

Several ISAPREs have implemented a type of managed care using networks of preferred private health providers paid on a fee-for-service basis. In some cases, ISAPRE affiliates are also referred to public health facilities, in which case the ISAPRE must reimburse the public sector for the care.

The Chilean health care system is subject to adverse selection, as seen from the income distribution between FONASA and the ISAPREs. In 2003, FONASA covered 90.9% of individuals in the first (poorest) income quintile, compared to 33.2% in the fifth (wealthiest) quintile. This trend is reversed for the ISAPREs, which cover just 1.6% of the population in the first quintile compared to 51.2% in the wealthiest, according to analyses of the Chilean Socioeconomic Household Survey (CASEN).

Managed Care within Developed Health Care Systems

For a number of decades some market-oriented policymakers within most developed nations have suggested that competing health insurance plans, patterned after U.S. MCOs, would offer certain benefits to most socialized models of care. In addition, even without the introduction of competing MCO-like plans, many policymakers believe there are many opportunities to learn from the methods applied by private health insurance and managed care organizations.

Over the last several decades, the belief that efficiency in health care can be improved through competition has led several nations to introduce elements of competition via what is sometimes termed "internal markets." According to this school of thought, properly regulated competition leads to more efficient use of resources, controls health care expenditures, and improves quality.[2,3] For example, in a national health system, independent or semi-independent plans or sickness funds could offer additional services, price reductions, and/or higher quality services on top of mandated benefits.

One difficulty with the introduction of such competition is the temptation for "cream-skimming" or "gaming" to attract healthier members than average. Recent experience in Israel revealed that instead of focusing on improving clinical quality and efficiency, the competing sickness funds emphasized improvements in customer amenities and overly aggressive marketing tactics.[15] In Germany, when the sickness fund playing field was made more competitive, the health plans with the lowest premium costs (and not necessarily the most comprehensive services) had the largest increase in members.[16] This event lead to the introduction of a risk-adjusted transfer of revenue between sickness funds to account for adverse risk selection.

For several reasons, the results of introducing competition into government-sponsored health care have not been as dramatic as proponents might have hoped.[3] First, because the allocation of monies by government is based on average cost, unless risk adjustment is put in place (as Germany and Netherlands have done) sickness funds try to select members with the lowest risk, threatening the integrity of the system. Second, there is limited opportunity to influence quality and efficiency of health care because provider payments and practices are heavily regulated and thus plans may not be able to offer appropriate incentives to clinicians. In other words, to achieve efficiency and effectiveness gains, these competing health insurance plans ideally need the flexibility to influence providers in a number of ways. This flexibility may be limited by system structure, such as the availability of providers, the mix of doctor specialties, and lack of non-inpatient alternatives (*eg*, ambulatory surgery).[3] Finally, the higher administrative costs of a system with multiple competing plans is often troublesome to policymakers. These extra transaction costs need to ultimately be shown to translate to added value, if the devolved competing plans are to be accepted within socialized settings.

To experienced U.S. MCO managers or observers, none of these issues is new; they all are on the list of real or perceived challenges faced over the last few decades in the United States. The good news is that the U.S. managed care community can offer other nations—such as Germany, the United Kingdom, or Israel—some solutions to these issues as they move forward with delivery and financing models that involve alternative risk-bearing health plans or MCO-like entities.

Managed care and health insurance also have considerable international potential, even for those nations with little interest in competing plans. This includes the role of private insurance as a complement, supplement, or even partial substitute for existing government-sponsored systems and also as a source of care management expertise.

In the European Union, private health insurance accounts for less than 5% of total health expenditures but may play a more significant role in individual member states, as illustrated previously in Table 29-2. In France, for example, in 2000 more than 90% of the population had complementary private insurance, which covers services that are excluded or not fully reimbursed by the public system. In the Netherlands, higher-income families, which represent about a quarter of the population, are not eligible to participate in the public system and must purchase private health insurance as a substitute. Finally, those European consumers wanting faster access to elective services and freedom from restrictions can often purchase supplementary private insurance, as more than 10% of the British population do.[17]

Despite the many potential roles for private plans and MCOs outside the United States, in most nations there is more than a bit of anxiety associated with the question of how to balance this privatization with a national commitment to equity and access for all. In part because of this challenge and also because of the limited market potential and other political barriers, few U.S. MCOs have elected to operate independent supplementary or complementary plans as an overlay to the national health program. Rather, U.S. insurers' forays abroad have tended to focus on substitute plans. Another option for managed care companies is not to offer risk-bearing insurance services at all. For example, they can enter into collaborative arrangements where they contract with government agencies (or their agents) to provide management or even clinical services. Given that all nations have a long way to go before they reach optimal care efficiency and effectiveness, appropriate use of managed care may offer some solutions to these issues.

Recent Experience of U.S. Managed Care Abroad

In terms of actual experience, over the past few decades most U.S. MCOs and health insurance companies have found that exporting their product overseas has proved to be extremely challenging. In the late 1990s, faced with a saturated domestic market, many companies looked for markets abroad as a source of growth. During that period, as many as 13 U.S. MCOs had significant business abroad;[4] today only a few still operate those businesses and are now often targeted at U.S. expatriates or for employees working for U.S. companies.

Companies have found that the challenges confronting them abroad are complex and require careful analyses and preparation. They have generally learned to be wary of such an uncertain enterprise and the resource commitment that may be required for success. This section summarizes some of the experiences and lessons learned from the executives and individuals involved in managed care enterprises abroad.

It has been suggested that at the most basic level, prerequisites for success abroad by U.S. companies in the managed care/health insurance domain include the need for health insurance/managed care to be a dedicated line of business (and not a sideline to a broader insurance or financial services offering), strong incentives for local providers to participate, adequate middle-income population of target market consumers, and the ability to collect adequate premiums to build a reasonable infrastructure.[18]

Other experts have suggested a number of other factors that should be considered when developing products for a specific nation. These include the state of the existing provider and health information infrastructures, consumer expectations and preferences, regulatory barriers, and local culture and perceptions associated with private insurance and managed care.[19]

Some of the strengths of U.S. MCOs are claims processing, utilization management, care management, quality improvement, and the design and implementation of provider payment schemes. But implementing these programs is a significant challenge when overlaid onto existing complex systems found in other nations. For example, in most other countries (at least those not yet using electronic medical records), there are few standardized codes that describe services provided. In Argentina, for example, a U.S./local managed care joint venture decided it would be easier to incorporate the Argentine service/procedure coding system into the MCO's claims processing system rather than try to change systems or "translate" between the local and international system.[20] However, the lack of a usable coding infrastructure created great difficulty in getting clinical information from providers and limited the ability of the MCO to implement even the most basic functions of managed care.

The tactical decision of the Argentine joint venture to use the local coding system rather than trying to be an "agent of change" illustrates the importance of recognizing existing institutional power and resistance to change. In Latin America, MCOs often experienced resistance from providers, unions, and political organizations.[21,22] One of the most important sources of power and resistance is the provider community. In the first place, there must be enough providers to support the managed care plans. In addition, plans must be able to build relationships and offer meaningful financial incentives. For example, in many low- and middle-income countries an informal economy (*ie*, off the books) provides sources of income for many providers and other stakeholders; thus, a more formal payment system introduced by an MCO might represent a serious threat to their livelihood. MCOs that fail to take these societal factors into account may face strong resistance from providers.

Like other cross-national business or social policy exchange, cultural sensitivity is essential to export managed care concepts or products successfully. Historically, failures have often been caused by lack of understanding of all facets of the market, often because the local context was viewed through a North American frame of reference.[23] For example, one of the features of managed care is that it frequently requires restrictions on services or consumer choices in exchange for lower costs. If consumers are not ready for this or do not see the benefit of this trade-off, MCO models are not likely to succeed. Although social trade-offs are the norm for many international social welfare programs, some consumers in those settings are wary of such trade-offs in the corporate context. It is not uncommon for international consumers to be uncomfortable with a shift from a view that health care or health insurance is a public good to that of a market commodity.[21] U.S. MCOs doing business abroad must be completely cognizant that there is a delicate balance between corporate and social contexts when it comes to health care in most nations outside the United States.

To the extent that the introduction of managed care results in inequities in access, it may be perceived very poorly in countries that value solidarity. In Argentina, for example, a public hospital provided 1.25 million outpatient visits by elderly patients covered by a privately administered social insurance fund. These patients were denied access to private providers because of nonpayment by the private insurer and some bureaucratic confusion.[24]

Perhaps the greatest challenge MCOs have faced abroad is the negative public perception of managed care. Both internationally and domestically, this has been referred to as "managed care backlash." Even when great efforts are made to be a "good corporate citizen," things do not always go according to plans. For example, UnitedHealth Care engaged in careful analysis before entering the South African market. The MCO formed a joint venture and built up the necessary infrastructure. However this initiative was not successful in large part due to negative media reports promoted—some say for political reasons—by the local South African press. (For more information about this venture, refer to the section titled "Case Study: UnitedHealth Group in South Africa," which follows.)

Case Study: UnitedHealth Group in South Africa

In the early 1990s, UnitedHealth Care Corporation (now UnitedHealth Group) was enjoying domestic success and believed that "its expertise in successfully managing diverse health care systems was an exportable asset." United believed that it understood the importance of adapting to local conditions through its experience with acquiring regional health plans. United's success in this area was a result of its focus on three core competencies: (1) strong centralized financial management, (2) efficient and automated claims-driven data systems, and (3) a doctor-friendly but expert medical managed capability. Internationally, United believed that managed care could reduce costs by reducing the inefficiencies inherent in Western-style scientific and technical medicine and changing the mechanism of coverage decisions to one of medical appropriateness.

After much analysis, United selected South Africa for its foray into international managed care because it believed the health system was most similar to the United States.[22] United formed a joint venture with Southern Life, a South African insurance company, and Anglo American Corporation, a huge mining and financial services conglomerate in South

Africa. The plan for the joint venture was that the South African companies would provide local market expertise, actuarial experience, and local relationships, and United would contribute managed care systems and programs and expertise. At first, responsibilities would be shared, but eventually management would be transferred entirely to the South Africans.

Despite the careful planning and successful implementation of the information system for the new company Southern HealthCare Limited, the joint venture faced several insurmountable challenges, including negative physician response and bad press. When

Anglo American made an independent business decision to divest of its nonmining businesses, the joint venture was effectively abandoned. In the final analysis, several factors have been identified as contributing to the failure: (1) overcommitment of resources, (2) failure to recognize the importance of direct patient pay pharmaceuticals as a source of revenue for South African physicians (this was eliminated in the new plan), (3) failure to gain the support of employers, and (4) lack of cultural sensitivity to the complex racial divide in South Africa, which ultimately led to the failure to gain black physicians' support for the plan.

U.S. Managed Care Abroad

What Happened?

In the 1990s, many managed care companies—including Aetna, CIGNA, United, and several Blue Cross Blue Shield plans—formed joint ventures and attempted to export their managed care plans into other health care systems. They entered markets in Latin America, Asia, and Africa. Although some achieved a measure of success and are still in operation, most U.S. MCOs have abandoned their risk-bearing insurance operations in other nations. The reasons for this trend include the complexity of adapting to local conditions, provider resistance, and anti-American or anti–managed care political sentiment.

What Is Happening Now?

A few U.S. MCOs/insurers have maintained international operations, including CIGNA, and UnitedHealth Group. They offer consulting and administrative services and are involved in a series of local care provision partnerships with local concerns. Their insurance products are limited mainly to U.S. expatriates and those working for U.S. companies abroad. Since globalization of other industries leads to more Americans working abroad, this appears to be a growing business.

What Does the Future Hold?

Although the wholesale exportation of managed care plans has generally not been successful, U.S. MCOs still have a great deal to offer to health systems abroad. In particular, information technology expertise and applications, utilization and care management tools and techniques, and other managed care tools and methodologies that can be more readily adapted to local systems are in demand. Consulting services and smaller joint ventures that can exploit these opportunities will be valuable to MCOs.

MANAGED CARE INTERNATIONALLY: WHERE TO NOW?

Rather than the full-scale exportation of their risk-bearing health insurance product lines, recently MCOs have found more receptive markets for their expertise and managed care tools, such as information technology applications and care management quality-enhancing techniques.

Despite the rocky start that U.S. health insurers and MCOs have experienced with their international exportation attempts (see the box titled "U.S. Managed Care Abroad"), these companies have developed expertise and on-the-ground experience that is of considerable relevance abroad. Several U.S. MCOs are responding to a resurgence in interest in the application of managed care tools by offering global consulting and administrative services. Moreover, many top-notch administrative teams from other nations are developing their own home-grown managed care models based in no small part on the recent experiences of the U.S. companies.

What follows is a discussion of some potential future directions for managed care in a global context, including a framework for analyzing aspects of a nation's health system that are relevant to managed care functions and tools.

Managed Care Readiness and Orientation

As discussed in the first section of this chapter, the financing and organization of health systems can differ greatly from one country to the next. This has significant implications for ways that managed care tools may be integrated into a given nation's system. Table 29-3 provides an assessment of key organizational and structural components of the systems in a subset of nations. This table should be useful to readers who wish to compare and contrast the U.S. managed care and traditional fee-for-service systems to the six other nations in this table. It should also provide a useful framework for assessment that readers may wish to replicate for other nations not included on the list. Specifically, Table 29-3 provides a framework to analyze how selected countries may differ on the following dimensions.

- *Degree of central/regional government control:* Even among national health systems, the degree of control over the health care system that government managers and policymakers can or choose to exert can vary tremendously. This dimension provides an assessment of the extent of control that the central or regional government has over the health care system and care processes relative to other nations being considered here.
- *Current role of private insurance/organizations:* Although there is a variety of potential roles for private insurance plans, this dimension measures the extent to which private plans/organizations play a significant role within each country. The term *private* includes both nongovernmental social insurance funds as well as private insurance or managed care companies.
- *Choice of health plan:* For consumers, the extent of choice they have with respect to which health plans they join plays an important role, both in terms of their satisfaction with the plans and overall health system, and in terms of how plans can compete for larger market share.
- *Choice of provider:* Similarly, consumer choice of provider is an important factor in consumer satisfaction and also the degree to which providers may or may not be affected by market pressures. In most nations, consumers have some choice of a primary care/general practitioner (GP), even if they are limited in their choice of specialists. Thus, this dimension captures the degree to which there is free access to specialists. For example, U.S. MCOs would rate lower on this dimension than traditional fee-for-service indemnity plans would. Also, the

Table 29–3 Characteristics Associated with Managed Care Readiness and Orientation in Selected Nations

	Overall System Structure		Consumers		Providers		Managed Care	
	Degree of Central/Regional Government Control	Autonomy of Health Plan/Management Organization	Choice of Health Plan	Choice of Provider	Degree of Provider/Integration/Organization	Degree of Financial Controls/Incentives	Population Orientation	Use of UR/EBM and Care Management*
United States (FFS/MCO)**	-/-	+/++	++/++	++/+	+/++	+/++	-/++	+/++
United Kingdom	++	+	-	-	+	+	++	+
Chile	+	+	+	+	-	+	-	-
Canada	++	-	-	+	-	-	-	-
Sweden	++	-	-	-	+	+	+	-
Germany	+	-	+	++	-	+	-	-
France	+	-	+	+	-	-	-	-

Key: Relative to other nations:
++ Widespread/very strong.
+ Not uncommon/strong.
– Not widespread/weak.
— Uncommon/very weak.

EBM, evidence-based medicine (eg, practice guidelines); FFS, fee-for-service; MCO, managed care organization; UR, utilization review/utilization management.
*Care management includes disease management and case management programs.
**Note: In the case of the United States, both nonmanaged fee-for-service and MCO-based systems are summarized.

670

rating for Germany, where all consumers have direct access mainly to community-based specialists, is higher than other nations where consumers usually reach specialists via their GPs or have choice of only a handful of alternatives when they go to their regional hospital (where the specialists work on a salaried basis).

- *Degree of provider integration and organization:* The degree of interconnected cohesiveness of function (particularly between primary and specialty care, or ambulatory and hospital care) directly affects care efficiency and effectiveness and is a hallmark of managed care. This concept is not dissimilar to that of the integrated delivery system (IDS) discussed in Chapter 2. The degree to which clinicians and their support structures view themselves as integrated units with singular goals and leadership has great implications for how influential they can be relative to government and health plan administrators. Such organizations can also be primarily political, such as a physician's union that has considerable power or influence.

- *Degree of financial controls and incentives:* This dimension measures the extent to which provider payments and incentives are aligned with health system goals. Examples would include payments to foster preventive care, to minimize the use of medical technology when not clinically appropriate, or to maximize adherence to evidence-based medical guidelines. This dimension attempts to gauge the presence of payer incentives beyond the simple ratcheting down of fees to keep system outlays constrained.

- *Population orientation:* Economists often note the difficulty associated with distributing finite health resources among members of a population. This dimension measures the degree to which each country adopts a population orientation with respect to health care, and public health and epidemiologic principles are joined with economic ones, with the ultimate goal of maximizing benefits across the society (or at least the enrolled group). Population-based systems tend to emphasize primary, preventive, and community-based services and to minimize high-technology services without clear-cut benefit.

- *Use of utilization review, evidence-based medicine, and care management:* Finally, many MCOs and health care systems have adopted guidelines, coordinated (often nurse-led) interventions, and other quality improvement techniques as discussed in Part Three of this book. The ultimate goal is to offer the right services to the right persons in accordance with the best scientific evidence. This dimension gauges the extent to which each country has adopted such techniques.

The assessment along the eight managed care readiness dimensions on Table 29-3 is made both to offer readers more information on these six important countries and also to provide a framework that others can follow when they wish to take stock of the fit between a region's current health care system, relative to the essentials of managed care. This table and the approach it embodies can help identify priority areas or challenges for a nation wishing to adopt various managed care principles. For example the ratings for Canada show that although this system has relatively strong centralized control, very little control or incentives are exerted over providers and few measures have been implemented to integrate providers or manage care. Indeed, this table illustrates how very few countries are currently making full use of care management techniques and evidence-based medicine.

Last for U.S. readers, Table 29-3 provides some examples of where we can turn to learn from other nations; for example, the geographic population-based programs in Sweden and Britain, and the British pay-for-performance and evidence-based coverage and guidelines of care programs are often superior to those found in many U.S. managed care plans. Although not the explicit focus of this chapter, we certainly believe there are numerous lessons for Americans from these and other highly developed health care systems. The Suggested Readings section at the end of this chapter offers many such "lessons in reverse" discussions.

CONCLUSION

Looking forward, we summarize a few likely global trends and their key implications for both the United States and international health care communities.

Given that all high-income developed countries (other than the United States, of course) already provide health insurance for virtually all of their populace, most of the international growth in health insurance enrollment will take place within low- and middle-income nations, particularly where there is a growing middle class. This presents considerable opportunity for the expansion of private health plans in these settings. But this approach is not without controversy; some social policy analysts are troubled by the prospect of parallel delivery systems for those with and without means and by the potential waste associated with the overhead of multiple competing private plans. On the other hand, self-pay or employer-sponsored private health insurance plans may be more efficient and responsive than government programs are, and they can free limited public resources that can best be used to target the programs to those with the greatest need.

Now and forever, it is safe to say that even wealthy countries will never be able to collect enough taxes or insurance premiums to provide all of the health care services that their citizens may need or want. So, policymakers (or consumers) in at least some countries

with universal government-sponsored or mandated health plans are likely to come to the conclusion that supplementary or complementary private health insurance should be fostered (or at least tolerated). Such private sector expansions might represent a possible role for U.S. managed care companies or the transnational partnerships they form.

Even if a nation's health care leaders do not embrace secondary private health plans, with certainty they will still find many useful lessons and practical techniques from within the vast managed care tool kit described throughout this book. As described in this chapter, possible innovations can focus on the care management, provider payment models, or organizational structure. Each of these is a complex and challenging domain.

Although U.S. managed care firms have not had runaway success abroad because of the overwhelming dual challenges of cost containment and optimal quality attainment, the global need for managed care tools and principles remains considerable. The question is not whether managed care approaches will be implemented internationally, but rather which are the most relevant, what processes are required for their local adaptation and implementation, and what the role might be for U.S. managed care organizations.

Whatever the case, the goal of this chapter has been to facilitate the sharing of the tremendous trove of information contained in this book. We have done this by providing a quick comparison of the health care systems of many nations, reviewing recent history, and offering future-oriented paradigms and frameworks. Our intent is to help guide the way for those working toward the technically and culturally appropriate transfer of managed care innovations around the globe.

References

1. Weiner JP, deLissovoy G. Razing a tower of Babel: A taxonomy for managed care and health insurance plans. *J Health Polit Policy Law.* Spring 1993:18(1), 75–103.
2. Enthoven AC, Singer SJ. The managed care backlash and the task force in California. *Health Affairs.* July–August 1998:17(4), 95–110.
3. Dixon A, Pfaff M, Hermesse J. Solidarity and competition in social health insurance companies. In: Saltman B, ed. *Social Health Insurance Systems in Western Europe.* Berkshire, UK and New York, NY: Open University Press, 2004.
4. Katzman CN. Managed care poised to take Europe. *Mod Healthc.* 1998:28(44), 38–40.
5. Pauly MV, Zweifel P, Scheffler RM, Preker AS, Bassett M. Private health insurance in developing countries. *Health Affairs.* March–April 2006:25(2), 369–379.
6. World Bank. *World Development Indicators 2006.* Washington, DC: World Bank, 2006.
7. Weiner JP, Gillam S, Lewis R. Organization and financing of British primary care groups and trusts: Observations through the prism of U.S. managed care. *J Health Serv Res Policy.* January 2002:7(1), 43–50.
8. Sekhri N. Mexico. In: Wieners WW, ed. *Global Health Care Markets: A Comprehensive Guide to Regions, Trends, and Opportunities Shaping the International Health Arena.* San Francisco, CA: Jossey-Bass, 2000.
9. Bassett M. Background paper for conference on private health insurance in developing countries. World Bank; Wharton Business School, 2005.
10. Colombo F, Tapay N. *Private Health Insurance in OECD Countries: The Benefits and Costs for Individuals and Health Systems.* Paris, France: OECD Publishing, 2004. OECD Health Working Papers, No. 15.
11. Organisation for Economic Co-Operation and Development. *The Reform of Health Care: A Comparative Analysis of Seven OECD Countries.* Paris, France: Organisation for Economic Co-Operation and Development, Health Policy Studies, 2002.
12. Gwatkin DR. *Are Free Government Health Services the Best Way to Reach the Poor?* Washington, DC: World Bank, 2004. Health, Nutrition, and Population Discussion Paper.
13. Reverente B. Philippines. In: Wieners WW, ed. *Global Health Care Markets: A Comprehensive Guide to Regions, Trends, and Opportunities Shaping the International Health Arena.* San Francisco, CA: Jossey-Bass, 2000.
14. Baeza CC, Packard TC. *Beyond Survival: Protecting Households from the Impoverishing Effects of Health Shocks in Latin America.* Washington, DC: World Bank, 2005.
15. Gross R, Harrison M. Implementing managed competition in Israel. *Soc Sci Med.* 2001:52(8), 1219–1231.
16. Gress S, Groenewegen P, Kerssens J, Braun B, Wasem J. Free choice of sickness funds in regulated competition: Evidence from Germany and the Netherlands. *Health Policy.* 2002:60(3), 235–254.
17. Thomson S, Mossialos E. Private health insurance and access to health care in the European Union. *Euro Observer.* 2004:6(1), 1–4.
18. Beichl L, Gunnery L, Navarro JA. A formula for successfully competing in non-U.S. health insurance markets. *Manag Care Q.* 2003:11(2), 22–28.
19. Kahn H, Ware M. Critical issues in evaluating global markets. In: Wieners WW, ed. *Global Health Care Markets: A Comprehensive Guide to Regions, Trends, and Opportunities Shaping the International Health Arena.* San Francisco, CA: Jossey-Bass, 2000.
20. Wieners WW. Setting up camp . . . overseas. If you're thinking about a foray abroad, IT implementations in Latin America and elsewhere offer constructive lessons. *Healthc Inform.* 1999:16(2), 52–54, 56, 58.
21. Stocker K, Waitzkin H, Iriart C. The exportation of managed care to Latin America. *NEJM.* 1999:340(14), 1131–1136.
22. Gould BS. When managed care doesn't travel well: A case study of South Africa. In: Wieners WW, ed. *Global Health Care Markets: A Comprehensive Guide to Regions, Trends, and Opportunities Shaping the International Health Arena.* San Francisco, CA: Jossey-Bass, 2000.

23. Kahn H, Li L. Crossing borders: Considerations in delivering health insurance products and services. *Manag Care Q*. 1999:7(2), 57–64.

24. Iriart C, Frarone S, Quiroga M, Leone F. *Atencion Gerenciada en Argentina: Informe Final*. Buenos Aires, Argentina: Universidad de Buenos Aires, 1998.

Suggested Reading

Kane NM, Turnbull NC. *Managing Health: An International Perspective*. San Francisco: Jossey-Bass, 2003.

Organisation for Economic Co-operation and Development. Available at: http://www.oecd.org.

Powell FD, Wessen AF, eds. *Health Care Systems in Transition: An International Perspective*. Thousand Oaks, CA: Sage Publications, 1999.

Saltman RB, Busse R, Figueras J, eds. *Social Health Insurance Systems in Western Europe*. Berkshire, UK and New York, NY: Open University Press, 2004.

Wieners W, ed. *Global Health Care Markets. A Comprehensive Guide to Regions, Trends, and Opportunities Shaping the International Health Arena*. San Francisco, CA: Jossey-Bass, 2000.

World Health Organization. Available at: http://www.who.int.

Part 6

REGULATORY AND LEGAL ISSUES

A wise government knows how to enforce with temper or to conciliate with dignity.

—George Grenville
(1712–1770), speech against
expulsion of John Wilkes, in
Parliament [1769]

30

Legal Issues in Provider Contracting

Mark S. Joffe and Kelli D. Back

Study Objectives

- Understand the necessary steps and considerations in negotiating a managed care contract.
- Understand the typical format of a managed care contract.
- Understand common clauses and provisions in managed care contracts.
- Understand the key issues underlying the terms of a managed care contract.

Discussion Topics

1. Discuss the differences between a letter of intent and an agreement. What is the purpose of each?
2. Discuss why the "definitions" section of a contract is important and name a few definitions that should be carefully reviewed or drafted and why.
3. Describe and discuss important issues relating to payment that should be addressed in a managed care agreement.
4. Describe and discuss the importance of the "Hold Harmless" clause in managed care contracts.
5. Discuss the two general categories of termination grounds typically included in a managed care contract. Describe the advantages of each from a provider perspective and the types of instances in which they might be evoked.
6. Describe and discuss four provider obligations commonly included in managed care contracts.

The purpose of a managed care organization is to provide or arrange for the provision of health care services. Most managed care organizations such as health maintenance organizations (HMOs) or preferred provider organizations (PPOs) provide their services through arrangements with individual physicians, individual practice associations (IPAs), medical groups, hospitals, and other types of health care professionals and facilities. The provider contract formalizes the managed care organization-provider relationship. A carefully drafted contract accomplishes more than mere memorializing of the arrangement between the parties. A well-written contract can foster a positive relationship between the provider and the managed care organization. Moreover, a good contract can provide important and needed protections to both parties if the relationship sours.

This chapter is intended to offer to the managed care organization and the provider a practical guide to reviewing and drafting a provider contract. In the appendices that follow the chapter are a managed care organization-primary care physician agreement and a managed care organization-hospital agreement. The authors have annotated these contracts, which have been provided solely for illustrative purposes. The operational aspects of network development (physician, hospital, and ancillary services), credentialing, reimbursement issues, and the like are addressed in Chapters 5 through 7.

Contracts need not be complex or lengthy to be legally binding and enforceable. A single-sentence letter agreement between a hospital and a managed care organization that says that the hospital agrees to provide access to its facility to enrollees of the managed care organization in exchange for payment of billed charges is a valid contract. If a single-paragraph agreement is legally binding, why is it necessary for managed care organization-provider contracts to be so lengthy? The answer is twofold. First, many terms of the contract, although not required, perform useful functions by articulating the rights and responsibilities of the parties. Because managed care is an important revenue source to most providers, a clear understanding of these rights and responsibilities is important. Second, a growing number of contractual provisions are required by state licensure regulations (eg, a hold harmless clause) or by government payer programs, such as Medicare and Medicaid.

An ideal contract or contract form does not exist. Appropriate contract terms vary depending on the issues of concern and objectives of the parties, each party's relative negotiating strength, and the desired degree of formality. Although the focus of this chapter is explaining key substantive provisions in a contract, the importance of clarity cannot be overstated. A poorly written contract confuses and misleads the parties. Lack of clarity increases substantially the likelihood of disagreements over the meaning of contract language. A contract should not only be written in simple, commonly understood language but should be well organized so that either party is able to find and review provisions as quickly and easily as possible.

The need for clarity has become more important as contracts have become increasingly complex. Many managed care organizations may act as an HMO, PPO, and a third-party administrator. Those health care plans will frequently enter into a single contract with a provider to provide services in all three capacities. In addition, this single contract may obligate the provider to furnish services not only to the managed care organization's enrollees but also to enrollees of a number of affiliates or nonaffiliates of the managed care organization.

The following discussion is designed to provide a workable guide for managed care organizations and providers to draft, amend, or review contracts. Much of the discussion is cast from the perspective of the managed care organization, but some points are also highlighted from the provider's perspective. Most of the discussion relates to contracts directly between the managed care organization and the provider of services. When the contract is between the managed care organization and an IPA or medical group, the managed care organization needs to ensure that the areas discussed later are appropriately addressed in both the managed care organization's contract and the contract between the IPA or medical group and the provider.

GENERAL ISSUES IN CONTRACTING

Key Objectives

The managed care organization should divide key objectives into two categories: those that are essential and those that, although not essential, are highly desirable. Throughout the negotiations process a managed care organization needs to keep in mind both the musts and the highly desirable objectives. Not infrequently, a managed care organization or a provider will suddenly realize at the end of the negotiation process that it has not achieved all its basic goals. The managed care organization's key objectives will vary. If the managed care organization is in a community with a single provider of a particular specialty service, merely entering into a contract on any terms with the provider may be its objective. On the other hand, the managed care organization's objectives might be quite complex, and it may demand carefully planned negotiations to achieve them.

"Must" objectives may derive from state and federal regulations, which may require or prohibit particular clauses in contracts. Managed care organizations need to be aware of these requirements and make sure that their contracting providers understand that these provisions are required by law.

Beyond the essential objectives are the highly desirable ones. Before commencing the drafting or the negotiation of the contract, the managed care organization should list these objectives and have a good understanding of their relative importance. This preliminary thought process assists the man-

aged care organization in developing its negotiating strategy.

Annual Calendar

Key provider contracts may take months to negotiate. If the contemplated arrangement with the provider is important to the managed care organization's delivery system, the managed care organization will want to avoid the diminution of its bargaining strength as the desired effective date approaches.

The managed care organization should have a master schedule identifying the contracts that need to be entered into and renewed. This schedule should include time lines that identify dates by which progress on key contract negotiations should take place. Although such an orderly system may be difficult to maintain, it may protect the managed care organization from potential problems that may arise if it is forced to operate without a contract or to negotiate from a weakened position.

Letter of Intent Compared to Contract

The purpose of a letter of intent is to define the basic elements of a contemplated arrangement or transaction between two parties. A letter of intent is used most often when the negotiation process between two parties is expected to be lengthy and expensive. A letter of intent is a preliminary, nonbinding understanding that allows the parties to ascertain whether they are able to agree on key terms. If the parties agree on a letter of intent, the terms of that letter serve as the blueprint for the contract. Some people confuse a letter of intent with a letter agreement. Because a letter of intent is not a legally binding agreement, regulators will not consider the provider in evaluating whether a managed care organization has made available and accessible the full range of services. Therefore, the use of a letter of intent should be limited to identifying the general parameters of a future contract.

Negotiating Strategy

Negotiating strategy is determined by objectives and relative negotiating strength. Depending on the locale or market dynamics, either the managed care organization or the provider may have greater negotiating strength. Except in circumstances in which the relative negotiating strength is so one-sided that one party can dictate the terms to the other party, each party should identify for itself before beginning negotiations the negotiable issues, the party's initial position on each issue, and the extent to which it will compromise. Because a managed care organization may use the same contract for many providers, the managed care organization needs to keep in mind the implications of amending one contract, for example, whether the plan will be able to administer that contract differently from all its other provider contracts.

A recurring theme presented at conference sessions discussing provider contracting and provider relations is the need to foster a win-win relationship, where both parties perceive that they gain from the relationship. The managed care organization's objective should be fostering long-term, mutually satisfactory relationships with providers. When managed care organizations have enough negotiating strength to dictate the contract terms, they should exercise that strength cautiously to ensure that their short-term actions do not jeopardize their long-term goals.

CONTRACT STRUCTURE

As mentioned previously, clarity is an important objective in drafting a provider contract. A key factor affecting the degree of clarity of a contract is the manner in which the agreement is organized. In fact, many managed care organization contracts follow fairly similar formats. The contract begins with a title describing the instrument (eg, "Primary Care Physician Agreement"). After this is the caption, which identifies the names of the par-

ties and the legal action taken, along with the transition, which contains words signifying that the parties have entered into an agreement. Then, the contract includes the recitals, which are best explained as the "whereas" clauses. These clauses are not intended to have legal significance but may become relevant to resolve inconsistencies in the body of the contract or if the drafter inappropriately includes substantive provisions in them. The use of the word whereas is merely tradition and has no legal significance.

The next section of the contract is the "definitions" section, which includes definitions of all key contract terms. The definitions section precedes the operative language, including the substantive health-related provisions that define the responsibilities and obligations of each of the parties, representations and warranties, and declarations. The last section of the contract, the closing or testimonium, reflects the assent of the parties through their signatures. Sometimes, the drafters of a provider contract decide to have the signature page on the first page for administrative simplicity.

Contracts frequently incorporate by reference other documents, some of which will be appended to the agreement as attachments or exhibits. As discussed further later, managed care organizations frequently reserve the right to amend some of these referenced documents unilaterally.

The contract's form or structure is intended to accomplish three purposes: to simplify a reader's use and understanding of the agreement, to facilitate amendment or revision of the contract where the contract form has been used for many providers, and to streamline the administrative process necessary to submit and obtain regulatory approvals.

Clarity and efficiency can be attained by using commonly understood terms, avoiding legal or technical jargon, using definitions to explain key and frequently used terms, and using well-organized headings and a numbering system. The ultimate objective is that any representative of the managed care organization or the provider who has an interest in an issue be able to find easily the pertinent contract provision and understand its meaning.

Exhibits and appendices are frequently used by managed care organizations to promote efficiency in administering many provider contracts. The managed care organization, to the extent possible, could design many of its provider contracts or groups of provider contracts around a core set of common requirements. Exhibits may be used to identify the terms that may vary, such as payment rates and provider responsibilities. This approach has several advantages. First, it eases the administrative burden in drafting and revising contracts. Second, if an appendix or exhibit is the only part of the contract that is being amended and it has a separate state insurance department provider number, the managed care organization need only submit the amendment for state review. Third, when a contract is under consideration for renewal and the key issue is the payment rate, having the payment rate listed separately in the appendix lessens the likelihood that the provider will review and suggest amending other provisions of the contract.

COMMON CLAUSES, PROVISIONS, AND KEY FACTORS

Names

The initial paragraph of the contract will identify the names of the parties entering into the agreement. It is always a good idea to ensure that the parties named in the opening paragraph are the parties who are signing the agreement. If one organization is signing the agreement on behalf of affiliates, you may want to have the signing party represent and warrant that it is authorized to sign on behalf of the nonsigning party or parties. This is also the case where a physician group or intermediate entity is signing on behalf of its member physicians. If the nonsigning party is much stronger financially than the signing party is, it would be worthwhile to

have a representation directly from the nonsigning party that the signing party may enter into the agreement on its behalf. In reviewing a contract, providers should be particularly sensitive to the responsibilities of nonparties to the agreement. If a managed care organization is signing the agreement on behalf of a self-insured employer, is the self-insured employer a party to the agreement? If not, what assurances does the provider have that the self-insured employer will fulfill its responsibilities under the agreement?

Recitals

A contract will typically contain in rather legalistic prose a series of statements describing who the parties are and what they are trying to accomplish. These statements are called "recitals" and are relatively unimportant because they should not contain substantive contractual obligations. However, managed care organizations and providers should review these statements to confirm their accuracy and that each party is not assuming any unintended responsibilities.

Table of Contents

Although a table of contents has no legal significance, the reader will be greatly assisted in finding pertinent sections in a long contract. One common failing in contract renegotiations is neglecting to update the table of contents after the contract has been amended.

Definitions

The definitions section of a contract plays an essential role in simplifying the structure and the reader's understanding of a contract. The body of the contract often contains complicated terms that merit amplification and explanation. The use of a definition, although requiring the reader to refer back to an earlier section for a meaning, simplifies greatly the discussion in the body of the agreement. A poorly drafted contract will define unnecessary terms or define terms in a manner that is inconsistent with their use in the body of the agreement.

Defined terms are frequently capitalized in a contract to alert the reader that the word is defined. Definitions are almost essential in many contracts, but their use may complicate the understanding of the agreement. Someone who reads a contract will first read a definition without knowing its significance. Later, when he or she reads the body of the contract, he or she may no longer recall a term's meaning. For this reason, someone reviewing a contract for the first time should read the definitions twice: initially and then in the context of each term's use. Definitions sections tend to err on the side of containing too many definitions. A term that is used only once in a contract need not be defined. On the other hand, a critical reader of a contract will identify instances in which the contract could be improved by the use of additional definitions.

In reviewing a contract, managed care organizations and providers should not underestimate the importance of the definitions section. A provider's right to payment may depend on how such terms as *emergency*, *covered services*, or *medical necessity* are defined. It is very important to review the definitions section of a contract initially as well as in the context of the terms' usage in the body of the contract.

An occasional defect in some contracts is that the drafter includes substantive contract provisions in definitions. A definition is merely an explanation of a meaning of a term and should not contain substantive provisions. This does not mean that a definition that imposes a substantive obligation on a party is invalid. In reviewing a contract, if a party identifies a substantive provision in a definition, the party should ensure that its usage is consistent with the corresponding provision in the body of the contract.

Terms that are commonly defined in a managed care context are *member, subscriber, medical director, provider, payer, physician, member, primary care physician, emergency,*

medically necessary, and *utilization review program.* Some of these terms, such as *medically necessary*, are crucial to readers' understanding of the parties' responsibilities and should be considered carefully in the review of a contract. In many managed care agreements, payers other than the managed care organization are responsible for payment under the contract. In this case, who is a payer and how they are selected and removed become very important to the provider. The definition of *member* or *enrollee* is also important. The contract should convey clearly who is covered under the agreement and whom the managed care organization can add in the future. The managed care organization and provider should ensure that these terms are consistent, if appropriate, with those in other contracts (*eg*, the group enrollment agreement).

It's important to note that a number of the definitions in the contract may be controlled by state or federal law. For example, Medicare and Medicaid law and a number of state laws set forth a definition of *emergency services*. In addition, Medicare law and an increasing number of states set forth standards for *medical necessity*. The contracting parties should be aware of the law and should, at a minimum, ensure that the definitions in the contract are consistent with such law.

Provider Obligations

Provider Qualifications and Credentialing

Provider contracts should include the provider's representations and warranties that the provider meets the managed care plan's applicable requirements for network participation. These representations and warranties should include, at a minimum, that the provider has a valid license, has not been excluded from participation in any federal health care program, and/or in the case of an institutional provider, meets any relevant accreditation standards and Medicare conditions for participation. As discussed later in this chapter, it is important that the provider be obligated to notify the managed care plan if any of this information changes.

In addition, the contract should include a provision requiring the provider to comply with any of the managed care plan's policies and procedures for credentialing and recredentialing of providers.

Provider Services

Because the purpose of the agreement is to contract for the provision of health services, the description of those services in the contract is important. As mentioned earlier, the recitation of services to be furnished by the provider could be either set out in the contract or set out in an exhibit or attachment. An exhibit format frequently allows the party more flexibility and administrative simplicity when it amends the exhibited portion of the agreement, particularly when the change requires regulatory approval.

Contracts may use the term *provider services* to denote the range of services that is to be provided under the contract. Managed care organizations frequently adapt physician contracts to apply to ancillary providers. In so doing, the managed care organization may not revise language that applies only to physicians.

The contract needs to specify to whom the provider is obligated to furnish services. Although the answer is that the provider furnishes services to covered enrollees, the contract needs to define what is meant by a *covered enrollee*, explain how the provider will learn who is covered, and assign the responsibility for payment if services are furnished to a noncovered person. Managed care organizations and providers frequently disagree on this issue. The providers' view is frequently that, if the managed care organization represented that the individual was covered, the managed care organization should be responsible for payment. In contrast, the managed care organization frequently asserts that it should not be responsible for the costs of services provided

to noncovered enrollees and that the provider should seek payment directly from the individual. This issue is particularly important when the enrollee population includes Medicaid beneficiaries who are unlikely to be able to pay the provider for services. Oftentimes, the issue is resolved based on relative negotiating strength.

Provider contracts should also cover adequately a number of other provider responsibilities, including their responsibilities to refer or to accept referrals of enrollees, the days and times of days the provider agrees to be available to provide services, and substitute on-call arrangements, if appropriate. Provider contracts may also specify the qualifications necessary for the provider of backup services when the provider is not available. Some of these requirements may be posed as ability to participate in public programs, such as the ability to receive payment under the Medicare program.

If the provider is a hospital, the contract will include language identifying the circumstances in which the managed care organization agrees to be responsible or not responsible for services provided to nonemergency patients. A fairly common provision in hospital contracts states that the hospital, except in emergencies, must, as a prerequisite to admit, have the order of the participating physician or other preadmission authorization. The hospital contract also should have an explicit provision requiring that the managed care organization be notified within a specified period after an emergency admission. A particularly sensitive issue is whether the managed care organization's coverage of emergency medical services meets state and/or federal requirements for such coverage. Medicare, Medicaid, and a number of state laws require managed care plans to pay for screening and stabilization services in situations in which a prudent layperson reasonably believed that an emergency medical condition existed. A related policy and contracting issue is whether such a law automatically entitles a hospital to reimbursement for performing the initial screen that is required when a patient goes to the emergency room.

A good provider contract must be supplemented by a competent provider relations program to ensure that problems that arise are resolved and that the providers have a means to answer questions about their contract responsibilities. Providers will be frequently given the opportunity to appeal internally claim denials and decisions of nonmedical necessity by the managed care organization.

Nondiscriminatory Requirements

Provider agreements frequently contain clauses obligating the provider to furnish services in the same manner as the provider furnishes services to nonmanaged health care patients (*ie*, not to discriminate on the basis of payment source). In addition, a clause is used to prohibit other types of discrimination on the basis of race, color, sex, age, disability, religion, and national origin. Government contracts may require the use of specific contract language, including a reference to compliance with the Americans with Disabilities Act and the Rehabilitation Act of 1973. As an alternative, the managed care organization and provider may want to add a second contract clause that requires compliance with all nondiscrimination requirements under federal, state, and local law. These obligations may also apply to subcontractors of the provider.

Compliance with Utilization Management and Quality Improvement Programs

The success of the managed care organization is dependent on its providers being able and willing to control unnecessary utilization. To do so, the providers need to follow the utilization review guidelines of the managed care organization. The contract needs to set out the provider's responsibilities in carrying out the managed care organization's utilization review program. The managed care organization's dilemma is how to articulate this obligation in the contract when the utilization review program may be quite detailed and frequently is updated over time. One op-

tion used by a few managed care organizations is to append the utilization review program to the contract as an exhibit. Another option is merely to incorporate the program by reference or to generally require the provider to comply with the managed care plan's policies and procedures and to include utilization review requirements in those policies and procedures. In either case, it is important for the managed care organization to ensure that the contract allows it to amend the utilization review standards in the future without the consent of the provider. If the managed care organization does not append a cross-referenced standard, the managed care organization should give each provider a copy of the guidelines and any amendments. Without this documentation, the provider might argue that he or she did not agree to the guidelines or subsequent amendments.

The contract needs to inform providers of their responsibilities to cooperate in efforts by the managed care organization to ensure compliance and the implications of the provider not meeting the guidelines. Contracts differ on whether the managed care organization is seeking the provider's "cooperation" or "compliance." Providers generally favor an obligation to cooperate rather than to comply with these programs because a requirement to comply with the programs decisions seems to preclude the right to disagree.

The same basic concepts and principles apply to the provider's acceptance of the managed care organization's quality assurance program. Some managed care organizations tend to equate their utilization review and their quality assurance programs. This attitude not only reflects a misunderstanding of the objectives of the two programs but is likely to engender the concern or criticism of government regulators who view the two programs as being separate. In the last several years, as managed care organizations have placed greater emphasis on their quality assurance/quality improvement programs, provider compliance responsibilities have correspondingly increased. To provide some guidance on the nature of these responsibilities, a few managed care organizations have appended summaries of these quality programs to the contracts to give providers a better idea of their responsibilities.

The contract should include a provision requiring the provider to cooperate both in furnishing information to the managed care organization and in taking corrective actions, if appropriate.

Acceptance of Enrollee Patients

A provider contract, particularly with a physician or physician group, will need a clause to ensure that the provider will accept enrollees regardless of health status. This provision is more important when the risk-sharing responsibilities with the providers are such that the physician has an incentive to dissuade high utilizers from becoming part of his or her panel. Some provider contracts with primary care physicians also include a minimum number of members that the physician will accept into his or her panel (*eg*, 250 members). The contract should also include fair and reasonable procedures for allowing the provider to limit or stop new members added to his or her panel (at a point after the provider has accepted at least the minimum number of members) and a mechanism to notify the managed care organization when these changes take place. The managed care organization needs to have data regarding which providers are limiting panel size to comply with regulatory requirements concerning access to care.

The contract should also specify the circumstances in which the provider, principally in the case of a primary care physician, can cease being an enrollee's physician. Examples may be abusive behavior or refusal to follow recommended course of treatment. This contract language would need to be consistent with language in the member subscriber agreement and in compliance with licensure requirements and/or federal health care program requirements, which frequently identify the grounds in which a physician may end the physician-enrollee relationship.

Enrollee Complaints

The contract should require the provider to cooperate in resolving enrollee complaints and to notify the managed care organization within a specified period of time when any complaints are conveyed to the provider. The provider should also be obligated to advise the managed care organization of any coverage denials so that the managed care organization might anticipate future enrollee complaints. To the extent governmental payer programs require special enrollee grievance procedures, the language in the contract should be written sufficiently broadly to ensure provider cooperation with those procedures.

Maintenance and Retention of Records and Confidentiality

Provider contracts should require the provider to maintain both medical and business records for specified periods of time. For example, these agreements could provide that the records must be maintained in accordance with federal and state laws and consistent with generally accepted business and professional standards as well as whatever other standards are established by the managed care organization. If the managed care organization participates in any public or private payer program that establishes certain specific records retention requirements, those requirements should be conveyed to the providers. The contract should state that these obligations survive the termination of the contract.

The managed care organization also needs a legal right to have access to books and records. The contract will want to state that the managed care organization, its representatives, and government agencies have the right to inspect, review, and make or obtain copies of medical, financial, and administrative records. The provider would want the availability of this information to be limited to services rendered to enrollees, after reasonable notice, and during normal business hours. The cost of performing these services is often an issue of controversy. If there are no fees for copying these records, the contract should state so. When the managed care organization is acting on behalf of other payers, it is desirable to have language acknowledging that the other payers have agreed to comply with applicable confidentiality laws.

In addition to the availability of books or records, the managed care organization might also want the right to require the provider to prepare reports identifying statistical and descriptive medical and patient data and other identifying information as specified by the managed care organization. If such a provision is included in the contract, the managed care organization should inform the provider of the types of reports it might request to minimize any future problems. Finally, the provider should be obligated to provide information that is necessary for compliance with state or federal law.

An often neglected legal issue is how the managed care organization obtains the authority to access medical records. Provider agreements periodically contain an acknowledgment by the provider that the managed care organization is authorized to receive medical records. The problem with this approach is that the managed care organization might not have the right to have access to this information, and, if it does not, an acknowledgment of that right in the contract has no legal effect. While the federal Health Insurance Portability and Accessibility Act (HIPAA; see also Chapter 32) gives providers and managed care plans the right to use and disclosed protected health information for purposes of treatment, payment, and health care operations, some state laws give insurers and HMOs, as payers, a limited right of access to medical records. This right may arise if the managed care organization is performing utilization review on behalf of an enrollee. Managed care organizations should review their state law provisions, and any applicable federal law provisions, on this issue and their plan's procedures for obtaining the appropriate consents of their members to have access to this information. Many managed care organizations obtain this information through signatures that are part of the initial enrollment materials. These consents could also be obtained at the time health services are rendered.

Managed care organizations frequently include provisions in contracts in which the provider acknowledges that the managed care organization has the right of access to enrollee records. The provider should be reluctant to agree to this provision without consulting state law. Although the clause acknowledging the right of access may make it easier to persuade a reluctant provider to release an enrollee's medical records, the managed care organization needs to remember that statement, or for that matter similar statements in the group enrollment agreement, do not confer that right. Finally, the contract should explicitly state that the provisions concerning access to records should survive the termination of the agreement.

A related provision almost always included in provider contracts is a requirement that the provider maintain the confidentiality of medical records. A common clause is a provision that will only release the records in accordance with the terms of the contract, in accordance with applicable law, or upon appropriate consent. As previously noted, federal privacy law generally allows use and disclosure of identifiable health information for purposes of payment, treatment, and health care operations. However, states may have laws that are more restrictive regarding the use and disclosure of such information. These laws are not preempted by federal law, and managed care organizations and providers must abide by stricter state law restrictions. Managed care organizations and providers need to be particularly sensitive to confidentiality concerns with regard to minors, incompetents, and persons with communicable diseases for which there are specific state confidentiality statutes governing disclosure of information.

If a managed care organization delegates to a provider responsibilities other than simply furnishing health care services to the managed care organization's members and the managed care organization is disclosing to the provider protected health information or the provider is obtaining such information on the managed care organization's behalf, the contract between the parties must include a "business associate agreement." Under HIPAA, a business associate agreement is required if a party will perform services involving the use or disclosure of protected health information on behalf of an entity subject to the HIPAA provisions concerning privacy and security of protected health information (known as a covered entity). Such services may include, but are not limited to, utilization review or claims processing, tasks often performed by IPAs. Both health care providers and managed care plans are covered entities under HIPAA. A model business associate agreement is included at the end of this chapter.

Payment

In General

The payment terms of the agreement often represent the most important provision for both the provider and the managed care organization. As mentioned earlier, the payment terms are frequently set forth in an exhibit appended to the contract and are cross-referenced in the body of the agreement. A number of payment issues should be covered in the contract. For example, who will collect the copayments? Another issue concerns the managed care organization's payment responsibilities for uncovered services. A provision needs to state that unauthorized or uncovered services are not the responsibility of the managed care organization. To avoid members receiving unexpected bills from providers for noncovered services, contracts may say that the provider must first inform the member that a service will not be covered by the health plan prior to providing the service. Moreover, to avoid any debates about whether a member was informed that the service would not be cov-

ered, the best practice is to require the provider to obtain the member's written acknowledgment of financial liability before the services are rendered. In addition, the contract may preclude the provider from ever billing an enrollee when the managed care organization has determined that the service is not medically necessary.

From the provider's perspective, he or she needs a clear understanding of what is necessary for a service to be authorized. If the provider submits claims to the managed care organization, the contract should set out the manner in which the claim is to be made and either identify the information to be provided in the claim or give the managed care organization the right to designate or revise that information in the future. If the contract specifies the information to be included in a claim, the managed care organization should also have the unilateral right to make changes in the future. If the provider submits claims electronically, both the provider and the managed care organization will be obligated to comply with the provisions of HIPAA concerning standard transactions, as discussed in Chapter 17.

The agreement should also obligate the provider to submit claims within a specified period and the managed care organization to pay claims within a certain number of days. The latter requirement should not apply to contested claims. The parties should ensure that the number of days for claims payment set forth in the contract is consistent with any applicable state or federal laws regulating such payment. Although Medicare Advantage law does not set forth a specific time frame in which contracting providers must be paid, it does require that Medicare Advantage organizations set forth in their provider contracts a "prompt payment" provision as negotiated by the contracting parties. Special provisions regarding timing of payment will apply to claims for which another carrier may be the primary payer. A common way to address the coordination of benefits issue in a balanced manner is to allow a 2-month period for collection from the purported primary carrier after submission of the bill to the primary carrier. If unsuccessful, the managed care organization would pay while awaiting resolution of the dispute.

At issue is the time in which the managed care organization is required to pay on claims. Contracts frequently identify a specific time period, for example, 30 to 60 days, during which payment on clean claims is to be made. Provider contracts rarely impose an interest penalty for late payment unless required by law, reflecting the greater bargaining strength of the managed care organization. Some contracts require the managed care organization to make a good faith effort to pay within a specified period. From the provider's perspective, the weakness of this provision is that "good faith" is probably too ambiguous to be enforceable. Many states have laws requiring insurers and HMOs to pay interest on late claims.

The contract needs also to address reconciliations to account for overpayments or underpayments. A managed care organization may wish to recoup previously paid amounts from a provider for a number of reasons, for example, the payment amount was incorrectly calculated or the plan discovered that the individual was not eligible to be a member of a health plan at the time the service was rendered. A provider may also request additional payment if the provider determines that it has been underpaid by the managed care organization. A number of states have laws limiting the time period during which a managed care organization can recoup previously paid amounts from its providers or providers can request additional payment. Even in instances where such laws are not applicable, the contract should set forth the period during which a reconciliation or recoupment may be requested for the parties to avoid liability for claims they thought were settled years ago. Provider contracts frequently provide that the managed care organization can subtract overpayments to providers from amounts due to the provider. From a provider's perspective, it is important

that the contract require the managed care plan to provide prior notice of its intent to recoup, specifying the basis for the recoupment and that the provider may appeal a recoupment decision.

Risk-Sharing Arrangements

The most complex aspects of provider contracts are often the risk-sharing arrangements such as those discussed in Chapter 6. Risk can be shared with providers in significantly varying degrees depending on the initial amount of risk transferred, the services for which the provider is at risk, and whether the managed care organization offers stop-loss protection. Risk pools with complicated formulas determining distributions are frequently used when services are capitated or payments are based on a fee schedule. Although the primary objective of these arrangements is to create incentives to discourage unnecessary utilization, the complexity of many of these arrangements has confused providers and engendered their distrust when their distribution falls below expectations. Some managed care organizations that had complex risk-sharing arrangements are now realizing that simpler, more understandable arrangements are preferable. If the arrangement designed by the managed care organization is somewhat complex, the provider's understanding will be greatly enhanced by the use of examples that illustrate for providers the total payments they will receive in different factual scenarios.

Managed care plans should be aware of and comply with any state and/or federal laws that regulate risk-sharing arrangements. For example, under the Medicare and Medicaid managed care programs, and as discussed in Chapter 6, managed care plans must comply with the requirements for physician incentive plans (PIPs). The PIP requirements impose stop-loss obligations on managed care plans when payment arrangements for the provision of services to Medicare or Medicaid beneficiaries puts a physician or physician group at risk for more than 25% of total potential payments for services the physician or group does not directly provide (*ie,* referral services). Moreover, managed care plans providing services to commercial enrollees with Medicare as a secondary payer may also need to comply with the PIP obligations to qualify for an exception from the compensation prohibitions under the personal services exception to the federal physician self-referral law (also known as Stark II).

Payment and PHOs

In some situations, a managed care plan may have negotiated to pay a physician-hospital organization a percentage of the managed care organization's payment from a payer in return for agreeing to provide all or a substantial portion of the organization's health care services. In developing these relationships, the parties need to identify very carefully the obligations of the provider organization. The agreement needs to clearly identify the services that will be covered and not be covered under the agreement. Will the managed care organization have the right to have the services performed by other providers if it is not satisfied with the contracted provider's performance? What assumptions have been made regarding the demographics and health needs of the covered population?

Other-Party Liability: Subrogation and Coordination of Benefits

Provider contracts should contain provisions to address situations in which a party other than the enrollee or managed care organization is financially responsible for all or part of the services provided to an enrollee.

Such provisions should set forth the provider's obligation to assist the managed care organization in identifying other parties that are responsible for paying for, or providing, services to an enrollee. In addition, the provision should identify the party with the responsibility for billing another payer and indicate the party to which the payment belongs. Some managed care organizations allow their providers to collect and keep third-party recoveries, whereas others will re-

quire that the information be reported and deducted. Often, the specific procedure depends on how the provider is paid, for example, on a fee-for-service basis, a capitation basis, or by some other mechanism.

A sensitive issue is the potential liability of a managed care organization if a provider collects from Medicare inappropriately when the managed care organization had primary responsibility under the Medicare secondary payer rules. Under the regulations of the Centers for Medicare & Medicaid Services (CMS), the managed care organization is legally responsible and may be forced to pay back CMS even if the payment was received by the provider without the knowledge of the managed care organization. Managed care organizations should include a contract provision transferring the ultimate financial liability to the provider in this circumstance.

Another issue that should be addressed in the contract is the responsibility of the managed care organization as a secondary carrier if the provider collects from the primary carrier an amount greater than the amount the provider would have received from the managed care organization. From the managed care organization's perspective, it will want a contract provision relieving the managed care organization of any payment responsibility if the provider has received at least the amount he or she would have been entitled to under the managed care organization-provider contract. It is important, however, to ensure that this practice is permissible under the state's coordination of benefits law. From the provider's perspective, the provider should try to negotiate payment by the secondary payer that will supplement the payment made by the primary payer so that the provider will receive the primary payer's entire allowable amount.

Other Payment-Related Issues

In recent years, providers for managed care organizations are becoming more sophisticated in analyzing and evaluating payment arrangements and are more aware of the ability or inability of managed care organizations to produce the volume of patients promised in exchange for a discount from the provider's charges. This is particularly true as managed care organizations offer larger provider panels and open network products to members and employers.

A few other payment-related issues that should be addressed in a contract are as follows: What if services are provided to a person who is no longer eligible for enrollment? What if services are provided to a nonenrollee who obtained services by using an enrollee's membership card?

Hold-Harmless and No Balance Billing Clauses

Virtually all provider contracts contain a hold-harmless clause under which the provider agrees not to sue or assert any claims against the enrollee for services covered under the contract, even if the managed care organization becomes insolvent or fails to meet its obligations. A no balance billing clause is similar (and may be used synonymously) and states that a provider may not balance bill a member for any payment owed by the plan, regardless of the reason for nonpayment; the provider may bill the member for any amount that the member is required to pay, such as copayment or coinsurance, or for services not covered under the schedule of benefits (eg, cosmetic surgery). Many state insurance departments (or other agencies having regulatory oversight in this area) will not approve the provider forms without inclusion of a hold-harmless clause with specific language. CMS also requires hold-harmless clauses for Medicare Advantage organizations, preferring language that was approved by the National Association of Insurance Commissioners.

Relationship of the Parties

Provider contracts usually contain a provision stating that the managed care organization and the provider have an independent contractual arrangement. The purpose for this provision is to refute an assertion that the provider serves as an employee of the managed care organization. The reason is that under the legal theory of *respondeat superior* the managed care organization would automatically be liable for the negligent acts of its employees. Although managed care organizations frequently include a provision such as this in their provider contracts, it has limited value. In a lawsuit against the managed care organization by an enrollee alleging malpractice, the court is likely to disregard such language and to focus on the relationship between the managed care organization and the provider and the manner in which the managed care organization represented the provider in evaluating whether the managed care organization should be vicariously liable.

A related clause frequently used in provider contracts states that nothing contained in the agreement shall be construed to require physicians to recommend any procedure or course of treatment that physicians deem professionally inappropriate. This clause is intended, in part, to affirm that the managed care organization is not engaged in the practice of medicine, an activity that the managed care organization may not be permitted to perform. Another reason for this clause is to protect the managed care organization from liability arising from a provider's negligence.

Use of Name and Proprietary Information

Many provider contracts limit the ability of either party to use the name of the other. This is done by identifying the circumstances in which the party's name may or may not be used. Contract clauses may allow the managed care organization the right to use the name of the provider in the provider directory or other documents listing the plan's participating providers. They may furnish the provider with the right to advise patients of their affiliation with the health plan. Otherwise, one party needs the written approval of the other party. The limitations on use apply not only to the name but to any symbol, trademark, and service mark of the entity.

In addition, the managed care organization and the provider will want to ensure that proprietary information is protected. The contract should require that the provider keep all information about the managed care organization confidential and prohibit the use of the information for any competitive purpose after the contract is terminated. With medical groups frequently switching managed care affiliations, this protection is important to the managed care organization.

Notification

The managed care organization needs to ensure that it is advised of a number of important changes that affect the ability of the provider to meet his or her contractual obligations. The contract should identify the information that needs to be conveyed to the managed care organization and the time frames for providing that information. For example, a physician might be required to notify a managed care organization within 5 days (or less) upon loss or suspension of his or her license or certification, loss or restriction of full active admitting privileges at any hospital, issuance of any formal charges brought by a government agency, change in or loss of liability insurance coverage, and/or the initiation of a civil action by an enrollee. Although specific events should be identified in the contract, a broad catch-all category should also be included, such as an event that if sustained would materially impair the provider's ability to perform the duties under the contract. The contract should require immediate notification if the provider is sanctioned under a federal health care program. If the managed care organization is contracting with a provider who has been sanctioned, the organization may no longer be eligible to receive federal funds.

In a hospital contract, the corresponding provisions would be when the hospital suffers from a change that materially impairs its ability to provide services or if action is taken against it regarding certifications, licenses, or federal agencies or private accrediting bodies.

The provider should ensure that the contract requires the plan to provide prior notification of any substantive changes to policies and procedures with which the provider is bound to comply, for example, to the plan's provider manual.

Insurance and Indemnification

Insurance provisions in contracts are fairly straightforward. The obligations in the contract may be for both professional liability coverage and general liability coverage. The managed care organization wants to ensure that the provider has resources to pay for any eventuality. The contract will state particular insurance limits, provide that the limits will be set forth in a separate attachment, or leave it up to the managed care organization to specify. A hospital agreement may require only that the limits be commensurate with limits contained in policies of similar hospitals in the state. From the managed care organization's perspective, it will probably want a specific requirement to ensure adequate levels of insurance. A provision should also be included requiring the provider to notify the managed care organization of any notification of cancellations of the policy. Another needed notification in a physician context is notification of any malpractice claims. From the provider's perspective, it is also important to ensure that the managed care organization maintains adequate insurance to cover its liabilities.

Cross-indemnification provisions in which each party indemnifies the other for damages caused by the other party are common in contracts. One weakness of the clause is that some professional liability carriers will not pay for claims arising from these clauses because of general exclusions in their policies for contractual claims. Although these clauses are frequently used, this limitation and the fact that the provider and the plan should still be liable for their own negligent acts suggest that these indemnification clauses are not essential.

Term, Suspension, and Termination

One section of most contracts identifies the term of the contract and the term of any subsequent contract renewals. Many contracts have automatic renewal provisions if no party exercises its right to terminate within a specified time period before the renewal date. Both managed care organizations and providers should give careful thought to the length of the contract and the renewal periods.

Some contracts give a right of suspension to the managed care organization. In suspension, the contract continues, but the provider loses specific rights. For example, if a provider fails to follow utilization review protocols a specified number of times, the provider will not be assigned new HMO members or perhaps will receive a reduction in the amount of payment. The advantage of a suspension provision is that total termination of a contract might be counterproductive for the managed care organization, but a suspension might be sufficiently punitive to persuade the provider to improve.

Termination provisions fall into two categories: termination without cause, and termination with cause. The value of having a provision that allows the managed care organization to terminate without cause is that the managed care organization need not defend a challenge by the provider on the substantive issue of whether the specified grounds for termination were met. A 90-day notice period is fairly common for termination without cause. However, managed care plans should be aware that state or federal law may affect a managed care plan's ability or procedures for terminating without cause. For example, the Medicare Advantage regulations require at least 60 days prior notice be-

fore terminating without cause. If the managed care organization has the right to terminate without cause, frequently the provider will also be given that right. Another regulatory issue to be aware of is that some state laws require providers to continue to provide services for a specified period of time after their contract has terminated. Such provisions commonly apply where the providers are furnishing a course or treatment to an individual with a terminal or chronic illness or to a pregnant woman. Such provisions are intended to ensure continuity of care for persons being treated by a provider at the time of the provider's termination.

Continuation of care requirements may also relate to the state's requirements for the managed care organization to have protections against insolvency and have to be reflected in the contract. If a managed care plan includes a requirement to continue care in the contract, it should ensure that the provider will continue meeting the contractual requirements with regard to the services for which the plan continues to cover after the termination. Specifically, the provider should continue to meet the managed care plan's hold-harmless requirements, reporting requirements, and quality assurance requirements.

Terminations with cause may allow the health plan to terminate faster and should be used in situations where the managed care organization needs to act quickly. The contract might establish two different categories: one for immediate termination upon notice and another for termination 30 days after written notice is provided. Many contracts give either party a period of time to cure any contract violations prior to termination. This time period, although useful to the managed care organization if it has allegedly violated the agreement, extends the period of time in which it can terminate the contract. Grounds for termination for cause may be suspension or revocation of license, loss of hospital privileges, breach of the contract, failure to meet accreditation and credentialing requirements, failure to provide services to enrollees in a professionally acceptable manner, bankruptcy, and refusal to accept an amendment to the contract agreement.

A provision allowing for termination if the provider takes any actions or makes any communications that undermine or could undermine the confidence of enrollees in the quality of care provided by the managed care organization may be included in a provider contract. However, a managed care plan should be aware that such provisions are sensitive and may be interpreted as a "gag clause." So-called gag clauses, which prohibit physicians from fully discussing a patient's treatment options and medical conditions, are prohibited under federal health care programs and a number of state laws. If the managed care plan elects to use such a provision, the clause should make clear that the intent is to prohibit disparagement of the managed care plan and that a physician remains free to advise his or her patients regarding all medically indicated treatment options, regardless of whether such treatments are covered under the managed care plan, to discuss the patient's medical condition, and to make medical recommendations within the scope of the provider's licensure.

The contract should give the managed care plan the right to immediately terminate the contract upon the occurrence of certain events, including the provider's loss of licensure or accreditation or exclusion from a federal health care program. A good contracting practice is to include a general provision, which allows for immediate termination of the contract if, in the opinion of the managed care organization, continuation of the contract would endanger the health or well-being of the managed care plan's members. Such a clause would allow the managed care organization the flexibility to terminate the contract immediately in the case of an unforeseen contingency of sufficient gravity to endanger the managed care plan's enrollees.

The contract should be clear that a provider, upon termination, is required to cooperate in the orderly transfer of enrollee care, including records, to other providers. The provider also should agree to cooperate in resolving any disputes. Finally, the provider should continue to furnish services under the terms of the contract until the services being rendered to enrollees are complete or the managed care organization has made appropriate provisions for another provider to assume the responsibility. The contract should also be clear that the provider is entitled to compensation for performing these services. In general, too little consideration has been given to preparing for contract terminations. When the provider and the managed care organization enter into a contract, little thought is given to what will occur when the contract ends. Often, relationships end acrimoniously, and it is in both parties' best interest to consider how their interests will be protected in the event the contract is terminated.

Medicare Advantage law requires a Medicare Advantage plan to furnish physicians with detailed written notice of an adverse participation decision (*eg*, a termination or suspension) and the right to appeal. The notice must specify the grounds for the action and the majority of the panel that decides the appeal must be peers of the affected physician. Some states also have laws furnishing providers with the right to appeal managed care organization terminations and set forth requirements for such appeal procedures.

"Flow Down" Clauses and Provider Subcontracts

A managed care plan may be obligated to "flow down" certain clauses that are included in the contract between the managed care plan and the payer. For example, if a managed care plan has a contract with CMS to offer a Medicare Advantage plan, the plan's contracts with providers must include certain provisions that are applicable to the Medicare Advantage organization, such as the obligation to retain records, documents and information related to the contract and services furnished under the contract for a period of at least 0 years and an acknowledgement that such records and documents are subject to inspection by HHS, the Comptroller General or their designees. The managed care plan should be aware of any contract provisions that must be flowed down to its contractors. Moreover, the managed care plan should carefully note whether those provisions must be included in the contracts of all downstream providers, that is, subcontractors entering into agreements to provide services to the managed care organization's members.

In addition to clauses that must be flowed down from the plan/payer contract, if a provider will be a subcontractor to another provider that contracts directly with the managed care plan, the contract between the managed care plan and the first-tier provider should include a provision that sets forth the requirements that must be included in the downstream subcontracts. This provision may set forth the terms of the provider's contract that must be included in any of the provider's subcontracts. Medicare Advantage policy specifically identifies a number of contract provisions that must be included in downstream contracts to provide services to members of Medicare Advantage organizations. Managed care plans should make sure that they comply with similar requirements under other federal or state laws.

In addition, if the provider will be subcontracting, the contract should specify whether the managed care plan or the provider will credential any subcontracting providers. If the managed care plan delegates its credentialing function, it should generally state the standards under which the provider will be credentialing its subcontractors. The managed care plan may want to reserve the right to approve, suspend, or deny the participation of any of the provider's subcontractors.

Declarations

In declarations, the parties provide answers to a number of "what if" questions. These clauses are common to all contracts.

A force majeure clause relieves a party of responsibility if an event occurs beyond its control. In a provider contract, this instance is more likely to arise if the provider is no longer able to provide services. In considering force majeure clauses, the parties need to distinguish between events that are beyond a party's control and those that disadvantage a party but for which the party should still be obligated to perform the contract's responsibilities.

A choice of law provision identifies the law that will apply in the event of a dispute. Absent a violation of public policy in the state in question, a court will apply the agreed-upon law. Frequently, lawyers draft contracts using the state in which their client is located without consideration of the advantages and disadvantages of the underlying law. In provider contracts where the managed care organization and the provider are located in the same state, this clause has little relevance.

A merger clause specifies that only the language in the agreement shall constitute the contract. Such a clause prevents a party from arguing that oral conversations or other documents not included in the contract modify the contract's terms.

A provision allowing or not allowing parties to assign their rights is frequently included in contracts. Provider contracts usually prohibit a provider from assigning its rights under a contract. Some contracts are silent on the right of the managed care organization to assign the contract. Silence would generally allow the managed care organization to assign the contract. An option is to allow the managed care organization to assign the contract only to an affiliate or a successor without the written consent of the provider.

A clause identifying how the contract will be amended is almost always included in a provider contract. A contract will frequently give the managed care organization the unilateral right to amend the contract absent an objection by the provider. This procedure is necessary when the managed care organization has a large provider panel, and it is administratively difficult to obtain the signatures of all the providers.

A severability clause allows the contract to continue if a court invalidates a portion of the contract. This is a common provision in a contract, but it is unlikely that the problem will arise.

Contracts also set forth a notice requirement identifying how notices are provided to parties and to whom. The manner in which notice is provided is important. If a notice requires that the communication be conveyed by certified mail with return receipt requested, an alternative form of delivery is not valid. Parties should consider what is administratively feasible before agreeing on how notice will be given.

Closing

Both parties need to confirm that the parties identified at the beginning of the contract are the parties that sign the contract. Also, if a corporation is one of the parties, the signatory needs to be authorized on behalf of the corporation to sign the agreement.

CONCLUSION

The provider contract establishes the foundation for the working relationship between the managed care organization and the provider. A good contract is well-organized and clearly written and accurately reflects the full intentions of the parties. In drafting and reviewing provider contracts, the managed care organization and the provider need to keep in mind their objectives in entering the relationship, the relationship of this contract to other provider contracts and agreements, and applicable regulatory requirements.

The appendices to this chapter contain two sample provider contracts and a sample business associate agreement. In the sample provider contracts, the author has annotated each contract to point out strengths and weaknesses of the provisions. These two contracts are provided for illustrative purposes and are not represented as ideal agreements.

Appendix 30-A
Sample Physician Agreement

AGREEMENT BETWEEN

_____

AND

PRIMARY CARE PHYSICIAN

THIS AGREEMENT, made and entered into the date set forth on the signature page hereto, by and between _____, Inc., a _____ corporation (hereinafter referred to as "MCO"), which is organized and operated as a managed care organization under the laws of the State of _____ and the individual physician or group practice identified on the signature page hereto (hereinafter referred to as "Primary Care Physician").

WHEREAS, MCO desires to operate a managed care organization pursuant to the laws of the State of _____;

WHEREAS, Primary Care Physician is a duly licensed physician (or if Primary Care Physician is a legal entity, the members of such entity are duly licensed physicians) in the State of _____, whose license(s) is (are) without limitation or restriction;[1] and

WHEREAS, MCO has as an objective the development and expansion of cost-effective means of delivering quality health services to Members, as defined herein, particularly through prepaid health care plans, and Primary Care Physician concurs in, actively supports, and will contribute to the achievement of this objective; and

WHEREAS, MCO and Primary Care Physician mutually desire to enter into an Agreement whereby the Primary Care Physician shall provide and coordinate the health care services to Members of MCO.

NOW, THEREFORE, in consideration of the premises and mutual covenants herein contained and other good and valuable consideration, it is mutually covenanted and agreed by and between the parties hereto as follows:

PART I. DEFINITIONS

A. Covered Services means those health services and benefits to which Members are entitled under the terms of an applicable Health Maintenance Certificate which may be amended by MCO from time to time.[2]

B. Emergency Services means those Medically Necessary services provided in connection with an "Emergency," defined as a sudden or unexpected onset of a condition requiring medical or surgical care which the Member secures after the onset of such condition [or as soon thereafter as care can be made available but which in any case not later than twenty-four (24) hours after onset] and in the absence of such care the Member could reasonably be expected to suffer serious physical impairment or death. Heart attacks, severe chest pain, cardiovascular accidents, hemorrhaging, poisonings, major burns, loss of consciousness, serious breathing difficulties, spinal injuries, shock, and other acute conditions as MCO shall determine are Emergencies.[3]

C. Encounter Form means a record of services provided by Physician to Members in a format acceptable to the MCO.[4]

D. Health Maintenance Certificate means a contract issued by MCO to a Member or an employer of Members specifying the services and benefits available under the MCO's prepaid health benefits program.

E. Health Professionals means doctors of medicine, doctors of osteopathy, dentists, nurses, chiropractors, podiatrists, optometrists, physician assistants, clinical psychologists, social workers, pharmacists, occupational therapists, physical therapists, and other professionals engaged in the delivery of health services who are licensed, practice under an institutional license, and are certified or practice under other authority consistent with the laws of the State of _____.

F. Medical Director means a Physician designated by MCO to monitor and review the provision of Covered Services to Members.

G. Medically Necessary services and/or supplies means the use of services or supplies as provided by a hospital, skilled nursing facility, Physician, or other provider required to identify or treat a Member's illness or injury and which, as determined by MCO's Medical Director or its utilization review committee, are: (1) consistent with the symptoms or diagnosis and treatment of the Member's condition, disease, ailment, or injury; (2) appropriate with regard to standards of good medical practice; (3) not solely for the convenience of the Member, his or her physician, hospital, or other health care provider; and (4) the most appropriate supply or level of service which can be safely provided to the Member.[5] When specifically applied to an inpatient Member, it further means that the Member's medical symptoms or condition requires that the diagnosis or treatment cannot be safely provided to the Member as an outpatient.[6]

H. Member means both a Subscriber and his or her eligible family members for whom premium payment has been made.[7]

I. Participating Physician means a Physician who, at the time of providing or authorizing services to a Member, has contracted with or on whose behalf a contract has been entered into with MCO to provide professional services to Members.

J. Participating Provider means a Physician, hospital, skilled nursing facility, home health agency, or any other duly licensed institution or Health Professional under contract with MCO to provide professional and hospital services to Members.

K. Physician means a duly licensed doctor of medicine, osteopathy or podiatry.

L. Primary Care Physician means a Participating Physician who provides primary care services to Members (e.g., general or family practitioner, internist, pediatrician, or such other physician specialty as may be designated by MCO) and is responsible for referrals of Members to Referral Physicians, other Participating Providers, and if necessary non-Participating Providers. Each Member shall select or have selected on his or her behalf a Primary Care Physician.

M. Referral Physician means a Participating Physician who is responsible for providing certain medical referral physician services upon referral by a Primary Care Physician.

N. Service Area means those counties in _____ set forth in Attachment A and such other areas as may be designated by MCO from time to time.

O. Subscriber means an individual who has contracted, or on whose behalf a contract has been entered into, with MCO for health care services.

PART II. OBLIGATIONS OF MCO

A. Administrative Procedures. MCO shall make available to Primary Care Physician a manual of administrative procedures (including any changes thereto) in the areas of record-keeping, reporting, and other administrative duties of the Primary Care Physician under this Agreement. Primary Care Physician agrees to abide by such administrative procedures including, but not limited to, the submission of MCO Encounter Forms documenting all Covered Services provided to Members by Primary Care Physician.[8]

B. Compensation. For all Medically Necessary Covered Services provided to Members by Primary Care Physician, MCO shall pay to Primary Care Physician the compensation set forth in Attachment B.[9] Itemized statements on MCO Encounter Forms, or approved equivalent, for all Covered Services rendered by Primary Care Physician must be submitted to MCO within ninety (90) days of the date the service was rendered in order to be compensated by MCO. The purpose of the risk-sharing/incentive compensation arrangement set forth in Attachment B is to monitor utilization, control costs of health services, including hospitalization, and to achieve utilization goals while maintaining quality of care.

C. Processing of Claims. MCO agrees to process Primary Care Physician claims for Covered Services rendered to Members. MCO will make payment within thirty (30) days from the date the claim is received with sufficient documentation. Where a claim requires additional documentation, MCO will make payment within thirty (30) days from date of receipt of sufficient documentation to approve the claim.[10]

D. Eligibility Report. MCO shall provide Primary Care Physician with a monthly listing of eligible Members who have selected or have been assigned to Primary Care Physician.

E. Reports. MCO will provide Primary Care Physician with periodic statements with respect to the compensation set forth in Attachment B and with utilization reports in accordance with MCO's administrative procedures. Primary Care Physician agrees to maintain the confidentiality of the information presented in such reports.

PART III. OBLIGATIONS OF PRIMARY CARE PHYSICIAN

A. Health Services. Primary Care Physician shall have the primary responsibility for arranging and coordinating the overall health care of Members, including appropriate referral to Participating Physicians and Participating Providers, and for managing and coordinating the performance of administrative functions relating to the delivery of health services to Members in accordance with this Agreement. In the event that Primary Care Physician shall provide Member non-Covered Services, Primary Care Physician shall, prior to the provision of such non-Covered Services, inform the Member:

1. of the service(s) to be provided,
2. that MCO will not pay for or be liable for said services, and
3. that Member will be financially liable for such services.[11]

   For any health care services rendered to or authorized for Members by Primary Care Physician for which MCO's prior approval is required and such prior approval was not obtained, Primary Care Physician agrees that in no event will MCO assume financial responsibility for charges arising from such services, and payments made by MCO for such services may be deducted by MCO from payments otherwise due Primary Care Physician.[12]

B. Referrals. Except in Emergencies or when authorized by MCO, Primary Care Physician agrees to make referrals of Members only to Participating Providers, and only in accordance with MCO policies. Primary Care Physician will furnish such Physicians and providers complete information on treatment procedures and diagnostic tests performed prior to such referral. Upon referral, Primary Care Physician agrees to notify

MCO of referral. In the event that services required by a Member are not available from Participating Providers, non-Participating Physicians or Providers may be utilized with the prior approval of MCO. MCO will periodically furnish Primary Care Physician with a current listing of MCO's Participating Referral Physicians and Participating Providers.

C. Hospital Admissions. In cases where a Member requires a non-Emergency hospital admission, Primary Care Physician agrees to secure authorization for such admission in accordance with MCO's procedures prior to the admission. In addition, the Primary Care Physician agrees to abide by MCO hospital discharge policies and procedures for Members.[13]

D. Primary Care Physician's Members. The Primary Care Physician shall not refuse to accept a Member as a patient on the basis of health status or medical condition of such Member, except with the approval of the Medical Director. Primary Care Physician may request that he/she does not wish to accept additional Members (excluding persons already in Primary Care Physician's practice that enroll in MCO as Members) by giving MCO written notice of such intent thirty (30) days in advance of the effective date of such closure. Primary Care Physician agrees to accept any MCO Members seeking his/her services during the thirty (30) day notice period. Primary Care Physician agrees to initiate closure of his/her practice to additional Members only if his/her practice, as a whole, is to be closed to additional patients or if authorized by MCO. A request for such authorization shall not be unreasonably denied. MCO may suspend, upon thirty (30) days prior written notice to Primary Care Physician, any further selection of Primary Care Physician by Members who have not already sought Primary Care Physician's services at the time of such suspension.

In addition, a physician who is a Participating Provider may request, in writing to MCO, that coverage for a Member be transferred to another Participating Physician. Participating Physician shall not seek without authorization by MCO to have a Member transferred because of the amount of services required by the Member or because of the health status of the Member.

E. Charges to Members. Primary Care Physician shall accept as payment in full, for services which he/she provides, the compensation specified in Attachment B. Primary Care Physician agrees that in no event, including, but not limited to, nonpayment, MCO insolvency, or breach of this Agreement, shall Physician bill, charge, collect a deposit from, seek compensation, remuneration, or reimbursement from, or have any recourse against Subscriber, Member, or persons other than the MCO acting on a Member's behalf for services provided pursuant to this Agreement. This provision shall not prohibit collection of copayments on MCO's behalf made in accordance with the terms of the Health Maintenance Certificate between MCO and Subscriber/Member.

Primary Care Physician agrees that in the event of MCO's insolvency or other cessation of operations, services to Members will continue through the period for which the premium has been paid and services to Members confined in an inpatient hospital on the date of insolvency or other cessation of operations will continue until their discharge.

Primary Care Physician further agrees that:

1. this provision shall survive the termination of this Agreement regardless of the cause giving rise to termination and shall be construed to be for the benefit of the MCO Member, and that

2. this provision supersedes any oral or written contrary agreement now existing or hereafter entered into between Primary Care Physician and Member, or persons acting on their behalf.[14]

Any modifications, addition or deletion to these provisions shall become effective on a date no earlier than 15 days after the _____ Department of Insurance has received written notice of such proposed changes.

F. Records and Reports.

1. Primary Care Physician shall submit to MCO for each Member encounter an MCO Encounter Form that shall contain such statistical and descriptive medical and patient data as specified by MCO. Primary Care Physician shall maintain such records and provide such medical, financial, and administrative information to MCO as the MCO determines may be necessary for compliance by MCO with state and federal law, as well as for program management purposes. Primary Care Physician will further provide to MCO and, if required, to authorized state and federal agencies, such access to medical records of MCO Members as is needed to ensure the quality of care rendered to such Members. MCO shall have access at reasonable times, upon request, to the billing and medical records of the Primary Care Physician relating to the health care services provided Members, and to information on the cost of such services, and on copayments received by the Primary Care Physician from Members for Covered Services. Utilization and cost data relating to a Participating Physician may be distributed by MCO to other Participating Physicians for MCO program management purposes.

2. MCO shall also have the right to inspect, at reasonable times, Primary Care Physician's facilities pursuant to MCO's credentialing, peer review, and quality assurance program.

3. Primary Care Physician shall maintain a complete medical record for each Member in accordance with the requirements established by MCO. Medical records of Members will include the recording of services provided by the Primary Care Physician, specialists, hospitals, and other reports from referral providers, discharge summaries, records of Emergency care received by the Member, and such other information as MCO requires.[15] Medical records of Members shall be treated as confidential so as to comply with all federal and state laws and regulations regarding the confidentiality of patient records.[16]

G. Provision of Services and Professional Requirements.

1. Primary Care Physician shall make necessary and appropriate arrangements to ensure the availability of physician services to his/her Member patients on a twenty-four (24) hours per day, seven (7) days per week basis, including arrangements to ensure coverage of his/her Member patients after hours or when Primary Care Physician is otherwise absent, consistent with MCO's administrative requirements. Primary Care Physician agrees that scheduling of appointments for Members shall be done in a timely manner. The Primary Care Physician will maintain weekly appointment hours which are sufficient and convenient to serve Members and will maintain at all times Emergency and on-call services. Covering arrangements shall be with another Physician who is also a Participating Provider or who has otherwise been approved in advance by MCO. For services rendered by any covering Physician on behalf of Primary Care Physician, including Emergency Services, it shall be Primary Care Physician's sole responsibility to make suitable arrangements with the covering

Physician regarding the manner in which said Physician will be reimbursed or otherwise compensated, provided, however, that Primary Care Physician shall ensure that the covering Physician will not, under any circumstances, bill MCO or bill Member for Covered Services (except copayments), and Primary Care Physician hereby agrees to indemnify and hold harmless Members and MCO against charges for Covered Services rendered by physicians who are covering on behalf of Primary Care Physician.

2. Primary Care Physician agrees:
   (a) not to discriminate in the treatment of his/her patients or in the quality of services delivered to MCO's Members on the basis of race, sex, age, religion, place of residence, health status, disability, or source of payment, and
   (b) to observe, protect and promote the rights of Members as patients. Primary Care Physician shall not seek to transfer a Member from his/her practice based on the Member's health status, without authorization by MCO.

3. Primary Care Physician agrees that all duties performed hereunder shall be consistent with the proper practice of medicine, and that such duties shall be performed in accordance with the customary rules of ethics and conduct of the applicable state and professional licensure boards and agencies.

4. Primary Care Physician agrees that to the extent he/she utilizes allied Health Professionals and other personnel for delivery of health care, he/she will inform MCO of the functions performed by such personnel and that such personnel shall meet applicable licensure or certification and supervision requirements applicable to the services performed.

5. Primary Care Physician shall be duly licensed to practice medicine in _____ and shall maintain good professional standing at all times. Evidence of such licensing shall be submitted to MCO upon request. In addition, Primary Care Physician must meet all qualifications and standards for membership on the medical staff of at least one of the hospitals, if any, which have contracted with MCO and shall be required to maintain staff membership and full admission privileges in accordance with the rules and regulations of such hospital and be otherwise acceptable to such hospital. Physician agrees to give immediate notice to MCO in the case of suspension or revocation, or initiation of any proceeding that could result in suspension or revocation, of his/her licensure, hospital privileges, or participation under a Federal health care program or the filing of a malpractice action against the Primary Care Physician.

H. Insurance. Primary Care Physician, including individual Physicians providing services to Members under this Agreement if Primary Care Physician is a legal entity, shall provide and maintain such policies of general and professional liability (malpractice) insurance as shall be necessary to insure the Primary Care Physician and his/her employees against any claim or claims for damages arising by reason of personal injuries or death occasioned, directly or indirectly, in connection with the performance of any service by Primary Care Physician. The amounts and extent of such insurance coverage shall be subject to the approval of MCO. Primary Care Physician shall provide memorandum copies of such insurance coverage to MCO upon request.[17] Primary Care Physician agrees to notify MCO within five (5) days of any reduction to or cancellation of such insurance coverage.

I. Administration.

1. Primary Care Physician agrees to cooperate and participate in such review and service programs as may be established by MCO, including utilization and quality assurance

programs, credentialing, sanctioning, external audit systems, administrative procedures, and Member and Physician grievance procedures. Primary Care Physician shall comply with all determinations rendered through the above programs.

2. Primary Care Physician agrees that MCO may use his/her name, address, phone number, picture, type of practice, applicable practice restrictions, and an indication of Primary Care Physician's willingness to accept additional Members, in MCO's roster of physician participants and other MCO materials. Primary Care Physician shall not reference MCO in any publicity, advertisements, notices, or promotional material or in any announcement to the Members without prior review and written approval of MCO.

3. Primary Care Physician agrees to provide to MCO information for the collection and coordination of benefits when a Member holds other coverage that is deemed primary for the provision of services to said Member and to abide by MCO coordination of benefits and duplicate coverage policies. This shall include, but not be limited to, permitting MCO to bill and process forms for any third-party payer on the Primary Care Physician's behalf for Covered Services and to retain any sums received. In addition, Primary Care Physician shall cooperate in and abide by MCO subrogation policies and procedures.

4. Primary Care Physician agrees to maintain the confidentiality of all information related to fees, charges, expenses, and utilization derived from, through, or provided by MCO.

5. In the event of:
   (a) termination of this Agreement,
   (b) the selection by a Member of another Primary Care Physician in accordance with MCO procedures, or
   (c) the approval by MCO of Primary Care Physician's request to transfer a Member from his/her practice,

   Primary Care Physician agrees to transfer copies of the Member's medical records, X-rays, or other data to MCO when requested to do so in writing by MCO, at the reasonable, customary, and usual fee for such copies.

6. Upon termination of the Agreement, the Primary Care Physician shall not use any information obtained during the course of the Agreement in furtherance of any competitors of the MCO.

7. Primary Care Physician warrants and represents that all information and statements given to MCO in applying for or maintaining his/her MCO Primary Care Physician Agreement are true, accurate, and complete. The MCO Physician application shall be incorporated by reference into this Agreement. Any inaccurate or incomplete information or misrepresentation of information provided by Primary Care Physician may result in the immediate termination of the Agreement by MCO. Primary Care Physician shall notify MCO as soon as possible, but no more than five (5) days after, of any changes to the information provided in the MCO Physician application.

8. Primary Care Physician shall cooperate with MCO in complying with applicable laws relating to MCO.

PART IV. MISCELLANEOUS

A. Modification of This Agreement. This Agreement may be amended or modified in writing as mutually agreed upon by the parties. In addition, MCO may modify any provision of this Agreement upon thirty (30) days prior written notice to Primary Care Physician.

Primary Care Physician shall be deemed to have accepted MCO's modification if Primary Care Physician fails to object to such modification, in writing, within the thirty (30) day notice period.[18]

B. Interpretation. This Agreement shall be governed in all respects by the laws of the State of _____. The invalidity or unenforceability of any terms or conditions hereof shall in no way affect the validity or enforceability of any other terms or provisions. The waiver by either party of a breach or violation of any provision of this Agreement shall not operate as or be construed to be a waiver of any subsequent breach thereof.

C. Assignment. This Agreement, being intended to secure the services of and be personal to the Primary Care Physician, shall not be assigned, sublet, delegated, or transferred by Primary Care Physician without the prior written consent of MCO.

D. Notice. Any notice required to be given pursuant to the terms and provisions hereof shall be sent by certified mail, return receipt requested, postage prepaid, to MCO or to Primary Care Physician at the respective addresses indicated herein. Notice shall be deemed to be effective when mailed, but notice of change of address shall be effective upon receipt.[19]

E. Relationship of Parties. None of the provisions of this Agreement is intended to create nor shall be deemed or construed to create any relationship between the parties hereto other than that of independent entities contracting with each other hereunder solely for the purpose of effecting the provisions of this Agreement. Neither of the parties hereto, nor any of their respective employees, shall be construed to be the agent, employer, employee or representative of the other, nor will either party have an express or implied right of authority to assume or create any obligation or responsibility on behalf of or in the name of the other party. Neither Primary Care Physician nor MCO shall be liable to any other party for any act, or any failure to act, of the other party to this Agreement.

F. Gender. The use of any gender herein shall be deemed to include the other gender where applicable.

G. Legal Entity. If Primary Care Physician is a legal entity, an application for each Physician who is a member of such entity must be submitted to and accepted by MCO before such Physician may serve as a Primary Care Physician under this Agreement.

H. Term and Termination. The term of this Agreement shall be for three (3) years from the "effective date" set forth on the signature page. This Agreement may be terminated by either party at any time without cause by prior written notice given at least sixty (60) days in advance of the effective date of such termination. This Agreement may also be terminated by MCO effective immediately upon written notice if Primary Care Physician's (or if a legal entity, any of the entity's physicians') medical license, participation under a Federal health care program or hospital privileges are suspended, limited, restricted, or revoked, or if Primary Care Physician violates Part III(E), (G)(3), (G)(5), (H), (I)(1), or (I)(4) herein. Upon termination, the rights of each party hereunder shall terminate, provided, however, that such action shall not release the Primary Care Physician or MCO from their obligations with respect to:

1. payments accrued to the Primary Care Physician prior to termination,
2. the Primary Care Physician's agreement not to seek compensation from Members for Covered Services provided prior to termination, and
3. completion of treatment of Members then receiving care until continuation of the Member's care can be arranged by MCO.

In the event of termination, no distribution of any money accruing to Primary Care Physician under the provisions of Attachment B shall be made until the regularly scheduled date for such distributions. Upon termination, MCO is empowered and authorized to notify Members and prospective Members, other Primary Care Physicians, and other persons or entities whom it deems to have an interest herein of such termination, through such means as it may choose.

In the event of notice of termination, MCO may notify Members of such fact and assign Members or require Members to select another Primary Care Physician prior to the effective date of termination. In any event, MCO shall continue to compensate Primary Care Physician until the effective date of termination as provided herein for those Members who, because of health reasons, cannot be assigned or make such selection during the notice of termination period and as provided by MCO's Medical Director.

IN WITNESS WHEREOF, the foregoing Agreement between _____ and Primary Care Physician, is entered into by and between the undersigned parties, to be effective this _____ day of _____, 20_____.

PRIMARY CARE PHYSICIAN   _____

_____   By: _____
(Name of Individual Physician or of Group Practice—Please Print)

_____   _____
(Mailing Address)   (Date)

_____
(City, State, ZIP)

_____
(Telephone Number)

_____
(Taxpayer Identification Number)

_____
(DEA#)

_____
(Signature)

_____
(Name and Title if signing as authorized
representative of Group Practice)

_____
(Date)

Notes to Appendix 30-A

1. Although there is nothing wrong with having a statement here that the primary care physician's license is not restricted, the body of the contract, as is the case in this contract in Section IV.H, needs to contain this requirement and provide that the failure to maintain the license is grounds for termination.

2. This definition notes the MCO's right to revise the covered services that the primary care physician is required to provide. If the physicians were capitated for those services, a mechanism would need to be available to revise the capitation rate accordingly. If the services were not limited to MCO enrollees [*eg,* covered persons under an administrative services only (ASO) arrangement with a self-insured employer], this definition would have to be written more broadly.

3. The definition for emergency services would be coordinated with the definition used in the MCO's group enrollment agreement. In many instances, the definition of emergency services is regulated under state or federal law. Examples are a useful method of illustrating the types of conditions that are considered emergencies. Some contracts will exclude deliveries during the last month of pregnancy while the mother is traveling outside the service area.

4. By stating that the encounter form must be acceptable to the MCO, the contract allows the MCO to change its requirements in the future.

5. This clause gives the MCO the authority to deny coverage for a medically appropriate procedure where another procedure is also appropriate. Although this clause does not explicitly address the subject, it is intended to give the MCO the right to cover the most cost-effective, medically appropriate procedure. An alternative way of addressing the issue is to state explicitly as one of the criteria that the procedure performed is the least costly setting or manner appropriate to treat the enrollee's medical condition.

6. This last sentence is a good addition to the definition. It makes clear the preference of outpatient care over inpatient care.

7. Member is usually regarded as synonymous with enrollee. The definition of member should be consistent with the definition used in the group enrollment agreement.

8. This paragraph allows the MCO to designate and amend the information, including the claims form, that the primary care physician provides the MCO without obtaining the prior approval of the primary care physician.

9. This contract reimburses primary care physicians on a fee-for-service basis. Attachment B also sets forth alternative language if an MCO pays its primary care physicians on a capitated basis.

10. Prompt payment time frames are usually set forth in state law. The time frames in the contract must meet those legal requirements. This paragraph allows the MCO to delay payment to the physician while waiting for sufficient documentation.

11. This prior notification requirement is an important requirement and often required by state law.

12. It is important for the MCO to make sure that the physicians know the circumstances or conditions for which prior MCO approval is required.

13. Here, again, it is important for the MCO to ensure that the primary care physicians have full notice of all the requirements for prior authorization and discharges.

14. State regulatory agencies often dictate the precise language of this clause.

15. This paragraph contains an important requirement. The primary care physician serves as a gatekeeper and the coordinator of care for this MCO. To serve this function, the primary

care physician needs information from referral providers. There, of course, needs to be a requirement in the contracts with referral physicians that this information be provided to the applicable primary care physician.

16. For this sentence to be effective, the MCO needs to ensure that its staff and the primary care physician understand state and federal confidentiality laws. Special requirements often arise in some areas, such as for acquired immunodeficiency syndrome and mental health and substance abuse services.

17. The MCO should have this insurance information on file. Thus, the MCO, as a matter of course, should request this information and require notification of changes in the insurance coverage.

18. This is a common provision and useful in simplifying the administrative work associated with amending the agreement. Needless to say, it is important for the MCO to explain clearly the nature of the amendment to the primary care physician. From a provider's perspective, it is desirable to obtain a provision that allows the provider to object to any unilateral amendment. Further, providers should obtain an exception that would not allow the MCO to unilaterally decrease the payment rate set forth in the agreement.

19. Before adopting this paragraph, an MCO should consider whether it is necessary to require that all notifications be sent by certified mail, return receipt requested. If the MCO has a large provider panel, it might prefer the right to send information by regular mail.

ATTACHMENT B
COMPENSATION SCHEDULE
PRIMARY CARE PHYSICIAN AGREEMENT

I. Services Rendered by Physicians

For Covered Services provided by Primary Care Physician in accordance with the terms of this Agreement, MCO shall pay Primary Care Physician his/her Reimbursement Allowance, less any applicable copayment for which the Member is responsible under the applicable Health Maintenance Certificate, and less the Withhold Amount, as described below. "Reimbursement Allowance" shall mean the lower of (i) the usual and customary fee charged by Primary Care Physician for the Covered Service, or (ii) the maximum amount allowed under the fee limits established by MCO.

II. Withholds from Reimbursement Allowance

MCO shall withhold from each payment to Primary Care Physician a percentage of the Reimbursement Allowance ("Withhold Amount") and shall allocate an amount equal to such withhold to an MCO Risk Fund. MCO shall have the right, at its sole discretion, to modify the percentage withheld from Primary Care Physician if, in its judgment, the financial condition, operations, or commitments of the MCO or its expenses for particular health services or for services by any particular Participating Providers warrant such modification.

III. Withhold Amount Distributions

MCO may, at its sole discretion, from time to time distribute to Primary Care Physician Withhold Amounts retained by MCO from payments to Primary Care Physician, plus such additional amounts, if any, that MCO may deem appropriate as a financial incentive to the provision of cost-effective health care services. MCO may, from time to time, commit or expend Withhold Amounts, in whole or in part, to assure the financial stability of or commitments of the MCO or health care plans or payers with or for which the MCO has an agreement to arrange for the provision of health care services, or to satisfy budgetary or financial objectives established by MCO.

Subject to MCO's peer review procedures and policies, a Primary Care Physician may be excluded from any distribution if he/she does not qualify for such distribution, for example, if he/she has exceeded MCO utilization standards or criteria. No Primary Care Physician shall have any entitlement to any funds in the MCO Risk Fund.

IV. Accounting

Primary Care Physician shall be entitled to an accounting of Withhold Amounts from payments to him/her upon written request to MCO.

ATTACHMENT B (ALTERNATE)
CAPITATION PAYMENT
PRIMARY CARE PHYSICIAN AGREEMENT

Compensation

I. Capitation Allocation

The total monthly amounts paid to Primary Care Physician will be determined as follows:

For each Member selecting Primary Care Physician ("selecting" also includes Members assigned to a Primary Care Physician), 90% of the monthly Primary Care Service capitation set forth below for Primary Care Services shall be paid by MCO to Primary Care Physician by the fifth day of the following month. The capitation shall be set according to the particular benefit plan in which each Member is enrolled. Where the capitation is not currently adjusted for age and/or sex, MCO reserves the right to make such age and/or sex adjustment to the capitation rates upon thirty (30) days notice. In consideration of such payments, Primary Care Physician agrees to provide to Members the Primary Care Services set forth in Attachment C hereto.

Health Plan shall allocate the remaining 10% of the monthly capitation payments to a Risk Reserve Fund which fund is subject to the further provisions of this Attachment. The capitation payments to Primary Care Physician for Primary Care Services, subject to the above withhold, are as follows:

Coverage Plans

Age/Sex	Commercial Plan___ Capitation Payment	Commercial Plan___ Capitation Payment	Commercial Plan___ Capitation Payment
0–24 Months/M/F	$ _____	$ _____	$ _____
2–4 Years/M/F	$ _____	$ _____	$ _____
5–19 Years/M/F	$ _____	$ _____	$ _____
20–39 Years/F	$ _____	$ _____	$ _____
20–39 Years/M	$ _____	$ _____	$ _____
40–49 Years/F	$ _____	$ _____	$ _____
40–49 Years/M	$ _____	$ _____	$ _____
50–59 Years/F	$ _____	$ _____	$ _____
50–59 Years/M	$ _____	$ _____	$ _____
>60 Years/F	$ _____	$ _____	$ _____
>60 Years/M	$ _____	$ _____	$ _____

Primary Care Physician is financially liable for all Primary Care Services rendered to Members under the above capitation. If Primary Care Physician fails to do so, MCO may pay for such services on behalf of Primary Care Physician and deduct such payments from any sums otherwise due Primary Care Physician by MCO.

Appendix 30-B
Sample Hospital Agreement

MANAGED CARE ORGANIZATION
PARTICIPATING HOSPITAL AGREEMENT[20]

THIS AGREEMENT, made and entered into the date set forth on the signature page hereto, by and between _____ (the "Hospital"), a facility duly licensed under the laws of the State of _____ and located at _____, and _____ ("MCO"), a corporation organized under the _____ law, and located at _____.

WHEREAS, MCO provides a plan of health care benefits (the "Plan") to individuals and their eligible family members and dependents who contract with MCO or who are the beneficiaries of a contract with MCO for such benefits ("Members"), and in connection with such Plan, arranges for the provision of health care services, including Hospital Services, to such Members; and

WHEREAS, the Hospital desires to provide Hospital Services to Members in accordance with the terms and conditions of this Agreement as hereinafter set forth; and

WHEREAS, MCO desires to arrange for the services of the Hospital for the benefit of the Members of the Plan.

NOW, THEREFORE, in consideration of the foregoing recitals and the mutual covenants and promises herein contained and other good and valuable consideration, receipt and sufficiency of which are hereby acknowledged, the parties hereto agree and covenant as follows:

PART I. DEFINITIONS

A. Covered Services means those health services and benefits to which Members are entitled under the terms of the applicable Health Maintenance Certificate, which may be amended by MCO from time to time.

B. Emergency Services means those Medically Necessary services provided in connection with an "Emergency," defined as a sudden or unexpected onset of a condition requiring medical or surgical care which the Member receives after the onset of such condition [or as soon thereafter as care can be made available but not more than twenty-four (24) hours after onset] and in the absence of such care the Member could reasonably be expected to suffer serious physical impairment or death. Heart attacks, severe chest pain, cardiovascular accidents, hemorrhaging, poisonings, major burns, loss of consciousness, serious breathing difficulties, spinal injuries, shock, and other acute conditions as MCO shall determine are Emergencies.

C. Health Maintenance Certificate means a contract issued by MCO to a Member or an employer of Members specifying the services and benefits available under the MCO's prepaid health benefits program.

D. Hospital Services means all inpatient services, emergency room, and outpatient hospital services that are Covered Services.

E. Medical Director means a Physician designated by MCO to monitor and review the provision of Covered Services to Members.

F. Medically Necessary services and/or supplies means the use of services or supplies as provided by a hospital, skilled nursing facility, Physician or other provider required to identify or treat a Member's illness or injury and which, as determined by MCO's Medical Director or its utilization management committee, are: (1) consistent with the symptoms or diagnosis and treatment of the Member's condition, disease, ailment, or injury; (2) appropriate with regard to standards of good medical practice; (3) not solely for the convenience of the Member, his/her Physician, hospital, or other health care provider; and (4) the most appropriate supply or level of service which can be safely provided to the Member. When specifically applied to an inpatient Member, it further means that the Member's medical symptoms or condition requires that the diagnosis or treatment cannot be safely provided to the Member as an outpatient.

G. Member means both an MCO subscriber and his/her enrolled family members for whom premium payment has been made.

H. Participating Physician means a Physician who, at the time of providing or authorizing services to a Member, has contracted with or on whose behalf a contract has been entered into with MCO to provide professional services to Members.

 I. Participating Provider means a Physician, hospital, skilled nursing facility, home health agency, or any other duly licensed institution or health professional under contract with MCO to provide health care services to Members. A list of Participating Providers and their locations is available to each Member upon enrollment. Such list shall be revised from time to time as MCO deems necessary.

J. Physician means a duly licensed doctor of medicine, osteopathy or podiatry.

K. Primary Care Physician means a Participating Physician who provides primary care services to Members (*eg,* general or family practitioner, internist, pediatrician, or such other physician specialty as may be designated by MCO) and is responsible for referrals of Members to referral Physicians, other Participating Providers, and if necessary, non-Participating Providers.

PART II. HOSPITAL OBLIGATIONS

A. Hospital shall provide to Members those Hospital Services that Hospital has the capacity to provide. Such services shall be provided by Hospital in accordance with the provisions of its Articles of Incorporation and bylaws and medical staff bylaws and the appropriate terms of this Agreement.

B. Hospital shall render Hospital Services to Members in an economical and efficient manner consistent with professional standards of medical care generally accepted in the medical community. Hospital shall not discriminate in the treatment of members and, except as otherwise required by this Agreement, shall make its services available to Members in the same manner as to its other patients.[21] In the event that an admission of a Member cannot be accommodated by Hospital, Hospital shall make the same efforts to arrange for the provision of services at another facility approved by MCO that it would make for other patients in similar circumstances. In the event that Hospital shall provide Member non-Covered Services, Hospital shall, prior to the provision of such non-Covered Services, inform the Member:

 1. of the service(s) to be provided,
 2. that MCO will not pay for or be liable for said services, and
 3. that Member will be financially liable for such services.

C. Except in an Emergency, Hospital shall provide Hospital Inpatient Services to a Member only when Hospital has received certification from MCO in advance of admission of such

Member. Services which have not been so approved or authorized shall be the sole financial responsibility of Hospital.[22]

D. If, and to the extent that, Hospital is not authorized to perform preadmission testing, Hospital agrees to accept the results of qualified and timely laboratory, radiological, and other tests and procedures that may be performed on a Member prior to admission. The Hospital will not require that duplicate tests or procedures be performed after the Enrollee is admitted, unless such tests and procedures are Medically Necessary.

E. In an Emergency, Hospital shall immediately proceed to render Medically Necessary services to the Member. Hospital shall also contact MCO within twenty-four (24) hours of the treatment of the emergency treatment visit or emergency admission. MCO has twenty-four (24) hour on-call nurse coverage for notification of Emergency Services or admits.

   If Hospital fails to notify MCO within the required time period, neither MCO nor the Member shall be liable for charges for Hospital Services rendered subsequent to the required notification period that are deemed by MCO not to be Medically Necessary.[23]

F. Hospital shall cooperate with and abide by MCO's programs that monitor and evaluate whether Hospital Services provided to Members in accordance with this Agreement are Medically Necessary and consistent with professional standards of medical care generally accepted in the medical community. Such programs include, but are not limited to, utilization management, quality assurance review, and grievance procedures. In connection with MCO's programs, Hospital shall permit MCO's utilization management personnel to visit Members in the Hospital and, to the extent permitted by applicable laws, to inspect and copy health records (including medical records) of Members maintained by Hospital for the purposes of concurrent and retrospective utilization management, discharge planning, and other program management purposes.

G. Hospital shall cooperate with MCO in complying with applicable laws relating to MCO.

PART III. LICENSURE AND ACCREDITATION

Hospital represents that it is duly licensed by the Department of Health of the State of _____ to operate a hospital, is a qualified provider under the Medicare program, and is accredited by the Joint Commission on the Accreditation of Healthcare Organizations ("Joint Commission"). Hospital shall maintain in good standing such license and accreditation and shall notify MCO immediately should any action of any kind be initiated against Hospital which could result in:

1. the suspension or loss of such license,
2. the suspension or loss of such accreditation, or
3. the imposition of any sanctions against Hospital under a Federal health care program.

Hospital shall furnish to MCO such evidence of licensure, Medicare qualification, and accreditation as MCO may request.

PART IV. RECORDS

A. Hospital shall maintain with respect to each Member receiving Hospital Services pursuant to this Agreement a standard hospital medical record in such form, containing such information, and preserved for such time period(s) as are required by the rules and regulations of the _____ Department of Health, the Medicare program, and the Joint Commission. The original hospital medical records shall be and remain the property of

Hospital and shall not be removed or transferred from Hospital except in accordance with applicable laws and general Hospital policies, rules, and regulations relating thereto; provided, however, that MCO shall have the right, in accordance with paragraph (B) below, to inspect, review, and make copies of such records upon request.

B. Upon consent of the Member and a request for such records or information, Hospital shall provide copies of information contained in the medical records of Members to other authorized providers of health care services and to MCO for the purpose of facilitating the delivery of appropriate health care services to Members and carrying out the purposes and provisions of this Agreement, and shall facilitate the sharing of such records among health care providers involved in a Member's care. MCO, and if required, authorized state and federal agencies, shall have the right upon request to inspect at reasonable times and to obtain copies of all records that are maintained by Hospital relating to the care of Members pursuant to this Agreement.

PART V. INSURANCE AND INDEMNIFICATION

A. Hospital shall secure and maintain at its expense throughout the term of this Agreement such policy or policies of general liability and professional liability insurance as shall be necessary to insure Hospital, its agents, and employees against any claim or claims for damages arising by reason of injury or death, occasioned directly or indirectly by the performance or nonperformance of any service by Hospital, its agents, or employees. Upon request, Hospital shall provide MCO with a copy of the policy (or policies) or certificate(s) of insurance which evidence compliance with the foregoing insurance requirements. It is specifically agreed that coverage amounts in general conformity with other similar type and size hospitals within the State of _____ shall be acceptable to MCO and be considered satisfactory and in compliance with this requirement.[24]

B. Hospital and MCO each shall indemnify and hold the other harmless from any and all liability, loss, damage, claim, or expense of any kind, including costs and attorney's fees, arising out of the performance of this Agreement and for which the other is solely responsible.

PART VI. MEDICAL STAFF MEMBERSHIP

Notwithstanding any other provision of this Agreement, a Participating Physician may not admit or treat a Member in the Hospital unless he/she is a member in good standing of Hospital's organized medical staff with appropriate clinical privileges to admit and treat such Member.[25]

PART VII. MCO OBLIGATIONS

A. MCO shall provide to or for the benefit of each Member an identification card which shall be presented for purposes of assisting Hospital in verifying Member eligibility. In addition, MCO shall maintain other verification procedures by which Hospital may confirm the eligibility of any Member.

B. MCO shall provide thirty (30) days advance notice to Hospital of any changes in Covered Services or in the copayments or conditions of coverage applicable thereto.

C. MCO will, whenever an individual, admitted or referred, is not a Member, advise Hospital within thirty (30) days from the date of receipt of an invoice from Hospital for services to such an individual. In such cases, Hospital shall directly bill the individual or another third-party payer for services rendered to such individual.

D. In the event continued stay or services are denied after a patient has been admitted, MCO or its representative shall inform the patient that services have been denied.

PART VIII. USE OF NAME

Except as provided in this paragraph, neither MCO nor Hospital shall use the other's name, symbols, trademarks, or service marks in advertising or promotional material or otherwise. MCO shall have the right to use the name of Hospital for purposes of marketing, informing Members of the identity of Hospital, and otherwise to carry out the terms of this Agreement. Hospital shall have the right to use MCO's name in its informational or promotional materials with MCO's prior approval, which approval shall not be unreasonably withheld.

PART IX. COMPENSATION

Hospital will be compensated by MCO for all Medically Necessary Covered Services provided to Members in accordance with the provisions of Attachment A annexed hereto and incorporated herein.[26]

PART X. PAYMENT TO HOSPITAL BY MCO

For Hospital Services rendered to Members, Hospital shall invoice MCO at Hospital's current charges. [Alternative: For Hospital Services rendered to Members, Hospital shall invoice MCO.[27]] Except for Hospital Services which MCO determines require further review under MCO's utilization management procedures, or when there are circumstances which are beyond the control of MCO, including submission of incomplete claims, MCO shall make payment of invoices for Hospital Services within thirty (30) calendar days after the MCO's receipt thereof. MCO authorized copayments shall be collected by the Hospital from the Member and the Member shall be solely responsible for the payment of such copayments. All billings by Hospital shall be considered final unless adjustments are requested in writing by Hospital within sixty (60) days after receipt of original billing by MCO, except for circumstances which are beyond the control of Hospital.[28] No payment shall be made unless the invoice for services is received within sixty (60) days after the date of discharge of the Member or date of service, whichever occurs later. Hospital shall interim bill MCO every thirty (30) days for patients whose length of stay is greater than thirty (30) days.

PART XI. PROHIBITIONS ON MEMBER BILLING

Hospital hereby agrees that in no event, including, but not limited to, nonpayment by MCO, MCO's insolvency, or breach of this Agreement, shall Hospital bill, charge, collect a deposit from, seek compensation, remuneration, or reimbursement from, or have any recourse against a Member or persons other than MCO acting on a Member's behalf for services provided pursuant to this Agreement. This provision shall not prohibit collection of copayment on MCO's behalf in accordance with the terms of the Health Maintenance Certificate between MCO and Member.

Hospital agrees that in the event of MCO's insolvency or other cessation of operations, services to Members will continue through the period for which the premium has been paid and services to Members confined in an inpatient hospital on the date of insolvency or other cessation of operations will continue until their discharge.

Hospital further agrees that:

1. this provision shall survive the termination of this Agreement regardless of the cause giving rise to termination and shall be construed to be for the benefit of the Member, and

2. this provision supersedes any oral or written contrary agreement now existing or here-after entered into between Hospital and Member, or persons acting on their behalf.

Any modifications, addition or deletion to these provisions shall become effective on a date no earlier than 15 days after the _____ Department of Insurance has received written notice of such proposed changes.

PART XII. INSPECTION OF RECORDS

Upon request, and at reasonable times, MCO and Hospital shall make available to the other for review such books, records, utilization information, and other documents or information relating directly to any determination required by this Agreement. All such information shall be held by the receiving party in confidence and shall only be used in connection with the administration of this Agreement.

PART XIII. COORDINATION OF BENEFITS

Hospital agrees to cooperate with MCO toward effective implementation of any provisions of MCO's Health Maintenance Certificates relating to coordination of benefits and claims by third parties. Hospital shall forward to MCO any payments received from a third-party payer for authorized Hospital Services where MCO has made payment to Hospital covering such Hospital Services and such third-party payer is determined to be primarily obligated for such Hospital Services under applicable Coordination of Benefits rules. Such payment shall not exceed the amount paid to Hospital by MCO. Except as otherwise required by law, Hospital agrees to permit MCO to bill and process forms for any third-party payer on Hospital's behalf, or to bill such third party directly, as determined by MCO. Hospital further agrees to waive, when requested, any claims against third-party payers for its provision of Hospital Services to Members and to execute any further documents that reasonably may be required or appropriate for this purpose. Any such waiver shall be contingent upon MCO's payment to Hospital of its (MCO's) obligations for charges incurred by Member. This paragraph shall not be interpreted as a waiver of Medicare beneficiary cost-sharing obligations to the extent that such waiver is in violation of Federal law.

PART XIV. TERM AND TERMINATION

A. This Agreement shall take effect on the "effective date" set forth on the signature page and shall continue for a period of 1 year or until terminated as provided herein.

1. Either party may terminate this Agreement without cause upon at least ninety (90) days written notice prior to the term of this Agreement.

2. Either party may terminate this Agreement with cause upon at least thirty (30) days prior written notice.

B. MCO shall have the right to terminate this Agreement immediately by notice to Hospital upon the occurrence of any of the following events:

1. the suspension or revocation of Hospital's license,
2. the suspension, revocation, or loss of the Hospital's Joint Commission accreditation or Medicare qualification, or
3. breach of Part II(E) or Part XI of this Agreement.

C. MCO shall continue to pay Hospital in accordance with the provisions of Attachment A for Hospital Services provided by Hospital to Members hospitalized at the time of termination of this Agreement, pending clinically appropriate discharge or transfer to an MCO designated hospital when medically appropriate as determined by MCO. In continuing to provide such Hospital Services, Hospital shall abide by the applicable terms and conditions of this Agreement.

PART XV. ADMINISTRATION

Hospital agrees to abide by and cooperate with MCO administrative policies including, but not limited to, claims procedures, copayment collections, and duplicate coverage/subrogation recoveries. Nothing in this Agreement shall be construed to require Hospital to violate, breach, or modify its written policies and procedures unless specifically agreed to herein.

PART XVI. MEMBER GRIEVANCES

Hospital agrees to cooperate in and abide by MCO grievance procedures in resolving Member's grievances related to the provision of Hospital Services. In this regard, MCO shall bring to the attention of appropriate Hospital officials all Member complaints involving Hospital, and Hospital shall, in accordance with its regular procedure, investigate such complaints and use its best efforts to resolve them in a fair and equitable manner. Hospital agrees to notify MCO promptly of any action taken or proposed with respect to the resolution of such complaints and the avoidance of similar complaints in the future. The Hospital shall notify the MCO after it has received a complaint from an MCO Member.

PART XVII. MISCELLANEOUS

A. If any term, provision, covenant, or condition of this Agreement is invalid, void, or unenforceable, the rest of the Agreement shall remain in full force and effect. The invalidity or unenforceability of any term or provision hereof shall in no way affect the validity or enforceability of any other term or provision.
B. This Agreement contains the complete understanding and agreement between Hospital and MCO and supersedes all representations, understandings, or agreements prior to the execution hereof.
C. MCO and Hospital agree that, to the extent compatible with the separate and independent management of each, they shall at all times maintain an effective liaison and close cooperation with each other to provide maximum benefits to Members at the most reasonable cost consistent with quality standards of hospital care.
D. No waiver, alteration, amendment, or modification of this Agreement shall be valid unless in each instance a written memorandum specifically expressing such waiver, alteration, amendment, or modification is made and subscribed by a duly authorized officer of Hospital and a duly authorized officer of MCO.
E. Hospital shall not assign its rights, duties, or obligations under this Agreement without the express, written permission of MCO.

F. None of the provisions of this Agreement are intended to create nor shall be deemed to create any relationship between MCO and Hospital other than that of independent entities contracting with each other hereunder solely for the purpose of effecting the provisions of this Agreement. Neither of the parties hereto, nor any of their respective employees shall be construed to be the agent, employer, employee, or representative of the other.

G. This Agreement shall be construed in accordance with the laws of the State of _____.

H. The headings and numbers of sections and paragraphs contained in this Agreement are for reference purposes only and shall not affect in any way the meaning or interpretation of this Agreement.

I. Any notice required or permitted to be given pursuant to the terms and provisions of this Agreement shall be sent by registered mail or certified mail, return receipt requested, postage prepaid, to:

_____

_____

_____

_____

_____

_____

and to Hospital at:

_____

_____

_____

_____

_____

IN WITNESS WHEREOF, the foregoing Agreement between _____ and Hospital is entered into by and between the undersigned parties, to be effective the _____ day of _____, 20_____.

By: _____

Title: _____

Date: _____

HOSPITAL

By: _____

Title: _____

Date: _____

ATTACHMENT A
PARTICIPATING HOSPITAL COMPENSATION

Subject to the terms and conditions set forth in this Agreement, MCO shall pay Hospital _____ (_____ %) of Hospital's schedule of charges effective _____ as submitted and approved by MCO, for Medically Necessary Covered Services provided to Members.

ATTACHMENT A (ALTERNATE)
PARTICIPATING HOSPITAL COMPENSATION

Subject to the terms and conditions set forth in this Agreement, MCO shall pay Hospital, as follows:

Service	Type of Reimbursement	Total Reimbursement
Inpatient care		
Nonmaternity—secondary	Per Diem	$_____
Nonmaternity—tertiary	Per Diem	$_____
Maternity	Per Diem	$_____
Psychiatric	Per Diem	$_____
Well newborn children	Per Diem	$_____
Outpatient care		
Other than outpatient surgery	Percentage Discount	_____%
Outpatient surgery		Hospital will be reimbursed (1) the percentage discount stated above, (2) any guaranteed maximum "global" rate program adopted by the Hospital for ambulatory surgical procedures,[29] or (3) 125%[30] of the per diem payment amount had the Enrollee been admitted to the Hospital, whichever is least.

Notes to Appendix 30-B

20. For consistency, the MCO has used the same definitions for this agreement and the preceding primary care physician agreement. This agreement also uses some of the same provisions as in the primary care physician agreement. Comments made to those provisions in the primary care physician agreement will not be repeated here.

21. This requirement serves the same purpose as its counterpart in the primary care physician agreement of requiring the hospital to treat MCO members in the same manner as fee-for-service patients.

22. A growing issue, not addressed in this provision, is the MCO's responsibility for hospital charges incurred to provide a medical screening examination, as required by Section 1867 of the Social Security Act, to enrollees seeking care from the hospital's emergency department. The hospital may want to seek an explicit statement requiring the MCO to cover the cost of that examination.

23. To avoid disputes, the hospital and MCO need a common understanding of the meaning of the term *Medically Necessary*. The definition of that term used in this contract favors the MCO by allowing for its interpretation.

24. This paragraph reflects the difference in relative bargaining strength that the MCO has with hospitals and physicians. Although the MCO-primary care physician agreement gives the MCO the right to approve malpractice coverage, no such right is contained in the MCO-participating hospital agreement. Another factor may be that the concern of inadequate coverage may be greater for a physician than a hospital.

25. Requiring the MCO's physicians to comply with the hospital's medical staff requirements is important and reasonable.
26. Attachment A provides for payment as a percentage of charges. By structuring the agreement in this manner, the MCO is able to negotiate different payment arrangements with hospitals without revising the body of the agreement.
27. This broader alternative language along with the cross-reference to Attachment A in the preceding paragraph allows the body of the contract to be used for any type of payment arrangement. An alternative Attachment A is offered that establishes per diem rates for inpatient stays and a percentage of charges for outpatient services.
28. To avoid potential disputes, the hospital and the MCO should have some general understanding of the meaning of the term beyond the control of Hospital.
29. If Medicare adopts a global fee for reimbursement of outpatient hospital costs, an increasing number of MCO-hospital contracts are likely to adopt a similar approach.
30. This percentage commonly varies from 100% to 125%.

Appendix 30-C
Sample Business Associate Addendum

BUSINESS ASSOCIATE ADDENDUM

I. DEFINITIONS

As used in this Addendum, the following terms have the meanings assigned to them below:

A. Agreement. "Agreement" shall mean the Provider Service Agreement.

B. Business Associate. "Business Associate" shall mean Provider.

C. Covered Entity. "Covered Entity" shall mean MCO.

D. Individual. "Individual" shall have the same meaning as the term "individual" in 45 CFR §160.103 and shall include a person who qualifies as a personal representative in accordance with 45 CFR §164.502(g).

E. Privacy Rule. "Privacy Rule" shall mean the Standards for Privacy of Individually Identifiable Health Information at 45 CFR Part 160 and Part 164, Subparts A and E.

F. Protected Health Information. "Protected Health Information" shall have the same meaning as the term "protected health information" in 45 CFR §160.103, limited to the information created or received by Business Associate from or on behalf of Covered Entity.

G. Required By Law. "Required By Law" shall have the same meaning as the term "required by law" in 45 CFR §164.103.

H. Secretary. "Secretary" shall mean the Secretary of the Department of Health and Human Services or his designee.

Any other terms used, but not otherwise defined, in this Addendum shall have the same meaning as those terms in the Privacy Rule.

II. PERMITTED USES AND DISCLOSURES

A. Except as otherwise limited in this Addendum, Business Associate may use or disclose Protected Health Information to perform functions, activities, or services for, or on behalf of, Covered Entity as set forth in the Agreement, provided that such use or disclosure would not violate the Privacy Rule if done by Covered Entity.

B. Covered Entity shall not request Business Associate to use or disclose Protected Health Information in any manner that would not be permissible under the Privacy Rule if done by Covered Entity, except as set forth in Sections II.C and II.D herein.

C. Business Associate may use Protected Health Information for the proper management and administration of the Business Associate or to carry out the legal responsibilities of the Business Associate.

D. Business Associate may disclose Protected Health Information for the proper management and administration of the Business Associate, provided that disclosures are Required By Law, or Business Associate obtains reasonable assurances from the person to whom the information is disclosed that it will remain confidential and used or further disclosed only as Required By Law or for the purpose for which it was disclosed to the person, and the person notifies the Business Associate of any instances of which it is aware in which the confidentiality of the information has been breached.

E. Business Associate may use Protected Health Information to provide Data Aggregation services to Covered Entity as permitted by 45 CFR §164.504(e)(2)(i)(B).

F. Business Associate may use Protected Health Information to report violations of law to appropriate Federal and State authorities, consistent with §164.502(j)(1).

III. OBLIGATIONS AND ACTIVITIES OF BUSINESS ASSOCIATE

A. Business Associate agrees to not use or disclose Protected Health Information other than as permitted or required by this Addendum or as Required By Law.

B. Business Associate agrees to use appropriate safeguards to prevent use or disclosure of the Protected Health Information other than as provided for by this Addendum.

C. Business Associate agrees to report to Covered Entity any use or disclosure of the Protected Health Information not provided for by this Addendum of which it becomes aware.

D. Business Associate agrees to ensure that any agent, including a subcontractor, to whom it provides Protected Health Information received from, or created or received by Business Associate on behalf of Covered Entity agrees to the same restrictions and conditions that apply through this Addendum to Business Associate with respect to such information.

E. Business Associate agrees to provide access to Covered Entity, within 10 business days of a request of Covered Entity, to Protected Health Information in a nonduplicative Designated Record Set, in order to meet the requirements under 45 CFR §164.524.

F. Business Associate agrees to make any amendment(s) to Protected Health Information in a Designated Record Set that the Covered Entity directs or agrees to pursuant to 45 CFR §164.526 within 10 business days of a request from Covered Entity.

G. Business Associate agrees to make internal practices, books, and records, including policies and procedures and Protected Health Information, relating to the use and disclosure of Protected Health Information received from, or created or received by Business Associate on behalf of, Covered Entity available to the Covered Entity, or to the Secretary, in a reasonable time and manner requested by Covered Entity or the time and manner designated by the Secretary, for purposes of the Secretary determining Covered Entity's compliance with the Privacy Rule.

H. Business Associate agrees to document such disclosures of Protected Health Information and information related to such disclosures as would be required for Covered Entity to respond to a request by an Individual for an accounting of disclosures of Protected Health Information in accordance with 45 CFR §164.528.

I. Business Associate agrees to provide to Covered Entity, within 10 business days of a request from Covered Entity, information collected in accordance with Section III.H. of this Addendum, to permit Covered Entity to respond to a request by an Individual for an accounting of disclosures of Protected Health Information in accordance with 45 CFR §164.528.

J. Business Associate agrees to implement administrative, physical, and technical safeguards that reasonably and appropriately protect the confidentiality, integrity, and availability of the Electronic Protected Health Information that it creates, receives, maintains, or transmits on behalf of Covered Entity as required by 45 CFR 164 Subpart C and ensure that any agent, including a subcontractor, to whom Business Associate provides such information agrees to implement reasonable and appropriate safeguards to protect it.

K. Business Associate agrees to report to Covered Entity any security incident of which it becomes aware.

IV. OBLIGATIONS OF COVERED ENTITY

A. Covered Entity shall notify Business Associate of any limitation(s) in its notice of privacy practices of Covered Entity in accordance with 45 CFR §164.520, to the extent that such limitation may affect Business Associate's use or disclosure of Protected Health Information.

B. Covered Entity shall notify Business Associate of any changes in, or revocation of, permission by Individual to use or disclose Protected Health Information, to the extent that such changes may affect Business Associate's use or disclosure of Protected Health Information.

C. Covered Entity shall notify Business Associate of any restriction to the use or disclosure of Protected Health Information that Covered Entity has agreed to in accordance with 45 CFR §164.522, to the extent that such restriction may affect Business Associate's use or disclosure of Protected Health Information.

V. TERM AND TERMINATION

A. Term. The provisions of this Addendum shall terminate when all of the Protected Health Information provided by Covered Entity to Business Associate, or created or received by Business Associate on behalf of Covered Entity, is destroyed or returned to Covered Entity, or, if it is infeasible to return or destroy Protected Health Information, protections are extended to such information, in accordance with the termination provisions in this Section.

B. Termination for Cause. Upon Covered Entity's knowledge of a material breach by Business Associate, Covered Entity shall either:

   1. Provide Business Associate 30 days to cure the breach or end the violation. If Business Associate fails to cure the breach within 30 days, this Addendum and all provisions of the Agreement that require the exchange of Protected Health Information to implement shall be terminated,

   2. Immediately terminate this Addendum and all provisions of the Agreement that require the exchange of Protected Health Information to implement if Business Associate has breached a material term of this Addendum and cure is not possible, or

   3. If neither termination nor cure are feasible, Covered Entity shall report the violation to the Secretary.

C. Effect of Termination.

   1. Except as provided in paragraph (b) of this section V.C. of this Addendum, upon termination of this Addendum, for any reason, Business Associate shall return or destroy all Protected Health Information received from Covered Entity, or created or received by Business Associate on behalf of Covered Entity. This provision shall apply to Protected Health Information that is in the possession of subcontractors or agents of Business Associate. Business Associate shall retain no copies of the Protected Health Information.

   2. In the event that Business Associate determines that returning or destroying the Protected Health Information is infeasible, Business Associate shall provide to Covered Entity notification of the conditions that make return or destruction infeasible. Upon the Parties' agreement that return or destruction of Protected Health Information is infeasible, Business Associate shall extend the protections of this Addendum to such Protected Health Information and limit further uses and disclosures of such Protected Health Information to those purposes that make the return or destruction infeasible, for so long as Business Associate maintains such Protected Health Information.

VI. MISCELLANEOUS

A. <u>Regulatory References.</u> A reference in this Addendum to a section in the Privacy Rule means the section as in effect or as amended.

B. <u>Amendment.</u> The Parties agree to take such action as is necessary to amend this Addendum from time to time as is necessary for Covered Entity to comply with the requirements of the Privacy Rule and the Health Insurance Portability and Accountability Act of 1996, Pub. L. No. 104-191.

C. <u>Survival.</u> The respective rights and obligations of Business Associate under Section V.C. of this Addendum shall survive the termination of the Agreement and this Addendum.

D. <u>Interpretation.</u> Any ambiguity in this Addendum shall be resolved to permit Covered Entity to comply with the Privacy Rule.

E. <u>Indemnification.</u> Business Associate will indemnify and hold harmless Covered Entity and any of its officers, directors, employees, or agents from and against that portion of any claim, cause of action, liability, damage, cost or expense, including attorneys' fees, arising solely out of any nonpermitted or violating Use, Disclosure, or request for Protected Health Information or other breach of this Addendum by Business Associate.

Covered Entity will indemnify and hold harmless Business Associate and any of its officers, directors, employees, or agents from and against that portion of any claim, cause of action, liability, damage, cost or expense, including attorneys' fees, arising solely out of any nonpermitted or violating Use, Disclosure, or request for Protected Health Information or other breach of this Addendum by Covered Entity.

31

ERISA AND
MANAGED CARE

Jacqueline M. Saue and Gregg H. Dooge

Study Objectives

- Understand how ERISA regulates employee-benefit plans.
- Understand the differences between insured benefits and self-insured benefits.
- Understand ERISA preemption of state laws for self-funded benefits plans.
- Understand when ERISA does or does not preempt different types of legal liability.
- Understand the documentation, reporting, and disclosure requirements under ERISA.
- Understand how benefits plan design is and is not regulated under ERISA.
- Understand the fiduciary duties required under ERISA.
- Understand what ERISA requires and does not require regarding challenges to benefits claims denials.
- Understand ERISA's enforcement scheme and remedies.

Discussion Topics

1. Describe ERISA preemption of state insurance laws and mandates. Discuss the implications of this preemption.
2. Discuss when an employer would or would not choose to self-fund a health benefits plan for employees.
3. Describe the fiduciary responsibility aspect of ERISA. Discuss the implications of those responsibilities.
4. Describe how a benefits claims denial may be challenged under ERISA. Discuss how a benefits plan might avoid successful challenges, and the implications of such actions.
5. Discuss why ERISA came into being in the first place, and how it has evolved over the years.

INTRODUCTION

Few federal laws have a greater impact on the operations of managed care organizations (MCOs) than the Employee Retirement Income Security Act (ERISA) of 1974, as amended.[1] Although ERISA does not directly regulate MCOs, it does regulate most employer-sponsored employee benefit plans to which MCOs market their products. ERISA will affect the nature, design, and administration of such products by MCOs. Moreover, ERISA will determine what state laws can be applied to such products as well as what legal challenges can be made to the administration of such products.

This chapter is designed to provide MCOs with a working knowledge of the provisions of ERISA that are likely to affect their operations. Topics addressed include ERISA's documentation, reporting, and disclosure requirements; benefit plan design considerations; the amendment of benefit plans; the duties of ERISA fiduciaries, which may include MCOs; challenges to benefit denials; ERISA's civil enforcement scheme and remedies; and the effect of ERISA preemption of state laws and causes of actions on MCOs' operations.

DOCUMENTATION, REPORTING, AND DISCLOSURE REQUIREMENTS

A plan maintained by a nongovernment employer that provides health care or health care benefits to employees (including plans providing coverage or benefits through a managed care arrangement) generally constitutes an employee benefit plan subject to ERISA.[2] Such plans must meet the documentation, reporting, and disclosure requirements set forth in ERISA.

Plan Document

Every employee benefit plan governed by ERISA is required to be set forth in a written plan document (or documents) that detail the operative provisions governing benefits un-der the plan.[3] In the case of health care benefits that are provided through an insurance contract or a contract with an MCO, the sponsoring employer might maintain a simple plan document that describes certain of the plan's rules, such as a description of the plan's eligibility and amendment provisions, but that otherwise refers to the insurance or managed care contract for the description of plan benefits.

Summary Plan Description

A summary plan description is a booklet that describes the operative provisions of a plan in lay language. The Department of Labor has prescribed the types of information that are required to be included in the summary plan description.[4] For insured or managed care plans, employers often use the booklet published by the insurance company or MCO as the basis for the summary plan description, although the employer generally will have to add certain administrative information to comply with the Department of Labor requirements concerning summary plan descriptions. In some cases, a health care plan contains detailed benefit schedules that are difficult to summarize. In lieu of repeating the benefit schedules, the summary plan description may provide a general description of the types of benefits provided if the summary informs participants that the complete schedules are available for their review.[5]

The summary plan description must be distributed to participants within 120 days after the date on which the plan is adopted or made effective (or, in the case of an employee who becomes a participant after the adoption or effective date of the plan, within 90 days after the date on which the employee becomes a participant).[6] In general, a new summary plan description must be issued every 5 years, although if there have been no amendments to the plan, distribution of a new summary plan description can be made every 10 years.[7]

Summary of Material Modifications

If there are changes in the plan that affect the information provided in the summary plan description at a time when the plan sponsor is not required to publish a new summary plan description, the employer must publish a summary of material modifications.[8] The summary of material modifications explains the plan changes and acts as a supplement to the summary plan description until a revised summary plan description is distributed. Generally, the summary of material modifications must be distributed to plan participants within 210 days after the close of the plan year in which the plan amendment is adopted, although in the case of an amendment that constitutes a "material reduction in covered services or benefits" under a group health plan, the summary of material modifications, with limited exceptions, must be distributed within 60 days after adoption of the amendment.[9] Alternatively, the plan sponsor may at any time publish an updated summary plan description in lieu of the summary of material modifications.

Discrepancies in Plan Documentation

"Although the summary plan description and summary of material modifications are intended, as their names suggest, as summaries of the actual plan document, some courts have held that the summaries override the terms of the plan where the plan and the summaries conflict.[10] Thus, where the summary plan description provides for benefits in a situation not covered under the formal plan document, the summary plan description might govern, particularly if there is a direct conflict between the summary plan description and the underlying plan document,[11] and if the participant or beneficiary is able to demonstrate reliance on or prejudice as a result of the faulty summary plan description.[12] However, the courts have not always agreed on the question of reliance, or

whether prejudice in the absence of detrimental reliance, is sufficient to sustain a claim.[13]

Government Reporting Requirements

The plan administrator of an ERISA welfare benefit plan (including plans that provide benefits pursuant to a managed care contract) must file a variety of documents with either the Department of Labor or the Internal Revenue Service. Each year, the plan administrator must file an annual return unless the plan is exempt from filing.[14] Generally, an annual return (filed on Form 5500) is required for plans that have more than 100 participants as of the first day of the plan year. Plans with fewer than 100 participants as of the first day of the plan year generally are exempt from filing if benefits are provided through insurance contracts, the premiums for which are paid from the plan sponsor's general corporate assets, if benefits are provided directly by the plan sponsor out of general corporate assets, or a combination of the two.[15] Plans in which benefits or insurance premiums are payable through a trust and certain plans that receive employee contributions do not qualify for the exception, and an annual return is required to be filed even though the plans might have fewer than 100 participants.[16]

Some health plans are operated in conjunction with a "flexible spending arrangement" or "cafeteria plan" under Section 125 of the Internal Revenue Code. A simple example would be a health plan in which the employer requires its employees to pay a portion of the premium. The employer then establishes a plan under Section 125 that enables a plan participant to make so-called salary reduction contributions; that is, the participant reduces his or her salary in exchange for the employer's payment of the employee premium contribution. Historically, even if the Section 125 arrangement covers fewer than 100 participants, an annual report was required.[17] In 2002, the Internal Revenue Service suspended the annual reporting requirement for Section 125 arrangements.[18] However, even though the Internal Revenue Service has suspended the Form 5500 reporting requirement with respect to the Section 125 arrangement, a Form 5500 series annual report still might be required with respect to the underlying plan that is funded through the Section 125 arrangement, unless a different exemption applies.

The annual return is due on or before the last day of the seventh month after the close of the plan year, although certain extensions are possible.[19] The return is filed with the Internal Revenue Service and is provided by the Service to the Department of Labor. The annual return is not distributed to plan participants as a general matter, although a plan participant must be allowed to review and make copies of the annual return.[20]

PLAN DESIGN CONSIDERATIONS

Plan sponsors have considerable flexibility with respect to the design of their welfare benefit programs, owing to the fact that ERISA provides limited substantive regulation of welfare benefit plans yet ERISA preempts most state law regulation of benefit plans.

Substantive Regulation under ERISA

ERISA provides relatively little regulation of the content of employee welfare benefit plans (a category that includes health benefit plans), although recent ERISA amendments have begun to regulate the content of employee welfare benefit plans more extensively. In contrast to the regulation of pension plans, where ERISA provides detailed and generally comprehensive requirements, ERISA regulation of employer-sponsored health plans has been piecemeal and is limited to the following:

- An employer-sponsored health plan is required to comply with the terms of a qualified medical child support order. A qualified medical child support order is a court order or court-approved property settlement agreement that is entered pursuant to state domestic relations law or certain state Medicaid laws and that provides for health insurance coverage for a child of an employee.[21]
- A group health plan, if it otherwise provides coverage for dependent natural children, is required to provide identical coverage for children who are placed for adoption with the covered employee.[22]
- A group health plan may not reduce its coverage of pediatric vaccines below the level of coverage that it provided as of May 1, 1993.[23]
- A plan of an employer with 20 or more employees is required to provide employees and their covered dependents whose coverage under the plan would otherwise cease as a result of termination of employment or certain other "qualifying events" the opportunity to purchase continued coverage under the plan for a limited period of time.[24] (State law insurance continuation rules may also apply.)
- A group health plan generally may exclude coverage for preexisting conditions (whether physical or mental) only for those conditions that were diagnosed or for which the participant received treatment within 6 months prior to enrollment and the exclusion generally cannot extend for more than 12 months after enrollment. Further, a group health plan generally must credit periods of prior coverage toward the 12-month exclusion period unless there exists a 63-day or greater gap between the prior coverage and the participant's coverage under the group health plan.[25] In addition, a group health plan may not treat pregnancy as a preexisting condition,

and a group health plan may not impose a preexisting condition limitation with respect to a newborn who is enrolled in the plan within 30 days of birth or with respect to a child who is adopted or placed for adoption and who is enrolled in the plan within 30 days of adoption or placement for adoption.[26]

- A group health plan may not establish eligibility rules (or require a higher premium contribution) based upon an individual's health status, medical condition, claims experience, receipt of health care, medical history, genetic information, evidence of insurability, and/or disability.[27]

- A group health plan that is a multiemployer plan or a multiple-employer welfare arrangement may not, with certain exceptions, deny an employer who participates in the plan and whose employees are covered under the plan, continued access to the plan.[28]

- A group health plan may not, with certain exceptions, restrict hospitalization benefits for the delivering mother or newborn child to less than 48 hours for normal vaginal deliveries or 96 hours following a cesarean section.[29]

- A group health plan with 50 or more employees generally may not place lower annual and/or aggregate dollar limits on mental health care benefits as compared to limits place upon medical and surgical benefits.[30] Currently, this provision is scheduled to expire on December 31, 2006,[31] although it may be extended. Congress has, on several occasions, extended the "sunset" date and might do so again.

- A group health plan that provides medical and surgical benefits for mastectomies must also provide benefits for breast reconstruction, prostheses, and all physical complications related to a mastectomy.[32] Notice of this rule must be provided as part of any yearly informational packet sent to plan participants or beneficiaries.[33]

- A group health plan must provide "special enrollment rights" in certain situations in which the participant acquires a new dependent or coverage under another group health plan terminated.[34] The special enrollment rights permit enrollment in the group health plan notwithstanding plan provisions that would otherwise restrict enrollment to a date or dates during the plan year.

Despite the limited regulation of the content of employee welfare benefit plans, ERISA's impact is considerable.

ERISA Preemption of State Insurance Laws Affecting Plan Design

As is explained in more detail in the section devoted to ERISA preemption, ERISA broadly preempts all state law (and state law causes of action) that relate to ERISA plans.[35] Although limited exceptions exist for state laws that regulate insurance, banking, or securities as well as for certain generally applicable laws, ERISA's preemptive scope provides plan sponsors with great flexibility with respect to the design of their benefit programs because ERISA generally will preempt state law attempts to regulate the terms and conditions of ERISA plans. Examples of such state laws are discussed in Chapter 33.

Distinction between Insured and Self-Insured Plans

The exception for state laws that regulate the "business of insurance" creates an interesting distinction between health benefit plans that purchase insurance and those for which the plan sponsor self-insures (or self-funds) the benefits. So-called mandated benefits laws—that is, state laws that mandate that health insurance contracts subject to the state's jurisdiction provide coverage or benefits for certain conditions or illnesses—constitute laws that regulate the business of insurance and are saved from preemption.[36] A self-insured (or self-funded) plan does not purchase insurance, however, and a provision of ERISA known as the "deemer clause" prevents a state from directly applying its insurance regulation to the employee benefit plan.[37] The result is a significant distinction between insured and self-insured plans. Although a state may not directly regulate an employee benefit plan, the state may indirectly regulate the content of an insured plan by regulating the terms and conditions of the insurance contract that the plan purchases. A state may not, however, directly or indirectly regulate the terms and conditions of a self-insured plan.

When is a Plan Self-Insured?

Historically, most managed care programs were insured arrangements, although today a growing number of plan sponsors have adopted self-insured arrangements that incorporate a preferred provider organization (PPO), point-of-service (POS) product, or other feature generally associated within the rubric of managed care. Because of the significance of the distinction between insured and self-insured plans, courts and state regulators have been called upon to determine whether certain plans are insured or self-insured.

This issue typically arises when the plan claims to be self-insured, but the plan or the plan sponsor then purchases stop-loss or excess loss insurance to protect the plan or plan sponsor from large losses. Stop-loss or excess loss insurance provides reimbursement to the plan or plan sponsor in the event that benefits paid by the plan to or on behalf of a plan participant or all plan participants as a group exceed thresholds established in the insurance policy. Stop-loss coverage is written with either or both a specific or individual attachment point and an aggregate attachment point. Above the specific or individual attachment point, the plan or plan sponsor is entitled to reimbursement for claims paid during the policy year with re-spect to a single plan participant. Above the aggregate attachment point, the plan or the plan sponsor is entitled to reimbursement for claims paid during the policy year with respect to all plan participants.

Plans that purchase stop-loss or excess loss insurance coverage generally have been considered self-insured for the purposes of the preemption rules described previously so that a state is not allowed to regulate the plan indirectly through application of its mandated benefit or other health insurance laws to the terms and conditions of the insurance contract.[38] Rather, the stop-loss or excess loss contract typically is viewed as property and casualty insurance that is subject to the state's rules and regulations for such insurance. This characterization is subject to two caveats.

First, the plan participant should have no rights to claim benefits directly against the stop-loss or excess loss insurer. Stop-loss or excess loss insurance is intended to provide reimbursement to the plan or the plan sponsor for losses incurred beyond certain thresholds. If the plan participant has a direct claim against the insurer, however, the stop-loss or excess loss contract arguably constitutes a direct health insurance contract that the state could regulate as such.

Second, the thresholds at which the insurance company reimburses the plan or the plan sponsor should be sufficient so that the plan or the plan sponsor bears substantial risk for the provision of benefits under the plan (other than the risk of the insurance carrier's bankruptcy). Although courts have generally held that ERISA preempts application of a state regulation to the effect that stop-loss insurance with an attachment point below a prescribed minimum would be treated as health insurance,[39] one court has suggested that, if the thresholds are set so low that they constitute a disguised deductible, the insurance contract, even though treated by the parties as providing stop-loss or excess loss coverage, might be treated as direct health insurance.[40]

Limits on ERISA Preemption

ERISA's preemptive reach is extremely broad. For example, state community property laws, although traditionally an area of recognized state law concern, have been determined to be preempted by ERISA where the law attempts to regulate the benefits provided by the plan or the manner in which those benefits are provided.[41] However, ERISA preemption is not all encompassing. For example, a New York law that imposed surcharges on hospital bills was not preempted by ERISA.[42] Although the surcharges undoubtedly had an impact on a self-insured plan by increasing the cost of the benefits provided by the plan, the New York surcharge system did not relate to ERISA plans and therefore was not preempted. Similarly, a Kentucky law that prohibited health maintenance organization (HMO) plans from discriminating against providers willing to meet the HMO's financial terms and conditions qualified as law regulating insurance and thus was saved from preemption.[43] Although these indirect impact and insurance laws may survive preemption, a state law that attempts to regulate the benefits provided by the plan will be preempted unless saved, in the case of an insured plan, as a law regulating the business of insurance. Thus, plan sponsors have significant flexibility with respect to the design of health benefit plans free from most state law.

Other Federal Laws Affecting Plan Design

Although ERISA grants plan sponsors considerable flexibility with respect to the design of their health care plans, other federal laws may restrict a plan sponsor's discretion to some extent. For example, a plan may not discriminate on the basis of age or other protected classification.[44] Moreover, a plan may not discriminate on the basis of disability in a manner that violates the Americans with Disabilities Act (ADA).[45]

The ADA contains several rules that generally were designed to protect employee benefit plans. For example, the ADA does not prohibit an insurer, HMO, hospital, or medical service company from underwriting risks, classifying risks, or administering risks in a manner that is not based on or not inconsistent with state law.[46] Similarly, the ADA does not prohibit a person or organization from establishing, sponsoring, observing, or administering the terms of a bona fide benefit plan that is not subject to state laws that regulate insurance (*ie,* a self-insured plan).[47] In all cases, however, the protection provided under these provisions of the ADA is not available if the practice or plan provision is used as a subterfuge to evade the purposes of the ADA.[48]

The Equal Employment Opportunity Commission has indicated that the ADA does not prohibit broad limitations on the nature and scope of services covered under the plan, such as a general exclusion on preexisting conditions or a separate annual or lifetime maximum on the amount of benefits payable for nervous and mental disorders.[49] (Although not prescribed by the ADA, a separate annual or lifetime maximum on the amount of benefits payable for nervous and mental disorders generally *would* violate the mental health parity provisions of ERISA.)[50] These broad limitations affect plan participants generally whether or not the plan participant is disabled within the meaning of the ADA. By contrast, health-related distinctions that are based on disability may violate the ADA. A plan provision is disability based if it (1) singles out a particular disability, such as human immunodeficiency virus infection, (2) addresses a discrete group of disabilities, such as cancers, muscular dystrophies, or kidney diseases, or (3) excludes disabilities in general, such as not covering any condition that substantially limits a major life activity.[51]

Provisions in employer-sponsored group health plans that discriminate on the basis of disability are not always clear cut. For example, in *Henderson v. Bodine Aluminum, Inc.,* the U.S. Court of Appeals for the Eighth Circuit issued an injunction preventing the defendant company from denying coverage for expenses incurred by a cancer patient in connection with high-dose chemotherapy treatments.[52] The health plan in question excluded coverage of high-dose chemotherapy for certain types of cancer, an exclusion that the Eighth Circuit Court concluded might violate the ADA. However, several other cases have determined that the ADA does not necessarily require that the benefits provided by a plan with respect to a particular disability be equivalent to the benefits provided with respect to another disability.[53]

AMENDMENT OF PLANS

ERISA requires that every employee benefit plan provide a procedure for amending the plan and for identifying the persons who have authority to amend the plan.[54] Generally, a plan sponsor reserves for itself the power and authority to amend (or even terminate) a plan. The employer's reserved amendment authority and the process by which the employer exercises that authority has been the subject of considerable debate.

Benefit Reductions

Many employers provide health plan coverage to former employees who retired after attaining a certain age and after completing a minimum period of service specified in the plan (eg, age 55 and 10 years of service). Traditionally, the employer had few retirees relative to active employees, and health care costs were reasonable. As health care costs escalated, however, and as the employer's population shifted to include a greater number of retirees relative to active employees, employers began to modify (and in some cases terminate) the coverage provided to retirees.

Predictably, retirees whose coverage was modified or eliminated challenged many of the benefit cutbacks. Although early cases were far from uniform—some favoring the employer, some applying a rebuttable presumption in favor of the retiree—more recent cases, although still not entirely uniform, have become more homogenous in their approach, at least with respect to nonbargaining unit retirees. In particular, the cases have rejected a per se rule and have instead viewed the issue as a question of plan interpretation. Where the employer (plan sponsor) has reserved to itself the authority to amend, modify, or terminate the plan, the employer's exercise of that right has been upheld, even where the coverage is described as lifetime coverage.[55] Where the employer has not reserved for itself the authority to amend, modify, or terminate the plan, however, or if the plan language is ambiguous, the courts will seek to ascertain the parties' intent when creating the plan (ie, did the employer or, in the case of a collectively bargained arrangement, the parties to the contract intend to create vested benefit rights that cannot thereafter be modified by the employer?).[56] The starting point, however, is the plan language concerning the employer's right to amend the plan.

Where the coverage is provided pursuant to a collective bargaining agreement, the court often is asked to determine whether the employer's obligation to provide the retiree coverage is limited to the term of the collective bargaining agreement, or whether the parties intended the employer's obligation to extend beyond expiration of the collective bargaining agreement. In some circuits, the courts have suggested that the context in which labor management negotiations take place might, in conjunction with supporting evidence of intent, provide an inference of intent to create vested benefit rights that are not dependent upon future negotiations.[57] Other circuits have rejected such an inference.[58] Also, one court has indicated that if eligibility for retiree welfare benefits is tied to eligibility for retirement pension benefits, this might suggest an intent to create lifetime benefits that extend beyond the term of the collective bargaining agreement.[59]

Even where the plan documents reserve to the employer the right to amend, modify, or terminate the plan, the employer might be estopped from implementing the change as a result of prior assurances provided to plan participants. For example, in a case involving Unisys Corporation retirees, the U.S. Court of Appeals for the Third Circuit permitted a retiree challenge to proceed based on a breach of fiduciary duty theory despite the fact that the plan document had at all times reserved to the employer the right to amend, modify, or terminate benefits.[60] The retirees alleged that plan fiduciaries had violated their fiduciary duties by consistently misrepresenting to plan participants over a period of years that retiree benefits were lifetime benefits. Similarly, the Third Circuit permitted a retiree challenge to proceed where the retirees alleged that the employer induced the employees to accept early retirement based upon the assurance of lifetime benefits without specific disclosure of the employer's reserved right to modify or terminate coverage.[61]

Amendment Procedure

Even where a plan document does reserve the right of the employer to amend the plan, employees and retirees have challenged the process by which amendments have been adopted. In *Schoonejongen v. Curtiss-Wright Corp.*, the employer terminated a retiree health insurance program.[62] The plan reserved to the employer the right to amend or terminate the plan but did not specify the process by which amendments could be adopted or the persons or person with the authority to amend the plan. The U.S. Court of Appeals for the Third Circuit held that the plan amendment procedure, and thus the amendment terminating the plan, was invalid under ERISA.

The Third Circuit position was short-lived. The U.S. Supreme Court reversed, holding that the plan amendment procedure was valid even though it did not specifically identify the person or persons with the authority

to amend the plan.[63] Also, the U.S. Court of Appeals for the Seventh Circuit refused to set aside an amendment terminating a retiree welfare plan even though the plan did not contain an adequate amendment procedure under ERISA.[64] It would thus appear that the courts will not easily set aside plan changes communicated by the employer to plan participants. Nevertheless, a plan sponsor would be well advised to avoid the issue altogether by specifying the amendment procedure in the plan document and, having done so, to follow that procedure.

FIDUCIARY DUTIES

ERISA imposes special duties on plan fiduciaries. ERISA's definition of *fiduciary* is functional, that is, a person, regardless of formal title or position, is a fiduciary to the extent that he or she exercises discretionary authority and control over the operation or administration of the plan, exercises any control over plan assets, or renders investment advice for a fee.[65]

ERISA prescribes the minimum standard of conduct applicable to fiduciaries, the so-called fiduciary duties. A fiduciary with respect to a plan must discharge his or her obligations with respect to a plan solely in the interests of the plan participants and beneficiaries and for the exclusive purpose of providing benefits to plan participants and their beneficiaries and defraying reasonable expenses of administering the plan.[66] Furthermore, the fiduciary must act in accordance with the plan documents (except to the extent that the documents are themselves inconsistent with ERISA) and with the care, skill, and diligence that a prudent person familiar with such matters would use in a similar enterprise.[67] Finally, if the plan is funded, plan investment must be diversified to minimize the risk of large losses.[68]

Often, a plan fiduciary is also an officer of the sponsoring employer, raising the question of when such a person is wearing his or her "fiduciary hat," and thus is required to act in the sole interest of plan participants and their beneficiaries, and when the fiduciary is wearing his or her "corporate hat," and thus is able to act in the best interests of the plan sponsor. Although the distinction is not always clear, the authority to amend or even terminate the plan is a "settlor function," that is, an employer is not acting in a fiduciary capacity when deciding to amend or terminate a plan.[69] Thus, an employer might prospectively amend its group health plan to eliminate certain coverages (assuming that such elimination does not violate the ADA), and this action, although detrimental to plan participants, does not implicate the fiduciary's obligations under ERISA. Similarly, the decision to terminate a plan is a "settlor" or business decision of the plan sponsor. Although certain aspects of the termination process might constitute fiduciary functions, the decision to terminate does not.[70]

The distinction between fiduciary functions and nonfiduciary settlor functions has blurred to some extent. Although the decision to amend a plan is a settlor function, the Supreme Court has indicated that providing information about likely future plan benefits falls within ERISA's definition of a fiduciary act.[71] Although the duty not to misinform or misrepresent is well established, the courts have been more reluctant to impose upon plan fiduciaries an affirmative duty to inform absent specific questions by participants, or to provide information beyond that required under ERISA's statutory disclosure rules.[72] However, in appropriate circumstances, and in particular where a participant or beneficiary has made a general inquiry regarding his or her situation, some courts have determined that a fiduciary must do more than simply not misinform, but rather, the fiduciary has an affirmative obligation to provide all material information regarding the situation.[73]

Another area in which a number of courts have held that plan fiduciaries have an obligation to disclose information about proposed plan amendments as soon as the proposal is under "serious consideration."[74] Generally,

these courts have determined that serious consideration does not exist until (1) a specific proposal (2) is being discussed for the purpose of implementation (3) by management with the authority to implement the change.[75]

Other cases have viewed the "serious consideration" test as part of a broader question of whether the plan fiduciary is in receipt of material information, and whether the fiduciary's duty of loyalty to plan participants and beneficiaries requires that material information relevant to a plan participant or beneficiary be disclosed.[76]

In addition to ERISA's general fiduciary responsibility rules, ERISA also prohibits a plan fiduciary from engaging in a number of transactions known as prohibited transactions.[77] There are two sets of prohibited transactions. The first set prohibits a plan fiduciary from causing a plan to engage in certain transactions (such as sale or lease of property or extension of credit) between a plan and a party in interest. A party in interest includes a fiduciary with respect to the plan, persons who perform services for a plan, and other persons or entities related to such fiduciaries or service providers.[78] Unless advance approval is obtained from the Department of Labor, this type of related party transaction is prohibited without regard to the economic benefits of the transaction to the plan.

A second branch of the prohibited transaction rules proscribes a fiduciary from acting in certain conflict of interest situations or from receiving compensation from a third party in connection with a transaction involving the assets of the plan. For example, a fiduciary with respect to the plan may not cause the plan to retain the fiduciary (or a related party) to perform additional services for a fee. Where a fiduciary uses the authority, discretion, and control that makes him or her a fiduciary to cause the plan to pay an additional fee to the fiduciary, the fiduciary has engaged in a prohibited act of self-dealing.[79]

CHALLENGES TO BENEFIT DENIALS

Dispute resolution, both at the administrative (plan) level and through litigation, has become an increasingly important topic.

Claims Procedure

Every employee benefit plan under ERISA is required to establish a procedure whereby a plan participant or beneficiary may challenge a denial of his or her claim for benefits.[80]

A claims procedure will be deemed reasonable if a plan participant's or beneficiary's claim is answered in writing, with explanation of the reasons for the decision and references to pertinent plan provisions (including internal rules and guidelines), within 90 days. A description of the plan's review procedures, including the time limits for filing an appeal, and a statement of the participant's or beneficiaries right to bring a court action following an adverse decision on appeal, must also be provided.

If the claim is denied and the plan participant or beneficiary wishes to pursue the matter further, an appeal may be filed with the appropriate fiduciary designated by the plan. In general, the appeal must be answered in writing, again with explanation of the reasons for the decision and references to pertinent plan provisions (including internal rules and guidelines), within 60 days after the date on which the appeal is filed. In certain cases, the 90-day initial review period and 60-day appeal review period can be extended if the plan participant or beneficiary is notified of the need for additional time before expiration of the initial period.[81]

Special Standards for Group Health Plans and Disability Benefit Claims

However, group health plans and benefit claims involving disability benefits are governed by more stringent rules. The time by which the plan must make and communicate its decision varies with the type of claim presented. For example, urgent care claims must be decided in as little as 72 hours, while so-called postservice claims may be decided in 30 days.

In addition, with respect to group health and disability benefit claims, the plan must provide a claimant a minimum of 180 days during which to appeal an adverse benefit determination.

Claimants must be able to review all relevant documents, whether or not such documents or records were actually relied upon in making determination, including all documents and reports created or received during the review process (*eg,* expert identities and/or reports).

A claimant must be provided the opportunity for a full and fair review (appeal) of denied claims. Full and fair review must include a review of the adverse determination by an appropriate named fiduciary who was not involved in the initial determination and who is not a subordinate of someone involved in the initial determination. No deference is to be given to the initial determination as part of the review process, and the review is to take into account all comments, documents and records. Any appeal of a claim involving urgent care must be conducted on an expedited basis. Appeals of adverse determinations on urgent care claims must be decided and communicated to the claimant, as soon as possible but not later than 72 hours after receipt of request for review.

The review of any determination that is based on medical judgment must be conducted in consultation with a health care professional who is independent of the health care professional involved in the initial determination.

Standard of Review in Court Action

If the plan participant is not satisfied with the disposition of his or her claim at the plan level, he or she can file suit in state or federal court. An important threshold question involves the standard of review that the court will apply in reviewing the plan administrator's denial of the plan participant's claim.

In *Firestone Tire & Rubber Co. v. Bruch*, the U.S. Supreme Court determined that, in accordance with established principles of trust law, a plan participant's or beneficiary's challenge to a denial of benefits is to be reviewed under a de novo standard—that is, the court independently reviews and weighs the evidence and makes its decision accordingly, without deference to the decision made by the plan administrator—unless the plan document grants to the plan administrator or other appropriate fiduciary the discretionary authority and control to determine eligibility for benefits or to construe the terms of the plan.[82] Where the plan grants the administrator such discretionary authority and control, the court is to review the benefit denial under the more deferential arbitrary and capricious standard of review. Under this standard, the court reviews the evidence but overturns the plan administrator's decision only if it represents a clearly unreasonable interpretation or construction of the plan.

The Supreme Court's decision, although based upon principles of trust law, is puzzling to many. Although the general rule is de novo review, the Supreme Court's decision creates an exception that potentially eliminates the general rule. By including appropriate language in the plan document, a plan sponsor changes the standard of review that a court will apply in the event that a plan participant challenges a benefit denial. More generally, why should a plan sponsor be allowed to select the standard of review through its decision to include or not include certain language in the plan document?

In the years after the Supreme Court's *Bruch* decision, the lower federal courts have struggled with the implications of the decision, often with potentially conflicting results. In a number of decisions, plan language was determined to be sufficient to support the more deferential arbitrary and capricious standard of review. For example, in *Kennedy v. Georgia-Pacific Corp.*, plan language to the effect that the plan administrator "shall be solely responsible for the administration and interpretation" of the plan was found to be sufficient.[83] In other cases, courts have applied the de novo standard even though the document contained evidence that the plan administrator (or other fiduciary) was intended to have considerable authority and control with respect to the plan. For example, in *Michael Reese Hospital & Medical Center v. Solo Cup Employee Health Benefit Plan*, even though the plan document gave the administrator "the authority to control and manage the operation and administration of the plan," it was held that the plan demonstrated insufficient intent to grant to the administrator discretionary authority to determine eligibility or to construe the terms of the plan.[84]

In other cases, particularly those involving self-funded arrangements for which benefits are payable from the plan sponsor's general corporate assets, courts have focused on the conflict of interest under which a plan fiduciary may operate because a denial of benefits is directly beneficial to the plan sponsor's treasury. In some conflict of interest cases, courts have applied a less deferential standard of review than the arbitrary and capricious standard that would normally be applicable.[85] In other cases, the courts have continued to apply the arbitrary and capricious standard, but have indicated that the fiduciary's conflict of interest is a factor to be taken into account in determining whether the fiduciary's actions were arbitrary and capricious.[86] By whichever route, the courts are cognizant of and treat a fiduciary's conflict of interest as a relevant consideration. The potential conflict of interest is present even if the employer retains a third-party claims administrator to initially determine claims, so long as the employer is the fiduciary with the ultimate authority to decide claim appeals.[87]

Some courts have established a "default condition" under which the plan administrator is not entitled to the arbitrary and capricious standard unless the administrator can show the plan clearly gives it discretionary authority and control over plan interpretation and benefit decisions.[88] One court has even gone so far as to publish safe harbor language to obtain the arbitrary and capricious standard of review: "Benefits will be paid under this plan only if the plan administrator decides in his discretion that the applicant is entitled to them."[89] Although not mandatory to obtain the arbitrary and capricious standard, the safe harbor language certainly places a plan sponsor or administrator on notice as to the type of clear language that the court would prefer to see from where the arbitrary and capricious standard of review is being claimed.

Additional State Law Review Procedures

In addition to the claim and appeal procedures required under ERISA, insurance companies (including HMOs) may be subject to additional dispute resolution procedures under state law. Although insurers and HMOs have argued that the additional state law procedures are preempted by ERISA, an Illinois law that required an HMO to provide an independent second opinion where the HMO had denied a request for medical treatment recommended by the insured individual's primary care physician was held to be saved from ERISA preemption as a law regulating insurance.[90]

Right to Jury Trial

Most courts have held that ERISA does not provide a right to a jury trial, reasoning that benefit claims under ERISA are equitable in nature.[91] The decisions are not uniform, however, and a minority of courts have found a right to jury trial on the basis that certain claims have both legal and equitable components.[92]

ERISA'S CIVIL ENFORCEMENT SCHEME AND REMEDIES

In addition to suits for benefits brought by a plan participant or beneficiary, ERISA authorizes a plan participant, beneficiary, fiduciary,

or the secretary of the Department of Labor to bring a variety of civil actions. Among the more important suits are those that involve the right of a plan participant, beneficiary, fiduciary, or the secretary to bring an action for breach of fiduciary duty under §502(a)(2) of ERISA.[93] Also, a plan participant, beneficiary, or fiduciary may bring an action under §502(a)(3) of ERISA to enjoin any act or practice that violates (or to enforce the provisions of) Title I of ERISA or the terms of the plan or to obtain other appropriate equitable relief.[94]

Although ERISA authorizes a variety of civil actions, the remedies that are available to a successful plaintiff have been quite limited. An action for breach of fiduciary duty under §502(a)(2) of ERISA is an action brought on behalf of the plan and all recovery runs in favor of the plan. Accordingly, the U.S. Supreme Court in *Massachusetts Mutual Life Insurance Co. v. Russell* held that a plan participant or beneficiary could not recover extracontractual or punitive damages.[95] Later, the Supreme Court in *Mertens v. Hewitt Associates* held that §502(a)(3) authorizes only traditional forms of equitable relief, not monetary damages.[96]

The Supreme Court's restrictive interpretation of §502(a)(2) and §502(a)(3) takes on added significance in light of ERISA's preemption of state laws and state law causes of action that relate to ERISA-governed employee benefit plans. Because of ERISA's preemptive reach, plaintiffs may not forgo ERISA's civil enforcement scheme in favor of state law remedies, which might, if not preempted, include punitive or extracontractual damages.[97]

After the Supreme Court's holding in *Russell* and *Mertens*, the courts have struggled to attempt to provide meaningful remedies to plan participants and beneficiaries in actions brought under §502(a)(3) of ERISA. For example, in *Watkins v. Westinghouse Hanford Co.*, the U.S. Court of Appeals for the Ninth Circuit ruled that a plan participant could not recover under §502(a)(3) benefits allegedly due the plan participant as a result of a misrepresentation.[98] More recently, however, a number of decisions have embraced the possibility of monetary relief in connection with equitable claims of reinstatement or restitution. The Supreme Court, in *Varity Corp. v. Howe*, approved reinstatement of participant benefits following a fiduciary's break of duty.[99] Further, Seventh Circuit, in a case denying the plaintiffs' claim, nevertheless determined that not all monetary relief is damages, thus suggesting that the remedies available under §502(a)(3) may not be as narrow as once thought. According to the Seventh Circuit, "[e]quity sometimes awards monetary damages or the equivalent and restitution is both a legal and equitable remedy that is monetary yet is distinct from damages."[100] Similarly, the Fourth Circuit determined that a court could award, as equitable relief, a pension equivalent to the pension to which an employee would have become entitled if the employer had not breached its fiduciary duty.[101]

One area in which the distinction between legal and equitable relief has frequently arisen involves a plan's ability to recover prior benefit payments pursuant to the plan's subrogation and reimbursement provisions, such as where a medical plan pays benefits and the participant later recovers from a third party. In 2002, in *Great-West Life & Annuity Ins. Co. v. Knudson*,[102] the Supreme Court determined that a benefit plan's reimbursement claim could not proceed under §502(a)(3) because it sought legal rather than equitable enforcement of the plan's rights. However, in 2006, the Court, in *Sereboff v. Mid Atlantic Medical Services, Inc.*,[103] clarified that the reimbursement claim in *Knudson* did not fail simply because it sought money, but rather because it did not seek to recover money due it from a particular fund held by the other party. So, the Supreme Court determined that if the plan seeks equitable enforcement of its subrogation or reimbursement rights, the claim may proceed under §502(a)(3), even though the ultimate recovery is money.

ERISA PREEMPTION

Arguably, no provision of ERISA has more of an effect on the operations of MCOs than ERISA's preemption clause. This section explains the general principles of preemption and discusses the impact of preemption on the following activities of MCOs: the provision of health care services, either directly or by contract; utilization review determinations; the establishment of provider networks; representations of eligibility and coverage to health care providers; and the provision of administrative and other noninsurance services to ERISA plans.

General Principles of Preemption

There are two types of ERISA preemption: conflict or ordinary preemption under §514(a) of ERISA, and complete preemption under §502(a) of ERISA.[104]

Conflict or Ordinary Preemption under §514(a) of ERISA

When Congress enacted ERISA, it intended to make the regulation of employee benefit plans an exclusively federal concern. Congress, however, also did not want to divest the states of their traditional power to regulate insurance. Pursuant to this scheme, Congress enacted three clauses relating to the preemptive effect of ERISA:

- *The preemption clause:* This clause provides that ERISA supersedes any and all state laws insofar as they may relate to any employee benefit plan subject to ERISA, except to the extent that such laws may be "saved" from preemption by the savings clause.[105]
- *The savings clause:* This clause preserves from preemption any law of any state that regulates insurance, banking, or securities except as provided in the deemer clause.[106]
- *The deemer clause:* This clause provides that an employee benefit plan shall not

be deemed to be an insurance company or other insurer, bank, trust company, or investment company or to be engaged in the business of insurance or banking for the purposes of any law of any state purporting to regulate insurance companies, insurance contracts, banks, trust companies, or investment companies.[107]

The Preemption Clause

As noted earlier, §514(a) of ERISA preempts "any and all State laws insofar as they may now or hereafter relate to any employee benefit plan." A law relates to an employee benefit plan if it has "a connection with or reference to such a plan."[108] In application, the preemption clause has been "conspicuous for its breadth," preempting not only state laws that are specifically designed to affect employee benefit plans but also those that may affect such plans only indirectly.[109,110] Those state laws that courts have found not to be preempted under §514(a) were generally limited to laws of general applicability that only tangentially affected ERISA plans.[111]

In recent years, however, the U.S. Supreme Court narrowed the preemptive force of §514(a) in a trio of cases: *New York State Conference of Blue Cross & Blue Shield Plans v. Travelers Insurance Co.* ("*Travelers*"), followed by *De Buono v. NYSA-ILA Medical and Clinical Services* ("*De Buono*"), and *California Division of Labor Enforcement v. Dillingham Construction N.A., Inc.* ("*Dillingham*").[112] In *Travelers*, the Supreme Court refused to preempt a New York State statute requiring surcharges on hospital bills of patients covered by commercial carriers and on HMOs based on the number of Medicaid enrollees, warning against utilizing an "uncritical literalism" when deciding the reach of ERISA preemption and stressing that preemption under ERISA was to be determined with reference to ERISA's statutory objectives.[113] The *Travelers* decision identified three categories of state laws that Congress intended to preempt: state laws that mandated employee benefit structures or their adminis-

tration; state laws that provided alternative enforcement mechanisms; and state laws that bound plan administrators to a particular choice.[114] The Supreme Court in *De Buono* declined to preempt a New York state tax on the gross receipts of health care facilities operated by a trust fund established to administer an ERISA plan, emphasizing that health and safety matters were within the historic police powers of the states and that ERISA's "relate to" language was not intended to modify the starting presumption that Congress did not intend to supplant state law that fell within areas of traditional state regulation.[115] Finally, in *Dillingham,* the Supreme Court, refusing to preempt California's prevailing wage law, found that preemption would have been warranted only if the state law acted "immediately and exclusively upon ERISA plans . . . or where the existence of ERISA plans is essential to the law's operation."[116] Following the lead of *Travelers, De Buono,* and *Dillingham*, lower courts have begun to whittle away at the broad parameters of ERISA preemption.

The Savings Clause

A state law that relates to an ERISA plan may be saved from preemption if it falls within §514(b)(2)(A), which excepts from preemption those state laws that "regulate insurance." In *Kentucky Ass'n of Health Plans, Inc. v. Miller*,[117] the Supreme Court ruled that a state law regulates insurance, and will be saved from ERISA preemption, if (1) the law is limited to the insurance industry, and (2) the law has a substantial effect on the risk-pooling arrangement between the insurer and the insured.

The Deemer Clause

The deemer clause exempts from any direct or indirect state regulation self-funded employee benefit plans.[118] All power to regulate insurance reserved to the states under the savings clause is taken away with respect to self-insured plans under the deemer clause. The language of the deemer clause, according to the U.S. Supreme Court, is either coextensive with or broader, not narrower, than that of the savings clause.[119] Thus, state laws that relate to employee benefit plans but that are saved from preemption under §514(b)(2)(A) are still preempted as applied to self-funded ERISA plans. The Supreme Court's recent revisions regarding application of the insurance savings clause, and how that clause should be applied, did not change its previously announced interpretation of the deemer clause.[120] As discussed earlier in regard to the benefit design of ERISA plans, this interpretation of the insurance savings and deemer clauses establishes a disparity between the regulation of insured and uninsured plans, the Supreme Court has determined that such a dichotomy was the intent of Congress when it enacted the statute.[121]

Complete Preemption Under §502(a) of ERISA

The U.S. Supreme Court has held that any state law cause of action that duplicates, supplements, or supplants ERISA's civil enforcement remedy conflicts with the clear congressional intent to make that remedy exclusive, and thus is both removable to federal court and completely preempted under §502(a) of ERISA.[122]

Vicarious Liability for Medical Malpractice

Of the various tort theories used to impose liability on MCOs for the medical malpractice of health care providers to whom they refer patients, none has generated more litigation than that of vicarious liability for medical malpractice based on the theories of implied agency and/or apparent or ostensible agency. Although the elements of apparent or ostensible agency vary from jurisdiction to jurisdiction, a common allegation is that the patient reasonably relied upon actions or representations of the MCO, which "held out" the negligent provider as its employee or agent, the degree of reliance required of the patient being subject to judicial debate.[123]

ERISA preemption has played a crucial role in determining whether an MCO will be vicariously liable for the malpractice of health care providers. Although, early cases were split as to whether ERISA preempted medical malpractice claims against MCOs based on vicarious liability theories, recent federal Circuit Court decisions demonstrate the current judicial trend against preemption.

The U.S. Court of Appeals for the Tenth Circuit in the case of *Pacificare of Oklahoma, Inc. v. Burrage* identified four categories of laws that "related to" an employee benefit plan: laws that regulated the type of benefits or terms of ERISA plans; laws that created reporting, disclosure, funding, or vesting requirements for ERISA plans; laws that provided rules for the calculation of the amount of benefits to be paid under ERISA plans; and laws and common law rules that provided remedies for misconduct growing out of the administration of ERISA plans.[124] The Tenth Circuit held that a claim that an HMO was vicariously liable for the malpractice of one of its primary care physicians did not involve the administration of benefits or the level or quality of benefits promised by the plan; it merely alleged negligent care by the physician and an agency relationship between the physician and the HMO. The court pointed out that ERISA would not preempt the malpractice claim against the physician and concluded that ERISA should similarly not preempt the vicarious liability claim against the HMO if the HMO held the physician out as its agent. Reference to the ERISA plan to resolve the agency issue did not "implicate the concerns of ERISA preemption."[125]

In *Dukes v. U.S. Healthcare, Inc.*, the U.S. Court of Appeals for the Third Circuit addressed the issue of whether vicarious malpractice liability claims against the defendant HMO were completely preempted by ERISA and, thus, could be removed from the state court to federal court.[126] The lower federal courts had allowed such a removal, and then had dismissed the claims, holding that they were preempted by ERISA. The Third Circuit reversed, holding that removal was improper where plaintiffs were merely attacking the quality of the benefits received and were not claiming that the ERISA plans had erroneously withheld benefits that were due or were not seeking to enforce rights under the terms of their respective plans or to clarify rights to future benefits. The court expressly distinguished the situation where the HMO denied benefits in its utilization review role.[127,128]

The Third Circuit further refined its distinction between the quantity of benefits due under an ERISA plan and the quality of the benefits provided under such plan in *Pryzbowski v. U.S. Healthcare, Inc.*[129] and *DiFelice v. Aetna U.S. Healthcare.*[130] Adopting terminology used by the U.S. Supreme Court in the case *Pegram v. Herdrich,*[131] the Third Circuit held that claims that challenged the quality of benefits received—that is, "treatment decisions"—would not fall within §502(a) and so would not be completely preempted. Conversely, claims that challenged the quantity of benefits received, focusing on the administration of the plan—that is, "eligibility decisions"—would be completely preempted.[132] The Third Circuit opined that the deciding factor was whether the claim could have been the subject of a civil enforcement action under §502(a).[133]

The U.S. Court of Appeals for the Ninth Circuit has joined the Third and Tenth Circuits in holding that ERISA does not preempt claims against MCOs involving allegations of negligence in the provision of medical care.[134]

Negligent Utilization Review Decisions

The majority rule is that utilization review decisions by MCOs, even when they involve medical decisions, are an integral part of the administration of ERISA plans and, thus, are preempted by ERISA.

For example, in *Pryzbowski v. U.S. Healthcare, Inc.*, a plan beneficiary filed a negligence action against his HMO and his

primary care physicians based on their alleged failure to timely authorize his referral to out-of-network providers.[135] The U.S. Court of Appeals for the Third Circuit held that such allegations fell within the realm of the administration of benefits and, therefore, were completely preempted under §502(a) of ERISA.[136]

In *Jass v. Prudential Health Plan, Inc.*, plaintiff sued her treating physician, the plan administrator of her husband's benefit plan ("PruCare"), and a nurse employee of PruCare.[137] Plaintiff alleged that her treating physician had been negligent when performing knee replacement surgery, and that the nurse employee of PruCare had negligently failed to authorize physical therapy to rehabilitate the plaintiff's knee, resulting in plaintiff's premature discharge from the hospital. The U.S. Court of Appeals for the Seventh Circuit held that ERISA preempted plaintiff's claim that PruCare was vicariously liable for the alleged negligence of both its nurse employee and the treating physician based on actual or ostensible agency theories.

The U.S. Court of Appeals for the Sixth Circuit reached a similar conclusion in the case of *Tolton v. American Biodyne, Inc.*, the coadministrators of the estate of a mental patient who had committed suicide sued, among others, the patient's ERISA plan administrator, the plan's mental health utilization review company, and the psychologists performing utilization review on behalf of the utilization review company, alleging that the plan administrator wrongfully denied benefits for inpatient psychiatric care based upon the utilization review company's refusal to authorize such care.[138] Plaintiffs' state law claims based on such utilization review decision included wrongful death, improper refusal to authorize benefits, medical malpractice, and insurance bad faith. The court held that such claims clearly related to the ERISA plan and were preempted by ERISA.

In reaching its decision, the *Tolton* court relied on an earlier opinion of the U.S. Court of Appeals for the Fifth Circuit, *Corcoran v.*

United Healthcare, Inc.[139] In *Corcoran*, the utilization review decision at issue was the refusal by the defendant utilization review company to precertify hospitalization for a high-risk pregnancy despite the recommendation of the patient's physician. Instead, the defendant authorized 10 hours per day of home nursing care. The patient, who had already been admitted to the hospital, returned home when she learned that the expenses for her hospitalization would not be covered. At a time when no nurse was on duty, her fetus went into distress and died. The patient and her husband then sued the defendant, alleging wrongful death and medical malpractice. The Fifth Circuit in *Corcoran* acknowledged that utilization reviewers make medical decisions despite any disclaimers to the contrary in policy manuals or promotional materials. The court found, however, that the medical decisions made by the defendant were inseparable from its determinations regarding what benefits were available under the plan. The court found that the wrongful death claim related to a denial of benefits under the plan and so was preempted by ERISA.[140]

In 2004, the U.S. Supreme Court decided the case of *Aetna Health, Inc. v. Davila*.[141] *Davila* involved an HMO's denial of coverage for an extended hospital stay. The discharged plan beneficiary had sued the HMO, alleging that the denial of coverage violated the Texas Health Care Liability Act ("THCLA"), which imposed a legal duty on the HMO to exercise ordinary care. The Supreme Court held that the plan beneficiary's THCLA cause of action was completely preempted by ERISA's civil enforcement scheme, stating that "[t]he fact that a benefits determination is infused with medical judgments does not alter this result."[142]

At least two federal circuit courts have relied upon the *Davila* decision in holding that utilization review decisions are completely preempted by ERISA. In *Cicio v. Does*, the Second Circuit completely preempted a malpractice claim against an HMO based upon its denial of preauthorization for the treatment of multiple myeloma with high-dose

chemotherapy/autonomous stem cell transplant.[143] In *Land v. CIGNA Healthcare*, the Eleventh Circuit completely preempted a malpractice claim against an HMO based upon its decision to authorize outpatient, instead of inpatient, treatment for a plan beneficiary's infected finger.[144]

Negligent Selection of Health Care Providers

Like the analogous duty imposed on hospitals to exercise reasonable care in the selection and granting of privileges to its medical staff, an MCO has a duty to conduct a reasonable investigation of the qualifications and competence of the health care providers to whom they refer patients.[145,146] Courts have declined to describe what will constitute a reasonable investigation of a provider's credentials, stating that its scope will vary from case to case.[147] Recent cases have focused not on the nature or extent of the investigation of a provider's qualifications, but on whether a claim that an MCO was negligent in the selection of health care providers is preempted by ERISA. The courts have split on this issue.

A representative case holding in favor of preemption is *Kearney v. U.S. Healthcare, Inc.*[148] In *Kearney*, plaintiff filed wrongful death and survival claims against an HMO, alleging that decedent's primary care physician failed to diagnose properly decedent's condition or to refer decedent to a hospital for specialized treatment. Plaintiff claimed that the HMO breached its contract to provide needed specialized care by limiting or discouraging the use of specialists, hospitalization, and state-of-the-art diagnostic procedures; misrepresented the primary care physician's competence; and was negligent in selecting and supervising the primary care physician. Plaintiff also claimed that the HMO was vicariously liable for the malpractice of the primary care physician. The court held that a "claim that an operator or administrator of a plan failed to use due care in selecting those with whom it contracted to perform services relates to the manner in which benefits are administered or provided and is preempted."[149] The court dismissed not only plaintiff's claims of negligent selection, but also the claim for misrepresentation and breach of contract. However, the court held that plaintiff's claim that the HMO was vicariously liable for the malpractice of the primary care physician on ostensible agency grounds was not preempted.

In *Bui v. AT&T*, the estate of an employee who had died following heart surgery in a foreign country sued his employer, alleging that his employer had been negligent in the selection of the service provider providing emergency medical advice and evacuation services.[150] The U.S. Court of Appeals for the Ninth Circuit held that such negligent selection claims were "purely administrative" and, therefore, preempted.[151]

Although other courts have agreed with the preemption of negligent selection claims,[152] there is authority to the contrary. For example, the U.S. Court of Appeals for the Third Circuit in *In re U.S. HealthCare, Inc.*, held that a claim that an HMO was negligent in selecting and supervising a physician who had allegedly discharged a newborn infant prematurely was not completely preempted under ERISA.[153]

In *Jackson v. Roseman*, plaintiff brought a medical malpractice case against his physicians and the HMO with which they contracted.[154] Plaintiff alleged that the HMO was vicariously liable for the negligence of his physicians in allowing the growth and ultimate metastasis of a malignant cancer in his mouth. The court noted that the complaint could also be read as asserting a claim of direct negligence on the part of the HMO for negligent hiring and supervision of its contracting physicians.[155] Although the court declined to address the merits of whether a negligent hiring and/or supervision claim went to the heart of the benefit plan's administration, the court indicated that it agreed with the reasoning of the U.S. Court of Appeals for the Second Circuit in *Lupo v. Human Affairs Int'l, Inc.*, a case involving claims of negligent hiring and/or supervision of a psy-

chologist.[156] In that case, the Second Circuit rejected defendant's argument that claims of negligent hiring and supervision of health care providers so resembled a denial of benefits or a denial of some other plan-created right as to support the removal of such claims from state court to federal court.[157]

Provider Claims of Negligent Misrepresentation and/or Breach of Contract

Whether claims by a provider that an MCO misrepresented the existence or extent of coverage or breached its direct contract with such provider are preempted by ERISA may hinge on whether the provider is suing in its own capacity or as an assignee of the MCO's insured or member. A majority of courts have held that state law causes of action brought by a provider suing in its own capacity are not preempted by ERISA, even though such causes of action would be preempted if the provider were suing in a derivative capacity as assignee for the insured or member.

For example, in the influential case of *Memorial Hospital System v. Northbrook Life Insurance Co.*, the plaintiff hospital had treated a patient after the hospital had called the employer of the patient's husband and verified that the patient had coverage under a group insurance policy issued and administered by defendant insurer.[158] Subsequently, the patient and her husband assigned their benefits to the hospital. Upon the hospital's request for payment, however, defendant insurer informed the hospital that the patient had not been eligible for benefits on the date of her hospitalization and denied benefits. The hospital subsequently sued, alleging that the employer had acted as defendant's agent in verifying coverage, and asserting state law causes of deceptive and unfair trade practices under the Texas insurance code, breach of contract, negligent misrepresentation, and equitable estoppel. Upon appeal of the dismissal of the deceptive and unfair trade practices claim by the lower court, the U.S. Court of Appeals for the Fifth Circuit held that such claim was not sufficiently related to the employee benefit plan at issue so as to be preempted. The court noted that the provider did not have independent standing to seek redress under ERISA, and stated that it could not believe that "Congress intended the preemptive scope of ERISA to shield welfare plan fiduciaries from the consequences of their acts toward non-ERISA health care providers when a cause of action based on such conduct would not relate to the terms or conditions of a welfare plan, nor affect—or affect only tangentially—the ongoing administration of the plan."[159]

The Fifth Circuit had occasion to expound upon its reasoning in *Memorial Hospital System* in a subsequent case, *Cypress Fairbanks Medical Center, Inc. v. Pan-American Life Insurance Co.*[160] In *Cypress*, plaintiff was admitted to the defendant hospital after the hospital received assurances from plaintiff's insurer that he was covered under an ERISA plan, and he incurred charges of $178,215.44. Ultimately, the insurer refused to pay on the ground that plaintiff's "coverage was rescinded as to the effective date."[161] The Fifth Circuit held that its decision in *Memorial Hospital System* controlled, and pointed out that prior cases where it had found ERISA preemption "had two unifying characteristics: (1) the state law claims address areas of exclusive concern, such as the right to receive benefits under the terms of an ERISA plan; and (2) the claims directly affect the relationship among the traditional ERISA entities—the employer, the plan and its fiduciaries, and the participants and beneficiaries."[162] The court found that the claims of the hospital fell into neither category and concluded that ERISA did not preempt a provider's state law claims if such claims were "premised on a finding that the beneficiary is not covered at all by an existing ERISA plan."[163]

Other courts have adopted the reasoning of the *Memorial Hospital System* line of cases and refused to insulate ERISA plans, their sponsors, or their administrators from liability when they mistakenly verify eligibility or coverage to a health care provider.[164]

A majority of courts have also refused to preempt breach of contract claims where the health care provider has sued, not as an assignee of the plan beneficiary, but on a direct contract with the MCO. For example, the U.S. Court of Appeals for the Ninth Circuit in *Blue Cross of California v. Anesthesia Care Associates Medical Group, Inc.* held that claims by physicians contracting with the health plan that the health plan had breached the fee schedule provisions of its participating physician agreements were not preempted under either §502(a) or §514(a) of ERISA.[165] Similarly, the U.S. District Court for the District of Maryland has refused to completely preempt claims by a hospital that a health plan breached its contract with the hospital to timely pay for services provided to plan beneficiaries.[166]

Preemption of Any Willing Provider Laws

One of the hottest legal battles in the managed care arena has been the fight between states and MCOs over the applicability of so-called "any willing provider" (AWP) laws to networks that contract with ERISA plans. Although the terms of AWP statutes differ from state to state as discussed in Chapter 33, AWP statutes require that MCOs and other entities establishing provider networks not discriminate against a provider so long as the provider meets the network's general qualifications and is willing to be compensated at the network's reduced payment rate.

"Proponents of AWP laws argue that AWP laws protect patient choice and that the identity of the treating provider is a part of the overall package of benefits. According to such proponents, consumers should not be forced to accept providers chosen by an MCO by a threat of reduced levels of benefits.

The problem with AWP laws from the managed care industry's viewpoint is that they significantly diminish the means by which MCOs persuade providers to accept lower rates of compensation for their services. The attraction of MCOs for health care providers, despite the reduced compensation, is the increased volume of patients that can be generated through limiting the network of participating providers. By preventing MCOs from differentiating between participating and nonparticipating providers, providers cannot be assured of a certain number of patients, thereby markedly reducing the leverage with which MCOs bargain for lower rate of payment.

Because of the runaway costs of health care and the concerted effort to find means by which to curb health care expenses, there are also strong policy reasons for finding ERISA preemption of AWP laws. As discussed previously, if MCOs are prohibited from closing their networks, they can no longer ensure a certain volume of business. In this manner, AWP laws eliminate any leverage MCOs may have had to bargain with providers for reduced rates of compensation, effectively eliminating the benefits of establishing a provider network.

As explained earlier, under the traditional conflict preemption analysis, the first issue to be addressed is whether the state law or regulation "relates to" the ERISA plan. If so, the law or regulation will be preempted unless it is "saved" from preemption because it "regulates insurance." The nature of the activity that the state is seeking to regulate, however, must constitute "insurance"; it is not sufficient that the services are being provided by an insurance company or other entity subject to insurance regulation or that the state law or regulation is part of the insurance code. However, even if the statute regulates insurance, it will nevertheless be preempted if applied directly to a self-funded ERISA plan.

The federal circuit courts had split as to whether particular AWP laws regulated insurance and, thus, were saved from preemption. One of the first AWP laws to be challenged by the managed care industry was in Virginia.[167] Virginia's AWP statute allowed insurers to form PPOs and establish terms and conditions that physicians, hospitals, or other providers had to meet to qualify as a preferred provider. The statute, however, prohibited insurers from both unreasonably discriminating against and

among such providers and from excluding providers willing to meet the terms and conditions for participation in the PPO. The challenge to the Virginia statute arose after a PPO established by Aetna, which provided services exclusively to employee benefit plans, refused to allow a hospital to participate in its network. Instead, the PPO only contracted with hospitals that were already participants in Aetna's HMO. In *Stuart Circle Hospital Corporation v. Aetna Health Management,* the hospital sued Aetna for failing to comply with the AWP statute and excluding it from the PPO network for the sole reason that it was not a member of Aetna's HMO.[168] Aetna defended on the ground that the statute was preempted by ERISA.

In the *Stuart Circle* case, the U.S. Court of Appeals for the Fourth Circuit first found that the AWP statute "related to" ERISA plans. The court noted that the statute not only expressly provided that it applied to health benefit programs offered or administered by insurers but also restricted the ability of an insurer to limit the choice of providers that would otherwise confine the plan participants of an ERISA plan to those preferred by the insurer. However, the court went on to hold that the statute was saved from preemption because it regulated the "business of insurance" and consequently fell within the ERISA savings clause. Applying the three-prong test for the "business of insurance" set forth in the McCarran-Ferguson Act, the court found that the statute spread policyholder risk because insurers whose benefits otherwise would be reduced or denied if they sought treatment from nonparticipating providers would receive full benefits under the statute. In addition, the court asserted, the statute affected an integral part of the relationship between the insurer and the insured because the statute affected the provision for treatment and cost. Finally, the Virginia statute was explicitly limited to entities within the insurance industry, thus satisfying the third McCarran-Ferguson prong. Consequently, the court held that Virginia AWP statute was not preempted by ERISA.[169]

However, the U.S. Court of Appeals for the Fifth Circuit reached the opposite conclusion in two cases: *CIGNA Healthplan of Louisiana, Inc. v. Louisiana ex rel. Ieyoub*[170] and *Texas Pharmacy Ass'n v. Prudential Insurance Co.*[171] The Fifth Circuit held that the AWP laws in Louisiana and Texas, respectively, were preempted because they bound employers or plan administrators to particular choices by requiring the ERISA plan to purchase benefits of a particular structure, that is, a structure that includes any willing providers.[172] The U.S. Court of Appeals for the Tenth Circuit also preempted the Arkansas AWP law.[173]

In the 2003 landmark case of *Kentucky Ass'n of Health Plans, Inc. v. Miller*, the U.S. Supreme Court sided with the opponents of preemption.[174] Kentucky had enacted two AWP laws, which prohibited any health insurer from discriminating against any provider who was willing to meet the terms and conditions for participation established by the insurer, and which required a health benefit plan that included chiropractic benefits to permit any licensed chiropractor who agreed to abide by the terms and conditions of the plan to serve as a participating primary chiropractor. Several HMOs and their association had sued the Kentucky insurance commissioner, asserting that the AWP laws were preempted by ERISA. The Supreme Court disagreed, finding that the AWP laws were saved from preemption as laws "regulating insurance." Making a "clean break" from application of the McCarran-Ferguson factors, the Supreme Court held that for a state law to be deemed a law that regulated insurance, it must satisfy two requirements: (1) the state law must be specifically directed toward entities engaged in insurance; and (2) the state law must substantially affect the risk-pooling arrangement between the insurer and the insured.[175] The Supreme Court found that the Kentucky AWP laws satisfied both requirements and, thus, were saved from preemption.[176]

CONCLUSION

ERISA can affect many of the core functions of an MCO, from product design to administration to issues of legal liability. Accordingly, MCOs would be well advised to acquire proficiency with respect to the requirements of this far-reaching statute and the rapidly developing and ever-evolving body of case law interpreting it.

References and Notes

1. 29 U.S.C. §1001 *et seq.*
2. 29 U.S.C. §§1002(1), 1002(3), 1003.
3. 29 U.S.C. §1102.
4. 29 U.S.C. §1022; 29 C.F.R. §2520.104b-2.
5. 29 C.F.R. §2520.102-3(j).
6. 29 U.S.C. §1024.
7. *Id.*
8. *Id.*
9. *Id.*
10. *See, e.g., Bergt v. Ret. Plan for Pilots Employed by Mark-Air, Inc.* 293 F.3d 1139 (9th Cir. 2002); *Aiken v. Policy Mgmt. Sys. Corp.,* 13 F.3d 138 (4th Cir. 1993); *Edwards v. State Farm Mut. Auto. Ins. Co.,* 851 F.2d 134 (6th Cir. 1988).
11. *Koons v. Aventis Pharmaceuticals, Inc.,* 367 F.3d 768 (8th Cir. 2004).
12. *See, e.g., Liberty Life Assurance Co. of Boston v. Kennedy,* 358 F.3d 1295 (11th Cir. 2004); *Marolt v. Alliant Techsystems, Inc.,* 146 F.3d 617 (8th Cir. 1998); *Fallo v. Piccadilly Cafeterias, Inc.,* 141 F.3d 580 (5th Cir. 1998).
13. *Compare Burke v. Kodak Ret. Income Plan,* 336 F.3d 103 (2d Cir. 2003) and *Gridley v. Cleveland Pneumatic Co.,* 924 F.2d 1310 (3d Cir. 1991), *cert. denied,* 501 U.S. 1232 (1991).
14. 29 U.S.C. §1024.
15. 29 C.F.R. §2520.104-20.
16. Dep't Labor Adv. Op. 92-24A (Nov. 6, 1992) and ERISA Technical Release 92-01, 57 Fed. Reg. 23272 (June 2, 1992), as extended by Pension and Welfare Benefits Administration

Notice issued August 23, 1993, 58 Fed. Reg. 45359 (August 27, 1993).

17. 26 U.S.C. §6039D.

18. Internal Revenue Service Notice 2002-24, 2002-1 C.B. 735 (2002).

19. 29 U.S.C. §1024.

20. *Id.*

21. 29 U.S.C. §1169.

22. *Id.*

23. *Id.*

24. 29 U.S.C. §§1161–1168.

25. 29 U.S.C. §1181.

26. *Id.*

27. 29 U.S.C. §1182.

28. 29 U.S.C. §1183.

29. 29 U.S.C. §1185.

30. 29 U.S.C. §1185a.

31. *Id.*

32. 29 U.S.C. §1185b.

33. *Id.*

34. 29 U.S.C. 1181.

35. 29 U.S.C. §1144.

36. *Metropolitan Life Ins. Co. v. Mass.,* 471 U.S. 724 (1985).

37. *FMC Corp. v. Holliday,* 498 U.S. 52 (1990).

38. *Bill Gray Enterprises, Inc. Employee Health & Welfare Plan v. Gourly,* 248 F.3d 206 (3d Cir. 2001); *Drexelbrook Eng'g Co. v. Travelers Ins. Co.,* 891 F.2d 280 (3d Cir. 1989); and *United Food & Commercial Workers & Employers Ariz. Health & Welfare Trust v. Pacyga,* 801 F.2d 1157 (9th Cir. 1986).

39. *Am. Med. Sec. Inc. v. Bartlett,* 111 F.3d 358 (4th Cir. 1997), and *Assoc. Indus. of Mo. v. Angoff,* 937 S.W.2d 277 (Mo. Ct. App. 1996).

40. *Brown v. Granatelli,* 897 F.2d 1351 (5th Cir.), *cert. denied,* 498 U.S. 848 (1990).

41. *Egelhoff v. Egelhoff,* 532 U.S. 141 (2001); and *Boggs v. Boggs,* 520 U.S. 833 (1997).

42. *De Buono v. NYSA-ILA Med. & Clinical Servs. Fund,* 520 U.S. 806 (1997); *N.Y. State Conference of Blue Cross & Blue Shield Plans v. Travelers Ins. Co.,* 514 U.S. 645 (1995).

43. *Kentucky Ass'n of Health Plans v. Miller,* 538 U.S. 329 (2003).

44. *See, e.g.,* Age Discrimination in Employment Act of 1967, as amended, 29 U.S.C. §621 *et seq.*

45. 42 U.S.C. §12101 *et seq.*

46. 42 U.S.C. §12202.

47. *Id.*

48. *Id.*

49. 29 C.F.R. Part 1630, EEOC Interpretative Guidance on Title I of the Americans with Disabilities Act. *See also Chaudhry v. Neighborhood Health P'ship, Inc.,* 2006 WL 1117962 (11th Cir. Apr. 26, 2006).

50. 29 U.S.C. §1185a.

51. EEOC Interim Enforcement Guidance Part III(B).

52. 70 F.3d 958 (8th Cir. 1995).

53. *See, e.g., Weyer v. Twentieth Century Fox Film Corp.,* 198 F.3d 1104 (9th Cir. 2000); and *Ford v. Schering-Plaugh Corp.,* 145 F.3d 601 (3d Cir. 1998).

54. 29 U.S.C. §1102.

55. *See, e.g., Boyer v. Douglas Components Corp.,* 986 F.2d 999 (6th Cir. 1993); and *Sprague v. General Motors Corp.,* 133 F.3d 388 (6th Cir. 1998), *cert. denied,* 524 U.S. 923.

56. *Id.*

57. *Yolton v. El Paso Tennessee Pipeline Co.,* 435 F.3d.571 (6th Cir. 2006); and *Int'l Union Auto, Aerospace and Agr. Implement Workers of Am. (UAW) v. Yard-Man, Inc.,* 716 F.2d 1476 (6th Cir. 1983), *cert. denied,* 465 U.S. 1007 (1984).

58. *Rosetto v. Pabst Brewing Co.,* 217 F.3d 539 (7th Cir. 2000); and *UAW v. Skinner Engine Co.,* 188 F.3d 130 (3d Cir. 1999).

59. *McCoy v. Meridian Auto. Sys., Inc.,* 390 F.3d. 417 (6th Cir. 2004); and *Golden v. Kelsey-Hayes Co.,* 73 F.3d 648 (6th Cir. 1996).

60. *In re Unisys Corp. Retiree Med. Benefit "ERISA" Litigation,* 57 F.3d 1255 (3d Cir. 1995), *cert. denied,* 517 U.S. 1103 (1996).

61. *Adams v. Freedom Forge Corp.,* 204 F.3d 475 (3d Cir. 2000).

62. 18 F. 3d 1034 (3d Cir. 1994).

63. *Curtiss-Wright Corp. v. Schoonejongen,* 514 U.S. 73 (1995).

64. *Murphy v. Keystone Steel & Wire Co.,* 61 F.3d 560 (7th Cir. 1995); *see also Ross v. Rail Car America Group Disability Income Plan,* 285 F.3d 735 (8th Cir. 2002).

65. 29 U.S.C. §1002(21).

66. 29 U.S.C. §1104.

67. *Id.*

68. *Id.*

69. *Curtiss-Wright Corp. v. Schoonejongen,* 514 U.S. 73, (1995); *see also Lockheed Corp. v. Spink,* 517 U.S. 882 (1996).

70. Department of Labor Adv. Opn. 2003-3A.

71. *Varity Corp. v. Howe,* 516 U.S. 489 (1996); *see also Watson v. Deaconess Waltham Hosp.,* 298 F.3d 102 (1st Cir. 2002).

72. *Bins v. Exxon Co. USA, Inc.,* 220 F.3d 1042 (9th Cir. 2000) (*reh'g en banc*).

73. *Mathews v. Chevron Corp.*, 362 F.3d 1172 (9th Cir. 2004); *In re Unisys Corp. Retiree Med. Benefit ERISA Litig.*, 57 F.3d 1255 (3d Cir. 1995), and *Eddy v. Colonial Life Ins. Co.*, 919 F.2d 747 (D.C. Cir. 1990).

74. *See, e.g., Fischer v. Philadelphia Elec. Co.*, 96 F.3d 1533 (3d Cir. 1996), *cert. denied*, 520 U.S. 1116 (1997).

75. *Id.*

76. *Ballone v. Eastman Kodak Co.*, 109 F.3d 117 (2d Cir. 1997); *see also Caputo v. Pfizer, Inc.*, 267 F.3d 181 (2d Cir. 2001).

77. 29 U.S.C. §1106.

78. 29 U.S.C. §1002(14).

79. 29 C.F.R. §2550.408b-2.

80. 29 U.S.C. §1133.

81. 29 C.F.R. §2560.503-1.

82. 489 U.S. 101 (1989).

83. 31 F.3d 606 (8th Cir. 1994).

84. 899 F.2d 639 (7th Cir. 1990).

85. *See, e.g., Stratton v. E.I. DuPont De Nemours & Co.*, 363 F.3d 250 (3d Cir. 2004); and *Peruzzi v. Summa Med. Plan*, 137 F.3d 431 (6th Cir. 1998).

86. *See, e.g., Calvert v. Firstar Fin., Inc.*, 409 F.3d 286 (6th Cir. 2005); *Chambers v. Family Health Plan*, 100 F.3d 818 (10th Cir. 1996); *Pagan v. NYNEX Medical Pension Plan*, 52 F.3d 438 (2d Cir. 1995).

87. *Williams v. Bellsouth Telecommunications, Inc.*, 373 F.3d 1132 (11th Cir. 2004).

88. *Sandy v. Reliance Standard Life Ins. Co.*, 222 F.3d 1202 (9th Cir. 2000) and *Herzberger v. Standard Ins. Co.*, 205 F.3d 327 (7th Cir. 2000).

89. *Herzberger v. Standard Ins. Co.*, 205 F. 3d at 331.

90. *Rush Prudential HMO, Inc. v. Moran*, 536 U.S. 355 (2002).

91. *See, e.g., Thomas v. Or. Fruit Prods. Co.*, 228 F 3d 991 (9th Cir. 2000); *Cox v. Keystone Carbon Co.*, 894 F.2d 647 (3d Cir.), *cert. denied*, 498 U.S. 811 (1990); *Chilton v. Savannah Foods & Indus., Inc.*, 814 F.2d 620 (11th Cir. 1987).

92. *Blue Cross & Blue Shield v. Lewis*, 753 F. Supp. 345 (N.D. Ala. 1990).

93. 29 U.S.C. §1132(a)(2).

94. 29 U.S.C. §1132(a)(3).

95. 473 U.S. 134 (1985).

96. 508 U.S. 248 (1993)

97. *See, e.g., Pilot Life Ins. Co. v. Dedeaux*, 481 U.S. 41 (1987).

98. 12 F.3d 1517 (9th Cir. 1993).

99. 516 U.S. 489 (1996).

100. *Clair v. Harris Trust & Sav. Bank*, 190 F.3d 495 (7 Cir. 1999); *see also Allison v. Bank One-Denver*, 289 F 3d 1223 (10th Cir. 2002).

101. *Schaffer v. Westinghouse Savannah River Co.*, 2005 WL 567812 (4th Cir. 2005).

102. 534 U.S. 204 (2002).

103. 126 S.Ct. 1869 (2006).

104. *Aetna Health, Inc. v. Davila*, 542 U.S. 200 (2004).

105. Section 514(a) of ERISA; 28 U.S.C. §1144(a).

106. Section 514(b)(2)(B) of ERISA; 29 U.S.C. §1144(b)(2)(A).

107. Section 514(b)(2)(B) of ERISA; 29 U.S.C. §1144(b)(2)(B).

108. *Shaw v. Delta Air Lines, Inc.*, 463 U.S. 85, 96–97 (1983).

109. *FMC Corp. v. Holliday*, 498 U.S. 52, 58 (1990).

110. *Ingersoll-Rand Co. v. McClendon*, 498 U.S. 133 (1990); *United Wire, Metal & Mach. Health & Welfare Fund v. Morristown Mem'l Hosp.*, 995 F.2d 1179 (3d Cir.), *cert. denied*, 510 U.S. 944 (1993) (a state law may be preempted even though it has no direct nexus with ERISA plans if its effect is to dictate or restrict the choices of ERISA plans with regard to their benefits, structure, reporting, and administration).

111. *See FMC Corp.*, 498 U.S. at 58; *Shaw v. Delta Air Lines, Inc.*, 463 U.S. 85, 100 n. 21 (1983) (some state actions may affect employee benefit plans in "too tenuous, remote, or peripheral a manner to warrant a finding that the law 'relates to' the plan"); *Mackey v. Lanier Collection Agency & Serv., Inc.*, 486 U.S. 825 (1988).

112. *New York State Conference of Blue Cross & Blue Shield Plans v. Travelers Ins. Co.*, 514 U.S. 645 (1995); *California Div. of Labor Enforcement v. Dillingham Constr. N.A., Inc.*, 519 U.S. 316 (1997); *De Buono v. NYSA-ILA Medical & Clinical Servs.*, 520 U.S. 806 (1997).

113. 514 U.S. at 656.

114. 514 U.S. at 658–660.

115. 520 U.S. at 814.

116. 519 U.S. at 325.

117. 538 U.S. 329 (2003).

118. *FMC Corp. v. Holliday*, 498 U.S. at 64-65.

119. *Id.*

120. *Prudential Ins. Co. v. HMO Partners, Inc.*, 413 F.3d 897 (8th Cir. 2005).

121. *Id.* ("Our interpretation of the deemer clause makes clear that if a plan is insured, a State may regulate it indirectly through regulation of its insurer and its insurer's insurance contracts; if the plan is uninsured, the State may not regulate it").

122. *Aetna Health, Inc. v. Davila*, 542 U.S. 200 (2004).

123. *See Petrovich v. Share Health Plan*, 188 Ill.2d 17, 719 N.E.2d 756 (1999); *Jones v. Chicago HMO Ltd., 191 Ill.2d 278, 730 N.E.2d 1119 (2000); Raglin v. HMO Ill., Inc.*, 230 Ill. App.3d 642, 595 N.E.2d 153 (1992); *McClellan v. Health Maint. Org.*, 413 Pa. Super. 128, 604 A.2d 1953, *appeal denied sub nom. Health Maint. Org. v. McClellan*, 532 Pa. 664, 616 A.2d 985 (1992); *Boyd v. Albert Einstein Med. Ctr.*, 377 Pa. Super. 609, 547 A.2d 1229 (1988).

124. 59 F.3d 151 (10th Cir. 1995).

125. *Id.* at 155; *see also Prudential Health Care Plan, Inc. v. Lewis*, 77 F.3d 493 (10th Cir. 1996); *Negron v. Patel*, 6 F. Supp. 2d 366 (E.D. Pa. 1998); 57 F.3d 350 (3d Cir. 1995), *cert. denied sub nom. U.S. Healthcare, Inc. v. Dukes*, 516 U.S. 1009 (1995).

126. 57 F.3d 350 (3d Cir. 1995), *cert. denied sub nom. U.S. Healthcare, Inc. v. Dukes*, 516 U.S. 1009 (1995).

127. The Third Circuit acknowledged that the distinction between the quantity of benefits due under an ERISA plan and the quality of those benefits would not always be clear. The court recognized that there could be cases where the quality of care rendered was so low as to constitute a denial of benefits or the ERISA plan had described a benefit in terms related to the quality of services and the plan participant was claiming damages resulting from a failure to provide services of the promised quality. The court also noted that an employer and an HMO could agree that a quality of care standard articulated in their contract could replace standards that would otherwise be supplied by applicable state tort law but declined to express an opinion as to whether such an agreement would be enforceable. 57 F.3d at 358-359.

128. *Id.* at 360–361. The Seventh and Second Circuit Courts also have held that a vicarious liability professional malpractice claim was not removable to state court. *Rice v. Panchal*,

65 F.3d 637 (7th Cir. 1995); *Lupo v. Human Affairs Int'l, Inc.*, 28 F.3d 269 (2d Cir. 1994); *see also Muller v. Maron*, No. 94-5052, 1995 WL 605483 (E.D. Pa. Oct. 13, 1995).

129. 245 F.3d 266 (3d Cir. 2001).

130. 346 F.3d 422 (3d Cir. 2003).

131. 530 U.S. 211 (2000). The *Pegram* decision did not involve a claim that an HMO was vicariously liable for the medical malpractice of its network providers. However, in holding that an HMO was not a fiduciary to the extent that it made "mixed eligibility decisions acting through its physicians," the Supreme Court opined that ERISA was not enacted "in order to federalize malpractice litigation." Id. at 231, 236.

132. 346 F.3d at 446–447.

133. *Id.*

134. *Bui v. AT&T*, 310 F.3d 1143, 1147 (9th Cir. 2002).

135. 245 F.3d 266 (3d Cir. 2001).

136. *Id.* at 273.

137. 88 F.3d 1482 (7th Cir. 1996).

138. 48 F.3d 937 (6th Cir. 1995).

139. 965 F.2d 1321 (5th Cir.), *cert. denied*, 506 U.S. 1033 (1992).

140. *Id.; see also Kuhl v. Lincoln Nat'l Health Plan*, 999 F.2d 298 (8th Cir. 1993), *cert. denied*, 510 U.S. 1045 (1994) (ERISA preempted a wrongful death claim based on a delay in precertification of surgery because the precertification decision related to the administration of benefits); *Rodriguez v. Pacificare of Tex., Inc.*, 980 F.2d 1014 (5th Cir.), *cert. denied*, 508 U.S. 956 (1993); *Garrison v. Northeast Ga. Med. Ctr., Inc., 66 F. Supp. 2d 1336* (N.D. Ga. 1999); *Silva v. Kaiser Permanente*, 59 F. Supp. 2d 597 (N.D. Tex. 1999); *Bailey-Gates v. Aetna Life Ins. Co.*, 890 F. Supp. 73 (D. Conn. 1994).

141. 542 U.S. 200 (2004).

142. *Id.* at 219.

143. 385 F.3d 156 (2d Cir. 2004).

144. 381 F.3d 1274 (11th Cir. 2004); *see also Mayeaux v. La. Health Serv. & Indem. Co.*, 376 F.3d 420 (5th Cir. 2004).

145. *See Johnson v. Misericordia Comty. Hosp.*, 99 Wis.2d 708, 301 N.W.2d 156 (1981).

146. *See Shannon v. McNulty*, 718 A.2d 828 (Pa. Super. 1998); *McClellan v. Health Maint. Org.*, 413 Pa. Super. 128, 604 A.2d 1053, *appeal denied sub nom. Health Maint. Org. v. McClellan*, 532 Pa. 664, 616 A.2d 985

(1992); *Harrell v. Total Health Care, Inc.*, No. W.D. 39809, 1989 W.L. 153066 (Mo. Ct. App. Apr. 25, 1989), *aff'd on other grounds*, 781 S.W.2d 58 (Mo. 1989).

147. *See Harrell v. Total Health Care, Inc.*, No. W.D. 39809, 1989 WL 153066 (Mo. Ct. App. Apr. 25, 1989), *aff'd on other grounds*, 781 S.W.2d 58 (Mo. 1989).

148. 859 F.Supp. 182 (E.D. Pa. 1994).

149. *Id.* at 187.

150. 310 F.3d 1143 (9th Cir. 2002).

151. *Id.* at 1151.

152. *See, e.g., Butler v. Wu*, 853 F. Supp. 125 (D.N.J. 1994); *Elsesser v. Hosp. of the Philadelphia Coll. of Osteopathic Med.*, 802 F. Supp. 1286 (E.D. Pa. 1992); *Altieri v. CIGNA Dental Health, Inc.*, 753 F. Supp. 61 (D. Conn. 1990); *Dalton v. Peninsula Hosp. Ctr.*, 164 Misc.2d 912, 626 N.Y.S.2d 362 (N.Y. Sup. Ct. 1995).

153. 193 F.2d 151 (3d Cir. 1999), *cert denied sub nom. U.S. Healthcare, Inc. v. Bauman*, 530 U.S. 1242 (2000).

154. 878 F. Supp. 820 (D. Md. 1995).

155. *Id.* at 824 n. 6.

156. *Lupo v. Human Affairs Int'l, Inc.*, 28 F.3d 269 (2d Cir. 1994).

157. *Id.; see also Wirthlin v. Jarvis*, No. C-1-99-477, 2001 WL 1842473 (S.D. Ohio Jan. 12, 2001); *Herrera v. Lovelace Health Sys.*, 35 F. Supp. 2d 1327 (D. N.M. 1999); *Santitoro v. Evans*, 935 F. Supp. 733 (E.D. N.C. 1996); *Villazon v. Prudential Health Care Plan, Inc.*, 843 So.2d 842 (Fla. 2003); *McClellan v. Health Maint. Org.*, 413 Pa. Super. 128, 604 A.2d 1053, *appeal denied sub nom. Health Maint. Org. v. McClellan*, 532 Pa. 664, 616 A.2d 985 (1992).

158. 904 F.2d 236 (5th Cir. 1990), *reh'g denied*, No. 89-2513, 1990 U.S. App. LEXIS 13227 (5th Cir. July 16, 1990).

159. *Id.* at 249–250.

160. 110 F.3d 280 (5th Cir.), *cert. denied sub nom. Pan-American Life Ins. Co. v. Cypress Fairbanks Med. Ctr., Inc.*, 522 U.S. 862 (1997).

161. *Id.* at 281.

162. *Id.* at 283.

163. *Id.* at 283.

164. *See Home Health, Inc. v. Prudential Ins. Co.*, 101 F.3d 600 (8th Cir. 1996); *The Meadows v. Employers Health Ins.*, 47 F.3d 1006 (9th Cir. 1995); *Lordmann Enters., Inc. v. Equicor, Inc.*, 32 F.3d 1529 (11th Cir. 1994), *cert. denied sub nom. Equicor, Inc. v. Lordmann Enters., Inc.*, 516 U.S. 930 (1995); *Hospice of Metro Denver, Inc. v. Group Health Ins. of Okla., Inc.*, 944 F.2d 752 (10th Cir. 1991); *St. Luke's Episcopal Hosp. v. Great West Life & Annuity Ins. Co.*, 38 F. Supp. 2d 497 (S.D. Tex. 1999); *Davis v. United Healthcare Ins. Co.*, 34 F. Supp. 2d 1044 (S. D. Miss. 1998); *Jefferson Parish Hosp. Serv. Dist. No. 2 v. Ruby Tuesday's Inc.*, No. 97-2722, 1998 U.S. Dist. LEXIS 767 (E.D. La. Jan. 23, 1998); *Variety Children's Hosp., Inc. v. Blue Cross/Blue Shield of Fla.*, 942 F. Supp. 562 (S.D. Fla. 1996); *Memorial Hosp. Sys. v. John Hancock. Mut. Life Ins. Co.*, 952 F. Supp. 449 (S.D. Tex. 1996); *Rehabilitation Inst. v. Group Adm'rs, Ltd.*, 844 F. Supp. 1275 (N.D. Ill. 1994); *Hoag Memorial Hosp. v. Managed Care Adm'rs*, 820 F. Supp. 1232 (C.D. Cal. 1993); *Gaston Mem'l Hosp. Home Health Servs., Inc. v. Bridgestone/Firestone, Inc.*, 830 F. Supp. 287 (W.D.N.C. 1993); *Suburban Hosp., Inc. v. Sampson*, 807 F.Supp. 31 (D. Md. 1992).

165. 187 F.3d 1045 (9th Cir. 1999).

166. *Peninsula Regional Med. Ctr. v. Mid Atlantic Medical Services, LLC*, 327 F. Supp. 2d 572 (D. Md. 2004); *Johns Hopkins Hosp. v. CareFirst of Md., Inc.*, 327 F. Supp. 2d 577 (D. Md. 2004); *see also Children's Hosp. Corp. v. Kindercare Learning Ctrs., Inc.*, 360 F. Supp. 2d 202 (D. Mass. 2005); *Tenet Healthsytem Hosp., Inc. v. Crosby Tugs, Inc.*, No. 04-1632, 2005 WL 1038072 (E.D. La. Apr. 27, 2005); *Baylor Univ. Med. Ctr. v. Epoch Group, L.C.*, No. 3:03-CV-2392, 2004 WL 2434290 (N.D. Tex. Oct. 29, 2004); *River Parishes, Inc. v. Aetna U.S. Healthcare, Inc.*, No. 00-3380, 2001 WL 277938 (E.D. La. Mar. 20, 2001).

167. *Stuart Circle Hosp. Corp. v. Aetna Health Management*, 995 F.2d 500 (4th Cir.), *cert. denied sub nom. Aetna Life Ins. Co. v. Stuart Circle Hosp. Corp.*, 510 U.S. 1003 (1993).

168. *Id.*

169. *See also Blue Cross & Blue Shield v. Bell*, 798 F.2d 1331 (10th Cir. 1986); *Blue Cross & Blue Shield of Va. v. St. Mary's Hosp. of Richmond, Inc.*, 245 Va. 24, 426 S.E.2d 117 (1993); *Blue Cross Hosp. Serv., Inc. v. Frappier*, 698 S.W.2d 326 (Mo. 1985).

170. 82 F. 3d 642 (5th Cir. 1996).

171. 105 F.3d 1035 (5th Cir. 1997).

172. 82 F.3d at 648; 105 F. 3d at 1037.
173. *Prudential Ins. Co. v. National Park Med. Ctr.,* 154 F.3d 812 (8th Cir. 1998).
174. 538 U.S. 329 (2003).
175. *Id.* at 341–342.
176. *Id.; see also Prudential Ins. Co. v. National Park Med. Ctr., Inc.,* 413 F.3d 897 (8th Cir. 2005) (Arkansas AWP law was saved from conflict preemption, but ERISA's civil enforcement provision completely preempted civil penalties provision of AWP law with respect to suits that could have been brought under ERISA).

32

HIPAA AND MANAGED HEALTH CARE

Leigh C. Riley and Peter R. Kongstvedt

Study Objectives

- Understand the meaning of administrative simplification and be able to explain why it is an important term in the health care industry.
- Understand the term "protected health information" (PHI).
- Understand the security requirements included in HIPAA's administrative simplification provisions.
- Understand the privacy requirements under HIPAA.
- Understand the meaning of the term "electronic data interchange" (EDI).
- Understand the standards for electronic business transactions that are included in administrative simplification.
- Understand the standards for electronic transmission of code sets.

Discussion Topics

1. Describe what is included under the administrative simplification portion of HIPAA. Why is it important to the health care industry?
2. Describe the electronic transactions performed in the health care industry and how they are affected by HIPAA. Discuss the positive and negative consequences and implications of this.
3. Describe the code set requirements in HIPAA. Discuss the positive and negative consequences and implications of this.
4. Discuss how HIPAA privacy requirements might differ from state laws about confidentiality of health information. Discuss when either HIPAA requirements or state requirements might prevail.
5. Explain why confidentiality of health information has been a controversial public policy issue.

INTRODUCTION

One of the most important federal laws having a major effect on managed care organizations (MCOs) and health care providers is the Health Insurance Portability and Accountability Act of 1996 (HIPAA), as amended.[1] Though initially promoted as a vehicle for improving the portability of health insurance, other aspects were added as well. When first passed, HIPAA had five major sections, or "titles":

Title I: Health Care Access, Portability, and Renewability

Title II: Preventing Fraud and Abuse; Administrative Simplification

Title III: Tax-Related Health Provisions (including the creation of Medical Savings Accounts, a forerunner of today's consumer-directed health plans)

Title IV: Application and Enforcement of Group Health Plan Requirements

Title V: Revenue Offsets

In the fall of 1996, just a few weeks after its initial passage, amendments regarding mandatory maternity length of stay benefits, mental health parity, women's health, cancer rights, and a few other items were added. A great deal of Titles I, III, IV, V, and parts of II are relatively arcane and, although important for compliance purposes, not appropriate for a review textbook such as this.

HIPAA's actual impact on the U.S. health care environment has been relatively modest with one major exception: Title II, Subsection F of HIPAA: "Administrative Simplification." The impact of Administrative Simplification has been and continues to be substantial, and this chapter focuses on that aspect as it applies to MCOs.

Regretably, the "portability" aspect of HIPAA has proven itself to be both complex and costly, with very little impact on most Americans. Health plans must comply with that provision of HIPAA, but the reader will need to access competent legal resources for further discussion of this aspect.

ADMINISTRATIVE SIMPLIFICATION

Administrative Simplification addresses four issues of widespread importance to health plans, providers, and indeed all covered entities (defined later). HIPAA regulates the following:

- How covered entities, which include insurers that provide health benefits such as MCOs as well as providers of health care and other related entities, may use and disclose certain items of information called "protected health information" (PHI)
- What security measures must be in place to protect the privacy of electronic PHI
- The mandated use of certain standards for a defined set of electronic transactions between covered entities
- The creation of a new National Provider Identifier (NPI)

Two other identifiers were created under HIPAA: a National Health Plan (Payer) Identifier and a National Health Identifier for Individuals. The U.S. Department of Health and Human Services (DHHS), that branch of government charged with creating and implementing the regulations under the Administrative Simplification provisions of HIPAA, has not issued any proposed standards for the National Health Plan Identifier at the time of publication. The National Identifier for Individuals was effectively stopped in its tracks because of privacy concerns and will not be implemented. A National Employer Identifier was also created, but its use is voluntary and will not be discussed in this chapter.

The HIPAA-mandated standards for electronic transactions became effective in May 2002 (May 2003, for small health plans; *ie,* insurers with premiums of less than $5 million per year).[2] The privacy regulations became effective in April 2003 (April 2004, for small health plans),[3] and the security regulations became effective in April 2005 (April 2006, for small health plans).[4] The NPI is scheduled to be phased in by May 23, 2007 (May 23, 2008 for small health plans).[5]

COVERED ENTITY UNDER HIPAA

The HIPAA requirements and standards subject to the Administrative Simplification regulations apply only to "covered entities." A covered entity includes a health plan,[6] which is defined as any individual or group plan that provides or pays the cost of medical care.[7] Insurers and health maintenance organizations (HMOs) are specifically included in the definition of a health plan.[8] Thus, MCOs are directly regulated by HIPAA. Examples of other covered entities include hospitals, physicians, psychologists, dentists, pharmacies, claims clearinghouses, and others that are not the focus of this chapter.

PRIVACY AND SECURITY

Privacy and security both relate to a covered entity's obligation to protect health information. Privacy refers to the need to keep such information private, and the policies and procedures necessary to ensure privacy. Security refers to the policies and procedures to ensure that privacy is maintained in electronic records and communications by covered entities.

Protected Health Information

Central to the privacy and security regulations is the concept of "protected health information," or PHI. Only information that falls within the definition of protected health information is subject to the regulations. All other information is outside the regulatory scope of HIPAA. Although the privacy and security provisions of HIPAA are separate, they are inextricably linked because of this.

PHI is individually identifiable health information that is transmitted or maintained in electronic media or in any other form or medium.[9] In other words, all electronic, paper, and oral information is covered. Health information is all information that is created or received by a covered entity and that relates to the past, present, or future physical or mental

health or condition of an individual, the provision of health care to an individual, or the past, present, or future payment for the provision of health care to an individual.[10] Information is "individually identifiable" if it either identifies the individual, such as by name, or if there is a reasonable basis to believe the information can be used to identify the individual, such as an address or Social Security number.[11] Protected health information is intended to be extremely broad and cover most of the information received by an MCO with respect to a health benefits contract.

Privacy Standards Applicable to Uses and Disclosures of Protected Health Information

Under the HIPAA privacy regulations, an MCO may not use or disclose PHI except as permitted in the regulations. Fortunately, the regulations permit MCOs to use and disclose PHI for almost all general functions needed to be performed by an MCO in the course of its business as an insurer of health benefits. The main categories of permitted uses and disclosures are the following:

- *For Payment, Treatment, and Health Care Operations:*[12] This is the largest category of permitted uses and disclosures and covers most routine functions needed to be performed by an MCO. Each of the terms *payment*, *treatment*, and *health care operations* is defined in the privacy regulations. *Payment* includes such activities as making determinations of eligibility for coverage, risk-adjusting premiums based on the enrollee's health status, billing, claims management, collection activities, and utilization review activities. *Treatment* includes the provision, coordination, and management of health care and related services by a health care provider and a third party, such as an MCO. *Health care operations* covers all other business operations, such as conducting quality assessment and improvement activities, underwriting, premium rating, and other activities related to the creation, renewal, or placement of a health insurance contract, and conducting or arranging for legal or auditing services.

- *To the Individual:*[13] The MCO must disclose PHI to the individual who is the subject of that information. In addition, the MCO must disclose PHI to the individual's personal representative.[14] In most instances, the parent of an unemancipated minor child is considered the child's personal representative.[15] However, the MCO may be prohibited by state law from disclosing certain PHI about a minor child to its parent.

- *For Legal, Public, and Similar Activities:*[16] The MCO may disclose PHI when required by law or for judicial or administrative proceedings, for law enforcement activities, for public health activities (such as to a disease control agency), to a health oversight agency, for research purposes, to avert a serious threat to health or safety, and for specialized government functions (such as military and veterans activities). An MCO may also disclose PHI to the extent required by state workers' compensation laws.

- *To Business Associates:* Often, a covered entity needs to utilize the services of third parties to run its business. These third parties might include consultants, auditors, lawyers, or subcontractors. If one of these third parties will be creating, receiving, or maintaining PHI on behalf of the covered entity in connection with its performance of services for the covered entity, the third party is considered a "business associate."[17] In such a case, the covered entity must ensure that the business associate enters into a business associate contract, which is an agreement that obligates the business associate to essentially act as if it were a covered entity with respect to PHI.[18] The HIPAA privacy regulations contain a detailed list of the items that are required

to be included in a valid business associate contract.[19]

- *To Plan Sponsors:* An MCO may disclose PHI to the employer or other entity that is sponsoring the group health plan for which the MCO is insuring benefits. There are no restrictions on the MCO's ability to disclose summary health information (which is PHI with some identifiers removed) to the plan sponsor if the plan sponsor needs the information for purposes of obtaining premium bids for health insurance coverage, or modifying or amending its group health plan, or on disclosing information about whether an individual is or is not enrolled for insurance coverage.[20] If the plan sponsor needs to obtain PHI beyond these limited items for purposes of performing plan administration functions however, the plan sponsor must amend its group health plan to provide that the plan sponsor will essentially act as a covered entity with respect to its plan's PHI, and the plan sponsor must certify that it will comply with the requirements set out in the plan amendment.[21] (The preambles to the regulations state that the purpose of the certification is to allow insurers such as MCOs to obtain the certification from the plan sponsor and be able to rely on it for purposes of disclosing PHI.) The plan sponsor is prohibited from using PHI for employment-related actions.

If a type of use or disclosure is not specifically permitted in the HIPAA privacy regulations, the MCO must obtain the individual's authorization to use or disclose his or her PHI. The authorization must meet certain requirements contained in the privacy regulations, such as a description of the information to be use or disclosed, an expiration date of the authorization, and certain required statements such as regarding the individual's right to revoke the authorization.[22] An MCO should not disclose PHI pursuant to an authorization unless it has confirmed that the authorization contains all of the elements required by HIPAA.

Individual Rights

HIPAA also grants rights to members of an MCO. Under HIPAA, an individual has the following rights:

1. Request a restriction on the use and disclosure of the member's PHI.[23] However, a covered entity is not required to agree to the restriction.
2. Receive communications containing PHI from the MCO by alternative means or at alternative locations, if the member clearly states that the disclosure of all or part of the information could endanger the individual.[24] For example, a member could request that an explanation of benefits form be sent via e-mail to the member's work e-mail address, or be mailed to a friend's house. If the request is reasonable, the MCO must accommodate the request.
3. Inspect or copy the member's PHI, except in very limited circumstances, such as information compiled in anticipation of a civil proceeding.[25] If access will be denied, the MCO must respond to the member in writing.[26] In general, the MCO must either provide notice of a denial or provide access within 30 days after receipt of the member's request.[27]
4. Amend the member's PHI. The MCO must determine whether to grant or deny the amendment request generally within 60 days of receipt of the request.[28] Whether the MCO approves or denies the request, it must provide written notice to the member.[29]
5. Receive an accounting of certain disclosures of the member's PHI. The MCO need not account for disclosures to carry out payment, treatment, and health care operations, to the member or others involved in the member's health care, made pursuant to an autho-

rization, or that were made more than 6 years earlier (or made earlier than the HIPAA effective date).[30] Some additional exceptions are listed in the regulations. The accounting must generally include the date of the disclosure, the name of the entity or person to whom the disclosure was made, a brief description of the PHI disclosed, and a brief statement of the purpose of the disclosure.[31]

Administrative Requirements

The HIPAA privacy provisions impose several administrative requirements on MCOs.

An MCO must provide a notice of privacy practices to its members.[32] The notice of privacy practices contains certain information, as specified in the HIPAA privacy regulations, intended to put members on notice about the potential uses and disclosures that may be made of their PHI and their individual rights.[33] The MCO must provide this notice initially when a member enrolls in the MCO and must provide an updated notice within 60 days of any material modification to the information contained in the notice.[34] In addition, every 3 years, the MCO must provide a notice reminding members of the availability of the notice.[35]

An MCO must establish policies and procedures addressing all of the privacy requirements[36] and must designate a privacy official who is responsible for the development and implementation of those policies and procedures.[37]

An MCO must train its workforce personnel about the HIPAA requirements[38] and apply sanctions against any workforce members who fail to comply with the MCO's HIPAA policies and procedures.[39]

An MCO must establish a process for receiving complaints about potential HIPAA violations.[40] An MCO must also mitigate, to the extent practicable, any harmful effects of a known HIPAA violation.[41]

An MCO must have in place appropriate administrative, technical, and physical safeguards to protect the privacy of PHI.[42] (The security regulations address in more detail these rules as they apply to electronic PHI.) An MCO may not retaliate against a member for exercising his or her rights or any other individual for opposing an action that the individual in good faith believes violates the privacy rules, filing a complaint, or assisting in an investigation or proceeding relating to a HIPAA violation.[43]

Finally, an MCO must maintain all written records, such as its policies and procedures and all written communications made to members, for 6 years from the date of the document's creation.[44]

Security Standards Applicable to Electronic Protected Health Information

Even though the HIPAA privacy provisions generally require covered entities to ensure the confidentiality of PHI by appropriately securing it, the HIPAA security rules require additional measures for *electronic* PHI. Electronic PHI is PHI that is transmitted or maintained in electronic media, which includes hard drives or computer disks, Internet, and e-mail.[45] Facsimile transmission, telephone, and paper PHI are not considered electronic PHI (though are still subject to the general privacy requirements as discussed earlier).

The HIPAA security rules generally require a covered entity to do the following:

1. Ensure the confidentiality, integrity, and availability of electronic PHI
2. Protect against any reasonably anticipated threats or hazards to the security and integrity of electronic PHI
3. Protect against any reasonably anticipated uses or disclosures of electronic PHI not permitted by the HIPAA privacy rules
4. Ensure compliance with the preceding by its workforce[46]

The security rules specify 18 different standards for complying with these general principles. For many of the standards, additional implementation steps (called specifications) are either required or addressable.[47] A required specification is just that: a covered entity must implement the specification. An addressable specification may or may not need to be implemented, depending on whether the covered entity determines that the specification is a reasonable and appropriate safeguard in its environment, when analyzed with reference to the likely contribution to protecting electronic PHI.[48] If a covered entity determines that an addressable specification need not be implemented, the covered entity must either document its determination or implement an equivalent alternative measure.[49]

The following summarizes the 18 standards of the HIPAA security rules and lists the required specifications:

1. *Security management process:* Implement policies and procedures to prevent, detect, contain, and correct security violations. The required specifications include conducting a risk analysis, implementing risk management measures, applying sanctions against noncompliant workforce members, and conducting a regular review of activities.[50]
2. *Assigned security responsibility:* Identify the security official who is responsible for development and implementation of the covered entity's security policies and procedures.[51]
3. *Workforce security:* Implement policies and procedures to ensure that all members of the covered entity's workforce have access as appropriate to electronic PHI, and to prevent those members of the workforce who do not have access from obtaining access.[52]
4. *Information access management:* Implement policies and procedures for authorizing access to electronic PHI.[53]
5. *Security awareness and training:* Implement a security awareness and training program for all workforce members.[54]

6. *Security incident procedures:* Implement policies and procedures to address security incidents. The required specification includes identifying and responding to suspected or known security incidents, mitigating the harmful effects of an incident, and documenting incidents and their outcomes.[55]

7. *Contingency plan:* Establish, and implement if needed, policies and procedures for responding to an emergency or other occurrence, such as a fire or natural disaster, that damages systems containing electronic PHI. The required specifications include creating and maintaining retrievable exact copies of the PHI, implementing procedures to restore lost data, ensuring continuation of critical business processes while operating in emergency mode, and periodically testing and revising contingency plans.[56]

8. *Evaluation:* Perform periodic evaluation of the procedures, in light of environmental or operational changes, to establish that the covered entity complies with the security standards.[57]

9. *Business associate contracts:* Obtain satisfactory written assurance from any business associate that creates, maintains, or receives electronic PHI that it will implement safeguards of electronic PHI similar to that required of the covered entity, that it will ensure its agents do likewise, and report to the covered entity any security incident of which it becomes aware. The business associate's written assurance is a required specification.[58]

10. *Facility access controls:* Implement policies and procedures to limit physical access to electronic PHI systems and the facility(ies) in which they are housed.[59]

11. *Workstation use:* Implement policies and procedures that specify the functions to be performed, the manner in which those functions are to be performed, and the physical attributes of

the surrounding of a specific workstation that can access electronic PHI.[60]

12. *Workstation security:* Implement physical safeguards for all workstations that access electronic PHI to restrict access to authorized users.[61]

13. *Device and media controls:* Implement policies and procedures that govern the receipt and removal of hardware and electronic media that contain electronic PHI into and out of a facility. Required specifications include addressing the final disposition of electronic PHI and/or the hardware on which it is used, and removal of electronic PHI from electronic media before the media is reused.[62]

14. *Access control:* Implement technical policies and procedures for systems that maintain electronic PHI to allow access only to those individuals or software programs that have been granted access rights. Required specifications include assigning a unique name and/or number for identifying and tracking user identity, and establishing procedures for obtaining necessary electronic PHI during an emergency.[63]

15. *Audit controls:* Implement hardware, software, and/or procedural mechanisms that record and examine activity in information systems that contain electronic PHI.[64]

16. *Integrity:* Implement policies and procedures to protect electronic PHI from improper alteration or destruction.[65]

17. *Person or identity authentication:* Implement procedures to verify that a person or entity seeking access to electronic PHI is the one claimed.[66]

18. *Transmission security:* Implement technical security measures to guard against unauthorized access to electronic PHI that is being transmitted over an electronic communications network.[67]

All of the policies and procedures described in the standards are required to be maintained for 6 years from the date of creation or when it was last in effect, whichever is later.[68]

Preemption of State Law

The HIPAA privacy and security regulations generally preempt all state laws that are contrary to HIPAA.[69] There are four exceptions:

1. The Secretary of the DHHS determines that the state law is necessary to regulate certain items, including state regulation of insurance.
2. The state law is more stringent than HIPAA, in which case, the covered entity would need to comply with the more stringent state law.
3. The state law applies to the reporting of disease or injury, child abuse, birth, or death, or certain public health activities.
4. The state law requires a health plan, including an MCO, to report or provide access to information for the purposes of management audits, financial audits, licensure, and the like.[70]

Compliance and Enforcement

The Secretary of DHHS has primary enforcement responsibility for the HIPAA privacy and security regulations.[71] The general principles for achieving compliance are cooperation and assistance.[72] In other words, DHHS will generally react to minor or inadvertent noncompliance issues with requests for the covered entity to comply and information and assistance on how compliance can be achieved.

DHHS has two mechanisms for discovering noncompliance. First, an individual who believes that there has been a HIPAA violation may file a complaint with the DHHS, and the DHHS may investigate the complaint.[73] Second, DHHS may conduct compliance reviews of covered entities.[74] Covered entities are required to provide records, permit access to records, and otherwise cooperate with DHHS during an investigation or compliance review.[75]

If noncompliance is discovered, the DHHS will first try to resolve the matter by informal

means.[76] If that is not possible, the DHHS will issue a written finding of noncompliance.[77] The DHHS may also seek to impose penalties on a covered entity that is not in compliance. If that happens, the DHHS is required to issue a written notice of intent to impose a penalty, and the covered entity has the right to request a hearing in front of an administrative law judge.[78] The potential penalties range in severity depending on the type of violation, as follows:[79]

- A civil penalty of $100 per each violation, capped at $25,000 per year for all violations or prohibitions of an identical nature. The penalty will be waived if it is found to be a result of reasonable cause (and not willful neglect) and is corrected within 30 days of the date the violation became known (or would have been known with the exercise of reasonable care).
- If a covered entity that knowingly and in violation of HIPAA uses or causes to be used a unique health identifier, obtains PHI relating to an individual, or discloses PHI to another person, the covered entity may be fined up to $50,000 and/or imprisoned for up to 1 year.
- If the preceding offense is committed under false pretenses, the penalty increases to up to $100,000 and/or imprisonment of up to 10 years.
- If the preceding offense is committed with intent to sell, transfer, or use PHI for commercial advantage, personal gain, or malicious harm, the penalty increases to up to $250,000 and/or imprisonment of up to 10 years.

TRANSACTIONS AND CODE SETS

Transactions refer specifically to certain business-related electronic transactions between covered entities, though the distinction between clinical information and business-related information is not distinct. Code sets refer to the types of standardized codes that must be used in the transactions as they apply to different types of clinical services, and are considered PHI.

Transactions

Much of the information contained in transactions is also considered PHI (for example, a member name or diagnosis). Transactions and code sets are actually separate though overlapping topics, but they are generally discussed as one topic because the law and regulations only apply to electronic transactions. HIPAA does not mandate that physicians or other providers use electronic connectivity, but it does mandate that if they do use electronic connectivity for these transactions, they must conform to these standards. HIPAA does not allow the use of any nonstandard electronic transactions in health care by covered entities if a standard has been designated as being applicable.

For transactions other than pharmacy claims, the transaction standards are those of the X12 (sometimes referred to as X12N) standards of the American National Standards Institute (ANSI).[80] When the mandated standards went into effect in 2002, version 4010 of the X12 standards was the one chosen. Newer versions now exist, but because of the need to maintain stability in standards so as to encourage adoption, the 4010 versions remain the standard at the time of publication. Migration to the 5010 version is expected to occur at some point in the future, but exactly when is not yet known. For pharmacy claims, the designated standards are those of the National Council for Prescription Drug Programs (NCPDP), Batch Standard Implementation Guide and Telecommunication Standard Implementation Guide.[81] Not all standards required under HIPAA have been finalized however; for example, at the time of publication, the standard for the claims attachment*

---

*A claims attachment is additional clinical information that an MCO might need to process a claim; such information is now usually provided by paper copy or non-standard electronic format such as a text file or electronic radiograph.

was proposed (but not officially designated) to be the 4050 version of ANSI 275 combined with the Clinical Architecture Document (CDA) standards from Health Level 7 (HL7), while the standard for First Report of Injury had not yet been proposed at all.

Table 32-1 lists the electronic transaction standards under HIPAA.

The standards themselves are subject to periodic updating. Under HIPAA, designated standards maintenance organizations (DSMOs) are charged with making recommendations to DHHS regarding updates to existing standards as well as the addition of new standards.[82] The following organizations are considered DSMOs under HIPAA:[83]

1. Accredited Standards Committee X12 (also known as the American National Standards Institute, ANSI)
2. Dental Content Committee of the American Dental Association
3. Health Level Seven (HL7)
4. National Council for Prescription Drug Programs (NCPDP)
5. National Uniform Billing Committee
6. National Uniform Claim Committee

Code Sets

The standardized code sets required under HIPAA are as follows:[84]

- *International Classification of Diseases,* 9th Edition, Clinical Modification (ICD–9–CM), Volumes 1 and 2 for the following conditions:

  (1) Diseases
  (2) Injuries
  (3) Impairments
  (4) Other health problems and their manifestations
  (5) Causes of injury, disease, impairment, or other health problems

- ICD-9-CM Volume 3, Procedures, for the following procedures or other actions taken for diseases, injuries, and impairments on hospital inpatients reported by hospitals:

Table 32–1 HIPAA Standardized Electronic Transactions

Transaction	Standard
Provider claims submission	ANSI X12 – 837 (different versions exist for institutional, professional, and dental)
Pharmacy claims	NCPDP
Eligibility	ANSI X12 – 270 (inquiry) ANSI X12 – 271 (response)
Claim status	ANSI X12 – 276 (inquiry) ANSI X12 – 277 (response)
Provider referral certification and authorization	ANSI X12 – 278
Health care payment to provider, with remittance advice	ANSI X12 – 835
Enrollment and disenrollment in health plan*	ANSI X12 – 834
Claims attachment (additional clinical information from provider to health plan, used for claims adjudication)	ANSI X12 – 275 (not finalized at the time of publication), and HL7 CDA
Premium payment to health plan*	ANSI X12 – 820
First report of injury	ANSI X12 – 148 (not yet issued)

*These are for voluntary but not mandatory use by employers, unions, or associations that pay premiums to the health plan on behalf of members.
Source: Compiled by author based on 45 CFR §160.920 and other sources at the Centers for Medicare and Medicaid Services (CMS) within the DHHS. Available at: http://www.cms.gov.

(1) Prevention
(2) Diagnosis
(3) Treatment
(4) Management

- National Drug Codes (NDC) for drugs and biologics
- Code on Dental Procedures and Nomenclature, as maintained and distributed by the American Dental Association, for dental services
- The combination of Health Care Common Procedure Coding System (HCPCS), as maintained and distributed by the DHHS, and *Current Procedural Terminology,* Fourth Edition (CPT–4), as maintained and distributed by the American Medical Association (AMA) for physician services and other health care services. These services include, but are not limited to, the following:

(1) Physician services
(2) Physical and occupational therapy services
(3) Radiologic procedures
(4) Clinical laboratory tests
(5) Other medical diagnostic procedures
(6) Hearing and vision services
(7) Transportation services including ambulance
(8) Orthotic and prosthetic devices
(9) Durable medical equipment

All of these heavily used code sets have been in existence for quite a while, though with periodic updating and modifications. At the time of publication, consideration is being given via the DSMOs to updating ICD-9 to ICD-10 (which would also incorporate many of the codes that are currently covered by HCPCS). The ICD-10 code set is approximately 10 times the size of the ICD-9 set, and will therefore require considerable modifications to provider and payer (both commercial and governmental) systems; the dates being discussed for implementation are 2010 or 2012, but when it will actually take place is not known. The AMA is currently undertaking a project to develop the CPT-5 code set, but there is no discussion at the time of publication as to when that would be generally adopted.

THE NATIONAL PROVIDER IDENTIFIER

The NPI is a new, uniform identifier that all providers will be required to use, and as noted early in the chapter is being phased in at the time of publication. The NPI is a 10-digit* number, with the 10th digit being a checksum. There is no embedded intelligence in the NPI.[85] In other words, nothing in the 10 digits will provide any additional information about the provider other than identifying who or what the provider is. An institutional provider may under some circumstances obtain a separate NPI for a "subpart" if the subpart is unique[86] (for example, a division of a hospital system that bills Medicare separately for distinct types of services).

---

*The NPI specifically uses digits, not alphanumeric symbols, which may seem an arcane difference, but it is potentially very significant depending on how an MCO's information system is set up.

The NPI will replace all other forms of provider identifiers such as the Medicare universal provider identification numbers (UPIN), Blue Cross and Blue Shield numbers, health plan provider numbers, TRICARE (see Chapter 28) numbers, Medicaid numbers, and so forth. The only provider numbers that are not affected are the taxpayer identifying number and the Drug Enforcement Administration (DEA) number for providers who prescribe or administer prescription drugs. The National Employer Identification Number (EIN) is not affected either, to the extent that a provider is also an employer. The NPI is unique and never ending in that once assigned an NPI, the provider will use that identifier for all transactions regardless of location, plan type, or anything else. Further discussion of the NPI is found in Chapter 5.

CONCLUSION

HIPAA is a law and set of regulations with far-reaching effect upon health plans and other covered entities. Though the initial focus of HIPAA was on other aspects of how health care is provided and made accessible to individuals, its most fundamental impact has been on how MCOs and other covered entities protect and secure the privacy of an individual's health information, and as a boost toward enabling more electronic connectivity between the various parties in the health care system.

References

1. P.L. 104-191.
2. 45 CFR § 162.900(b).
3. 45 CFR § 164.534(b).
4. 45 CFR § 164.318(a).
5. *Federal Register.* January 23, 2004;69(15).
6. 45 CFR § 160.102(a).
7. 45 CFR § 160.103.
8. Ibid.
9. Ibid.
10. Ibid.
11. Ibid.
12. 45 CFR § 164.506.
13. 45 CFR § 164.502(a)(i).
14. 45 CFR § 164.502(g)(1).
15. 45 CFR § 164.502(g)(2).
16. 45 CFR § 164.512.
17. 45 CFR § 160.103.
18. 45 CFR § 164.502(e).

19. 45 CFR § 164.504(e).
20. 45 CFR § 164.504(f)(1)(ii).
21. 45 CFR § 164.504(f)(2).
22. 45 CFR § 164.508.
23. 45 CFR § 164.522(a).
24. 45 CFR § 164.522(b).
25. 45 CFR § 164.524(a).
26. 45 CFR § 164.524(d).
27. 45 CFR § 164.524(b)(2).
28. 45 CFR § 164.526(b).
29. 45 CFR § 164.526(c).
30. 45 CFR § 164.528(a)(1).
31. 45 CFR § 164.528(b)(2).
32. 45 CFR § 164.520(a).
33. 45 CFR § 164.520(b).
34. 45 CFR § 164.520(c).
35. Ibid.
36. 45 CFR § 164.530(i).
37. 45 CFR § 164.530(a).
38. 45 CFR § 164.530(b).
39. 45 CFR § 164.530(e).
40. 45 CFR § 164.530(d).
41. 45 CFR § 164.530(f).
42. 45 CFR § 164.530(c).
43. 45 CFR § 164.530(g).
44. 45 CFR § 164.530(j).
45. 45 CFR § 160.103.
46. 45 CFR § 164.306.
47. 45 CFR § 164.306(d).
48. 45 CFR § 164.306(3).
49. Ibid.
50. 45 CFR § 164.308(a)(1).
51. 45 CFR § 164.308(a)(2).
52. 45 CFR § 164.308(a)(3).

53. 45 CFR § 164.308(a)(4).
54. 45 CFR § 164.308(a)(5).
55. 45 CFR § 164.308(a)(6).
56. 45 CFR § 164.308(a)(7).
57. 45 CFR § 164.308(a)(8).
58. 45 CFR § 164.308(b).
59. 45 CFR § 164.310(a).
60. 45 CFR § 164.310(b).
61. 45 CFR § 164.310(c).
62. 45 CFR § 164.310(d).
63. 45 CFR § 164.312(a).
64. 45 CFR § 164.312(b).
65. 45 CFR § 164.312(c).
66. 45 CFR § 164.312(d).
67. 45 CFR § 164.312(e).
68. 45 CFR § 164.316.
69. 45 CFR § 160.203.
70. 45 CFR § 160.203(a)–(d).
71. 45 CFR § 160.300.
72. 45 CFR § 160.304.
73. 45 CFR § 160.306.
74. 45 CFR § 160.308.
75. 45 CFR § 160.310.
76. 45 CFR § 160.312.
77. Ibid.
78. 45 CFR § 160.500–160.526.
79. P.L. 104-191, §§ 1176 and 1177.
80. 45 CFR § 160.920.
81. Ibid.
82. 45 CFR § 160.910.
83. 45 CFR § 162.920(a).
84. 45 CFR § 160.1002.
85. 45 CFR § 160.406.
86. 45 CFR § 160.408.

33

STATE REGULATION OF MANAGED CARE

Donna Horoschak and Samantha Silva*

Study Objectives

- Understand how various managed care organizations are regulated by state agencies.
- Understand the steps state regulators take to safeguard the interest of consumers.
- Understand how HMOs are licensed and recertified.
- Understand the problems associated with anti-managed care legislation.
- Understand the inter-relationship between state and federal regulation.
- Understand how regulation is driven by market segmentation and the challenges of maintaining a level regulatory playing field among various forms of managed care.

Discussion Topics

1. Discuss the most critical components of state oversight of HMO operations. How might this differ for different types of health plans?
2. Discuss when state regulation does and does not apply to health coverage sold by different types of managed care plans and arrangements.
3. Discuss how state regulation is driven by what is best for consumers and when it is driven by what is best for special interest groups.
4. Discuss possible ways to create a seamless regulatory system for all managed care organizations.

*The authors gratefully acknowledge the contributions of Kristin Stewart, M.H.A., and Betsy Pelovitz, J.D., Regional Director, at America's Health Insurance Plans.

INTRODUCTION

In our federal system of government, states have the principal responsibility for the regulation of managed care organizations (MCOs). In recent years, the scope of state regulation has expanded to intervene more directly in the structure and operations of MCOs. At the same time, the federal government has begun to play a more prominent role in the managed care market, both as a regulator and as a purchaser. Although federal regulation historically has tended to supplement rather than supplant state regulation of MCOs, there is growing congressional interest in legislative proposals that seek to streamline regulatory structures and, at the same time, shift the balance between federal and state oversight of MCOs.

In most cases, state regulation is triggered if an MCO has assumed insurance risk for the provision of medical services, or the MCO provides one or more services pursuant to a fully insured arrangement. The authority of states to regulate health benefits plans that do not involve insured products is circumscribed by the preemption provisions of the federal Employee Retirement Income Security Act of 1974 (ERISA). (See Chapter 31 for a detailed discussion about ERISA.)

This chapter highlights the role of the states in regulating MCO operations. In particular, it describes oversight of health maintenance organization (HMO) and preferred provider organization (PPO) operations, point-of-service (POS) products, and utilization management organizations (UMOs) (also referred to as utilization review organizations). Because space limitations preclude review of every state's laws, many of the regulatory issues detailed later are based on model acts adopted by the National Association of Insurance Commissioners (NAIC), which represents insurance departments in the 50 states and U.S. territories. One important NAIC document is the HMO Model Act, which was adopted by the NAIC in 1972 to clearly authorize the establishment of HMOs and provide for an ongoing regulatory monitoring system. This model legislation, or substantial portions thereof, has now been enacted by 31 states and the District of Columbia.[1] The remaining states also have adopted laws regulating HMOs, but these laws are not based on the NAIC HMO Model Act.

State regulation of PPOs is more varied, and states have applied provisions from several NAIC models to PPOs. In general, states permit insurers to enter into preferred provider arrangements that ensure reasonable access to covered services under the network and include mechanisms to control the cost of the health benefit plan.

The HMO Model Act is designed to operate in conjunction with, and as a companion to, other NAIC models that establish standards for the regulation of HMOs, including the Managed Care Plan Network Adequacy Model Act, the Quality Assessment and Improvement Model Act, the Health Care Professional Credentialing Verification Model Act, the Utilization Review Model Act, the Health Carrier Grievance Procedure Model Act, the Health Carrier External Review Model Act, the Health Information Privacy Model Act, the Privacy of Consumer Financial and Health Information Model Regulation, the Risk-Based Capital (RBC) for Health Organizations Model Act, and the Health Carrier Prescription Drug Benefit Management Model Act.

Some of these models are structured as requirements for licensure, while others—such as the model addressing external review—are structured as requirements independent of the licensure process. Some of the models apply only to HMOs and other MCOs, whereas others—such as the privacy of health information model—apply more broadly to health insurers.

STATE OVERSIGHT: THE REGULATORY PROCESS

The majority of the MCOs regulated by the states are designated as HMOs or PPOs. This section begins with a discussion of state oversight of HMOs and PPOs and is followed by a discussion of state oversight of other types of MCOs.

HMOs and PPOs

On the state level, HMOs usually are regulated by more than one agency. Typically, regulatory supervision is shared by the departments of insurance and health. Insurance regulators assume principal responsibility for the financial aspects of HMO operations and, in many states, for external review of adverse benefit determinations. Health regulators focus on quality of care issues, utilization patterns, and the ability of participating providers to provide adequate care. Although typical, this division of regulatory authority is not universal. For example, the Department of Managed Health Care oversees all aspects of HMO operations in California.

Risk-bearing PPOs are generally regulated by departments of insurance, either under the laws applicable to all insurance carriers or a special section of state insurance law.

Licensure

HMOs obtain licensure by applying for a certificate of authority. An organization may be incorporated for the sole purpose of becoming licensed as an HMO, or an existing company may sponsor an HMO product line through a subsidiary or affiliated organization. Applications usually are processed by the insurance department and, among other items, include the following documents: corporate bylaws, sample provider and group contract forms, evidence of coverage forms, financial statements, financial feasibility plan, description of service area, internal grievance procedures, and the proposed QA program. Payment of licensing fees is usually required, and about 25 states assess premium taxes against HMOs, while about another 10 impose some form of tax or fee on HMOs.*[2]

The licensure process provides state officials with a mechanism to ensure that the HMO is operating properly and is in compliance with all the applicable laws and regula-

---

*Other forms of taxation include imposition of income or franchise tax.

tions. In addition, the HMO Model Act provides for periodic reviews of whether a licensed HMO continues to meet the requirements for licensure; these reviews may occur "as often as is reasonably necessary for the protection of the interests of the people of this state but not less frequently than every five (5) years." If an HMO or other MCO fails to submit to this oversight, it probably will be considered by regulators as engaging in the unauthorized practice of insurance and may be subject to criminal and civil penalties.

Many states require PPOs to be licensed, registered, or certified. In the states with such a requirement, the standards imposed on PPOs tend to vary depending on whether the PPO is risk-bearing or not. Risk-bearing PPOs are likely to be subject to solvency and other requirements similar to those for HMOs and insurers. PPOs that do not bear risk may only have to register. Some states require the insurer with which a PPO contracts (most often an indemnity plan) to document that the PPO complies with certain state laws. Generally, the discussion of PPO regulation in this chapter focuses on risk-bearing PPOs.

Enrollee Information

The HMO Model Act sets forth requirements for communicating health plan information to HMO enrollees. Individual and group contract holders are entitled to receive a copy of their contracts. Each contract must contain basic information describing eligibility requirements, covered benefits, out-of-pocket expenses, limitations and exclusions, termination or cancellation of policies, claims processing, grievance procedures, continuation of benefits, conversion rights, subrogation rights, term of coverage, and grace period after nonpayment of premiums. Regulators require these documents to be filed with and approved by the regulatory body in charge of reviewing contracts.

In addition to individual and group contacts, the HMO Model Act requires HMOs to make other disclosures. Every enrollee is entitled to receive a document referred to as the evidence of coverage, which describes essential features and services of the HMO. Plans also must provide details about how services can be obtained through the HMO network and a telephone number at the plan for answers to additional questions. Upon enrollment or reenrollment, members receive a list of all health plan providers, and HMOs must notify enrollees in writing if their primary care provider's participation terminates. Within 30 days after a material change in the plan, HMOs are to notify enrollees of the change if it has a direct impact on them. Generally, the HMO Model Act allows the HMO to make required notices either in writing or by electronic means.

Many states require that insurers contracting with PPOs provide enrollees with a document that discloses the extent of coverage, the conditions for reimbursement, deductibles and co-insurance, and the process for addressing enrollee complaints, among other information. In addition, insurance policies offering PPO benefits must conform to the same disclosure and marketing requirements as are applicable to any other type of health insurance policy.[3]

Access to Medical Services

Under the HMO Model Act, HMOs must ensure the availability and accessibility of medical services. HMO patients should have access to medical care during reasonable hours; emergency care should be provided 24 hours a day, seven days a week. Regulators limit an HMO's certificate of authority to designated service areas (usually established by ZIP code regions or counties) where a determination has been made that the HMO has a sufficient provider network. Regulators also establish protocols governing HMO specialty referrals to ensure appropriate accessibility. In addition, most states require HMOs to offer an annual open enrollment period to prospective enrollees or in the event of another health plan's insolvency.

The NAIC Managed Care Plan Network Adequacy Model Act (Network Adequacy Model), which was adopted by the NAIC in 1996 and applies to HMOs as well as to insurers offering preferred provider arrangements, provides for states to choose among different ways of measuring network adequacy, including provider-enrollee ratios, geographic accessibility, waiting times, hours of operation, and the volume of technological and specialty services available in a plan's service area. It requires plans to file an access plan with the appropriate state agency to show how the plan will meet the access standard adopted by the state.[3] By 2005, 19 states had approved legislation or regulation based on, or related to, the Network Adequacy Model.*[4]

Provider Issues

The HMO Model Act requires organizations applying for state licensure to provide regulators with copies of provider contract forms for different classes of providers, as well as the names and addresses of all the providers with which it has contracts. It also requires each contract to include a hold harmless clause under which providers agree, as part of their contract with the HMO, not to bill HMO enrollees for covered services under any circumstance. (See Chapter 30 for additional detail on provider contracts, including sample contract language.) State officials review sample contracts to ensure that they do not create incentives that could compromise access to, or quality of, care.

In addition to the requirements in the HMO Model Act, the Network Adequacy Model includes several provisions relating to provider contracting, which apply more broadly to MCOs. First, MCOs are required to adopt standards for selecting participating providers and to make these standards available to the appropriate state agency for review. Second, MCOs must give at least 60 days notice before terminating a provider contract "without cause." Third, the act prohibits MCOs from offering "an inducement . . .

---

*Five states have enacted the model act or substantial portions of the act and 14 states have enacted related legislation or regulation.

to a provider to provide less than medically necessary services to a covered person" and from including in provider contracts any provision that would restrict provider-patient communications or limit a provider's ability to act as a patient advocate.

In recent years, states have enacted additional requirements for provider contracts used by MCOs beyond those found in the NAIC model acts. Provider contracting laws often specify terms or conditions that must or must not be included in a contract between a health insurance plan and provider. Some laws propose procedures that health insurance plans must follow when negotiating or terminating contracts with providers. Additionally, some states require disclosure of reimbursement methodology and fee schedules, while others establish procedures for amending contract provisions.[5]

Several states address how an MCO must reimburse providers who do not enter into a contract to participate in its network, but who provide services on an out-of-network basis to the MCO's enrollees. These laws may apply to either HMOs or PPOs, or both. By the end of 2005, 19 states had enacted laws or issued regulations that require MCOs to accept assignment of payment from or make direct payments to nonparticipating providers.[6] These so-called mandatory assignment of benefits laws may apply generally to health care providers or services or may apply only to subsets of providers or services. For example, Louisiana and South Dakota laws apply only to reimbursement to nonparticipating hospitals, whereas an Ohio law applies only to reimbursement for hospital-based emergency services.[7]

Over the last several years, states have moved to require health insurance plans to process claims within certain time frames. These "prompt pay" laws typically apply broadly to health insurers and MCOs directly reimbursing health care providers. At the end of 2005, 49 states and the District of Columbia had passed laws requiring insurers to process (pay or deny) reimbursement claims within time frames ranging from 15 days to 60 days, with some states establishing shorter time frames for claims submitted electronically.[7] These time frames usually only apply to "clean claims," that is, those claims that require no further information for processing. If claims are not paid within the prescribed time frames, interest may begin to accrue on all or a portion of the amount of the claim. Some states build a tolerance factor into their laws, recognizing that a 100% compliance rate may not be achievable. For example, Rhode Island requires that 95% of complete written claims be resolved in 40 days and that 95% complete electronic claims be resolved within 30 days.[7]

Another area state legislators have been addressing is health insurance plan cost sharing; specifically, restricting the percent differential a health insurance plan may impose on in-network and out-of-network benefits. For example, Florida prohibits annual deductibles for out-of-network services from exceeding four times the deductible amount for in-network services, whereas Massachusetts requires benefit levels for covered health care services provided by out-of-network providers to be at least 80% of the benefit levels for the same covered services by an in-network provider. By 2005, at least 15 states had enacted laws addressing these or similar cost-sharing issues.[8]

Reports and Rate Filings

State regulators employ a number of methods to ensure that licensed HMOs remain in compliance with the law. Generally, HMOs file an annual report with the insurance department. This report includes audited financial statements, a list of participating providers, an update and summary of enrollee grievances handled during the year, and any additional information that regulators deem necessary to make a proper review of the organization.

The HMO Model Act also specifies that HMOs file a schedule of premium rates or a methodology for determining premium rates with the insurance department. Some states require the regulator to approve rates before use, while others follow a more flexible file and use approach. Under the latter approach, an HMO may use its proposed rate if the regulator makes no objection within a certain time frame.[9] State laws generally provide that rates must not be excessive, inadequate, or unfairly discriminatory. Many states also apply specific rate requirements for certain products. For example, most states apply rating requirements to products sold to small employers. At the end of 2005, 48 states had laws governing rates for products sold to small employers.[10] PPOs that are offered as insured products are typically subject to state laws governing health insurer's rating practices.

In addition, states require HMOs to update regulators automatically if there are changes in documents that were part of the initial certificate of authority application filing (or part of the annual filings). Regulators keep permanent records, including primary care physician agreements, specialist provider contracts, group and individual contracts, certificate of coverage, and other pertinent information.

States may also require HMOs and other MCOs to report on quality and consumer satisfaction. For example, 25 states' laws require the reporting of some form of Health Plan Employer Data and Information Set (HEDIS) data and another 6 require reporting of such data if an HMO or MCO enters into a contract to provide coverage through a state program.[11] HEDIS is a set of standardized performance measures sponsored, supported, and maintained by the National Committee for Quality Assurance (NCQA), a national accreditation organization for MCOs and other entities.[11] (See Chapter 23 for additional information on quality and accreditation.)

Quality Assurance and Utilization Management

For the most part, states require an HMO to file a description of its internal quality assurance (QA) or quality management (QM) program and activities before obtaining a state license. Regulators review the description and, during site reviews, interview staff and check records to ensure that the description is accurate. Some states require accreditation by an independent external accrediting body and others recognize such accreditation as satisfying certain state regulatory requirements.[11] As noted in the preceding section, some states require HMOs and other MCOs to report certain quality information.

Under the HMO Model Act, HMOs are obliged to establish procedures to ensure that services meet reasonable standards for quality of care. These procedures must include an internal program to monitor and evaluate the quality of care provided. At a minimum, this program includes a written statement of goals and objectives, a written QA plan specifying who within the HMO is responsible for implementing the plan, systems for ongoing and focused evaluations, a system for credentialing and peer review of providers, and processes to initiate corrective action when deficiencies are identified. In addition, HMOs are required to record formal QA activities, develop an adequate patient record system, make clinical records available to determine compliance with QA standards, and periodically report QA program activities to the HMO's board, providers, and staff.

The NAIC has also adopted three quality-related model acts dealing in greater specificity with standards for QA, utilization management (UM) (sometimes also referred to as utilization review), and credentialing activities.

Under the NAIC Quality Assessment and Improvement Model Act, health carriers that offer managed care plans must have an internal system that identifies opportunities to improve care, measures the performance of participating providers and conducts peer review activities, collects and analyzes data on over- and underutilization of services, and ensures that providers have input on the quality improvement process. By 2005, 30 states had adopted legislation or regulation based on, or related to, the standards established in this model act.*[12]

---

*Two states have enacted the model act or part of the model act, and 28 states have enacted related legislation or regulation.

Under the Utilization Review and Benefit Determination Model Act (UR Model), HMOs, PPOs, and other health carriers subject to state regulation and that provide or perform UM services are required to use documented clinical review criteria that are based on sound clinical evidence, ensure that qualified health professionals administer the UM program, and abide by strict limits on the time period for all UM decisions. The model act prohibits compensation arrangements that encourage UM staff to make inappropriate determinations and provides for a process of appealing adverse UM decisions.

The Health Care Professional Credentialing Verification Model Act requires health carriers offering managed care plans to establish written policies and procedures for credentialing all health care professionals and apply them in a consistent manner. Among the information to be verified are licensure, status of hospital privileges, current professional liability coverage, specialty board status, and completion of educational programs. Most of this information is updated every 3 years. By 2005, 20 states had adopted legislation or regulations based on, or related to, this NAIC model act.*[13] Additionally, several of these states have adopted the standard credentialing application promoted by a voluntary alliance of carriers. (See Chapter 8 for more information on credentialing.)

States also regulate the QA and UM activities of PPOs. Sometimes they do so as part of laws that apply broadly to all health insurance carriers; in other cases, they have done so in PPO-specific legislation. Requirements range from filing a description of QA and UM programs to compliance with standards and certification requirements for those making UM decisions.

Grievance Procedures

The HMO Model Act specifies that HMOs have written procedures, approved by the ap-

propriate state agency, that are designed to ensure prompt and effective resolution of written grievances. A description of these procedures is to be included in the contract or evidence of coverage given to each enrollee. Such procedures must provide for the submission of written grievances on standard forms supplied by the HMO and for resolution of such grievances within 90 days of submission. A member's enrollment in the HMO generally may not be terminated while a grievance is pending. If binding arbitration is a condition of enrollment with an HMO, this fact must be disclosed in the individual's contract or evidence of coverage.

Adopted in 1996, the NAIC's Health Carrier Grievance Procedure Model Act (Grievance Procedure Model) and its UR Model include more detailed requirements in this area. Since the NAIC's adoption of these models, the U.S. Department of Labor (DOL), which administers Title I of ERISA, has promulgated a regulation establishing standards for benefit claims procedures of employee benefit plans governed by ERISA. The regulation, issued in November 2000, sets out specific requirements governing the time periods for making benefit determinations and deciding appeals, notice and disclosure requirements, standards of review, and the use of arbitration or other dispute resolution procedures. (See Chapter 31 for a discussion of ERISA.) Health carriers that contract with employers to provide insured health benefits for ERISA plans are subject to both state law requirements and the DOL claim procedures rule. In general, unless a state law "prevents the application of a requirement of the regulation," the state law will apply.[14]

After the issuance of the DOL regulation, the NAIC revisited both the Grievance Procedure Model and the UR Model and amended the models to follow the federal requirements more closely. However, the models continue to contain requirements in addition to those under the federal regulation. For example, the Grievance Procedure Model gives an enrollee the option of a second level of internal appeal, whereas the federal regulation permits, but

---

*One state has enacted the model act, and 19 states have enacted related legislation or regulation.

does not require, the health carrier to establish a second appeal level.

By 2005, 43 states had adopted laws or regulations addressing utilization review, and 39 states had laws pertaining to grievance procedures.*[15]

External Appeals

In 1999, the NAIC adopted the Health Carrier External Review Model Act. This model act provides procedures for the establishment and maintenance of external review procedures to ensure that covered persons have the opportunity for an independent review of an adverse coverage determination under a managed care program. The scope of the model includes all health carriers that provide UM. A unique approach has been developed to assist states in determining the extent of the insurance commissioner's role in the review process. Three options offer varying levels of administrative involvement for the state Department of Insurance (DOI): high DOI involvement allowing DOI to conduct a preliminary review, assign the independent review organization (IRO), and review the IRO decision; less involvement following all of the high-involvement steps except DOI review of the IRO decision; and low involvement allowing the health carrier to assign the IRO from a list of DOI-approved IROs.

Other key provisions include a relatively broad definition of *adverse determination* that triggers eligibility for review that includes denials for medical necessity, appropriateness, health care setting, and level of care or effectiveness; a standard of review that requires the IRO to consider a range of information, including "appropriate practice guidelines" that are defined to include "evidence-based" guidelines as well as "generally accepted"

practice guidelines; exhaustion of internal appeals requirement for all but expedited reviews for life-threatening cases; minimum qualifications established for IROs along with criteria for approving IROs by the state department of insurance; reporting requirements for IROs and health carriers; binding decisions on both parties; an optional $25 filing fee for the health plan member that is waived under certain circumstances; and a provision making the carrier bear the cost of the external review.*

By the end of 2005, 43 states and the District of Columbia had adopted legislation giving enrollees a right to appeal at least some cases involving a denial of care to an external review entity, such as a private organization approved by the state.[16] Although there are significant variations among the states in the details of these laws, external review mechanisms generally apply to coverage denials

---

*Since the adoption of the National Association of Insurance Commissioners external review model, the courts have established a distinction between the types of external review laws that survive ERISA "preemption" challenges and those that do not. In 2002, the Supreme Court upheld an Illinois external review law applicable to denials based on "medical necessity" grounds. In this case, the court held that ERISA did not preempt the law because it was "garden variety insurance regulation" and, therefore, "saved" from preemption (*Rush Prudential HMO v. Moran,* 122 S.Ct. 2151 [2002]). On the other hand, the court noted that a state external review law that is more like arbitration and less like a medical "second opinion" might be considered a separate vehicle to assert a claim for benefits outside of, or in addition to, the exclusive remedies provided under ERISA, and would be preempted. Based on the *Rush Prudential* decision and a later Supreme Court case (*Aetna Health Inc. v. Davila,* 124 S.Ct. 2488 [2004]), the Hawaii Supreme Court determined that Hawaii's external review law was impliedly preempted because it created remedies beyond those provided under ERISA (*Hawaii Management Alliance Association v. Insurance Commissioner,* 100 P.3d 952 [Hawaii 2004] [cert. denied]).

---

*Six states have enacted the UR and Benefit Determination Model Act, and 37 states have enacted related legislation or regulation; 4 states have enacted the Health Carrier Grievance Procedure Model Act or parts of the model, and 35 states have enacted related legislation or regulation.

based on medical necessity criteria or a determination that the service is experimental or investigational. Other provisions may require completion of the internal appeals process before external review occurs, selection of an independent reviewer by the plan from a list of reviewers approved by the state or by a state official (typically the insurance commissioner), no conflicts of interest for external reviewer, the plan to pay the costs of the external review process, and the external reviewer's decision to be binding on the plan.

Variations in the laws include requiring that the service in question meet a minimum dollar threshold, requiring the initiator of an external review to pay a filing fee, making the external reviewer's decision binding on the enrollee, and requiring a "pre-review" by the state regulator or external reviewer to determine that the claim meets specified requirements before it proceeds to a full external review.

Privacy of Medical Information

In 1998, the NAIC approved the Health Information Privacy Model Act (Privacy Model), a model developed to protect consumers' privacy and set forth standards for health carriers, including MCOs, in handling an individual's health information. The Privacy Model prohibits health carriers from collecting, using, or disclosing protected health information without an individual's authorization, except for certain purposes, such as claims payment, ongoing treatment, fraud detection, and rate-making activities. In addition, a health carrier that has collected protected health information pursuant to a valid authorization as described in the Privacy Model is permitted to use and disclose such information for other activities such as disease and case management, UM, and QA activities. The model also establishes requirements for health carriers with respect to notification of health information practices, safeguarding protected health information, and allowing individuals to access and amend their protected health information.

A few states formally enacted all or portions of the Privacy Model after it was adopted by the NAIC. Subsequently, federal privacy regulations promulgated in accordance with the Health Insurance Portability and Accountability Act (HIPAA) became effective April 14, 2003, and address many of the same issues detailed in the Model Act. (See Chapter 32 for more information on HIPAA privacy requirements.)

In 2000, the NAIC approved the Privacy of Consumer Financial and Health Information Regulation, a model regulation developed in response to the Gramm–Leach–Bliley Act (GLBA)—a federal law intended to modernize the financial services industry. The model regulation, like GLBA, governs the treatment of "nonpublic personal financial information" as well as "nonpublic personal health information" by all licensees of a state insurance department.

The NAIC model regulation prohibits the disclosure of nonpublic personal health information without an individual's authorization, except for the performance of "insurance functions," including claims administration, disease management, QA, and UM. In recognition of the overlap between the HIPAA and GLBA, the NAIC model regulation states that if a licensee is in compliance with HIPAA's federal privacy regulations, the licensee is not subject to the rules of the NAIC's GLBA model regulation relating to health information.

Management of Drug Benefits

To promote the appropriate use of prescription drugs and control costs, MCOs use various techniques to manage drug benefits, such as formularies, prior authorization requirements, and tiered structures. In 2003, the NAIC adopted the Health Carrier Prescription Drug Benefit Management Model Act (Drug Benefit Management Model), which establishes requirements pertaining to health carriers, including MCOs, for managing drug benefits.

Carriers typically develop formularies, lists of drugs a carrier uses for coverage purposes, through a pharmacy and therapeutics com mittee with health care professionals, such as physicians and pharmacists, as members of the committee. The Drug Benefit Management Model recognizes this practice and requires carriers to establish a process for such committees to follow in establishing a formulary. The model also sets forth procedures for carriers when considering requests for exceptions to a formulary and requires a carrier's decision on such a request to be based on sound clinical, medical, and scientific evidence. The information a carrier should provide to enrollees is a focus of the model, and it specifically requires disclosure of the following information:

1. Any formulary it uses
2. The process to obtain an exception from the formulary
3. Any appeal process
4. The out-of-pocket costs an enrollee may incur

Although no state has adopted the Drug Benefit Management Model as written, states have adopted laws that reflect portions of the model. Many states have adopted statutes specifically governing the use of formularies and the disclosure of information about formularies. States have also passed laws addressing drug benefits, including the use of mail-order pharmacies and generic substitutes that affect an MCO's ability to manage the benefits effectively. Other non-formulary-specific state statutes in areas such as UM and grievances and appeals may also indirectly apply to the use of formularies. (See Chapter 12 for a more complete discussion of drug benefit management techniques.)

Solvency Standards and Insolvency Protections

To prevent HMO insolvencies and protect consumers and other affected parties against the effects of insolvencies that do occur, the HMO Model Act establishes specific capital, reserve, and deposit requirements that all HMOs must meet. Before a certificate of authority is issued, an initial net worth of $3

million is required. After issuance, a minimum net worth must be maintained by the HMO equal to the greater of $2.5 million or an amount equal to the sum of 8% of annual health expenditures (except those paid on a capitated basis or a managed hospital payment basis) and 4% of annual hospital expenditures paid on a managed payment basis.

Early in 1998, the NAIC adopted a new, more flexible approach to determining how much capital MCOs must have. The product of a deliberative process that began in 1993, the Risk-Based Capital (RBC) for Health Organizations Model Act (RBC for Health Organizations Model) responds to the diversity of organizations and arrangements that provide health benefits coverage by codifying an approach under which capital and surplus requirements will vary from one MCO to another based on the specific nature and volatility of the organization's business. Also discussed in Chapter 24, the RBC formula permits state regulators to assess the specific risk profile of individual MCOs, give credit for provider contracting mechanisms (such as capitation and withholds) that reduce the risk borne by an MCO, and determine appropriate capital requirements based on these risk profiles.

To determine the specific capital requirements for a particular MCO, the RBC formula takes into account five different kinds of risk: the risk that the financial condition of an affiliated entity will cause an adverse change in the MCO's available capital (affiliate risk); the risk of adverse fluctuations in the value of the MCO's assets (asset risk); the risk that premiums will not be sufficient to pay claims (underwriting risk); the risk of reinsurers or capitated participating providers not fulfilling contractual obligations (credit risk); and the general risk of conducting business, including the risk that expenses will exceed budgeted amounts (business risk).

RBC information is reported to state regulators via annual financial statements (called blanks), which MCOs are required to file each March. Based on this information, an organization-specific capital requirement is computed and then compared with the MCO's total adjusted capital. If the MCO does not meet its capital requirement, it is subject to one of three levels of regulatory intervention: company action level, regulatory action level, and mandatory control level. These interventions range from requiring the submission of a corrective action plan to placing the MCO under the direct control of state regulators. As of 2005, 18 states had adopted an RBC law addressing health organizations.[17]

Although RBC may ultimately replace existing capital requirements in many states, it is not expected to displace other mechanisms for protecting enrollees in the event of insolvency, such as the deposits, hold harmless language, and other safeguards. For example, the HMO Model Act requires a minimum deposit of $1 million with the state insurance department. The deposit is considered an admitted asset of the HMO in the determination of its net worth, but it is used to protect the interests of HMO enrollees or to cover administrative costs if the HMO goes into receivership or liquidation. As previously discussed, most states also require HMOs to include hold harmless clauses in their provider contracts. In situations where the HMO fails to pay for covered medical care, such clauses prohibit providers from seeking collection from the enrollees. Some states, such as California and New York, have statutory hold harmless requirements protecting enrollees even in the absence of a contractual provision.

Several states also require that HMOs enter into reinsurance arrangements to cover liabilities in the event of an insolvency. And, aside from reinsurance arrangements, some states create a separate guaranty fund for HMOs or create a separate account for HMOs in a life and health guaranty fund. Under theses approaches, coverage for enrollees of an insolvent HMO is provided through the association or fund. These laws require HMOs to belong to the association or fund and allow the association or fund to assess member HMOs as necessary to provide coverage to an insolvent

HMO's enrollees. Another handful of states allow an assessment on solvent HMOs if necessary to provide coverage to enrollees of an insolvent HMO, without creating an association or fund to provide the coverage. In addition, some states require solvent HMOs in the market to provide coverage to enrollees of the insolvent HMO.*[18]

Alternative protections for consumers also have been adopted, including continuation of benefit provisions (requiring providers to continue to treat members of insolvent HMOs who are either undergoing an ongoing course of care or are in a designated trimester of pregnancy) and, as noted earlier, provider hold harmless agreements and increased net worth and statutory deposit requirements.

If necessary, insurance departments require HMOs to take further precautions to safeguard enrollee benefits. These additional measures might include purchasing additional insurance, entering into contracts obligating providers to continue delivering care if the HMO ceases operation, setting aside additional solvency reserves, or securing letters of credit.

If a regulator determines that an HMO's financial condition threatens enrollees, creditors, or the general public, the regulator usually has broad discretion to order the HMO to take specific corrective actions. Such actions may include reducing potential liabilities through reinsurance, suspending the volume of new business for a period of time, or

---

*Five states (Alabama, Florida, Illinois, Virginia, and West Virginia) create a separate guaranty fund for HMOs. Two states (Idaho and Wisconsin) create a separate account for HMOs in a life and health guaranty fund. Another five states, Iowa, Mississippi, Oklahoma, Texas, and Utah, and Washington, DC, allow an assessment on solvent HMOs if necessary to provide coverage to enrollees of an insolvent HMO, without creating an association or fund to provide the coverage. In addition, Mississippi, Oklahoma, Texas, and Utah require solvent HMOs in the market to provide coverage to enrollees of the insolvent HMO.

increasing the HMO's capital and surplus contributions.

Many states also require PPOs—particularly risk-bearing PPOs—to meet requirements relating to solvency and insolvency protections. Some have established PPO-specific requirements, such as posting a bond equal to 10% of the PPO's estimated aggregate reimbursement, whereas others require that risk-bearing PPOs abide by the solvency requirements applicable to HMOs or indemnity insurers. This latter approach has led to increasing use of RBC solvency standards for PPOs as more and more states adopt the RBC model.

Financial and Market Conduct Examinations and Site Visits

Regulators also can conduct specialized inquiries, which often examine HMO finances, marketing activities, and QA programs. In part, the objective of these regulatory reviews is to determine the HMO's financial solvency and statutory compliance and whether any trends can be identified that may cause problems in the future. For example, the HMO Model Act requires the insurance department to complete a detailed examination of the HMO's financial affairs at least once every 5 years. The NAIC's *HMO Examination Handbook* sets forth specific procedures for examining HMO balance sheet assets and liabilities. The goals are to verify ownership and stated asset amounts and to ensure the adequacy of the HMO's net worth to meet current and future liabilities. Examiners may review an HMO's cash resources; investments; premium receivables; interest receivables; prepaid expenses; restricted assets; leasehold arrangements; accounts payable; unpaid claims; unearned premiums; outstanding loans; statutory liability; building, land, equipment, and inventory lists; and other company assets and costs. If an HMO is undercapitalized or otherwise short of funds, regulators usually provide an opportunity for the HMO to take corrective action. Regulators take financial shortfalls seriously,

however, and will suspend or revoke an HMO's license if necessary to protect consumer interest. As previously noted, the RBC Health Organizations Model provides for a similar, multitiered approach to regulatory interventions.

State regulators are charged with evaluating compliance by MCOs and other regulated entities with statues and regulations. The NAIC's *Market Regulation Handbook* was developed as a collaborative effort by the states actively involved in conducting examinations of a company's statutory and regulatory compliance. The handbook establishes guidelines and best practices to assist states in developing their own market conduct examination procedures. The seven main areas that are reviewed as part of a market conduct examination are as follows:

1. Company operations and management
2. Complaint handling
3. Marketing and sales
4. Producer licensing
5. Policyholder service
6. Underwriting
7. Claims

The focus of these examinations is intended to be on general business patterns or practices and not on random or isolated errors. If an MCO is found to have engaged in unlawful market practices, regulators usually provide an opportunity for the MCO to take corrective and/or remedial action. Serious misconduct and consumer harm can result in the suspension or revocation of an MCO's license if necessary to protect the public from further harm.

As part of the examination process, regulators may conduct a site visit to see the MCO's operations firsthand, to review health plan documents, and to assess the efficiency and soundness of operations. The site visit may be relatively brief, or it can take place over a period of days or weeks. Occasionally, regulators contact participating providers and enrollees directly to determine how the MCO is operating.

HIPAA State Implementation

The federal Health Insurance Portability and Accountability Act of 1996 (HIPAA; see also Chapter 32) was designed by Congress to improve the availability and portability of health coverage by establishing federal minimum standards for access, portability, and renewability in both the group and individual coverage markets, with primary responsibility for implementation going to the states. To achieve these goals, HIPAA limits exclusions for preexisting medical conditions, provides rights that allow certain individuals to enroll in health coverage when they lose coverage or have a new dependant, and prohibits discrimination in employer group coverage in enrollment eligibility against employees and their dependants based on health status.

At the time of enactment, HIPAA established a new model of federal-state regulation by granting states primary responsibility for implementing the law. Prior to HIPAA's enactment, most states had approved and implemented health insurance reform laws that set forth requirements similar to those under the federal law. In many cases, particularly as applied to the group market, states' requirements exceeded the federal law. However, in other areas, most often in the individual market, some states' requirements fell short of the federal law. The new regulatory model recognizes that if state requirements did not already comply with federal requirements, they could be modified to come into compliance.

Point-of-Service Offerings

Under a point-of-service (POS) option, when a health plan member needs medical care, he or she chooses, at the time of service, whether to go to a provider within the plan's network or to seek medical care out of the network, in which case higher cost-sharing would apply. (See also Chapter 2.) When an HMO offers a POS product on its own by underwriting out-of-plan benefits, this is re-

ferred to as a standalone product. Some state laws, however, prohibit HMOs from offering a point-of-service product without entering into an agreement with an insurance company to cover the out-of-plan usage, referred to as a wraparound product.*

In the states that allow HMOs to offer POS products under their own license, the following provisions are typical:

- A limit on the percentage (10–20%) of total health care expenditures for enrollees who obtain services outside the plan
- Increased financial solvency requirements
- A tracking system to measure in-network and out-of-network utilization separately
- A mechanism for processing and paying for all out-of-plan service claims

Many states have adopted laws mandating that HMOs offer POS products in certain situations. In general, mandatory POS laws require HMOs to offer POS coverage (or PPOs, or any coverage arrangement allowing enrollees to access services outside the HMO) to either health coverage purchasers or health plan enrollees. If the mandatory offering is directed to purchasers, the purchaser decides whether to offer the POS option to employees. In addition, such laws usually include requirements that enrollees choosing the out-of-network option pay any higher premiums and cost-sharing amounts that result.

Multistate Operations

MCOs operating in more than one state must comply with the regulations of each jurisdiction. Other multistate MCOs can face the same regulatory challenge when complying with the rules in more than one state as well. Most states mandate that foreign MCOs meet

---

*Other state laws require an HMO to maintain additional surplus if out-of-plan usage causes payments to nonparticipating providers to exceed a certain threshold. Wis. Stat. §609.95.

the same requirements applicable to domestic MCOs. States also may require that out-of-state MCOs register to do business under the appropriate foreign corporation law and appoint an agent in the state for receipt of legal notifications.

Multistate operations can become expensive if plans are subject to numerous financial examinations and other regulatory requirements. To alleviate this concern, some states permit regulators who are considering the application of a foreign MCO to accept financial reports and other information from the MCO's state of origin. The NAIC also has established guidelines for coordinating financial examinations of MCOs licensed in more than one state. The coordinated examination is called for by the lead state, where the MCO is domiciled; other states where the MCO operates are encouraged to participate.

The concept of "domestic deference" described previously is one that the NAIC continues to consider for extension to market conduct examinations. The streamlining of market conduct examinations would form a cornerstone in state regulators' response to federal pressure to modernize the state regulatory system. In addition, the NAIC has established the Market Analysis Working Group (MAWG) that serves as a forum for coordinating market conduct activities among the states. State legislatures are also starting to consider market conduct examination streamlining, and at least one legislative group, the American Legislative Exchange Council (ALEC), has adopted model legislation codifying a domestic deference approach.[19]

Occasionally, regulations in one state may adversely affect or hinder the operations of an MCO licensed in another state. Historically, group insurance policies generally have been subject to the law of the state of issuance. A policy issued in state A would be subject to that state's insurance laws and regulations, including mandated benefits. This general rule has been eroded by extraterritorial application of a state's insurance laws. The laws of state B may require that any state B resident covered under a group health policy, even if issued in state A, receive the same coverage that would be required had the group policy been issued in state B.

Specialty HMOs

A specialty HMO is an entity that accepts a capitated payment to provide for (or arrange for the provision of) a limited set of medical service categories. The arrangement is a form of a carve-out. In some cases, a specialty HMO receives its capitation payment from a general HMO and in other cases (often involving dental services) directly from an employer. In 1989, the NAIC adopted the Prepaid Limited Health Service Organization Model Act (Limited HSO Model), which addresses these entities. The Limited HSO Model recognizes dental care, vision care, mental health, substance abuse, pharmaceutical, and podiatric care services as limited services offered by these specialty HMOs.[20]

General requirements under the model are similar to, but not as comprehensive as, those in the HMO Model Act. Requirements include licensure and issuance of a certificate of authority, filing of various documents, review of payment methodologies, development of a complaint system, periodic examinations, financial and investment guidelines, insolvency protections, oversight of agents, confidentiality rules, issuance of a fidelity bond for officers and employees, and provider contracting standards.[20] By 2005, at least 22 states had adopted laws addressing specialty HMOs.[20]

Utilization Management Organizations

The continuing demand by employers to manage utilization of health care services and to control costs has resulted in a steady proliferation over the past 15 years of independent utilization management organizations (UMOs). Many states regulate independent UMOs, and many also regulate HMOs' internal UM programs through state HMO acts or other statutes. It is important to note that some states apply standalone UM laws to independent UMOs *and* HMOs, and in some states the resulting combination of standalone UM laws and UM requirements in separate HMO laws can create confusion and be unnecessarily duplicative for HMOs.

By 2004, 45 states had enacted laws regulating either independent UMOs or UM activities by MCOs.[21] As discussed earlier, there are a number of provisions that are common to state UM laws. A prevalent requirement, included in 34 laws, is that organizations conducting UM must be licensed, registered, or certified prior to performing UM activities in the state.[21] In 39 states, specific clinical review criteria must be used when making a UM determination, and in 41 states, a physician or "clinical peer" must review all adverse coverage determinations.[21] In addition, 50 states and the District of Columbia require some type of initial appeals process for UM activities.[21] Other areas that are frequently governed by state laws include prohibitions against financial incentives that are tied to UM determinations, oversight of delegated UM, and requirements that UMOs be privately accredited.

If a UMO contracts on an exclusive basis with self-funded employers, its operations are regulated by ERISA, and state laws do not apply. ERISA itself regulates the appeals process for adverse coverage determinations. However, many state regulators argue that if a UMO has even one commercial contract where an MCO is assuming the insurance risk, all of the UMO's operations are subject to state laws.

Although UM laws share many common attributes, variations can create compliance problems for UMOs that operate in multiple states. One of the major compliance concerns facing multistate UMOs is the issue of same-state licensure for reviewers. Although most states require only that a reviewer be licensed in a state, but not necessarily the state in which the review takes place, as of 2005, 19 states required either reviewers or medical directors to be licensed in the state in which the review takes place.[21] As such, UMO reviewers or medical directors may be required to become licensed in multiple states.

Similar to state regulation, the federal regulatory environment for UM has changed significantly in recent years. The DOL's claims procedure regulation, issued in 2000, addresses, among other issues, time frames for prospective, concurrent, and retrospective claim determinations. (This federal regulation is discussed earlier in this chapter and in detail in Chapter 31.) State and federal regulations can and do differ, and stricter state regulation is typically not preempted by the federal regulation. This can result in UMOs and entities performing UM activities needing to comply with different requirements for the same activities.

Third-Party Administrators

A third-party administrator (TPA) is an organization that administers group benefits and claims for a self-funded company or group. The NAIC adopted the Third Party Administrator Statute (TPA Statute) in 1977 to address issues that arise in administering these benefits and claims.[22] A TPA normally does not assume any insurance risk and the definition under the TPA Statute excludes licensed insurers, including MCOs, and an affiliate of an insurer if it only provides administrative services to its affiliated insurer. Forty states require licensure or registration of TPAs and, of those, almost 30 states require the TPA to post a surety bond or some other form of evidence of financial responsibility.[23]

The TPA Statute contains provisions governing the following: the TPA's written agreement with insurers, including a statement of duties; payment methodology; maintenance and disclosure of records; insurer responsibilities, such as determination of benefit levels; fiduciary obligations when the TPA collects charges and premiums; issuance of TPA licenses and grounds for suspension or revocation; and filing of annual reports and payment of fees.

Self-Funded Plans

An employer may decide to finance its health plan through "self-funding." This is an arrangement under which an employer finances its employees' health coverage out of its general assets. Thus, the employer takes on some or all of the risk of paying for its employees' health benefits instead of shifting the risk to an insurance company or MCO. The risk of coverage can be shared with employees through deductibles and copayments. If an employer wants to limit its risk, it also may purchase insurance to cover losses beyond a certain stop-loss point. Most self-funded plans choose to purchase some form of stop-loss insurance to limit their risk.

Self-funded plans are regulated by the DOL under ERISA. (See also Chapter 31.) As such, these arrangements typically are beyond the state's insurance regulatory jurisdiction. However, self-funded plans may use a TPA to administer the plan and, as discussed earlier, the TPA could be subject to state regulation.

A small number of state insurance departments have focused on the point at which a self-funded plan's stop-loss insurance is triggered, contending that when the trigger point is very low, the plan is not actually self-funded, but instead is an insured health plan subject to state regulation. The NAIC has issued model legislation that sets specific and aggregate stop-loss attachment points, however, few states have adopted laws in this area.

Many employers self-funding health benefits rely on managed care arrangements for the delivery of health benefits. MCOs that otherwise have state-licensed products usually can offer services or products under or with self-funded arrangements in at least three ways:

1. *Administrative services only:* Regulated entities such as insurance companies and MCOs can offer a self-funded man-

aged care product under an administrative services-only arrangement with an employer who assumes the financial risk of the benefits plan. The MCO handles administrative functions for the employer group, which can include utilization management.

2. *Use of MCO provider networks:* Under these arrangements, a self-funded employer can contract with an MCO to use its provider panel. The employer pays the MCO on a fee-for-service basis for medical services rendered to avoid transfer of insurance risk from the employer to the MCO or providers.

3. *Health plan choice:* Many employers who offer a self-funded health benefit plan also offer employees an option to be covered under a plan sold by an MCO. This is particularly true for large employers (200 or more workers), with 78% of covered employees in large firms having a choice of health plans.[24]

MANAGED CARE LEGISLATION

This section discusses select areas of MCO operations that have been addressed in state legislative and regulatory proposals.

Overview

MCOs were designed as a response to quality and cost-containment concerns experienced by traditional indemnity insurance. To address these issues, MCOs developed techniques such as QA procedures, UM programs, and selective contracting. In the past 15 years, as MCOs have gained a substantial foothold in the marketplace, states have moved toward redefining the ground rules and altering principles that differentiate MCOs from indemnity insurance.

Any Willing Provider

The creation of selective provider panels is a cornerstone of MCO operations. Many states, however, have enacted "any willing provider" (AWP) laws that prevent MCOs from selectively contracting with a limited group of providers. In most instances, however, AWP laws apply to specific categories of providers, such as pharmacists, rather than across the board to include all providers. Such laws generally require an MCO to accept into its network any nonparticipating provider willing to meet the terms and conditions of the MCO. MCOs have opposed such mandates because they could increase costs and prevent health plans from selectively choosing only the most highly qualified health care professionals.

Several studies have documented the potential costs of implementing AWP laws, attributing cost increases to the plans' reduced ability to obtain price discounts and conduct effective UM.* Additionally, the U.S. Federal Trade Commission (FTC) has weighed in on the implications of AWP proposals, in one opinion letter stating: "Although the law may be intended to assure consumers greater freedom to choose where they obtain services, it appears likely to have the unintended effect of denying consumers the advantages of cost-reducing arrangements and limiting their choices in the provision of health care services."[25] The National Governors Association has repeatedly reaffirmed its opposition to AWP legislation as first articulated in a 1994 policy statement and adopted at successive annual meetings.†[26]

---

*See Barents Group LLC, McLean, VA. *Impacts of Four Legislative Provisions on Managed Care Consumers: 1999–2003.* Chicago. Arthur Andersen and Company, 1998. *Cost Estimates Related to the Impact of Any Willing Provider Requirements in the State of Washington.* Arthur Andersen and Company, 1997. Arthur Andersen and Company. *Florida Health Security Program: Actuarial Report.* Chicago, Ill: Arthur Andersen and Company; 1994.

†This position was most recently adopted at the Winter Meeting 2005 of the National Governors Association and is effective from the Winter Meeting 2005 through Winter Meeting 2007.

By the end of 2005, approximately half of the states had adopted AWP laws affecting MCOs. The vast majority of these laws are limited to pharmacists and require health plans to accept into the plan's network non-participating pharmacists willing to meet the terms and conditions of the MCO. In some of these states, HMOs receive full or partial exemptions from such open pharmacy requirements.[27]

State AWP laws have been legally challenged on the basis of federal preemption under the federal HMO Act, ERISA, and the Federal Employees Health Benefits Act. However, in 2003, the U.S. Supreme Court, in a unanimous decision, found that Kentucky's AWP law was not preempted by ERISA and, therefore, was allowed to stand.[28]

Collective Bargaining/Physician Antitrust

Competition is crucial to keeping health care costs under control in the private and public sectors, and to inspire innovative means of improving and measuring quality. However, over the last several years, competing physicians have sought legislative antitrust exemptions that would permit them to engage in collective activity that would otherwise be illegal under antitrust laws. Although most states have rejected such legislation, as of the end of 2005, Alaska, New Jersey, and Texas had laws permitting competing providers to collectively negotiate contract terms and conditions with health insurance plans under certain circumstances.[29]

State legislatures rely upon the "state action doctrine" in carving out collective activity, which would otherwise be illegal, from the federal antitrust laws. The state action doctrine exempts private parties from antitrust liability for actions that are undertaken within the context of a state regulatory program. The basis for the doctrine is that the federal antitrust laws do not, by themselves, limit the states from exercising their sovereignty to engage in economic regulation, and do not prohibit acts of state government. Under the state action doctrine, private parties may engage in activity that would otherwise violate antitrust laws when the following requirements, as established by the U.S. Supreme Court, are satisfied: (1) the state must articulate (usually through legislation) a clear policy to displace competition with regulation, and (2) the state must actively supervise the activity in question.[30]

In 1996, the Department of Justice (DOJ) and the Federal Trade Commission (FTC) issued antitrust guidelines articulating that physicians who participate in a broad range of joint ventures have the ability to engage in collective activity and have been accorded "safety zones" by the federal government when conducting these activities. In July 2004, the DOJ and the FTC released *Report on Health Care Competition* after 2 years of hearings by interested parties.[31] The report affirmed that physician networks can enter into joint negotiations with health insurance plans, as long as the networks are either financially (*eg*, accepting risk) or clinically integrated (*eg*, value-based purchasing). The DOJ/FTC report identified various ways in which health care provider collective bargaining could likely harm consumers and other participants in the health care system, including higher prices for health insurance coverage, which could lead to reduced benefits and an increase in the number of uninsured.

Health Plan Liability

In all states, MCOs can be held liable based on the same principles of liability applied to hospitals, including vicarious liability and direct corporate liability, for such acts as the negligent hiring and supervision of physicians, the failure to provide adequate facilities and equipment, and consumer fraud and misrepresentation. In 1997, Texas became the first state to expand MCO liability beyond these principles. The Texas statute holds health plans to a standard of "ordinary care" when making "health care treatment decisions."[32] Although in the late 1990s several states introduced legislation similar to the Texas law, by the end of 2005, only nine states had enacted laws expanding health plans' liability.[*][33] In many of these states, the changes have been made to states' tort laws that expose health plans to liability for their coverage determinations and UM activities.

MCOs have raised concerns that an expansion of liability would increase costs, thereby adding to the number of uninsured Americans, and diminish quality of care. The cost impact of expanded liability has been studied by various research groups and government agencies. Many of these studies have examined not only the direct costs of litigation but also the indirect costs of "defensive medicine." *Defensive medicine* refers to the phenomenon characterized by the ordering of unnecessary tests that do not benefit patients to avoid costly litigation. A recent survey of Pennsylvania providers in six specialties revealed that 93% reported practicing defensive medicine.[34] One source estimated that the direct costs of litigation and the widespread practice of defensive medicine increase health care spending by as much as 10%.[35]

MCOs are also concerned that quality, too, could be harmed by expanded health plan liability, as plans are compelled to tailor care management activities to jury verdicts—which have little correlation to actual negligence—rather than to medical facts. In fact, a survey of physicians found that 76% felt that concerns about malpractice litigation have hurt their ability to provide quality care.[36] Moreover, the current liability system as applied to physicians was identified by the President's Advisory Commission on Consumer Protection and Quality in the Health Care Industry as "perhaps the most significant deterrent to the identification and reduction of

---

*Nine states (Arizona, California, Georgia, Maine, New Jersey, North Carolina, Oklahoma, Texas, and Washington) have expanded health plan liability. Two additional states (Oregon and West Virginia) have limited liability expansion to instances when the health plan fails to comply with an external review decision.

[medical] errors," and the American Medical Association has pointed out that the current system inhibits medical innovation.[37]

Mandates

State laws governing HMOs require that their enrollees be offered comprehensive health care services. In fact, the industry's ability to provide broad coverage has been one of its distinctive trademarks. Nevertheless, many states now require coverage of specialty services, too. Most mandated benefits are specific to certain conditions. Such benefits include coverage for clinical trials, congenital defects, phenylketonuria, *in vitro* fertilization, temporomandibular joint syndrome (TMJ), autologous bone marrow transplants, and Lyme disease, to name a few. In the late 1960s, state legislatures had passed only a handful of mandated benefits; today, there are more than 1,800 mandated benefits and providers with more on their way.[38]

When state legislatures mandate coverage of expensive services a point of diminishing returns is quickly reached. A persistent concern is whether less money will be spent on basic health care as funds are rerouted to cover the mandates. Another concern is that health plans have to raise premiums to compensate for cost increases resulting from these mandates. An analysis by the Lewin Group, a private health services research firm, found that each 1% real increase in health care premiums is associated with an estimated 300,000 individuals losing health coverage.[39] Mandated benefits also reduce HMOs' flexibility in structuring benefit packages to suit the needs of a particular group and sometimes even result in harmful, unintended consequences for consumers.

One case study of the unintended consequences of mandates concerns the use of autologous bone marrow transplant (ABMT) as a treatment for breast cancer. In the mid-1990s, there was considerable interest within the medical and consumer communities surrounding ABMT for the treatment of breast cancer. Despite the lack of adequate scientific studies to prove its effectiveness, ABMT coverage was mandated in 10 states and for all federal employees covered by the Federal Employees Health Benefits Program. Because of these mandates, there was little incentive for women to participate in clinical trials to test the treatment's effectiveness. This lack of participation delayed the completion of the clinical trials necessary to evaluate the effectiveness of ABMT for the treatment of breast cancer. Clinical trials ultimately found that ABMT was no more effective than standard therapy and actually placed women who received this treatment at greater risk for complications, compromised health status, and even death. Thousands of women underwent this extremely painful, sometimes fatal, yet ineffective procedure. In the absence of these mandates, clinical trials would have been completed in a more timely manner and shown that this treatment provided little to no benefit to women with breast cancer.[40] Given the length of time it took to repeal many of these mandates and the fact that some have yet to be repealed, this experience shows the inflexible, static nature of mandates because they cannot, in a timely manner, reflect changes in the practice of medicine, new medical technology, or other medical advances or knowledge that may make the mandate obsolete or even harmful to patients.

Uncertainty about the implications of mandating health care benefits without knowing the possible impact on quality, cost, and utilization has moved many legislatures to create commissions to study mandates. As of year-end 2005, 24 states have enacted laws requiring an examination of the consequences of either existing or proposed health care mandates.*[41] Two states, Kansas and

---

*Twenty-four states (Arizona, Arkansas, California, Colorado, Florida, Georgia, Hawaii, Indiana, Kansas, Kentucky, Louisiana, Maine, Maryland, Massachusetts, New Hampshire, New Jersey, North Dakota, Ohio, Pennsylvania, South Carolina, Tennessee, Virginia, Washington, and Wisconsin) have passed legislation addressing the review of existing or proposed mandated benefits.

North Dakota, require any new benefit mandate to be implemented on a pilot basis for 1 year in the state employee health benefits program. A state employee benefits commission must submit a report to the legislature after the year's end, assessing the mandate's impact on the state employee benefit program, including data on utilization and costs of coverage.[41] Another less usual approach is the passage of a moratorium on the adoption of new mandated benefit laws for a specified period of time.[41]

Furthermore, to address health care premium increases over the last few years, attributable in large part to increasing health care costs stemming from the provision of mandated health benefits, states have made efforts to permit health insurance plans to offer flexible health benefit plans that are exempt from some or all state-mandated benefits. As of year-end 2005, 11 states had mandate waiver laws that allow health insurance plans to offer benefit plans absent some or all benefit and/or provider mandates.[42]

REGULATION BY MARKET SEGMENT

Although the focus of this chapter is on state regulation, it is important to note that, because regulation is driven by market segments, a typical MCO is regulated by several entities, depending on the combination of product lines it offers. The primary regulatory bodies responsible for protecting consumers include the following entities.

State Insurance and Health Departments

State departments of insurance and health regulate most HMOs. In most states, the insurance departments typically regulate the financial aspects of an HMO, such as solvency requirements and rate filings. Health departments usually regulate HMO activities and policies, such as UR and QA. However, in a few states a single department is primarily responsible for regulating health plan operations.

As previously discussed, employee health benefit plans sponsored by private employers are regulated by the DOL under ERISA, although states retain regulatory jurisdiction over the insured products purchased by employee benefit plans. Accordingly, health care coverage purchased by individuals, provided to employees of a business where the health plan retains the risk, or offered to state employees must meet state law requirements.

U.S. Department of Labor

As noted earlier, the DOL regulates employer-sponsored health benefit plans under ERISA. When employers offer coverage through a self-funded multiple employer welfare arrangement (MEWA), the DOL coordinates regulation with the states pursuant to a 1982 amendment to ERISA. Under this coordinated approach, the states have primary responsibility for overseeing the financial soundness of MEWAs and the licensing of MEWA operators and the DOL enforces ERISA's fiduciary provisions against MEWA operators to the extent a MEWA is an ERISA plan or is holding plan assets.[43] Under Title I of ERISA, DOL has responsibilities with respect to benefit claims procedures of employee benefit plans. In addition, DOL has been active in implementing changes to ERISA through regulatory work and participation in an *amicus curiae* program through the DOL solicitor's office. (See Chapter 31 for detailed discussion of federal regulation under ERISA.)

U.S. Department of Health and Human Services

Located in the U.S. Department of Health and Human Services (DHHS), the Centers for Medicare and Medicaid Services (CMS) is the primary federal agency that oversees the Medicare and Medicaid programs and the State Children's Health Insurance Program (SCHIP). MCOs that participate in the Medicare managed care program, known as Medicare Advantage, must comply with rules and regulations established by CMS. These rules preempt state laws and other standards related to benefits requirements, inclusion or treatment of providers in networks, and coverage determination, including appeals and grievance processes, in cases in which state laws are inconsistent with federal Medicare Advantage requirements. The federal rules also prohibit states from imposing taxes on payments that health plans receive under the Medicare Advantage program. (See Chapter 26 for detailed discussion of Medicare managed care.)

CMS's role in overseeing Medicaid managed care and SCHIP, which was established by the 1997 Balanced Budget Act, differs somewhat from its responsibility for the Medicare Advantage program. For these two programs, CMS provides general rules and frameworks under which states must administer their programs and ensure MCOs' compliance with rules and regulations.

State Medicaid Departments

State social service or welfare departments, in conjunction with CMS, regulate state Medicaid programs. Medicaid is a joint federal-state program under which states receive federal matching funds to defray part of the cost of providing medical assistance to targeted, low-income populations. CMS reviews state plans for assurances that the state will require participating MCOs to meet standards set in the federal statute. This statute includes standards that Medicaid managed care plans must meet and requires preapproval by CMS for every Medicaid managed care plan contract over a threshold dollar amount. (See Chapter 27 for detailed discussion of Medicaid managed care.)

U.S. Office of Personnel Management

The Office of Personnel Management (OPM) regulates coverage offered to federal employees within the Federal Employees Health Benefits Program (FEHBP). In designing the federal employee program, Congress took steps to ensure uniformity of benefits by ex-

plicitly preempting state laws that are inconsistent with the contract between the program and the plan, as well as state premium taxes.[44] Although ERISA does not apply to FEHBP plans, the program imposes limits similar to those under ERISA on the remedies that are available to an enrollee.

OPM manages the health benefits of more than 8 million enrollees (not including covered dependants).[45] Regulatory responsibilities include determining which plans will be part of the FEHB program, communicating information to plan members, requiring participating plans to perform administrative tasks, negotiating premium rates, and auditing the plans periodically. In 2005, there were 279 health plan choices offered to federal employees, retirees, and their dependants.[46] The FEHBP does not include a standard benefit package, however, OPM requires the benefit packages of participating plans to include certain core benefits.[46] Each spring, OPM sends all plan providers its "call letter," a document that specifies, among other things, the types of benefits that must be available to plan participants as well as the cost goals and procedural changes that the plans need to adopt. OPM key initiatives for the FEHBP in 2007 include encouraging proposals for Health Savings Accounts, the use of health information technology, and transparency in health care costs.

U.S. Department of Defense

The Department of Defense (DOD) regulates coverage delivered through its military health services system (MHSS), a worldwide health care system composed of some 75 hospitals and 461 clinics serving an eligible population of approximately 9 million.[47] In addition to covering members of the armed services on active duty and their dependants, DOD also offers health care benefits to inactive armed services personnel and their dependants. The Civilian Health and Medical Program of the Uniformed Services (CHAMPUS) program was established in 1967 to provide health insurance to active duty personnel's dependants, retirees, and dependants of retirees. Under CHAMPUS, beneficiaries would be reimbursed for portions of the cost of health care from a civilian provider. The introduction of TRICARE health benefits in the 1990s allowed beneficiaries the option of enrolling in a DOD-managed HMO, a PPO, or CHAMPUS (now called the TRICARE Standard).

Under TRICARE, each military commander, or lead agent, in each of three geographic regions, is charged with managing care provided by military medical facilities. Additionally, the lead agent must contract with private providers through a competitive bidding process to ensure that the medical needs within each geographic region are met. The idiosyncratic mix of private and public coverage under MHSS means that it faces issues different from most other purchasers.[47] (See Chapter 28 for details on TRICARE.)

CONCLUSION

The regulatory structure for MCOs faces daunting challenges in the years ahead. Historically state-centered, the system increasingly is characterized by overlapping state and federal regulation. There are serious unanswered questions about whether such a regime will produce regulation that is workable for MCOs and offers value to consumers. As mentioned previously, some federal legislators are examining ways to streamline the regulatory structure.

Further, as the debate escalates at both the federal and state levels about the best way to provide coverage for all citizens, it will be important to recognize the key role MCOs have played and continue to play in arranging for affordable, quality care. Many states have recognized the value of MCOs in offering health coverage options in the context of their government health programs and, likewise, private employers have consistently turned to MCO coverage options for their workers. As MCOs continue to form an integral part of the health care system, it should be recognized that the policies and practices of physicians, nurses, and other health care professionals and hospitals and other institutional providers play central and independent roles in determining how well the health care system works. To make real progress in solving the U.S. health care system's cost and quality problems and making coverage available to all citizens, policymakers and regulators should view the role and regulation of MCOs from a system-wide perspective that recognizes the unique role of each system participant.

References

1. National Association of Insurance Commissioners (NAIC). *Health Maintenance Organizations Model Act*. Updated 2005. www.naic.org.
2. National Association of Insurance Commissioners. Premium taxation of HMOs. In: *Compendium of State Laws on Insurance Topics*. Updated 2005. www.naic.org.
3. American Association of Health Plans (AAHP). *The Regulation of Health Plans*. Washington, DC: American Association of Health Plans, 1998:29.
4. National Association of Insurance Commissioners. *Managed Care Plan Network Adequacy Model Act*. October 2005. www.naic.org.
5. America's Health Insurance Plans (AHIP). *Provider Contracting: Summary of Selected 2004 Legislation*. Washington, DC: America's Health Insurance Plans, December 31, 2004.
6. America's Health Insurance Plans. *Assignment of Benefits: Summary of State Laws*. Washington, DC: America's Health Insurance Plans, December 31, 2005.
7. America's Health Insurance Plans. *Prompt Payment: Summary of State Laws and Selected 2005 State Legislation*. Washington, DC: America's Health Insurance Plans, December 31, 2005.
8. America's Health Insurance Plans. *Out-of-Network Cost-sharing Requirements: Summary of State Laws*. Washington, DC: America's Health Insurance Plans, January 2005 (unpublished).

9. National Association of Insurance Commissioners. Filing requirements health insurance forms and rates. In: *Compendium of State Laws on Insurance Topics*. Updated 2005. www.naic.org.

10. America's Health Insurance Plans. *Small Group Premium Rating Rules: Summary of State Laws*. Washington, DC: America's Health Insurance Plans, December 31, 2005.

11. National Committee for Quality Assurance (NCQA). The NCQA Public Policy Programs state recognition of NCQA accreditation page. Updated April 2006. Available at: http://www. ncqa.org/Programs/publicpolicy/staterecognition. htm#State%20Recognition%20of%20NCQA%20Accreditation. Accessed November 28, 2006.

12. National Association of Insurance Commissioners. *Quality Assessment and Improvement Model Act*. Washington, DC: National Association of Insurance Commissioners, October 2005.

13. National Association of Insurance Commissioners. *Health Care Professional Credentialing Verification Model Act*. Washington, DC: National Association of Insurance Commissioners, October 2005.

14. American Association of Health Plans. *The ERISA Claim Procedures Rule: Enforcement and Penalties*. Washington, DC: American Association of Health Plans, June 24, 2002. AAHP Regulatory Brief.

15. National Association of Insurance Commissioners. *Utilization Review and Benefit Determination Model Act and Grievance Procedures Model Act*. Washington, DC: National Association of Insurance Commissioners, October 2005.

16. America's Health Insurance Plans *Independent Medical Review: State Laws and Regulations*. Washington, DC: America's Health Insurance Plans, December 31, 2005.

17. National Association of Insurance Commissioners. Capital and surplus requirements for companies. In: *Compendium of State Laws on Insurance Topics*. Washington, DC: National Association of Insurance Commissioners, 2005.

18. America's Health Insurance Plans. *HMO Guaranty Fund Coverage and Insolvency Assessments: Summary of State Laws, Regulations, and Selected 2005 State Legislation*. Washington, DC: America's Health Insurance Plans, December 31, 2005.

19. American Legislative Exchange Council (ALEC). *Market Conduct Surveillance Model Act*. Approved January 2006. www.alec.org.

20. National Association of Insurance Commissioners. *Prepaid Limited Health Service Organization Model Act*. Washington, DC: National Association of Insurance Commissioners, October 2005. www.naic.org

21. URAC. *Utilization Management Guide*. 3rd ed. Washington, DC: URAC, December 2004.

22. National Association of Insurance Commissioners. Third Party Administrator Statute. In: *Model Laws, Regulations and Guidelines*. Washington, DC: National Association of Insurance Commissioners, 2001. www.naic.org.

23. National Association of Insurance Commissioners. Third party administrator licensure and bond requirements. In: *Compendium of State Laws on Insurance Topics*. Washington, DC: National Association of Insurance Commissioners, August 2005. www.naic.org.

24. Kaiser Family Foundation and Health Research and Educational Trust. *Employer Health Benefits, 2005 Annual Survey*. Washington, DC: Kaiser Family Foundation and Health Research and Educational Trust, 2005.

25. U.S. Federal Trade Commission. Opinion Letter to Attorney General of Montana Regarding Any Willing Provider Law [Mont. Code Ann. §33-22-17 (1991)], February 4, 1993.

26. National Governors Association. *Private Sector Health Care Reform Policy*. Washington, DC: National Governors Association, 2005. Policy Position HHS-22.

27. National Conference of State Legislators (NCSL). Health policy tracking services. December 2003 and WAshington, DC, America's Health Insurance Plans, March 2005.

28. *Kentucky Association of Health Plans v. Miller*, 123 S.Ct. 1471 (2003).

29. America's Health Insurance Plans *Antitrust Exemptions for Physicians: Summary of State Collective Negotiation Laws*. Washington, DC: America's Health Insurance Plans, December 31, 2005.

30. *Parker v. Brown*, 317 U.S. 341 (1943) and *California Retail Liquor Dealers Association v. Midcal Aluminum, Inc.*, No. 79-97, 445 U.S. 97 (1980).

31. Federal Trade Commission and U.S. Department of Justice. *Improving Health Care: A Dose of Competition*. Washington, DC: Federal Trade Commission and U.S. Department of Justice Publisher, July 2004.

32. Tex. Code Ann. §§88.001 through 88.003.

33. America's Health Insurance Plans *Health Plan Liability: Summary of State Laws.* Washington, DC: America's Health Insurance Plans, December 31, 2005 and America's Health Insurance Plans.

34. *JAMA.* David M. Studdert, Michelle M. Mello, William M. Sage, Catherine M. DesRoches, Jordon Peugh, Kinga Zapert, Troyen A. Brennan. Defensive Medicine Among High-Risk Specialist Physicians in a Volatile Malpractice Environment. *JAMA* 2005 293: 2609–2617.

35. PricewaterhouseCoopers, prepared for America's Health Insurance Plans. *The Factors Fueling Rising Healthcare Costs 2006.* Washington, DC; January 2006. The 10% was adapted from Kessler and McClellan as sourced in Department of Health and Human Services, Office of the Assistant Secretary for Planning and Evaluation. *Addressing the New Health Care Crisis: Reforming the Medical Litigation System to Improve the Quality of Health Care.* Washington, DC, March 2003 and Centers for Medicare and Medicaid Services. Medical Economic Indices (www.cms.com). Kessler and McClellan estimate that the cost of defensive medicine was in the range of 5% to 9% of medical costs. The direct cost of medical liability insurance is roughly 2%. This suggests that total medical liability costs are in the 7% to 11% range.

36. Harris Interactive. April 2002. Taylor, Humphrey. Most Doctors Report Fear of Malpractice Liability Has Harmed Their Ability to Provide Quality Care: Caused Them to Order Unnecessary Tests, Provide Unnecessary Treatment and Make Unnecessary Referrals. Place of publication Rochester, NY. Available at www.harrisinteractive.com/hari_poll/index.asp?PID = 300.

37. President's Advisory Commission on Consumer Protection and Health Care Quality. Reducing errors and increasing safety. In: *Final Report and Recommendations.* p. 2; American Medical Association, testimony presented to U.S. House of Representatives, Committee on Ways and Means, Subcommittee on Health; May 20, 1993.

38. Council for Affordable Health Insurance (CAHI). *State Health Insurance Mandates.* Alexandria, Va: Council for Affordable Health Insurance; 2006.

39. Lewin Group LLC. Letter to AAHP on Estimate of Impact of Health Care Premium Increase on Insured Americans. Falls Church, Va: Lewin Group LLC, November 1997.

40. Mello M., and Brennan T. The controversy over high-dose chemotherapy with autologous bone marrow transplant for breast cancer. *Health Affairs.* September/October 2001. Vol 20, Issue 5: 101–117.

41. America's Health Insurance Plans. *Mandate Review: Summary of State Laws.* Washington, DC: America's Health Insurance Plans, December 31, 2005.

42. America's Health Insurance Plans. *Flexible Benefit Plans: Summary of State Laws and Mandated Coverage.* Washington, DC: America's Health Insurance Plans, December 31, 2005.

43. U.S. Department of Labor, Employee Benefits Security Administration. *MEWA Enforcement.* Washington, DC: U.S. Department of Labor, Employee Benefits Security Administration, April 2006.

44. Academy for Healthcare Management. *Managed Care Organizations: Governance and Regulation.* Washington, DC: Academy for Healthcare Management, 1998:8–15.

45. Office of Personnel Management (OPM) and Federal Employee Health Benefits Program (FEHBP). Insurance Services Programs. 2006. Available at: http://www.opm.gov/insure/. Accessed November 28, 2006.

46. Government Accountability Office (GAO). *Early Experience with a Consumer Directed Plan.* Washington, DC: Government Accountability Office, November 2005.

47. Congressional Research Service (CRS). *Military Medical Care Services: Questions and Answers.* Washington, DC: Congressional Research Service, March 23, 2006.

Glossary of Terms and Acronyms*

Words are not as satisfactory as we should like them to be, but, like our neighbors, we have got to live with them and must make the best and not the worst of them.

—Samuel Butler
(1835–1902)
Samuel Butler's Notebooks [1851]

24/7: Slang term that means something is available 24 hours per day, 7 days per week. For example, the nurse advice line is available 24/7.

AAHC: American Accreditation HealthCare Commission; a name once used by URAC, but no longer. *See also* URAC.

AAPCC: Adjusted average per capita cost. The best estimate of the Centers for Medicare and Medicaid Services (CMS) of the amount of money it costs to care for Medicare recipients under fee-for-service Medicare in a given area. The AAPCC is made up of 142 different rate cells; 140 of them are factored for age, sex, Medicaid eligibility, institutional status, working age, and whether a person has both Part A and Part B of Medicare. The two remaining cells are for individuals with end-stage renal disease. This was and is used to

calculate payments to Medicare health plans, but is being replaced with a system that is based on severity of illness among beneficiaries specifically enrolled in the health plan.

Access fee: A fee charged by a managed care organization (MCO) for access to its provider network, including its reimbursement terms, by an employer or another MCO. *See also* Rental PPO.

Accrete: The term used by CMS for the process of adding new Medicare enrollees to a plan. *See also* Delete.

Accrual: The amount of money that is set aside to cover expenses. The accrual is the plan's best estimate of what those expenses are and (for medical expenses) is based on a combination of data from the authorization system, the claims system, the lag studies, and the plan's prior history.

---

*These are working definitions of common terms and acronyms in the managed health care industry and related health care sectors. In an industry this dynamic, it is not possible to list every term or acronym in use because new ones come into use faster than any publication can keep up with. Other terms will become obsolete or fall out of use while this book is still in print (this is especially so for governmental agencies and programs). Some definitions in this glossary may also be disputed by others in the industry; the editor is open to receiving communication from any such nitpickers.

ACGs: Ambulatory care groups. ACGs are a method of categorizing outpatient episodes. There are 51 mutually exclusive ACGs that are based on resource use over time and modified by principal diagnosis, age, and sex. *See also* ADGs; APCs; APGs.

ACR: Adjusted community rate. Used in the past by Medicare managed care plans. It is being phased out and replaced with an acuity-based methodology.

ACS contract: *See* ASO.

Actuarial assumptions: The assumptions that an actuary uses in calculating the expected costs and revenues of the plan. Examples include utilization rates, age and sex mix of enrollees, and cost for medical services.

ADGs: Ambulatory diagnostic groups. ADGs are a method of categorizing outpatient episodes. There are 34 possible ADGs. *See also* ACGs; APGs.

Adjudication: The management and processing of claims by an MCO or health insurance company.

Admitted asset: A financial asset of a health plan that can be converted to cash on short notice. *See also* Net worth; Nonadmitted asset; Risk-based capital (RBC).

Adverse selection: The problem of attracting members who are sicker than the general population (specifically, members who are sicker than was anticipated when the budget for medical costs was developed).

AHIP: American's Health Insurance Plans. The primary trade organization of managed care organizations. Its areas of focus include legislative and lobbying efforts, education, certification of training in managed health care operations, and representation of the health insurance industry to the public. Initially there were three groups: the Group Health Association of America (GHAA), the American Managed Care and Review Association (AMCRA), and the Health Insurance Association of America (HIAA). These predecessor organizations represented different types of health plan constituencies. GHAA and AMCRA merged to form the American Association of Health Plans (AAHP), which in turn merged with HIAA to form AHIP.

AHP: *See* Association health plan.

AHRQ: The Agency for Healthcare Research and Quality.

Allowed charge: The maximum charge that an MCO or other payer (such as Medicare or Medicaid) will pay for a specific service, even if the amount billed is greater than the allowed charge. This does not mean that it will be paid, however; cost sharing by the member or beneficiary may still apply, for example, a deductible or co-insurance.

ALOS: *See* LOS/ELOS/ALOS.

Alternative medicine: *See* CAM.

Ancillary services: Health care services that are ordered by a physician but provided by some other type of provider; for example, diagnostic testing or physician therapy. Does not apply to inpatient care, ambulatory procedures, or pharmacy.

Annual limit: The maximum amount of coverage that a health plan will provide in a year. This may apply to either the aggregate of all costs in a year (*eg*, coverage stops when costs exceed $1 million in a year), or it may apply to a specific service (*eg*, no more than 20 behavioral health visits are covered in a year). Does not carry over into the next year. Some health maintenance organizations (HMOs) do not have annual limits on charges in the aggregate.

ANSI: The American National Standards Institute. ANSI develops and maintains standards for electronic data interchange. HIPAA mandates the use of ANSI × 12N standards for electronic transactions in the health care system.

APC: Ambulatory patient classification. This is the method settled on by CMS to use for implementing the PPS for ambulatory procedures. Like the other methods, this is a way of clustering many different ambulatory procedure codes into groups for purposes of payment.

APG: Ambulatory patient group. A reimbursement methodology developed by 3M Health Information Systems for the CMS but also used by some commercial health plans. APGs are to outpatient procedures what DRGs are to inpatient days. APGs provide for a fixed reimbursement to an institution for outpatient procedures or visits and incorporate data regarding the reason for the visit and patient data. APGs prevent unbundling of ancillary services. *See also* ACGs; ADGs; APCs.

ASO: Administrative services only. A contract between an insurance company and a self-funded plan where the insurance company performs administrative services only and does not assume any risk. Services usually include claims processing but may include other services such as actuarial analysis, utilization review, and so forth. *See also* ERISA.

Assignment of benefits: The payment of medical benefits directly to a provider of care rather than to a member. Generally requires either a contract between the health plan and the provider or a written release from the subscriber to the provider allowing the provider to bill the health plan.

Association health plan: An association made up of smaller businesses that group together for purposes of providing health benefits to employees. This may be done by purchasing group health insurance in which all of the businesses in the association participate equally, or it may be done by creating a pool of employees sufficiently large so as to self-insure, thereby avoiding benefits mandates and premium taxes. *See also* MET; MEWA.

Authorization: In the context of managed care, authorization refers to the need to obtain authorization before certain types of health care services are covered. Most commonly used in "gatekeeper" type HMOs in which a PCP must authorize a referral to a specialist or the HMO will not pay for the specialist visit. Sometimes referred to as preauthorization or preauth. Sometimes used synonymously with precertification (*see*

Precertification); though no clear distinction is actually made, by convention authorization is applied more often to specialty referral services, whereas precertification is applied more often to facility-based services.

AWP: Any willing provider. This is a form of state law that requires an MCO to accept any provider willing to meet the terms and conditions in the MCO's contract, whether or not the MCO wants or needs that provider. Considered to be an expensive form of anti–managed care legislation.

AWP: Average wholesale price. Commonly used in pharmacy contracting, the AWP is generally determined through reference to a common source of information.

Back office: An informal term describing the administrative processes of a health plan; for example, claims processing or contract management.

Balance billing: The practice of a provider billing a patient for all charges not paid for by the insurance plan, even if those charges are above the plan's UCR or are considered medically unnecessary. Managed care plans and service plans generally prohibit providers from balance billing except for allowed co-pays, co-insurance, and deductibles. Such prohibition against balance billing may even extend to the plan's failure to pay at all (*eg*, because of bankruptcy).

BBA '97: Balanced Budget Act of 1997. A sweeping piece of legislation, part of BBA '97 created the Medicare+Choice program (since replaced by Medicare Advantage) as well as demonstration MSAs.

BD/K: Bed days per thousand members. A common measure of inpatient utilization, it may be applied to differing time periods such as a single day, month-to-date, and year-to-date.

Behavioral shift: A change in the behavior of an individual with health insurance or managed care coverage based on either the existence of the coverage itself, a change in benefits coverage, or as a result of the influence of the health plan.

Best practices: If you do not know what these are, it is suggested that you turn to page 1, begin reading, and work your way back to this point.

BPO: Business process outsourcing. A form of outsourcing to a third party that focuses on one or more administrative processes of an MCO such as claims or enrollment.

Bridge: *See* Doughnut hole.

Cafeteria plan: An informal term for a flexible benefits plan; *see also* Flexible benefits plan.

CAHPS: Consumer Assessment of Healthcare Providers and Systems. Begun by the federal government for use in Medicare and Medicaid managed care plans, it is now also used by commercial health plans. Maintained by the AHRQ and required as part of the NCQA accreditation process. Its initial focus was on managed health care plans, but is being expanded to ambulatory providers, hospitals, and the Medicare prescription drug program.

Call center: *See* Contact center.

CAM: Complementary and alternative medicine. This is a general term that covers treatment modalities other than traditional allopathic medicine. Examples include acupuncture, chiropractic medicine, homeopathy, and various forms of "natural healing."

Capitation: A set amount of money received or paid out; it is based on membership rather than on services delivered and usually is expressed in units of PMPM. May be affected by such factors as age and sex of the enrolled member.

CAQH: Council for Affordable Quality Healthcare. A not-for-profit alliance of health plans, networks, and trade associations, to foster industry collaboration on initiatives that simplify health care administration, including credentialing of providers.

Carve-out: Refers to a set of medical services that are "carved out" of the basic arrangement. In terms of plan benefits, may refer to a set of benefits that are carved out and contracted for separately; for example, mental health/substance abuse services may be separated from basic medical/surgical. May also refer to carving out a set of services from a basic capitation rate with a provider; for example, capitating for cardiac care, but carving out cardiac surgery and paying case rates for that.

Case management: A method of managing the provision of health care to members with high-cost medical conditions. The goal is to coordinate the care so as to both improve continuity and quality of care as well as lower costs. This generally is a dedicated function in the utilization management department. The official definition according to the Certification of Insurance Rehabilitation Specialists Commission (CIRSC) is: "Case management is a collaborative process which assesses, plans, implements, coordinates, monitors, and evaluates the options and services required to meet an individual's health needs, using communication and available resources to promote quality, cost-effective outcomes" and "occurs across a continuum of care, addressing ongoing individual needs" rather than being restricted to a single practice setting. When focused solely on high-cost inpatient cases, may be referred to as large case management or catastrophic case management.

Case mix: The mix of cases in an inpatient setting, accounting for differences in potential or real cost and outcomes. Case mix adjustment refers to a methodology of using case mix to evaluate performance of a provider or project potential costs.

CCIP: *See* Chronic care improvement program. (CCIP)

CCP: *See* Coordinated care plan (CCP).

CCO: Corporate compliance officer. *See* Corporate compliance.

CDH/CDHP: *See* Consumer-directed health plan (CDH/CDHP).

Certificate of Authority: The license required by an HMO that is issued by the state after the HMO meets regulatory requirements. A form of state license.

Certificate of coverage: *See* EOC.

CHAMPUS: Civilian Health and Medical Program of the Uniformed Services. The old term for the federal program providing health care coverage to families of military personnel, military retirees, certain spouses and dependants of such personnel, and certain others. Now called TRICARE. *See also* TRICARE; Military Health System.

Chargemaster: The list of charges a hospital has for each and every thing it can charge for on a pure, FFS basis. Also called a charge master.

Chest pain unit: The term used to describe a specialized unit, usually either in or associated with the emergency department. The purpose of the chest pain unit is to rapidly identify an evolving cardiac event and initiate treatment as early as possible to decrease morbidity and mortality. The other (lesser) primary value of the unit is to rapidly identify chest pain that is noncardiac in origin so as to avoid unnecessary hospitalization. Other terms that may be used include chest pain emergency room, chest pain evaluation unit, short-stay ED CCU, and ED monitored observation beds.

Chronic care improvement program (CCIP): A requirement of the MMA, the CCIP of an MA plan identifies enrollees with multiple or sufficiently severe chronic conditions who meet the criteria for participation in the program and have a mechanism for monitoring enrollees' participation. A form of a disease management program under MA.

Churning: The practice of a provider seeing a patient more often than is medically necessary, primarily to increase revenue through an increased number of services. Churning may also apply to any performance-based reimbursement system where there is a heavy emphasis on productivity (in other words, rewarding a provider for seeing a high volume of patients whether through fee-for-service or through an appraisal system that pays a bonus for productivity).

Claims: The term used to describe a bill for services from a health care provider to the organization or person responsible for payment. Claims can be paper or electronic.

Claims clearinghouse: A company that accepts claims or other transactions from providers, formats them into HIPAA-compliant standards, and electronically transmits them to the payer.

Claims repricing: An activity in which a rental PPO (*see* Rental PPO) receives claims submitted by the participating providers, reprices them using the PPO fee schedule, and then transmits the repriced claim to the MCO or insurance company for final processing.

CLM: Career limiting move. A boneheaded mistake by a manager. What this book is designed to try to prevent.

Closed panel: A managed care plan that contracts with physicians on an exclusive basis for services and does not allow those physicians to see patients for another managed care organization. Examples include staff and group model HMOs. Could apply to a large private medical group that contracts with an HMO.

CMP: Competitive medical plan. A now archaic federal designation that allowed a health plan to obtain eligibility to receive a Medicare risk contract without having to obtain qualification as an HMO. Requirements for eligibility were somewhat less restrictive than for an HMO. Replaced by certain types of Medicare Advantage plans.

CMS: The Centers for Medicare and Medicaid Services. The federal agency that oversees all aspects of health financing for Medicare and (in conjunction with states) Medicaid. Part of DHHS.

CMS-1450: A paper claim form used by hospitals and facilities, standardized by CMS.

The older name was UB-92, though the older name is still widely used. Does not apply to electronic claims.

CMS-1500: A paper claims form used by professionals to bill for services. Developed for Medicare, but also used in the commercial sector.

CMS-hierarchical condition categories system (CMS-HCC): A system that is based on diagnoses made in inpatient and outpatient settings as well as physician settings of care and is used to adjust payments to MA plans.

COA: Certificate of authority. The state-issued operating license for an HMO.

COB: Coordination of benefits. An agreement that uses language developed by the National Association of Insurance Commissioners and prevents double payment for services when a subscriber has coverage from two or more sources. For example, a husband may have Blue Cross Blue Shield through work, and the wife may have elected an HMO through her place of employment. The agreement gives the order for what organization has primary responsibility for payment and what organization has secondary responsibility for payment. The respective primary and secondary payment obligations of the two coverages are determined by the Order of Benefits Determination (OOBD) Rules contained in the National Association of Insurance Commissioners (NAIC) Model COB Regulation, as interpreted and adopted by the various states.

COBRA: Consolidated Omnibus Reconciliation Act. A portion of this act requires employers to offer the opportunity for terminated employees to purchase continuation of health care coverage under the group's medical plan. *See also* Conversion.

Code sets: Sets of codes used by providers to bill for services. As a practical matter, it is used when discussing the official codes that must be used for any electronic transaction covered under HIPAA. These code sets are ICD-9-CM, CPT-4, NDC, HCPCS, and the Code on Dental Procedures and Nomenclature. Official code sets change over time.

Co-insurance: A provision in a member's coverage that limits the amount of coverage by the plan to a certain percentage, commonly 80%. Any additional costs are paid by the member out-of-pocket.

Commercial health insurance: Health insurance or HMO coverage for subscribers who are not covered by virtue of a governmental program such as Medicare, Medicaid, or SCHIP. May be group or direct-pay.

Commission: The money paid to a sales representative, broker, or other type of sales agent for selling the health plan. May be a flat amount of money or a percentage of the premium.

Community rating: The rating methodology required of HMOs under the laws of many states, and occasionally of PPOs and indemnity plans under certain circumstances. When required, it usually applies only to the small group market. The HMO must obtain the same amount of money per member for all members in the plan. Community rating may allow for variability by allowing the HMO to factor in differences for age, sex, mix (average contract size), and industry factors; not all factors are necessarily allowed under state laws, however. Such techniques are referred to as community rating by class and adjusted community rating. *See also* Experience rating.

Complementary and alternative medicine: *See* CAM.

Compliance: *See* Corporate compliance.

CON: Certificate of need. The requirement that a health care organization obtain permission from an oversight agency before making changes. Generally applies only to facilities or facility-based services. Varies on a state to state basis.

Concurrent review: Refers to utilization management that takes place during the provision of services. Almost exclusively applied to inpatient hospital stays.

Consumer-directed health plan (CDH/CDHP): A type of health plan that combines a high-deductible health insurance policy with a pre-tax fund such as an HRA or an HSA. The HRA or HSA is used to pay for qualified services on a first-dollar basis, but is not large enough to cover the entire deductible, the so-called doughnut hole. CDHPs also provide information such as cost data and decision-support tools to consumers to promote greater involvement on the part of the consumer in making health care choices.

Contact center: That place within an MCO that supports inbound inquiries across a broad array of media (though most frequently, inbound telephone calls), blended with outbound contact and outreach transactions.

Contract year: The 12-month period that a contract for services is in force. Not necessarily tied to a calendar year.

Contributory plan: A group health plan in which the employees must contribute a certain amount toward the premium cost, with the employer paying the rest.

Conversion: The conversion of a member covered under a group master contract to coverage under an individual contract. This is offered to subscribers who lose their group coverage (*eg*, through job loss, death of a working spouse, and so forth) and who are ineligible for coverage under another group contract. *See also* COBRA.

Coordinated care plan (CCP): Medicare Advantage plans that include HMOs, PPOs (both regional and local), provider-sponsored organizations that operate like HMOs, and HMOs with point-of-service products. CCPs can require enrollees to use a network of providers for coverage of Medicare services. Other than in an emergency, a CCP has no obligation to cover the cost of care if a non-network provider is used, even if the care would have been covered in fee-for-service Medicare.

Copayment: That portion of a claim or medical expense that a member must pay out-of-pocket. Usually a fixed amount, such as $5 in many HMOs.

Corporate compliance: The function in a health plan or provider charged with ensuring compliance with federal rules and regulations. There are many compliance areas for Medicare, and specific compliance requirements exist for privacy and security under HIPAA and financial requirements under Sarbanes-Oxley. Regulations for Medicare and HIPAA also require the existence of a corporate compliance officer (CCO).

Corporate Practice of Medicine acts or statutes: State laws that prohibit a physician from working for a corporation; in other words, a physician can only work for him- or herself or another physician. Put another way, a corporation cannot practice medicine. Often created through the effort on the part of certain members of the medical community to prevent physicians from working directly for managed care plans or hospitals.

Cost sharing: Any form of coverage in which the member pays some portion of the cost of providing services. Usual forms of cost sharing include deductibles, co-insurance, and co-payments.

Cost shifting: When a provider cannot cover the cost of providing services under the reimbursement received, the provider raises the prices to other payors to cover that portion of the cost.

CPT-4: *Current Procedural Terminology,* 4th edition. A set of five-digit codes that apply to medical services delivered. Frequently used for billing by professionals. *See also* HCPCS.

Credentialing: The most common use of the term refers to obtaining and reviewing the documentation of professional providers. Such documentation includes licensure, certifications, insurance, evidence of malpractice insurance, malpractice history, and so forth. Generally includes both reviewing information provided by the provider as well as verification that the information is correct and complete. A much less frequent use of the term applies to closed panels and medical groups and refers to obtaining hospital privileges and other privileges to practice medicine.

Critical paths: Defined pathways of clinical care that provide for the greatest efficiency of care at the greatest quality. Critical paths are also an ever-changing activity as science and medicine evolve. This term is being replaced through common usage with the term *clinical guidelines*.

CRM: Customer relationship management. Originally the term was used to describe all of the processes and information systems used by an organization as regards its interactions with its customers, such as telephone calling systems and customer databases. It is now used more broadly to include the use of the same processes and technology as regards any external constituency, such as an MCO's nonroutine interactions with its providers.

CSR: Customer service representative. An individual who interfaces directly with members in the member services function of an MCO.

Custodial care: Care provided to an individual that is primarily the basic activities of living. May be medical or nonmedical, but the care is not meant to be curative or as a form of medical treatment, and is often lifelong. Rarely covered by any form of group health insurance or HMO.

Customer services: *See* Member services.

CVO: Credentialing verification organization. This is an independent organization that performs primary verification of a professional provider's credentials. The managed care organization may then rely on that verification rather than subjecting the provider to provide credentials independently. This lowers the cost and "hassle" for credentialing. NCQA (*see* NCQA) has issued certification standards for CVOs.

CWW: Clinic without walls. *See also* Group practice without walls.

Date of service: Refers to the date that medical services were rendered. Usually different from the date a claim is submitted.

DAW: Dispense as written. The instruction from a physician to a pharmacist to dispense a brand name pharmaceutical rather than a generic substitution.

Days per thousand: A standard unit of measurement of utilization. Refers to an annualized use of the hospital or other institutional care. It is the number of hospital days that are used in a year for each thousand covered lives.

Defined benefit: A term of insurance that refers to an employer (or governmental agency that provides benefits to employees) providing a benefit that is the same regardless of the cost (though cost sharing with employees is not a part of the definition of defined benefit). In other words, an employee knows what type(s) of insurance or managed health care plans are offered and what the benefits are under each, and the employer's contribution to the cost of that coverage is a function of how expensive that coverage is. This is the most common form of employee health insurance benefit as of early 2000.

Defined contribution: A term of insurance that refers to an employer designating a fixed amount of money for use in purchasing health insurance, but not requiring the employee to use only those health plans chosen by the employer. In other words, here's your money, now go find some health insurance.

DCG: Diagnostic care group. A methodology commissioned by the CMS to look at how to adjust prospective payments to health plans based on retrospective severity. Replaced by the CMS-Hierarchical Condition Categories.

Death spiral: An insurance term that refers to a vicious spiral of high premium rates and adverse selection, generally in a free-choice environment (typically, an insurance company or health plan in an account with multiple other plans, or a plan offering coverage to potential members who have alternative choices, such as through an association). One plan ends up having continually higher premium rates such that the only members who stay with the plan are those whose medical costs are so high (and who cannot change because of provider loyalty or benefits restrictions such as preexisting conditions) that they far exceed any possible premium revenue. Called the death spiral because the losses from underwriting mount faster than the premiums can ever recover, and the account eventually terminates coverage, leaving the carrier in a permanent loss position.

Deductible: That portion of a subscriber's (or member's) health care expenses that must be paid out-of-pocket before any insurance coverage applies, commonly $100 to $300. May apply only to the out-of-network portion of a point-of-service plan. May also apply only to one portion of the plan coverage (*eg*, there may be a deductible for pharmacy services or hospital care, but not for anything else).

Delete: The term used by CMS for the process of removing Medicare enrollees from a plan. *See also* Accrete.

Demand management: Services or support that an MCO provides members to lower the demand for acute care services. Includes self-help tools, nurse advice lines, and preventive services.

Dental Content Committee of the American Dental Association: A DSMO under HIPAA that focuses on coding standards for dental procedures.

Dependant: A member who is covered by virtue of a family relationship with the member who has the health plan coverage. For example, one person has health insurance or an HMO through work, and that individual's spouse and children, the dependants, also have coverage under that contract.

Designated standards maintenance organizations (DSMOs): Organizations designated in HIPAA that are charged with making recommendations to DHHS regarding updates to existing standards as well as the addition of new standards to the transactions and code sets.

DHHS: The United States Department of Health and Human Services. This is the cabinet-level federal agency that oversees many programs, including the CMS which is responsible for Medicare and Medicaid (in conjunction with individual states), as well as oversight of HIPAA and other related federal legislation.

DHMO: Dental health maintenance organization. An HMO organized strictly to provide dental benefits.

Direct access: *See* Open access.

Direct contract model: A managed care health plan that contracts directly with private practice physicians in the community, rather than through an intermediary such as an IPA or a medical group. A common type of model in open panel HMOs.

Direct contracting: A term describing a provider or integrated health care delivery system contracting directly with employers rather than through an insurance company or managed care organization. A superficially attractive option that occasionally works when the employer is large enough. Not to be confused with direct contract model (see below).

Direct-pay subscriber: An individual subscriber to a health plan who is not covered under a group policy, but rather pays the health plan directly. May be a commercial member who has passed underwriting screening, or may be a conversion plan holder (*see also* Conversion). Is not used to describe Medicare or Medicaid subscribers by convention; even though such subscribers are enrolled individually, part or all of their premiums are paid via a governmental agency.

Discharge planning: That part of utilization management that is concerned with arranging for care or medical needs to facilitate discharge from the hospital.

Disease management: The process of intensively managing a particular disease. This differs from large case management in that it goes well beyond a given case in the hospital or an acute exacerbation of a condition. Disease management encompasses all settings of care and places a heavy emphasis on prevention and maintenance. Similar to case management, but more focused on a defined set of diseases.

Disenrollment: The process of termination of coverage. Voluntary termination would include a member quitting because he or she simply wants out. Involuntary termination would include leaving the plan because of changing jobs. A rare and serious form of involuntary disenrollment is when the plan terminates a member's coverage against the member's will. This is usually only allowed (under state and federal laws) for gross offenses such as fraud, abuse, nonpayment of premium or copayments, or a demonstrated inability to comply with recommended treatment plans.

Dispensing fee: The fee paid to a pharmacy for that part of the cost of a prescription that is not the ingredient cost. Usually a flat dollar amount, not tied to the cost of the drug.

Distribution channel: An informal term used to describe the various ways that an MCO sells its products; for example, brokers, consultants, employed sales force, electronic sales portals, and so forth.

DME: Durable medical equipment. Medical equipment that is not disposable (*ie*, is used repeatedly) and is only related to care for a medical condition. Examples would include wheelchairs, home hospital beds, and so forth. An area of increasing expense, particularly in conjunction with case management.

DOL: U.S. Department of Labor. Regulates coverage offered to employees when employers retain the insurance risk (*ie*, self-funding pursuant to ERISA), either on a stand-alone basis or through a multiple-employer welfare arrangement.

Doughnut hole: The term applied to the difference between when first-dollar coverage stops and insurance then begins. Also referred to as a bridge. May be applied in a CDHP to the gap between the HRA or HSA and when the high-deductible insurance plan starts to cover costs. Also exists in the basic Medicare Part D drug benefit passed under the MMA, at least at the time of publication. A term that may not necessarily have great persistency.

Dread disease policy: A peculiar type of health insurance that only covers a specific and frightening type of illness, such as cancer. Uncommon.

DRG: Diagnosis-related groups. A statistical system of classifying any inpatient stay into groups for purposes of payment. DRGs may be primary or secondary, and an outlier classification also exists. This is the form of reimbursement that the CMS uses to pay hospitals for Medicare recipients. Also used by a few states for all payers and by many private health plans for contracting purposes. DRGs are being replaced by MS-DRGs in 2008–2009. See also MS-DRG.

DSM-IV: *Diagnostic and Statistical Manual of Mental Disorders*, 4th edition. The manual used to provide a diagnostic coding system for mental and substance abuse disorders. Far different from ICD-9-CM.

DSMO: *See* Designated standards maintenance organization.

Dual choice: An archaic term, sometimes also referred to as Section 1310 or mandating. That portion of the original federal HMO regulations that required any employer with 25 or more employees that reside in an HMO's service area, pays minimum wage, and offers health coverage to offer a federally qualified HMO as well. The HMO had to request it. This provision "sunsetted" in 1995.

Dual eligibles: Individuals who are entitled to both Medicare and Medicaid coverage.

Dual option: This once referred only to offering of both an HMO and a traditional insurance plan by one carrier. It now refers to offering two different health plans, regardless of type.

Duplicate claims: When the same claim is submitted more than once, it is usually because payment hasn't been received quickly. Can lead to duplicate payments and incorrect data in the claims file.

DUR: Drug utilization review.

EAP: Employee assistance program. A program that a company puts into effect for its employees to provide them with help in dealing with personal problems such as alcohol or drug abuse, mental health or stress issues, and so forth.

Earned premium: That portion of the premium paid to an MCO for coverage for a time period that has already passed. Premium that is paid in advance is considered unearned premium until the entire time period that the premium is meant to cover has passed, on a proportionate basis.

e-Business: *See* e-Commerce.

e-Commerce: A term that refers to the use of electronic communications to conduct business. Also called e-business. By convention, e-commerce applies to the use of the Internet for such transactions. Also by convention, the *e* is almost always lowercase (and who knows why?). ee cummings would approve.

ED: Emergency department. That location or department in a hospital or other institutional facility that is focused on caring for acutely ill or injured patients. In earlier times, this was often a room or set of rooms, hence the older designation emergency room, or ER. These days, at least in busy urban and suburban hospitals, volume is high, physicians are specially trained and certified in emergency care, and it has grown to be an entire department.

EDI: Electronic data interchange. A term that refers to the exchange of data through electronic means rather than by using paper or the telephone. Prior to the rise of the Internet, EDI was applied primarily to direct electronic communications via proprietary means. EDI may now encompass electronic data exchange via both proprietary channels as well as the Internet; but by common usage, EDI is most often used for proprietary channels, whereas the term *e-commerce* is used most often for Internet-based electronic exchanges.

Effective date: The day that health plan coverage goes into effect or is modified.

EFT: Electronic funds transfer. Getting paid by electronic transfer of funds directly to one's bank instead of receiving a paper check.

Electronic health record: A more expansive type of electronic record encompassing more than the care provided by a single provider or entity to a single patient.

Electronic medical record: An electronic version of the type of health record that a physician or a hospital keeps on a single patient.

Eligibility: When an individual is eligible for coverage under a plan. Also used to determine when an individual is no longer eligible for coverage (*eg*, a dependant child reaches a certain age and is no longer eligible for coverage under his or her parent's health plan).

EHR: *See* Electronic health record.

EMR: *See* Electronic medical record.

EMTALA: The Emergency Medical Treatment and Active Labor Act. 1986. 42, USC 1395 dd (1986) Pub. L. No. 99-272, 9121. "Antidumping" legislation dictates that all patients presenting to any hospital emergency department must have a medical screening exam performed by qualified personnel, usually the emergency physician. The medical screening exam cannot be delayed for insurance reasons: either to obtain insurance information or to obtain preauthorization for examination. Specific language in EMTALA states: "An emergency medical condition means a medical condition manifested by acute symptoms of sufficient severity (including severe pain) that the absence of immediate medical attention could reasonably be expected to result in: a) placing the patient's health in serious jeopardy; b) serious impairment to bodily functions; or c) serious dysfunction of any bodily organ or part."

Encounter: An outpatient or ambulatory visit by a member to a provider. Applies primarily to physician office visits, but may encompass other types of encounters as well. In fee-for-service plans, an encounter also generates a claim. In capitated plans, the encounter is still the visit, but no claim is generated.

Enrollee: An individual enrolled in a managed health care plan. Usually applies to the subscriber or person who has the coverage in the first place rather than to their dependants, but the term is not always used that precisely.

EOB: Explanation of benefits (statement). A statement mailed to a member or covered insured explaining how and why a claim was or was not paid; the Medicare version is called an EOMB (*see also* ERISA).

EOC: Evidence of coverage; also known as a certificate of benefits. The EOC is a document that describes the health care benefits covered by the health plan and provides the member with some form of documentation that he or she in fact does have health insurance and what that insurance covers and how it works.

EPO: Exclusive provider organization. An EPO is similar to an HMO in that it often uses primary physicians as gatekeepers, often capitates providers, has a limited provider panel, and uses an authorization system, and so forth. It is referred to as exclusive because the member must remain within the network to receive benefits. The main difference is that EPOs are generally regulated under insurance statutes rather than HMO regulations. Not allowed in many states that maintain that EPOs are really HMOs.

ePrescribing: When a physician uses electronic means to prescribe drugs.

Equity model: A term applied to a form of for-profit vertically integrated health care delivery system in which the physicians are owners.

ER: Emergency room; *see* ED.

ERISA: Employee Retirement Income Security Act. One provision of this act allows self-funded plans to avoid paying premium taxes, complying with state-mandated benefits, or otherwise complying with state laws and regulations regarding insurance, even when insurance companies and managed care plans that stand risk for medical costs must do so. Another provision requires that plans and insurance companies provide an explanation of benefits (EOB) statement to a member or covered insured in the event of a denial of a claim, explaining why the claim was denied and informing the individual of his or her rights of appeal. Numerous other provisions in ERISA are very important for a managed care organization to know.

ESRD: End-stage renal disease. Although no other particular clinical definitions are found in this glossary, this one is only because Medicare treats beneficiaries with ESRD differently from other types for purposes of enrollment in MA plans.

Ethics in Referrals Act: *See* Stark regulations.

Evidence of insurability: The form that documents whether or not an individual is eligible for health plan coverage when the individual does not enroll through an open enrollment period. For example, if an employee wants to change health plans in the middle of a contract year, the new health plan may require evidence of insurability (often both a questionnaire and a medical exam) to ensure that it will not be accepting adverse risk.

eVisit: Electronic visit, referring to an interaction between a provider (usually a physician) and a patient, using a secure electronic communications channel rather than face-to-face or via a telephone call.

Exclusion: As used in managed care and health insurance, exclusions refer to those services or conditions for which there will be no (or very limited) coverage. The most common is an exclusion in an individual direct-pay policy for preexisting conditions, in which there will be no coverage for conditions that existed at the time the policy was issued; there is also usually a time limit for this type of exclusion, for example, after 2 years coverage will apply. An exclusion may also be a complete one, such as no coverage for experimental or scientifically unproven care.

Experience rating: The method of setting premium rates based on the actual health care costs of a group or groups.

Experimental and investigational treatment: The term used by MCOs and insurance companies to refer to medical care that is not yet proven, or that may be the subject of clinical investigation. Most plans will not cover costs for this unless the patient is enrolled in a qualified investigational trial.

Extracontractual benefits: Health care benefits beyond what the member's actual policy covers. These benefits are provided by a plan to reduce utilization. For example, a plan may not provide coverage for a hospital bed at home, but it is more cost effective for the plan to provide such a bed than to keep admitting a member to the hospital.

FAR: Federal acquisition regulations. The regulations applied to the federal government's acquisition of services, including health care services, excluding Medicare (*see also* FEHBARS).

Fast-track ED: A pathway in the ED allowing minor ailments to be managed quickly, at lower cost, often by nonphysician practitioners.

Favored nations discount: A contractual agreement between a provider and a payer stating that the provider will automatically provide the payer the best discount it provides anyone else. Prohibited in many states.

Federal qualification: A term once applied to HMOs and CMPs that met federal standards regarding benefits, financial solvency, rating methods, marketing, member services, health care delivery systems, and other standards. No longer used.

Fee schedule: May also be referred to as fee maximums or as a fee allowance schedule. A listing of the maximum fee that a health plan will pay for a certain service, based on CPT billing codes.

FEHBARS: Federal Employee Health Benefit Acquisition Regulations. The regulations applied to OPM's purchase of health care benefits programs for federal employees.

FEHBP: Federal Employee Health Benefits Program. The program that provides health benefits to federal employees. *See also* OPM.

FFS: Fee-for-service. A patient sees a provider, and then the provider bills the health plan or patient and gets paid based on that bill.

Fiscal intermediary: A company that processes the administrative transactions on behalf of Medicare, though the term may also be used by similar types of companies providing services to state Medicaid programs. May be limited to adjudication and payment of claims or may encompass other activities as well.

Flexible benefits plan: A benefits plan at a company that allows an employee to select from different options up to a set amount of money and always includes an FSA. Also called a cafeteria plan or a Section 125 plan.

Flexible spending account (FSA): A financial account funded with pre-tax dollars via payroll deduction by an employer. Funds may be used to reimburse the employee for qualified expenses not covered under insurance. FSAs exist for health care and, separately, for child care services. Unused FSA funds do not roll into following years; they are "use it or lose it."

Formulary: A listing of drugs that a health plan provides coverage for, but almost always at differing levels. For example, drugs considered Tier 1 in the formulary may be covered with a $5 copay, Tier 2 at a $20 copay, Tier 3 at a $50 copay. May also list drugs that require precertification for coverage or that are subject to other coverage limitations.

Foundation: A not-for-profit form of integrated health care delivery system. The foundation model is usually formed in response to tax laws that affect not-for-profit hospitals or in response to states with laws prohibiting the corporate practice of medicine (*see also* Corporate Practice of Medicine acts or statutes). The foundation purchases both the tangible and intangible assets of a physician's practice, and then the physicians form a medical group that contracts with the foundation on an exclusive basis for services to patients seen through the foundation.

FPP: Faculty practice plan. A form of group practice organized around a teaching program. It may be a single group encompassing all the physicians providing services to patients at the teaching hospital and clinics, or it may be multiple groups drawn along specialty lines (*eg*, psychiatry, cardiology, or surgery).

Fraudandabuse: A term with its roots in a description applied to fraud and/or abuse by health care providers or intermediaries in the provision of services to Medicare and Medicaid beneficiaries. Since that time nobody, and I mean nobody, uses either term separately, and it has taken on a generic meaning applied to any form of perceived skullduggery on the part of a provider or health plan doing business with the government. *See also* Waste, fraud, and abuse.

FSA: *See* Flexible spending account.

FTE: Full-time equivalent. The equivalent of one full-time employee. For example, two part-time employees are 0.5 FTE each, for a total of 1 FTE.

Full professional risk capitation: A loose term used to refer to a physician group or organization receiving capitation for all professional expenses, not just for the services it provides itself; does not include capitation for institutional services (*see* Global capitation). The group is then responsible for sub-capitating or otherwise reimbursing other physicians for services to their members.

Gag clause: A clause in a provider contract that prevents a physician from telling a patient about available clinical treatment options; that is, a "gag." This clause was much like the Sasquatch: big, hairy, and scary, but hard to actually find. The federal government conducted a review of managed care physician contracts and was unable to find any examples. Gag clauses have been banned by many states. Most or all contracts between MCOs and physicians do contain clauses that prohibit the physician from revealing business secrets such as reimbursement schedules, but this is a different matter. In some cases in the past, contracts also required a physician to contact the MCO before initiating a treatment option, which may have been interpreted or treated as such a clause, but the majority of contracts actually require the physician to actively discuss options with the patient.

Gatekeeper: An informal, though widely used term that refers to a primary care case management model health plan. In this model, all care from providers other than the primary care physician, except for true emergencies, must be authorized by the primary care physician before care is rendered. This is a predominant feature of most (but not all) HMOs.

Generic drug: A drug that is equivalent to a brand-name drug, but usually less expensive. Most managed care organizations that provide drug benefits cover generic drugs but may require a member to pay a higher copay for a brand name drug.

Glass–Steagall Act of 1933: *See* Gramm–Leach–Bliley Act of 1999.

Global capitation: The term used when an organization receives capitation for all medical services, including institutional and professional.

Grace period: The amount of time that an MCO or insurance company must allow a group or individual who hasn't paid the premium to make good on the payment before the plan can cancel the policy. If the delinquent company or individual pays up during the grace period, the policy is said to be reinstated and coverage is considered unbroken.

Gramm–Leach–Bliley Act of 1999: The Gramm–Leach–Bliley Act (S.900/H.R. 10) repealed the Glass–Steagall Act of 1933 that had been passed in the aftermath of the crash of 1929. Glass–Steagall prohibited most U.S. commercial banks from performing investment banking activities such as bringing new debt and equity issues to market, or other such underwriting, and from functioning as insurance companies. In addition to the repeal of Glass–Steagall, Gramm–Leach–Bliley also allows affiliations between securities firms, banks, and insurance companies.

Group: The members who are covered by virtue of receiving health plan coverage at a single company.

Group health insurance: A commercial health insurance policy (or HMO coverage policy) that is sold to an employer to provide coverage to employees. Does not apply to a conversion policy or a direct-pay policy, nor to Medicare or Medicaid plans.

Group model HMO: An HMO that contracts with a medical group for the provision of health care services. The relationship between the HMO and the medical group is generally very close, although there are wide variations in the relative independence of the group from the HMO. A form of closed panel health plan.

Group practice: The American Medical Association defines group practice as three or more physicians who deliver patient care, make joint use of equipment and personnel, and divide income by a prearranged formula.

Group practice without walls (GPWW): A group practice in which the members of the group come together legally but continue to practice in private offices scattered throughout the service area. Sometimes called a clinic without walls (CWW).

HCFA: Health Care Financing Administration. The older term for CMS; no longer used.

HCFA-1500: *See* CMS-1500.

HCPCS: Healthcare (previously HCFA) Common Procedural Coding System. A set of codes used by Medicare that describes services and procedures. HCPCS includes CPT codes, but also has codes for services not included in CPT such as DME and ambulance. Although HCPCS is nationally defined, there is provision for local use of certain codes.

HDHP: High-deductible health plan; *see* High-deductible health insurance.

Health care: You probably think you know what this means, eh? Well, maybe, maybe not. The term is generally used to refer to the services that a health care professional or institution provide (eg, services from a physician, at a hospital, from a physical therapist, and so forth); it is this use of the term that is universally used when discussing care management. There is a broader definition, however, that encompasses services from nontraditional providers and, more important, the health care that individuals self-administer (which is actually the majority of health care anyone receives). When individuals use the broad sense of the term *health care*, they frequently use *medical care* to refer to what is considered the narrow meaning noted previously. Broad or narrow: it's your choice depending on the context.

Health Reimbursement Account/Arrangement (HRA): A financial account associated with a CDHP and used to pay for first-dollar qualified health care expenses up to a preset limit using pre-tax funds provided by an employer. Unused HRA funds may roll into the next year, but they do not follow an individual when they change employment. Always associated with a high-deductible health insurance policy.

Health Risk Appraisal (HRA): Instrument designed to elicit or compile information about the health risk of any given individual. Initially, these tools were fairly uniform, but they have now become quite specialized and targeted toward particular populations with distinctive risk profiles (eg, Medicare, Medicaid, underserved, commercial population, and so forth).

Health Savings Account (HSA): Created under the MMA, an HSA is a financial account of pre-tax dollars for current or future qualified medical expenses, retirement, or long-term care premium expenses. Unused funds roll into following years. Funding may come from an employer and/or an individual and does follow an individual when he or she changes employment. Always associated with a qualified, high-deductible health insurance policy.

Healthcare Integrity and Protection Data Bank: An electronic databank established under HIPAA that records information about providers around fraud and abuse, criminal convictions, civil judgments, injunctions, licensure restrictions, and exclusion from participation in any governmental programs.

HEDIS®: Health Plan Employer Data Information Set. Developed by NCQA with considerable input from the employer community and the managed care community, HEDIS® is an ever-evolving set of data reporting standards. HEDIS® is designed to provide some standardization in performance reporting for financial, utilization, membership, clinical data, and more. Employers and consumers then can compare performance between plans, if the plan reports HEDIS® data. The initial focus was on HMOs, but it has become much more varied.

HHS: Health and Human Services; *see* DHHS.

High-deductible health insurance/high-deductible health plan: Just what it sounds like, a health insurance policy with a very high deductible, such as $1,500 or even $5,000 per year. The deductible for an individual will be different from an aggregate deductible for a family. Associated as well with MSAs, HRAs, and HSAs, high-deductible insurance is a mainstay in a typical CDHP.

HIPAA: Health Insurance Portability and Accountability Act. Enacted in 1997, this act creates a rather vaguely worded set of requirements that allows for insurance portability (ie, the ability to keep your health insurance even if you move or change jobs), guaranteed issue of all health insurance products to small groups (but only if they have met requirements for prior continuous coverage) and mental health parity (ie, the dollar limits on mental health coverage cannot be less than that for medical coverage; it is silent, however, on the issues of differential visit limitations, differential co-insurance requirements, or restrictions on networks). More important HIPAA also contains significant provisions regarding "administrative simplification" and standards for privacy and security. Administrative simplification also mandated the use of certain standards for types of electronic transactions (eg, electronic claims) and code sets.

HL7: Health Level 7. A DSMO under HIPAA, HL7 focuses on electronic connectivity standards for clinical information.

HMO: Health maintenance organization. The definition of an HMO has changed substantially. Originally, an HMO was defined as a prepaid organization that provided health care to voluntarily enrolled members in return for a preset amount of money on a PMPM basis. With the increase in self-insured business, or with financial arrangements that do not rely on prepayment, that definition is no longer accurate. Now the definition needs to encompass two possibilities: a licensed health plan (licensed as an HMO, that is) that places at least some of the providers at risk for medical expenses, and a health plan that utilizes designated (usually primary care) physicians as gatekeepers (although there are some HMOs that do not). Many in the field have given up and now use the broader term *MCO* because it avoids having to make difficult definitions like this one.

Hold harmless clause: A contractual clause between a provider and an MCO that prohibits the provider from balance billing a member even in the event the MCO fails to pay the provider; that is, the provider holds the member harmless.

HOS: Health Outcomes Survey. The HOS is a survey that health plans with a Medicare Advantage risk contract must conduct to look at clinical outcomes of covered Medicare beneficiaries. CMS arranges and pays for administration of the CAHPS survey, whereas Medicare Advantage health plans are responsible for administering the HOS survey.

Hospice: A program or facility dedicated to palliative care at the end of life. May be a combination of a home-care program, an outpatient facility, and/or an inpatient facility.

Hospitalist: A physician who concentrates solely on hospitalized patients. In an MCO or medical group, this physician may specialize in hospital care, or the duties may be undertaken on a rotating basis. May also be employed by the hospital. This model allows the other physicians to concentrate on outpatient care, while the hospitalist focuses on the care of all the plan's or group's patients in the hospital.

HRA: An acronym that means either Health Risk Appraisal or Health Reimbursement Account, depending on circumstances. *See also* Health Risk Appraisal; Health Reimbursement Account.

HSA: *See* Health Savings Account.

IBNR: Incurred but not reported. The amount of money that the plan had better accrue for medical expenses that it knows nothing about yet. These are medical expenses that the authorization system has not captured and for which claims have not yet hit the door. Unexpected IBNRs have torpedoed more managed care plans than any other cause.

ICD-9-CM: *International Classification of Diseases,* 9th revision, *Clinical Modification.* The classification of disease by diagnosis codified into six-digit numbers. It will eventually be replaced by ICD-10, which is approximately 10 times the size of ICD-9.

IDN: *See* IDS.

IDS: Integrated delivery system; also referred to as an integrated health care delivery system. Another acronym that means the same thing is IDN (integrated delivery network). An IDS is an organized system of health care providers to span a broad range of health care services. Although there is no clear definition of an IDS, in its full flower an IDS should be able to access the market on a broad basis, optimize cost and clinical outcomes, accept and manage a full range of financial arrangements to provide a set of defined benefits to a defined population, align financial incentives of the participants (including physicians), and operate under a cohesive management structure. *See also* Equity model; Foundation model; IHO; IPA; MSO; PHO; Staff model.

Imputed premium: Applies to self-funded plans where no actual premium is paid (other than reinsurance premium). Because the self-funded plan pays costs via a system of electronic lockboxes, there is no pool of premium dollars that is regularly replenished. However, even a self-funded plan must budget for expected costs and must also determine the amount that should be deducted from an employee's paycheck for the employee's portion of the cost of the plan; therefore, an imputed premium is calculated for these purposes.

Indemnity insurance: Insurance that "indemnifies" the policy holder from losses. In health insurance, this applies to providing financial coverage for health care costs, with little or no attempt to manage that cost (other than, perhaps, a precertification program); most important, it is not based on a contracted network of providers, unlike a service plan that may otherwise appear the same. Indemnity insurance plans do limit the amount they will pay for a professional service, however, based on some form of fee scale; such limits are rarely in place for institutional costs, however. Once common, indemnity plans are quite rare now because of high cost.

Independent review organization: An independent group that an MCO contracts with to provide a secondary external review of coverage denials based on medical reasons. Required in some states, which may also require that a designated IRO be approved by the state's department of insurance.

Individual policy: *See* Direct pay.

Informatics: A loosely defined term that refers to using data mining to create usable reports. It is intended to imply a more sophisticated approach to obtaining and using data than is used for routine operations. The term is preferentially used by many MCOs for the function and/or department that analyzes medical data.

Insourcing: Bringing back into the MCO a process or activity that was once outsourced.

Intensivist: A type of hospitalist (physician) who focuses solely on care provided in the intensive (or critical) care unit.

Intermediary: *See* Fiscal intermediary.

Investigational treatment: *See* Experimental and investigational treatment.

IPA: Independent practice association. An organization that has a contract with a managed care plan to deliver services in return for a single capitation rate. The IPA in turn contracts with individual providers to provide the services either on a capitation basis or on a fee-for-service basis. The typical IPA encompasses all specialties, but an IPA can be solely for primary care or may be single specialty. An IPA may also be the "PO" part of a PHO.

IRO: *See* Independent review organization.

ISAR: Intraservice area rate adjustment. This serves to "correct" erroneous projections regarding the county of origin by adjusting the bid of an MA plan based on the relationship among the local MA payment rates of the individual counties that are included in the bid.

IT: Information technology. A blanket term referring to all of the computer hardware and software systems that support the operations of a health plan. Virtually all operational functions of a health plan are supported by IT in one way or another.

JCAHO (Joint Commission): Joint Commission for the Accreditation of Healthcare Organizations. A not-for-profit organization that performs accreditation reviews primarily on hospitals, other institutional facilities, and outpatient facilities. Most managed care plans require any hospital under contract to be accredited by the Joint Commission.

Lag study: A report that tells managers how old the claims are that are being processed and how much is paid out each month (both for that month and for any earlier months, by month) and compares these to the amount of money that was accrued for expenses each month. A powerful tool used to determine whether the plan's reserves are adequate to meet all expenses. Plans that fail to perform lag studies properly may find themselves staring into the abyss.

Lag table: The tool used by finance to manage the lag study.

Lapse: To drop coverage. This may refer to an individual who stops paying premium, thereby allowing her or his policy to lapse, subject to a grace period (*see* Grace period). When used as a ratio, it is the opposite of a persistency ratio; that is, the percentage of commercially enrolled groups that drop the health plan.

Legend drug: A drug that can be provided only with a prescription from a licensed provider.

Line of business: A health plan (*eg*, an HMO, EPO, or PPO) that is set up as a line of business within another, larger organization, usually an insurance company. This legally differentiates it from a freestanding company or a company set up as a subsidiary. It may also refer to a unique product type (*eg*, Medicaid) within a health plan.

LOS/ELOS/ALOS: Length of stay/estimated length of stay/average length of stay.

Loss ratio: *See* Medical loss ratio.

MA Local plan: A Medicare Advantage managed care plan that does not provide services throughout the entire designated region. The older Medicare+Choice HMOs (and, though not common, PPOs) mostly became MA Local plans unless they were able to expand to cover the entire region, which was rare.

MA MSA: A Medicare Advantage MSA plan. MSA plans are not network plans in the sense of being able to limit coverage to a network. Enrollees of such plans have the right to expect the plan to cover the cost of care at any provider willing to accept the individual as a patient, consistent with the rules of the plan regarding coverage (*eg*, an MSA plan has no coverage before a deductible is met). *See also* MSA.

MA Regional plan: A Medicare Advantage PPO-type plan that provides services throughout the entire designated region.

MAC: Maximum allowable charge (or cost). The maximum, although not the minimum, that a vendor may charge for something. This term is often used in pharmacy contracting; a related term, used in conjunction with professional fees, is fee maximum.

Managed behavioral health care organization (MBHO): A third party that manages the behavioral health services benefits for an MCO. It may also contract directly with an employer. An MBHO may be at financial risk, or it may manage the services under an administrative contract only. A form of clinical outsourcing.

Managed health care: A regrettably nebulous term. At the very least, it is a system of health care delivery that tries to manage the cost of health care, the quality of that health care, and access to that care. Common denominators include a panel of contracted providers that is less than the entire universe of available providers, some type of limitations on benefits to subscribers who use non-contracted providers (unless authorized to do so), and some type of authorization or pre-certification system. Managed health care is actually a spectrum of systems, ranging from so-called managed indemnity, through CDHPs, POS, PPOs, open panel HMOs, and closed panel HMOs. For a better definition, the reader is urged to read this book and formulate his or her own idea.

Mandated benefits: Benefits that a health plan is required to provide by law. This is generally used to refer to benefits above and beyond routine insurance-type benefits, and it generally applies at the state level (where there is high variability from state to state). Common examples include in vitro fertilization, defined days of inpatient mental health or substance abuse treatment, and other special-condition treatments. Self-funded plans are exempt from most mandated benefits under ERISA, but even the federal government gets into the act with mandatory 2-day length of stay for childbirth and mental health parity provisions under HIPAA that apply to both insured and self-funded plans.

Mandatory external review: The requirement that an MCO provide a means for a physician or member who appeals a decision about medical coverage to obtain a second opinion from an unbiased external reviewer, a physician in a specialty appropriate for the clinical condition. This process has been mandated in some states and is widely undertaken on a voluntary basis in any event.

Master group contract: The actual contract between a health plan and a group that purchases coverage. The master group contract provides specific terms of coverage, rights, and responsibilities of both parties.

Maximum out-of-pocket cost: The most amount of money a member will ever need to pay for covered services during a contract year. The maximum out-of-pocket includes deductibles and co-insurance. Once this limit is reached, the health plan pays for all services up to the maximum level of coverage. Applies mostly to non-HMO plans such as indemnity plans, CDHPs, PPOs, and POS plans.

MBHO: *See* Managed behavioral health care organization.

MCO: Managed care organization. A generic term applied to a managed care plan. In the past decade or so, some initially used the term MCO to refer to an HMO simply because they thought that there was less negative connotation. However, it now encompasses plans that do not conform exactly to the strict definition of an HMO (although that definition has itself loosened considerably) and may also apply to a PPO, EPO, CDHP, IDS, or even an OWA.

Medical informatics: *See* Informatics.

Medical loss ratio: The ratio between the cost to deliver medical care and the amount of money that was taken in by a plan and can vary from around 85% to around 92%. The medical loss ratio is dependent on the amount of money brought in as well as the cost of delivering care; thus, if the rates are too low, the ratio may be high, even though the actual cost of delivering care is not really out of line.

Medical policy: Policies of a health plan regarding what will be paid for as medical benefits. Routine medical policy is linked to routine claims processing and may even be automated in the claims system; for example, the plan may pay only 50% of the fee of a second surgeon or may not pay for two surgical procedures done during one episode of anesthesia. This also refers to how a plan approaches payment policy for experimental or investigational care and payment for noncovered services in lieu of more expensive covered services.

Medically necessary: The term used to refer to whether or not a clinical service or supply (*eg*, a drug or a device) is actually necessary to protect or preserve the health of an individual, based on evidence-based medical knowledge or practices. Not always easy to define in any particular circumstance.

Medicare: Social health insurance provided by the federal government for citizens over the age of 65 as well as some others, such as individuals with end-stage renal disease. Regular Medicare is an FFS type of insurance; Part A covers hospital care and Part B covers professional services. Medicare now also provides a drug benefit under Part D, passed un-

der the MMA. Traditional FFS Medicare is administered by intermediaries performing on behalf of CMS, while Medicare Advantage uses various forms of private health plans.

Medicare Advantage (MA): Created as part of the MMA, MA replaced and expanded other forms of Medicare managed care. MA plans may be HMOs, PPOs, or PFFS plans; they may also be local or regional. Special needs plans (SNPs) were also created to focus on specific types of beneficiaries. MA MSAs are also overseen under MA. Replaced the older Medicare+Choice program.

Medicare+Choice: The old name for Medicare private insurance options. See Medicare Advantage.

Medicare Modernization Act of 2003 (MMA): The federal act originally titled the *Medicare Prescription Drug Improvement and Modernization Act of 2003*. The MMA is the basis for both the Medicare Part D drug benefit and for the variety of Medicare Advantage (MA) plans described elsewhere, including MA Local, MA Regional, and MA PFFS.

Medigap insurance: A form of state-licensed health insurance that covers whatever Medicare doesn't. Medigap policies are subject to minimum standards under federal law and have been further restricted under the MMA.

Member: An individual covered under a managed care plan. May be either the subscriber or a dependant.

Member months: The total of all months that each member was covered. For example, if a plan had 10,000 members in January and 12,000 members in February, the total member months for the year to date as of March 1 would be 22,000.

Member services: The department, as well as the actual services, that support a member's needs, not including the actual provision of health care. Examples of such member services include resolving problems, managing disputes by members about coverage issues, managing the grievance and appeals processes, and so forth. Member services also function in a proactive manner, reaching out to members with educational programs, self-service capabilities, and the like. Also known as customer services.

Mental Health Parity Act: Passed by Congress in 1996, it requires group health plans that offer mental health coverage benefits to apply the same annual and aggregate lifetime dollar limits to mental health coverage as those applied to coverage of other services. The federal law applies to fully insured and self-insured plans, including state-regulated plans. However, states may enact requirements more stringent than those contained under the federal law.

Messenger model: A type of IDS that simply acts as a messenger between an MCO and the providers participating in the IDS as regards contracting terms. Does not have the power to collectively bargain, thus avoiding antitrust violations.

MET: Multiple employer trust. *See* MEWA.

MEWA: Multiple employer welfare association. A group of employers who band together for purposes of purchasing group health insurance, often through a self-funded approach to avoid state mandates and insurance regulation. By virtue of ERISA, such entities are regulated little, if at all. Many MEWAs have enabled small employers to obtain cost-effective health coverage, but some MEWAs have not had the financial resources to withstand the risk of medical costs and have failed, leaving the members without insurance or recourse. In some states, MEWAs and METs are no longer legal. *See also* Association health plan.

Military Health System (MHS): A large and complex health care system designed to provide, and to maintain readiness to provide, medical services and support to the armed forces during military operations and to provide medical services and support to members of the armed forces, their dependants, and others entitled to Department of Defense (DOD) medical care. *See also* TRICARE.

MIS: Management information system. An older term for the computer hardware and software that provides the support for managing the plan. *See also,* the more commonly used term, IT.

Mixed model: A managed care plan that mixes two or more types of delivery systems. This has traditionally been used to describe an HMO that has both closed panel and open panel delivery systems.

MLP: Midlevel practitioner. Physician's assistants, clinical nurse practitioners, nurse midwives, and the like. Nonphysicians who deliver medical care, generally under the supervision of a physician but for less cost.

MMA: *See* Medicare Modernization Act.

MMI: Master member index. The MMI is used in physician practice profiling to identify in a reliable manner each patient receiving care from a particular physician. Subject to the privacy and security provisions under HIPAA.

Moral hazard: An old term of insurance that remains applicable today. Loosely defined for purposes of this glossary, moral hazard refers to the concept of providing insurance to a market in which it is certain that financial losses will occur. A bit more accurately, it has several aspects, such as an insured individual knowing things about his or her risk that the insurance company does not know and cannot observe, therefore causing a negative financial outcome for the insurance company. It may also refer to the provision of insurance causing an individual to incur costs that would not have been incurred if insurance wasn't provided and to a greater degree than the insurance company could predict.

MS-DRG: Medicare Severity Diagnosis-Related Groups. Implemented by Medicare to replace traditional DRGs. MS-DRGs are based not only on txhe diagnosis and procedures performed, but also take into account other chronic conditions and co-morbidities, including major chronic conditions and co-morbidities. With the advent of MS-DRGs in 2008–2009, fewer cases will qualify as outliers.

MSA: Medical Savings Account. Created as a demonstration under BBA '97, MSAs are specialized savings accounts into which a consumer can put pre-tax dollars for use in paying medical expenses in lieu of purchasing a comprehensive health insurance or managed care product. MSAs require a catastrophic health insurance policy as a "safety net" to protect against very high costs. They still exist, in both commercial form and for Medicare, but have been supplanted by CDHPs that are similar in approach but have additional features that make them more attractive to the market.

MSO: Management service organization. A form of integrated health delivery system. Sometimes similar to a service bureau (see below), the MSO often actually purchases certain hard assets of a physician's practice, and then provides services to that physician at fair market rates. MSOs are usually formed as a means to contract more effectively with managed care organizations, although their simple creation does not guarantee success.

MTF: Military treatment facilities. *See* Military Health System.

Multispecialty group: Just what it sounds like: a medical group made up of different specialty physicians. May or may not include primary care.

Mutual company: A type of not-for-profit health insurance company or Blue Cross Blue Shield plan that is legally owned by the policy holders, not the community nor private investors.

NAHMOR: National Association of HMO Regulators.

NAIC: National Association of Insurance Commissioners.

National Practitioner Data Bank: A data bank established under the federal Health Care Improvement and Quality Act of 1986, it electronically stores information about physician malpractice suits successfully litigated or settled and disciplinary actions upon physicians. Accessible by hospitals and health plans under controlled circumstances as part of the credentialing process. Hospitals and health plans must likewise report disciplinary actions to the databank.

NCPDP: National Council for Prescription Drug Programs. The NCPDP developed and maintains accepted electronic data interchange standards for pharmacy claims transmission and adjudication, which accelerated the adoption of pharmacy e-commerce. This standard permits the submission of pharmacy claims and the adjudication of those claims in a real-time interactive mode. Recognized by ANSI and addressed under HIPAA.

NCQA: National Committee on Quality Assurance. A not-for-profit organization that performs quality-oriented accreditation reviews on HMOs and similar types of managed care plans. NCQA also now accredits CVOs, PPOs, certain types of DM programs, and so forth. NCQA developed and maintains the HEDIS standards.

NDC: National drug code. The national classification system for identifying prescription drugs.

Net worth: For purposes of health insurance and managed care, net worth is what a health plan has in assets that can readily be converted into cash in the event of plan failure, such as unrestricted cash or investments or other equally liquid and unencumbered assets. States have net worth minimum requirements for licensed health plans that vary with the size of the potential liability. *See also* Nonadmitted asset; Risk-based capital.

Network model HMO: A health plan that contracts with multiple physician groups to deliver health care to members. Generally limited to large single or multispecialty groups. Distinguished from group model plans that contract with a single medical group, IPAs that contract through an intermediary, and direct contract model plans that contract with individual physicians in the community.

NIO: Noninvestor owned. A term preferred by some not-for-profit health plans, including some Blue Cross and Blue Shield plans, because they are taxed as though they are for-profit health insurance companies, not as though they are charitable organizations.

Nonadmitted asset: An asset owned by an MCO that does not count toward its net worth by the insurance department. Varies from state to state, but usually is applied to assets that cannot be readily converted into cash in the event of a health plan failure. It may also apply only to a portion of such an asset; for example, no more than 5% of a plan's net worth can consist of such assets as computers, real estate, and so forth.

Nonpar: Short for nonparticipating. Refers to a provider that does not have a contract with the health plan.

NPI: National Provider Identifier. The NPI is mandated under HIPAA and will replace almost all other types of provider (broadly defined) identifiers regardless of customer (*ie*, commercial health plan, Medicare, Medicaid, TRICARE, and so forth) in 2007 (2008 for small health plans). The NPI is a 10-digit number, with the 10th digit being a checksum that can help detect keying errors. It contains no embedded intelligence; that is, it contains no information about the health care provider such as the type of health care provider or state where the health care provider is located. The NPI does not replace the DEA number or the tax ID number of a provider, however.

NPlanID: The National Health Plan Identifier mandated under HIPAA. These will be the identifiers used by health plans (broadly defined) when conducting all transactions, regardless of the type of customer (*eg*, commercial health plan, Medicare plan, and so forth) or provider. At the time of publication, neither the standards for the NPlanID nor an implementation date has been announced.

Observation unit: A treatment room usually adjacent to the ED where rapid evaluation and stabilization of a medical problem can be managed, resulting in discharge of the patient to home, for example, from chest pain unit.

OCR: Optical character recognition. A system of hardware and software that is able to recognize written characters scanned in from a paper source and convert those characters into standard data. Used in any processing systems in which paper forms may be submitted; claims and enrollment forms are the most common. OCR works well with typed or printer-generated documents, but less well with hand-written documents. OCR accuracy and effectiveness is enhanced when standard forms are used (*eg*, the HCFA 1500-R or the UB-92), and even more when specialized forms (*eg*, those that use red "drop-out" ink to print the form) are used to eliminate the need for the OCR system to scan and read the characters on the form itself. Data scanned in via OCR is usually checked by clerks for accuracy and to correct errors; however, it is still more efficient than keying the data in manually.

OIG: The Office of the Inspector General. This is the federal agency responsible for conducting investigations and audits of federal contractors or any system that receives funds or reimbursement from the federal government. There are actually several OIG departments in different federal programs; examples pertinent to managed health care would include TRICARE, CMS, and the FEHBP.

OMC: Office of Managed Care. Once used as the name for the federal agency that oversaw federal qualification and compliance for HMOs. Even older names were Health Maintenance Organization Service (HMOS), Office of Health Maintenance Organizations

(OHMO), Office of Prepaid Health Care (OPHC), and the Office of Prepaid Health Care Operations and Oversight (OPHCOO). Now used primarily by states for that function that oversees state-licensed MCOs.

OOBD: Order of benefits determination. *See* COB.

Open access: A term that refers to an HMO that does not use a primary care physician "gatekeeper" model for access to specialty physicians. In other words, a member may self-refer to a specialty physician rather than seek an authorization from the PCP. HMOs that use an open access model often have a significant copayment differential between care received. May also be called direct access.

Open enrollment period: The period when an employee may change health plans; usually occurs once per year. A general rule is that most managed care plans will have around half their membership up for open enrollment in the fall for an effective date of January 1. A special form of open enrollment is still law in some states. This yearly open enrollment requires an HMO to accept any individual applicant (*ie*, one not coming in through an employer group) for coverage, regardless of health status. Such special open enrollments usually occur for 1 month each year. Many Blue Cross Blue Shield plans have similar open enrollments for indemnity products.

Open panel HMO: A managed care plan that contracts (either directly or indirectly) with private physicians to deliver care in their own offices. Examples would include a direct contract HMO and an IPA.

OPL: Other-party liability. *See* COB.

OPM: Office of Personnel Management. The federal agency that administers the FEHBP. This is the agency with which a managed care plan contracts to provide coverage for federal employees.

Outlier: Something that is well outside of an expected range. May refer to a provider who is using medical resources at a much higher rate than their peers, or to a case in a hospital that is far more expensive than anticipated, or in fact to anything at all that is significantly more or less than expected.

Outsourcing: Having a process or activity that an MCO provides done by a contracted third party. For example, contracting with an offshore company to manually enter data from images of paper claims.

OWA: Other weird arrangement. A general acronym that applies to any new and bizarre twist to a health plan or benefit design.

Package pricing: Also referred to as bundled pricing. An MCO pays an organization a single fee for all inpatient, outpatient, and professional expenses associated with a procedure, including preadmission and postdischarge care. Common procedures that use this form of pricing include cardiac bypass surgery and transplants.

Par provider: Shorthand term for participating provider (*ie*, one who has signed an agreement with a plan to provide services). May apply to professional or institutional providers.

Part D: The drug benefit created under the MMA. May be provided by a private, freestanding prescription drug plan or included in an MA plan.

Patient Bill of Rights (PBOR): A law or policy describing what rights a patient has regarding his or her health care and how patients should be treated; it may be applied to either a provider or a payer. A voluntary PBOR is often posted by hospitals. Some states (but not the federal government at the time of publication, despite vigorous efforts in past years by various legislators) also have passed PBOR legislation regarding health plans.

Pay and pursue: Also referred to as "pay and chase." The antonym is pursue and pay, or "chase" and pay. A term commonly used in OPL or COB, this refers to the order in which a health plan will deal with claims that may be the principal liability of another insurance company or managed health care plan. Pay and pursue refers to the health plan paying for the claim and then trying to recover all or some of the costs from the other insurance company. Pursue and pay refers to the plan transferring the claim to that insurance carrier that is primarily responsible for the cost and not paying the claim unless the primary carrier does not cover the cost in full, in which case the secondary plan will cover that portion of the costs that were not covered by the primary insurer. *See also* COB.

Pay-for-performance (P4P): The term applied to providing financial incentives to providers (hospitals and/or physicians) to improve compliance with standards of care and to improve outcomes and patient safety.

PCCM: Primary care case manager. This acronym is used in Medicaid managed care programs and refers to the state designating PCPs as case managers to function as "gatekeepers," but reimbursing those PCPs using traditional Medicaid fee-for-service, as well as paying the PCP a nominal management fee such as $2 to $5 PMPM.

PCP: Primary care physician. Generally applies to internists, pediatricians, family physicians, and general practitioners and occasionally to obstetrician/gynecologists.

PDP: Prescription drug plan. A private, freestanding plan providing drug coverage to Medicare beneficiaries under MA. Does not provide coverage for other services.

PEL: Provider excess loss. Refers to a stop-loss insurance policy purchased by risk-bearing provider organizations, full-risk-bearing medical groups, or IDSs to limit exposure to catastrophic claims costs.

Pended/suspended claims: Although the terms *pend* and *suspend* are often used synonymously, some MCOs differentiate between claims that examiners place on hold (pends) and those that are placed on hold automatically by one or more systems edits (suspends).

PEPM: Per employee per month. Like PMPM, but rolls the unit up to the level of the employee or subscriber, rather than measuring based on all members (subscribers plus dependants).

Per diem reimbursement: Reimbursement of an institution, usually a hospital, based on a set rate per day rather than on charges. Per diem reimbursement can be varied by service (*eg*, medical/surgical, obstetrics, mental health, and intensive care) or can be uniform regardless of intensity of services.

Persistency: Also called a persistency ratio. The term refers to a commercial group staying with an MCO from year to year. A persistency ratio of 90 would mean that 90% of groups enrolled do not change health plans.

PHI: Protected health information. That information that reveals medical information or data about an individual. PHI is addressed specifically by HIPAA in the Privacy and Security sections.

PHO: Physician–hospital organization. These are legal (or perhaps informal) organizations that bind hospitals and the attending medical staff and were developed for the purpose of contracting with managed care plans. A PHO may be open to any members of the staff who apply, or they may be closed to staff members who fail to qualify (or who are part of an already over represented specialty).

Periodic interim payment: A method of advancing money from a payer to a provider before an exact accounting of claims is done. For example, an MCO may make a monthly PIP to a hospital, and then reconcile every quarter. This used to be common between BCBS plans and hospitals but no longer is. Because of the time value of money, a PIP is usually used now only when the MCO or payer is unable to process claims quickly and correctly but needs to pay the providers in the meantime.

Personal health record: A record, usually created by a health plan, of an individual's health-related data. The sources of that data include claims from providers, prescription drugs the plan paid for, demographic data, and so forth. Clinical data such as results of diagnostic lab tests or imaging may be provided if the plan has access to it, and the member can add additional data such as drug allergies or the results of a health risk appraisal. The purpose is to provide at least a usable subset of important health-related information in an electronically portable or transmittable format to improve continuity of care and emergency care.

PFFS: *See* Private fee-for-service plan.

PHR: *See* Personal health record.

Physician incentive program: A generic term referring to a reimbursement methodology under which a physician's income from an MCO (or an IDS) is affected by the physician's performance or the overall performance of the plan (*eg*, utilization, medical cost, quality measurements, member satisfaction, and so forth). This term has a very specific usage by the CMS, which limits the degree of incentive or risk allowed under a Medicare HMO (refer to PIP regulations at 42 CFR 422.208/210 of the June 26, 1998, regulations that implement Medicare Part C). CMS essentially bans "gainsharing" via a PIP altogether in an IDS receiving reimbursement under Medicare. Some states also now have laws and regulations regarding limits on PIPs and requirements for disclosure of incentives to members enrolled in MCOs. *See also* SFR.

PIP: *See* Periodic interim payment; *see also* Physician incentive program.

PIP/DCG: Principal inpatient diagnostic cost group. A methodology that CMS used looking at inpatient stays as a predictor of total Medicare expenditures for an individual so as to apply to risk-adjusted payments to Medicare risk plans. Since replaced by the CMS-Hierarchical Condition Categories system.

PMPM: Per member per month. Specifically applies to a revenue or cost for each enrolled member each month.

PMPY: Per member per year. The same as PMPM, but based on a year.

POD: Pool of doctors. This refers to the plan grouping physicians into units smaller than the entire panel but larger than individual practices. Typical PODs have between 10 and 30 physicians. Often used for performance measurement and compensation. The POD is often not a real legal entity, but rather a grouping. Not to be confused with the pod people from *Invasion of the Body Snatchers*.

POS: Point-of-service. A plan where members do not have to choose how to receive services until they need them. The most common use of the term applies to a plan that enrolls each member in both an HMO (or HMO-like) system and a PPO or an indemnity plan. These plans provide a difference in benefits (*eg*, 100% coverage rather than 70%) depending on whether the member chooses to use the plan (including its providers and in compliance with the authorization system) or go outside the plan for services.

PPM: Physician practice management company. An organization that manages physician's practices and in most cases either owns the practices outright or has rights to purchase them in the future. PPMs concentrate only on physicians and not on hospitals, although some PPMs have also branched into joint ventures with hospitals and insurers. Most PPMs failed spectacularly, but some still exist, particularly for single specialties.

PPO: Preferred provider organization. A plan that contracts with independent providers at a discount for services. The panel is limited in size and usually has some type of utilization review system associated with it. A PPO may be risk bearing, such as an insurance company, or may be non-risk bearing, such as a physician-sponsored PPO that markets itself to insurance companies or self-insured companies via an access fee.

PPS: *See* Prospective payment system.

Preauthorization: *See* Authorization. *See also* Precertification.

Precertification: Also known as preadmission certification, preadmission review, and precert. The process of obtaining certification or authorization from the health plan for routine hospital admissions or for ambulatory procedures. Often involves appropriateness review against criteria and assignment of length of stay. Failure to obtain precertification often results in a financial penalty either to the provider or the subscriber.

Preexisting condition: A medical condition for which a member has received treatment during a specified period of time prior to becoming covered under a health plan. May have an effect on whether treatments for that condition will be covered under certain types of health plans.

Premium: The money paid to a health plan for coverage. The term may be applied on an individual basis or a group basis. Recognized by the health plan as premium revenue. *See also* Earned premium revenue; Unearned premium revenue; Imputed premium.

Premium tax: A tax levied by a state on health insurance premiums for policies sold in that state. Employers that self-fund their health benefits plan, as well as Medicare Advantage plans, are not subject to premium taxes.

Prepaid or prepayment: Payment for services before they are incurred. Capitation is a form of prepayment because the provider is paid before the month that services will be provided. HMOs were once called prepaid health plans because premiums were paid in advance of the HMO providing the service. Can also be applied to the prepayment of any type of insurance premium, though health plans sometimes prefer to call it unearned premium revenue. Never applies to self-funding except when self-funded plans fund capitation to providers.

Preventive care: Health care that is aimed at preventing complications of existing diseases or preventing the occurrence of a disease. Often misspelled as "preventative," which is not a word.

Private fee-for-service plan (PFFS): A type of Medicare Advantage plan in which a private insurance company accepts risk for enrolled beneficiaries, but pays providers on an FFS basis that does not have any risk component to the provider. PFFS plans are not network plans in the sense of being able to limit coverage to a network and must cover the cost of care from any provider willing to accept the individual as a patient, consistent with the rules of the plan regarding coverage.

Private inurement: What happens when a not-for-profit business operates in such a way as to provide more than incidental financial gain to a private individual; for example, if a not-for-profit hospital pays too much money for a physician's practice or fails to charge fair market rates for services provided to a physician. Prohibited by the IRS.

PRO: Peer review organization. The old name for organizations charged with reviewing quality and cost for Medicare. Since replaced by QIOs.

Profiling: Measuring a provider's performance on selected measures and comparing that performance to similar providers. Usually applied to physicians. May be used for purposes of network selection or tiering, feedback reports, and/or P4P programs. Very complicated to perform properly.

Prospective payment system (PPS): Medicare's terminology for determining fixed pricing for reimbursement of hospitals and facilities for care. The most well known example of PPS is DRGs, but also includes APCs. Prospective payment may be used by commercial plans as it applies to payment of facilities using the same methodologies.

Prospective review: Reviewing the need for medical care before the care is rendered. *See also* Precertification.

Provider: The generic term used to refer to anyone providing medical services. In fact, it may even be used to refer to any*thing* that provides medical services, such as a hospital. Most often, however, it is used to refer to physicians. How physicians migrated from being called physicians to being called providers is not very clear cut, and certainly not embraced by physicians, but it is a term in general use, including in this book.

Prudent layperson: *See* Reasonable Layperson Standard.

PSA: Professional services agreement. A contract between a physician or medical group and an IDS or MCO for the provision of medical services.

PSO: Provider-sponsored organization. An entity allowed under the BBA '97 Medicare+ Choice. A PSO is a risk-bearing managed care organization that contracts directly with CMS for Medicare enrollees, but unlike an HMO, the PSO is made up of the providers themselves, and the providers bear substantial risk for expenses. The rules for financial solvency are somewhat different for a PSO as compared to an HMO, and if a PSO is not licensed by the state, provisions exist to seek licensure directly from the CMS. PSOs are the result of the belief by providers and legislators that there were fat profits to be had by "cutting out the middle man" in the form of removing the HMO from the equation. A few PSOs actually got started under a demonstration program, and a few more came into being under BBA '97. Most failed utterly and are defunct, though a few remain.

PTMPY: Per thousand members per year. A common way of reporting utilization. The most common example is hospital utilization, expressed as days per thousand members per year.

Pursue and pay: *See* Pay and pursue.

QA or QM: Quality assurance (older term) or quality management (newer term).

QIO: *See* Quality improvement organization.

QIP: Quality Improvement Program. The program put in place by CMS for Medicare Advantage plans of all types. The QIP uses data from HEDIS, HOS, and CAHPS, as well as financial and member disenrollment data. Accreditation by NCQA is also considered under the QIP.

QISMC: Quality Improvement System for Managed Care. The now discontinued CMS program regarding quality of care and member satisfaction for Medicare risk plans. Replaced by the Quality Improvement Program (QIP).

Quality improvement organization: An organization under contract to CMS to conduct quality reviews of providers, respond to beneficiary complaints about care, measure and report performance of providers, ensure that payment is made only for medically necessary services, and other functions. Applies to all types of plans and services, not just managed care.

Qui tam sui: A provision in tort law that allows a citizen to file suit on behalf of the (federal) government and to collect one third of the proceeds of that lawsuit. Such suits are usually also subject to treble damages, making success a lucrative endeavor. The point of this is to encourage citizens with knowledge of deliberate wrongdoing to blow the whistle on the transgressor because the government cannot always know when fraud is occurring. In the context of this book, *qui tam sui* applies to health insurance programs paid with federal funds (*ie*, Medicare, Medicaid, TRICARE, and the FEHBP).

Rate: The amount of money that a group or individual must pay to the health plan for coverage. Usually a monthly fee. Rating refers to the health plan developing those rates.

RBC: *See* Risk-based capital.

RBRVS: Resource-based relative value scale. This is a relative value scale developed for the CMS for use by Medicare. The RBRVS assigns relative values to each CPT code for services on the basis of the resources related to the procedure rather than simply on the basis of historical trends. The practical effect has been to lower reimbursement for procedural services (*eg*, cardiac surgery) and to raise reimbursement for cognitive services (*eg*, office visits).

Reasonable Layperson Standard: This means that the judgment of a reasonable nonclinician should be applied in determining if a service is warranted or not. This standard is almost always focused on the use of emergency or urgent care, when a layperson has good reason to believe that a medical problem must be addressed immediately, even if a trained provider may not feel that it was urgent. The specific language most often used, and addressed directly in the Balanced Budget Act of 1997 as pertaining to Medicare and Medicaid recipients is: "*Health plans should provide payment when a consumer presents to an emergency department with acute symptoms of sufficient severity: including severe pain: such that a "prudent layperson" could reasonably expect the absence of medical attention to result in placing health in serious jeopardy, serious impairment to bodily functions, or serious dysfunction of any bodily organ or part.*"

Rebundlers: Software programs that roll up and reprice fragmented bills as well as apply industry-standard claims adjudication conventions.

Reinstatement: When an insurance or managed care policy is reinstated after payment for delinquent premiums during a defined grace period. *See* Grace period.

Reinsurance: Insurance purchased by a health plan to protect it against extremely high cost cases (*see also* Stop loss).

Rental PPO: A PPO network owned and managed by a third party that rents access (and often services such as claims repricing) to an MCO or health insurance company. Not the same as a risk-bearing PPO that combines a network with the insurance function.

Reserves: The amount of money that a health plan puts aside to cover health care costs. May apply to anticipated costs such as IBNRs or may apply to money that the plan does not expect to have to use to pay for current medical claims but keeps as a cushion against future adverse health care costs.

Reserves can be made up only of admitted assets. Also called statutory reserves because the accounting is done per Statutory Accounting Principles (SAP), not Generally Accepted Accounting Principles (GAAP), allowing the state insurance department greater leeway in deciding what counts toward net worth based on the liquidity of the assets. *See also* Admitted assets; Nonadmitted assets; Risk-based capital.

Retail care clinic: A small clinic, usually associated with a retail store such as a pharmacy or grocery store, staffed by non-physician providers. These clinics diagnose and treat a variety of low-acuity medical conditions at costs that are substantially lower than what a physician would charge.

Retention: A term with two meanings depending on context. Retention is used to describe that portion of a health insurance premium that is for administrative costs, not medical claims cost. Retention may also less commonly be used as a synonym for persistency; *see* Persistency.

Retrospective review: Reviewing health care costs after the care has been rendered. There are several forms of retrospective review. One form looks at individual claims for medical necessity, billing errors or fraud. The other form looks at patterns of costs, rather than individual cases.

Rider: An add-on to the core insurance or HMO policy; for example, coverage for dental or optometry services. Surprisingly, most regular drug benefits are provided via a rider and are not part of the main medical-surgical policy, whereas coverage for injectable drugs (including specialty pharmacy drugs) may be part of the main policy.

Risk adjustment: A methodology to account for the health status of patients when predicting or explaining costs of health care for defined populations or for evaluating retrospectively the performance of providers who care for them. Also known as severity adjustment and acuity adjustment. Case mix is related, but applies only to inpatient care.

Risk-based capital (RBC): A formula embodied in the Risk-Based Capital for Health Organizations Model Act, created under the auspices of the NAIC. RBC takes into account the fluctuating value of plan assets; the financial condition of plan affiliates; the risk that providers may not be able to provide contracted services; the risk that amounts due may not be recovered from reinsurance carriers; and general business risks (ie, expenses may exceed income). The RBC formula gives credit for provider payment arrangements that reduce underwriting risk, including capitation as well as provider withholds, bonuses, contracted fee schedules, and aggregate cost arrangements. Although not required in all states, RBC is the agreed-upon standard for an insurance department to determine whether or not a health plan meets minimum financial solvency requirements.

Risk contract: Also known as a Medicare Risk Contract; an informal but widely used term. A contract between a health plan and the CMS under Medicare Advantage under which the health plan provides services to Medicare beneficiaries and receives a monthly payment for enrolled Medicare members and is on an at-risk basis.

Risk corridor: The upper and lower limits of financial risk for a health plan or provider that is at risk for medical costs. Both limits must exist to be considered a risk corridor. A risk corridor of 20%, for example, would mean that the plan or provider can have financial losses or gains of no more than 10% of the baseline payment.

Risk management: Management activities aimed at lowering an organization's legal and financial exposures, especially to lawsuits.

Risk pool: This term can have two different meanings as applied to managed care, though both are related to medical care costs. In one case, it refers to a pool of funds that may be drawn against to cover medical costs, with any unused funds being paid to a provider or providers under capitation. The other meaning refers to the group of individuals (eg, employees or Medicare enrollees) for which premiums are paid to an MCO or health insurance company; the money paid by or on behalf of healthier people then being used to cover the costs of sicker people; that is, spreading out the risk by pooling the money. See also Rule of small numbers.

Rule of small numbers: The notion that predictions that are based on large numbers (eg, a population of 2 million lives) have little relevance when the numbers are small (eg, 100 lives); chance then plays a far more important role.

RVU: Relative value unit. A number used as a multiplier to calculate the payment to a provider. The RVU is determined based on the procedure, and then is used by a plan to multiply against a value for each RVU to determine total payment to the provider. Not consistent or uniform, the RVU is often a combination of negotiation and national standards. See also RBRVS.

Safe harbor: The circumstances under which a hospital or other health care entity can provide something to a physician or other health entity and not violate the anti-kickback portion of the Stark regulations. See also Stark regulations.

Schedule of benefits: The listing of what is and what is not covered by a health plan, and under what circumstances.

SCHIP: State Children's Health Insurance Program. A program created by the federal government to provide a "safety net" and preventive care level of health coverage for children, funded through a combination of federal and state funds and administered by the states in conformance with federal requirements.

SCP: Specialty care physician; that is, a physician who is not a PCP. SCP is not used as an acronym nearly as often as is PCP.

Second opinion: An opinion obtained from another physician regarding the necessity for a treatment that has been recommended by one physician. May be required by some health plans for certain high-cost procedures. Once commonly used, now uncommon.

Section 1115 waiver: That section of federal law that provides for a state to opt out of the standard Medicaid fee-for-service program and adopt a managed care approach to financing and providing health care services to Medicaid-eligible recipients. Usually requires that some of the savings be applied to broaden coverage of who is eligible for Medicaid.

Section 125 Plan: *See* Flexible benefits plan.

Self-care: The series of steps "lay" individuals take to assess and treat an illness or injury, typically without the benefit of higher levels of training in the theory or science of medicine and with little or no consultation with a medical professional.

Self-insured or self-funded plan: A health plan where the risk for medical cost is assumed by the company rather than an insurance company or managed care plan. Under ERISA, self-funded plans are exempt from state laws and regulations such as premium taxes and mandatory benefits. Self-funded plans often contract with insurance companies or third-party administrators to administer the benefits (*see also* ASO).

Sentinel effect: The phenomenon that when it is know that behavior is being observed, that behavior changes, often in the direction the observer is looking for. Applies to the fact that utilization management systems and profiling systems often lead to reductions in utilization before much intervention even takes place, simply because the providers know that someone is watching.

Service area: The geographic area in which an HMO provides access to primary care. The service area is usually specifically designated by the regulators (state or federal), and the HMO is prohibited from marketing outside of the service area. May be defined by county or by ZIP code. It is possible for an HMO to have more than one service area and for the service areas to either be contiguous (*ie*, they actually border each other) or noncontiguous

(*ie*, there is a geographic gap between the service areas).

Service bureau: A weak form of integrated delivery system in which a hospital (or other organization) provides services to a physician's practice in return for a fair market price. May also try to negotiate with managed care plans but generally not considered to be an effective negotiating mechanism.

Service plan: A health insurance plan that has direct contracts with providers but is not necessarily a managed care plan. The archetypal service plans are traditional (*ie*, non-managed care) Blue Cross and Blue Shield plans, though a few non-Blue service plans do exist. The contract applies to direct billing of the plan by providers (rather than billing of the member), a provision for direct payment of the provider (rather than reimbursement of the member), a requirement that the provider accept the plan's determination of UCR and not balance bill the member in excess of that amount, and a range of other terms. May or may not address issues of utilization and quality.

SFR: Significant financial risk. A term used by the CMS that refers to the total amount of a physician's income at risk in a Medicare HMO. Such financial risk is considered "significant" when it exceeds a certain percentage of the total potential income that physician could receive under the reimbursement program. SFR most commonly is defined as any physician incentive payment program that allows for a variation of more than 25% between the minimum and the maximum amount of potential reimbursement.

Shadow pricing: The practice of setting premium rates at a level just below the competition's rates whether or not those rates can be justified. In other words, the premium rates could actually be lower, but to maximize profit the rates are raised to a level that will remain attractive but result in greater revenue. This practice is generally considered unethical and, in the case of community rating, possibly illegal.

SHMO: Social health maintenance organization. An HMO that goes beyond the medical care needs of its membership to include their social needs as well. A relatively rare form of HMO.

Shock claim: Also referred to as a catastrophic claim. A shock claim is an extraordinarily expensive total cost of health care for an individual patient. Shock claims are taken into account by actuaries when they determine the trends for medical costs because shock claims have a certain amount of randomness to them because they are infrequent and costly, unlike routine care that is predictable.

Shoe box effect: When an indemnity-type benefits plan has a deductible, there may be beneficiaries who save up their receipts to file for reimbursement at a later time (*ie*, saves them in a shoe box). Those receipts then get lost, or the beneficiary never sends them in, so the insurance company never has to pay.

Silent PPO: A term that is now rarely used because it is considered either unethical or illegal. A silent PPO was a form of rental PPO (*see* Rental PPO) in which the MCO or health insurance company did not clearly identify what was being used when a member received services (by having the PPO's logo on the ID card somewhere, for example). This led to unanticipated reductions in payments as a result of PPO reimbursement policies being applied after the fact.

Single point of entry: A relatively new term that means that an individual uses the same system to access both group health medical benefits and benefits for work-related medical conditions.

Single specialty hospital: A hospital that provides services focusing on a single specialty such as cardiac procedures or orthopedics. Physicians often have a small equity interest in them.

Slice business: A term referring to more than one MCO or health insurance company

offering plans to the employees of one company.

SNP: *See* Special needs plan.

Special needs plan: A type of MA plan. This type of plan may exclusively enroll, or enroll a disproportionate percentage of, special needs Medicare beneficiaries. Individuals with special needs include beneficiaries entitled to both Medicare and Medicaid ("dual eligibles"), institutionalized beneficiaries, and individuals with severe or disabling chronic conditions.

Specialty network manager: A term used to describe a single specialist (or perhaps a specialist organization) that accepts capitation to manage a single specialty. Specialty services are supplied by many different specialty physicians, but the network manager has the responsibility for managing access and cost and is at economic risk. A relatively uncommon model.

Specialty pharmacy: Injectable drugs that are almost always proteins created through recombinant DNA. These specialty drugs (unlike insulin, which would otherwise meet the criteria) focus on relatively uncommon but very costly conditions. They also almost always have only one single source.

Specialty pharmacy distributor (SPD): A company that distributes specialty pharmacy, from the manufacturer to the provider and/or directly to the patient, to address the unique distribution, storage, and utilization issues around these types of injectable drugs. May be part of a PBM or a separate company.

Staff model HMO: An HMO that employs providers directly, and those providers see members in the HMO's own facilities. A form of closed panel HMO. A different use of this term is sometimes applied to vertically integrated health care delivery systems that employ physicians but in which the system is not licensed as an HMO.

Stark regulations: Named after Fortney "Pete" Stark, congressional representative from California. The so-called Stark regulations are actually two sets of regulations: Stark I and Stark II, stemming from the Ethics in Referrals Act. These regulations are not for amateurs to handle, and competent legal counsel is required for any provider system doing business with federal or state governments.

State licensure: The license or certificate of authority issued by a state to a health plan that allows the plan to write business in the state. May be based on having a license in a different state; *see* State of domicile.

State of domicile: The state that an insurance company or MCO is licensed in as its primary location. For example, an MCO may have its state of domicile in Virginia but might also be licensed and doing business in Maryland and the District of Columbia. In many states, the insurance commissioner will defer primary regulation to the insurance department in the state of domicile as long as all minimum standards of the state are met.

Statutory reserves: *See* Reserves.

Stop loss: A form of reinsurance that provides protection for medical expenses above a certain limit, generally on a year-by-year basis. This may apply to an entire health plan or to any single component. For example, the health plan may have stop-loss reinsurance for cases that exceed $100,000. After a case hits $100,000, the plan receives 80% of expenses in excess of $100,000 back from the reinsurance company for the rest of the year. Another example would be the plan providing a stop loss to participating physicians for referral expenses over $2,500. When a case exceeds that amount in a single year, the plan no longer deducts those costs from the physician's referral pool for the remainder of the year. Specific coverage refers to individual cases, whereas aggregate coverage refers to the total costs rather than a specific case.

Subacute care facility: A health facility that is a step down from an acute care hospital. May be a nursing home or a facility that provides medical care but not surgical or emergency care. Some confine use of the term to services that are a step up from conventional skilled nursing facility intensity of services, adding RNs around the clock and intravenous medications.

Subordinated note: Essentially a promise from a lender that a health plan can borrow money up to the limit of the note if it must to pay claims, and that the holder of the note will not be repaid before all claims costs are settled. This subordination allows the plan to claim it for purposes of net worth because it may be so used. A note or loan for which the plan must pay the note holder regardless of the plan's inability to pay claims is not subordinated and cannot be counted as part of its net worth.

Subrogation: The contractual right of a health plan to recover payments made to a member for health care costs after that member has received such payment for damages in a legal action.

Subscriber: The individual or member who has the health plan coverage by virtue of being eligible on his or her own behalf rather than as a dependant.

Sutton's law: "Go where the money is!" Attributed to the Depression-era bank robber Willy Sutton, who, when asked why he robbed banks, replied, "That's where the money is." Sutton apparently denies ever having made that statement. In any event, it is a good law to use when determining what needs attention in a managed care plan.

Taft–Hartley Plan: A type of health plan provided by a union to its members, usually using funds contributed by more than one employer or company. Also eligible to be a type of MA plan.

TANF: Temporary Assistance to Needy Families. Administered by DHHS, TANF provides assistance and work opportunities to needy families by granting states the federal funds and wide flexibility to develop and implement their own welfare programs. TANF replaced the older term AFDC.

TAT: Turnaround time. The amount of time it takes a health plan to process and pay a claim from the time it arrives.

TEFRA: Tax Equity and Fiscal Responsibility Act. One key provision of this act prohibits employers and health plans from requiring full-time employees between the ages of 65 and 69 to use Medicare rather than the group health plan.

Termination date: The day that health plan coverage is no longer in effect.

Tiering: A term that applies to categorizing something into different tiers for purposes of benefits differentials. When used in pharmacy, Tier 1 drugs require lower copays than Tier 2, Tier 3, and so forth. When applied to providers, members accessing Tier 1 providers likewise have less (or even no) cost sharing than if they use a Tier 2 provider.

Time loss management: The application of managed care techniques to worker's compensation treatments for injuries or illnesses to reduce the amount of time lost on the job by the affected employee.

Total capitation: *See* Global capitation.

TPA: Third-party administrator. A firm that performs administrative functions (*eg*, claims processing, membership, and the like) for a self-funded plan or a start-up managed care plan (*see also* ASO).

Transparency: Refers to making data available to the public. Also called pricing transparency when such data is the price for services from different providers of care.

Triage: The origins of this term are grizzly: the process of sorting out wounded soldiers into those who need treatment immediately, those who can wait, and those who are too severely injured to even try and save. In health plans, this refers to the process of sorting out requests for services by members into those who need to be seen right away, those who can wait a little while, and those

whose problems can be handled with advice over the phone.

TRICARE: The Department of Defense's worldwide managed health care program. TRICARE was initiated in 1995, integrating health care services provided in the direct care system of military hospitals and clinics with services purchased from civilian providers for anybody eligible for coverage (*eg*, retirees and dependants). There are various different TRICARE benefits programs. The non-MTF portion of TRICARE is administered by private managed care companies in three regions in the United States. *See also* Military Health System.

Triple option: The offering of an HMO, a PPO, and a traditional insurance plan by one carrier.

Twenty-four-hour care: An ill-defined term that essentially means that health care is provided 24 hours per day, regardless of the financing mechanism; applies primarily to the convergence of group health, workers' compensation, and industrial health, all under managed care. Not commonly used anymore.

UB-92: *See* CMS-1450.

UCR: Usual, customary, or reasonable. A method of profiling prevailing fees in an area and reimbursing providers on the basis of that profile. One archaic method is to average all fees and choose the 80th or 90th percentile, although in this era a plan will usually use another method to determine what is reasonable. Sometimes this term is used synonymously with a fee allowance schedule when that schedule is set relatively high.

Unbundling: The practice of a provider billing for multiple components of service that were previously included in a single fee. For example, if dressings and instruments were included in a fee for a minor procedure, the fee for the procedure remains the same, but there are now additional charges for the dressings and instruments.

Underwriting: In one definition, this refers to bearing the risk for something (*ie*, a policy is underwritten by an insurance company). In another definition, this refers to the analysis of a group that is done to determine rates and benefits, or to determine whether the group should be offered coverage at all. A related definition refers to health screening of each individual applicant for insurance and refusing to provide coverage for preexisting conditions.

Unearned premium: *See* Earned premium.

Upcoding: The practice of a provider billing for a procedure that pays better than the service actually performed pays. For example, an office visit that would normally be reimbursed at $45 is coded as one that is reimbursed at $53.

UPIN: Universal Provider Identification Number. An identification number issued by CMS for use in billing Medicare. The UPIN is being replaced by the NPI in 2007; in fact, all provider identification numbers are being replaced by the NPI. *See* NPI.

URAC: A not-for-profit organization that performs reviews on external utilization review agencies (freestanding companies, utilization management departments of insurance companies, or utilization management departments of managed care plans). Its primary focus is MCOs, though it has expanded its accreditation activities; for example, accrediting health-related Web sites. States often require certification by URAC for another accreditation organization to operate. URAC once stood for the Utilization Review Accreditation Commission, but now is known only as URAC. URAC was also once known as the American Accreditation HealthCare Commission (AAHC), but that name is no longer used either.

URO: Utilization review organization. A freestanding organization that does nothing but UR, usually on a remote basis, using the telephone and paper correspondence. It may be independent or may be part of another company such as an insurance company that sells UR services on a stand-alone basis.

Waste, fraud, and abuse: Not the name of a law firm or a rock band, this troika is used to cast blame for greedy and sometimes illegal behavior on the part of either providers or health plans, usually by the government, but possibly by private purchasers of health care benefits as well. *See also* Fraudandabuse.

Workers' compensation: A form of social insurance provided through property-casualty insurers. Workers' compensation provides medical benefits and replacement of lost wages that result from injuries or illnesses that arise from the work place; in turn, the employee cannot normally sue the employer unless true negligence exists. Workers' compensation has undergone dramatic increases in cost as group health has shifted into managed care, resulting in workers' compensation carriers adopting managed care approaches. Worker's compensation is often heavily regulated under state laws that are significantly different from those used for group health insurance and is often the subject of intense negotiation between management and organized labor. *See* Time loss management; Twenty-four-hour care.

Wraparound plan: Commonly used to refer to insurance or health plan coverage for copays and deductibles that are not covered under a member's base plan. This is often used for Medicare.

Zero down: The practice of a medical group or provider system distributing all of the capital surplus in a health plan or the group to the members of the group, rather than retaining any capital or reinvesting it in the group or plan.

INDEX

Note: Page numbers followed by an italicized *t* or *f* indicate a table or figure on that page, respectively.